Introduction to Nursing Practice

Introduction to Nursing Practice

ARLYNE B. SAPERSTEIN, M.N., R.N.

ASSISTANT PROFESSOR
DIVISION OF NURSING STUDIES
CURRY COLLEGE
MILTON, MASSACHUSETTS

MARGARET A. FRAZIER, M.S., R.N.

ASSISTANT PROFESSOR
DIRECTOR, LEARNING RESOURCES LABORATORY
BOSTON UNIVERSITY SCHOOL OF NURSING
BOSTON, MASSACHUSETTS

F. A. DAVIS COMPANY • Philadelphia

**Library of Congress Cataloging in
Publication Data**

Main entry under title:
Introduction to nursing practice.

  Includes bibliographies and index.
  1. Nursing. I. Saperstein, Arlyne B.
II. Frazier, Margaret A. [DNLM: 1. Nursing.
WY100.3 S24li]
RT41.I59   610.73   79-17422
ISBN 0-8036-7729-4

This book is dedicated with love to

my parents, Ben and Sylvia Barnett
  and
my son, Richard Steven Saperstein

A.B.S.

my parents, James Alexander and Ann Elizabeth Frazier
  and
my husband, Kevin Thomas Plodzik

M.A.F.

PREFACE

This book is intended to serve as a basic text for students studying the fundamentals of nursing and as a reference throughout their later studies and careers. Its purpose is to introduce the student to the practice of nursing and to provide a sound knowledge base upon which to implement the decision-making process and perform appropriate procedures for the provision of optimum health care. The focus of this text is on the client as an individual and the nursing care required to meet his particular health needs. The client is presented as an active participant in his health care rather than merely a passive recipient. The role of the nurse is presented as that of a person with the necessary knowledge base and skills to assess the client's health care needs; coordinate health care efforts and resources; and plan, implement, and evaluate health care measures to meet the client's needs, including client education and acting as a client advocate.

The text is presented in five parts, each part forming the basis for the next: Concepts about the Client, Concepts about Health and Illness, Aspects of the Health Care System, Individualizing Health Care Needs, and Providing Basic Health Care. We have tried to provide the necessary balance and integration of theory and skills, and of psychosocial aspects and physiologic considerations throughout the text.

In chapters where new terminology is introduced, glossaries are provided. For frequently used procedures, a table format is utilized which describes the procedure, the scientific principle or rationale, and special client considerations. An extensive drug classification chart and numerous illustrations are provided to aid the student.

The reader will note that the student and the nurse are referred to as "she," while the client is usually referred to as "he." This is done merely for the purpose of simplicity and to avoid confusion. We recognize that all nurses are not female. However, to avoid the cumbersome "he/she," and since more than 90 percent of nurses are female, it was our decision to use the feminine pronoun. Also, although we prefer the use of the term "client," the terms "patient" and "client" are used interchangeably in the text.

Arlyne B. Saperstein
Margaret A. Frazier

vii

ACKNOWLEDGMENTS

There are too many people involved in the planning, writing and publication of a book to mention all of them individually. We, therefore, wish to express our heartfelt thanks to everyone who assisted or supported us in even the smallest way.

We are especially grateful to our contributors, without whom this text would not have been possible; to the editors and staff of F.A. Davis Company, including Judith M. Kim, Mary Helen Jacob, Jane Edwards, Nancy W. Schmidt, Phyllis Spagnolo, and Don Stengel; to typists, Judy True, Donna Silva, Diane O'Brien, Fanny Chung, and Mary Beth Howe; and to illustrators/photographers, Wadsworth Hine, Al Uckerman, and Ed Zides.

Six very special people, because of either their encouragement and support or the impact they made on our professional development will always be thought of with gratitude and warmth. They are Dr. Milton Shuch, Dr. Marcia Curtis, R.N., Dr. Gene Phillips, the late Dr. Blanche Urey, R.N., Elsie Duddy, R.N., and Rosy Doherty, R.N.

A.B.S.
M.A.F.

CONTRIBUTORS

SHERRY BAME, M.S., R.N.
   Doctoral Candidate
   University of Michigan
   Formerly, Coordinator of Staff Development
   Washtenaw County Health Department and
      VNA
   Ann Arbor, Michigan

BARBARA A. BEEKER, Ed.D., R.N.
   Professor and Chairperson
   Department of Professional Nursing
   University of Vermont
   School of Nursing
   Burlington, Vermont

BARBARA BIHM, M.S.N., B.S.N.
   Instructor of Nursing
   University of Southwestern Louisiana
   Lafayette, Louisiana

TANYA L. BODO, M.N., R.N.
   Assistant Professor
   University of Florida
   College of Nursing
   Gainesville, Florida

ELLEN CHRISTIAN, M.S., R.N.
   Assistant Professor
   Southeastern Massachusetts University
   School of Nursing
   North Dartmouth, Massachusetts

CARL J. COOPER, Ph.D.
   Professor of Psychology
   Chairman, Division of Behavioral
      Sciences and Education
   Curry College
   Milton, Massachusetts

MAUREEN CUSHING, J.D., B.S.N.
   Lecturer in Health Care Law
   Private Law Practice
   Boston, Massachusetts

VINCENT J. DeFEO, Ph.D.
   Professor of Anatomy and Reproductive Biology
   University of Hawaii at Manoa
   John A. Burns School of Medicine
   Honolulu, Hawaii

DOROTHY DeMAIO, Ed.D., R.N., F.A.A.N.
Associate Professor
Rutgers University
School of Nursing
Graduate MCH Program
Newark, New Jersey

SUE A. DRISCOLL, M.S., R.N.
Clinical Nurse Specialist
Pulmonary Diseases
University of Wisconsin Hospitals
Center for Health Sciences
Madison, Wisconsin

LINDA G. DUMAS, M.S., M.A., R.N.
Instructor
Boston University
School of Nursing
Boston, Massachusetts

M. PATRICIA FASCE, M.S., R.N.
Associate Professor
Berkshire Community College
Pittsfield, Massachusetts

BEVERLY C. FINEMAN, M.Ed., R.N.
Doctoral Candidate
Columbia University
Formerly, Assistant Professor
Columbia University
School of Nursing
New York, New York

GENEVIEVE FITZPATRICK, M.S., R.N.
Assistant Professor
Baccalaureate Coordinator
Division of Nursing Studies
Curry College
Milton, Massachusetts

MARGARET A. FRAZIER, M.S., R.N.
Assistant Professor
Director, Learning Resources Laboratory
Boston University
School of Nursing
Boston, Massachusetts

JACQUELINE F. FREITAS, M.S., R.N.
Associate Chief, Nursing Service for Education
Veterans Administration
Medical Center
Boston, Massachusetts

ANITA GIOVANNETTI GALWAY, M.S., R.N.
Assistant Professor
Saint Anselm's College
Manchester, New Hampshire

MARY BETH HANNER, M.P.H., R.N.
Assistant Professor
Russell Sage College
Troy, New York

CAROL V. HAYES, M.Ed., R.N.
Associate Professor
University of Florida
College of Nursing
Gainesville, Florida

MARION ISAACS, M.S., R.N.
Assistant Professor
Graduate Division: Community Health Nursing
Boston University
School of Nursing
Boston, Massachusetts

LINDA L. JARVIS, M.S.N., R.N.
Assistant Professor
Boston University
School of Nursing
Boston, Massachusetts

ELISE D. NAVRATIL-KLINE, M.S., R.N.
Assistant Professor
Division of Nursing Studies
Curry College
Milton, Massachusetts

ELIZABETH C. KUDZMA, M.S., R.N.
Doctoral Candidate
Boston University
Associate Professor
Division of Nursing Studies
Curry College
Milton, Massachusetts

JO ANN LENOCKER, M.S., B.S.N.
Formerly, Instructor
University of Florida
College of Nursing
Gainesville, Florida

RAMONA MAE LESLIE, M.S., R.N.
Instructor
Russell Sage College
Troy, New York

CLAIRE D. MARANDA, M.S., R.N.
Doctoral Candidate
Boston College
Associate Professor
Division of Nursing Studies
Curry College
Milton, Massachusetts

MARYA SAMPSON MARTHAS, Ed.D., R.N.
Clinical Specialist
McLean Hospital
Belmont, Massachusetts

DIANE O. McGIVERN, Ph.D., R.N.
Associate Dean and Director of the Undergrad-
uate Program
University of Pennsylvania
School of Nursing
Philadelphia, Pennsylvania

MAUREEN O'BRIEN MODESTY, M.S., R.N.
Assistant Professor
University of Maryland
School of Nursing
Baltimore, Maryland

CHRISTINE S. PAKATAR, M.S., R.N.
Assistant Professor, Nurse Practitioner
Russell Sage College
Troy, New York

SARAH B. PASTERNACK, M.A., R.N.
Assistant Professor
Boston University
School of Nursing
Boston, Massachusetts

PATRICIA CHEHY PILETTE, Ed.D., M.S., R.N.
Nursing Consultant
Co-Director Humanistic Nursing Consultant
Services
Boston, Massachusetts

PEARL P. ROSENDAHL, Ed.D., R.N.
Adult Nurse Practitioner
Associate Professor
Boston University
School of Nursing
Boston, Massachusetts

GAIL J. SANZONE, M.S., R.N.
Assistant Professor
Russell Sage College
Troy, New York

ARLYNE B. SAPERSTEIN, M.N., R.N.
Assistant Professor
Division of Nursing Studies
Curry College
Milton, Massachusetts

DOROTHY C. SILVER, M.Ed., R.D.
Director of Nutritional Care and the Dietetic In-
ternship
Mount Auburn Hospital
Cambridge, Massachusetts

MAJOR FAITH STERLING, M.S., R.N.
Nurse Advisor to the Reserve Component to the
Headquarters of the U.S. Readiness Region
VIII
Denver, Colorado

MARY ELLEN SULLIVAN, M.S., R.N.
Assistant Professor
Division of Nursing Studies
Curry College
Milton, Massachusetts

NANCY S. SYPERT, M.N., R.N.
Assistant Professor
University of Florida
College of Nursing
Gainesville, Florida

JO JOYCE TACKETT, M.P.H., R.N.
  Assistant Professor of Nursing
  Blackhawk Community College
  Kewanee, Illinois

PAMELA GAHERIN WATSON, M.S., R.N.
  Assistant Professor
  Boston University
  School of Nursing
  Boston, Massachusetts

ROBIN YOUNG WOOD, M.S., R.N.
  Assistant Professor
  Boston University
  School of Nursing
  Boston, Massachusetts

KATHLEEN F. ZAGATA, M.S., R.N.
  Psychiatric Nurse Clinician
  Massachusetts General Hospital
  Boston, Massachusetts

CAROL ZIMMERN, M.A., R.N.
  Assistant Professor
  University of Miami
  Miami, Florida

CONTENTS

PART 1: CONCEPTS ABOUT THE CLIENT

In the world of business, a manufacturer who wishes to sell a product or a service must consider several things. Is there a need for the product, and obviously, who is the consumer who will purchase it? To determine the salient characteristics of the potential consumer and the type of environment in which he lives, the manufacturer initiates a marketing research project. From the data collected, he establishes criteria on which to base decisions concerning the appearance, packaging, and advertising of the product to complement the needs, desires, and motivations of this consumer. Without serious consideration of the potential consumer, "product managers" would have little sense of what and how to deliver their merchandise in a manner likely to be successful.

Similarly, health care is a service which a system or providers wish to distribute to as many "consumers" as possible. To understand the consumer of this service—that is, the client—the "providers" must understand a number of general characteristics which apply in one way or another to the recipient.

The nursing student may find some of the concepts presented in the following four chapters familiar from her studies of behavioral and social sciences. These studies along with those in the natural sciences provide a base of information which will be useful in understanding the consumers who are in need of health care services. A look at growth and development will give the reader basic information about clients of all ages and stages of maturity (Chapter 1); a description of the various types of family units and their functions provides background information pertaining to different life styles (Chapter 2); concepts of human sexuality apply to all human beings and have significance to the health worker in understanding certain aspects of the client as well as themselves (Chapter 3); and finally, a description of who a client is gives the reader an introduction to the consumer of health care services as he assumes the role of client (Chapter 4).

CHAPTER 1

Human growth and development occur as a consequence of a series of both quantitative and qualitative changes. Quantitiative changes which include increases in age, height, and weight, are probably the easiest to recognize and measure. They encompass most of the developmental manifestations in growth and development tables. Qualitative changes, which include differences in vocabulary, speech, and motor control at various ages, are harder to measure and trace; however, they can significantly affect individual performance, capabilities, life patterns, and choices.

Theorists have described individual patterns of human development. In psychoanalytic theory, Freud stressed the importance of early childhood experiences on later adult development and suggested several childhood periods—the oral, anal, phallic, and latency phases.[1] He emphasized the deterministic nature of childhood experiences which negated the value of later adult intervention.

Erikson, whose description of human growth and development was an outgrowth of Freudian theory,

GROWTH AND DEVELOPMENT

Elizabeth C. Kudzma, M.S., R.N., and
Claire D. Maranda, M.S., R.N.

suggested that the individual progresses through an epigenetic* conception of ego development.[2] He defined the following eight developmental stages, each with its associated specific crisis: (1) basic trust versus mistrust, (2) autonomy versus shame and doubt, (3) initiative versus guilt, (4) industry versus inferiority, (5) identity versus role confusion, (6) intimacy versus isolation, (7) generativity versus stagnation, and (8) ego integrity versus despair.[3] These stages suggest critical periods of decision-making between progression and regression and indicate that each phase is systematically related to other phases. Progression or regression in any stage may facilitate or hinder development in future stages. Of particular significance is Erikson's belief in growth throughout the entire life cycle; he emphasized all life periods, not just the early ones.

*"In embryology, the theory that parts of an organism arise by a process of progressive development, from simple to complex structures. . . ." (*Taber's Cyclopedic Medical Dictionary*, 13th ed., edited by Thomas, C. L., Philadelphia, F. A. Davis Company, 1977.)

Piaget, a renowned theorist of human growth and development, suggested that intellectual development is a continuous process of organization of mental structures and that each subsequent intellectual stage represents a reorganization of the prior stage. The individual becomes aware of his environment through the processes of "assimilation" and "accommodation."[4] Assimilation includes utilization and incorporation of objects from the environment. Accommodation is the resulting change in the individual's cognitive structures due to the prior process of assimilation. The two processes interact continuously, and the balance between them represents the adaptation of the individual to his environment.

Piaget also believes that the child passes through several patterns of thinking as he matures; a child's thought processes are very different from adult reasoning because human beings reason differently at different ages. The child has his own concept of reality which serves as a reference point from which to compare, test, and redefine new experiences.[5,6]

Piaget's developmental modes of reasoning are: (1) sensorimotor, (2) preoperation, (3) concrete operational, and (4) formal operational.[7,8] Although various environmental conditions can alter the pace at which each stage is achieved, the sequence of stages is consistent, and stages cannot be skipped. At any stage, modes of reasoning characteristic of earlier stages are often present, and the child may be capable of reverting to earlier levels of reasoning.

This chapter on growth and development represents a summary of current theory. While individual growth and development will be traced using Erikson's eight basic stages, the beliefs of other theorists are examined. The current interest in growth and development in all stages of life, not merely childhood and adolescence, is perhaps best exemplified by the popularity of Sheehy's book, *Passages*, which describes crises in adult life.[9]

INFANT

Rapid growth and development characterize the period of infancy (newborn to 1 year). At birth, the infant depends on reflex activity, such as sucking, and the nurturance of others for survival. By the age of 12 months, the infant has developed behaviors (albeit primitive) that permit him to be somewhat independent—mobility, self-feeding, speech, and the ability to interact meaningfully with adults. In addition, his birth weight has tripled, and he will have gained approximately 8 to 10 inches in height. Except for growth in utero, the child grows more rapidly during infancy than in any other period in the life cycle.

Psychosocially, he develops a sense of trust which is necessary for resolution of all the other developmental crises as defined by Erikson. Freud termed this period of development the oral stage, because the infant's primary source of pleasure and exploration of the world is through his mouth.[10]

Psychosocial Development

The main thrust of psychosocial development during the first year of life aims at the attainment of Erikson's sense of basic trust.[11] The infant first develops a sense of trust in the mother* and then

---

*Mother is used throughout to refer to the main caretaker with the understanding that in today's society, the biological mother may not be the major caretaker or that there may be more than one.

other significant people in his environment. Healthy maternal-infant bonding must occur very early in the life of the newborn for normal development to occur. A child will never gain a sense of trust in his mother unless there is a strong relationship established in the newborn period. Klaus and Kennell state:

> This original mother-infant bond is the wellspring for all the infant's subsequent attachments and is the formative relationship in the course of which the child develops a sense of himself. Throughout his lifetime, the strength and character of this attachment will influence the quality of all future bonds to other individuals.[12]

Because bonding occurs as a result of the mother seeing, touching, and caring for her infant, the nurse must make it possible for the mother to have early contact with the newborn even if premature or ill. When the mother provides consistent, high quality care which includes feeding, cuddling, playing, rocking, keeping him dry and clean, and providing warmth, the infant soon learns that his needs will be met. The trust that he gains in the nurturer will later be extended to others. According to Stone and Church, the infant learns "whether the world is a good and satisfying place to live or a source of pain, misery, frustration, and uncertainty."[13]

This is not meant to imply that the baby must have all of his needs met the instant they occur. If consistent and loving care is provided, the infant will learn to wait for a few minutes to have a need met. Instant gratification of all of the infant's needs is not necessary and could lead to future problems.

Socially, the infant first responds to the mother with a smile. The first social smile occurs around the age of 6 weeks but may often be preceded by facial behaviors that resemble a smile. A social smile is a response of the infant to seeing his mother. The infant responds well to adult company and will engage in play with adults. Social games like pat-a-cake become important toward the end of the first year. Fear of strangers may occur around the age of 8 months, especially after the infant recognizes the mother as the caretaker. This recognition, which comes before 8 months, is exhibited by different behavior in the presence of his mother than in the presence of strangers. According to Erikson, the infant's first social achievement is "his willingness to let the mother out of sight without undue anxiety or rage, because she has become an inner certainty as well as an outer predictability."[11]

Infant Feeding

Nutrition and feeding methods are important for the infant who is undergoing rapid physical growth. There is no universally accepted manner of feeding or introducing new foods during the first year of life. The following is an attempt to summarize the current theories on infant feeding.

Breast-feeding, which has many advantages over formula feeding, is gaining in popularity. Breast-fed infants have fewer allergies and obtain many valuable antibodies from mother's milk which prevent certain diseases during the first few months of life. This type of feeding eliminates formula preparation and assures that the feeding is at the proper temperature. The breast-fed infant usually spends more time feeding than the bottle-fed infant. Therefore, the breast-fed infant sucks longer and has more opportunity to establish maternal-infant bonding.

Even though breast-feeding has many advantages, the nurse should recognize that bottle-feeding provides good nutrition and is frequently the most acceptable form of feeding. There are many types of infant formulas, but discussion of these is beyond the scope of this text. The nurse working with infants must familiarize herself with common formulas used in clinical practice.

Infants are born with the ability to suck, but they must learn to eat solid foods and to drink from a cup. There is no magical time framework for the accomplishment of these tasks, and pediatricians vary greatly as to appropriate timing. The following are general principles applicable to most infants:

1. Introduce only one new food at a time. This will assist in identification of food allergies.
2. Gradually increase the consistency of new foods. Cereal is diluted with formula in varying amounts.
3. The progression of foods introduced is: cereal, fruit, vegetables, meat, and egg yolks. Egg whites are reserved for the end of the first year or the beginning of the second since many infants are allergic to albumin.
4. Fruit juices are introduced diluted, and gradually the infant is given more concentrated juices. Fruit juices are not warmed since vitamin C is destroyed by heat. Babies who tend to have allergies probably should receive their vitamin C in the form of a vitamin supplement instead of in fruit juices.
5. Avoid introducing new foods when the infant is very hungry since this may be very frustrating.
6. Finger foods may be started when the infant can grasp these easily and usually when he starts to teethe (around 6 months).
7. Table foods are introduced when the child begins to teethe and should be selected carefully as to texture and consistency.
8. If mothers choose to buy baby foods they should be instructed to read labels carefully. Commercial foods may contain additives that are not desirable, and also one may be confused by labeling practices. The main ingredient in canned products is the first one listed.
9. Mothers may make their own baby foods and freeze them in individual portions using ice trays. Home prepared foods tend to contain more calories than canned foods; the infant will, therefore, need a smaller quantity due to the difference in quality.
10. Cup-feeding is frequently introduced with juices between feedings or when the infant demonstrates a lack of interest in the bottle or breast. Usually, it is wise to replace nursing with a cup for only one feeding at a time.
11. Do not allow an infant to go to bed with a bottle of juice or milk even if he can hold the bottle well. Once the infant's teeth have erupted, the sugars in the juices and in the milk, if allowed to stay on the teeth all night, will cause serious dental caries. This is often referred to as "bottle mouth syndrome."
12. Mothers should not discontinue formula feedings until instructed by the pediatrician. Too early introduction of whole milk may cause severe anemia in some babies, and the use of skim milk may not provide the infants with needed fats.

Good nutrition is crucial to the infant's growth and development. The feeding experience is as crucial as the quality of the nutrients offered. Meals are pleasurable for infants when their needs for sucking and for being fondled are met. Much of the babies sense of trust is gained through the feeding experience. Mothers who reject the feeding experience or who see it as messy and unpleasant may potentiate a syndrome called "failure to thrive." This refers to infants who are lethargic and refuse to feed adequately.

Cognitive and Intellectual Development

Learning occurs basically through the use of the senses. During the first year, the infant will pass through and attain Piaget's four stages of sensorimotor cognitive development. Briefly, these four stages are defined as follows (ages are approximate):

1. Reflex activity (newborn to 6 weeks): Three important reflexes dominate the infant's learning: sucking, eye movements, and palmar grasp.
2. Primary circular reactions (6 weeks to 4 to 5 months): Learning occurs through reactions that involve only the infant's own body; for example, the infant brings his hand before his face repeatedly.
3. Secondary circular reactions (4 to 9 months): Three major behaviors enhance learning: intentional grasping, secondary circular reactions, and differentiation between means and ends. Secondary circular reactions involve reactions which include repeating chance discoveries.
4. Coordination between means and goals (9 to 12 months): Piaget's concept of intelligence is defined "as the use of certain means to reach certain goals."[14] The infant can now use previously learned experiences and connect them with a desired goal.[7,14]

Between the ages of 6 and 8 months, the infant gains a sense of object permanence; that is, he now realizes that objects still exist when out of sight. Prior to this, if an object was taken away from an infant, he believed that it no longer existed (Fig. 1-1).

Language development begins early. Development starts when the infant's cry becomes differentiated at about 2 months; that is, the nature of the cry of the child indicates to the mother the reason for crying (i.e., hunger, pain, or anger). The first noises made by the infant except for crying is

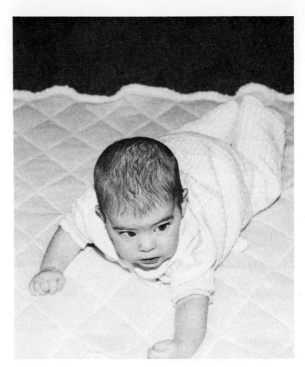

FIGURE 1-1. The infant is alert to his surroundings.

a cooing noise which is followed by babbling. Infants babble prior to the age of 6 months. Babbling is followed by the utterance of recognizable sounds ("da-da," "ma-ma"), and the first real word is usually uttered at about 12 months. Parents should not be concerned if this does not occur until the second year. Controversy exists regarding the way children learn to talk, but it is believed that much learning occurs through imitation of adults. The infant not only derives pleasure from listening to adults, but also learns to speak; infants who hear little adult speech often have delayed language development.

Physical and Motor Development

The infant grows very rapidly during the first 12 months of life. Most infants will double their birth weight by 6 months and triple it by 1 year. At no time in the life span will growth occur as quickly.

Physical and motor development proceeds in two directions—cephalocaudal and proximodistal. Cephalocaudal growth (from head downwards) is illustrated by the infant who first learns to lift his head off the bed, then his chest, and only much later learns to sit up. Proximodistal growth (from the center outward) is illustrated by the infant, who at first randomly moves his arms, but gradually learns motor control until he finally learns to control the fine muscles of the hand.

Milestones are used to indicate the mean age at which children should demonstrate certain behaviors. These apply to all aspects of development but are particularly applicable to the infant's physical and motor development. One must caution the reader that these refer to mean or average behaviors; individual differences do occur. Some of the most important physical and motor developmental milestones seen in the first year of life are listed in Table 1-1.

Accidents are often related to the child's development. The infant will roll over and fall off a table if left unattended or unrestrained. He will reach out and grasp at objects which are dangerous (hot liquids). He can slip in the bath tub before he learns to sit well without support. (Even after he can sit well, however, he cannot be trusted in the tub.) He will tug at cords to see what is at the other end when he is able to reach them by crawling or hitching (electrical coffee pots are frequently pulled over). He will explore objects by putting them in his mouth (aspiration of small objects), and he pokes his fingers into anything (electrical sockets). Accident prevention must start early even before the child has learned a particular behavior that can lead to trouble; for example, the infant should be restrained on a dressing table long before he learns to turn over.

Nurses need to assess infants and children for growth and developmental level. Iowa Growth

Charts are useful to evaluate physical height and weight. Charts with head circumferences are used to evaluate head size. The Denver Developmental Screening Test assesses personal (social, fine motor), adaptive, language, and gross motor skills in infants, toddlers, and preschoolers. (The Denver Developmental Screening Test is further discussed in Part 4, Chapter 22, "Child Health Assessment."

Implications for Nursing

1. Consistency in providing nursing care will help the infant maintain a sense of trust.
2. Physical needs must be satisfied if the infant is to maintain or gain a sense of trust.
3. The nurse should provide the infant with opportunities to suck.
4. The nurse should spend time rocking, cuddling, and talking to infants.
5. The nurse should provide play opportunities and appropriate toys for the infant.
6. Good observation of reflex activity is necessary for proper evaluation of infants.
7. Since infancy is a period of rapid growth, the nurse must be aware that infants have a high metabolic rate and therefore need more calories and fluids per body weight than adults.
8. The safety needs of infants must always be considered. Infants undergo rapid change in motor ability and cannot assume responsibility for themselves.
9. To promote appropriate muscular development, the nurse should provide opportunities for the infant to use his developing muscles.
10. Because early maternal attachment is of prime importance, mothers who cannot care for their infant shortly after birth must be allowed to see their child, and to help care for him within limitations imposed by the nature of the separation.
11. Maternal separation is difficult for infants after the age of 6 months. In the pediatric unit, the nurse should encourage mothers to stay or to visit frequently, and to participate in the care of the infant.
12. Nurses must know the principles that apply to good nutrition and apply this knowledge in their care and teaching of mothers.

TABLE 1-1. Common Developmental Milestones

Age (Months)	Milestones
1	Raises head slightly off the bed.
3	Reaches out at objects.
4	Can sit propped up for short periods of time.
6	Can roll completely over.
6—7	Can sit unsupported.
7—8	Thumb apposition.
9—10	Crawls (pulls self on abdomen) and creeps (moves on hands and knees with trunk above floor).
12	Walks with help (many walk alone).

TODDLER

Learning skills necessary to promote a sense of independence or autonomy keep the toddler (ages 1 to 3 years) very busy. Some of these skills are walking, talking, self-feeding, and toilet training. As a means of learning, toddlers busily explore their environment, but these activities often get them into difficulty. Accidents involving ingestion and falls are common during this period. Rituals and favorite toys become very important for toddlers who need some objects or activities which remain stable in their world of constant change. Negative behavior and temper tantrums may be frequent and a cause of frustration for the parents.

The rapid physical growth of infancy slows down during this period and the toddler may demonstrate a loss of appetite called physiological anorexia—a normal characteristic of toddlerhood.

Psychosocial Development

Most authorities on growth and development describe the toddler's quest for autonomy and his need for increasing independence. Erikson viewed this period as the time when the child "begins to experience the whole critical opposition of being an autonomous creature and being a dependent one."[15] The child during this period will often say "me do it" whether or not he can do the task at hand. This may lead to frustration for both the child and the parent. If frustration and failure prevails in the struggle, irrespective of the core problem, the result will be attainment of shame and doubt instead of a sense of autonomy.

Attainment of a sense of autonomy involves the social modalities of "holding on" and "letting go."[16] The child during this period learns many new behaviors. Control of bowel and bladder is the major skill frequently attributed to this age group, but this is only one of the behaviors that the toddler must learn. Other areas of development include learning to talk, increasing mobility (walking, climbing up and down stairs, jumping), learning to undress, and socialization skills. This period corresponds with the Freudian anal phase in which satisfaction is sought through excretory functions.[10]

Parents need to exert controls to protect the child. Erikson, in discussing the use of control, stated: "As his environment encourages him to 'stand on his own feet'; it must protect him against meaningless and arbitrary experiences of shame and of early doubt."[17] Temper tantrums may result from frustration or from controls inconsistently applied. The negative behavior that is characteristic of toddlers is often difficult for both parents and nurses. Frequently the "no" of the toddler does not really mean "no." For example, it is not uncommon to call a toddler and get a response of "no" while he runs toward the caller.

Favorite toys and ritualistic behavior especially at bedtime seem to provide stability for the young child and are sources of comfort during struggles to gain independence and yet maintain dependence. Separation from the mother is especially traumatic. Toddlers learn that the mother can go away and will return, but any prolonged separation can have long lasting negative effects. Fear of abandonment may prevent the toddler from forming any lasting relationships in later years.

Toddlers often will not play with other toddlers even if in the same room. They engage in what is called parallel play which involves two or more children playing side by side with very little interaction. They will play with adults, and they do enjoy a variety of activities. Water play (supervised), sand boxes, and push toys are only a few examples of appropriate play activities, and materials.

Cognitive, Intellectual, and Language Development

The toddler in his second year of life continues in the sensorimotor phase of development, but he now enters Piaget's stages 5 and 6.

5. Tertiary circular reaction (12 to 18 months): This stage is also referred to as the stage of discovery of new means. Groping leads to the discovery of the use of intermediary object as a means to attain an end; that is, the child discovers that a stick will help to reach a distant object.
6. Intervention of new means (18 to 24 months): New means are discovered with a lot less groping. He begins to show evidence of mental representation of events.[7,18]

During this second year, the child begins to imitate. Early imitation requires the presence of a model, but in the second half of the year, the toddler can remember and imitate an event that took place a few days before.

At 2, the child begins the preoperational phase of development. This phase ends at about 7 years of age. The child begins to cope with more than one event at a time, and he proceeds to symbolic and perceptual levels of function. Language, symbolic play, and imitation are acquired during this time. Egocentric thinking characterizes the thoughts of the toddler. The toddler thinks mostly about himself. Toward the end of the toddler period, the child will begin to pose questions (who, what, where, when, and why) about events and his environment; these questions may be repeated time after time.

Most toddlers by the end of their second year have a repertoire of approximately 300 words, but they understand much more than they actually speak. It is at this period that one should worry about the child who is not speaking (aphasia). Deafness is frequently the cause of aphasia in children, particularly if other areas of development are proceeding at a normal pace.

Physical and Motor Development

There are no considerable changes in height and weight between the years of 1 to 3 as compared with the first year. By 24 months, the toddler should weigh approximately 26–28 pounds, and will have grown 3 to 4 inches. The anterior fontannel closes by 18 months. (Many children have closed anterior fontannels by the age of 12 months.)

The child walks alone usually before 14 months; he learns to run, jump, walk up and down stairs. He learns to feed himself, hold a cup (by 15 months), and control a spoon (by 18 months). By 2 years, he can drink from a cup and spoon-feed himself. He learns to stack blocks, and by the age of 3, he should be able to build a tower of nine or 10 blocks. He also learns to copy a straight line and to throw a ball (Fig. 1-2).

As the child becomes more mobile, he is much more likely to have accidents. Safety precautions are important, especially those which prevent the ingestion of foreign objects. In their quest for

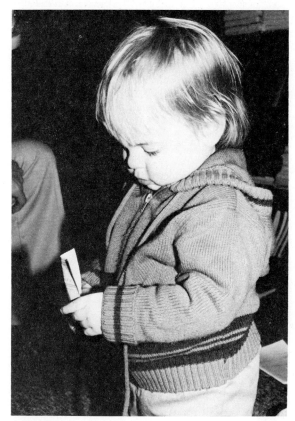

FIGURE 1-2. The toddler begins to use fine motor coordination.

knowledge, toddlers are very likely to test noxious materials if these are in accessible areas. It is important to emphasize that toddlers can run, climb, and move very quickly.

Implications for Nursing

1. The toddler needs opportunities to practice newly developed skills to maintain a sense of autonomy and independence.
2. Efforts must be made by nursing personnel to help the hospitalized child to maintain sphincter control once established. This does not mean punishing any child who has accidents, particularly if they are sick.
3. Nurses are in a position to help parents cope with the various behaviors—negativism, rituals, and temper tantrums—of toddlers.
4. Opportunities for appropriate and safe play must be provided.

5. Toddlers who are ill should face a minimum amount of separation from their mother.
6. Toddlers need controls on their behavior since they do not know their limits.
7. Nurses must educate the public regarding accident prevention, especially those related to ingestions, falls, and motor vehicles.
8. Toddlers need to practice newly acquired language.
9. Toddlers need simple answers to the questions who, where, what, when, and why; the child may ask these questions over and over again.
10. The nutritional requirements of toddlers decline due to slower rates of growth.

PRESCHOOLER

The preschooler (3 to 6-years-old) delights everyone with his creativity and his imagination. Separating fantasy from reality as well as understanding adult reasoning may at times be difficult. Egocentric thinking affects his relations with others and his view of the world, even though cooperative play emerges during this period. Contact with peers begins to gain in importance and will become increasingly important for many years to come. Sexual curiosity and exploration occur and may positively or negatively affect later behavior. Moral realism rather than subjective morality is seen in his evaluation of misdeeds.

Psychosocial Development

The child begins the preschool period with an established sense of trust and autonomy, and he must now achieve a sense of initiative so as to avoid gaining a sense of guilt. Erikson defined initiative as that which

> adds to autonomy the quality of undertaking, planning and attacking a task for the sake of being active and on the move, where before self-will, more often than not, inspired acts of defiance or, at any rate, protested independence.[19]

The danger as described by Erikson is a sense of guilt, "over the goals contemplated and the acts initiated in one's exuberant enjoyment of new locomotor and mental power . . ."[19]

The preschooler learns about his environment and other people by doing; he is constantly busy with many projects. At the same time conscience develops, and he must learn to control and assert himself. If successful, he will gain a sense of initiative, and if he fails, he will develop a sense of guilt.

Development of the rudiments of conscience is evident during this period. The child recognizes that an action is "bad" but is unable to differentiate circumstances that affect the amount of guilt associated with the act. For example, accidental breaking of 12 cups is considered worse than the deliberate breaking of one cup because the child associates guilt with magnitude not intent. The child knows that his actions may result in punishment.

Guilt can be the result of sexual activities. Freud refers to this period as the phallic phase.[10] Children learn that there is a difference between the two sexes; and frequently, they explore each others bodies. In addition, many if not all children masturbate during this period of development. Masturbation releases tension and is often engaged in when the child is tired and tense (i.e., at bedtime). Castration fears may be associated with sexual exploration of the preschooler. The child may fear that his genitals will be harmed as a result of masturbation. Therefore, surgery involving the genitals may be traumatic for preschoolers.

Play is associative at the beginning of the period, but it eventually becomes cooperative. Associative play involves participating in the same play activity of other children without any interaction. Individual children play with blocks, but no cooperation is seen in the building activities. Cooperative play contributes to the socialization process by forcing children to share and communicate with each other. Dramatic play is common. By imitating adults, the child learns various roles. Because of the child's vivid imagination, few props are necessary. A hat or a piece of clothing is usually all that is needed to act various roles—fireman, nurse, or policeman. A box may be an engine, a rocket, or furniture. Expensive toys are not necessary; in fact, they may even be detrimental, since creativity should be encouraged (Fig. 1-3).

Cognitive, Intellectual, and Language Development

According to Piaget, the preschooler continues in the preoperational stage of development. This

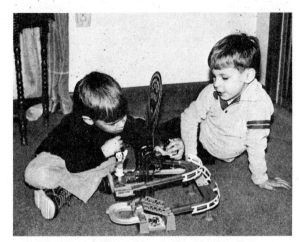

FIGURE 1-3. Preschoolers sharing during play.

stage starts around the age of 2 and continues into the early school age period. By now the child has mental representations, and he can internalize thoughts. His world often becomes dominated by symbolism. Marlow states: "with symbolism, a mental event can stand for something in the real world."[20] The child cannot reason but is able to associate two events accurately. He does not yet link cause and effect.

His concept of the world is based on animism, realism, and artificialism.[21] In animism, the child considers material objects as alive; a toy bear may be thought to feel, hear, and see. Realism is characterized by confusion between physical and psychological realities. For example, nightmares may be perceived as reality. Artificialism follows animism. Stone and Church define artificialism as "the assumption that all events are to be explained by the actions of some humanlike agent, entity, or force which wills things to happen in fulfillment of some purpose of its own."[22] This concept of the world leads the preschooler to the continual asking of who, why, when, where, and what—questions which were initiated in the toddler period, but now become pronounced.

Language development progresses very rapidly during this stage. The child learns approximately 600 words per year from ages 2 to 6. A vocabulary of 2100 words by the age of 5 is considered average.[23] This rapid language development aids in the socialization process that is taking place, especially as it relates to peer group associations.

Calling this the preschool period is a misnomer in some respects, especially in the United States where so many children attend nursery school and even prenursery school. Many school systems now provide kindergarten classes, and in some parts of the country provisions must be made so that every child has this opportunity.

The availability of preschool education has many implications for nursing. This is a time in which many health problems can be identified; the nurse can be instrumental in prevention, early identification, and early treatment of problems seen in children. Selection of a particular preschool educational program is important since programs and objectives vary; not all these programs will meet the needs of all children.

Physical and Motor Development

Growth continues at a rate of approximately 5 pounds and 2½ inches per year. Loss of body fat will change body appearance.

Dental care is necessary to maintain the primary dentition which is completed at 24 months and to promote good dental health necessary for the permanent teeth. By the age of 6 the child will cut his first permanent molars and probably lose the primary lower central incisors.

The preschooler develops both growth and fine motor coordination. For example, he learns to ride a tricycle, to master a jungle gym, and to make recognizable shapes (circles, squares, and triangles); some may even learn to print letters and their names. The child gains mastery in the use of finger paints, crayons, and enjoys working with colors.

Safety continues to be a consideration for anyone caring for preschoolers. As they gain in motor ability they become more likely to have accidents related to their newly acquired skills. Motor vehicle accidents continue to be the major source of problems; that is, they are not only the result of being a passenger in a car but are frequently related to the activities in which the child participates—for example, riding a tricycle or playing in the street.

Implications for Nursing

1. Children in this age group may associate illness with punishment for a misdeed or even a wish they may have had.
2. Moral development is beginning, but it is in

its earliest stage. This affects the child's reaction to punishment and his feelings of guilt.

3. Their understanding and view of illness may be colored by fantasy.
4. Play activities for these children must reflect the child's interest in dramatic and cooperative play.
5. The preschooler's thought is egocentric. The preschooler understands only how phenomena affects him; he is oblivious to effects on others.
6. Because the preschooler is gaining a sense of initiative, he is usually very occupied doing and creating. Nurses must not discourage these activities.
7. Preschoolers have a good command of the language and communicate their needs, but they are unable to reason or to abstract.
8. Preschoolers need to be permitted to ask questions and may repeatedly ask the same question. They need simple answers to their questions of why, who, when, what, and where.
9. Sexual curiosity is normal, and *simple* answers are helpful.
10. Masturbation is normal, and nurses should ignore this behavior.
11. Because motor coordination is rapidly increasing and children need a chance to practice newly acquired skills, the nurse should provide play activities, if possible, that will enhance motor development.
12. Anticipatory guidance for parents regarding accident prevention is important.
13. It is important to educate parents about appropriate dental care for the preschooler. Children can learn how to brush their teeth properly. They should also learn that going to the dentist is important and necessary and not an experience that should be feared.

SCHOOLCHILDREN

The entrance of the child into school (ages 6 to 10) is a central experience in the next stage of growth and development. School is an important factor in growth and development because: (1) the child must regularly go outside his home into a wider environment; (2) he must constantly interact with peers; and (3) he is subject to authoritative adults other than his parents. Also, during this time, the child begins to gain a sense of competence which will continue throughout his schooling.

In all cultures, children of school age receive some instruction in cultural values. In preliterate and semiliterate societies, the focus in early learning is on the most general types of instruction which will lead to the widest option in terms of future careers. This usually includes, but is not limited to, instruction in reading, writing, and arithmetic.

Psychosocial Development

Jackson suggested that the importance of elementary schooling in the life of the child cannot be underestimated because of the frequency of trivial classroom events, the standardization of the school environment, and the compulsory nature of school attendance.[24] During elementary schooling, the young child learns to cope with institutional life and develops adaptive strategies that form the basis for later education and life. The central characteristics of the elementary school classroom environment, "delay, denial, interruption, and social distraction" must be overcome in order for learning to occur.[25] The child must learn to cope with rules, regulations, and routines of the school.

Development of a sense of industry in this stage refers to the initiation and amplification of new capacities promoted by classroom learning in the child. Rewards for accomplishments completed at a satisfactory level are important for total development of the child's self-concept. Inferiority may result if a sense of inadequacy is developed through constant detrimental comparison with peers or through negative feedback from teachers, parents, and other significant individuals.[26]

This period corresponds to Freud's latency period so termed because sexual interests appear quiescent, only to emerge later during adolescence.[10] Though most of the child's activities are directed toward developing cooperative peer relationships, certain elements of a sexual nature may still interest the child such as curiosity about the birth process. The birth of additional siblings may also stimulate sexual questions.

Cognitive and Intellectual Development

The school years are a period of rapid intellectual change, especially with regard to language acquisition. Language skills are learned and refined within this period. At this time, girls may appear to progress faster than boys in academic areas, especially in vocabulary development and sentence structure. Stimulation in the home environment and easy access to newspapers and books further language acquisition.

In cognitive development, the child is progressing into concrete operational thought;[7] this is distinguished by the ability to order lower classes from higher classes, by understanding the reversibility of classes, by an understanding of conservation, or that quantities may be of the same volume or weight yet occupy very different dimensions. The child learns to operate with the symbol systems of language and mathematics. The capacity of the child to add, multiply, and divide is acquired at this time. In language, the child can organize words to form classes within greater classes; for example, blackbirds are a smaller class within a greater class of birds.

Physical and Motor Development

The average height of schoolchildren ranges from 44 to 54 inches, and the average weight is between 45 and 71 pounds. Height, weight, and nutritional status are indicators of adequate growth and development. Steady, rapid increases in physical growth are normal in the healthy child. It is not uncommon for some parts of the body to grow more slowly than others. Arms and legs, for example, may temporarily grow out of proportion to the rest of the body.

Other characteristics of adequate growth, development, and nutritional status are clear skin, shiny hair, firm muscles, and straight posture. Normal appearance of eyes, gums, and teeth are also indicators. Growth charts are useful as criteria to gauge an individual's growth; however, heredity, nutrition, and culture may make the application of growth charts variable.

Play with peers is a central characteristic of this age group. Activities with repetitive motor actions such as bicycling and swimming are particularly enjoyed. Actual motor control is fairly clumsy and uncoordinated at age 6, but proceeds toward greater coordination by age 10. The child develops an interest in organized sports and competitive activities, such as baseball. Indoor games, checkers, and cards, now become interesting as reading and numerical abilities improve. Organized groups with adult leadership, such as scouting, are preferred.

Accidents are a leading cause of injury and death to children. Most accidents occur near the home, in school, or on streets and highways adjacent to both places. Accident prevention is directed toward educating children to environmental hazards and checking objects and playthings which may be a source of injury.

Implications for Nursing

1. School is a central feature in the child's life. Assessment should be directed at determining whether the school experience is a pleasant one. It may be helpful to determine the climate of the classroom environment (relaxed, open, rigid, or formal), the interaction of the child with his peers, and any differences in behavior between the child being observed and other children.
2. Facial expressions and posture are important. They may give many clues to the child's feelings. Is the face and mouth relaxed, rigid, or taut? Are the shoulders drooped and weary? Emotional concerns may be reflected in the child's physical expressions and mannerisms.
3. Motor skills are undergoing refinement through various activities including manipulation. What types of play and games does the child enjoy? At what physical activities does the child excel, and at what play activities is he uncoordinated?
4. Table games and play activities are important diversions in the institutional (hospital) setting.
5. The child needs directions from adults whether in playing or following hospital routines.
6. Accidents, especially motor vehicles, are a major cause of death and injury. Accident

prevention and education should be initiated.

7. Ill children frequently associate illness with punishment for imagined or real misdeeds.
8. When children are ill, the nurse should encourage peer contact. For example, cards and papers from classmates are welcomed and enjoyed.
9. The schoolchild needs to feel competent. Therefore, persons responsible for their care should provide some activities in which they can succeed.

PREADOLESCENCE AND ADOLESCENCE

The preadolescent period, roughly ages 10 to 13, is a time of rapid physical growth and development. It is also thought to be a time of personality reintegration prior to the formation of the more adultlike personality patterns in adolescence. Preadolescence is frequently a difficult time for parents and teachers, as various types of behavior which were not exhibited during childhood surface. Irritating activities such as physical restlessness, dirty jokes, baby talk, and stubbornness exhibited toward parents and siblings may occur frequently or periodically. Manners and courtesy appear to be forgotten. The preadolescent becomes engrossed in interaction with his peer group, and the formation of groups which manifest antiadult behavior is common.

The onset of puberty is considered the beginning of adolescence, and this period extends to early adulthood, or the time when early adult responsibilities are assumed. The adolescent stage is most pronounced in Western societies, where there is an extended period between childhood and adult responsibilities. However, there is some variance among authorities as to the duration of adolescence. Education is continued through this period as more years of formal schooling are required to meet the needs of advanced technological and industrial societies. Adolescents are, therefore, dependent on adults, economically, socially, and intellectually for an extended period.

This extended adolescent period is compounded by the general state of physical maturity in adolescents which has been accelerated by better nutritional practices. Accelerated sexual maturity, a potential conflict for the high school student, is exacerbated by societal prescriptions which ordain that sexual activity and marriage be delayed until secondary schooling is completed.

Psychosocial Development

Adolescence is also a period of decision-making. There are many choices to be made about the future, including choice of life style, career, family structure, and artistic expression.[27] Adolescents are individuals in transition with choices to make and needs for love, adventure, and self-discovery.

The adolescent has special needs for dependence and independence. Although he is still dependent on adults for education, housing, food, and other necessities, he experiments with adult roles. This requires some development and allowance for independence. Independent functioning is acquired gradually through fluctuations between regressive, dependent behavior, and self-reliant behavior. When adolescents exhibit more assertiveness, they are frequently showing more mature independent behavior. Encouraging adolescents to become more knowledgeable about their own needs and desires is the first step in clarifying autonomy. Adolescents frequently have difficulty dealing with authority. Because they are striving for independence and like to feel in control of their lives, their refusal to cooperate and angry or rebellious behavior may indicate feelings of a loss of control.

Adolescence is characterized by the development of a sexual, social, and intellectual identity, and an integration of childhood identifications. The opposite of identity is role confusion or diffusion. Diffusion results from inability to define an identity for the self.[28] Adolescence in psychoanalytic theory corresponds to the genital phase[29] or a time when complete organization of individual instincts is supposed to occur.

In their search for identity, adolescents may over identify with heros or famous people. They may fall in love in an attempt to see their own self-image reflected through the views of another individual. They frequently form cliques and exclude those who do not conform to the perceived identities of those in the favored group.

The adolescent may be characterized as an individual who does not have his behavioral personality coordinated. His childhood identity is changed but his adult identity is not defined or mature.

Physical Development

Adolescence is characterized by increased physical growth and development of secondary sexual characteristics. Both sexes increase in size (height and weight); some individuals undergo marked changes within as little as 3 months. In girls, a period of great growth often appears prior to menarche. The pituitary gland (located in the brain) is responsible for most of the growth as it secretes gonadotropic hormones which act primarily on the gonads; this stimulates the adrenal cortex, and the growth of secondary sexual characteristics begins to occur. Before total growth is curtailed, secondary sexual characteristics are usually present.

Secondary sexual characteristics are promoted by the ovarian and testicular hormones—estrogen and androgen. In any individual, the amount and timing of gonadal hormones may vary, causing the wide variation of height, build, and body contour commonly seen in adolescents and adults. Sex hormones are responsible for increases in growth and organ sensitivity. With boys, the androgens promote masculine sexuality and stimulate sexual fantasy and organ arousal. In girls, the estrogens promote female sexuality and increase receptivity. Behavior is also modified, resulting in the grooming, flirtation, courtship, and seduction that is characteristic of adolescents. Eventually, the adolescent integrates his new bodily changes into his self-image. This is assisted by his peers and adults who reflect back to the teenager what they perceive as his changed outward image. Eventually, the teenager adjusts to his changed self-image. For example, boys perceive themselves as tenors or baritones, not sopranos, and girls adopt more feminine adult clothing, such as long dresses, bikini bathing suits, and nylon stockings.

The adolescent is extremely concerned with his body and feels that even minor blemishes are serious. He worries about his past and future physical growth, height, sexual maturation, and development of secondary sexual characteristics. Adolescents are concerned with things they can see, for example, big feet or a nose that is perceived to be out of proportion. Some of these exhibited phenomena may be misinterpreted as characteristic of

disease or defect. The adolescent is afraid he might not be normal, but has difficulty in discriminating average from normal. (The presence of acne may be normal for adolescents; however, all adolescents do not have acne.) Unfortunately, commenting that many of these problems will pass with time does not help the problem. To the adolescent, outgrowing his perceived defects may take forever.

Cognitive and Intellectual Development

Most adolescents have reached and are beginning to reason with formal operational thought[30]—that is, they are now capable of using mathematical and algebraic symbols and can reason philosophically. Adolescents can now not only reason about concrete entities (characteristic of prior cognitive stages) but also abstract ideas and concepts.

At this time, adolescents are also able to formulate hypotheses and test them against fact and personal experiences. The isolation of variables and construction of all possible combinations of variables are possible. Combinations, triads, and permutations of different variables take on added interest. Adolescents may become engrossed in the double meanings of various words; word puns and the double-entendre may delight peers but aggravate parents and teachers.

Implications for Nursing

1. Physical appearance is very important to the adolescent. Is the adolescent generally satisfied with his appearance? How does he perceive himself? Is his perception very different from that of his peers? Does he look more mature or less mature than others of his age?
2. The secondary sexual characteristics that develop in adolescence should be assessed. In girls, these include presence, frequency, and duration of menstruation, breast development, and presence of pubic hair. In boys, these include pubic hair, increase in size of testes and penis, and deepening of the voice. Chest and facial hair occurs relatively late.
3. Interaction with peers should be assessed. How does the adolescent behave with individuals of the same or opposite sex? Does he frequently exhibit angry or rebellious behav-

ior? Is he moody or sullen? Does he belong to a particular group? Are his friends rebellious and likely to lead him into trouble?

4. Cognitively, the adolescent should be capable of reasoning abstractly. He can problem solve and formulate hypotheses. He can reason from the general to the specific and back again.

5. Adolescents have many decisions to make about future careers. What type of career is he interested in? What kinds of education will be needed for a career? Do his abilities approximate those required to achieve the desired occupation?

6. In the hospital setting the privacy of adolescents should be respected. Sports injuries and car accidents are a frequent cause of hospitalization.

7. Due to rapid growth, adolescents have big appetites and particular food likes and dislikes. If nutritional intake is affected or diminished, food that adolescents like should be offered.

8. When ill, the adolescent should be allowed to phone or visit with his friends.

YOUNG ADULTS

The major events occurring during young adulthood are career preparation, selection of a partner, and achievement of parenthood. During this time, educational preparation for a career is usually completed, and the first job is obtained. The first job may represent a severe disruption in the individual's life pattern; it may signal a break with friends known through school, a move to a new location away from family and friends, and the necessity to develop financial independence. Success on the first job and subsequent jobs is needed to achieve economic independence and successful wage earner status.

Selection of a partner proceeds from and out of behavior initiated in adolescence. There is wide variation in the time period during which a mate might finally be chosen. Some of this may depend on career preparation, but there appears to be a current trend toward delay of marriage. This has probably occurred because the identity of being "single" is more accepted and because women as well as men desire more advanced educational and occupational opportunities.

Psychosocial Development

Young adults are characterized by development of intimacy, the capability of commitment to associations and relationships, and the ethical sense to support these commitments.[31] Intimacy is found in close friendships, physical contact, assertive behavior, and in sexual activity. True sexuality develops during this period, for sexual life prior to this time was of an identity-seeking nature.[32] Earlier, immature modes of sexuality are eventually integrated into a full, mature sexual life. The opposite of intimacy is isolation; that is, contacts which would mean eventual intimacy are avoided.

The birth of the first child heralds a significant change in life style for the parents. The actual time of pregnancy acts as a preparatory period for parenthood. During pregnancy, there may be much fantasizing, playacting, or daydreaming about parental roles. Usually the idea of parent has been thought about earlier, but the true reality of the pregnancy speeds up the preparatory process. The parents must now assume the responsibility for care of an infant. This infant requires feeding, holding, clothing, bathing, and attention to individual needs and emotions. The needs of the parents must be temporarily subsumed to the needs of the child.

Common concerns during early parenthood center around the capacity to be "good parents" and the early infant-parent relationships. Some may be concerned for the physical condition of the infant or that economic or social position is now diminished. These concerns may be compounded by the absence of family, grandparents, aunts, and uncles who might have formerly provided some support and positive intervention.

While the role of nurturer and caretaker of children has traditionally been associated with the mother, fathers are currently expanding their roles to incorporate some of the tasks previously relegated to the mother. Fathers are participating in prenatal classes, labor, and delivery care; however, participation varies according to the institution. Early contact between the father and his offspring may promote paternal behavior.[33] Early introduction of the father and baby may also encourage greater participation and concern in the child's physical and emotional development.[34] Phillips and Anzalone report:

> Over and over again fathers reported themselves to be profoundly affected by the birth of their infants and to experience a great feeling of satisfaction with themselves for sharing in the birth experience. These men's basic nurturing instincts seemed to allow them to find fathering both stimulating and gratifying. In fact, most of these fathers were just as involved as the mothers in interacting with their infants, although they often left the caretaking responsibilities to the baby's mother.[35]

Psychological concepts of child care are an outgrowth of the parent's own experience with parent figures. This explains why it is possible to inherit the ability to provide emotional support and concern and pass this to subsequent generations. It is significant to note that the experience of "basic trust"[11] or mutuality in the child must be achieved at the same time his parents are achieving the parallel stage of intimacy. If the adult is not capable of close affiliations and relationships, he may subsequently cause impairment of the child's comfort, confidence, and reliance on outside providers.

Cognitive and Intellectual Development

Intellectual development tends to center around completing career preparation and finding a suitable occupation. Appropriate jobs and upward mobility in the adult world are important for fiscal security. High achievement in school is necessary for entrance into certain professions.

Cognitive development occurring in young adulthood is characterized by further extension of formal operational thought. While adolescents become capable of reasoning formally, during young adulthood further increases in reasoning capacities are noted, especially in those individuals who seek advanced education.

Physical and Motor Development

Once the individual has reached adulthood, physical changes are slower and of lesser magnitude. Adults of both sexes are at the maximum devel-opment of physical attractiveness, energy, and vigor. Hospitalizations at this time are frequently related to surgery or the result of trauma.

Implications for Nursing

1. Anticipatory guidance should be provided which is related to physical, social, and psychological changes associated with young adulthood.
2. Instruction about childbearing and child-rearing should be available.
3. Young adults have many questions about childrearing practices. These questions are probably most evident when children are sick or are not attaining normal milestones. At these times, nurses can provide information, or direct the parents to other individuals who can answer their questions.
4. The nurse should maintain and contribute to a positive inpatient environment which fosters early parental-infant bonding.
5. Nurturing, a task of young adulthood, may have to be learned especially by young adults who did not receive adequate nurturing themselves.
6. Completion or augmentation of appropriate education should be encouraged.
7. Guidance should be provided to assist individuals in this developmental phase to achieve independence.
8. Hospitalization for young adults may be a threat to their economical and psychological security.

MIDDLE YEARS

Middle years are variously defined as the years between 30 and 55,[36] 40-60,[37] and 45-65.[23] Major physical and psychological changes are occurring that may be characterized by crises for some individuals. Hargreaves stated that "mid-life can be a mourning period for both men and women."[38] It does not have to be and is not a continuous crisis for many, especially if one has achieved each developmental goal at the appropriate time. The middle years are certainly a time of change, but more importantly, they are fruitful years where one can see and enjoy the results of labor. If the individual acquires the sense of generativity during the middle years, he or she will find satisfaction and happiness rather than regret for the things that they did not accomplish as young adults. Physical changes occur in both men and women, but more emphasis is placed on the menopause; however the middle years involve more than the menopause.

Psychosocial Development

The core struggle of the middle years is a quest to achieve a sense of generativity and thus prevent a sense of stagnation. This core struggle is identical for all adults in their middle years regardless of their state of life. Single as well as married people may demonstrate achievement in this area of development. Having a family is not solely equated to generativity as defined by Erikson. He stated:

> Generativity, then, is primarily the concern in establishing and guiding the next generation, although there are individuals who, through misfortune or because of special and genuine gifts in other directions, do not apply this drive to their own offspring. And, indeed, the concept generativity is meant to include more popular synonyms and productivity and creativity, which, however, cannot replace it.[39]

Murray and Zentner explained generativity "as a concern about providing for others that is equal to the concern of providing for the self."[40] They went on to state that biological parents do not necessarily achieve a sense of generativity by being parents "and the unmarried person or the person without children can be quite generative."[40]

The generative person feels that he is doing a good job, and he or she is realistic about accomplishments. They are interested in helping others; they can give to others; they are creative and innovative; they feel needed and know they are meaningfully contributing to society; and they accept themselves as they are.

The person who in the middle years is preoccupied with self and is unable to give to others, has not gained a sense of generativity. He has, in fact, achieved the opposite—a sense of stagnation or self-absorption. Self-absorption may lead to all types of physical and psychological problems. Erikson stated that if generativity fails then "regression to obsessive need for pseudointimacy takes place often with a pervading sense of stagnation and personal impoverishment."[39] Murray and Zentner described this person as "withdrawn, resigned, isolated, introspective, and rebellious, and because of his own preoccupations with self, he is unable to give of himself to others."[41]

Changing body images may cause emotional upheaval in some individuals, men or women, who adhere to the assumption of our society that "young" is beautiful. Certainly, the physiological changes are real. It is possible that some of the psychological upheavals relate to hormonal changes.

After the children leave home, the husband and wife must adjust to being alone once again. This may be difficult if they have invested all their energies in rearing children, in their jobs, or have grown apart. Some couples seek counseling at this time if they have difficulties relating to each other.

Sexually the wife may be more active after the menopause since she has no more fear of pregnancy, while the husband may become less active. Sexual relations may change but should not be less satisfying than they were in the past.

Leisure time now that the children are grown may cause some difficulty for those individuals who have not maintained any interests outside the home during the period of childrearing. For these individuals, especially the women, they will have to cope with the depression associated with the "empty-nest syndrome." Murray and Zentner summarize this period by stating:

> Although there is much discussion in the literature about the crisis of menopause and the "empty-nest" menopause and middle age, for women and men, may bring an enriched sense of self and enhanced capacity to cope with life. It is a crisis in that behavioral changes are necessary but not a crisis in the negative sense of incapacitation[42] (Fig. 1-4).

Cognitive and Intellectual Development

Much learning can take place during the middle years. Frequently, individuals have more leisure time and thus can spend more energy in learning new things. Career changes may occur for women. This is seen in nursing as well as in many other

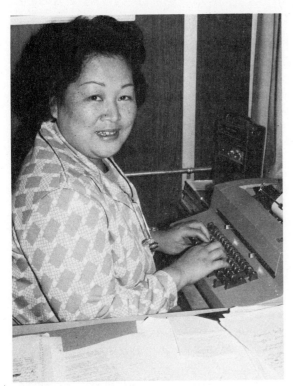

FIGURE 1-4. Outside-of-home activities are important to the middle aged adult.

fields. Nursing provides many opportunities for women and men in their middle years.

Individuals who return to school often excel. They may be more mature and committed to learning. Cognitive function does not decrease in the middle years; in fact, the experiences of life may expand the ability to learn.

Physical Considerations

Physical and physiologic changes occur both in men and women during the middle years. In the literature more emphasis is placed on women because of the menopause which refers to the time when menstruation stops. Although this is frequently called "change of life," this term seems to be an unfortunate one. Hargreaves stated:

Women experience many injustices, but one of the cruelest is use of the phrase "change of life" for the menopause. It has a ring of abruptness and finality that just is not true. The Germans use a much more meaningful term, *die Wechseljahre* which means "the changing years." The French use *le retour d'age*, which implies a return to youth and carefree days.[43]

Physical changes in the menopause are related to changes in hormonal level, that is, a decrease of estrogen in the female. Replacement of estrogen is not always successful since the side effects are often more serious than the beneficial results. These changes include vasomotor instability characterized by hot flashes, palpitations, paresthesia, headaches, menstrual irregularities, osteoporosis, coronary atherosclerosis (prior to the menopause women are less likely than men to suffer coronary insufficiency), loss of skin turgor, dry skin, and vaginal atrophy which may cause painful intercourse. In addition, androgens remain at a constant level while the estrogens drop. Some degree of masculinization may occur which may be detrimental if one already has a poor self-image due to the process of aging.

While men do not have a "menopause," they do develop signs of aging and they do have a decrease of testosterone resulting in shrinking of testes and formation of less sperm. Libido may also decrease.

Presbyopia, dental problems, and the tendency to gain weight may affect both men and women. For some individuals, the necessity of bifocals is very traumatic.

Implications for Nursing

1. Anticipatory guidance should be provided related to the physical, social, and psychological changes associated with middle years.
2. Diet instruction may prevent weight gain associated with the middle years.
3. Sexual counseling should be provided if needed, and if any serious problems are encountered in this area, the couple should be referred to the proper agencies.
4. Information should be provided to individuals regarding the importance of having activities outside of the home.
5. Preventive medical and dental care should be encouraged.
6. These years can be viewed as positive experience for the individuals in this age group.

7. Hospitalized individuals should be assisted to maintain a positive self-image.
8. Individuals may be encouraged to continue education if they show interest and desire.
9. Appropriate education could eliminate the many myths associated with the menopause.

LATER MATURITY

Retirement usually signals the onset of later maturity. For some, retirement is welcomed for the freedom to devote more time for enjoyed activities; for others, retirement represents loss of social contacts and decrease in occupational livelihood and status.

The elderly population is becoming a larger and more influential segment of society. Responding to increased political pressure, federal, state, and local governments have provided more medical, educational, nutritional, and social services for the elderly; examples are provision of hot meals or places for social interaction. The elderly person is often deprived of the usual opportunities for socialization. Facilitating socialization is important for maintenance of orientation and perceptual acuity. The problem is that one could force a socialization pattern on an elderly person that he considers undesirable or of little interest.

Many of the particular needs of the elderly are centered around provision of an adequate monthly income. Retirees receiving social security and enrolled in private pension plans are relatively lucky and may be able to enjoy travel and entertainment. For many, the realities of living on a fixed income are eroded by increasing inflation. Hospitalization and fear of illness are common concerns. Although many retirees may be enrolled in Medicare or some type of medical insurance, the thought of a lengthy or catastrophic illness causes much anxiety. Even cumulative daily medication costs may tax a limited income.

Adequate housing is also a problem. The home or apartment in which elderly clients may have been living for years may now be inadequate for their present needs. There may be no nearby grocery, clinic, or church, and without an automobile or the capacity to drive, they are isolated. The neighborhood in which they have always lived may have deteriorated, and lighting and security may be critical factors.

Psychosocial Development

Reminiscing is characteristic of aging. The importance of memories and sharing them with others has been underestimated by the helping professions. Reminiscing can be a gift which the elderly person can offer another. The elderly individual requires an attentive person to reinforce his perception of himself as an interesting person.[44]

Bereavement is frequent in this age group. The loss of a spouse may precipitate an extended grief reaction. Frequently, the nature of the loss is hard to define. The death of a spouse may represent loss of a companion, sexual partner, accountant, house and property caretaker, listener, or income provider.[45] Bereavement may affect physical health; somatic complaints are common.

After bereavement, social activities with other widows or widowers should be encouraged to aid in the redevelopment of individual autonomy and to counteract withdrawal. Some communities make provisions for the special needs of widows and widowers by providing places to meet, talk, and learn from others in similar circumstances. Counseling groups may assist the withdrawn individual to make the transition into active society (Fig. 1-5).

This period is characterized by ego integrity, the ego's natural tendency toward accrued order and meaning.[46] It is distinguished by acceptance of one's past life and life cycle. In opposition to ego integrity is despair that the remaining life may be too short, or that a new life pattern cannot be initiated.[47] The older person seeks satisfaction in the choices and alternatives he made during his lifetime.

Nursing homes care for individuals who need continuous monitoring and assistance with daily activities. Frequently, there may be instruction on the adjustment to various disabilities and ways to increase functional capacities.[48] The decision to send a family member to a nursing home can cause extreme anxiety. Hospitalization insurance may pay for only a portion of the costs, and individuals may be forced to deplete their resources and those of their families, or be forced to seek public assistance.

Cognitive and Intellectual Development

Apparent cognitive diminution is caused by sensory and perceptual changes related to aging.[49] For this

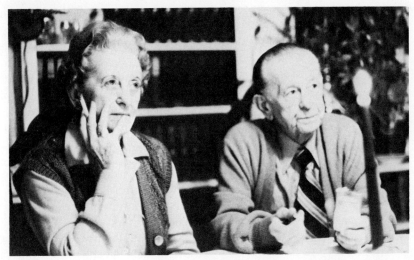

FIGURE 1-5. Social activities provide for companionship and stimulation in later years.

reason, caretakers need to guard the older person from injury. The caretaker must discriminate between sensory loss and cognitive decline. Better lens refraction or improved hearing aids may remedy sensory loss. Greater precision in the measurement of mental capacities could achieve better quality of life for the elderly client.

A consistent repeated routine is important for the older person who has memory lapses. The impact of recent memory losses can be diminished by accumulation of safe daily habits. Reminders of daily reality, familiar objects, clocks, family photographs, all may reinforce personal orientation.

Physical Considerations

Aging is an inevitable and continuous process. From birth, individuals are involved in a continuum when wear and tear is always increasing on the human body. Aging is, however, accompanied by varied adaptations which allow the individual to survive and to readjust his life style.

Age brings gradual slowing of metabolism; this means there is a decrease in cellular division or the building up and breaking down of cells. Healing takes place more slowly, and the body's reaction to infection is less rapid. There is general loss of elasticity of the connective tissue and osteoporosis. The rib cage may also be less elastic making the elderly person prone to lung congestion. All of these changes cause general decrease in speed of response and strength. In addition, arteriosclerosis

(thickening and loss of elasticity in the arterial walls) may cause periods of dizziness, shortness of breath, and tendency to tire easily.

The elderly are a diverse group with varied needs. While some may need complete assistance in provision for their daily living, others who may be chronologically older, may be entirely independent. The challenge is to determine and discriminate the unique abilities and capacities of the elderly individual (Fig. 1-6).

Implications for Nursing

Education about physical performance is frequently required.

1. The older person takes longer to respond to various stimuli. Accidents can result from decreased response.
2. The older client is almost always at a financial disadvantage. Savings and social security may not be adequate to provide for rising costs, health needs, and taxes.
3. Opportunities for socialization are decreased. Friends die, move away, or are unable to travel. Social outlets may be uninteresting and limited.
4. Housing is frequently too large, in poor areas, in poor condition, or has too many sets of stairs. Elderly people in good health require their own familiar home setting.
5. Some sensory loss is inevitable with old age. Adequate health screening could eliminate

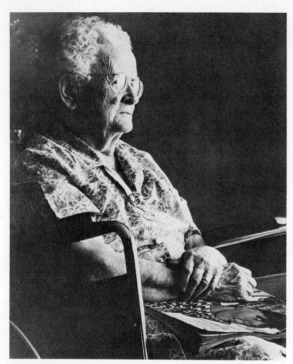

FIGURE 1-6. Dignity and contentment displayed in the elderly adult who has attained ego identity.

distress from glasses and hearing aids that do not function properly.

6. Illnesses and hospitalizations are more common in later life. The elderly person frequently requires professional services, drugs, and appliances more often and for a longer period. Chronic illnesses are more common.

7. A slow unhurried manner is most appropriate when working with the elderly. The nurse may need to inquire about what the patient likes, or if he has good or poor recent memory.

8. Nutrition is often forgotten in the elderly. Meals should be routine with well prepared, easily digested food. Fluid intake should be encouraged and adequate protein intake provided.

SUMMARY

It should be apparent as the reader nears the end of this chapter, that several principles guide application of growth and development theory for nursing. Some of the most important principles are repeated in the following paragraphs.

First, the direction of development is usually cephalocaudal (head to foot) and proximodistal (inner to outer). Therefore, the child learns to control his head before his feet, and the muscles of his leg before the finer muscles of his toes and feet. In addition, anatomical structures which support development must be completed before any functioning can occur. Therefore, the fine muscles in the hand must develop before the toddler can begin to use the hand.

Second, children must learn simple tasks prior to learning complex ones; that is, a child learns to scribble before he can copy simple figures or print letters.

Third, development is gradual and dependent on development in earlier stages and prior experience. Individuals do not suddenly change from one stage to another or completely miss a period. Development is dependent on the resolution of the earlier stage (positive or negative) and experiences which supported growth through that period. Enrichment of experiences at any stage promotes optimal growth and development and health.

Fourth, individuals should be provided with experiences and activities appropriate for their stage in development. Assessment of the individual's readiness for learning is important. For example, an infant should not be given small green toy soldiers to play with because (1) these toys are not colorful and have little texture, and (2) because they are small, they could be swallowed. The elderly individual should not be called "grandma" (unless this is desired) and spoken to in a childish or paternalistic manner. In addition, experiences or activities which challenge the individual are needed at all ages to increase and amplify mental abilities.

Fifth, each individual should be recognized as separate and unique. The actual growth and developmental pattern of any individual is contingent on many factors, such as rate of maturation, heredity, nutrition, experience, and environment. While each individual moves through the same stages, and factors can be identified which hinder or enhance development, the stages are age related, and there is an upward limit on acceleration of development. Nurses can increase the individuality and uniqueness of their clients by identifying hindrances to development and providing opportunities for positive experiences, activities, and skills to optimize and amplify growth.

REFERENCES

1. Freud, S.: *An Outline of Psycho-Analysis.* Edited by Strachey, J., New York, W. W. Norton Company, 1949, p. 1013.
   Freud, S.: *New Introductory Lectures in Psychoanalysis.* Edited by Strachey, J., New York, W. W. Norton Company, 1933, pp. 97–102.
2. Erikson, E.: *Childhood and Society,* 2nd ed. New York, W. W. Norton Company, 1963, p. 270.
3. *Ibid.*, p. 273.
4. Piaget, J.: The genetic approach to the psychology of thought, in *Critical Features of Piaget's Theory of the Development of Thought,* by Murray, F. B., New York, MSS Information Corporation, 1972, p. 54.
5. Piaget, J.: *The Child's Conception of the World.* Totowa, N.J., Littlefield Adams and Company, 1929, pp. 31–32.
6. Piaget, J.: *The Child's Conception of Physical Causality.* London, Routledge and Kegan Paul Ltd., 1930, pp. 237–305.
7. Piaget, J.: *The Psychology of Intelligence.* London, Routledge and Kegan Paul Ltd., 1950, pp. 87–155.
8. Piaget, J.: Development and learning, in *Critical Features of Piaget's Theory of the Development of Thought,* by Murray, F. B., New York, MSS Information Corporation, 1972, pp. 58–59.
9. Sheehy, G.: *Passages: Predictable Crises of Adult Life.* New York, Bantam Books, Inc., 1976.
10. Freud, *An Outline of Psycho-Analysis,* pp. 10–11.
11. Erikson, *op. cit.*, p. 247.
12. Klaus, M., and Kennel, J. H.: *Maternal-Infant Bonding.* St. Louis, C. V. Mosby Company, 1976, pp. 1–2.
13. Stone, L. J., and Church, J.: *Childhood and Adolescence,* 3rd ed. New York, Random House, 1973, p. 101.
14. Gruber, H., and Voneche, J.: *The Essential Piaget.* New York, Basic Books, 1977, pp. 216–218.
15. Erikson, *op. cit.*, p. 271.
16. *Ibid.*, p. 251.
17. Erikson, *op. cit.*, p. 252.
18. Gruber and Voneche, *op. cit.,* pp. 218–219.
19. Erikson, *op. cit.*, p. 255.
20. Marlow, D.: *Textbook of Pediatric Nursing,* 5th ed. Philadelphia, W. B. Saunders Company, 1977, p. 611.
21. Piaget: *The Child's Conceptions of the World,* pp. 33–60, 169–252, 350–388.
22. Stone and Church, *op. cit.*, p. 305.
23. Murray, R., and Zentner, J.: *Nursing and Assessment and Health Promotion through the Life Span.* Englewood Cliffs, N.J., Prentice Hall, 1975, p. 107.
24. Jackson, P.: *Life in Classrooms.* New York, Holt, Rinehart and Winston, 1968, p. 5.
25. *Ibid.*, p. 17.
26. Erikson, *op. cit.*, p. 260.
27. Lystad, M.: The adolescent image in American books for children: then and now. *Child Today* 6:35, 1977.
28. Erikson, *op. cit.*, pp. 261–262.
29. Freud: *Outline of Psycho-Analysis,* p. 12.
30. Piaget, J.: *Judgement and Reasoning in the Child.* New York, Harcourt, Brace, and Company, 1928, pp. 62–95.
31. Erikson, *op. cit.*, p. 263.
32. *Ibid.*, p. 264.
33. Phillips, C., and Anzalone, J. T.: *Fathering: Participation in Labor and Birth.* St. Louis: C. V. Mosby Company, 1978, p. 14.
34. *Ibid.*, p. 15.
35. *Ibid.*, p. 145.
36. Peplau, H.: Mid-life crises. *Am. J. Nurs.* 75:1791, 1975.
37. Diekelman, N., et al.: The middle years—A special supplement. *Am. J. Nurs.* 75:993, 1975.
38. Hargreaves, A.: Making the most of the middle years. *Am. J. Nurs.* 75:1773, 1975.
39. Erikson, *op. cit.*, p. 267.
40. Murray and Zentner, *op. cit.*, p. 266.
41. *Ibid.*, p. 267.
42. *Ibid.*, p. 254.
43. Hargreaves, *op. cit.*, p. 1774.
44. Burnside, I.: Listen to the aged. *Am. J. Nurs.* 75:1801, 1975.
45. Prock, V.: The mid-stage women. *Am. J. Nurs.* 75:1021, 1975.
46. Erikson, *op. cit.*, p. 268.
47. *Ibid.*, p. 269.
48. Schwab, M.: Nursing care in nursing homes. *Am. J. Nurs.* 75:1812, 1975.
49. Hirschfeld, M.: The cognitively impaired older adult. *Am. J. Nurs.* 76:1982, 1976.

BIBLIOGRAPHY

Brown, M. S., and Murphy, M. A.: *Ambulatory Pediatrics for Nurses.* New York, McGraw-Hill Book Company, 1975.

Diekelman, N., and Galloway, K.: A time of change. *Am. J. Nurs.* 75:993, 1975.

Freud, S.: *The Basic Writings of Sigmund Freud.* Translated and edited by Brill, A. A., New York. Modern Library, Inc., 1938.

Hardin, D.: The school-age child and the school nurse, in *Care of the Well Child—A Special Supplement.* *Am. J. Nurs.* 74:1476, 1974.

Galloway, K.: The change of life. *Am. J. Nurs.* 75:1006, 1975.

Jackson, P. W.: *Life in Classrooms.* New York, Holt, Rinehart, and Winston, Inc., 1968.

Klaus, M. H., and Kennell, J. H.: *Maternal-Infant Bonding.* St. Louis, C. V. Mosby Company, 1976.

Pasternack, S. B.: Annual well child visit, in *Care of the Well Child—A Special Supplement. Am. J. Nurs.* 74:1472, 1974.

Roberts, F. B.: *Perinatal Nursing.* New York, McGraw-Hill Book Company, 1977.

Thomas C. L. (ed.): *Taber's Cyclopedic Medical Dictionary.* 13th ed. Philadelphia, F. A. Davis Company, 1977.

CHAPTER 2

In some way, each of us has been a part of a family system. We are individuals with our own inimitable ways of perceiving, interpreting, acting upon, or responding to life events. And yet, we are social animals. We are a part of a larger society with a sense of our own limitations and capabilities and with an idea of where we would like to go with our lives. How did we learn characteristic patterns of behavior which allow us to fit into society? In the following pages, we will find that many of our behavior patterns were learned from the smallest but one of the most important social units—the family.

Social changes over the past 20 years have given rise to a variety of alternative styles of marriage and childrearing: from communal families to multiple marriages. The more traditional forms are the nuclear and the extended family. The nuclear family is composed of two partners and their offspring interacting in a common environment. The extended family includes the nuclear family plus grandparents, uncles, aunts, and cousins, interacting within a common environment. Murdock proposed that the nuclear family was the universal unit. In other

THE FAMILY

Elise D. Navratil-Kline, M.S., R.N.

words, even in multigenerational or extended families, there are nuclear family units.[1] The same principle may be applied to groups who consider themselves families or a single parent family who adds a new member. The theoretical content of this chapter, while focusing on the nuclear family, can also be applied to other types of families.

This chapter treats the family as a dynamic, changing system which adapts to the needs of its members and yet, modifies itself to the demands of a rapidly changing society. It is viewed from an historical, sociological, and finally, a systems perspective. Family systems will be explored in terms of these structures and processes. This chapter concludes with a brief discussion of future trends for the family and the implications for the health professional.

HISTORICAL PERSPECTIVES OF AMERICAN FAMILIES

In its effort to remain a viable social category, let us look at the changes the American family has undergone within the last two centuries. Technologically, the societal changes have been rapid and striking, moving from an agricultural to an industrial society. But has our social framework made such rapid advances?

If we look at the colonial family system in terms of the formation and structure, of the patterns of mate selection, and the family's relationship to other institutions, we can see that it differs from our present family unit. Adams[2] felt that the trend toward a nuclear family unit was bolstered by European tradition. Naturally, too the movement of settlers across the continent helped weaken ties with extended families as aunts, uncles, and grandparents stayed in Europe or on the Atlantic coast while their sons and daughters and their families moved across the unsettled territory.

In Europe, mate selection in the aristocracy was arranged primarily for political purposes and for continuity of blood lines. In lower socioeconomic levels, however, marriage was most frequently with a partner of personal choice. This is not to say that the parents or family of the potential partner had no influence on the choice. Frequently, the looked for matches offered economic betterment for their offspring. These European values were brought to the colonies by the early settlers who, for the most part, were from a lower socioeconomic stratum. Yet, the process of mate selection was changed by the ascendency of the concept of romantic love, which meant choosing a mate not for increasing economic security or for political purposes but for love alone. This concept may have evolved because of the scarcity of European women in the colonies and the large number of men who planned to settle there, since scarcity of an item on the market may enhance the desire for it.[3]

Once the couple married, the male, who was the acknowledged head of the family, dominated family decision-making. The wife's role was to bear and raise the children, and "keep the home fires burning." Legally her property became her husband's when she married. Children were taught respect for authority and elders, while religion served to reinforce the repression of sinful childish inclination. It was the parent's responsibility to set the children on the right path. Thus, the roles within the family were well defined. Because the family was largely self-sufficient, producing the necessities of life, each member was an active contributor to the family work force.

Due to its central importance as the activity center, the family was only partially tied to the various institutions at that time. Indeed, the family itself fulfilled many of the functions of these institutions. For example, education, both religious and secular, was carried out in the home; medicine frequently consisted only of "home remedies," and protection depended on the family's own resources.[4]

The greatest change in courtship patterns, as mentioned earlier, was the concept of romantic love, as it increasingly formed the basis for mate selection. Other influences on mate selection were, and are, value systems and residential patterns. In Victorian times, norms prohibited premarital sex, especially for women. Since the 1920's, however, there has been progressively more open questioning of this value.[5]

Today, the size of the family has decreased, and roles are no longer so clearly delineated. The husband usually is not the sole decision-maker of the family as the wife's influence has steadily risen. Thus, the present trend is away from the Colonial and Victorian patriarchies. Over the years, women's roles have changed as women have made legal, educational, and political gains. Roles have also changed as women have entered the labor force and become contributors to the family income.

Children's roles have also changed as have attitudes toward child-rearing. Since the family is no longer the basic production component of the economy, the child is no longer relegated to the status of an economic inferior. Whereas children tended to be perceived as small adults in the colonial family's labor structure, today's parents lack both the economic labor authority and the commitment to rigid moral absolutes shared by Victorian and colonial parents. The modern family views the child as a developing person, not a small adult.

One of the greatest agents for change in the structure of the family and its relation to society was the Industrial Revolution. As mentioned before, economic production moved out of the home and into the factory. Health care and educational institutions became more specialized, and many of the tasks formerly performed by the family were transferred to these institutions. Through increasing exposure to public media, values and norms were influenced and changed. Even recreation became more specialized, requiring special facilities, and family protection is now assumed by police forces.[6]

Thus, there have been changes within the family in response to social and technological changes. Yet surprisingly, the family structure or unit has been fairly constant through the years. What is it about the family that keeps it viable and adaptive within society? In spite of the myth of the disintegration of the modern family, why do people continue to establish family units? Perhaps these questions can be explored and answered in the following sections.

SOCIOLOGICAL PERSPECTIVES OF AMERICAN FAMILIES

There are two schools of thought concerning how and why the family unit has remained viable. One is the "universal functionalists" approach and the other is the "orderly-replacement" approach. According to Farber, the universal functionalists attempt to explain the phenomenon of the family in terms of the tasks it carries out to insure the continuity of society.[7] Reiss feels that the major function of the family is the rearing, maintenance, and socialization of offspring.[8] Other theorists feel that the family units have remained viable because they carry out the functions of reproduction, biological maintenance, socialization, economic cooperation, and ascription of status in society.

Granted, the family does perform many of the tasks mentioned; however, other institutions have successfully carried out many of these functions. Educational institutions and mass media help socialize children, and children are biologically maintained in some health care facilities. This approach does not, however, fully explain how the family has persisted through the generations.

The orderly-replacement approach attempts to explain how family patterns are transmitted through generations. This process has been explored by characterizing the family unit as ''closed'' or ''open.'' The closed family unit is isolated from social contacts. Members of this system have a strong sense of belonging and are in close communication with each other. Culture is transmitted over the years without change. Rules governing family interaction are simple and nonconflicting. Existing values, rules, and traditions are the only ones known and are considered sacred. Family members remain together for generations. Parents and family elders are responsible for the socialization of the young. Finally, these patterns are reinforced by the emotional ties the younger generation have with the older.[9]

A hypothetical example would be an extended family of approximately 60 people who inhabit an isolated area high in the mountains. They are all related through generations of intermarriage. Social contact and communication with the rest of the world is almost impossible because of the altitude of the mountains, rockslides, and deep snow, which makes the mountains impassable in winter. This family speaks a dialect of English which would have been comprehensible to an early colonist but to modern ears is difficult to understand. Techniques for meeting basic needs have remained unchanged for generations. Mothers teach daughters sewing, cooking, child-rearing, and preparation of home remedies. Fathers teach sons hunting, building, and raising and protecting livestock. Elders recite family histories, exploits, traditions, and laws to the youngsters in the evening. Thus, traditions and values remain constant, for the wisdom of the elders is unquestioningly accepted and respected. Except in death, no one leaves the group.

The open family, on the other hand, is characterized by rapid change and increased exposure to other social patterns. Rules governing family life can be complex and conflicting. Old values are examined and sometimes discarded in favor of new ones. One way of thinking is not regarded as sacred because others are known. There is a faster turnover of family members and greater movement toward change. For instance, children grow up and relocate to other geographic areas, or parents may divorce or separate with one parent moving to another area. Social conditions considered verboten in the closed family, such as divorce, may be acceptable in the open family.[10]

An example of an ''open'' family is the family of Marsha. She has been divorced for 2 years and has two small sons. Her family life is rather chaotic because of the difficulties involved in raising her sons alone and working full-time. Her ex-husband has moved to another state and has remarried, while Marsha's mother, father, and sister also live in another state. They have had difficulty accepting her new life style, especially her divorce, since for religious reasons, they believe divorce to be an unacceptable resolution to their daughter's marriage. Marsha disagrees with her family's traditional view of marriage and also with their religious beliefs. Despite the chaos and family pressure, she is happy with the alternatives her new life style offers her.

Since many elements of the open family social system can be applied to the American family, a more thorough examination of the family as a system is in order.

SYSTEMS FRAMEWORK FOR FAMILIES

The word ''unit'' or ''system'' has frequently been used to describe families. How is the family considered to be a system? What is a system? A system has been described as a group of parts (people) interacting with one another on a cause and effect basis. For instance, if a person within a system says or does something, other persons within that system will in some degree be affected. Each part of the system is linked with another part for a period of time in some form of uniform relationship.[11]

More simply, a person is part of a family for a number of days, months, or years and has a role or function within that family. A chief characteristic of a system is that it responds to input from within and from outside the system.[11] When a young child brings home a note from school saying he has been disruptive in class, in all probability his parents are going to react.

"System" implies the dynamics of change and adaptation in response to internal and external stimuli. The mechanism allowing this adaptive response to occur is called the "feedback loop." Feedback is the process enabling the system to communicate with its parts allowing appropriate response to a stimulus; it facilitates productive or nonproductive methods of carrying out functions necessary for adaptation.

Negative feedback within a system maintains harmony, equilibrium, or steadiness within the system in response to external and internal environmental changes. A child praised for the housework done to help mother will continue to behave in the same manner.

On the other hand, positive feedback facilitates deviation and change within the system. Although the terms "negative feedback" and "positive feedback" appear to be contradictory in their use here, they are the appropriately used vernacular and should not be confused or misinterpreted. The terms refer to the *outcome* of the communication (i.e., harmony or change). In other words, feedback may serve to increase or continue the systems disequilibrium. Again, it must be emphasized that the function of positive feedback is to produce change *within* the system. Two siblings might fight with one another in a dispute over who does the most work in their home, resulting ultimately in a more realistic redistribution of the work load.

How does the systems model apply to families? Most simply defined, a family is a collection of people who are connected to each other by interpersonal ties (biologic, emotional, or traditional ties).[12] This interrelationship of parts is governed by interpersonal communication and feedback. Families are generally described as open systems since they change, adapt, and are influenced by their environment. They can reinforce or diminish behaviors within the system via negative or positive feedback. Finally, small amounts of input, either energy or matter, in one part of the system can result in a flurry of activity in the other components of the system. The family, as a whole, or its members, respond to or are affected by stimuli from within and without.

In summary, systems theory applied to families implies that the family is a dynamic, adapting organism that responds to internal and external environmental stimuli in such a way as to ensure survival of the family unit. Thus, the picture of a family unit emerges in such a way that family structure and process assume dynamic, yet comprehensible functions as components of family change and adaptation.

FAMILY STRUCTURE

Family structure can best be described as the way a family is dynamically organized. Family organization depends on many factors: structure and function of the subsystems within the family, family interface and boundaries, roles of the family members, and type of family system which may describe a particular family. It is important to reiterate that the material that follows represents theoretical constructs which are useful in explaining facets of family structure.

Subsystems

Within the overall family system structure are subsystems (i.e., family members) which enable families to meet their operational needs. Each subsystem has levels of power, interrelationships, and different skills ascribed to it. Division of the family into subsystems also reveals mechanisms for maintaining personal differentiation within groups.[14] For example, within families a particular member is a "daughter," the "youngest," as well as a "female," and a "sister." No one else in the family fits into all these particular categories, and no one else possesses the skills relating to each category. The major subsystems in nuclear families are the spouse subsystem, parental subsystem, and the sibling subsystem.[15]

The spouse subsystem develops when two adults merge and form a family. This subsystem has specific tasks ascribed to it which are intrinsic to the functioning of the system. The major skills necessary for carrying out these tasks involve compromise and mutual accommodation. Couples must learn to merge their behavior patterns to allow them to support each other's functions. Patterns of accommodation may, however, be positive or negative; two people may complement the best or worst characteristics of each other. For example, dependent-protector patterns may develop in which one member remains dependent allowing the other member the role of protector. Finally, this subsystem must develop flexible boundaries which protect it from the needs and mandates of other systems; a couple may run into trouble if their in-laws continuously interfere with their relationship.

The second subsystem is the parental subsystem.[16] This develops with the addition of children. Couples must maintain mutual support and accommodation while functioning in such a manner that they are also nurturing, guiding, and controlling children. As families develop, the quantity of these socializing elements depends on both the child's need for independence and guidance and the parents' ability to modify their own behaviors to meet the child's developmental needs. This subsystem requires boundaries which are flexible enough to keep children apart from the spouse subsystem without cutting off access to both parents.

The third subsystem, the sibling subsystem, is one in which children learn to relate to peers,[17] developing skills in competition, cooperation, and so on. The boundaries of this subsystem must be developed to protect children from excessive parental control while maximizing opportunity for autonomy and exploration.

Boundaries and Roles

The system's boundaries are the rules which govern who interacts and how. If at the end of an evening, Dad looks at his watch and says, "Ok kids, it's time to go to bed," the roles in the power hierarchy are clearly defined; each member knows what behaviors are expected of him. Boundaries must be clear enough so that members can carry out their functions, yet allow for contact with members of other systems and subsystems.

"Interface" describes an area where two or more boundaries meet.[18] An example of a boundary interface occurs when a mother joins the Parent-Teachers' Association at her child's grammar school; there her boundaries as a representative of her family meet with the boundaries of the community.

Two opposite types of family boundaries are the enmeshed family and the disengaged family.[19] In enmeshed family systems, subsystem boundaries are diffuse. Behaviors of one member quickly affect behaviors of another. Variations in family behavior are responded to quickly and intensely. In many cases, blurred edges of subsystem boundaries can, however, discourage autonomy among family members. For example, in an enmeshed family, when the baby does not eat his pablum, the parents respond by becoming angry. On the other hand, in disengaged families the boundary system is rigid; only a very high level of stress will bridge the gap between the family subsystems to elicit a response. Members often function independently, have little sense of belonging to the family system, and have diminished skills necessary to interdependence. In such a family, for example, parents might be almost totally unaffected by their child's delinquency.

Interactional Patterns

Kantor and Lehr describe interactional patterns of families in terms of roles. The four major roles observed among family members are "mover," "opposer," "follower," and "bystander."[20]

The mover is the person within a system who initiates action toward some family goal. He establishes the framework for family response. For example, Jimmy, the eldest son, says to his family, "Why don't we all play baseball today?" The opposer is the family member who challenges or blocks the mover's direction. The function of the opposer (reactor) is to curb the energies and direction of the mover, thus imposing checks and balances on the system. His reaction opens up communication for debate and the development of more productive strategies for moving toward family goals. In response to Jimmy's statement his older sister says, "Oh, you always want to play baseball. I hate baseball. Let's go on a picnic instead. Then, you can play baseball, and we can do what we want." In this case, the family goal might have been some activity that would bring the system closer together. Jimmy, as the mover, initiated activity in that direction. His sister, as the opposer, blocked it but opened up the topic for debate.

In the role of the follower, the family member

can support either the mover, the opposer, or both. He does not initiate action, but he can shift allegiance quickly, and thus, has the ability to control action by regulating his support. This strengthens the follower's position in the system. The follower sometimes places himself in a difficult situation through what Kantor and Lehr call "communication double speak," that is, giving support to two or more incompatible positions. For example, Michael (Jimmy's brother) would be a follower if he were to say, "Yeah, let's all go out. But I'm not sure whether or not I want a picnic or baseball."

The fourth and final role is that of the bystander. The bystander avoids direct action and makes no alliances with the mover, opposer, or follower. These three may try to maneuver him into assuming a position (e.g., "Hey, Mom, what do you think?"), or to block him out if they feel opposition. The bystander can stay on the fence, maintaining neutrality until he decides what to do. He has three options: he can leave the field, continue to observe the interactions of the others, or act as mediator. Mom may finally say, "Well, I think your overall idea for us to do something together is good. But isn't it too cold outside for either?" Then, she may switch to the role of mover and say, "Why don't we work out something to do together here at home?"

In all four roles, each member made suggestions on the best way to reach a family goal—in this case, more interpersonal closeness within the system. The mover initiated the action; it was challenged by the opposer; the follower supported both; and the bystander moved closer to the conflict and served as mediator. Each member can also switch roles just as the mother switched from bystander to mover.

Types of Family Systems

Kantor and Lehr have described three types of family systems: closed, open, and random.[21] These systems are examined in terms of their utilization of space, time, and energy (Fig. 2-1).

CLOSED FAMILY SYSTEM

The key word in describing the closed family system is "stability." The power hierarchy is clearly defined; interpersonal and family "spaces" are fixed, boundaries are set by authority figures. Interpersonal space might be achieved by observing how close or distant family members get emotionally; it may also be evidenced by how close emotionally an outsider can get to the family. In a closed family, the implied or stated message to a visitor might be, "You are a guest." Should he attempt to get closer to the family, the message would become, "You are prying and invading our territory." The external space of the family is exemplified by the limits of the family property, the block, or the neighborhood. The goals of establishing this space include preservation of territory, self-protection, and privacy.

Family systems differ in their orientation to time; they can reflect past, present or future. They may also differ in their organization of time, that is, in their daily, monthly, or yearly schedules. In the closed family, the members tend to keep to a standard daily schedule. The orientation of this family tends not only toward the past and preserving the status quo but also toward the future (i.e., in which direction lies the achievement of some family goal).[21]

The concept of energy applied to family systems describes those elements which power activities within the family system. Energy can be of a physical nature, such as money, food, or clothing; or it may be emotional, such as nurturing, support, or love. In the closed family, the energy is usually delegated formally, in a prescribed manner.[21] Rules for how, when, and where to obtain energy are well defined. For example, in a closed family food shopping might be done at a specific market on a particular day by certain family members. If it is spiritual energy the family needs, the closed family may go to a specific church on Sunday, with the whole family required to attend.

As mentioned previously, "stability" is the family byword: family members who develop deviant patterns which interfere with the stability of the family system are not tolerated. Limits are set on the members' behavior, and if aberrant behavior continues, that member may be eliminated from the system so that the system can return to stable functioning.[21] The following is an example of a closed family.

The father of the Weitz family died when the children were fairly young. The mother became

PATTERNS OF INTERFACE IN THREE FAMILY TYPES

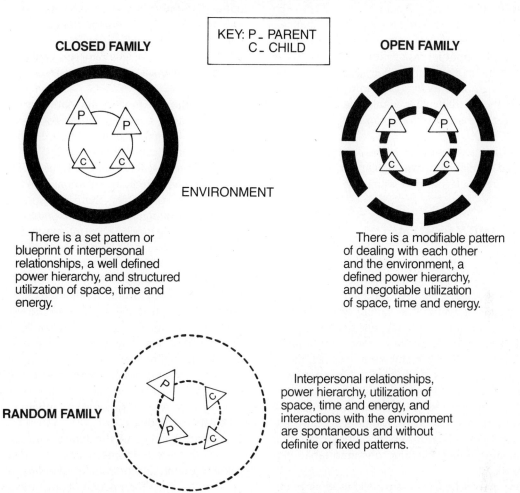

CLOSED FAMILY

KEY: P - PARENT
C - CHILD

OPEN FAMILY

ENVIRONMENT

There is a set pattern or
blueprint of interpersonal
relationships, a well defined
power hierarchy, and structured
utilization of space, time and
energy.

There is a modifiable pattern
of dealing with each other
and the environment, a
defined power hierarchy,
and negotiable utilization
of space, time and energy.

RANDOM FAMILY

Interpersonal relationships,
power hierarchy, utilization of
space, time and energy, and
interactions with the environment
are spontaneous and without
definite or fixed patterns.

FIGURE 2-1. Family members (in each type of family) usually will relate to one another in the same manner that they relate to the environment. For example, in the closed family there are set ways for one member to relate to another member. In addition, there are definite patterns for each member to follow in relating to the environment.

the authority figure in the family and was responsible for raising her five children.

Financial debts incurred by her husband's long illness left the family monetarily crippled. Consequently, the mother attempted to pay the bills by opening a dressmaking shop. The oldest son, who had dreams of becoming a doctor, was forced to leave school and work in a factory to help support the family. As the three daughters grew older, they also left school to work in the family shop. The life goal of the family was to send the youngest son to school in hopes that he would become the hoped-for professional in the family.

Family space was confined primarily to the house, shop, and neighborhood. The neighborhood consisted primarily of Jewish people, and the family was cordial but closed to outsiders. Within the family, interpersonal space remained fairly fixed. The mother tolerated some closeness with her children, but for the most part, she maintained a distance from them. The family time schedule revolved around running the shop and the youngest son's schooling. The family frequently spoke of the past, their father, and their religious heritage.

The other portions of time were spent in talking of the future and the youngest son's progress in medical school. Energy for the family was derived from the financial gains of the shop; each family member received his share of the finances, although most of the money went into running the family. Spirtual input into the family came from a traditional source, their synagogue. Each family member was expected to worship on the Sabbath and difficulties within the family were brought to the Rabbi for counseling.

Typical of a closed system, in this family the space was fixed, family time was regular and scheduled, and energy levels into and within the family were stable.

OPEN FAMILY SYSTEM

In the open family system, the key word is "negotiation." Space within and without is movable, time schedules are variable, and energy sources and delegation within the family are flexible.[21] Boundaries around the family are open, allowing outsiders to enter. Absence of members is tolerated, permitting family members to distance themselves emotionally and physically. Closeness and distancing are allowed as long as they stay within the family's negotiated guidelines. For example, the teenage son may stay in his room, away from the family, as long as he does not do it for so long that the family members become uncomfortable with his absence.

Family time schedules are usually used as guidelines, not as blueprints.[21] The daily schedules are modifiable, so, for example, the family does not always have to eat dinner at 6:00. The life plan of the family—its schedule for achieving overall family goals—is similarly modifiable. The emphasis is on the present and on everyday events.

Energy is flexibly distributed to family members. If the youngest daughter is feeling blue because she does not have a date for the senior prom, the family can be supportive until her inner energy level is raised. Also, the open family can obtain energy in a greater variety of ways. If the daughter became severely depressed, the family might consider professional help instead of prayer. However, while the open family has many sources for energy, these are not unlimited. If the energy needed was in the form of money, for example, there are a variety of ways of getting it, but ways which would not be acceptable to the family would be theft or prostitution. The family's expenditure of energy is also open to more variety; energy does not have to be expended in a prescribed manner as it would in a closed family system. The Simpson family illustrates the open family system.

Although the mother and father are the authority figures most family decisions are negotiated by all family members, including husband, wife, teenage son and daughter.

The space of the family is flexible. There are periods when family members are close to each other, and conversely, there are periods when the son or daughter need their privacy and distance from the family. They frequently bring their friends home to visit. Family time is flexible and schedules modifiable. When mother works late, the children are responsible for making dinner, or they wait to eat until mother gets home. The major "rule" that the family sticks to regarding time is that Sundays are for the family, and so, on that day they stay at home. The major goal is education, but again this goal is modifiable: the two children do not have to go to college; it is their choice. The mother recently returned to school, and again, the family members modified their time schedules.

Energy sources of the family are not fixed. During a period of family crisis, the mother was able to obtain outside sources of energy through psychotherapy. For a period of time, the son was interested in karate and oriental philosophy. His family encouraged him in this pursuit. When they no longer could afford to pay for his lessons, the issue was negotiated, and it was decided he could continue karate lessons if he was willing to pay for them.

Interpersonal spaces in this family type have movable boundaries; time schedules are variable and flexible to suit family needs. Energy is allocated to family members, expended and obtained relative to the needs of the family.

RANDOM FAMILY SYSTEM

The key word in describing the random type family system is "spontaneous." Interpersonal and territorial spaces are dispersed: each person within the system develops his own boundaries. No person in the power hierarchy regulates these spatial boundaries.[21] Membership within the family is nonobligatory: if a family member chose to leave the system to go across the country, the random system would not be threatened. Time within this family is irregularly divided. A daily schedule may exist but it is up to each family member whether or not to adhere to it. The family's orientation toward the past, present, future, and "routine" is nonspecific: unlike the closed family system, where orientation is toward the past and future, or the open system whose emphasis is on the present, the random family's orientation is to all three. They live in the present, but do not shape it out of family guidelines; the present merely develops out of everyday experiences. There is no long-term family life plan; a short-term life plan develops out of life experiences.[21]

The family can seek out all potential sources of energy without official family limits. Under ordinary circumstances there is no set structure for delegating energy within the family; indeed, there is a propensity for family members to disperse. There is, however, usually one member who in times of stress can impose his own guidelines on the family, holding it together temporarily. A family situation illustrating this point occurs when the youngest member of the family, while playing, falls down, badly cutting his hand. Everyone in the family reacts with horror and distress, moving in different directions while the child stands crying. After a few moments of utter chaos, the mother says, "Get a towel," "Get the car started. We'll take him to the hospital." She then picks the child up to wash his hand and see how badly he was cut.

The random family system is illustrated by the Zigmonds.

The father has separated from the family and lives several miles away. He stays with the family, however, every few days and then leaves. This pattern of behavior is very acceptable to his wife and children. The children have the freedom to establish their own boundaries in the neighborhood as long as the mother has a general idea of where they will be.

Time within the family is fairly unstructured. The children have to get up to go to school. They are responsible for getting their own breakfasts while their mother, an artist, organizes the materials she plans to show in a flea market.

Energy sources also are variable. The father is a school teacher with a fixed income. Mother adds to this income with the profits from what she sells at the flea market. When business is slow, she supplements their income by teaching ceramics. All potential emotional energy sources can be used. Both mother and father in times of stress have been involved in couples therapy, group therapy, individual therapy, and consciousness-raising groups. In addition, they have strong support systems set up with their friends in the community. Organizing energy within the family also is variable, and each member can receive input according to his need and the family's supply.

The major characteristic of the random system is spontaneity. Space, both extrafamilial and intrafamilial, is dispersed. Time is irregular with no single orientation to past, present, or future. Finally, energy for the family fluctuates, sources are unlimited, delegation of energy to members is variable, and expenditure of energy within and outside of the family is random.

FAMILY PROCESS

An adaptable organism, the family system changes in response to internal and external stimuli. This movement or response within the family is called "process." Family process in the simplest usage describes "what goes on within the family;" it is the action and interaction of family members within the system and along the family's interface with its environment. Each family has its own strategies for interaction among its members; each family changes and adapts to attain its goals through manipulation of space, time, and energy. Finally, all families have communication patterns which provide the input and feedback which bring about systemic change.

Family strategies are defined as the intentional actions of two or more people within a social-biological system which moves the family toward a goal.[22] Family members are aware at some cognitive level of the roles that they are expected to play. For example, if one family member sensed a need for the family to become closer emotionally, he might suggest that they do something together. Other family members could share in this strategy by assuming their expected roles, so that ultimately each participant would share responsibility for the outcome. A family member involved in a strategy may be a free agent, shifting his position at will; he may have restrictions in his role, or he may have the freedom to reject the role or move assigned.[22]

There are three different types of strategies: maintenance, stress, and repair. Maintenance strategies are those which attempt to keep the system as it is, such as an attempt to maintain emotional closeness by setting aside time to talk and be together. Stress strategies increase tension, generating confusion and turmoil within the family. For instance, siblings may be encouraged to compete with each other in academic achievement because one family goal is improved education for the children. The third strategy, repair, involves those interactions offering a chance to regroup or change to preserve viability as a system. An example is the fighting couple who arranges a truce to discuss and attempt to change disruptive behavior in order to live more harmoniously.

Family Goals

Process implies movement and change in a specific direction. Family interactions are based on this process and are a cause or response to family movement toward or away from family goals. These family goals or targets fall within three dimensions: affect, power, and meaning.[23,24]

In family interactions, the affective goal is the proper regulation of emotional distance. The primary targets are intimacy or closeness, and nurturance or support. The ideal family satisfies each member's need for closeness and caring.[25]

Two conditions which can be found in families are affective fusion and emotional alienation.[26] Affective fusion may occur when closeness between two or more family members is so intense that emotional boundaries disappear. Emotional alienation occurs when the separation is so great that family members are locked into positions which block all moves toward regaining closeness. These two conditions are the extreme ends of a continuum. Most interactions occur between these extremes, with constant shifting or manipulation to gain emotional closeness or distance.

Another target is power.[27] Overall, power within the family system is the ability to guide the system to its goals. Members learn and exercise specific disciplinary skills.[27] A family rewards and sets limits on its members to shape their movement and ultimately that of the system itself. The ideas of property, rights and responsibilities, dominance and submission, are all power issues which develop within a family and require negotiation. A member's position in the family hierarchy may determine his influence on all these issues. A typical exercise of power is seen when parents set limits on their children's playtime by sending them to their rooms to study.

The final target dimension is that of meaning.[28] A family's primary goal here is to provide identity and self-knowledge for individuals as well as the entire family while accurately conveying that identity to others. Members should be able to say, "I know who I am, and I know what I'm part of." Family systems have attitudes, values, world views, religious beliefs, and a sense of right and wrong, which are communicated to those inside and outside the family. Again, two poles exist: (1) absolute conformity or (2) intellectual irrelevance. Both create conceptual isolation. A family seeking meaning in the former manner may be so rigid that it creates distance between itself and outsiders. A family's search for meaning becomes irrelevant when one of its members or groups of members emphasize unshared meaning to such an extent that they become isolated from, or opposed to, the values and ideals held by the rest of the family or community.

Distance Regulation and Time Structures

Distance regulation is one of the dominant forces in family process. A system's "space" can be internal and external. It may be concrete, raising issues such as "Do we have large enough rooms for our children?"—quite a serious problem for a family of eight who live in a three room apartment. But spatial concepts may also apply to more abstract issues such as "How can I become closer emotionally to my parents?" or "What are the emotional boundaries between family members?" Within each system, there is constant negotiation of space with movement toward and away from members at different times.

Negotiation of external space for a family system involves its relationship to the environment. Each family develops regulations for who may enter or leave the boundaries of the system. What are the boundaries—the driveway, backyard, block, neighborhood, or town? Boundaries, for example, for some inner city dwellers extend only as far as the apartment door.

Space, both internal and external, is defined as those areas which are safe for its members. The system develops regulatory means for developing, protecting, and maintaining boundaries. All of these issues are intrinsic parts of the family's methods of distance regulation.

Time, in relation to family process, has been broken down by Kantor and Lehr into two different types: (1) daily experience: play baseball, come home for dinner, or go to bed, and (2) the family's history of their progress in the system's life cycle, which involves the direction in which the system has been moving or hopes to move.

Two descriptive terms applied to the family's time structures are "in-phase" and "out-of-phase."[30] When families are in-phase, there are similarities or concurrent use of time within a family (i.e., meals, work schedules, and bed times). When a family is out-of-phase, meals and work schedules are erratic and dissimilar. Families may also use their time to foster differences in space regulation. Time can be used to bring the family closer (dinner together) or further apart ("I'm too busy, I can't be with you now"). The system's regulation of time directly affects family process.

Energy and Communication

Energy, both static and kinetic, is another medium through which the system affects movement toward its goals. Static energy pertains to reservoirs of stored energy, and kinetic energy, the expenditure of these stores. Energy for a system can be food, money, clothing, and community resources or abstract forces such as interpersonal sharing and emotional support. Usually, the more energy that is expended, the more intense the experience.

Energy may also be viewed within the system in terms of supply and demand. Does that particular family have enough energy to meet the demands of the family, or does it have enough demands to consume the supplies? Does the family overextend itself in relation to having enough energy to meet its needs? Do family members have outlets for the expenditure of their energy? In times of stress, a family might find energy stores nonexistent or depleted. In such a case, what resources are available to that system to adapt to the situation? The concept of energy is a highly relevant issue in terms of stress and adaptation determining survival of the system in a changed or unchanged form.

Process in relation to family systems implies movement in some direction. Family feedback systems allow for regulation and facilitation of this movement. Without internal and external communications, there can be no family strategies or effective regulation of space, time, and energy, or movement toward family goals.

Verbal and nonverbal communications are primary feedback loops within the family and between the family and the world, providing information about other people and their relationships to the family and expected behaviors of family members and others.[31] Communication helps to regulate family process. Family members send, receive, and interpret information. Interpretation may depend on the denoted verbal communication (literal meaning) or on the connotated communication (emotional meaning assigned to the word).[31] The more abstract the message communicated, the more unclear the interpretation may be. Satir describes functional communication between family members as a series of verbal interactions in which messages are mutually clarified and qualified which serve to decrease confusion or generalized interpretation of those messages.[32]

Communication patterns occur on two different levels. They are "denotative" and "meta communicative."[33] The denotative level on which communication occurs is the literal context of what is said. "Gee, I really love a house full of mice." The meta communication level involves the message about the denotative (literal) message but also concerns a message on the nature of the relationship of the people the message involves. Mother pats father on the hand and says, "Gee, I really love a house full of mice," and grimaces. This message is very different from the literal message which was sent. What she was really saying was "Let's get rid of those mice!" In other words, the meta communication was a message about a message. A meta communication can transmit attitudes about the message sent, attitudes about the sender, and attitudes regarding the sender toward the receiver. The receiver now has the job of comparing the nonverbal and verbal communication and contrasting them with the literal message. When the communication and meta communication do not go together, the receiver has the job of fitting them into a single message. "Oh, you don't like the mice."

Congruent communication is when two or more messages are given at different levels but do not contradict each other.[34] Father groans saying, "I hate doing my income tax every year," as he breaks his pencil. Incongruent communication occurs when two or more messages are sent at different levels, and they contradict each other.[34] Father groans, then smiles, saying, "I love doing the income tax—next year, you do it." The degree in which messages become incongruent differs with the degree the messages do not correlate. The freedom the receiver has to clarify and qualify enhances his interpretation of the messages.

In summary, family feedback creates or diminishes movement toward goals. If a family member believes there is a need for more movement toward intimacy (affect), she might put her arm around Mom and say, "Why don't we all go out someplace?" The system's movement toward or away from its goals occurs through its use of space, time, and energy. Mom might pull away slightly and say, "Gee, I don't know if we can go out. Everyone is so busy lately, and we really don't have the money." Mom, on the other hand, might not feel the need for closeness, but she might feel a need for family movement in the area of meaning. In this case, in the area of religion. So she goes on to say to her daughter, "Look, one way for all of us to be together is if we all go to church this Sunday. We can all talk about it tonight at dinner." What can be identified here is the movement of a system toward or away from family goals, or family process. Family strategies or patterns of behavior facilitate or block this movement. Space, time, and energy are the dimensions in which family process occurs. Communications from within the family, and from its outer environment, provide feedback which regulates, enhances, or retards its dynamically changing state.

FUTURE OF THE AMERICAN FAMILY

At this point, it is quite relevant to ask what is the future of the nuclear family? New types of experimental families have appeared (i.e., the Kibbutz communal type unit, single parent families, and homosexual unions). Will new family systems replace the nuclear family? With the marked rise in divorce rates, families headed by women, new methods of contraception, and population control, will the nuclear family remain functional?

Putting aside the crystal ball, it is more appropriate to examine the trends. Women's roles in the family as a labor force are changing. How will this affect the family? If the family is viewed as an economic unit which utilizes paid and unpaid time of its members for market and home produced goods and services, the family must define the amount of time members spend on these tasks and decide whether to consume commercially or home produced goods.[35] More simply, if the mother works, the family has to decide how they are to allocate time to cook and clean house. The emphasis on time allocation is not only in terms of economics but also can be seen as time relegated to love, leisure, companionship, and consumption as well as materially productive work.[36] These allocations help shape the character of marriage and the family. Industrialization has streamlined the extended family into the present nuclear form. Smaller families are more mobile and less of an economic strain for family breadwinners. There is, presently, little market production within the home, but the family continues to serve as a redistributor of resources within the system.[36]

It has been predicted that a major shift will develop within families due to the continued impact of technology, especially with advances in birth control.[37] A greater equality between sexes is foreseen; one with companionship marriages, and families operating as income-pooling units.[37] There is increasing concern over population and the changing values regarding large families and women's roles. In the future, women will no longer be socialized into "traditional" roles; men will be freed from full family support. Children will still require cost in time and money, but there will be fewer of them, and they may be reared for the satisfactions they bring. A child's upbringing will be a shared family responsibility rather than falling into the woman's "domain."[37] It is speculated that the growing independence of women will affect decisions regarding marriage, childbearing, and family formation. With the rise in divorce, there will be an increase in single parent families. However, the present trend is also toward remarriage. Families will continue to form and reform based on personal satisfaction because they are likely to provide greater satisfaction for those involved.

Implications for Health Professions

Aside from providing a theoretical framework from which a family may be assessed, the implications of an understanding and application of family theories are more far reaching. As health professionals, all of us have contact with family members and their respective families. When family members are ill, they usually seek the services of health professionals which is generally our initial contact with them. They are treated at home, at a clinic, or in the hospital. With minor medical or emotional problems, the impact of the family member's illness might not be as traumatic for that particular family system. In some family systems, however, family members may assume a "sick" role. In other words, a family member may have a sick role assigned to him, which he accepts. This may be his characteristic role, or one which is assumed when the family system is stressed. It is at this point that an understanding of family systems becomes vital. It is essential in the delivery of health care because should the client be treated (whether or not the symptoms abate) and returned to that family system, he will again assume his role as "sick member." With this type of client, a more effective long-range approach would be to intervene with the entire family. This method of treatment would change family patterns of interaction in such a way that the family member would no longer need to be "sick" to maintain the system's equilibrium. The family will have learned alternate patterns of interaction to maintain its steady state. The sick member role can be seen in the following example.

A 22-year-old male was treated on an inpatient basis for acute pancreatitis. He developed pancreatitis following a 3 day alcoholic drinking binge. He was treated, released, then was readmitted 2 weeks later with a recurrence of the same symptoms. He again admitted to drinking heavily. Further assessment of his problem revealed that he usually drank after quarrels at home with his parents. These quarrels generated from conflicts within his family over his inability

and unwillingness to find a job to help support the family.

In response to this information, the medical team working on his case referred this individual and his family to a community based counseling service. The family was treated as a whole, eventually learning more productive ways of dealing with stressors; thus, he no longer needed to assume the "sick" role.

For the health practitioner, this implied an increased need for depth and understanding of family systems so strategies for change may be developed within the family system.

From a microscopic perspective, involvement with family systems may occur on a variety of levels, be it with primary, secondary, or tertiary care. Practitioners' roles are changing. A family-centered care approach is developing which utilizes interdisciplinary strategies attempting to increase personalized care. A major health trend is toward preventive medicine. If this trend is to be effective, Sussman[38] believes that the traditional role of the practitioner to the family must be changed.

People are becoming more aware of positive health not only as a goal but as a right. On a macroscopic level, the involvement of health care practitioners must be on a community level. If a systems approach to families is applied, and the family is seen as responding not only to the inner process of its members, but also to the environmental (community and society) processes, then environmental changes might also need to be effected. Sussman[38] suggested that agency programs—that is, client centered programs where conditions and communities are designed around families—might be utilized. This is an alternative to the present method of fitting families into communities on a least-cost economic principle with nearsighted professional expertise. This would necessitate developing health care delivery systems which approach the community as a system and abandoning our present highly specialized and controlled methods.

We may attempt to change societal stimuli, but on the other hand, societal demands also elicit a change in the health care delivery system. Ford[39] stressed that people are growing tired of fragmentation in service, high costs, and the unresponsiveness of the health care system. Societal needs and demands should eventually engender a change within the health care delivery network. Positive health may be a goal within our society, and if it is seen as a human right, the implications for health professionals, are indeed far-reaching.

REFERENCES

1. Reiss, I. L.: *The Family System in America.* New York, Holt, Rinehart, and Winston, 1971, p. 18.
2. Adams, B. N.: *The American Family.* Chicago, Markham Publishing Company, 1971, p. 59.
3. *Ibid.*, pp. 59–60.
4. *Ibid.*, pp. 60–64.
5. *Ibid.*, pp. 67–70.
6. *Ibid.*, pp. 68–71.
7. Farber, B.: *Family: Organization and Interaction.* San Francisco, Chandler Publishing Company, 1964, p. 24.
8. Reiss, *op. cit.*, p. 18.
9. Farber, *op. cit.,* pp. 29–32.
10. *Ibid.*, pp. 32–33.
11. Kantor, D., and Lehr, W.: *Inside the Family.* San Francisco, Jossey-Bass Publishers, 1976, p. 10.
12. *Ibid.*, p. 14.
13. Minuchin, S.: *Families and Family Therapy.* Cambridge, Mass., Harvard University Press, 1974, p. 52.
14. *Ibid.*, p. 53.
15. *Ibid.*, p. 56.
16. *Ibid.*, p. 57.
17. *Ibid.*, p. 59.
18. Kantor and Lehr, *op. cit.*, p. 23.
19. Minuchin, *op. cit.*, p. 55.
20. Kantor and Lehr, *op. cit.*, pp. 180–192.
21. *Ibid.*, pp. 119–137.
22. Kantor and Lehr, *op. cit.*, p. 15.
23. *Ibid.*, pp. 20–21.
24. *Ibid.*, p. 37.
25. *Ibid.*, p. 47.
26. *Ibid.*, p. 48.
27. *Ibid.*, p. 49.
28. *Ibid.*, pp. 51–52.
29. *Ibid.*, pp. 66–102.
30. *Ibid.*, p. 43.
31. Satir, V.: *Conjoint Family Therapy.* Palo Alto, Calif., Science and Behavior Books, Inc., 1967, p. 64.
32. *Ibid.*, p. 70.
33. *Ibid.*, pp. 75–76.
34. *Ibid.*, p. 82.
35. Ross, H. L., and Sawhill, I. V.: *Time of Transition:* *The Growth of Families Headed by Women.* Washington, D.C., The Urban Institute, 1975, p. 166.
36. *Ibid.*, p. 177.
37. *Ibid.*, p. 169.
38. Sussman, M. B.: Family systems in the 1970s: analysis, policies, and programs, in *Family Health Care.* New York, McGraw-Hill Book Company, 1973, p. 31.
39. Ford, L.: The development of family nursing, in *Family Health Care*, New York, McGraw-Hill Book Company, 1973, pp. 10–11.

BIBLIOGRAPHY

Adams, B. N.: *The American Family: A Sociological Interpretation.* Chicago, Markham Publishing Company, 1971.

Boszormany-Nagy, I., and Framo, J. (eds.): *Intensive Family Therapy.* New York, Harper and Row, 1965.

Burgess, E. W., and Locke, H. J.: *The Family from Institution to Companionship.* New York, American Book Company, 1945.

Bynne, S.: Nobody home: the erosion of the American family. *Psychol. Today* 10:40, 1977.

Fuchs, L. J.: *Family Matters.* New York, Random House, 1972.

Haley, J., and Hoffman, L.: *Techniques of Family Therapy.* New York, Basic Books, Inc., 1967.

Hope, K., and Young, N. (eds.): *Momma: The Source Book for Single Mothers.* New York, New American Library, 1976.

Hymonich, D. P., and Barnard, P. U.: *Family Health Care.* New York, McGraw-Hill Book Company, 1973.

Landis, J. T. (ed.): *Readings in Marriage and the Family.* New York, Prentice-Hall, Inc., 1952.

Miller, J. C.: Systems theory and family psychotherapy. *Nurs. Clin. North Am.* 6:395, 1971.

Otto, H. A. (ed.): *The Family in Search of a Future.* New York, Appleton-Century-Crofts, 1970.

Queen, S. A., and Haberstein, R. W.: *The Family in Various Cultures.* New York, J. B. Lippincott Company, 1967.

Rodman, H.: *Marriage, Family, and Society: A Reader.* New York, Random House, 1965.

Sobol, E. G., and Robischon, P.: *Family Nursing: A Study Guide.* St. Louis, C. V. Mosby Company, 1970.

Wells, J. G. (ed.): *Current Issues in Marriage and the Family.* New York, Macmillan Publishing Company, Inc. 1975.

CHAPTER 3

Our feelings are facts! They are real and need to be acknowledged at least to ourselves if we are to remain humanistic in our interactions with one another. As health professionals, with a responsibility for patients, failure to "listen to our feelings" may undermine that which we say we wish to accomplish. It is a matter of, "I can't get there from here unless I know where I really am." In this chapter, I wish to encourage you to become aware of whatever feelings may be elicited.

THOUGHTS, FEELINGS, AND BEHAVIORS

Let us spend a few moments with Figure 3-1. The notion is a simple one—that is, that thoughts, feelings, and behaviors are related—and it is not difficult to get from one to the other. The following examples illustrate this point:

1. Imagine (thought) someone canceling a date with you at the last minute after you have

HUMAN SEXUALITY

Vincent J. DeFeo, Ph.D.

gone through considerable effort in preparation. Are there any feelings associated with that thought? Would your subsequent behavior toward that individual be influenced by such feelings?

2. Think of a sexual experience (behavior) in which you have participated. What feelings are elicited by the thoughts of that behavior? Are the feelings comfortable or uncomfortable ones?

3. Imagine examining your own genitals in a hand mirror. What kinds of feelings might you get? Would you feel curious, cautious, anxious, pleased, turned on or off, shocked, afraid, disgusted, happy, disappointed? If you have never looked, has the thought ever occurred to you? If it has, what did you do about it and why?

4. Imagine entering a private room to take a patient's morning temperature and discovering that the patient is masturbating. What feelings do you think you would have? How would

those feelings affect your behavior in that situation? Suppose the patient were: (1) male instead of female; (2) young instead of old; or (3) attractive instead of unattractive. How might these affect your feelings and behavior? Would you behave the same in all circumstances or situationally and why?

Actually, there are no right or wrong ways in which to feel. Feelings, like clouds, drift in upon us, depending upon the circumstances; we have no real control over them. We therefore need not feel ashamed or guilty, or good or bad, or pleased or "anything" about our feelings. It is important though that we pay attention to them and recognize their presence because they can influence our behavior, and our behavior is something that we can do something about. While we are not responsible for having feelings, we are responsible for what we do with them. Recognition of our feelings enables us to take charge and to direct ourselves into an appropriate behavior which is neither threatening

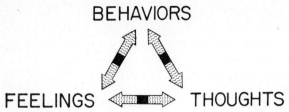

BEHAVIORS

FEELINGS ⟷ THOUGHTS

FIGURE 3-1. Thoughts, feelings, and behaviors can flow into one another. While we are not responsible for our feelings and thoughts—they just happen, we are responsible for what we do or do not do with them.

nor destructive to our own or another person's *self-esteem.*

REPRODUCTION VERSUS SEX

Each of us probably has different values regarding the relationship between reproduction and sex. Some of the ways in which we might indicate their relative importance are illustrated in Figure 3-2.

Does any given combination speak for you? If not, how would you depict the relationship? How would you have depicted it 10 years ago, and what do you think it might look like 30 years from now? How similar are your views to those of your parents? How about to your clients? Can you appreciate the fact that some of them might think just like you while others may not? There are no right ways or wrong ways for all of us; there is only how *each* person feels about it.

The diagrams in Figure 3-2 reflect not only cultural, religious, and moral values, but also some technological realities. From an evolutionary standpoint, both systems are interdependent. However, in these modern times, pregnancy can occur without sexual intercourse (artificial insemination) and because of contraception, sexual intercourse only infrequently gives rise to reproduction. Even in the reduction of the gonadal hormones, sex can and does occur with enjoyment. This is true for postcastrates, postmenopausal females, octogenarians of both sexes as well as prepubertal children and in-

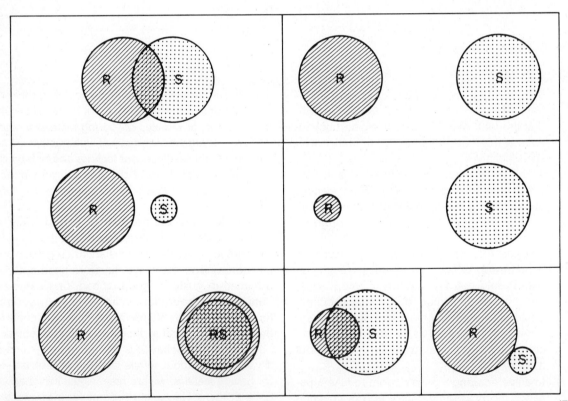

FIGURE 3-2. Do any of these diagrams adequately express the relative importance of sex (S) to reproduction (R) for you, at this time?

fants in which orgasmlike responses are associated with genital stimulation.

Aside from these facts about our biological capabilities as humans, it is important to realize that many people do perceive a close association between their reproductive and sexual abilities. It is therefore not uncommon for a woman faced with the prospects of a hysterectomy to have concerns about the possible loss of her sexual feelings. The effect of a mastectomy on self-esteem is not surprising in our media dominated culture. Thus, cosmetic surgery utilizing mammary gland prosthesis (Fig. 3-3) is easy to understand. Some women regard each reappearance of the menstrual flow as a sign of their womanliness, whereas some meno-

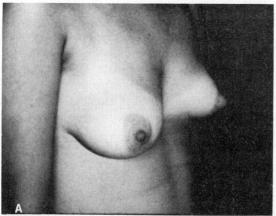
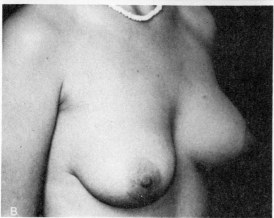

FIGURE 3-3. In most cultures, the mammary glands, regardless of size, constitute a "badge of femininity." A, This person's left gland did not develop as fully as the one on her right. She felt "weird" and breast sensations were unpleasant. B, Following bilateral mammoplasty, her self-image improved and her breasts responded erotically. (Photograph courtesy of Richard Siegel, M.D.).

pausal women whose intervals between menstrual periods are growing progressively longer may experience doubts about themselves during this transition period. Some individuals even have an association of sexuality with their menstrual period since they usually experience a heightened sexual awareness during the menstrual phase of the reproductive cycle. (It has been suggested that this may be related to the accompanying pelvic engorgement.) For males, the expulsion of semen appears to be important, perhaps because changes in ejaculatory volume, in the same individual, are associated with orgasms of varying intensity. In retrograde ejaculation into the bladder, which may accompany diabetes or prostatic surgery, absence of an ejaculate may be of such concern to the client that he may discount the orgasmic sensations that do exist. In most cases, proper counseling is both reassuring and beneficial to the recovery of sexual feelings.

Reproductive Bias

Ours, like many other cultures, possesses a "reproductive bias."[1] By this is meant that only those individuals whose sexual activities may lead to a *socially approved pregnancy* receive social acceptance of their sexual behavior. Others do not and are therefore disapproved of or ignored. Individuals receiving this social acceptance can be regarded as the "sexually elite," and those denied the acceptance can be regarded as the "sexually oppressed."[1] Into which of these categories, elite or oppressed, would you place the following classes of individuals: the married, the single, the divorced, the widows (widowers), the children, the teenagers, the old, the young adult, the rich, the poor, the physically handicapped, heterosexuals, homosexuals, ethnic minorities, prisoners, the unattractive, the educated, the uneducated, the glamourous?

As a nation, we are probably more preoccupied than other Western countries with creating and maintaining laws that specify which sexual behaviors are legal (moral) and which are not. More than 30 of our states have such restrictive laws which occasionally are still enforced. All such laws which focus on the sexual practice itself are derivatives of the reproductive bias. Our attempt to desexualize the aged and the handicapped by treating them like asexual children is also part of the same bias.

Evolution of Reproduction and Sex

Animal species can be regarded in terms of whether or not they are sexually dimorphic, that is, whether the male and female of the species are distinguishable by their physical characteristics. Animals which are not sexually dimorphic resemble each other more closely in stature and body mass, plumage, and hair distribution. There are several attributes of sexual dimorphism that are of interest here since they apply to the human species as well, and as with other animals, it has probably contributed to human evolutionary process through natural selection. The attributes are (1) *attractiveness*, (2) *competitiveness*, and (3) *polygyny*.[2] The differences between the sexes contribute to relative degrees of attractiveness of one partner for the other. Such attractiveness of the female sets up a competitiveness among the males for her favors.* The polygynous nature of the human male is well known even though societal mores might dictate otherwise. Studies, on approximately 185 cultures around the world, have indicated that polygynous behavior is the rule rather than the exception.[2] A modern expression of this in our own culture is the serial marital or nonmarital relationships that are now more apparent. (In this case, one can also regard the human female as asserting her social equality through serial polyandry.)

The offspring of sexually dimorphic species, other than the human, have been able to survive polygynous behavior on the part of the species because the females did not need the male to care for the young. She could do it all by herself. How then has the human race survived given our polygynous evolutionary nature and the fact that the human child has a long period of dependence because of the incomplete and slow development of its nervous system? The answer may lie in the nature of human sexuality which by being more varied, more interesting, more frequent, and probably more pleasurable than in any other species, contributes

---

*The human female is unique and has evolved mammary glands which are responsive to estrogen during puberty. Hence, she is unlike those of other species of mammals in which the glands do not develop until late in pregnancy. This is regarded as evidence of sexual dimorphism for enhancing attractiveness.[2] The notion has its support from studies of many primitive cultures and is not just a reflection of our media, although the media does distort and create artificial standards of attractiveness.

to the formation of pair-bonding and thus keeps the couple together. One should also note the uniqueness of human female sexuality. Unlike other animals which are dependent upon the state of ovarian activity (ovulation) for acceptance of the male, the human female can become interested in sexual activity at any time. Furthermore, the human female is endowed with the capacity for one or more orgasms which may contribute to her interest in the relationship, thus enhancing desirability and maintenance of the bond. (Though one might expect it to occur, there is no good evidence at present that orgasm exists in the females of other species.[2])

There is something to be said about the value of encouraging pair-bonding, even in the absence of dependent children. If we were to think of this as a "pleasure-bonding" as Masters and Johnson[3] refer to it, then we can see that it is this which tends to keep a relationship together. When two individuals are willing to bring pleasure to one another through touch, through words, or through however they wish to demonstrate it, then it is a beautiful human attribute that should be socially encouraged, rather than discouraged. We all need people who show that they care about us. Isolation and loneliness can be painful, and it is dehumanizing when we ignore this need for closeness or obstruct it. It is not uncommon for a hospital patient who wishes to be close to a visitor and really needs that kind of physical reassurance, to hold back for fear of embarrassment should the nurse walk in. This does not refer to overt or heavy sexual activity but the demonstration of simple closeness or embracing which may become awkward in the hospital setting. The following case illustrates the fact that more could be done in a hospital setting if nurses were more sensitive to the needs of their patients.

CASE. A young paraplegic female and quadraplegic male who met as long-term patients in a hospital decided to get married. The initial reaction on the part of both the staff and the clergy was "Why marry when they are unlikely to have children anyway?" But the couple did marry, were assigned the same hospital room and, of course, separate beds. A system was provided for holding the beds together for their wedding night and for a few days thereafter, but that was it. They were married for almost a year, and none of the staff anticipated the fact that the patients wanted those beds back together again at least on some recurring basis. The couple felt too embarrassed and even guilty for asking people to do the extra work involved in bringing the beds together. Yet, they felt hurt and ignored as a couple and lacked sufficient closeness. They felt no privacy, even with the door closed, since people did not knock before entering. The couple really desired some time to be physically close and to experience more than just hand and genital caressing. They were both sexually inexperienced and even though he was capable of erection, they had not sufficient opportunity to experience sexual intercourse. However, when the situation improved, their relationship improved, but only after an outsider interceded on their behalf and brought the attention of the nursing staff to the problem.

If you worked in such a setting as part of the nursing staff, what problems do you see, and how do you think you would deal with them?

Our life span which is becoming increasingly longer creates an unprecedented situation in evolutionary history. It requires new ways of looking at our society of aging humans, who while they have grown apart and independent of the basic family unit, still desire and require human contact, both socially and physically, if they are to remain mentally healthy. The existence of sexual feelings, however one defines them, among the aged is real. Some institutions may need to become more realistic regarding "patient rights."[4] Excessive control, ridicule, denigrating comments, and gossip can contribute to further client isolation and loneliness.

PLEASURE AND ATTACHMENT

For the formation of a pair-bond that provides for the development of the biologically dependent human infant, one can consider, in addition to social pressures, the existence and availability of pleasure as a natural motivator. As simplistic as it may seem, I would like to suggest that the physical pleasures which a couple gives to one another may have had their biological origin in the early maternal-infant interactions which led to attachment behaviors.

Attachment is "an intrinsic capacity that is developed under appropriate circumstances; it is not willed into being after a calculation of its advantages."[5] Attachment seems to develop regularly in marriage so long as the spouse is adequately *accessible* and *attentive*.[5] Once developed, the attachment persists even after separation, divorce, or death of a partner. The attachment thus has an imprinted quality, and the attachment figure can again elicit attachment feelings, until he or she is understood to have become intrinsically different.[5] Studies on maternal-infant bonding discuss the effect of early separation on family development and devote considerable attention to the phenomenon of attachment in the human, mainly at the maternal-infant level.[6] Some of the evidence suggests that a mother or nurse caring for a premature infant will form a close attachment to only *one* infant at a time. Furthermore, it is not easy for the process of attachment and detachment to occur *simultaneously*. When parents grieve from the loss of a close family relative, they are unable to adequately care for their newborn. It appears that grieving must be finished before new close attachments can be adequately formed.

The components leading to reciprocal interaction between mother and infant are crucial to the attachment process.[6] Not only does the infant attach to the mother, but the mother also attaches to the infant; each triggers and involves the other by way of touch, voice, and eye-to-eye contact through the *en face* position. The infant within the first few days of birth becomes *attentive*, particularly to the mother's voice, and responds by body movement according to the elements of speech (the language is not important). The infant's responses reward the mother and stimulate her to continue. It is as if the two were engaged in a kind of dance with each responding to the other's speech and movement. In an unresponsive infant, such as a blind one, attachment is more difficult, and other forms of stimulation must be encouraged.[6]

These principles and descriptions of maternal-infant interactions leading to attachment are not too different from those that exist in adult interactions (e.g., a couple involved in a sexual embrace). Each of them is obtaining pleasure at the sight, the sound, the movement, and responsiveness of the other with the result that there is an escalation of the "dance," which can culminate in orgasm. The "dance" is probably most interesting when it is creative and spontaneous, giving it the quality of playfulness. It is difficult to form a close attachment, or to sustain a sexual interest, in someone who is unresponsive, bored, tired, indifferent, or "just not there." Disappointment is inevitable when one looks to the partner for signs of willing participation and a desire for mutual pleasure and finds a lack of interest. Changes in the level of sexual responsiveness of a partner are clear signals that something has happened between them, such as increased anxieties or unresolved anger, that may require improved communication and sometimes counseling.

WILLINGNESS TO BELIEVE

One of the qualities that we share as humans and that characterizes us from the rest of the animal kingdom is the "willingness to believe." We are born with this capacity and are capable of surviving as long as we "continue to believe." I am not referring to anything complicated like a whole system of beliefs but rather something simple and even more inclusive. I would say that all the knowledge or information that we acquire through others, unless it is also something that we have experienced, is a "belief" and exists in a state of quasireality. For pragmatic purposes, however, we are inclined to treat it just as if it were real, and we then behave accordingly. Our beliefs are constantly shaped and updated by our culture, and it is interesting how through ridicule, punishment, or rewards we learn to give up existing beliefs and acquire new ones. The whole educational process itself, including the one you are in at this very moment, is evidence of what I am saying. We have taught people to pay attention to what other people write and say and to accept it. On the other hand, there are circumstances when we have judged or ridiculed others for having accepted what other people wrote or said! Not to believe what others believe can be threatening, and believing that which others do not believe can sometimes be frightening and may take courage.

Is there a place called Paris? Is there a place called Hana? How do you know? It is easy to believe the existence of something when there are many people who will say, in many different ways, that "it exists." What would it take for you to believe in the existence of Hana? All that it takes is *someone* that we are willing to believe in. If a source, a person, has credibility, it is very easy to

believe in what he says. A book, a journal, or even a newspaper can be very powerful in this regard. I confess to being a "believer" of the scientific articles that I read, when they are presented in a convincing manner that satisfies my standards. However, I am vulnerable because what I read sounds like it could be correct, but I have to trust the judgment of others (i.e., the editors of the journals and the referees whom they select). Thus, the ability to believe is based on the trust that I have developed for people.

Health professionals can be powerful in terms of their ability to contribute to, or alter, the beliefs of clients and others who seek information. It is often useful to explore a client's beliefs in order to correct misconceptions because with them may lie some of the problem. The beliefs that a person has can sometimes predispose him to symptoms or can relieve them (the placebo effect).

CASE. An adult married male who has just been diagnosed as having diabetes began reading actively about the subject in a medical text and learned that impotence was one of the side effects. That night, when he attempted intercourse with his wife, sure enough, he discovered that he was impotent. The next day he called his doctor who expressed his regret and confirmed his symptom of impotence as a known side effect of diabetes. The client soon became severely depressed, and his wife encouraged him to seek psychotherapy. The therapist began by asking questions such as, "Do you ever experience an erection at times other than with intercourse, for example, a morning erection or with masturbation?" The client immediately responded yes, whereupon the therapist told him that it was impossible for him to be classified as impotent due to a diabetic neuropathy. That was all the client needed to know. He was reassured and soon regained potency with his wife during their sexual activity.

Not all cases of impotence associated with diabetes are psychogenic in origin. There clearly can be neuropathies involved, and male diabetics show more problems than do females.[7] The above example merely illustrates the principle that beliefs themselves can become self-fulfilling prophesies. It is important to realize that old beliefs are constantly being replaced by new ones throughout life. Today, changes occur so quickly that giving up a belief and acquiring a more realistic one become essential to our adaptability and survival.

EXERCISES. Think of some of the beliefs you grew up with, concerning sex. Where are you now with those beliefs? Can you recall the moment in which you may have transformed or given up the belief? Mentally list some beliefs that you now hold regarding some "objectionable" sexual practices. How did you acquire those beliefs? Are those beliefs shared by a large number of people, or only a few? Does your belief about that sexual practice protect you from anything? Do you make anyone right, or do you make anyone wrong, through this belief?

The opportunity to examine beliefs allows for the rejection of beliefs that no longer serve a purpose. They may have been valuable at an earlier time but may no longer be applicable, perhaps as a result of increased competence and capabilities. Some beliefs can be readily given up while other beliefs are important for a long time; it is perfectly all right to retain them. A belief is usually not given up unless it can be replaced with one of greater value!

Sometimes a person may request an opinion as to whether a thought, a feeling, or a behavior is right or wrong for him. The following statement is sometimes helpful: "I really don't know whether it is right or wrong for *you*. It appears that you have been listening to a number of opinions, and maybe it is time to begin to listen to yourself. How do *you* really feel about this?" This provides an opportunity to be supportive without being judgmental and enables a person to get at some of his beliefs and anxieties. It is very reassuring for people to know that they are not alone and that others feel the way they do, that is, they are "normal."

CASE. In the course of a history taking, a sophomore medical student discovered considerable loneliness in a 65-year-old widow who had been admitted for a medical problem. In pursuing it further, he learned that this woman was feeling very anxious and guilty over her sexual feelings since her husband's death 2 years ago. In the discussion, the student was able to reassure her of the naturalness of her sexual feelings and was then able to discuss masturbation with her, something which she had never explored for herself.

What does it take to enable someone to believe in us? Whether the person is a patient or not, whether the person is a child, a lover, a relative, an elderly person, or a friend—it is all the same. What did this medical student have that the attending physician apparently was not able to provide and which seemed to be an important aspect of her problem? What the student provided was an element that was "attachmentlike." He was *accessible* and *attentive* in addition to knowledgeable, and he used his "gift of time" to establish a rapport in which trust occurred. Trust which may take some time to build is at the heart of any healthy relationship, whether or not it is a therapeutic one. With trust we expose our "willingness to believe in someone" and are open to change. We are also potentially vulnerable and are therefore taking a risk.

Trust

Trust can be defined in many ways. What would you consider to be the ingredients of a trusting relationship? There are three elements of trust that I have found useful and that I like to share with students.[8] All three are essential to a trusting relationship and a reduction of any one will limit the capacity for trust. On the other hand, an abundance of all three qualities in an individual contributes to a very enriching and loving relationship. The elements of trust are: (1) *integrity*, (2) *competence*, and (3) *a well-meaning intention*. Integrity refers to honesty, to being direct, and not giving conflicting messages. Competence refers to real ability, to skill, and to knowledge, as well as recognizing one's own limitations. Well-meaning intention refers to the notion of a genuine interest and concern for the other person's well-being; it implies caring. It means no ego trip; it means no manipulation; it means no attempt to impress or to demean someone. What do you see as the intention when people indulge in gossip? This activity creates difficulty in establishing the kind of trust that makes for cooperation and pleasant working conditions.

What does any of this have to do with the area of sexuality? It is the very core of it. Without going further, pause for a moment to think of different ways within a sexual relationship in which trust may be diminished as a result of damage to *integrity, competence,* or a *well-meaning intention.* With which element of trust are each of the following related. (1) She or he will not talk about what is going on between them. (2) She or he always has a need to be in control of the situation. (3) She or he is mechanical and unimaginative. (4) She or he is unwilling to learn what turns you on. (5) She or he says it is unimportant and discounts your feelings that it *is* important. (6) He ejaculates too fast all the time, then goes right to sleep. (7) She or he does not care whether or not you have an orgasm because "that is your responsibility." (8) She or he is unfaithful in a relationship which is based on sexual exclusivity and gets caught. (9) She or he ridicules, teases, or belittles areas of your body that you are sensitive about (Fig. 3-4). (10) She or he is unwilling to seek help on a marital or sexual problem. These examples are all negative ones and have a deleterious influence on the maintenance of trust. A couple with all those problems really needs some help. If, however, there was a willingness on the part of both partners to try to change things, for the better, then that willingness itself is what trust is all about—a reaffirmation of the well-meaning intention which shows that they still care about the relationship and each other. The unwillingness to do that creates doubts, erodes the trust, and often leads to disappointment, anger, and perhaps ultimately to the termination of the relationship.

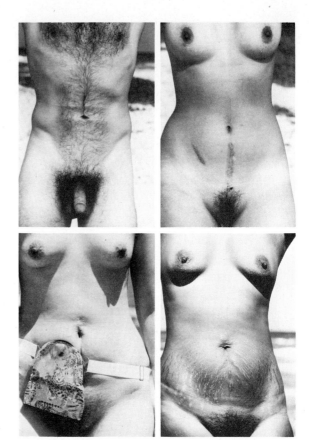

FIGURE 3-4. Life brings changes to the human body which challenge self-esteem and the ability to cope. These four individuals feel *positive* about their bodies and are competent to form and maintain close relationships.

CASE. A male sought help because he and his wife wanted to have a baby, but they were unable to because during their 4 years of marriage, they had never experienced vaginal penetration. The problem was that he ejaculated very quickly. He only had to kiss his wife or have her touch his penis, and ejaculation would be almost immediate. Although he had no prior sexual experience, she did and was orgasmic with penis penetration by several lovers in her past. Whenever she made him aware of this, he would feel inadequate and a failure as both a man and a husband. (She once told him "If you knew you were going to have this problem, why did you ever want to marry me?") His problem continued to create frustrations and disappointments for both of them, and they minimized the importance of sex in their relationship. Nothing was done about the problem until they decided to have a baby and wanted to have it "the right way." A treatment for premature ejaculation was initiated and proceeded effectively to the point where it was necessary to involve the wife in the next stage of treatment. It was at this point that the wife was not fully cooperative and indeed would sabotage the treatment. It was apparent that she had a need to keep him in this state of incompetence. It was not until his overbearing, patronizing attitude toward her was worked on and changed, that she became cooperative. Treatment for his prematurity continued successfully. She became vaginally orgasmic and within a year had their baby.

The point of this example is that a sexual problem may exist indirectly through unresolved relationship problems. There were mutual losses of trust in this relationship. What were they and which elements were being destroyed? A couple often needs help from the outside in order to see what is going on and what they are doing to one another in response to the loss of trust each has developed toward the other. A willingness to recommit themselves to the relationship with the implied desire to make things work better gives a relationship a new start and the success that may then be achieved begins to rebuild the trust. In therapy, sexual problems are often a useful presenting symptom for getting at the most basic problems in a relationship.

Touching

Touching, when used appropriately, can contribute to the development of trust or when used inappropriately, to the destruction of trust. It is a matter of intention of the person doing the touching as well as his (her) sensitivity and timing. Touching is a most important human gift, one that many people have been taught to fear or even abandon. It is a precious gift, both to others *and* to ourselves, for when *we touch someone else, we have simultaneously touched ourselves!* To have that touch accepted and appreciated is an enhancement of our own self-esteem. We feel worthy, valued, approved of, desired, all those nice words that give us a good feeling.

We sometimes forget that our self-esteem is really an emotion. It is a feeling about ourselves. Is it any wonder that the sense of touch can do so much to help that feeling when it comes along with caring or that it can do so much to destroy that feeling when it comes abusively as with hostility. As infants, our sense of touch probably contributed very strongly to the development of our self-esteem long before we were able to acquire a vocabulary and understanding. Through touch, reassurance becomes much simpler. Communication was direct, and we did not have to read between the lines. The need for touching persists into adulthood; some individuals prefer to be the "givers," and others prefer to be the "receivers"—but it is all the same.

Studies indicate that some women wish to be held more than they wish to have genital sex and will thereby use sex mainly to obtain cuddling.[9,10] In some of these cases, the need is so great that the individual may engage in promiscuous behavior, including prostitution. Inhibitions of holding and touching can be related to sexual dysfunctions.[11] Indeed, the first step toward improvement of many of the sexual dysfunctions in both males and females is through the use of the sensate focus technique which utilizes pleasurable but nongenital touching.[12] With such treatment, it is perhaps the involvement of the functional partner as a pleasure-giver that re-establishes the feeling of nurturance and the enhancement of self-esteem in the sexually dysfunctional partner.

GENITALS

Much has been made of the messages which we have been given as boys or girls concerning permission to touch genitals. It is usually felt that parents are much more permissive toward boys in giving positive reinforcement for being able to handle their penises in a proficient manner regarding direction of the urine stream into the pot or commode. (Some credit is deserved because it is not always easy to direct a urine stream, especially in the presence of an erection.) The penis also takes on a social function in boys as they may share in the task of putting out a campfire or carving their initials in the snow or engaging in urinary or ejaculatory contests. Girls, on the other hand, tend to be more private and "ladylike." Some of the early scripts which are learned carry well into adulthood, for example, "Don't show your panties!" It is okay, however, to show a bikini, which can be smaller than panties and which just covers the genitals. Also, it is okay to allow the genitals to be seen during a pelvic examination, but it is not okay for the *panties* to be seen by just anyone. The last time you prepared for your pelvic examination, what did you do with your panties? Did you leave them on top of your clothes because they were the last item to be removed, or did you find it necessary to hide them somewhere in your other clothing?

The results of these early conditionings probably contribute to young men having learned to have orgasms more spontaneously than young women due to greater genital awareness and acceptability. It is not surprising that there are many women, who even as adults, have yet to visualize their own gen-

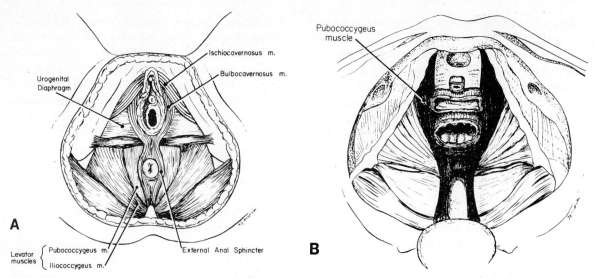

FIGURE 3-5. A, Diagram of the perineum showing part of the pubococcygeus (PC) muscle. B, Diagram of the pubococcygeus muscle seen in its entirety, from above. Note that the muscle is separated by the urethra, the vagina and the rectum. The vaginal portion of the muscle is easily palpated, at "4 and 8 o'clock," by a fingertip inserted into the vagina.

itals. It seems strange that the thought should never even have occurred to them, or if it had, it needed to be suppressed. In association with her pelvic examination, the client is often encouraged to visualize her genitals in a hand mirror and to ask the nurse or physician any questions she may wish to about her anatomy or its function, including the lack of "vaginal feeling."[13,14] It is an excellent opportunity to correct misconceptions, to emphasize the normal variations that exist, and to teach the Kegel exercises. The exercises consist of a series of contractions that strengthen the pubococcygeus muscle through which the vagina passes (Figs. 3-5 and 3-6). Enhancing her own self-acceptance of

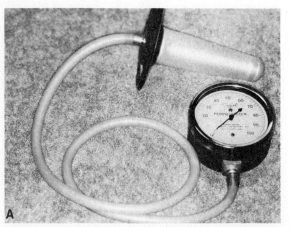
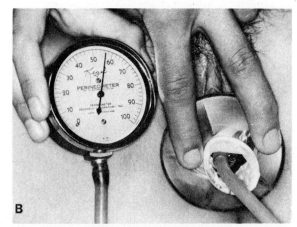

FIGURE 3-6. A, The Kegel perineometer which is used to measure the strength of pubococcygeus muscle contraction. B, A reading of 57 units is elicited in this individual following a quick contraction of the PC muscle (noncontracting muscle reading for this individual is 15 units). Training of this muscle increases genital awareness and improves vaginal perception.[13] Some women have become orgasmic with penile stimulation following use of the exercises.

this area of her body can contribute to an improved sexual relationship with her partner. In Figures 3-7 and 3-8 some vulvar variations are presented. Some of the differences regarding the vulva which are easily apparent are: (1) The amount of hair on the mons and the labia majora can vary. (2) The longitudinal extent of the labia minora can also vary (Figs. 3-7 and 3-8), that is, they can posteriorly extend to the fourchette, three-quarters of the way, or half way. (3) The extent of protrusion of the labia minora is in some cases rather extensive, and the labia can be folded back along each side (Fig. 3-7B). It is interesting that some cultures, unlike our own, have adopted the lovely name "butterfly" (*mariposa*—Mexican; *cho-cho*—Japanese) for this configuration. (4) The size of the clitoris, particularly the glans, is sometimes of concern (Fig. 3-9). Its only known biological function in the human is as a pleasure-inducing organ. Size has nothing to do with orgasmic capability. Furthermore, a recent review on the clitoris recalls histological data indicating a lack of receptors in one specimen among the eight clitorises studied.[15] In that individual, however, the labia minora were well endowed with re-

ceptors. The location of sensitive (responsive) areas can be determined by a couple during a mutual "sexological examination." This is a good way for partners to learn about each other.

Questions of female circumcisions sometimes arise and usually refer to a loosening or removal of some of the clitoral prepuce. This is quite different from the so-called "circumcision" performed in primitive cultures where the clitoris itself may actually be removed, and the labia minora are brought together and sutured, except for a small opening to allow for passage of urine and menstrual fluid.[15] This procedure is more accurately described as infibulation.

Among sexologists, the hymen (Fig. 3-10) is receiving renewed attention as a result of recent studies.[16] Some cases of vaginismus (pain with attempted penetration) may have an anatomical basis in the form of a persistent hymenal thread (septate hymen) running in an anterior-posterior direction across the vaginal orifice. The thread may escape routine physical examination since it may be stretched somewhat and displaced to either side of the orifice. When vaginismus is correlated with

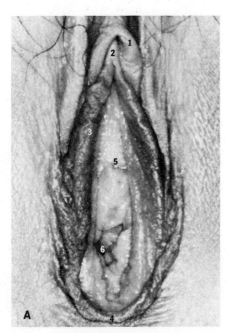 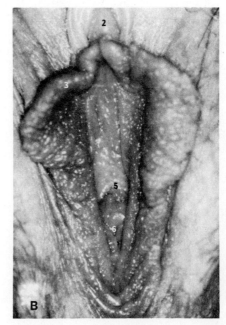

FIGURE 3-7. Examples of differences between vulvas. A, Note how far the labia minora extend toward the fourchette. B, Note the degree of labial protrusion. This protrusion is unrelated to parity, sexual activity, or even masturbation. Labia are sometimes asymmetrical either in length or in thickness. 1 = prepuce; 2 = glans clitoris; 3 = labia minora; 4 = fourchette; 5 = urethral orifice; 6 = vaginal orifice (closed in B).

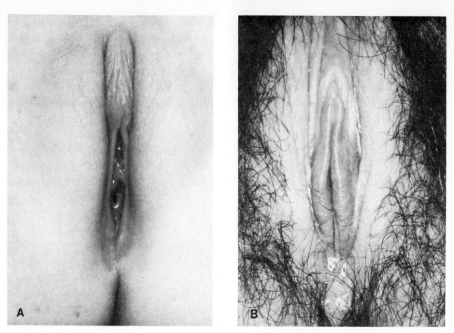

FIGURE 3-8. Compare (A) the vulva of a prepubertal individual (age 12) with that of (B) the vulva of an adult (age 19). What similarities and differences are you aware of? Compare these with Figure 3-7, and discuss your observations with your colleagues.

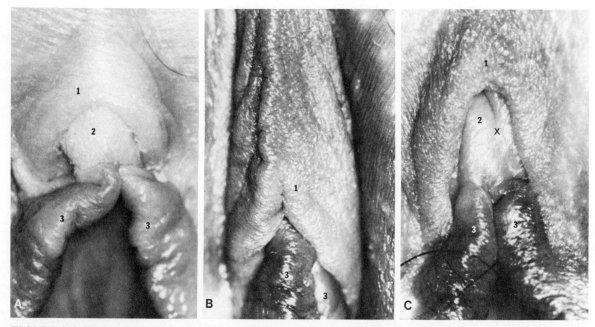

FIGURE 3-9. Normal clitorises and prepuces in the sexually nonaroused state. A, The prepuce (1) is drawn upward to expose the glans clitoris (2). The labia minora (3) are attached to the glans clitoris and contribute to the prepuce as well (also see Fig. 3-8A). B , Note that the prepuce completely covers the glans clitoris which is exposed (C) upon its retraction. This individual has an area of slight clitoral adhesion to the prepuce (X), but contrary to some opinion shows no orgasmic difficulty with either clitoral or vaginal stimulation.

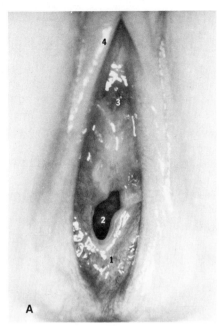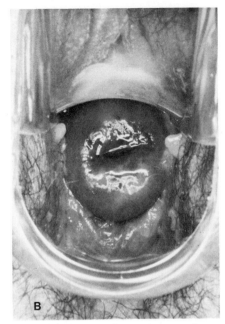

FIGURE 3-10. A, The hymenal area in a prepubertal individual (see Fig. 3-8A). 1 = hymen; 2 = vaginal orifice; 3 = urethral orifice; 4 = labia minora. B, Vaginal examination—adult: note the remnants of the hymen ("hymenal tabs" at 3 and 9 o'clock) and the cervix in the background.

this type of hymen, it can readily be treated simply by clipping the hymenal strand. The source of pain is thus eliminated. It is suggested that routine examination of the neonate for the presence of a septate hymen and treatment at that time should be done to eliminate subsequent problems.[16] (Some sex educators also encourage young women to take the responsibility for dilation of their own hymen, using their own fingers.)

Male genitals also show variety. The chief difference (Fig. 3-11) is in regard to circumcision versus the natural state of noncircumcision. In our culture, males are sometimes confused as to the meaning of the term "circumcised," and it is not surprising for a male who is circumcised to think of himself as uncircumcised until he learns the difference.

The decision to circumcise is one which mothers-to-be may forget to make until they are asked their preference at the hospital. In this country, most often the decision is for circumcision. Estimates of 69–97 percent have been given.[17] As American health professionals, however, we should realize that most males in the world today are probably *uncircumcised*, including most Europeans, Central and South Americans, and Asians. It is important

for nurses to become familiar with the pros and cons of the practice. The American Academy of Pediatrics recently stated, "There are no valid medical indications for circumcision in the neonatal period."[18] Although it is regarded as minor surgery, significant complications may occur in 1 of 500 circumcised newborns.[19] It has been suggested that the value of the prepuce in early life is to protect the glans penis from ammonia in the baby's diapers.[20] An excellent objective overview on circumcision is that of Kaplan[21] who raises the interesting question of cost. Extrapolations based on San Diego County suggest that the costs to the American public of routine, newborn circumcision might be almost $60,000,000 a year.

The size and distribution of veins in the skin of the penis also create differences in appearance. Some penises may be very smooth, particularly in the erect state (Fig. 3-12A), whereas others are not. Sometimes the skin will show tiny elevations along the entire length of the shaft (Fig. 3-12B). These elevations are derived from sebaceous glands related to vestigial hairs and are probably similar to those associated with the areola.

The importance of penis size is often a recurring

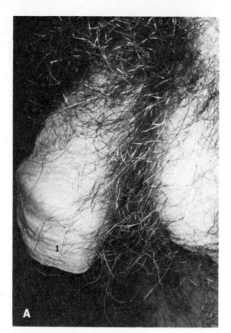 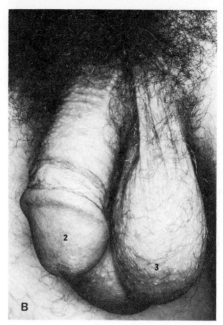

FIGURE 3-11. A, Adult uncircumcised penis in the nonerect state. Note (1) the extension of the skin (prepuce) which covers the glans penis (compare with Fig. 3-9B). B, Adult circumcised penis in nonerect state. The glans penis (2) is always exposed. The difference in skin tone, just above the glans, is due to the original circumcision. The differences in elevation of the scrotum (3) between these individuals is due to ambient temperature. Which one was subjected to the cooler temperature?

question especially to males. In an ongoing study on *perception* of penis sizes by males and females, using a series of six latex penis models, it appears that heterosexual males have very limited experience with other erect penises except in porno films. It is perhaps this limited experience which contributes to self-devaluation. The males in our study tended to exaggerate what they believed women would choose as an effective penis and if these males had a chance, they would prefer to have a penis somewhat larger than their own. Females, by the time they had 10 partners, seem to have experienced a variety of penis sizes. The preferred sizes, in this study consisting mainly of nulliparas, are those which exclude the extremes. It also appears that women who have a single sexual partner prefer the same penis size as that of their current partner (i.e., if the partner has a penis toward the smaller end of the scale, then that is the one preferred, whereas if it is toward the larger end of the scale, then that is the size preferred). This suggests again what women often say (i.e., "The person plays a more important part of the sexual relationship than does the size of his penis"). Yet, some males still have difficulty accepting the fact that "It is the magician that makes the magic and not the wand." Our study tends to indicate that part of the problem may be related to the idea that a male may not have the same perception of his own penis as his partner has.

Masturbation

Although there are cultural and religious attitudes associated with masturbation, many individuals, particularly the younger generation, are becoming more comfortable and accepting of this natural behavior. This is in sharp contrast to the attitude which prevailed earlier in the century in which harness type devices were proposed and used as treatment for this "disturbing and unhealthy practice."[22] How could any human being in the process of self-exploration as an infant or child not have discovered that there are certain areas of the body that produce more pleasant sensations than others? It is a built-in part of the biological system that obviously has had survival-value for us as a race, possibly through the development of the pleasure-

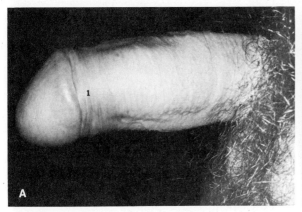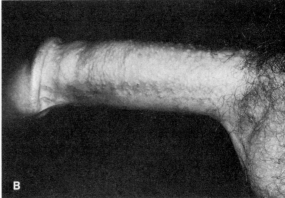

FIGURE 3-12. A, Erection of the adult uncircumcised penis shown in Figure 3-11A with prepuce (1) retracted. B, Erection of the circumcised penis shown in Figure 3-11B. The elevations on the penile skin of this individual are due to sebaceous glands; the appearance of the skin presents no problem whatsoever to the individual or to his partner.

bond as first discovered within ourselves. As Woody Allen says, "Don't knock masturbation. It's having sex with someone I deeply love."

Although it is now a matter of historical interest, it is worth noting that the objectionableness of masturbation was once a commonly held medical belief that pervaded our society. This demonstrates both the power of medical opinion and the fact that beliefs can and do change with time. A survey conducted less than 10 years ago on 500 students in six medical schools showed that 22 percent of the students still believed that masturbation was etiologically related to mental illness.[23] (It was also interesting to note that a significant number of the faculty of these medical schools held similar beliefs.)

Masturbation still causes considerable anxiety for some individuals, regardless of age. It is an excellent area, however, in which parents upon discovery of this stage of natural development in their child can accept and endorse the child's right to experience pleasure and at the same time guide the child, in order to value the experience as something for a private setting. To deal with this area comfortably may sound ideal, but it can be accomplished. Furthermore, the relationship between parent and child becomes enhanced through trust building, and the child's self-esteem is preserved. Each of us can help parents through reassurance of the naturalness of masturbation while also being aware that there may be other concerns, too. We should also keep in mind that the reasons individuals masturbate are varied. From your knowledge,

what would you add to the following list of reasons for masturbation?

1. A personal pleasure—a treat during a state of well-being.
2. To avoid pregnancy (i.e., a substitute for intercourse).
3. A cheer-up during the "blues."
4. A sedative, bringing on a good night's sleep.
5. An anxiety reliever. (Students sometimes report increased frequencies of masturbation when studying for exams.)
6. To relieve loneliness or sexual longing for a loved one. (The practice was actually recommended by marriage counselors on military bases during periods of marital separation associated with military tours of duty, e.g., Vietnam war.)
7. To bring relief (orgasm) after sexual arousal.
8. To reduce testicular swelling and aching after prolonged sex play.
9. To "check the system" after surgery (e.g., herniorrhaphy).
10. To relieve premenstrual tension or menstrual cramps.
11. To reduce social tension. (A secretary reported that when she became upset in her office, due to misdirected and unfair anger toward her, she went to the restroom and masturbated quickly and easily and with very little sexual feeling. Within a few minutes she was back at her desk, calm and able to continue with her work.)

12. To learn how to become orgasmic. (Since orgasm is a learned response, masturbation is often part of the therapeutic procedure recommended for preorgasmic women.)

13. To teach a partner what is desired in the way of stimulation. (This is not always easy, and it usually requires a high level of trust between partners in order for each person to demonstrate to the other, that which it is okay to do only in private. It is interesting how it is far more acceptable for a couple to engage in intercourse, whereas it is very threatening to simply let a partner see what one does during masturbation. Couples often find that to share this experience enriches the feelings of closeness in their relationship. Furthermore, the sharing itself can become highly erotic.)

What problems do you anticipate regarding patient masturbation in a hospital setting? Would you defend a patient's right to privacy? How would you feel about or deal with your discovery of a child masturbating (stroking the genitals)? What if it were an adolescent, an adult, or an elderly person? Would it make any difference whether the person were of your own or of the opposite sex? How do you feel about being regarded as a "sexual fantasy-object" by a client of either sex? How would you regard the client who extends an invitation, verbal or nonverbal, for you to caress his or her genitals? Would it make any difference whether or not you found the client attractive? What if the client was a male recovering from a spinal cord injury? Would it make a difference? Is there any circumstance under which you would consider it appropriate to handle a client's genitals in a manner that may be pleasurable to him or her?

It is something useful to keep in mind that sexual awareness on the part of a client is often a positive sign to the client—a sign of improvement of health and well-being. To be able to acknowledge it comfortably, especially if it takes the form of a compliment to you, may require skill, time, and the development of a genuine *self-appreciation*. To attack the self-esteem of clients through ridiculing them, embarrassing them, commanding, lecturing, or ignoring them while walking off in disgust is not an appropriate solution. Such a nurse could really use some time for self-examination as to the true nature

of the problem. Is it with the client, the nurse, or both, and what can be done to improve the situation?

LEARNING ABOUT HUMAN SEXUALITY

Recently Gebhard[24] compared a small sample of college students with unpublished data from the original Kinsey studies of a generation ago on the acquisition of basic sex information. He found that children and young people are now learning the basic facts of life at a considerably younger age than did their parents and grandparents. Furthermore, this was true for girls as well as boys. While same sex peers remain the dominant educators, they are losing some of their importance to other sources of information, especially mothers. Other studies on adolescents and their parents also note that fathers are not usually mentioned among the sources of information for either sex unless the father has a professional occupation.[25] Schools and the media constitute an additional source of information even though the latter may be superficial and not always very factual. The lack of access to good information is responsible for the epidemic of teenage pregnancy each year.[26] Some sex educators believe that there is a positive correlation between sex education and an adolescent's willingness to postpone that first sexual intercourse. Yet, many school systems are still opposed to the teaching of human sexuality even though 8 out of 10 adults favor it.[26] Often, they do not realize that most boys and girls between the ages of 8 and 13 already know about coitus[24] and in addition, over 50 percent of teenagers between the ages of 15 and 19 have already experienced it.[26] By providing good information, nurses can help parents promote healthy sexual adjustment in their children.[27]

Among professional schools, the teaching of human sexuality is steadily appearing in the curriculum. Less than 10 years ago, there were only about 15 medical schools in the United States which had a course in the subject, and by 1980, it is anticipated that most schools will have included it. Furthermore, one state (California) requires evidence of coursework in this area for state relicensing of physicians. In a recent study of nursing programs by Woods and Mandetta[28] in which replies were received from 69 percent of 218 baccalaureate programs, the institutions agreed that graduates of their programs should be able to minimize the incidence of sexual dysfunction by educating adults and should be able to counsel clients regarding their sexual problems after surgery or illness. In most instances, however, the authors found a deficit between what the curriculum provided and the actual knowledge and competencies of the graduates.[28] Eventually the deficits are bound to be corrected in such programs.

In the meantime, what can students do? I suggest that they not automatically avoid the sexual implications of a medical or surgical problem but start by acknowledging it and dealing with it by learning about it. Good use can be made of nursing journals which are increasing their coverage of sexual topics related to nursing care. The suggestions included in many of these articles are valuable because they are practical and to the point. As professionals, nurses must know the latest facts and information regarding the sexual implications of a health related problem. It is also natural to be curious, without feeling ashamed, apologetic, or embarrassed. As long as our basic intention is to benefit the client, then we can be helpful even when a client's value system differs from our own. We also can learn from problems which clients themselves are solving, and these can later be suggested to others. We can learn from one another, too, by sharing information which has been acquired in the course of training, reading, or working with clients and their sexual concerns or problems. Remember that feelings are real for all of us. They need to be heard and respected, not ridiculed, minimized, or discouraged. Our sexuality is often closely related to our self-esteem. By focusing on our intentions and working toward trust we can enhance a client's self-esteem and our own as well for having been helpful to them.

A useful model which has been proposed for the brief treatment of sexual problems is that of Annon.[29] It is referred to as the PLISSIT model and is mentioned here because it works. It consists of the following four components: P = permission, LI = limited information, SS = specific suggestions, and IT = intensive therapy. Most sex-related concerns can be addressed through the first three components of the model, and only certain problems require intensive therapy. Common sexual dysfunctions can also be effectively treated through the first three components. Often clients simply seek per-

mission to be "just the way they are." Knowing that they are not alone in their thoughts, their feelings, or their behaviors is very reassuring for it means that they are not unusual and that a precedent already exists which seems to be working for others. The following is an abbreviated example of Annon's permission-giving, together with some limited information, for a client that has revealed a concern about his masturbation.

Annon: If I hear you correctly, you feel that you have an ideal relationship with your wife in a number of areas, including sex, yet you're concerned because you also masturbate.

Client: Obviously something must be wrong with my feelings toward her, otherwise why would I have to masturbate?

Annon: You feel that somehow it's wrong, or not right, to have a good sexual relationship with your wife and yet also want to enjoy masturbation?

Client: Well, isn't it?

Annon: Only you can decide what is right or wrong for you. All I can tell you is that what you describe is really quite normal. In fact, many married men do exactly the same thing as you are doing, not to mention married women as well.

Client: No kidding? You mean . . . you mean it's really normal? . . . It's . . . other people masturbate when they're married?

Annon: Well, let me put it this way. In a recent survey it was found that more than 7 out of 10 married men masturbate, and they reported that it did not diminish their sexual satisfaction in other areas . . . Now, if masturbation was causing a direct problem in your relationship with your wife, then such activity might not be helpful. However, in your case, it is not causing a problem for you.

Client: (Lets out a long, even sigh and sinks back in his chair.) You don't know how relieved I feel. It's kind of nice to know that you're normal—just like everyone else.

Permission for sexual *thoughts and fantasies* about people other than their partner can be given by pointing out how common and natural such thoughts are, thereby relieving much anxiety and guilt. Permission to have *feelings* in response to tactile stimulation is also helpful. For example, it is quite common for a woman who is breast-feeding her baby to experience some degree of sexual arousal. Indeed, some women also experience orgasm with their breast-feedings. (This could perhaps be regarded as a very nice fringe benefit.)

We also give permission for *behaviors* that are common but that the client does not know about. As an example, a woman who reaches orgasm within a few minutes worries that she is a "nymphomaniac," whereas a woman who requires 20 minutes of direct stimulation worries that there is something wrong with her! In these cases, the problem comes from the pressure to be like everyone else, instead of appreciating the way we are. An exploration of the problems associated with "the way we are" may clarify and eliminate the anxious feelings accompanying the pressure for change. Clients with spinal cord injury, and usually lacking genital sensations, may be given permisision to explore alternative means (hands, mouth, tongue) for sexual gratification. *There is no area of the body that cannot be used for sexual expression.*[30]

An important aspect of permission-giving is "to oneself." It is important to have permission not to be an expert and to be able to say that we do not know the answer when we do not. No one can be a true *expert* in this field. However, we can always try to respond as a true person, that is, as someone who is willing to listen and to respect without judgment or labeling.

In order to assist people in the area of permission-giving, it is helpful to have information based on research. For example, the sexual thought patterns of almost 3500 adults across the United States were studied, and it was found that in general, young adults think about sex at least once every 10 minutes; middle-aged adults think about sex at least once every 35 minutes; and an elderly individual thinks about sex at least once an hour.[31] Is it any wonder that thoughts of sex happen to occur to hospital patients from time to time, particularly as they are getting well?

The second component of the PLISSIT model, *limited information*, differs from permission-giving in that specific factual information relevant to the concern is presented. Often this may take the form of providing anatomical or physiological information. Information on the variations in the female genitalia as a follow-up of a pelvic examination can provide reassurance. Information about the nature of the prepuce and its attachment to the glans for a number of months, in the uncircumcised infant, can relieve the mother who would find that she is unable to pull back the prepuce. It also protects the infant from developing a phimosis.[20] Information as to the appropriateness of sexual intercourse during menstruation, during pregnancy, after delivery, after surgery, or after a coronary is highly desirable.

The third component, *specific suggestions*, differs from permission and limited information in that direct attempts are made to help the client change behavior in order to reach the stated goals. In the case of an individual seeking sex therapy, a *sex problem* history is essential because no specific suggestions are appropriate until one has obtained information about the client and the unique circumstances of the problem.[29] This *refers* to problems such as impotence, failure to experience orgasm, or vaginismus. While the examples are not too relevant for this discussion, the principle is nevertheless valid. The nurse is in a special setting and situation in which she is in a position to offer *specific suggestions* for actual or potential sexual problems relating to an existing medical problem. This cannot be handled by a psychotherapist or general sex therapist. Often, a client will not express a sex-related concern because it is not a serious problem compared to the other problems with which a hospital staff is involved. Yet the handling of sexual concerns and how to solve the problems that may arise, including the fears of those problems, may be very important to a client's well-being and improvement of health. A diabetic male may be more concerned with his impotence than his diabetes. If a trusting relationship has developed, a nurse is in an excellent position to give permission to the client to talk about those sexual concerns—to become a special and real person because you have taken the initiative to bring up the subject.

While it may be presumptuous to assume that all clients have sexually-related concerns with their medical problem, it would also be presumptuous to assume that no client does. Unless the client brings it up as a genuine concern, the only way you would know about it is to ask. For example, "Some clients have questions about ___ as it relates to their sexuality. Has anyone discussed this with you? Is there anything that you would like to ask about ___?" Whether questions have been brought up at this time or not, keep the possibility open that the client may want to continue later. Extend an invitation to "feel free to bring up any questions or problems whenever they should come up." In some cases the client may be asking for *permission*, may need *limited information*, or is ready for *specific suggestions* in the handling of a problem which is unfamiliar because it simply has not existed before. "How do I have intercourse while wearing a urethral catheter?" "Will my partner become infected, since my urine is infected?" "How can I have sex if I have an ileal conduit?" "Can I remove my catheter and then replace it?" "What can I do about the severe headache I get when my genitals are stimulated?" "How can I have sex without getting out of the wheelchair?" (There are answers to these simple and direct questions dealing with the client with a spinal-cord injury.[30,32,33])

Think of the kinds of sexual concerns that could exist with regard to each of the following conditions. Would this be a concern of the client, of the spouse (partner), or both? For each of the concerns, what would you be providing—*permission, limited information,* or *specific suggestions*? You may wish to discuss your responses with those of a colleague(s). Sexual concerns associated with: (1) a first versus a fifth pregnancy,[36,37] (2) nursing an infant, (3) a mild versus a severe coronary,[34,35] (4) mastectomy,[38,39] (5) cervical carcinoma,[40,41] (6) renal dialysis,[42,43] (7) ostomy,[44,45] (8) diabetes,[46] (9) recurrent cystitis or vaginal infection,[47,48] (10) alcoholism,[49] (11) osteoarthritis,[50] (12) prostatectomy,[51] (13) hysterectomy, (14) emphysema,[52] (15) a 70-year-old woman or man,[53,54] (16) vaginal anesthesia,[13,14] (17) tuberculosis,[55] or (18) spinal cord injury.[33]

The following examples taken from an article by Picconi[56] are an indication of the ways in which a nurse may give permission for the discussion of sexual concerns. For a *coronary* patient: "Many patients after a heart attack express concern about how sexual activity will affect their hearts. Do you have any questions about this?" For an *ostomy* patient: "Some patients are afraid that their device

will become dislodged during sexual activity, and that could be embarrassing for both partners. Do you know what you can do to prevent this?" For a patient with a *spinal cord-injury*: "It's possible to have vaginal intercourse with a catheter in place. Would you like to know how to go about this?" For an *emphysema* patient: "When you first get home you may feel too tired to have intercourse. Are you aware of positions that might be less tiring?" For a *radical hysterectomy* patient: "Your doctor probably told you that you would be able to resume sexual activity in a few weeks, but did he mention that intercourse may feel different? May I explain to you why this is so?"

We also need to be aware that in any type of counseling work there is a risk that good intentions may be unknowingly subverted by the client. In some cases, sexual dysfunction may be welcomed as a "weapon" or as a justification to avoid sex. There are many interesting sexual problems uncovered by therapists which give a fascinating insight into the power of relationships and the effect that two people have on each other. I mention a few, even though they are not necessarily related to nursing practice, in order to give an appreciation that there are more complicated and time consuming problems that you may uncover that go beyond the good nursing practice which you offer. It would be wise in this case to give permission or encouragement to the individual (or couple) to seek additional help with the *relationship problem*. Your efforts even might extend to recommendations of community resources. Here are examples of some problems of this type: (1) The male did not realize that he had developed his premature ejaculation in response to unresolved anger toward his partner. (2) In the "unconsummated marriage" in which a couple have not experienced intercourse, even after several years, it is not unusual for the wife to have vaginismus and for the husband to develop impotence in collusion with her. Hence, both avoid sexual intercourse. (3) A husband who cared devotedly for his terminally ill wife and now, a year after her death, finds himself impotent when he begins a new relationship. (4) A male who believes he is weakened after ejaculation and so withholds it from his partner except on weekends when he can sleep late. She feels guilty about her sexual "aggressiveness," regards his ejaculate as a "gift," and feels angry toward him.

Sources of Information about Sexuality for Nursing

Within recent years the nursing profession, at least through its journals, has been addressing itself with increasing effectiveness to the topic of human sexuality as just another part of nursing care to be considered as one would any other system of the body. Nurses deserve to be commended for this move. Some of the topics which I have read in preparation for this chapter are quite illuminating, especially for their high level of practicality and problem-solving orientation. Many physicians, unfortunately, are still either unprepared or unwilling to become involved in an area which they feel to be too time-consuming. This attitude is often communicated to the client. (It is appalling when only 10–12 percent of surgeons are willing to discuss the sex related implication of a mastectomy with their patient.[38])

As a nurse, there is a valuable role which you may fill at whatever level of the health-care system you may find yourself. In the meantime, prepare, for you have a right to know and to obtain the answers to sexually related medical problems from professional colleagues in your own and other disciplines. As long as your intentions are well-meaning and you are helping clients to cope more effectively with their present and subsequent levels of reality, you are practicing good nursing care. The time is right and the needs exist. Clients have been waiting a long time for those with professional abilities to recognize and show caring for the sexual aspect of their human nature as well.

REFERENCES

1. Gochros, H. L., and Gochros, J. S.: *The Sexually Oppressed.* New York, Association Press, 1977.
2. Austin, C. R., and Short, R. V.: *Reproduction in Mammals. The Evolution of Reproduction.* New York, Cambridge University Press, 1976.
3. Masters, W. H., and Johnson, V. E.: *The Pleasure Bond.* Boston, Little, Brown and Co., 1975.
4. Downey, G. W.: The next patient right: sex in the nursing home. *Mod. Health Care* 1:56, 1974.
5. Weiss, R. S.: *Marital Separation.* New York, Basic Books, Inc., 1975.
6. Klaus, M. H., and Kennell, J. H.: *Maternal-infant Bonding.* St. Louis, C.V. Mosby Co., 1976.
7. Ellenberg, M.: Sex and the female diabetic. *Med. Aspects Hum. Sex.* 11(12):30, 1977.
8. Crasilneck, H. B., and Hall, J. A.: *Clinical Hypnosis.* New York, Grune and Stratton, 1975.
9. Hollender, M. H.: Women's wish to be held: sexual and non-sexual aspects. *Med. Aspects Hum. Sex.* 5(10):12, 1971.
10. Hollender, M. H., and McGehee, J. B.: The wish to be held during pregnancy. *J. Psychosom. Res.* 18:193, 1974.
11. Lief, H. I.: Holding and touching as part of sexual behavior. *Med. Aspects Hum. Sex.* 11(10):87, 1977.
12. Masters, W. H., and Johnson, V. E.: *Human Sexual Inadequacy.* Boston, Little, Brown and Co., 1970.
13. Barbach, L. G.: *For Yourself: The Fulfillment of Female Sexuality.* New York, Doubleday and Co., 1975.
14. Weisberg, M.: Vaginal anesthesia. *Med. Aspects Hum. Sex.* 11(3):81, 1977.
15. Lowry, T. P., and Lowry, T. S.: *The Clitoris.* St. Louis, Warren H. Green, Inc., 1976.
16. Sarrel, P. M.: *Biological Aspects of Sexual Function—The Hymenal Strand.* Presented at International Congress of Sexology, Montreal, 1976.
17. Leitch, I. O. W.: Circumcision: a continuing enigma. *Aust. Paediatr. J.* 6:59, 1970.
18. Thompson, H. C. et al.: Report of the ad hoc task force on circumcision. *Pediatrics* 56:610, 1975.
19. Gee, W. F., and Ansell, J. S.: Neonatal circumcision: a ten-year overview: with comparison of the gomco clamp and the plastibell device. *Pediatrics* 58:824, 1976.
20. Howat, J. M.: Circumcision. *Nurs. Times* 72(37):1434, 1976.
21. Kaplan, G. W.: Circumcision—an overview. *Curr. Probl. Pediatr.* 7:1, 1977.
22. Schwarz, G. S.: Devices to prevent masturbation. *Med. Aspects Hum. Sex.* 7(5):141, 1973.
23. Lief, H. I.: Obstacles to the ideal and complete sex education of the medical student and physician, in *Contemporary Sexual Behavior: Critical Issues in the 1970's,* edited by Zubin, J., and Money, J., Baltimore, Johns Hopkins Press, 1973.
24. Gebhard, P. H.: The acquisition of basic sex information. *J. Sex Res.* 13:148, 1977.
25. Welbourne, A. K.: *The Relation of Parental Sexual Knowledge and Attitudes and Communication about Sexual Topics with their Early Adolescent Children.* Doctoral Dissertation, New York University, 1977.
26. Alan Guttmacher Institute: *11 Million Teenagers, What Can Be Done about the Epidemic of Adolescent Pregnancies in the United States.* New York, Planned Parenthood Federation of America, 1976.
27. Rybicki, L. L.: Preparing parents to teach their children about human sexuality. *M.C.N.* 1(3):182, 1976.
28. Woods, N. F., and Mandetta, A. F.: Sexuality in the baccalaureate nursing curriculum. *Nurs. Forum* 15(3):294, 1976.
29. Annon, J. S.: *Behavioral Treatment of Sexual Prob-*

lems: *Brief Therapy*. New York, Harper and Row, 1976.

30. Mooney, T. O., Cole, T. M., and Chilgren, R. A.: *Sexual Options for Paraplegics and Quadriplegics.* Boston, Little, Brown and Co., 1975.

31. Cameron, P., et al.: *Consciousness: Thoughts about World and Social Problems, Death, and Sex.* Paper presented at the Kentucky Psychological Association Convention, Louisville, 1970.

32. Cole, T. M.: Sexuality and the spinal cord injured, in *Human Sexuality: A Health Practitioner's Text,* edited by Green, R., Baltimore, Williams and Wilkins Co., 1975.

33. Eisenberg, M. and Rustad, L.: *Sex and the Spinal Cord Injured: Some Questions and Answers.* (Stock No. 5100-00076) Washington, D.C., U.S. Gov. Printing Office, 1974.

34. Puksta, N. S.: All about sex . . . after a coronary. *Am. J. Nurs.* 77(4):602, 1977.

35. Scheingold, L. D., and Wagner, N. N.: *Sound Sex and the Aging Heart.* New York, Human Science Press, 1974.

36. Lief, H. I.: Sexual desire and responsivity during pregnancy. *Med. Aspects Hum. Sex.* 11(12):51, 1977.

37. Zalar, M. K.: Sexual counseling for pregnant couples, *M.C.N.* 1(3):176, 1976.

38. Ervin, C. V.: Psychologic adjustment to mastectomy. *Med. Aspects Hum. Sex.* 7(2):42, 1973,

39. Lief, H. I.: Sexual concerns of mastectomy patients. *Med. Aspects Hum. Sex.* 12(1):57, 1978.

40. Kistner, R.: Promiscuity and premalignant lesions of the cervix. *Med. Aspects Hum. Sex.* 6(9):15, 1972.

41. Jordan, J. A.: Sexual activity and cervical squamous carcinoma. *Nurs. Mirror* 143(15):48, 1976.

42. Hickman, B. W.: All about sex . . . despite dialysis. *Am. J. Nurs.* 77(4):606, 1977.

43. Levy, N. B.: Uremic sex (letters to the editor). *N. Engl. J. Med.* 297:725, 1977.

44. Pamphlets—"*Sex and the Male Ostomate,*" "*Sex, Courtship and the Single Ostomate,*" and "*Sex, Pregnancy and the Female Ostomate*" available through the United Ostomy Association, 1111 Wilshire Boulevard, Los Angeles, CA 90017.

45. Dlin, B. M., and Perlman, A.: Sex after ileostomy or colostomy. *Med. Aspects Hum. Sex.* 6(7):32, 1972.

46. Ellenberg, M.: Impotence in diabetics: a neurologic rather than an endocrinologic problem. *Med. Aspects Hum. Sex.* 7(4):12, 1973.

47. Marshall, S.: Cystitis and urethritis in women related to sexual activity. *Med. Aspects Hum. Sex.* 8(5):165, 1974.

48. Devanesan, M., et al.: Somatic expressions of sexual anxiety. *Med. Aspects Hum. Sex.* 11(12):84, 1977.

49. Paredes, A.: Marital-sexual factors in alcoholism. *Med. Aspects Hum. Sex.* 7(4):98, 1973.

50. Langmyhr, G. J.: Varieties of coital positions: advantages and disadvantages. *Med. Aspects Hum. Sex.* 10(6):128, 1976.

51. Steele, R.: Sexual factors in prostatic cancer. *Med. Aspects Hum. Sex.* 6(8):70, 1972.

52. Kass, I., Updegraff, K., and Muffly, R.: Sex in chronic obstructive pulmonary disease. *Med. Aspects Hum. Sex.* 6(2):33, 1972.

53. Easley, E. B.: Atrophic vaginitis and sexual relations. *Med. Aspects Hum. Sex.* 8(11):32, 1974.

54. Stanford, D.: All about sex . . . after middle age. *Am. J. Nurs.* 77:608, 1977.

55. Surawicz, F.: Sexual fears associated with non-venereal genital diseases. *Med. Aspects Hum. Sex.* 11(12):71, 1977.

56. Picconi, J.: Human sexuality. *Nurs. '77* 2:72D, 1977.

CHAPTER 4

Nursing aims to assist people in achieving their maximum health potential. Maintenance and promotion of health, prevention of disease, nursing diagnosis, intervention, and rehabilitation encompass the scope of nursing's goals. Nursing is concerned with people—all people—well and sick, rich and poor, young and old. The arenas of nursing's services extend into all areas where there are people: at home, at school, at work, at play, in hospital, nursing home, and clinic; on this planet; and now moving into outer space.[1]

As professionals involved in health care delivery, nurses have a responsibility to accept the concept of comprehensive care. This focuses the attention of all health professionals on the entire continuum of a person's health, with goals of maintaining purposeful adaptation and promoting wellness, rather than on an isolated episode of illness. What we do as health practitioners will depend on our view of health and on our established goals.

The patterns of health care delivery depend not only on our definition of health as professionals but

THE CLIENT AS A PERSON

Tanya L. Bodo, M.N., R.N., and
JoAnn Lenocker, M.S., R.N.

that of our clients as well. Consequently, as nurses, we must incorporate into our definition of health an understanding of how the layperson defines health and illness, how it is that he comes into contact with the health professional, and what happens when he assumes the role of patient or client.

LAYPERSON'S DEFINITION OF HEALTH AND ILLNESS

To understand the layperson's definition of health and illness better, the factors that influence that definition must be examined. As will become evident, these factors overlap as the individual becomes involved in the process of developing his or her concept of health and illness.

Social, Cultural, and Economic Factors

The layperson's definition of illness is determined socially and culturally rather than clinically or medically. What is considered normal, healthy, or un-healthy is determined by the society and culture in which the individual resides. This society may be defined as his family, community, social group, or a combination of all of these. Each society influences the development of "behavioral and biological norms" which are rules of conduct or social expectations that arise from mutually held values and beliefs within the group. Concepts of illness derive from these "norms" in that illness represents a deviation from expected standards of performance. An example of established behavioral norms is readily observed in the society formed around a small southern rural fishing village. The males over the age of 15 are expected to be up before dawn every morning and on the lake fishing until sundown. Deviations from this expected behavior are accepted only if the man's wife is in childbirth or if he or one of his children is critically ill.

There are several sociocultural elements involved in a layperson's definition of illness and his responses to it. These elements may derive from social class, ethnic orientation, or religious affiliation. They influence the person's view of his body, his knowledge of illness, his interpretation of pain and various other symptoms, and his attitude toward modern medicine.

Several studies have shown that an important relationship exists between a person's socioeconomic status and his health behavior. Socioeconomic status is usually measured by a composite index which reflects a combination of the person's occupation, education, income, and type of home or residential area. One study was conducted by Koos[2] who interviewed the following three classes of a community: the "pillars of the community," the "respected working people," and the "down and outers." This study revealed a consistent difference among members of these three classes in their attitudes toward illness, in their use of the physician and dentist, and in other aspects of health related behavior. It was found that the lower the individual's social class, the less likely he was to identify a given symptom (e.g., infection, blood in his urine, or back pain) as one which required treatment. Even when the symptom was identified as being abnormal, these individuals were not likely to seek treatment.

Generally in our society, education and affluence encourage stricter definitions of health and decrease tolerance for the discomfort of illness. This is attributed to the fact that persons of higher socioeconomic status and education often have more scientific notions of health and illness. They also tend to have life styles and values closer to those of health professionals than persons from other strata.[3]

Equally influential are the individual's perceptions of wellness and wellness behavior. Baumann,[4] in an analysis of lay definitions of health, found these definitions to be distinguished by three criteria: (1) a subjective feeling of well-being; (2) an absence of symptoms; and (3) a state of being able to perform those activities that a person in good health should be able to perform. Looking at this last criterion, one can see that what an individual selects as a symptom or indication of illness is influenced by his daily activities. If a person's "wellness role" does not require good visual ability, then beginning visual disturbances may go unnoticed and unattended.

For many, religion may not play an important role in everyday life; for others, it may be a sustaining factor. With the occurrence of illness or other stressful life situations, which often lead to a feeling of vulnerability or even a fear of the future, spiritual beliefs often provide solace. Murray and Zentner[5] addressed the need for coordination by health professionals of both the "medical-physical" and the "religious-spiritual" worlds:

> The attitude that medical science is superior to religion has affected us all. Yet religion is there as it always has been. Each culture has had some organization or priesthood to sustain the important rituals and myths of its people. Primitive man combined the roles of physician, psychiatrist, and priest. . . . In the midst of our specialized world, you must attempt again to bring the three areas together. Segmenting the person has not worked.

Environmental and Situational Factors

Another factor in the layperson's definition of health and illness is that of situational factors which make it more or less difficult to obtain medical attention. One interview conducted by Koos[2] exemplifies how influential situational factors can be: "I wish I really knew what you mean by being sick. Sometimes I have felt so bad I could curl up and die, but had to go on because the kids had to be taken care of, and besides, we didn't have the money to spend for a doctor—how could I be sick?—how do you know when you are sick, anyway? Some people can go to bed most any time with anything, but most of us can't be sick—even when we need to be."

In this case, financial status was the specific situational factor, but this can easily be broadened to include the cost of seeking medical help in terms of time, peer-group sanction, and availability and closeness of health care resources. The less available the resources are, the less likely they will be utilized except in cases of extreme need. In addition, if the use of such resources is met with peer-group disapproval or rejection, which often occurs in mental illness, these resources probably will not be used.

Personality Factors

As it has been pointed out, social, cultural, environmental, and situational factors influence the individual's definition of health and illness. An incorporation of these factors into the individual's past and present life experiences determines the unique personality factors which also influence perceptions of health and illness.

In assessing personality factors, we need to first focus our attention on the motivational characteristics of the individual. The pattern and strength of motivation determine how a person will react to a situation and how stressful or threatening it is for him. Situations will be appraised as threatening to the extent that they relate to the important personal goals. If the motive is weak, the threat is weak. If the motive is strong, then depending on the individual and environmental resources, the threat may be great. An example which reflects this motivational factor can be seen in a sociocultural goal which is typical of our nation. In this country, we value doing, and we fear failure to overcome obstacles; thus, we are very competitive. Getting old is a threat because it threatens our ability to "do." Similarly, the executive who suffers a heart attack or the laborer who loses the use of an arm is threatened in terms of the "high motivational factor," in this case work productivity, which is severely jeopardized. In short, every individual has his own motivational characteristics that determine how he will react to a given situation of altered functional ability.

An important personality factor often overlooked by health professionals is that of the individual's general belief system about transactions with the environment. General beliefs about the environment and the individual's capacity to deal with them influence a person's perception of threat, that is, whether an illness presents a major problem for him. For example, if a person sees himself as fairly helpless, he may see his environment as powerful and unmanageable. If he sees himself as masterful, he may see the environment as a subject to control. Erikson's discussion[6] of how a child develops attitudes of trust or distrust is pertinent here. Early specific experiences producing attitudes of trust or distrust may generalize to all later transactions and dispose the individual to expect support or treachery.

People who believe the environment is hostile and dangerous and feel powerless to manage it often experience chronic anxiety. Such anxiety disposes the individual to feel threatened in a variety of situations and renders them less capable of dealing with situations of nonhealth or stress. This attitude is reflected in the comment made by a 17-year-old female who was experiencing her second unwanted pregnancy. "I didn't need or want another baby, but I guess it was going to happen no matter what I did . . . the pills made me sick and my boyfriend didn't want me using anything up inside of me . . . what could I do anyway? Guess I was just meant to have babies even if I don't want them."

Intellectual resources, education, and sophistication can influence perceptions of health and illness. Lack of intellectual resources increases the prospect of incorrect evaluations of health situations by the layperson. Similarly, a lack of education and sophistication renders the person less able to seek out and utilize available resources.

INTERACTION WITH HEALTH CARE DELIVERY SYSTEM

In an attempt to expand the understanding of a layperson's involvement in his health, attention must be focused on the client's interaction with the health care delivery system. Consideration must be given to the route that a client might take from community to hospital and the lines of defense that exist between these two entities. This process was investigated by Tippin,[7] a psychiatric social worker who formulated the "pin-ball theory of admission," when he traced the route of rehospitalized psychiatric patients from the community back into the hospital.

The first line of defense for the client involves personal or interpersonal relationships. This includes family, friends, neighbors, fellow employees, employer, supervisor, clubs, or organizations. Although this structure is rather informal, people in it often rally around an individual in times of stress or crisis. However, some people either have not formed this line of defense, or they have alienated it by their behavior or their cry for help.

The second line of defense between the client and the hospital concerns the professional helping agencies. These include physicians, welfare departments, schools, vocational rehabilitation, church counseling services, and other voluntary social agencies. Asking for help from these agencies often requires more strength than the person has, or he is frightened off by the impersonalization of the intake process. Frequently, those in need of this help are least informed about the resources available. The weakest link in the secondary line of defense is the lack of interagency communication which sees the client bounced from agency to agency with little or no communication between them regarding goals and plans for the client.

The third line of defense concerns those agencies which act as back-up services. These include psychiatric day-care centers, psychiatrists, mental health clinics, psychiatric wings of general hospitals, and psychiatric outpatient services. Clients use these services either directly or on referral from professional helping agencies. The communication between the second and third lines of defense is crucial. When it breaks down, the system's defensive efforts break down, and the client again finds himself bounced from agency to agency.

The fourth line of defense is the legal system, which includes the court system, the police, the sheriff's office, probation, and parole. This often is the last line of defense through which the patient passes on his way back to the psychiatric hospital.

The first three lines of defense are voluntary in that the client may initiate involvement. It is important to realize that the lines of defense identified for psychiatric clients, particularly the first three, are also operational for clients with other than mental health problems.

Nurses may come in contact with the client at various points en route from community to hospital. It is ultimately necessary that nurses' energies insure open and continuous communication between themselves, the client, and other involved agencies. If this is accomplished, it is often possible to prevent the necessity of hospitalization through the provision of preventive and maintenance health care.

System's Expectations of the Client

It is frequently found that the client is put in the position of meeting certain "requirements" of the health care delivery system, requirements which he may or may not be able to meet.

PATIENCE. Patience is one of the primary requirements forced on the client. Professionals tell him what he needs and will pay for without trying to find out what *he* thinks he needs or wants, or how he wants it. Patience is required while he waits in line or sits in the waiting room of the hospital, clinic, or doctor's office. Patience is required when he schedules the "earliest appointment possible," which may be in 1 to 2 months and only during his working hours, or as he is shuffled from one agency to the next. He must certainly be patient when he has to fill out the insurance forms or apply for food stamps, disability or vocational rehabilitation, particularly when he does not understand exactly what information is requested.

SOPHISTICATION. Sophistication is another characteristic expected of the client. He must be able to read and write, understand professional jargon and lots of "big words." He must be able to verbally relate his needs in a concise, coherent manner, giving relevant details and leaving out the irrelevant. Finally, he must act "reasonably" which requires that he be cooperative, receptive, and appreciative.

MOTIVATION. Most of all, the "system" requires motivation. Murray[8] identified the single most difficult problem in community health as motivation. The client is expected to take responsibility for his care by seeking periodic checkups, and when sick, he is supposed to seek an examination and treatment. When the client, even if faced by a multitude of other pressing problems, does not do this, he is considered "unmotivated." So in order to utilize the health care system, the individual client or family, above all, must be motivated. He displays motivation when he makes and keeps all appointments, no matter how difficult; when he follows, exactly as instructed by the professional, directions regarding his diet, medication, and activity levels, even when those directions are not always understood. In other words, the client is often required to have the same values regarding his health care, or that of his family, as the professional, even though the professional's values have been influenced by specialized education ranging from 1 to 12 years.

CONFRONTATION WITH ILLNESS

To address the factors which influence a person's reaction to hospitalization, one has to move a step backward—to illness itself. The following report by a middle-aged father during a period of illness is taken from *The Psychology of the Sickbed*.[9] It should help to tune our sensitivity to the changes in life style and altered perceptions inherent in illness.

The horizon in time too is narrowed. The plans of yesterday lose their meaning and their importance; they have hardly any real value. They seem more complicated, more exhausting, more foolish and ambitious than I saw them from the day before. All that awaits me becomes tasteless, or even distasteful. The past seems saturated with trivialities. It appears to me that I hardly ever tackled my real tasks. Future and past lose their outlines; I withdraw from both, and I live in the confined presence of this bed which guards me against the things that were and those that will be. Under normal circumstances, I live in the future and in the past as far as the future draws upon it to prescribe my duties. Apart from a few special moments, I never really live in the present, I never think of it. But the sickbed does not allow me to escape from the present.

Each of us can probably recall a period of illness which enticed us to seek the comfort and solitude of our bed for a few days. This represented an attempt to close out the demands of the world with which our bodies and minds were unwilling and perhaps incapable to handle. But even so, we realized that this was a temporary condition, that soon we would step out of this suspended period of time and once more surround ourselves with life and its demands. This is not a luxury afforded those persons suffering a serious, prolonged illness. Van den Berg[9] captures the essence of this situation: "The beginning of every serious illness is a halt. Normal life is at an end. Another life takes its place, a life of a completely unknown nature. . . . It is an experience of complete surprise, hardly imaginable to a healthy person." Is it any wonder that illness, whether from disease or injury, is not readily accepted, and frequently its existence persistently denied? Along with all its other demands, illness dictates to the person a task for which he is seldom prepared; the confrontation with the vulnerability of his body and the transience of his life.

For most patients, particularly those suffering from a prolonged or chronic illness, there have been previous contacts with medical care facilities prior to entering the hospital. Frequently the hospital admission is the last resort in a series of visits to clinics or private physicians. The choice of private physician or clinic is most often determined by the person's economic status and the stage to which his illness has progressed, rather than by any preference he might have. As the early symptoms begin to interfere with earning capacity and monies are spent in search of medical help, diagnosis, and treatment, many patients find they have exhausted their resources. The frustrations encountered in dealing with the fragmentation of care and the depletion of economic resources have a profound influence on the way in which the client approaches hospitalization as well as on his response to medical care.

If nurses are to effectively meet the needs of a patient, when he is hospitalized, they must address his holistic nature and take into account all those qualities that comprise his uniqueness. They must consider all that has gone on before he sought the "last resort"—hospitalization. No matter how protracted the illness or how extensive the medical attention received, the need to enter the hospital almost invariably comes as a shock.

COMMUNITY TO HOSPITAL: PERSON TO CLIENT

When patient care was moved from the home to the hospital, the geographic boundaries of the sickroom ceased to be four walls. The patient's therapeutic environment became the wards, the corridors, the elevators, and the treatment and procedure rooms in various parts of the hospital. When patient-care was institutionalized, the patient was placed in "horizontal orbit". . . .[10]

When the illness journey culminates in hospitalization, the client must be turned into a patient. He must be prepared for "horizontal orbit." In an analysis of the "social dilemma" created by hospitalization, Taylor[11] identified three characteristics that differentiate people who are hospital patients from people who are not. Each person who becomes a patient has qualified as "hospital sick." Society interprets this as a "crisis," and thus most individuals arrive at the hospital believing they are the victims of crisis. Each person who becomes a hospital patient has been separated from his natural environment. He enters a world that is strange and unfamiliar without his accustomed support systems. The hospital patient has been accorded temporary membership in a hospital community.

Admissions Process: Initiation into Hospital Membership

The rites of membership required for entry into the hospital community are observed when one examines the admissions process of the hospital. When a client arrives at the emergency room, admissions office, or nurses' station to begin the admissions process, he is not usually his "real self." He is primarily a stranger among strange people, filled with dread and imaginings and uncertainty about what the future will hold. Frequently, he is met with a cold, clinical, unfeeling reception which serves to confirm his feelings of uneasiness. The illness or condition which has brought him to the hospital increased his vulnerability and weakened his defenses and ability to deal with stress. Even the ordinary and easy things, such as giving one's name and address, or following directions, become difficult. The most common worries on admission as identified by a group of clients in one study were those caused by separation from known faces and places on entering a strange environment.[12]

Another study group comprised of a number of women who had delivered in a busy maternity center were asked what would have made their entrance into the hospital less stressing.[13] They unanimously agreed that they would have felt more secure if they had been familiar with the location and layout of the hospital at the time they came in in labor. Expanding on this idea one woman added: "I think the one thing that any expectant mother wants to know is 'what's going to happen when she gets there?' She probably won't be as calm as otherwise, and she doesn't want to get to the wrong door . . . you want to know what's going to happen, without any anxiety while you're waiting—wondering . . . all these things are unanswered until you take a tour. Then you have a picture in your mind." The lack of familiarity with the hospital layout has been the nemesis of countless clients. There seems to be a trend, although slow moving, in hospitals across the nation to include a tour of the hospital prior to admission, particularly for children and expectant parents. Hopefully, nurses, doctors, and hospital administrators will soon realize the benefit that this provides the client and move to incorporate this practice into the services they offer.

The hospital remains, however, geared to action, speed, and the tyranny of the clock. They hurry the new client along at a speed which does not permit consideration of his emotional needs or even the requirements made by his physical condition. He moves from one step to the next in the transition from person to patient—and at each step a part of him is left behind. From the admissions desk to the hospital bed, this process is analyzed by Taylor[11] in an attempt to identify how it operates to reduce a person to a patient:

The procedures used to admit people to hospitals orient them to the role of hospital patient. When I first examined the dynamics of this process, it seemed to me to be similar to the process used by the Chinese to brainwash their prisoners during the Korean war. The duty of a captured soldier is to attempt escapes in order to tie up as much enemy manpower as possible. The Chinese brainwashed their prisoners in order to remove the desire to escape, and they did so in the following fashion. First the captured soldier's frame of reference was removed. Lectures, interrogations, and repeated written confessions gradually browbeat most captives of all nationalities, into rejections of the norms and values of their own societies. When this difficult task had been accomplished, the frame of reference of the enemy was imposed, and the prisoner had lost his desire to continue to fight a war no longer believed in. When this desired end was reached, the manpower required to retain prisoners in captivity became minimal.

The hospital patient is not a prisoner, although his role is similar to that of a prisoner. The patient role is mandated rather than chosen; it is a temporary role but the length of the 'sentence' being served cannot be stated as precisely as the sentences imposed by judges, and both patient and prisoner are expected to conform to the policies of the institution and accept, without question, the decisions and edicts of its staff. In the case of the hospital patient the admission procedures not only admit the patient to hospital records and a hospital bed, they also orient him to his position in the hospital hierarchy and his role as hospital patient.

Those who design hospital admission procedures and those who impose them on persons about to become hospital patients usually are not aware that the procedures they invent and invoke orient people to a new, and in some cases alien, role. Their purpose is to collect information needed by the institution and to see to it that the admittee is moved out of the admitting office into a designated hospital bed. During this process the hospital's interests are protected by removing the admittee's valuables for safekeeping. When the admission process is examined as a socialization process, orienting the sick to their inpatient role, its startling similarity to brainwashing emerges.

Persons about to become hospital patients are, at the least, in physical crisis and, in many cases, also in social crisis. Those who enter through the emergency room assume that the acute nature of their crises will enable them to bypass red tape; but hospitals rarely conform to these expectations and their failure to do so creates alarm and despondency in persons becoming patients, and alerts them to their low position in the hospital hierarchy. The person on a stretcher en route from the emergency room to surgery is interrogated during this journey about ability to pay, disposal of body, religious preference, and other information needed by hospitals. If hospital admission has been pre-arranged, prospective patients know the hospital is expecting them and assume that they will be treated as expected customers. However, the pre-arranged admission is kept waiting before being interrogated and, in many hospitals, the intimate information needed by the institution is extracted in what could be called a public confessional. It is common practice to ask for most of the information needed by the hospital, the answers to twenty or thirty questions, before admission to a hospital bed is mentioned. At this point the hospital has diminished the patient's physical crisis by ignoring it and suggesting there is a sicker patient down the hall; dismissed the patient's social crisis by failing to recognize it; and made it clear to the patient that admitting him to the hospital's files takes priority over admitting him to a hospital bed and dealing with the medical crisis which precipitated hospitalization.

Weakened by the hospital's interpretation of his situation the patient is relieved of the 'valuables' which support his identity—money, jewelry, and other valuables—and wheeled to his slot in the hospital's filing system, a hospital bed. If the patient is an emergency admission he or she will be detoured through intensive care or surgery and recovery during this process and before being admitted into the hospital's filing system of the patients. In either case the patient has been reduced during final filing.

The direct admission to a hospital bed has been wheeled to the desk on the floor in which he is to be filed. The female volunteer or male orderly transporting him has, in most cases, been cautioned about misinforming him. The consequence: a refusal to answer innocuous questions about 'Where am I going?' 'When will I be fed?' and the like; and a disoriented patient. The transporter hands the papers containing information about the patient to a person at the desk and withdraws. The desk enters information about the new patient into its processing system and eventually the patient's clothes are removed, the patient is encased in a hospital gown, labeled and inserted into a hospital bed.

At this point the patient's usual frame of reference has been removed, he now is low man on the hospital totem pole dependent on the hospital and its staff and submissive to their rules, regulations, and decisions. If the 'brainwashing' hidden in the admission procedures has been effective he has been prepared to become a 'good' patient.

Membership in the Hospital Community: Client's Needs and Expectations

LOSS OF PRIVACY AND CONTROL

Lack of privacy becomes obvious when one considers the admission procedures just described. Privacy is one of the most cherished possessions of all mankind, the right to his own thoughts and activities in isolation if he so chooses. Let us reflect for a moment on the nature of privacy as described by Schuster.[14]

Privacy is a comfortable condition reflecting a deserved degree of social retreat on the part of the person seeking it. It represents a valued, meaningful and purposeful withdrawal whose dimensions and duration are within the control of the one seeking privacy. It is a personal and internal state to the extent that privacy cannot be imposed from without. . . .

All aspects of privacy are contingent upon boundaries set by the individual. When there is an uninvited advance beyond this boundary, it is viewed as an invasion of privacy.

Boundaries set by the person governing privacy of life style are infringed upon when his preferences in day-to-day living are ignored. The hospital routine shows little consideration for this when meals are served—that is, by not trying to satisfy the patient's accustomed meal time, but by serving meals only on the standard 7 am, 12 noon, and 5 pm schedule. The patient is told when to go to bed, when to get up, when he may have visitors, when he will see the doctor, when his medications should be taken—all without regard for his privacy of life style. For many patients this can lead to a deterioration of their condition. Take for example, Mrs. S., an elderly woman, who suffered a mild stroke. Hospitalization was necessitated by the temporary paralysis which resulted from the stroke and the fact that Mrs. S. lived alone. Within a few days, however, her condition stabilized, and she was left with only a slight decrease in strength in her left arm and leg. The floor staff and physician were unable to find the cause for her lack of appetite and complaints of severe constipation. A particularly alert nurse found that those problems were hospital-induced. It seems that Mrs. S.'s routine of many years had been to arise early, go for a brisk walk, and upon returning home have a cup of hot tea, all of which assured a normal bowel pattern. Further, she never ate breakfast before 10 am because she would become nauseated and stay that way for the rest of the day. Needless to say her privacy of life style had been infringed upon with a resulting negative effect.

Privacy to carry out personal grooming and hygiene is severely limited in the hospital. Comments like these are often heard: "No sooner would I sit on the pot, than the nurse would come in to get the measuring container for another patient . . . or get undressed for a shower than someone would come tell me 'the doctor is here to see you.' When you're a patient, you might as well forget about privacy!"

The new client quickly learns that he has been robbed of all responsibility for decision-making concerning privacy of life style. In addition, he learns through experience that he has little control over meeting his own needs. New mothers require a period of concentrated sleep and rest immediately following delivery. However, many women can readily attest to the fact that this need is unmet if it conflicts with the ongoing routine. "The biggest objection I had was when the girls came down from the labor room, tired and wanting to sleep. If it happens to be during the day, they just don't get the chance because life goes on as usual. The visitors come as usual. I had the baby at 3 am and got to sleep about 4 and at 7 o'clock, of course, I was awakened for breakfast."[13]

LOSS OF INDIVIDUALITY

For the person to be transformed into a client, he is required to relinquish those things which have become a part of his identity. For one gentleman this occurred when he had to change into hospital attire. "When I took off my shoes and pants and put them in the drawer my identity went with them." Most clients find it disconcerting to shuffle around their room or down the hall in slippers with their gown flapping open behind them.

For the person, who has spent years developing independence of judgment and action, to suddenly find himself reduced to the anonymity of a horizontal position between the sheets is a severe jolt to his morale. For the housewife, whose identity revolves around commanding her household, the hospital removes those things which allowed expression of her individuality; she is now the one commanded. For the businessman, who carefully plans the day around meetings and deadlines which require decision-making and an ability to dictate tasks, it is disconcerting to have his total way of life reversed. The day's activities are now planned *for* him. The doctors and nurses now make the decisions over which he has little influence. If all of these things have not served to prove to the client that his individuality is insignificant, there are other occurrences that will, when he discovers that even his name is unknown to some of the staff who attend him, or that he is designated as the "occupant" of a particular room and bed, or by his disease condition, or type of treatment being received. How dehumanizing it is to hear oneself referred to as "Dr. Smith's gallbladder down in room 342." It is unfortunate that the technology and mechanization that dictate hospital routine have led to such depersonalization.

When one considers why this depersonalization takes place a number of factors come to mind. The hospital has evolved into an efficient machine, with time schedules and routines which have allowed the patient to become lost in its efficiency. This is reflected in the fact that health personnel often set as the criteria for judging their effectiveness those matters pertaining to plant and equipment, finances, and organization of staff, rather than the quality of client care. Physicians generally do not allow themselves to become emotionally involved with clients and resist anything which appears to threaten their ability to remain professionally detached. Barnes[12] feels that this characteristic of detachment is the result of the need to develop mental defenses strong enough to control major upset. The upset results when the knowledge of pathology and disease is combined with the implications for their clients' lives. Nurses have too often allowed themselves to become caught up in the "efficiency of the hospital machine," with decreasing attention given to learning more about their individual clients. Over the past few decades this trend has been reversing, and nursing is redirecting its focus exclusively on the client.

Individualizing information should accompany every new client to the floor, and nurses should make it their responsibility to familiarize themselves with this information. Brown[15] suggested that this information should be made immediately available to the floor staff by its inclusion on the face-sheet that precedes the new client. This would necessitate an expansion of the basic face-sheet data which could easily be accommodated during the admission intake procedure. She sees its usefulness in meeting many needs of health personnel as they attempt to individualize client care: ". . . what is equally needed is a method for utilizing this frame of reference that is simple enough for doctors, nurses, social workers and others to apply as a basis for making their initial assessment of who the pa-tient-person is. . . . More knowledge about who patients are as persons would hopefully stimulate interest in them, while the greater security that staff would gain from training in directed talking and listening to patients might relieve the often seemingly calloused attitudes that are probably rooted in discomfort as well as in disinterest." The data that Brown[15] suggested should be included on the face-sheet information have been adapted to Figure 4-1.

REGRESSION

When a person's illness is severe and requires immediate hospitalization, he is suddenly withdrawn from his source of strength and emotional support—that is, his home and family. The combination of the stress imposed by illness and the loss of support system imposed by admission to the hospital may result in the phenomenon of regression. The behaviors that may occur as a result of this regression are described by Brown:[16]

. . . emotional regression is likely to occur perhaps to such a degree that the patient obviously behaves very much like a child in his dependency upon parental figures, in his frequent complaints and insistence upon service, and in his generally noticeable satisfaction if warm person-

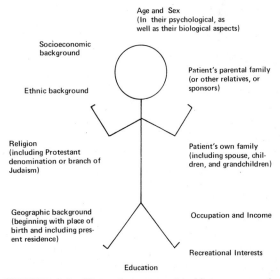

FIGURE 4-1. This information should appear on the face-sheet of each new client's record. It is the nurse's responsibility to become familiar with these data.

alized attention is given him. Fear, worries, loss of self-identity, discomforts and deprivation, ennui, and embarrassment because of aspects of the physical care he must accept may all combine to reduce him to psychological childhood. At the same time, he is aware that he is an adult and should not act like a child; this realization can create considerable conflict within him.

This same emotional regression is frequently seen in children who have been admitted to the hospital. It is distressing to parents when the developmental advances their child has made, such as the accomplishment of toilet training or self-feeding, seem to have been undone.

The behaviors described above are familiar to doctors and nurses. However, their manifestations are often overwhelming, and the client is labeled as "demanding" or "uncooperative"; attention is given instead to the "cooperative" client. In the end, this simply serves to intensify the insecurity felt by the client experiencing emotional regression.

LOSS OF INVOLVEMENT AND BELONGING

Man's involvement in and responsibility to society and his family are reflected in countless sayings: "Home is where the heart is," "A man's home is his castle," "Work is the businessman's balm," "He's the provider of the house," and "The Nation is built around its people." When a person enters the hospital, family, friends, and work associates release him from his responsibilities. Some accept this release from responsibility with gratitude; for others, it is grudgingly given up. The hospital further removes the person from his social environment and does not allow him to carry out social obligations regardless of whether he desires to or not. For many patients, this increases their stress and anxiety as it is closely associated with a loss of identity. Taylor[10] has identified those factors in the hospital that tend to decrease the client's "sense of social cohesion" and the measures which might be used to increase it (Table 4-1).

Some of the measures suggested are idealistic and far ahead of the current state of client care. The intent of Table 4-1 is to provide suggestions whose ramifications should be explored and adaptations considered when necessary.

VISITATION RIGHTS

The hospital allows the community members the privilege of limited intrusion on its affairs. Few contemplate that it is the community which has allowed the hospital to intrude on its affairs by removing its sick members.

Visitation rights vary significantly from hospital to hospital—from those which impose no restrictions at all to those which allow only an hour of visitation one day a week. Some clients are unable, physically or emotionally, to tolerate visitors. For others, it can be a severe deprivation to restrict visitation by their family and friends, particularly children. Even with all the scientific research indicating the critical need for a child to have parental contact, there are hospitals with very rigid visitation rules for parents.

The important deciding factor as to what the visitation rights should be rests with each individual client. What his needs are and how they might best be met should set the rules for his visitations.

LACK OF COMMUNICATION

Of all the areas disturbing to the client's peace of mind, the lack of communication ranks the highest. It is no wonder that many clients are convinced there is a secret plot to keep them uninformed and in the dark about their own bodies. Doctors perform their examinations and diagnostic tests and carry the "privileged information" off for deliberation or discussion with colleagues without the slightest hint to the client as to what has been discovered. The nurse obtains the client's blood pressure or gives him his medication without a second thought as to the client's interest in them. If asked she may divulge this "privileged information" or may simply reply "you'll have to ask your doctor," or "I'm not allowed to tell you that." And who thinks to tell the client what is expected of him or explains the floor routine. Again comments from clients help to illustrate this point. One client's roommate used the wrong route of administration for his medication: "The nurse never told him anything, she just left the capsule in the cup on his bedside. When she returned an hour or so later she asked him if the suppository had worked yet. Well at that point I said, 'not unless it works from either end.' " A new mother on the postpartum unit was fearful for her

TABLE 4-1 Factors Which Increase or Decrease Client's Sense of Social Cohesion During Hospitalization

Decreasing Factors	Increasing Factors
1. Physically removes patient from the various social groups of which he is a member.	1. Physical removal remains necessary, *but* the admission procedure could be modified.
2. Limits access to patient of other members of these groups.	2. Criteria for visitors allowed could be the expressed social needs of the patient rather than numbers and categories of visitors permitted by a universal hospital regulation. For example: socially insignificant, boring, and threatening visitors could be either excluded or rigorously limited; and significant visitors could be encouraged and included. Most hospitals exclude children below a specified age, and do not recognize the possibility that a sick person's most significant relationship might be a relationship with an animal.
3. Limits patient's ability to discharge group membership responsibilities.	3. The nurse might help the patient to identify his membership responsibilities and sort them into three categories: a. Those which have been either discharged or delegated—the patient may need reassurance. b. Those which can be discharged from the hospital bed—the patient may need help. c. Those which can be delegated to others—the patient may need help. d. Areas of a sense of excessive responsibility—the patient may need help and reassurance.
4. Membership in the hospital community offers the patient a limited sense of social cohesion. a. The treatment and care of patients are organized into the hospital as a number of separate tasks assigned to a number of different specialists and departments.	4. A systematic attempt could be made to increase the patient's sense of being a member of the hospital community. a. The care and treatment of the patient could be organized into the hospital as three separate but overlapping responsibilities assigned to three people, a nurse, a physician, and one administrative person. The single person from administration would handle all the hospital's business affairs with the patient. These three people would work together as the patient's basic hospital team.
b. Each staff member or hospital department has discharged his or its responsibility to the hospital as soon as the assigned patient task is completed. The patient may be on the receiving end of transactions with as many as 50 persons in a 24-hour period.	b. The physician, the nurse, and the administrative person could be made responsible for all hospital patient transactions within his or her area of competence. For example: the administrative person would be the only member of the hospital staff with whom the patient or his family would transact business: admission, insurance, billing, discharge, and so forth.
c. Patient participation, as a member of the hospital community, is limited to submitting to the rules and regulations of the hospital and to the decisions of hospital specialists.	c. The patient could participate as a member of the hospital community by becoming an active member of the health team. If his condition permits the patient might, for example, record information concerning those matters about which he alone has firsthand knowledge: in and out of bed, eating, eliminating, sleeping, activities, anxieties, and so forth.
d. Patients frequently fail to perceive the various categories of hospital specialists as a community. To the patient, the hospital community seems fragmented into groups of people who never communicate with each other.	d. If a determined effort were made to refrain from repeatedly asking the patient the same question, the patient might begin to believe that the hospital is a community of health specialists. He also might believe that he is being cared for by a health team. This could be done in a relatively simple manner, if, for example, the patient is *not* asked questions the answers to which already have been recorded in the chart.

This table has been reprinted with permission of Taylor, C.D.: *In Horizontal Orbit: Hospitals and the Cult of Efficiency.* New York, Holt, Rinehart, and Winston, 1970.

baby's well-being: "I kept waiting and waiting for them to bring my baby out for me to feed. When they didn't come and didn't come I began to wonder if she was ok or if something had gone wrong. Finally I was crying and in such a state I woke up my roommate. She was the one that told me 'they won't bring your baby out until in the morning if you don't ring the bell for her.' "

Not only must there be an attempt by all persons relating to the client to insure open communication, but also an awareness of the prerequisites for effective communication. Each person must put himself in the place of the other while maintaining his own identity. Only if one is willing and able to accept the attitudes of those with whom he communicates will the communication be effective.

CLIENT ALLIANCE— A SUSTAINING FACTOR

There develops among clients on a floor or in a ward a camaraderie which often becomes a sustaining factor in the attempt to adjust to the hospital community. If one is perceptive, he will soon realize the "we're all in this together" attitude that exists inside every hospital.

The hospital provides a singular situation, unlike any other event shared by adult individuals. The uniqueness is reflected in this client's words: "It's a feeling thing. I will never see him again in all my life because it's a one-time situation. We both shared the same room, both had the same problems and that was it. When it's over, it's over. Although I certainly wouldn't mind seeing him again."[14]

The friendship ties among clients develop very quickly and serve to make the person feel "at home." Soon after his arrival, after the staff have finished with him, the client is initiated to hospital life by his roommates. The topics which take priority are the floor routine, medical care, and the doctors. It is usually through information from these conversations that the timetable for activities is learned, who the staff members are that allow a little stretching of the rules, or which ones have a gentle hand and which ones should be avoided. It is likely that these friendships and the kindly support from fellow sufferers have the most positive effect on the newcomer's adaptation to the hospital community and his future memories of his hospital stay.

FAMILY NEEDS

All clients have families or those who are important in their lives outside of the hospital. Only through the inclusion of these family members in planning for client care will efforts be effective. They will be there to pick up where the hospital staff leave off as the client leaves the hospital to return to the community. The family's feelings, ambitions, and plans for the future are interrelated with those of the client. All of these may be, and often are, thwarted by the client's illness. Recognition of the family's attitudes is an important element in the facilitation or hindering of the client's progress. Unless the health care personnel intervene and assist the family in handling these problems, their feelings may find release at the client's expense as he becomes the focus of their ventilation. The best results are obtained when the family is included in rather than excluded from considerations for the client.

HOSPITAL TO COMMUNITY: CLIENT TO PERSON

"I will be discharging you from the hospital today Mrs. Smith." For some clients this is a long awaited word from their physician. Demands of the client role have been tolerated, but now all energies are eagerly focused on the return to the outside world. Family, job, friends, and personal interests suddenly resume their former status, and the associated responsibilities are gratefully received. Illness has given up its residence in the body, and the person now reclaims full control, with all the inherent rights and privileges to dictate its functionings. The family and society await with equal anticipation the client's return, at which time they bestow upon him his former duties and roles; they too have dispelled the sick role. This individual has successfully accomplished the transition from client back to person.

"Mr. Jones was doing so well. He was one of our *best* patients. Now that the doctor has told him he can go home, he's become demanding and has found all kinds of new complaints." On not a few occasions nurses, doctors, and social workers have observed this phenomenon when the client has been given the official release from the hospital community. The reasons for this hesitancy to release the "client-sick role" can be varied.

Fear that the medical or surgical condition which

necessitated hospitalization cannot be adequately monitored or controlled at home causes many clients to seek an extension to their hospital stay. The client who has been critically ill, requiring the use of special equipment to maintain and monitor the life systems for a prolonged period of time, may develop a psychological dependency upon them. One such client who had suffered a heart attack requiring close observation in an intensive care unit for several days was heard to make the following statement on the day he was to be discharged: "I know it sound ridiculous—but I'm really scared to leave the hospital. When I had problems here, the nurses knew it even before I did because the machines would show it. What if it (arrythmia) happens at home and I don't know about it till too late?" Anticipatory preparation through teaching by the hospital staff well before the projected day of discharge would help make this transition much less threatening for many clients.

There may be no home or family for the elderly person to return to or perhaps the family feels unable or is unwilling to take this individual into their home; the hospital has in fact become their home and the staff their surrogate family. Unless arrangements can be made through the help of the social worker or community agencies for a home for such persons their future is grim indeed.

In the past, one of the weaknesses with regard to the care of the client has been the lack of offering him the kind of assistance necessary to carry on once he leaves the hospital environment. More recently, professional nurses have integrated this aspect of client care into their overall care plan. Early in the hospitalization, efforts should begin to teach both the client and the family about his illness and what anticipated adaptations may need to be made prior to the client's return home.

The reassurance that there are resources for continued nursing support once back home has made this move an easier one for many clients. Through direct referrals, the hospital nurse is able to assure continuity of client care between the community health agencies. The public health nurse represents the long arms of the hospitals and clinics; her goals include: maintenance and functioning of the client and family, support of the patient's care regimen, maximizing the comfort and safety of the client, coordination of community and family efforts, and the reduction of client and family stress occasioned by illness.

Over the past several years, nursing has initiated a new and more fruitful approach to defining its professional role. The emphasis is shifting to a systematic study with clinical and research bases in which the client is the focus of attention. To this extent, nursing is becoming a flexible entity whose goal is designed to help the patient or client. This shift in emphasis holds many promises.

It encourages examination of who the patient is as a person with a psychological past, present, and future; it centers attention on what the client as an individual should have, not only in skilled nursing procedures and in health guidance but in comforts and satisfactions designed to check emotional regression and foster progression toward independence. In the consideration of comforts and satisfactions, nurses have begun to open the door to conscious evaluation of the significance of a variety of environmental factors.[16]

REFERENCES

1. Rogers, M. E.: *The Theoretical Basis for Nursing.* Philadelphia, F. A. Davis Co., 1970.
2. Koos, E. L.: *The Health of Regionville: What the People Thought and Did About It.* New York, Columbia University Press, 1954.
3. Friedson, E.: Client control and medical practice. *Am. J. Sociol.* 65:347, 1960.
4. Baumann, B.: Diversities in conceptions of health and physical fitness. *J. Health Hum. Behav.* 2:40, 1961.
5. Murray, R., and Zentner, J.: *Nursing Concepts for Health Promotion.* Englewood Cliffs, N.J., Prentice-Hall, Inc., 1975.
6. Erikson, E. H.: *Childhood and Society.* New York, W. W. Norton and Co., Inc., 1950.
7. Tippin, G.: Pin-ball theory of admission. Unpublished manuscript.
8. Murray, L.: The myth of the unmotivated family. *J. Psychiatr. Nurs.* 10:1, 1972.
9. van den Berg, J. H.: *The Psychology of the Sickbed.* Pittsburgh, Duquesne University Press, 1966.
10. Taylor, C. D.: *In Horizontal Orbit: Hospitals and the Cult of Efficiency.* New York, Holt, Rinehart and Winston, 1970.
11. Taylor, C. D.: Lecture presented to nursing students, University of Florida, Gainesville, 1976.
12. Barnes, E.: *People in Hospital.* New York, Macmillan and Co., Ltd., 1961.
13. Lesser, M. S., and Kean, V. R.: *Nurse-Patient Relationships in a Hospital Maternity Service.* St. Louis, C. V. Mosby Co., 1956.
14. Schuster, E. A.: Privacy, the patient and hospitalization. *Soc. Sci. Med.* 10:245, 1976.

15. Brown, E. L.: *Newer Dimensions in Patient Care: Patients as People*, part 3. New York, Russell Sage Foundation, 1964.
16. Brown, E. L.: *Newer Dimensions in Patient Care: The Use of the Physical and Social Environments of the General Hospital for Therapeutic Purposes*, part 1. New York, Russell Sage Foundation, 1961.

BIBLIOGRAPHY

Berhhard, R.: The dehumanized hospital hurts you and your patients. *Nurs. Digest* 5:39, 1977.

Bhanunathi, P. P.: Nurses' conception of 'sick role,' and 'good patient' behavior: a cross-cultural comparison. *Internat. Nurs. Rev.* 24:20, 1977.

Brown, B. J.: The role of nursing administrator in patient care delivery systems. *Nurs. Admin. Q.* 1:1, 1976.

Clark, E. L.: A model of nurse staffing for effective patient care. *J. Nurs. Admin.* 7(2):22, 1977.

Coser, R. L.: *Life in the Ward*. East Lansing, Michigan State University Press, 1962.

Field, M.: *Patients Are People: A Medical-Social Approach to Prolonged Illness*, 2d ed. New York, Columbia University Press, 1963.

Freeman, R.: *Community Health Nursing Practice*. Philadelphia, W. B. Saunders Co., 1970.

Hymovich, D., and Barnard, M.: *Family Health Care*. New York, McGraw-Hill Book Co., 1963.

Keywood, O.: I. The effects of an integrated service on standards of health care. *Nurs. Mirror* 143(10):63, 1976.

Kirchhoff, K.: Let's ask the patient: consumer input can improve patient care. *J. Nurs. Admin.* 6(12):36, 1976.

Krell, G.: Overstay among hospital patients: problems and approaches. *Health Soc. Work* 2:163, 1977.

Lake, G. M.: Hospitalization and personality change: recognition vital to nursing care. *Can. Nurse* 73(1):44, 1977.

Lutz, C.: Communication patterns of hospitalized patients. *Mich. Nurse* 50:8, 1977.

Marston, M. V.: Compliance with medical regimens: a review of the literature. *Nurs. Res.* 19:312, 1970.

McCormic, Rev. R. A.: The moral right to privacy. *Hosp. Prog.* 57:38, 1976.

Price, J. L. W.: The patient's morale. *Lancet* 1:533, 1977.

Rogers, L.: Reactions to social pressures. *Hosp. J.A.H.A.* 46:181, 1972.

Smith, R. K.: Depersonalization inexcusable. *Nurs. Outlook* 18(12):15, 1970.

Taylor, C. D.: The hospital patient's social dilemma. *Am. J. Nurs.* 65:96, 1965.

Wicker, I. B.: Overcoming cultural barriers. *Hosp. J. A. H. A.* 45:77, 1971.

PART 2: CONCEPTS ABOUT HEALTH AND ILLNESS

In Part 1, concepts about the client—that is, the consumer of health care services—were presented. Part 2 considers the status of this person's well-being. An understanding of what constitutes health and illness (Chapter 5), as well as the nebulous area between the two, and what they signify to the individual and his family are essential to adequately care for the client in any and all of the various conditions in which he is encountered.

After reviewing the definitions and descriptions of health and illness, homeodynamics and stress (Chapter 6) and crisis and intervention (Chapter 7)—factors which influence man's physical and emotional well-being or lack or it, are addressed. The responses of the client, his family, significant others, and those in his community to these states are also discussed.

Once one is aware of what health and illness are and what factors influence these states, then naturally, the next step is to consider how illness can be prevented or how interrupted health can be successfully restored. The last two chapters in this section (Chapters 8 and 9) focus on these issues, emphasizing the fact that maintenance of a healthy state for all human beings is now a major goal of health care today.

CHAPTER 5

A major responsibility of the nursing profession is to help clients evaluate the various medical care options available today. While most people take an interest in their health, they often try to "buy" it with over-the-counter medications, vitamins and nutritional aids, exercise equipment, or expensive visits to "health care experts." Newspapers, magazines, radio, and television are filled with competing advertisements for quick and easy home remedies for obesity, colds, fevers, aches, and pains. Product superiority is often claimed with vague and misleading statistics as well as personal testimonies. The extraordinary array of health aids offered to the consumer can be confirmed by a trip to any supermarket or drugstore or simply by a few hours in front of the television. Thus, an awareness of the impact that advertising has on health behaviors should alert health care personnel (health providers), to the importance of careful analysis of available health care products.

Increased mechanization, convenience foods, increased leisure time, and longer life spans have all

HEALTH AND ILLNESS

Linda L. Jarvis, M.S.N., R.N.

dramatically influenced the overall health and activity practices of most of us. Sedentary work is now common, and even the traditionally physical work, such as farming and industrial activity, is so mechanized that significant reductions in energy expenditure have resulted. These reduced activity levels are just as significant to overall health as the ingestion of a variety of health care products.

For a majority of the adult population, time for physical activity has to be carefully scheduled, which often results in short but excessive spurts of energy. Thus, the weekend athlete who feels compelled to make up for the inactivity during the week, is now frequently plagued with foot and leg problems, muscle spasms, cardiovascular disorders, and other injuries which often detrimentally affect his overall health. There are also those individuals who do not participate in any physical activity because of either busy work schedules, poor physical condition, or simply lack of interest. Although more insidious, the latter group is exposed to risks equally severe as the weekend athlete. Exercise in mod-

eration, however, could probably help to reduce the incidence of cardiovascular disease, obesity, and general deterioration.

Leininger states that reactions to illness, disease, treatments, health maintenance, daily activity, body discomforts, changes in life, and food preferences are linked to cultural beliefs, values, and previous experience.[1] Thus, finding reliable ways to interest individuals, families, or entire communities in health maintenance is the challenge of the future, and nurses are indeed in key positions to meet this challenge. However, only the careful assessment of populations, their cultures, beliefs, values, and experiences, as well as the re-evaluation of personal health habits by health providers and educators, will enable them to maintain or improve community health habits.

HEALTH-ILLNESS DEFINITIONS

Health and illness have different connotations for each individual. Health, for example, may mean simply the absence of disease, feeling good, or being productive at work or at home. Perceptions and influences on health states vary according to age, culture, geographic location, professional and personal responsibilities, and past experience with health or disease. Thus, family and individual histories are essential for a thorough understanding of health behaviors, allowing health care personnel to better establish both short and long-term nursing objectives and appropriate nursing interventions.

It must also be remembered that nurses have their own preconceived attitudes about health based on their personal, cultural, and educational experiences. Thus, an awareness of these attitudes and prejudices is essential for the proper and efficient delivery of health care.

To more thoroughly understand the concepts of health and disease, several definitions are presented in Table 5-1. It is apparent from this table that many definitions but no universal agreement exists.

Health and illness involve interactions among social, physical, psychological, and environmental factors; the critical factor, however, is the individual's adaptability to all of these influences. Reac-

tions depend on age, physical characteristics, body defenses, and cultural and social perceptions of health and illness. Attempts to effect change in health behaviors without a consideration of the relationship between the environment and the client will only lead to frustration. For example, if a dental health campaign proposed to reduce dental caries in urban fifth graders, a dental history of each student would be essential. This history should include the number of caries per child (filled and unfilled), brushing patterns, dental floss usage, nutritional habits, and frequency of dental checkups. The nutritional habits should include adherence to the Basic Four, between meal snacks, and sugar consumption. Water fluoridation is another variable that should also be considered. Cultural and growth and developmental characteristics must also be evaluated. These data would help to establish a baseline on dental health practices which could then be used as a guide for the educational program to be presented. Only after all of this information is compiled, will the design, implementation, and evaluation of an educational program be possible.

Although a single definition of health or illness

TABLE 5-1. Definitions of Health and Disease

Health	Disease
"a state of an organism with respect to functioning, disease, and abnormality at any given time."[2]	"an abnormal condition of an organism or part, especially as a consequence of infection, inherent weakness, or environmental stress that impairs normal physiological functioning."[8]
"a state of complete physical, mental, and social well-being and not merely the absence of disease or infirmity."[3]	"a reaction to a stress which extends beyond the bounds of individual reserve and adaptability."[9]
"a state of physical, mental, and social well-being and the ability to function and not merely the absence of illness or infirmity."[4]	"a dynamic process manifest in diseases, pathologic conditions, impairment of structure and function, psychosomatic disturbances and maladaptive behavior and personality changes. Disease is determined by multiple interacting genetic, environmental and individual variables, not by single factors acting alone."[10]
"it must be defined and measured in terms of adaptive capacity toward environmental circumstances and hazards. When adaptability fails, he is ill."[5]	"the maladjustment of the existing environment to the host."[11]
"optimal health is not a condition of an individual but a state of interaction between self and the environment. It is a ceaseless struggle between a basically hostile environment and a series of defenses we are endowed with and which we add to when necessary. The homeostatic balance of forces is our goal, and this may be accomplished by decreasing the threat of the environment or raising the capacity of the host to defend himself."[6]	

has not been identified in the preceding paragraphs, health care professionals are encouraged to formulate their own basic definitions, keeping in mind that perceptions and attitudes of nurses and clients invariably differ. These differences are more easily identified if there is a firm frame of reference from which to work. Most important, when studying health and illness, remember that they represent a dynamic state with sometimes complicated interrelationships among individuals, families, and the community.

HEALTH-ILLNESS BEHAVIORS

Nurses can have little impact on health behaviors unless they are aware of the variations of health-illness attitudes. Culture, religion, and socioeconomic factors play a major role in shaping health practices and attitudes. Although individuals within groups may differ, the examples that follow illustrate the type of attitudinal differences of which nurses should be cognizant.

Navajo Indians have the highest regard for the individual and his right to speak for himself.[12] It may, therefore, be difficult or impossible to obtain information about a client from family members. Because the Navajos believe that illness is a sign of disharmony with nature, rituals, chants, sacred food, sand painting, signs, and the medicine man are often used to restore health.[13] If health care professionals are consulted, their care is often supplemented with Navajo cures. Because the family is so important, many individuals may accompany the person who is ill, whether at home or in the hospital. Death is seen as a part of life with rituals carried out in traditional ways. Sharing is a hallmark of the American Indian in all aspects of life.[14]

Chicano families, which tend to be patriarchal, come first and the individual second.[15] The individual seeks help first from the family and only turns to outside help as a last resort. Since illnesses are viewed as coming from God, they are not always viewed negatively. Submission and acceptance is the secret of life with prayer used as an aid in accepting and enduring illness.[16] Health services come from healers such as espiritualists and curonderos.

The Chinese define health as a flow of energy called Yin (negative, dark, cold, and female) and Yang (positive, light, warm, and male). Any imbalance in Yin and Yang leads to disease. Because blood is thought to provide strength and be irreplaceable, blood tests are prohibited. The Chinese seek health through acupuncture, massage, spiritual healing, herbs, meditation, and philosophy.

The people of Appalachia are primarily Caucasian and fundamentalist in religious practices.[17] The extended family is of primary importance.[18] Orthodox health care is often sought for childbirth, emergencies, or to legitimize disability claims,[19] but otherwise faith healers or folk remedies are used.

Black families are often present-oriented with both husband and wife striving to help the family survive.[20] Children and the extended family are valued. Home cures may be tried before professionals are sought. Religion is important, and prayers and open expression of religious practices are common.

Specific religious practices also influence health behaviors; for example, orthodox Jewish clients require food preparation which is kosher; Jehovah's Witnesses do not approve of blood transfusions; and birth control (other than rhythm) is not sanctioned by the Catholic Church. Thus, familiarity with the specific practices of various religious groups is an important part of nursing education so that behavior and choice can be anticipated.

Health care is also influenced by socioeconomic factors. Utilization of services depends on payment consideration and kind of health provider utilized. Because there are long waits, overt and covert discrimination and dehumanization at busy clinics, emergency rooms are now frequented by individuals seeking primary care. Payment may come from out of pocket funds; third-party payers, such as insurance, medicare, medicaid; or prepayment plans such as health maintenance organizations. Access to care is dependent on financial status, availability, and transportation to services.

It is assumed that people have a variety of needs which must be met to attain a high quality of life. The list which follows contains the needs identified by Maslow as of paramount importance to the individual.

1. Physiological needs: food, sleep, and sex.
2. Safety needs: freedom of fear from injury or insult, familiar surroundings, and a secure job.
3. The belongingness and love needs: presence of friends, family, spouse, and affectionate relationships with people.

4. The esteem needs: self-respect; respect of others; desire for a stable, firmly based usually high evaluation of themselves; desire for strength, for achievement, for adequacy, for mastery and competence, for confidence in the face of the world and for independence and freedom; and desire for reputation or prestige, status, dominance, recognition, attention, importance, or appreciation.
5. The need for self-actualization: man's desire for self-fulfillment and the need for man to attain his potential.
6. The desire to know and to understand: seeking information, facts, synthesizing data, information, observations, curiosity, philosophy, experimenting, analysis, looking for relations and meanings, to construct a system of values.
7. The aesthetic needs: for beauty, avoidance of ugliness, order, symmetry, completion of an art.[21]

The list is hierarchical, and it is assumed that one must have the basic needs, such as physiological and safety, before the others can be met. If all of one's energies are spent in obtaining food, shelter, or a secure job, there is little chance that energy can be directed to self-actualization or the search for knowledge. Of course, several needs may be satisfied simultaneously, depending on past, present, and anticipated experiences. Mental and emotional impairments may well be the result of the absence of need fulfilling activities.

HEALTH-ILLNESS CONTINUUM

The health-illness continuum is a graduated scale for measuring a client's total health picture (Fig. 5-1). At one pole is optimal health and at the other, death. Terris noted that "disease can occur without illness. Health and illness are mutually exclusive, but health and disease are not."[4] Examples include diseases such as cancer, tuberculosis, hemophilia, or allergies which are found in apparently healthy individuals during routine examinations or screening programs. The individual, family, and community perceptions of their health state are directly influenced by subjective (feeling of well-being) and objective (ability to function) factors.[4] The following list is a summary of the assumptions that are im-

FIGURE 5-1. The health-illness continuum. (With permission from the author: Terris, M.: Approaches to an epidemiology of health. *Am. J. Public Health* 65(10):1039, 1975.)

portant to an understanding of the health-illness continuum. (1) Health is a dynamic state. (2) The perception of the health state is individualized. (3) Factors such as age, sex, culture, geographic location, and past experiences with health or illness influence one's perception of health and health behavior. (4) The nurse brings to every client interaction her own perceptions of health and illness. Each of these assumptions should be considered whenever assessing, planning, implementing, or evaluating nursing care.

The time interval defining the health-illness continuum is variable and individualized. It is influenced by the client's degree of natural resistance, age, normal progression of disease or trauma, perceived threat of the condition, and past experience with illness. It is possible for an individual to plateau at any point on the continuum or move up or down the gradient at any time during his lifetime. A chronic disorder, such as diabetes mellitus, when controlled with drugs and diet enables the individual to stay relatively symptom free, functional, and "healthy"; however, this is a life long health concern for this individual. On the other hand, an individual in optimal health who suffers bruises, lacerations, and a simple fracture will, barring complications, experience only temporary pain, dependency, and inconvenience. In 6 to 8 weeks, the injuries will be healed, rehabilitation completed, and the individual returned to his preaccident health state.

Dunn suggests that we view wellness and illness as a graduated scale, viewing wellness as an ever changing panorama of life itself inviting exploration of its every dimension including knowledge of one's inner self—a task from which many adults often seem to flee.[23] Health and illness are not separate entities but rather interrelated states through which individuals pass continuously through their lifetimes. To assume that one is totally ill or totally well at any given time does not take into account the enormous impact of social, psychological, and environmental factors which influence us at different times. Accepting this point of view clears the way for nurses to provide nursing interventions to a "healthy" population.

Nurses today have begun to turn their attention and practical skills to the concept of health. However, nursing care for healthy individuals can be frightening and threatening. In the absence of a pathological condition, what kind of nursing care can be provided? Dunn provides a brief guide for the nursing care of well populations. He advocates the assessment of the individual and family by the following criteria: (1) evaluation of the day-to-day functioning and emotional interrelationships of the family members; (2) description of the activities in which family members engage; (3) determination of the values that are important to the family and its individual members; (4) determination of the degree to which the illness or the wellness of an individual reflects the health status of the family unit.[24]

With this information, the nurse is in a position to collect as much data as possible. Short and long-term goals should be set, and nursing interventions initiated. What could be more rewarding than helping individuals, families, and communities maintain or strengthen positive health practices? It is conceivable that with a determined effort by health professionals, particularly nurses, to actively strengthen individual health behaviors, that within a short time their overall health status could be markedly improved, and we could begin to see a decline in some of the diseases and health practice problems we now face.

For example, if nurses began an aggressive anti-smoking campaign, the incidence of lung cancer, emphysema, and other respiratory problems would undoubtedly be affected.[25] Nurses could be influential in combating these conditions. Naturally some nurses would have to examine their own smoking behaviors (i.e., whether to quit smoking or not participate in the effort) as well as become more involved or aware of legislative action at all levels of government, to enable them to enforce anti-smoking codes and programs effectively. In hospitals, schools, and work areas, anti-smoking education would have to be an ongoing effort. Knowledge of the population in terms of values,

culture, beliefs, age, level of education, motivation, and concern over health behaviors would have to be assessed by the nurse and these data incorporated into the teaching programs.

Since 1968, there has been a reduction in the number of deaths related to heart disease,[26] partially because of concerted efforts to educate people about the benefits of a good diet and exercise, as well as the establishment of coronary care units, and the training of paraprofessionals to administer emergency first aid to heart attack victims. The same success could be realized with the respiratory diseases.

HEALTH BELIEF MODELS

During the 1950s and 1960s, from research supported by the Public Health Service on the concept of health came Rosenstock's Health Belief Model, which he applied to preventive health practices and illness related behavior.[27] This research has influenced the design of health care delivery and health education.

The Health Belief Model, when used to predict preventive health behavior, identifies the following three variables: (1) perceived susceptibility; (2) perceived seriousness; (3) perceived benefits or barriers to taking action. Perceived susceptibility concerns the individual acknowledgment of the possibility that he could be susceptible to a particular condition;[28] his reactions can vary from denial of any health risk, to stated concern that the condition will be contracted. Perceived seriousness concerns the varied ability of the individual to recognize the impact the condition could have on job, family, physical and mental status, and social relations.[28] Perceived benefits or barriers to taking action are influenced by the norms and pressures of the social group.[29] If the benefits outweigh the barriers or cost, the necessary action will be taken to reduce or modify the threat of the condition or vice versa.[29,30] The individual's perception is the critical factor in his preventive health behavior. Any efforts by health providers must take these factors into account before designing health delivery systems.

When the Health Belief Model is applied to sick role behavior, it can also be divided into three parts: (1) readiness to undertake sick role behavior; (2) modifying and enabling factors; and (3) actual sick role behaviors. Readiness to undertake recommended sick role behavior includes the following variables: (1) *motivations*, such as concerns about health matters in general and intention to comply; (2) *value of illness threat-reduction*, such as subjective estimates of susceptibility or resusceptibility, vulnerability to illness in general, and presence of symptoms; and (3) *probability that compliant behavior will reduce the threat*, such as subjective estimates of the proposed regimen's safety and efficacy.[31] Modifying and enabling factors include: demography, attitudes, and interactions.[31] With sick role behaviors, the focus is on compliance with prescribed regimens such as drugs, diets, and exercise.[31] In the sick role model, the individual's *perception* of factors is critical to explaining his behavior.

The Health Belief Model continues to provide a basis for research in health behavior. Application of this model in nursing helps to explain client behavior so that necessary changes in the delivery of health services can be made.

Concepts of Health

Motivations to seek health care are as varied as the individuals themselves. Lewis states, "the patient's theoretical concept of health, though he may have devoted little conscious time to such beliefs, has a direct bearing upon his health-illness behavior."[32] Milio further states, "human beings, professional or nonprofessional, provider or consumer, make the easiest choice available to them most of the time and not necessarily because of what they know is most healthful."[33] Both of these statements have sobering and far-reaching consequences for health care providers who must take steps to shape individual concepts of health in order that health promoting behavior results.

Milio has tried to pinpoint the formation of individual concepts of health by the following:

1. The health status of populations is the result of deprivation or excess of critical health sustaining resources.
2. Behavior patterns of populations are a result of habitual selection from limited choices, and these habits of choice are related to: (a) actual and perceived options available; (b) beliefs and expectations developed and refined over time by socialization, formal learning, and immediate experience.

3. Organizational behavior (decisions or policy choices made by governmental/nongovernmental, national/nonnational, for profit/nonprofit, formal/nonformal organizations) sets the range of options available to individuals for their personal choice-making.
4. The choices of individuals at a given point in time concerning potentially health promoting or health damaging selections is affected by their effort to maximize valued resources.
5. Social change may be thought of as changes in patterns of behavior resulting from shifts in the choice-making of significant numbers of people within a population.
6. Health education as a process of teaching and learning health supporting information can have little significantly extensive impact on behavior patterns, that is, on personal choice-making, without the easy availability of new or newly perceived alternative health-promoting options for investing personal resources.[34]

Each of these postulates must be correlated with existing circumstances in various communities, and then steps taken to strengthen or improve health care.

PROVIDING HEALTH CARE

Nurses, as client advocates, have a responsibility to provide the best health care possible. But how is this done? What happens to the woman who needs a gynecological examination and Pap smear but because of the cost and lack of child care does not receive it? What happens to the retired coal miner with emphysema who seeks health care via hospitalization because there are no community health nurses in his area? How does a young child obtain renal dialysis when he lives 500 miles from the nearest dialysis unit and no home based units are available? What is a nurse's role in bringing these people and services together? Of course, there are no easy answers; however, all efforts directed at changing attitudes, increasing client accountability, or offering increased services should be carried out with direct input from the public for whom the services are planned. The public should be made aware of existing legislation, funds, and availability of present resources before changes can be made in the distribution of health services.

Nurses have a responsibility to identify and observe health behavior patterns of individuals, families, and the community in which they work. With these data, they can be instrumental in designing new health care delivery systems, and in educating and modifying the behavior of the population toward improved health practices. A familiarity with the community groups that make decisions is invaluable in planning improved health care. However, regardless of the setting, the nurse has a responsibility to inform clients of the choices available to them and assist them in decision-making when necessary. At no time can the variety of factors that affect individuals, families, or communities be ignored. While the decision concerning health choice is ultimately the client's, the nurse must assess any given situation carefully to determine the multitude of factors which may be influencing the choice at any given time.

It is also important to remember that the client often makes decisions based on economics rather than on the health benefits. Let us take for example an individual who works in a factory. Although he has a small cavity which needs attention, it takes him 4 weeks to obtain an appointment because he does not have a regular dentist. Also, no sick leave is provided for this kind of health need; thus he must take time off without pay. The only day off he has is Wednesday, but this is the dentist's day off. Faced with these economic constraints, this individual will, in all likelihood, live with his cavity until it becomes a serious problem. It simply costs too much in time, money, and inconvenience to obtain the necessary care. Because many health choices are made in terms of time, inconvenience, transportation difficulties, money, real or anticipated pain, and fear, nurses must learn to structure their work settings so that health is not purchased at the expense of delay and nonattendance. Nonattendance or noncompliance is not necessarily the fault of the client or due to lack of client concern. Thus, the system in which nursing is provided must be evaluated in terms of those factors which affect client behavior.

From your studies of the social sciences, you have learned that attitudes, beliefs, and behaviors can be resistant to change. Thus, a nurse's task becomes one of identifying the variety of choices open to the client and then structuring critical aspects of the choices so that the desired health choice becomes available and attainable. This takes careful assessment, planning, implementation, and evaluation.

Lewis defines health behavior in three major areas:

1. *The individual and his self-maintenance*: an individual's own personal health, manner in which he manages self-maintenance and copes with problems related to his personal well-being.
2. *The individual and his involvement with the present health care system*: his relationship to sources of health care, the manner in which he utilizes the care available, appropriateness of his contact with the health care system, and the data he presents to the health care professional.
3. *The individual and his involvement in the community with reference to maintaining or improving services or facilities*: his relationship to the larger community and the health care system as a whole, active involvement in maintaining or improving facilities and programs as well as the environment of that community.[35]

Lewis sees health behavior in terms of an interrelationship between the individual and health care setting and the community. Thus, nurses must be observant and sensitive to overt and covert behavioral cues, and must understand the structure and function of community facilities to best assist the individual in meeting his health needs.

Entering the Health Care System

There are three primary entry points to the health care system: (1) *institutional entry*: hospitals, hospital-based clinics, emergency rooms, rehabilitation centers, and nursing homes; (2) *community entry*: neighborhood health centers, health maintenance organizations, screening programs, and referral from an individual or agency; and (3) *other entry*: employment health requirements, military screening programs, and school health.

Personal illness and injury are the most common ways to enter the system. In fact, in highly populated urban areas, individuals are often not seen until they are seriously ill or injured. Trauma and illness are treated in emergency rooms and then referred to other outpatient settings (clinics or personal health care providers) or hospitals.

Those who practice preventive health maintenance may enter the health care system through the required annual physical examinations and semiannual dental examinations by either health maintenance organizations or private physicians. (Routine mental health evaluations are not yet an accepted part of preventive health care.) The choices available to the consumer of either a private physician or enrollment in an HMO program are determined by the cost and convenience of services. However, the value of frequent visits required by these programs has recently been questioned by physicians who feel that all of their time should not be spent with people with no health complaints.

Referral for diagnostic evaluation, another way to enter the system, can be self-motivated, a result of health screening, or by the primary care provider when suspicious symptomatology is found. This service can be performed at many locations: private physician's offices, clinics, diagnostic centers, hospitals. The choice of location depends on the location of the facility, availability of transportation, and cost.

Health screening programs and health fairs are becoming increasingly popular, especially for diseases such as diabetes, glaucoma, cancer, and hypertension. A well-organized screening program should evaluate the individual against standard criteria and then have a means of referral for abnormal findings. The referral can be to the client's physician, a sponsoring clinic, or a hospital for further evaluation. Information on the screened condition as well as other general health information should be available. Availability of referral services and careful follow-up by letter or phone call to determine compliance is essential to any screening program. By careful coordination of the screening process, referral, and follow-up, perhaps health promoting choice-making behavior can be shaped as mentioned in Milio's sixth postulate.

Yearly physicals by a client's personal health care provider or the company health service are required by many organizations, particularly industrial settings, state employment, and high risk employment areas. Many industrial settings have established quite innovative health programs, including expanded roles for nurses.

School health requirements are instrumental in screening for health problems. Most states require that all children entering first grade have a physical examination and a completed immunization program. However, there has recently been a decline in the number of children with completed immunization schedules,[36] which has resulted in a recurrence of some childhood diseases for which innoculations are available. A renewed emphasis on good physical examinations and completed immunizations could be valuable in referring suspicious problems for early treatment and preventing the occurrence of many communicable childhood diseases.

SUMMARY

Nurses are in a position to provide improved health care. They are seen as health resource persons, teachers, and direct care providers. To meet professional responsibilities and to provide improved health care to the consumer, a clear understanding of health and health-related behavior, which is complex and variable, is necessary. Promotion of constructive health practices through the use of the nursing process to describe and plan for the population with whom you work, applying principles learned in the social sciences to health behaviors, and the involvement of the consumer in health care strategy from conception to completion of program are also a nurse's forte. The health practices of all of us can be improved and strengthened, but it will take time, effort, and patience.

REFERENCES

1. Leininger, M.: Cultural diversities of health and nursing care. *Nurs. Clin. North Am.* 12:5, 1977.
2. Morris, W. (ed.): *The American Heritage Dictionary of the English Language.* Boston, Houghton Mifflin Co., 1976, p. 607.
3. World Health Organization: *Constitution: World Health Organization.* Geneva, World Health Organization, 1971.
4. Terris, M.: Approaches to an epidemiology of health. *Am. J. Public Health* 65:1038, 1975.
5. Sargent, F.: Man-environment-problem for public health. *Am. J. Public Health* 62:631, 1972.
6. Besson, G.: The health-illness spectrum. *Am. J. Public Health* 57:1904, 1967.
7. Morris, op. cit., p. 656.
8. *Ibid.*, p. 377.
9. Francis, T., Jr.: Research in preventive medicine. *J. Am. Med. Assoc.* 172:994, 1960.
10. Hoyman, H. S.: Rethinking an ecologic system

model of man's health, disease, aging, death. *Am. J. Public Health* 65:516, 1975.

11. Reverley, S.: A perspective on the root causes of illness. *Am. J. Public Health* 62:1140, 1972.
12. Kniep-Hardy, M., and Burkhardt, M. A.: Nursing the Navajo. *Am. J. Nurs.* 77(1):95, 1977.
13. *Ibid.*, p. 96.
14. Primeaux, M.: Caring for the American Indian patient. *Am. J. Nurs.* 77(1):94, 1977.
15. White, E. H.: Giving health care to minority patients. *Nurs. Clin. North Am.* 12:(1):32, 1977.
16. *Ibid.*, p. 33.
17. Tripp-Reimer, T., and Friedl, M. C.: Appalachians: a neglected minority. *Nurs. Clin. North Am.* 12(1):42, 1977.
18. *Ibid.*, p. 46
19. *Ibid.*, p. 48.
20. White, *op. cit.*, p. 29.
21. Maslow, A. H.: *Motivation and Personality.* New York, Harper and Row, 1954.
22. Terris, *op. cit.*, p. 1037.
23. Dunn, H. L.: High level wellness for man and society. *Am. J. Public Health* 49:786, 1969.
24. *Ibid.*, p. 790.
25. Higgins, I. T. T.: Smoking and cancer-communication. *Am. J. Public Health* 66:159–160, 1956.
26. Luckman, J., and Sorenson, K. C.: *Medical-Surgical Nursing—A Psychophysiologic Approach.* Philadelphia, W. B. Saunders Co., 1974, p. 610.
27. Rosenstock, I. M.: Historical origins of the health belief model, in *The Health Belief Model and Personal Health Behavior*, edited by Becker, M. H., Thorofare, N. J.: Charles B. Slack, Inc., 1974, p. 1.
28. *Ibid.*, p. 3.
29. *Ibid.*, p. 4.
30. Becker, M. H., Drackman, R. H., and Kirscht, J. P.: A new approach to explaining sick-role behavior in low income populations. *Am. J. Nurs.* 64:206, 1974.
31. Becker, M. H.: The health belief model and sick role behavior, in *The Health Belief Model and Personal Health Behavior*, edited by Becker, M. H., Thorofare, N. J.: Charles B. Slack, Inc., 1974, p. 89.
32. Lewis, W. R.: Health behavior and quality assurance. *Nurs. Clin. North Am.* 9(2):359, 1974.
33. Milio, N.: A framework for prevention: changing health damaging to health generating life patterns. *Am. J. Public Health* 66:435, 1976.
34. *Ibid.*, pp. 436–437.
35. Lewis, *op. cit.*, pp. 359–360.
36. Markland, R., and Durand, D. E.: An investigation of sociopsychological factors affecting infant immunizations. *Am. J. Public Health* 66:169, 1976.

BIBLIOGRAPHY

Abdellah, F. G.: Nurse practitioners and nursing practice. *Am. J. Public Health* 66:245, 1976.

Beland, I. L., and Passos, J. Y.: *Clinical Nursing—Pathophysiological and Psychological Approaches*, 3rd ed. New York, Macmillan Publishing Co., Inc., 1975.

Donabidian, A.: An examination of some direction in health care policy. *Am. J. Public Health* 63:243, 1973.

French, R.: *The Dynamics of Health Care.* New York, McGraw-Hill Book Co., 1968.

Hart, S. E.: An overview of health—a conceptual model. *Natl. League Nurs. Pub.* No. 52-1472, 1973.

Hochbaum, G. M.: *Health Behavior.* Belmont, Calif., Wadsworth Publishing Co., Inc., 1970.

Johnston, M.: Folk beliefs and ethnocultural behavior in pediatrics. *Nurs. Clin. North Am.* 12(1):77, 1977.

Leininger, M.: An open health care system model. *Nurs. Outlook* 21:171, 1973.

Maiman, L., and Becker, M. H.: The health belief model: origins and correlates in psychological theory. In *The Health Belief Model and Personal Health Behavior*, edited by Becker, M. H., Thorofare, N. J., Charles B. Slack, Inc., 1974.

Milio, N.: Dimensions of consumer participation and national health legislation. *Am. J. Public Health* 64:357, 1974.

Milio, N.: A broad perspective on health: a teaching-learning tool. *Nurs. Outlook* 24:160, 1976.

Murphy, M. J.: The development of a community health orientation scale. *Am. J. Public Health* 65:1293, 1975.

Overfield, T.: Biological variation concepts from physical anthropology. *Nurs. Clin. North Am.* 12:819, 1977.

Schwartzer, S.: Incentives and the consumption of preventive health care services, in *Consumer Incentive for Health Care*, edited by Mushkin, S. J., New York, PRODIST, 1974.

Scott, J. M.: the changing health care environment—its implications for nursing. *Am. J. of Public Health* 64:364, 1974.

Sleeper, R.: Issues in health care. *Natl. League Nurs. Pub.* No. 14-1599, 1976.

Walsh, M. E.: Health issues of today—perspectives for tomorrow. *Natl. League Nurs. Pub.* No. 14-1613, 1976.

Weber, A., Jermine, C., and Grandjean, E.: Irritating effects on man of air pollution due to cigarette smoking. *Am. J. Public Health.* 66:672, 1976.

Wilson, F. A., and Neuhauser, D.: *Health Services in the United States.* Cambridge, Ballinger Publishing Co., 1974.

U.S. Department of Health, Education and Welfare: *Compendium of National Health Expenditure Data.* Social Security Division, Office of Research and Statistics, 1976.

Zubkoff, M., and Dunlop, D.: Consumer behavior in preventive health services, in *Consumer Incentives for Health Care*, edited by Mushkin, S. J., New York, PRODIST, 1974.

CHAPTER 6

A baby is born; an old man dies. This is life, and life is filled with stress, change, and growing. Man is constantly learning and changing. In this chapter, this changing—that is, the continuous exchange of energy between man and his environment (homeodynamics)—and the stress that may result, particularly as it relates to health and illness, will be explored.

HOMEODYNAMICS OR HOMEOSTASIS?

In the past, it was probably safe to assume that if a word was not in the dictionary, then it did not exist; however, this is no longer true. New words are being coined so rapidly that by the time they get into print, they may already be obsolete. The word homeodynamics, for example, replaces the older word homeostasis,[1] which was thought outdated and much of the literature concerning it, contradictory.

Homeo is defined in the *American College Dic-*

HOMEODYNAMICS AND STRESS

Carol Zimmern, M.A., R.N.

tionary as "a word element meaning similar or like."[2] Stasis is defined as "stagnation in the flow of fluids of the body, as of the blood in an inflamed area."[3] Homeostasis then describes "an organism in physiological equilibrium maintained by coordinated functioning of the brain, heart, liver, etc."[2] In other words, homeostasis is a balanced state of existence.

In the 1930s, Cannon first introduced the principle of homeostasis to indicate a relatively steady state of the internal operations in the living system.[4] We can interpret this to mean that man exists in a steady state—that is, in a state of equilibrium.

Laszlo defined steady state as that "state maintained in and by the organism. This is a dynamic balance of energies, and substances are always poised for action. It is never a plain equilibrium, such as the state a watch reaches when it has run down."[5] Laszlo also maintains that "man regulates his own internal environment."[6]

There is a certain amount of contradiction between Cannon and Laszlo. Cannon says that there

are *no changes* in the system. However, we know that this is not true. The pulse rate changes according to activities, emotions, and other factors. Laszlo says that the organism is always ready to interact and that the energy is dynamic (i.e., characterized by continuous change). If this is the case, then there is *constant* interaction between the internal and external environments. Therefore, a more accurate term is homeodynamics.

In *homeostasis*, man is constantly striving to maintain a state of equilibrium. Man is separate from his environment, which he views as trying to interfere with his steady state. Therefore, there is no mutual exchange of energy between the two. In other words, man adapts to his environment. Adaptation again implies a striving for equilibrium. Homeostasis was once thought to occur in a closed system; however, this concept is no longer considered valid. Because this theory of homeostasis is contradictory, the concept of homeodynamics has come into being.

Homeodynamics, on the other hand, suggests a

Homeodynamics and Stress 89

mutual interaction between man and his environment, involving a continuous exchange of energy, which denotes an open energy system. "Man is a unified whole, possessing his own integrity, and manifesting characteristics that are more than and different from the sum of his parts."[7] A brain, a limb, or a kidney does not signify man. Each man is unique and in a continuous state of becoming; he is not in a steady state at all.

A state of becoming is a growth process. Toffler says that "all things, from the tiniest virus to the greatest galaxy are in reality not things at all, but processes. There is no static point, no nirvana-like unchange, against which to measure change. Change is, therefore, necessarily relative."[8] Changes in man are inseparable from environmental changes because of the interaction between the two. With each change there is evidence of the growing complexity of the pattern and organization of man. The most obvious example is the growth and change from infancy to adulthood. Thus, the continuous repatterning and reorganization of both man and his environment reflect a nonsteady state—a state which homeodynamics describes. The concept of homeodynamics may be difficult to grasp because much of the mutual interaction may not be visible.

STRESS

The concept of stress is directly related to the concept of homeodynamics. Stress, either positive or negative, influences the homeodynamic state of the organism. Since each individual is unique, what is stressful for one individual is not always stressful for another. The degree of stress may also differ. A severely stressful situation may inhibit normal function, whereas a minimum amount of stress may enhance growth and productivity.

Nurses should be aware that the hospital environment can be a very stressful situation, causing some clients to withdraw and others to make the most of their new environment. The concept of stress is basic to the understanding of the practice of holistic nursing care.

Defining stress is not an easy task. Selye defined stress as "essentially the rate of wear and tear in the body,"[9] and equated it with the process of aging. However, stress should not be viewed as only a physiological process; it is an inherent part of living. A person can react either positively or negatively to stress. A positive experience might be a mild anxiety attack before taking an exam. The anxiety, in all likelihood, will increase the student's capability to study and learn, resulting in a high test score. Also, the anxiety experienced by an individual who has pain in his lower right quadrant may be severe enough to make him seek medical attention.

A negative experience with stress might be seen in the child who sees a parent killed. He may withdraw as a reaction to stress to escape reality. A negative reaction may also be encountered after the surgery and hospitalization for a mastectomy, an experience which may have been so completely stressful, that when a lump is found in the other breast, medical care is not sought.

Selye elaborates his definition of stress by stating that "Stress is the nonspecific response of the body to any demand made upon it.[10] It is immaterial whether the agent or situation we face is pleasant or unpleasant."[11] Although there is a specific response by the body to each demand which may be considered a local response, there is also a generalized or a nonspecific response to stress. An example might be the trembling, increased blood pressure, dilated pupils, and increased respirations that accompany fear (Fig. 6-1).

A specific response to stress would be shivering when a person is exposed to cold. This produces more heat, and the blood vessels in the skin contract to decrease heat loss from body surfaces. If exposed to danger, epinephrine is released to increase the pulse rate and blood pressure in response to the danger. All of these responses work in unison because man is in a homeodynamic state.

Selye identified three phases of stress—*alarm, resistance,* and *exhaustion*—which he called the *general adaptation syndrome* (GAS).[12] Because different amounts of energy are required for each phase, it is important for the nurse to distinguish between the phases, so that appropriate nursing interactions can be planned.

The alarm phase, also called fight or flight, is the red-alert warning, which is usually the result of either[12] a physiological stress, such as a burn, or a psychological stress, such as a divorce. Physiological processes are set in motion. Large amounts of epinephrine and cortisone are secreted into the blood stream by an activated autonomic nervous

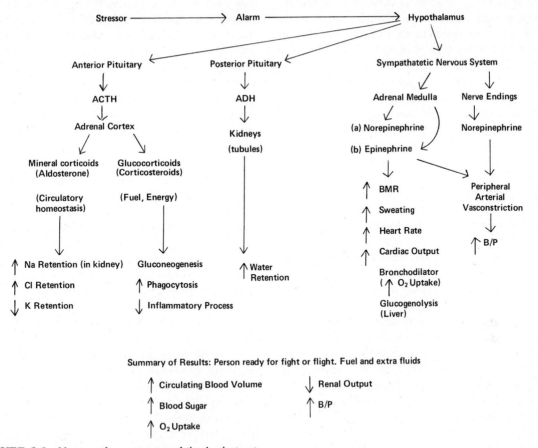

FIGURE 6-1. Nonspecific responses of the body to stress.

system. Typical signs of shock—pallor, increased respirations, drop in blood pressure, diaphoresis, cool and clammy skin—appear. This phase can last for a few minutes or for as long as 24 hours. However, "no living organism can be maintained continuously in a state of alarm."[12]

The resistance phase is the period of adjustment. The body uses its most appropriate channels to combat the stressor by limiting its effects to the smallest area of the body capable of dealing with it. Again, this can be a positive or negative situation. As the person learns to cope with the stressor, he can apply it in future situations.

Exhaustion is the final phase of GAS. The body's resources are depleted, and the homeodynamic state is decreasing. The stressed area can no longer be contained, and the entire body becomes stressed. The manifestations that appeared in the first phase reappear. The exhaustion phase, in some cases, can terminate in death. In other situ-

ations, the process can be reversed. For example, an elderly person with a history of heart disease, diabetes, and hypertension has an increased probability of going into the exhaustion phase if he develops pneumonia, whereas a young, healthy person with no history of a chronic illness is not likely to experience exhaustion with pneumonia. Older clients have a much longer and much more difficult recovery and rehabilitation period. According to Selye, life is really a protracted GAS which develops as a result of the stresses of living. Furthermore, life eventually ends in exhaustion and death.

In addition to the body's general response to stress, there also is a response to local stressors—*local adaptation syndrome* (LAS). Inflammation, manifested by heat, redness, edema, pain, or loss of function, is a local response to stress. If any of these signs are observed, a local adaptation syndrome is in process.

Engel defined stress as "any influence, whether

it arises from the internal environment or the external environment, which interferes with the satisfaction of basic needs or which disturbs or threatens to disturb the state of equilibrium."[13] This is a somewhat broader and yet more specific definition since it includes both our internal and external environments. Stress then can be seen as anything that has an influence on the organism in either a positive or negative sense. Reactions to stress depend in part on previous experience with a similar kind of stress and the abilities he has developed to cope. Stress can lead to increased self-actualization.

Nurses must be aware of the universality and variability of stress reactions in order to provide a high quality of health care. In order to determine how stress affects the homeodynamic state one must be able to identify a stressor and understand its influence. A stressor is an agent that intensifies the stress state,[13] which may or may not be apparent. Stressors may be: (1) physiologic—the normal changes occurring during pregnancy, puberty, and menstruation; (2) pathophysiologic—bacteria, viruses; (3) psychologic—decreased self-esteem, social pressures, marriage, jobs; (4) traumatic—injuries, burns, surgery; (5) socioeconomic—financial instability, changes in family relationships, divorce; and (6) cultural—moving from one place to another.[14] Usually stressors work simultaneously, and an individual responds holistically. For example, a rapid heart rate, increased respiration, and a raised basal metabolism often accompany a fever. However if a nurse is only concerned about the elevated temperature without considering the total system, ineffective and incomplete nursing care will result. In addition to aspirin and a sponge bath, the patient may need oxygen, four to five small meals instead of three regular meals, additional fluids, or more blankets to feel comfortable. Reactions to a stressor are not always predictable. In assessing a stressful situation, the nurse should consider the following interrelated factors: the nature of the stressor, the number of stressors operating simultaneously, time of exposure to the stressor, and past experience with similar stressors.[15]

Different kinds of stressors as well as the strength of each will cause varying degrees of response. If the responses are either excessive or insufficient to cope with the stressor, the stress state may intensify. Take for example a client who experiences severe chest pain after her physical examination. When encouraged to see her physician, she refused saying, "I don't want him to think I'm a hypochondriac." Her anxiety, respirations, and pulse increased in rate and intensity. Thus, the yearly physical was presumably not as great a stressor as the chest pain and seeing her physician between exams. Or take for example an individual who cuts his finger; he will use less energy to cope with his situation than a person who has multiple cuts all over his body. In the latter case, the stress state is intensified, and if the coping behaviors are not adequate, the stress state can become overwhelming.

Individuals are capable of coping successfully with a number of stressors at one time. However, when the stressors' demands for energy exceed the person's inner resources then he may need outside help or be so overwhelmed that death may result. Keep in mind though that death does not have to be the end result of the exhaustion phase. An individual must learn to set priorities for energy allocation.

The effect of multiple stressors is illustrated by the following example: a young woman became anxious because her mother had cancer. These anxieties increased as her mother's illness progressed, resulting in a less productive expenditure of energy. She had to increase the number of hours spent completing a chore, because of her diminished ability to concentrate. As a result, she got less sleep (a stressor) and ate sporadically (a stressor). Her work performance suffered as a result, and when asked a question (a stressor) by her employer, she burst into tears. This was not her normal response. The last stressor caused intensification of the stress state. When the stress state intensifies, the individual often becomes more vulnerable to additional stressors. If unable to allocate energies appropriately, there is a great risk that the state itself will become a stressor.

Exposure to a stressor over an extended period of time can deplete necessary resources which in turn reduces an individual's ability to resist the stressor's detrimental effects over time. When energy resources are depleted, exhaustion results. Imagine, for example, a person holding his breath until he faints from lack of oxygen. After fainting, normal breathing is restored, and the client revives when a sufficient amount of oxygen reaches the brain. When he fainted, the individual was in the exhaustion phase.

Previous experience with a stressor or similar stressor will influence a person's response. If a response to a prior stressor was positive, one could expect a positive result. However, if the response to the stressor was met with difficulty, the same difficulty may be encountered when the same stressor is encountered again. With a new stressor, the response is unpredictable.

No two individuals will react identically when exposed to the same stressor. Also, individual reactions to similar stimuli will differ. The nurse should attempt to determine whether the stressor will evoke positive or negative responses and to what degree intensification may occur.[16]

APPLICATION OF THEORY

Today, we live in a highly complex fast-moving society, in which great technological advances have been made. Travel from one end of the world to the other in a matter of hours is now possible. New drugs have been found to cure or prevent diseases. While all of these advances benefit man, they also create additional stress. If nurses are aware that stress exists and remember to watch for signs of it, then appropriate intervention can make it a positive experience.

In the above exploration of the concepts of homeodynamics and stress, we have accepted the assumption that man and environment are energy systems that continuously interact. To examine the relationship of the above theories to health and illness and their application to nursing practice, the nursing process, which consists of the following steps, can be applied: (1) assessment and data collection; (2) nursing diagnosis; (3) planning of care, implementation, and intervention; and (4) evaluation and revision (or termination or modification). This process may be implemented in any setting whether dealing with healthy or ill individuals. For a comprehensive study of the nursing process and all of its steps, see Part 4 of this text.

CASE. Tom is a 16-year-old adolescent, who lives with his parents and 21-year-old brother, David. His family lives in a private home in a suburb of a large metropolitan area. They are a middle-income, Protestant family. Tom has had the usual childhood diseases, is above average intelligence, and is considered a normal adolescent. He is a junior in high school and has recently passed his driving test.

Tom is now going through puberty, so that he is in a growth spurt with increased hair on his body, acne, and hormonal changes. He is aware of what to expect with the physiological changes because of a health education course he took in school. His parents always considered him an obedient child, but lately he has been challenging their decisions, wanting to make his own. He is spending more time with his peers and less with his family. His peer standards are very important to him. Tom is a chronic gum chewer. He is trying to decide which college he wants to go to and what to do with his life. There is a girl that he likes, but when he asks for a date she declines.

Following this rejection, Tom began to smoke, lost his appetite, became angry, had a fight with his mother, and was unable to complete his homework assignments. Several days later, Tom's brother introduced him to a new girl. His peers and family gave him encouragement, and he asked her for a date. She accepted and Tom became happy. He quit smoking, completed his homework assignments, and walked around the house whistling.

Although this is fairly typical adolescent behavior, collection of this data constitutes the first step of the nursing process. The influence (problem) would be that there is intensification of the stress state, validated by the changes in behavior following the first girl rejecting him. This would include his loss of appetite, smoking, irritability at home, and his inability to complete his homework. There may have been additional physiological changes if one actually observed him. The gum chewing is not significant because it is an established habit; however, in another individual, it might have indicated stress intensification. Thus, each individual's pattern of behavior must be established in the history.

After stating the specific problems, nursing actions must be planned. The specific problem in this situation was reaction to rejection. The stressor is the girl refusing to go out with Tom. Additional stressors are the physiological changes, decisions concerning college and career, and the struggle for independence. The resources Tom used with this particular stress situation were his brother, friends, the second girl, smoking, the defense mechanism of displacement, and internal resources that are not apparent, such as an increase in epinephrine. The major interaction was his family's and friends' encouragement to ask another girl for a date. The evaluation of the action was that it was effective, and no further intervention was needed. At that point, the crisis was past, and there is no longer intensification of the stress state.

The above example illustrates stress and homeodynamics in every day life. Stress also influences the maintenance or regaining of health. For example, a middle-aged woman was hospitalized for a myocardial infarction. She lived alone with her two cats. The nurse who admitted her observed that she was extremely restless, agitated, and withdrawn. Because she had been medicated for pain with 100 mg of meperidine hydrochloride (Demerol) and had received 10 mg of diazepam (Valium), she should have been resting fairly comfortably. Early in the morning, the nurse saw the patient crying. When asked if she could help, the woman blurted out, "I'm so worried about my cats. I live alone, and there is no one there to take care of them. They are the only family I have." The nurse asked a neighbor to care for the cats to reduce her client's anxiety.

In the initial analysis, the nurse may have automatically assumed that the woman feared for her life. Although this may have been a concern, it was not the overriding one. She was more concerned about her cats who were dependent on her. If the nurse only intervened with what appeared to be the problem, the stress would not be reduced, but rather increased. If the problem of who would take care of the cats had not been resolved, the stress would have directed the client's energy away from regaining her health, and thus would have become a destructive force. This ultimately, if not resolved, could have ended in death or a delay in regaining her health. The nurse must deal with her clients holistically, not in parts.

Although the overt signs of stress may not be visible, it must not be assumed that it does not exist. Another case comes to mind. Mary R. was 8 weeks pregnant when she went to her obstetrician to confirm her pregnancy. This was her first pregnancy. She kept her scheduled appointments, discussed her diet with the office nurse, gained 24 pounds during the entire pregnancy, and appeared happy and content. She gave birth to a full-term, six pound, four ounce, baby boy. She had a normal delivery and was discharged three days postpartum.

Mary R., however, did not return for her 6 week checkup. When the nurse called to find out why, she was told that Mary R. had been hospitalized for severe depression. Her husband said, "She never wanted the baby." In this case, no one was aware that the pregnancy was causing more than the normal amount of stress. Thus, no one intervened to reduce the stress. As a result, with the termination of the pregnancy and the birth of the infant, the stress state intensified and became overwhelming.

Assessment of Stress

In assessing the stress state, the nurse must keep in mind six categories that represent the behavioral changes that commonly occur when the stress state intensifies:[17] (1) accentuated use of a particular behavior pattern; (2) changes in various activities; (3) less organized behavior or organized at a lower level; (4) increased sensitivity to the environment; (5) existence of behaviors which show an alteration in usual physiologic activity; and (6) misinterpretation of "reality."[18]

These categories include a wide variety of behaviors that may occur when the stress state is intensified. There will be times when the same behavior will fall into more than one category, but this does not decrease the usefulness of the tool. To use this tool, you must look at a person holistically and compare previous and present physiologic and psychologic behaviors. By noting these changes, you can evaluate the influence of the intensified stress state on that individual. In the following paragraphs, each of these six assessment categories are discussed.

ACCENTUATED USE OF A PARTICULAR BEHAVIOR PATTERN. This may consist of one or more of the individual's usual behavior patterns, but there will be a more pronounced use, because more energy is being expended to decrease stress. A person who usually plays golf once a week may play every day when stress intensifies. In the case history presented previously, Tom began to adhere more rigidly to his usual schedule, thus becoming less flexible. One may also see inappropriate responses, such as a person crying hysterically when told he will be discharged from the hospital.

CHANGES IN VARIOUS ACTIVITIES. A person may either increase or decrease the activities he usually undertakes. In the case history presented previously, Tom lost interest in food. It is important to compare the present behavior to the previous behavior to see if there really are alterations. Often when a person is ill, he will delete some of his activities until he is feeling better. As activity levels become more normal, the stress state is probably decreasing in severity. When a 35-year-old woman, with two children, returned to school, she found it difficult to adjust, so her stress state intensified. She then became active with the PTA. Because she is well organized and able to set priorities for energy allocation, she found that increasing her activities helped her to deal with her intensified stress state.

LESS ORGANIZED BEHAVIOR OR ORGANIZED AT A LOWER LEVEL. The extent of organization varies from one person to the next, but each human being is productive at a particular organization level depending on his or her age and developmental level. Disorganization reflects poor use of energy resources. Activities may lack priority or purpose. An example of purposeless activity is an expectant father pacing aimlessly while waiting for his wife to give birth. A man going for a tax audit without taking his receipts shows a lack of attention to detail. In the case history, Tom was unable to complete his homework. The nurse must consider the level of behavior for her evaluation of the person's stress state. Frequently when people are under increased stress, they regress to an earlier stage of development. This is often seen with the hospitalized child—such as a 4-year-old who is toilet trained who regresses to bed wetting.

INCREASED SENSITIVITY TO THE ENVIRONMENT. When a person is in an intensified state of stress, his tolerence level decreases. Things that would not normally bother him now do. For instance, an individual who usually does not mind the radio playing might find it annoying when he is under increased stress. Irritation over seemingly minor things may indicate an intensifed stress state. In the case history, Tom ordinarily got along with his parents, but when stressed he argued with them.

EXISTENCE OF BEHAVIOR WHICH SHOWS AN ALTERATION IN USUAL PHYSIOLOGIC ACTIVITY. In Tom's case, one physiological change that should be noted was the increase in acne. Other people react to increased stress by having diarrhea or nausea.

MISINTERPRETATION OF "REALITY." When an individual is in an intensified stress state he may not hear what is being said. He may misinterpret or misunderstand the event or message. In Tom's case, he distorted the first girl's message, by taking it to mean that no girl would want to go out with him.

SUMMARY

We have discussed the theory and application of homeodynamics and stress. It is important to remember that stress is a normal reaction to the continuous interaction of man and his environment. Most human beings change and grow in response to these life experiences. Nurses should be as aware as possible of the universality and variability of reactions to stress, and its impact on each individual's homeodynamic state in order to help make each stress situation as positive an experience as possible.

REFERENCES

1. Rogers, M. E.: *An Introduction to the Theoretical Basis of Nursing.* Philadelphia, F. A. Davis Co., 1970, p. 102.
2. ———. *The American College Dictionary.* New York, Random House, 1964, p. 578.
3. *Ibid.*, p.1180.
4. Cannon, W. B.: *The Wisdom of the Body,* 2nd ed. New York, Norton Publishing Co., 1939.
5. Laszlo, E.: *The Systems View of the World.* New York, George Braziller, 1972, p. 43.
6. *Ibid.*, p. 41.
7. Rogers, *op. cit.*, p. 47.
8. Toffler, A.: *Future Shock.* New York, Bantam Books, 1970, p. 20.
9. Selye, H.: *The Stress of Life.* New York, McGraw-Hill Book Co., 1976, p. 1.
10. Selye, H.: *Stress Without Distress.* New York, New American Library, 1974, p. 14.
11. *Ibid.*, p. 15.
12. Selye, *The Stress of Life,* p. 37.
13. Engel, G. L.: A unified concept of health and disease. *Perspect. Biol. Med.* 3:459, 1960.
14. Byrne, M. J., and Thompson, L. F.: *Key Concepts for the Study and Practice of Nursing.* St. Louis, C. V. Mosby Co., 1972, p. 42.
15. Luckmann, J., and Sorenson, K. C.: *Medical-Surgical Nursing.* Philadelphia, W. B. Saunders Co., 1974, p. 10.
16. Byrne and Thompson, *op. cit.*, p. 48.
17. *Ibid.*, p. 52.
18. *Ibid.*, p. 59.

CHAPTER 7

Danger and opportunity. Though the two terms are seemingly contradictory, this translation of the Chinese characters representing the word crisis captures their meaning. The crisis situation poses difficulties, yet, if successfully resolved an individual or group may achieve a higher level of functioning. The purpose of this chapter is to provide an introduction and overview of the conceptual framework and intervention techniques one uses in achieving the potential of adaptive crisis resolution.

THEORETICAL CONCEPTS OF CRISIS

Historical Development

Assisting individuals in times of stress is not unique to modern times; however, the formal development of a crisis theory based on concomitant research has fairly recent origins and is intricately interwoven with the growth of preventive psychiatry. Preventive psychiatry advocates that the incidence, dura-

CRISIS AND INTERVENTION

Gail J. Sanzone, M.S., R.N.

tion, and incapacitation resulting from an emotional disorder can be reduced. With respect to a crisis model, a number of factors contributed to its development, including (1) the influence of military psychiatry and its implementation of the triage concept, (2) the studies of Lindemann and Caplan, (3) the community mental health movement with its recognition of the importance of primary prevention, and (4) the input from ego psychologists such as Erikson and Maslow.

The study of Lindemann[1] provided the impetus for the development of crisis theory. His classical work studied those bereaved by the Coconut Grove fire of 1943 in Boston. He outlined the grief and grieving process experienced with the loss of a significant other. After observing normal and pathological mourning reactions, he postulated that there were both adaptive and maladaptive ways of meeting life's hazardous situations, each having a definite effect on the individual's future coping ability and level of functioning. His future work on the concept of emotional crisis substantiated his belief

that failure to successfully master these inevitable events could lead to emotional problems.[2]

Erikson also contributed to the formulation of a crisis theory. His theory of development is rooted in the theoretical writings of Freud who believed that an individual's personality was formed in early childhood. In contrast, Erikson, who viewed personality development as spanning one's lifetime, defined eight stages in this maturation process. Each stage and its accompanying developmental tasks lays the groundwork for successful resolution of succeeding stages. Thus, a child who fails to develop trusting relationships in the first stage will experience difficulty in developing intimate relationships in the sixth stage. Due to the role changes and new behaviors that each phase requires, disturbances of a cognitive and affective nature are also present. At these times the individual is in a developmental crisis[3] as contrasted to Lindemann's focus on the situational crisis.

Influenced by the findings of Lindemann and Erikson, Caplan broadened the scope of crisis theory with his efforts in preventive psychiatry or community mental health. Since maladaptive coping in a situational or developmental crisis led to increased risk for the development of emotional disturbances and since all individuals, regardless of culture, experienced these events or stages, often achieving healthy resolution, Caplan believed that preventive measures could be identified which would forestall the pathological consequences.[4] Community psychiatry and its component of crisis, therefore, has essentially evolved from the search for the etiology of emotional disorders.

The U.S. Congress recognized the importance of this movement with the passage of the Comprehensive Community Mental Health Centers Act in 1963 (P.L. 88-164). In order to qualify for federal funding, centers are mandated to provide the following five essential services: inpatient, outpatient, partial hospitalization, 24-hour emergency service, and consultation and education. Though each may service clients in crisis, the latter two are particularly relevant to a crisis framework. The relevancy of emergency services is obvious. Through consultation and education, health professionals are practicing primary prevention which reduces the risk for the development of emotional problems.

Conceptual Framework

According to Caplan, a crisis is

> . . . when an individual faces an obstacle to important life goals that is, for a time insurmountable through the utilization of customary methods of problem solving. A period of disorganization ensues, a period of upset, during which many different abortive attempts at solution are made.[5]

More succinctly, it is a time of acute, emotional upset. A crisis state is different, however, from those of predicament and stress.

During a predicament, the person may not know which way to turn, but he is usually capable of resolving his dilemma. The same holds true for the state of stress, which in western society, is part of life. An inordinate amount of stress, however, may lead to a crisis situation. Holmes and Rahe developed a useful assessment tool which assigns nu-

merical values to life situations which nearly everyone experiences at one time or another.[6] These situations include changes relative to one's self, family, employment, school, or finances. If the total score of life changes over a time span of 1 year is 0 to 150, there is a 37 percent chance of becoming ill; 151 to 300, increases the chances to 51 percent, and if the score is 301 and over, there is an 80 percent possibility of becoming sick. It is important to note that the life change situation scale includes both positive and negative events. For example, marriage is assigned a mean value of 50 and outstanding personal achievement, 28. The determining factor is whether or not the life structure calls for a role or relationship change—that is, does it require the individual to deviate from the familiar and venture into the unknown.

Nursing students, for example, could have readjustment scores of about 276 within a year of graduating if they marry (50), have changes in finances (38), responsibilities (29), living conditions (24), personal habits (23), residence (20), recreation (19), social activities (17), sleeping patterns (16), eating habits (15), in addition to completing school (25). These scores would also apply to freshmen nursing students. It is important to remember that the total score is not a guarantee of illness, since successful coping may allay the crisis state.

DURATION

A crisis is time-limited, lasting from a few minutes to 6 weeks. It cannot continue indefinitely as the individual cannot withstand the disequilibrium and the accompanying anxiety for long periods of time. Caplan notes that by the end of a 6 week period, the individual adapts to achieve some form of equilibrium or homeostasis.[7] An important implication for clinicians is that intervention must be started as soon as possible. If a client has to wait 4 to 6 weeks to be examined, he may have already resolved the crisis but not always successfully.

A crisis may seem to last longer than 6 weeks. However, upon closer examination one can see that a second crisis is superimposed on the first. Due to the vulnerable state created by the initial crisis, the individual is more susceptible to developing other difficulties which, in turn, increases the duration of disequilibrium.

OUTCOMES

There are three possible outcomes in response to the crisis situation which may occur with or without intervention: (1) adaptation with growth, (2) return to precrisis level, and (3) maladaptation. The minimal therapeutic goal of crisis intervention is crisis resolution to the precrisis level of functioning. Achieving a higher level of functioning is the ideal aim of crisis intervention. Maslow provided the framework for this goal. Based on his research with normal, self-actualized individuals, he concluded that it was possible to grow psychologically as a result of crisis situations.[8] People who accomplish this goal tend to enrich their repertoire of problem-solving skills and are better able to re-establish equilibrium with the next crisis.

Maladaptive adjustments occur when the individual's level of functioning is lower than that of his precrisis state. This is the result of a number of factors, including personality, previous experience, and availability of support systems. Possible outcomes of poor adaptation are suicide, drug and alcohol abuse, and illegal activities. Polak believes that emotional disorders with subsequent psychiatric hospitalization are due to a series of poorly resolved antecedent crisis situations.[9]

FACTORS INFLUENCING OUTCOME. A number of forces are identifiable as influencing the aftermath of a crisis. These include the outcomes of previous crisis states, and the individual's available internal and external resources. These resources encompass the family, friends, health care professionals, agencies, or any support system available to the client in times of stress. Caplan maintains that though past experience influences outcome, external intervention at the appropriate time is more significant. Aquilera and Messick also believe that crisis intervention techniques are more effective with lower socioeconomic groups than long-term psychotherapy as it focuses on achieving only symptomatic relief and not basic personality reconstruction.

Classification

Traditionally, there are two major categories of crisis situations. These are the maturational crisis and the situational crisis. With both types, the individual perceives a stressful event as an obstacle and since his usual coping mechanisms are not sufficient to handle the disturbing event, a period of disorganization is a result of the individual's inability to maintain equilibrium.

MATURATIONAL CRISIS

As noted earlier, Erikson's theory[3] provides a framework for understanding the developmental or maturational crisis. Here, one experiences turmoil in the normal transitional states of growth and development. As the individual matures, there is a constant need to readjust. An interesting way to view the maturational crisis is in terms of gain and loss. For example, to gain independence the person loses dependency, and stress resulting from this situation yields the crisis state for the individual who must find new ways of relating. In each stage of the human life cycle, a new dimension of "social interaction" becomes possible—a new dimension between the individual and his environment. Each growth phase has its strengths and weaknesses, and failures at one stage can be rectified by successes at later stages. Erikson's eight stages of ego development in chronological order are: basic trust versus mistrust, autonomy versus shame and doubt, initiative versus guilt, industry versus inferiority, identity versus role confusion, intimacy versus isolation, generativity versus stagnation, and ego integrity versus despair.

The first stage, trust versus mistrust, extends through the first year of life. The infant, during this time, develops a relationship with his parents, especially his mother. The degree to which the child trusts the world and himself as a person depends on the quality of care given at this time. With this, as with all stages of personality development, the basic issue is not definitively resolved but arises at each subsequent stage of development.

Autonomy versus doubt spans the second and third year of life. Autonomy develops as the child gains a sense of control over his muscles and becomes increasingly adept with motor skills. The child takes pride in his accomplishments, and it is important that nurturers do not do everything for him as he will then come to doubt his ability to control himself and the surrounding environment.

The 4 and 5-year-old child will adaptively leave stage three, initiative versus guilt, if encouraged to function at his own level of ability. Successful completion is dependent upon parental response to his activities and questions.

Industry versus inferiority occurs during the elementary school years, ages 6 to 11. Here, the child begins to reason and adapt to rules. He is generally concerned about details, that is, how things are made and how they work. In this phase, school experiences and the home environment affect the child's sense of self-worth.

The fifth stage, identity versus role confusion, occurs from 12 to 18 and is generally a traumatic one, both from the teenager's perspective and that of his parents. The primary task is to integrate all he has been and knows about himself to develop an identity which carries over into adult life. The adolescent is also called upon to make career choices and if he entered this stage with feelings of shame, doubt, and inferiority, the youth is confused about his role.

The years between young adulthood and middle age are the setting for intimacy versus isolation stage. In addition to finding meaningful life work, the primary task is to develop and maintain an ability to share and care for another without losing one's self-identity in the process. Thus, the focus is on interpersonal relationships in marriage, with friends, or in productive work.

Generative versus self-absorption or stagnation occurs at mid-life. To be generative means the person is concerned with others beyond his immediate self and family and has concern for future generations and the environment they will live in. If this is not established, there is increasing emphasis and focus on self-concerns.

The final stage, integrity versus despair, is a time for reflection. Integrity arises from viewing past life with satisfaction and looking forward to what can be. Despair occurs when looking back with despondency over what might have been and viewing life with bitterness and seeing it as a series of mishaps. For a more detailed discussion of the stages of growth and development see Chapter 1.

Since experiencing these phases is pancultural, the stress resulting from such developmental events can be anticipated and thus, to a degree, prepared for. Williams[12] noted three reasons for dysfunction: (1) the individual may be unable to conceive of himself in the new role; (2) he may lack the resources to make the transition; and (3) there may be a refusal by others to see the individual in the new role. It should also be noted that because of the turmoil and deviation from the familiar, the individual is more insecure and thus more vulnerable to situational crisis states. The previously mentioned work of Holmes and Rahe[6] can be of use in assessing this risk.

SITUATIONAL CRISIS

According to Caplan,[13] situational crises stem from sudden, unpredictable events. They are simply life situations that bring on unplanned changes in one's capacity to function, including such role changes required by marriage, promotion, childbearing, and retirement. It is important to note that role changes affect not only the individual but all others involved in the relationship changes. For example, Caplan and his associates[14] examined the emotional reactions of expectant and new mothers delineating the role changes which transpired as a result of the pregnancy. They concluded that the perception and resolution of these changes influenced the quality of the mother-child relationship. Thus, the mother and the child are affected by the childbearing process, which in turn, may influence the outcome of Erikson's first stage of life for the infant.

Situational crises also include the loss or death of a loved one, premature birth of an infant, natural disasters, monetary losses and illness, whether of a physical or emotional nature. As with role changes, these crisis situations may affect more than one individual. In 1970, the destruction and deaths in Pennsylvania caused by Hurricane Agnes influenced not only the residents but also the families who lived in other areas of the country. President Kennedy's assasination in 1963 was an example of a national crisis.

With respect to illness, the work of Janis[15] has implications for nurses. He divided the responses of clients towards general surgery into three groups. The first group consisted of people who either appeared unconcerned or were relatively unconcerned. A moderate level of concern was manifested by the second group and the final group was composed of individuals highly concerned about the forthcoming surgery. Janis hypothesized that if the client knew what to expect this might alter his recovery phase.

Data was then given to all groups on their prospective surgery and their pre- and postoperative care. He found that the first group was not interested in the information and denied the need for it while the third group was too anxious to assimilate the information. In contrast, the second group requested more data, and their postsurgical course was altered in comparison to the other groups. They required fewer analgesics, progressed more rapidly, and were discharged 1 to 2 days earlier than patients in the other groups who had similar surgery. He concluded that the manner in which a client dealt with the diagnosis for surgery influenced his postsurgical response and that those with moderate anxiety and who did their "worry work" prior to surgery progressed faster. His findings emphasized the need for nurses to provide client teaching and thus provide successful intervention in a situational crisis.

Development of Crisis State

Caplan[16] describes four characteristic phases of crisis onset which help clarify the crisis situation and, hence, the intervention process. (1) Initially there is a rise in tension due to the problem situation which stimulates traditional problem-solving mechanisms. (2) If there is a lack of success in utilizing these mechanisms, the individual experiences an increase in anxiety and tension. (3) A further rise in tension, which may be highly uncomfortable for the individual, acts as a powerful motivator to mobilize all internal and external resources. These may include family, friends, and any supports the individual feels can assist in alleviating the discomfort. One means of avoiding the crisis state is for the person to redefine and change his goals which are dependent on his flexibility and ability to adapt. (4) Finally, if the problem is still unresolved and the usual coping mechanisms have not worked, there is a further rise in tension to the breaking point where the individual manifests the symptomatology of a crisis state.

INTERVENTION

Crisis intervention is a time-limited helping process which focuses on the resolution of the immediate problem. During this process, the clinician assists in mobilizing any resources to achieve this end.

Therefore, accurate assessment and awareness of personal, social, and environmental supports are essential to successful intervention.

Goal of Crisis Intervention

The minimal goal is achieving resolution of the immediate problem and restoration of the client to a precrisis level of functioning. Hopefully intervention will promote growth so that the individual adds to his repertoire of coping skills and thus achieves a higher level of functioning. Specific goals are situational and dependent on one's assessment of the crisis state.

Achieving the optimal aim is feasible due to a number of factors. As noted earlier, people in crisis are in disequilibrium and thus more open to change. Caplan[17] substantiates this by noting that one may achieve maximum results with minimal effort due to the instability created by the crisis. The experience of successful coping, for the individual, leads to an increased self-esteem and a transfer of new knowledge which helps the person in future stressful situations.

Length of Treatment

Since the duration of the crisis is usually 4 to 6 weeks, it is essential that intervention occur during this time span. Generally, one to six sessions or contacts via telephone or home visits lead to resolution of the immediate problem. In an acute care setting, it is especially important to respond as clients may be discharged in 1 or 2 weeks.

During the crisis period, the client may experience feelings of bewilderment and being overwhelmed. Hence, it is useful to inform them of the duration and that it is time-limited. It may also be important to visit the highly anxious client for short periods of time. The actual length of time, whether a few minutes or an hour, is dependent on the degree of anxiety and how this anxiety affects the individual's ability to understand and deal with the stressor.

Nurse's Role

Intervening in crisis situations is not restricted to the domain of professionals. Community mental health movements endorse the utilization of properly trained paraprofessionals or community workers and, in general, they have been effective. Caplan,[18] however, states that the nurse possesses the unique qualities of psychological and sociological closeness with her clients, which help to establish and maintain the working relationship one needs in crisis intervention.

Aquilera and Messick[19] also emphasize that the therapist's role is direct, that is, that of an active participant. Generally, the indirect approaches of psychoanalysis and the nondirective techniques of client centered counseling are ineffective in crisis situations. A frequent manifestation of the crisis state is poor decision-making capability; this, therefore, is the rationale for the clinician's active participation. Another justification is that the client contacts the therapist for assistance which, in effect, is saying "do for me what I currently cannot do for myself." If, however, the assessment reveals the client is not having decision-making impairment, the clinician has legal and ethical obligations to encourage this process.

Since everyone experiences crises throughout their life, the philosophy of crisis, that of normalcy should pervade the therapist's attitude, and the expectation one relates to clients should be one of hopefulness. To this end, it is useful to state that though things look bad now, the client will get better. Successful resolution definitely facilitates one's learning and growth as the individual feels more capable and in control of his life rather than feeling controlled by life.

Assessment

As with any problem situation, one of the initial tasks of the clinician is to perform an accurate assessment. The importance of this cannot be overemphasized. The research of Rosenbaum[20] highlights the hazards of inadequate assessment. In his study, researchers were admitted to a state hospital and were, generally, diagnosed as schizophrenic. When they revealed themselves, they were discharged. Following this, they contacted the hospital stating sane people were going to again seek admission. Though the institution's staff prepared for this follow-up visit, the researchers were again admitted. One interesting finding of the study was that though the staff was unable to detect the actors, the patients were able to identify them. Thus, accurate assessment is critical to successful intervention.

MANIFESTATIONS

Hansell,[21] who studied with Caplan, maintained that people in crisis experience a disruption of significant attachments to the world around the n. His basic thesis is that the life of each individual involves a stable transaction between the individual and his social, cultural, and psychological environment, and when these transactions or attachments are severed or about to be severed, one goes into crisis. He defined the following seven areas of attachment which the individual needs to maintain stability or equilibrium:

1. *Physical*: These are the basic needs for the individual to keep and maintain his orientation to the physical world (e.g., food and housing).
2. *Social*: The individual needs to have a meaningful social role (e.g., student, mother, wife, etc.) and to feel comfortable in this role. It is also necessary to assess how significant others react to this role and if it creates conflict. For example, if a husband objects to his wife working, this may create problems in their relationship.
3. *Community*: This means that the individual has a sense of roots, belonging. The suicidal individual frequently feels isolated and detached from the world around him.
4. *Intimacy*: This extends beyond sexual needs in that the person needs at least one individual in whom he can confide and count on for support. Again returning to the suicidal individual, he frequently has this support but perceives that he does not, which relates to his low self-esteem.
5. *Decision-making*: This deals with one's intellectual competence to handle problems in a way that is satisfying to him.
6. *Meaning*: Each individual operates by a set of values, which for him, mean his existence is worthwhile. This varies from person to person, and it is, therefore, necessary to ask what they view as important in their life. If a middle-income person loses his employment the impact may be greater than for the individual

who is periodically on public assistance, or if parents view college education as essential, but their offspring do not value or see the need for education.

7. *Economic*: This means that people need a way to survive economically within their community.

Assessment on a more personal and specific level includes exploring the individual's affective, cognitive, and behavioral manifestations of crisis. Affective relates to the feeling state of the individual, while cognitive refers to the person's thinking and perceptual processes, and behavioral to what he does and how he acts in response to the problem situation. Table 1 summarizes these manifestations.

AFFECTIVE MANIFESTATIONS. Affective symptomatology relates to the person's feelings of not being in control of the situation and includes feelings of panic and sadness. The latter needs to be differentiated from depression which may occur as an outcome of a maladaptively resolved crisis. Severe anxiety, of a physical and emotional nature, may also be present. The individual may also appear angry; this anger is usually directed inwardly for not being able to control the situation. At times, a divorce or death may precipitate anger at others for leaving. Frequently, the verbal manifestation of anger is "why is this happening to me."

Other affective signs, including guilt, are related to the feelings of anger. Lindemann identified and intervened with situations of survivor guilt where the person experienced anger at a person for leaving him. This, in turn, led to guilt feelings over this reaction and more significantly for surviving the catastrophe. Feelings of fear with a sense of isolation and self-worthlessness may also be present.

COGNITIVE MANIFESTATIONS. Cognitive or perceptual indications of crisis include confusion. As with anger, this may be expressed as "why is this happening to me." Poor decision-making ability with a short attention span and inability or difficulty concentrating may also be present. In addition, the client may manifest a distorted perception of reality and "tunnel vision" where the individual is unable to place the situation in proper perspective. It is important to distinguish this reality distortion from that found in psychotic disorders. Generally, the misperception present in crisis states does not have the systematic disorganization that occurs with underlying psychopathology, nor does the psychotic client portray the affective or behavioral manifestations that are apparent with a crisis situation.

BEHAVIORAL MANIFESTATIONS. Immobilization is a behavioral sign of crisis. In an attempt to resolve the problem, immobilization may lead to impulsive behavior where the client abuses drugs or alcohol and may become suicidal or homicidal. These actions are due to the person's effort to alleviate the discomfort that the crisis state creates for him. Crying may also be present but as with reality distortion, it is important to differentiate this from other problems. Again, a crisis probably does not exist if there is an absence of cognitive and affective dysfunction. Agitation, possibly in the form of pacing is a behavioral indicator of high anxiety.

CRISIS COMPONENTS

Throughout the assessment process, it has been highlighted that the clinician needs to ascertain if a crisis is present in the client. A useful framework to facilitate this process is one developed by Golen,[22] who adapted and refined Caplan's phases of crisis onset, maintaining that all four components are

TABLE 7-1. Individual Manifestations of Crisis

Affective:	Cognitive:	Behavioral:
Panic	Aborted decision-making	Immobilization
Sadness	Short attention span	Crying
Emotional lability	Distractibility	Agitation
High anxiety	Tunnel vision	Work-eating-recreation-rest
Anger	Reality distortion	Cycle disruption
Fear		
Guilt		
Isolation		
Worthlessness		

needed for identifying a situation as a crisis. These are the hazardous event, vulnerable state, precipitating factor, and state of active crisis.

The hazardous event is the initial external or internal circumstance which triggers the chain of events leading to the state of active crisis. A useful question to ascertain this stage is "What has been happening?" This type of inquiry provides a broad base from which to assess the client since it is general and open-ended.

The emotional and subjective reaction to the hazardous event is the vulnerable state. Asking the individual how he perceives the current problem provides an indication of the degree of stress. In addition, ascertaining the individual's typical response to problems, "What do you usually do when upset?" also provides information on vulnerability and the adequacy of his coping mechanisms.

The precipitating factor may, at times, be difficult to distinguish from the hazardous event but is usually the final straw. To help identify this disruptive blow stating "It looks like a lot of things have been happening; what occurred today?" is a means of focusing the interview. If the person responds that he does not know, asking "What were you thinking about just prior to calling or coming in?" may help delineate the precipitating factor. Assisting the individual to focus and identify the stressor is important, as people in crisis tend to feel overwhelmed and manifest circumstantial thought processes.

The state of active crisis occurs when the tension and anxiety has risen to an uncontrollable peak, and the individual manifests it with signs of a cognitive, affective, and behavioral nature. One key to determining if a crisis exists is assessing the degree of disruption in normal functioning. Therefore, ascertaining how the person views the problem as it affects him is necessary. Hence, it is also essential to find out what is normal for the individual, if similar situations occured in the past, and how he dealt with them. Though everybody requires a degree of anxiety to function, cognitive impairment requires prompt response. Without intervention, the individual may develop neurotic or psychotic symptomatology in an effort to cope with the problem.

DEVELOPING A PLAN

The initial plan is dependent on the therapist gathering enough data through the assessment process,

including information on factors influencing the client's disequilibrium and the manifestations of crisis. Particular emphasis is placed on identifying coping behaviors, determining the degree of disruption in everyday functioning, exploring the individual's perception, and ascertaining potential and actual resources. Thus, if the clinician realizes these elements are missing, his first plan might be to gather more information.

Aquilera and Messick refer to these as balancing factors. Figure 7-1 presents the effect of balancing factors in response to a stressful event. In contrast, Figure 7-2 portrays what happens when one or more of the balancing factors is absent.

With respect to identifying coping behavior, it is also necessary to assess whether or not it is healthy and realistic. Possible questions to facilitate this

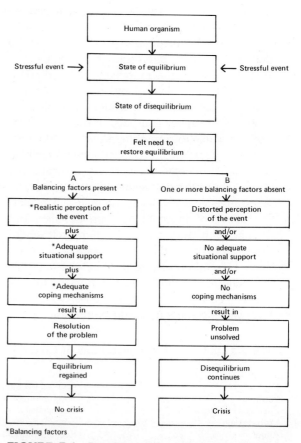

FIGURE 7-1. Paradigm: effect of balancing factors in a stressful event. (Reproduced with permission from Aquilera, D. C., and Messick, J. M.: *Crisis Intervention*, 3rd. ed. St. Louis, C. V. Mosby Co., 1978.)

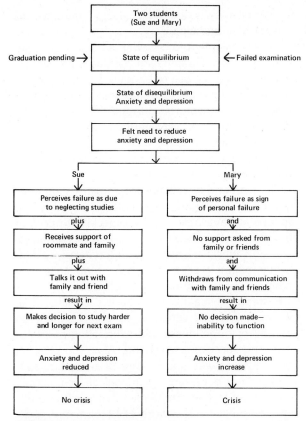

```
                    ┌─────────────────────┐
                    │   Two students      │
                    │   (Sue and Mary)    │
                    └─────────────────────┘
                               │
Graduation pending →  ┌─────────────────────┐  ← Failed examination
                      │ State of equilibrium│
                      └─────────────────────┘
                               │
                    ┌─────────────────────┐
                    │ State of disequilibrium│
                    │ Anxiety and depression │
                    └─────────────────────┘
                               │
                    ┌─────────────────────┐
                    │   Felt need to reduce  │
                    │  anxiety and depression│
                    └─────────────────────┘
                               │
              Sue  ───────────┴─────────────── Mary
```

Sue

Perceives failure as due to neglecting studies

plus

Receives support of roommate and family

plus

Talks it out with family and friend

result in

Makes decision to study harder and longer for next exam

Anxiety and depression reduced

No crisis

Mary

Perceives failure as sign of personal failure

and

No support asked from family or friends

and

Withdraws from communication with family and friends

result in

No decision made— inability to function

Anxiety and depression increase

Crisis

FIGURE 7-2. Paradigm applied to case studies. (Reproduced with permission from Aquilera, D. C., and Messick, J. M.: *Crisis Intervention*, 3rd. ed. St. Louis, C. V. Mosby Co., 1978.)

process include: "How do you respond when under stress?" "Can you think of other ways you could handle this situation?" "How did you act when similar situations occurred in the past?" and "How is this different?"

Knowledge on the extent of the disruption of everyday functioning may be assessed by exploring whether or not the client is able to carry on his routine activities such as school, work, and housework. Asking how he sees himself affecting others also sheds light on the degree of disequilibrium.

Exploring the client's perception of the situation's dynamics and his problem-solving skills may be accomplished by inquiring, "How do you think this situation came about?" and "Can you think of any way to handle the problem?" The therapist's goal in this case and throughout the intervention process

is to promote cognitive mastery; that is, in addition to widening his perception of the problem, the clinician also assists in comprehending intellectually the dynamics of the crisis state.

Finally, it is important to examine the individual's resources, noting who is mentioned and, more significantly, who is not included as a support system. If the client's family is not specified, it may be indicative of difficulty with them even if they appear irrelevant to the presenting problem. Therefore, it is necessary to verify this assumption by asking "I've noticed while we've been talking that you haven't mentioned your family. Tell me about them."

PLAN AND TECHNIQUES

Hoff[23] identified the following characteristics of the treatment plan which, in turn, clarify the intervention process: (1) problem-oriented, (2) realistic, (3) social network, (4) relevant to assessment, (5) collaboration, (6) time-limited and concrete, (7) dynamic and negotiable, (8) fosters a healthy outcome, (9) assesses risk of suicidal, homicidal, and impulsive behavior, (10) groundwork for long-term counseling, and (11) includes evaluation framework. These are attempts to resolve the immediate problem; they are not historically oriented. The clinician examines the individual's past life experiences only to ascertain how they influence the present. If chronic alcoholism leads to unemployment and subsequent eviction, the focus is on obtaining food and shelter for the client.

Interventions must also be realistic in that they match agency resources to client needs. If a telephone assessment reveals a client in acute distress and transportation is a problem, it would be inappropriate to ask the client to come for an immediate appointment. Instead, the worker needs to examine potential resources such as obtaining a ride from a friend or going to the client's home. To be realistic, the clinician must constantly validate and revalidate plans.

Interrelated with seeking validations is that efforts are mutually arrived at by the client and therapist. (This process is called contracting.) Collaboration is a cornerstone of the philosophy of crisis theory and intervention for it highlights the expectation of improvement. Delineating tasks and who is responsible for their completion also alleviates, to a degree, the client's feelings of worthlessness for it gives the person a sense of power and control. In addition, this process facilitates evaluation for it defines accountability.

Techniques also include involving the client's significant others and social network. As Hansell[19] emphasized, each individual is intricately involved with several areas of attachment and, therefore, others need to be included in actual interventions. If a client expresses discomfort about involving others, the clinician should convey an attitude that it is all right to seek help as we all need support at times. At the same time, the health professional must explore what it means for the person to seek help and what he thinks would happen if he did ask for assistance.

Efforts should also be relevant to the health professional's assessment of the client. Since affective manifestations tend to dominate, it is possible to counteract feelings of being overwhelmed and immobilized by emphasizing cognitive questions. Asking "What do you think is happening?" and "What are you basing this on?" assists in overcoming tunnel vision and tones down the emotionality of the situation.

It is also important for the health professional to be prepared to deal with feelings of anger, denial, and displacement. Since the crisis situation evokes many feelings of discomfort, it may be natural for someone to deny its impact. To overcome this state, perhaps some of the following questions could be asked: "I've noticed you haven't been discussing the implications of leaving school. Is it uncomfortable for you?" "What would it mean for you to think about this?" and "What do you think would happen?" If the client manifests anger or displacement, the health professional can respond with, "I hear your anger, let's discuss what's happening." By asking in this manner, the health professional is providing support, encouraging ventilation, and acting as a role model in how to deal with stress.

The plan and subsequent interventions must be time-limited and very concrete with regard to appointment times, place, length of contact, and who will be involved in the interview. The clinician must also be able to give his rationale for any plans with respect to the aforementioned items. For example, if the client is highly anxious with impaired activities of daily living (ADL) functioning, shorter sessions focusing on this, rather than having entirely verbal contact may be helpful.

Another element to consider is the threat of suicidal or homicidal behavior. Under what circumstances would the use of tranquilizers be appropriate? It is important to recognize that anxiety acts as a powerful motivator and though uncomfortable, medication will not alleviate the stress. Thus, motivation is maintained by anxiety, supportive concern, and personal investment in the problem-solving process.

The plan and techniques for implementing must also be dynamic and negotiable in that alternate options are available. This is especially important in counteracting the client's feelings of worthlessness and futility. Hence, if an intervention is ineffective, planning alternate actions in advance may minimize the risk of increased vulnerability.

Fostering a healthy outcome is the focus of all planning and interventions. As noted earlier, an attitude of hopefulness and contracting assists in achieving successful resolution. Also, the clinician needs to be aware that feelings of anger and sadness are not necessarily pathological for it is only when these feelings are denied that residual problems may occur. The work of Lindemann[1] highlights this point, and it is therefore useful to utilize techniques of encouraging ventilation and offering support. Distorted reality perception and subsequent suspiciousness or blaming may be dealt with by stating "I hear you saying that you think your husband hates you, yet I think it would be useful to examine what you are basing this on and what else is contributing to the problem." Though catharsis and ventilation do not, generally, resolve the problem, they provide a stepping stone as covert conflict becomes overt, thus facilitating resolution.

Evaluation and Anticipatory Guidance

Developing a viable plan of interventions requires that the health care provider build a framework from which to evaluate it. This then enables the clinician to review and alter only those actions that are ineffective. As noted earlier, active client participation helps allay feelings of powerlessness and also improves client compliance. Maluccio and Marlow[24] noted that contracting, when properly utilized, facilitates the achievement of client participation. Contracts are also helpful in keeping the focus on the "here and now" or immediate problem resolution.

Nelson and Mowry[25] also identified some benefits of contracting. They felt that it clarified role relationships thus providing structure, thereby, decreasing severe anxiety states. In addition, it defined the problems, responsibilities, and alternatives facing both the client and counsellor, thus facilitating the focus on the present. Contracting also minimizes the development of unhealthy dependency for it delineates the length of treatment and the participants' responsibilities. Since the client has a role in defining the problem, contracting minimizes the use of stigmatizing labels which would violate the philosophy of crisis methodology.

Though successful resolution is dependent on the specific situation, a number of responses are identifiable as guidelines for determining if interventions are effective or ineffective. Table 7-2 summarizes possible maladaptive and adaptive reactions.

Anticipatory guidance is planning with the individual to reduce the possibility of future crises. Decision counseling and summarization are part of this

TABLE 7-2. Evaluation Guidelines

Maladaptive:
1. Manifests excessive denial and withdrawal by retreating into fantasy which may overlay or replace reality.
2. Impulsive behavior possibly directing rage at vulnerable family members who allow scapegoating.
3. Dependency as demonstrated by excessive clinging or counter-dependency avoidance.
4. Emotions are often denied or overcontrolled with subsequent disruptive discharge.
5. "Helpless-hopeless" syndrome.
6. Ritualistic behavior which serves little or no purpose.
7. Continued work-rest cycle disruption.
8. Tendency to use alcohol, drugs, and food as cures.
9. Individual cannot evoke or invoke help.

Adaptive:
1. Able to deal simultaneously with the affective manifestations and the tasks confronting them.
2. Express emotions and is aware of painful emotions while engaging in constant catharsis.
3. Shows cognitive and situational mastery; demonstrates intelligent "worry-work."
4. Able to acknowledge and communicate increased dependency needs.
5. Can seek help, receive it, and utilize it.
6. Tolerates environmental uncertainty without resorting to impulsive actions.
7. Individual values—understanding, discovery, personal growth.

process. Stating "This is what you did in the past, this is what happened, and how else could you handle the situation?" assists the client to understand his role in the crisis. These techniques also may lay the foundation for long-term counseling if and when it is necessary. Though the clinician will not delve into examining the dynamics of alcoholism, he may, by helping with unemployment, food stamps, and housing, provide the groundwork for the client to seek psychotherapy. In turn, resolution of the underlying psychopathology reduces his vulnerability to future crises. Thus, termination following crisis intervention should always be accomplished with an open door where the client is encouraged to return for help in dealing with future crises or for long-term counseling.

SUMMARY

This chapter presented the major principles of crisis theory and intervention techniques. A crisis is a time-limited state of acute, emotional upset in which the usual coping patterns are ineffective. Turmoil occurs when there is a change in status from the familiar as the territory is uncharted, and the individual feels he does not have the skills to deal with the change. Resolution of the crisis may lead to a lower, same, or higher level of functioning. Thus, due to the disequilibrium, the individual is at a turning point in his life.

According to Caplan[26] there are three balancing factors that determine the state of equilibrium. These are the individual's perception of the event, available supports, and coping mechanisms. The counsellor directs intervention efforts at resolving the immediate problem, clarifying the individual's perception, mobilizing and using personal, social and environmental resources, and enhancing coping patterns. The basic process for this is one of ongoing problem-solving, assessing, planning, intervening, and evaluating. The disequilibrium also results in the individual being open to change with maximum results achieved with minimum effort.

Crisis intervention provides the opportunity to practice primary prevention, that is, reducing the incidence of mental disorder by effectively intervening in potentially hazardous circumstances. One needs to recognize that maturational and situational crises are not manifestations of illness but normal parts of everybody's life. They are crises that tax one's resources. A crisis is, therefore, not pathological but an opportunity for self-discovery and personal growth.

REFERENCES

1. Lindemann, E.: Symptomatology and management of acute grief. *Am. J. Psychiatry* 101:141–148, 1944.
2. Lindemann, E.: The meaning of crisis in individual and family. *Teachers College Record* 57:310, 1956.
3. Erikson, E.: *Childhood and Society*. New York, W. W. Norton and Co., 1950.
4. Caplan, G.: *Principles of Preventive Psychiatry*. New York, Basic Books, Inc., 1964.
5. Caplan, G.: *An Approach to Community Mental Health*. New York, Grune and Stratton, Inc., 1961, p. 18.
6. Holmes, T. H., and Rahe, R. H. J.: Life change and subsequent illness report. *Psychoso. Res.* 2:214, 1967.
7. Caplan, *op. cit., An Approach to Community Mental Health*, p. 41.
8. Maslow, A.: *Motivation and Personality*, 2d ed. New York, Harper and Row, 1970.
9. Polak, P. R.: The crisis of admission. *Soc. Psychiatry* 4:150, 1967.
10. Caplan, *op. cit., Principles of Preventive Psychiatry*, pp. 53–54.
11. Aquilera, D. C., and Messick, J. M.: *Crisis Intervention. Theory and Methodology*. St. Louis, C. V. Mosby Co., 1974, pp. 40–53.
12. Williams, F.: Intervention in maturational crises, in *Nursing of Families in Crisis*, edited by Hall, J., and Weaver, B., Philadelphia, J. B. Lippincott, 1974, pp. 43–50.
13. Caplan, *op. cit., Principles of Preventive Psychiatry*, pp. 38–39.
14. Caplan, *op. cit., An Approach to Community Mental Health*, pp. 65–132.
15. Janis, I.: *Psychological Stress*. New York, Wiley and Sons, 1958.
16. Caplan, *op. cit., Principles of Preventive Psychiatry*, pp. 40–41.
17. Caplan, *op. cit., Principles of Preventive Psychiatry*, p. 48.
18. Caplan, *op. cit., An Approach to Community Mental Health*, p. 177.
19. Aquilera and Messick, *op. cit., Crisis Intervention*, pp. 18–21.
20. Rosenbaum, D. L.: On being sane in insane places. *Science* 179:250–258, 1973.
21. Hansell, N.: *The Person in Distress: On the Biosocial Dynamics of Adaptation*. New York, Behavioral Publication Inc., 1976.
22. Golan, N.: When is a client in crisis. *Soc. Casework* 50:389–394, 1969.
23. Hoff, L. A.: Crisis intervention. Workshop sponsored by University of Cincinnati, June 13 and 14, 1977.
24. Maluccio, A. N., and Marlow, W. D.: The case for contract. *Soc. Work* 19:28–36, 1974.
25. Nelson, Z. P., and Mowry, D. D.: Contracting in crisis intervention. *Commun. Men. Health J.* 12:37–44, 1975.
26. Caplan, *op. cit. Principles of Preventive Psychiatry*. pp. 38–54.

CHAPTER 8

Prevention is a comprehensive topic that covers every aspect of the health care system; its personnel, its institutions, and its activities. In fact, prevention is now considered by some to be a specialty, largely because there is a specific and large body of knowledge that is directly concerned with preventive health care. There are even subspecialties within the field. This chapter presents an introduction to the field of prevention. A basic definition of preventive health care will be given within the conceptual framework that is the basis of epidemiology: host, agent, and environment. This framework is in turn based on the more fundamental concepts of health and disease.

A brief discussion will also be given regarding the implementation of preventive health care by health education and screening. Involvement of nursing personnel in prevention will be incorporated throughout the chapter. However, the reader is asked to consider the nurse's role in preventive health care as a philosophical commitment rather than a list of tasks or methodologies. Each nurse

PREVENTIVE HEALTH CARE

Sherry Bame, M.S., R.N.

can then creatively incorporate the goal of prevention into every aspect of health care. Whether the nurse works in a health department, nursing home, or an intensive care unit, preventive goals should always be considered part of the overall health care plan.

TREND TOWARD PREVENTION

Before discussing the definitions of prevention, let us look at what is currently going on that is making prevention a popular topic for everyone, not just those working in the health care field. As more attention is directed toward health care in general, inevitably someone asks, "What is being done to prevent this?" Whether it is smoking and heart disease, cancer and food additives, or general deterioration and physical fitness, there is currently a trend toward concern for the individual's state of health and the factors which influence it.

The mass *media*—that is, television, radio, newspapers, and magazines—have been both a boon

and a bomb regarding preventive health care. Sensational journalism often blows out of proportion the incidence or problem of a relatively rare disease. False reporting or misinformation may be more detrimental than no information at all. On the other hand, effective health education can be accomplished through the media. Motivation to practice prevention, dissemination of specific knowledge about the need for screening, and information about the availability of services have been very effectively handled by the media. No matter where one works or lives in the United States, television and radio have made viewers and listeners more aware of their health and the various threats upon it. Classic television "doctor" shows and afternoon "soap operas" expose a large number of people to medical information, jargon, and the health professionals who provide medical care. Thus, the public at large has become more aware of their own health and diseases and has some image of the care required to remedy and prevent problems.

A second factor that increases the focus on prevention is the *economics* of health care. The increasing costs of illness care is a great concern to everyone. The individual is not only forced to pay high insurance premiums, but also large income tax and social security deductions which help to fund federal health care programs. The President and Congress are continually considering legislation to curb the inflation in medical care. These economic factors are complex and certainly not within the scope of this chapter, but the financial pressure regarding the cost of illness has a major impact on increasing attention toward preventive health care. Very simply, it often costs less money to run a preventive screening or immunization program than it costs to pay for the medical and hospital care expenses to diagnose, treat, and rehabilitate the individuals who would actually contract the disease if not protected.

There are also social costs which indirectly affect financial evaluations of the benefits to preventive health care. The cost of a sick day subsequently affects the employer who either has to replace the sick employee or lose that work (service or product) for a period of time. The family bears the cost of the care in addition to the loss of income. The indirect financial effects spread to others if the individual's care is paid for through a third-party system (e.g., Blue Cross, Workmen's Compensation, Medicaid, Medicare, or a national health insurance). An exponential effect is felt if the disease is communicable. Exposure to others increases the social and financial costs to everyone involved.

Increased *technology* and the resulting increased specialization within the health care field have also contributed to the increased attention on prevention. More is actually known about diseases, their etiology, diagnosis, and treatment. Technology has enabled the medical profession to detect certain diseases at the benign stages. The specialist has refined knowledge about the early detection of certain conditions which has resulted in greater successes in treatment and management of these diseases. Therefore, prevention of the progression of disease and its complications becomes more feasible. In these stages, as well as in the initial detection of symptoms, the nurse plays a crucial role in assessment, observation, motivation, client education, and appropriate interventions.

Thus, due to the forces of the media, economics, and technological developments, more attention

has been directed toward prevention in health care. Underlying all these trends is a more fundamental social revolution in the United States in that health care is now seen as a *right* not a privilege. The same issues that concern our educational system are seen in the health care field. Other systems in our society are compared to health care organization in order to better understand the problems in the health care system. Inevitably, health care ends up standing out as unique. Solutions for other organizations do not work for hospitals. Community organizations have different concerns than ambulatory care organizations. Unlike any other system, the health care system affects everyone at some point in time, and those effects can be critical life and death decisions.

In an effort to mold the health care system to the needs of everyone, creative problem solving must be done in order that the system does not become overburdened and dysfunctional. Preventive health care can make a major contribution to alleviate the stress within the health care system. Primary prevention reduces the number of people in need of health or illness care. It also directs individuals to seek early intervention if needed. This takes less time, money, and personnel. Secondary prevention reduces the resources needed for delivery of acute care. Tertiary prevention is rehabilitative and returns the individual to a productive life, reduces the demand for chronic maintenance care, and reduces the social costs of the illness. Therefore, if health is truly a right for everyone, just as life, liberty, and the pursuit of happiness, then prevention is a necessary part of that "health package."

DEFINITIONS AND FRAMEWORK

Health is defined as more than just the absence of disease. Health involves psychological, emotional, and social considerations as well as physical factors. The World Health Organization includes in its charter this same perspective in its definition of health: "Health is a state of complete physical, mental, and social well-being and not merely the absence of disease or infirmity."[1] Although the World Health Organization defines health as "complete" well-being, health is actually a *relative* state, a "more or less healthy" condition. Factors in the environment that influence the individual result in a *dynamic, interactive* framework of health.

Health can be viewed as a continuum with the ideal "complete physical, mental, and social well-being" at one end and total infirmity or death at the other. Where an individual fits on the continuum is a result of subjective and objective physiological, psychological, and social factors at any point in time as compared to previous "health-illness status." The reader should refer back to Figure 5-1 in Chapter 5, "Health and Illness," which represents a simple line model of the health-illness continuum; however, what is really needed is a multidimensional figure taking into account all factors that influence the "health" of an individual, a family, or a community. However one defines the model subsequently influences how prevention is defined.

Disease

Just as health is the result of a dynamic interactive process, so too is *disease*, each following a *natural history* of its own. This process evolves as the result of *multiple causes*, each interacting and influencing the character of the resulting disease. The progression of this process is susceptible to *interruption* to limit further advancement or to slow or retard its progression.

Epidemiology is the study of the multiple causes of disease and their effects on the progression of the disease process. Three major factors are: (1) characteristics of the disease (*agent*), (2) the individual(s) exposure or susceptibility and their response to the disease producing stimuli (*host*), and (3) the context that facilitates susceptibility and development of the disease (*environment*).

When the host, agent, and environment are all conducive to potentiating each other, then the individual will become ill. This is illustrated in Figure 8-1 by the area where all three circles overlap. A hypothetical example might be a child who is fatigued, has an inadequate nutritional intake, and has no immunizations (host susceptible). It is springtime when measles are prevalent (*agent*), and other children in the class have recently contracted measles (*environment with the agent present*). The child has played and shared his soda with the other children who now have the measles (*host-agent-environment*). Because all three conditions are interacting, the likelihood that this child will come down with the measles is very high. If only two of

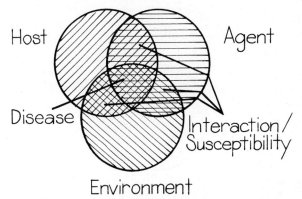

FIGURE 8-1. A model for epidemiology of disease. The degree of overlap of the three factors (host, agent, environment) indicates susceptibility or disease.

the three conditions were present, then the likelihood of the disease occurring is less. For example, if the child has been immunized against measles then his susceptibility is eliminated, and he would not become ill (Fig. 8-2). If the child had not been immunized, therefore was still susceptible, yet was rested and well nourished, then the risk of disease is present but less severe. The model is thus adjusted to show lesser susceptibility, yet still with a potential for disease (Fig. 8-3).

The same alterations can be done with each of the other two aspects of the situation: alteration of the disease agent and the environment. By viewing health care interventions at this level, one can begin to understand the complexity of prevention. How often can we actually alter all three conditions to insure health? Usually, a moderation or adjustment in only one factor is quite an accomplishment.

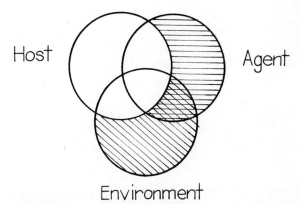

FIGURE 8-2. Prevention of disease by eliminating the susceptibility of one factor—the host.

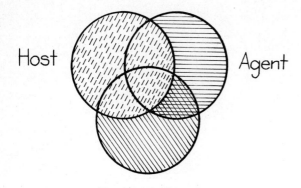

Host   Agent

Environment

FIGURE 8-3. Reducing the likelihood of disease by decreasing the susceptibility of the host.

Prevention

The above discussion focuses on disease and the factors which act to potentiate that disease. When one talks about "prevention," what is actually referred to is "prevention of disease." Disease is used here to mean any illness, injury, or condition which alters the individual's "health" status. Thus, we can refer to prevention of pneumonia, measles, as well as prevention of accidents within the same framework. The focus of preventive intervention efforts is directly related to the identifiable causes of each particular condition; to identify what preventive interventions are needed, one should sketch out the model of host, agent, and environment. Examining each factor for its characteristics in a particular condition gives an idea as to what components are involved. The following example concerning lead paint poisoning illustrates this idea.

Agent: Lead in the paint.
Host: Child with pica is left unsupervised at which time he chewed on furniture, painted materials, or peelings of paint on surfaces. Unknowledgeable about cause-effect of paint causing illness.
Environment: Painted furniture or surfaces that are accessible to the child. Peeling paint, accessible for consumption. Paint contains lead.

When any two factors interact (the overlapping of two circles), then the susceptibility of disease is present. Preventive intervention at this level in-

volves altering any one or more factors so that susceptibility is reduced or eliminated (Fig. 8-4).

Agent: Eliminating lead-based paint.
Host: Supervising the child at all times, and teaching the child about cause of this disease.
Environment: Eliminating paint chips and peeling paint. Painting surfaces at the height or reach of the child with nonlead based paint.

One needs to look at the true feasibility of carrying out these measures to guarantee elimination of the factor in the disease process. In this case, as in most situations, it is unreasonable to assume that the factor can be totally altered. Therefore, one looks at the interactions between factors and evaluates the possibility of reducing risk at this level (Fig. 8-5).

Host-agent: Children with pica should be carefully supervised and taught about the dangers of eating paint chips or chewing on painted surfaces or materials.
Host-environment: If the child has pica, special care should be taken to avoid peelings or chipped paint and when possible, nonlead-based paint used. If the child and environment are susceptible, an extreme measure would be to relocate the family to different living quarters.
Agent-environment: Living arrangements and play facilities where the likelihood of children being present should use nonlead-

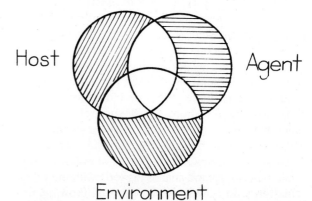

Host   Agent

Environment

FIGURE 8-4. Consideration of variables in each of the three factors (host, agent, environment) helps determine the potential for interaction and susceptibility to disease.

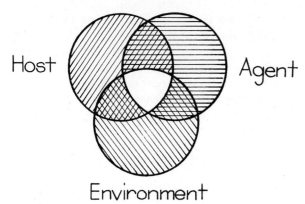

FIGURE 8-5. Focus for preventive care is to alter one or more factors so that susceptibility is reduced or eliminated.

based paint. Managers or builders of apartments or subdivisions which attract young families should be aware of this danger. Builders of play equipment should be knowledgeable about the potential of lead poisoning.

Although this example is abbreviated, hopefully the reader can begin to sense how to identify a model for prevention for any condition, whether it is a communicable disease, occupational disease, injury, carcinoma, or behavioral or psychological problem. By looking at each factor individually and then at the effects of interaction, one can identify specific actions that can be taken, thereby making the process manageable. Interventions at this level are identified as primary prevention.

When the situation is such that the three factors overlap, then the disease process begins (Fig. 8-6). Intervention at this phase is termed secondary prevention. The natural history of a disease or "non-health" condition is important in order to recognize the interventions which are appropriate for accurate diagnosis and treatment. A typical progression for disease is:

Subclinical:
   Disease present but cannot be detected.
   Laboratory abnormalities under stress.
   Laboratory abnormalities at rest.
Clinical:
   Clinical abnormalities under stress.
   Clinical abnormalities at rest.
   Patient feels ill: malaise, discomfort.

Interference with tasks.
Interference with roles.
Interference with mobility.
Death.[2]

Interventions are determined according to the stage of the illness. Preventive efforts are attempted as early as possible to halt and reverse the process. If effective therapeutic measures are not known, attempts are made to minimize the progression of disease. Screening attempts to diagnose subclinical cases at an early stage to avoid clinical onset of the disease or to set up a treatment program to minimize the effects of the illness. Therapeutic interventions at later stages may also stop the progression and restore the individual to a more independent state of functioning.

The multidisciplinary involvement in health care can also be viewed within this framework. The separate realms of the host, the agent, and the environment are influenced by researchers and educators in the fields of physiology, pathology, psychology, sociology, and by environmentalists, nutritionists, and health educators (Fig. 8-7). Medical, nursing, and social work involvement begins largely after interactions have occurred and suspicion is present that disease or "ill health" could develop. Activities center around minimizing or eliminating the risk of disease (Fig. 8-8).

The health care professional's involvement intensifies if the disease continues (Fig. 8-9). Other allied health professionals, such as physical therapists, occupational therapists, and dieticians become involved at this point to minimize the progressive ef-

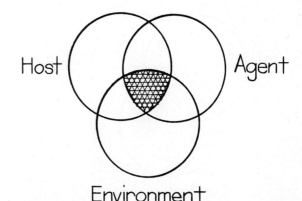

FIGURE 8-6. When all three factors interact, the disease process begins.

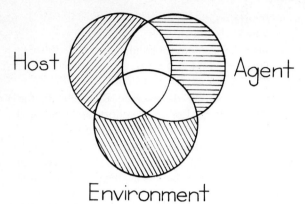

FIGURE 8-7. The focus of attention of researchers and educators is to understand the role each factor plays in the natural history of disease.

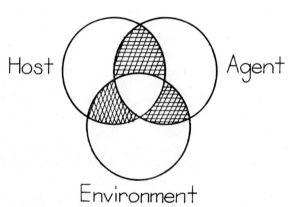

FIGURE 8-8. Activities of health professionals center on the areas of interaction, trying to minimize or eliminate the risk of disease.

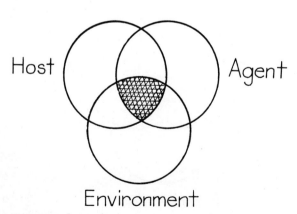

FIGURE 8-9. As disease develops, the health care professionals' involvement intensifies.

fect of the illness. Medical care centers around diagnostic, surgical, pharmaceutical, or other therapeutic interventions. Nursing is involved in facilitating the diagnostic and therapeutic processes as well as providing support and knowledge to the client and family to effectively cope with the illness and to move toward independence in management of the condition.

LEVELS OF PREVENTION

Primary Prevention

Primary prevention has been defined as intervention on the factors—host, agent, and environment—that cause disease. There are two categories within this stage: health promotion and specific protection. Health promotion involves those elements which potentiate "health" in a physical, psychological, and social sense. It is looking at the variables that can cause disease states and working to alter their effects in each of the three factors—host, agent, and environment (Fig. 8-10). Nursing's primary concern is with the individual or host. Education for a good standard of nutrition adjusted to the growth and development needs of the individual is health promotion to prevent susceptibility of the host to disease producing factors. The study of genetics and genetic counseling are primary prevention activities that examine physiological factors which act in the resistance or susceptibility toward disease (e.g., sickle cell anemia and malaria). Personality development involves families and groups

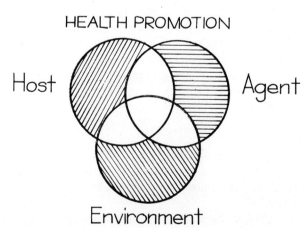

HEALTH PROMOTION

FIGURE 8-10. The shaded areas indicate the focus of attention for health promotion in primary prevention.

in the community to enable the individual to achieve emotional well-being. Provision of adequate housing, safe recreation facilities, and a safe work place is within the realm of primary prevention in the environment. Each of these factors influences the liability of the individual host toward susceptibility or potential for the development of disease. In other words, health promotion involves the elements within each of the three areas and their ability to upset the delicate equilibrium of a healthy state.

A second aspect in primary prevention is that of specific protection. This is concerned with the boundary lines between each of the three factors where factors overlap (Fig. 8-11). Specific protection activities are involved with reinforcements that can be implemented to strengthen each area and prevent or minimize overlap or risk. Examples of specific protection are immunization, personal hygiene, environmental sanitation, protection against occupational hazards, protection against accidents, use of specific nutrients, protection against carcinogens, avoidance of allergens, and fluoridation. The list goes on and on. Basically, changes are made in any combination of three factors—agent, host, or environment—with a particular focus to eliminate or alter specific disease-causing elements.

In carrying out health promotion and specific protection measures, there are three considerations to keep in mind: feasibility, cost, and social factors. First, is it possible? Do we have the knowledge and technology to actually implement prevention at this level? For most of the communicable diseases we do, but for diseases such as cancer or mental illness, we are limited and unable to provide prevention at this level.

The second consideration in implementation of primary prevention is the cost of the program. How many personnel are needed? How available are the materials needed, for example fluoride or immunogens? How expensive would it be to provide protection for everyone? How does this measure against the risk involved in the prevention program (e.g., anaphylactic reactions from immunizations)? Or is a sufficient measure of protection provided if certain groups who are more susceptible are given specific help? These high risk groups (target groups) derive the greatest benefit from the costs of the resources and energy spent on preventive measures (Fig. 8-12).

Another measure of cost/benefit is to identify the monitary and social resource costs in providing the preventive measure(s) as weighed against the potential cost of the disease or injury which could result. For example, the cost of safety goggles for every worker in the factory is measured against the cost of blindness for that worker, his family, and the employer.

An additional perspective to cost of primary prevention is to look at the extensiveness of the program and its worth in totally eradicating the problem. In other words, specific protection can be provided by interventions in any one or two factors, but to totally eliminate the disease, there must be intervention in all three factors. Are the costs of resources involved to do this worth the small re-

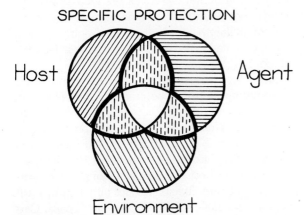

SPECIFIC PROTECTION

Host   Agent

Environment

FIGURE 8-11. Specific protection in primary prevention is concerned with reinforcing the boundaries of overlap to minimize interactions.

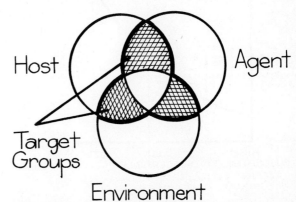

Host   Agent

Target Groups

Environment

FIGURE 8-12. High risk or target groups derive the greatest benefit from the costs of preventive measures.

duction in risk that is involved? Take for example the management of smallpox. For the risks of innoculation reactions, the susceptibility risk to smallpox in the United States is too small. Malaria management is another example. The cost of totally eradicating malaria as compared to the risk of contracting the disease is out of proportion. A hypothetical curve is presented in Figure 8-13 to illustrate this point.

The third consideration in the implementation of primary prevention measures is the social factors involved. Are there legal barriers which must be overcome in implementing the specific preventive measure? The controversy over fluoridation illustrates this factor. Are there beliefs, prejudices, and superstitions which affect implementation and utilization of specific prevention measures? Christian Scientists have a different belief system toward disease causation, and therefore immunizations are prohibited within their belief framework.

Enforcement of preventive measures may be needed and the rights of the individual ignored in order to "protect" the majority. Immunizations required for school entry are an example of this. The federal government imposes its standards on employers and employees in the enforcement of the Occupational Safety and Health Act (OSHA). The worker may not even be aware of hazards yet is forced to wear safety gear. For rat control programs, higher taxes may be levied for housing and

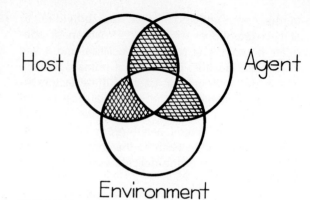

FIGURE 8-14. Specific protection of primary prevention.

neighborhood improvement, and perhaps even displacing some persons in the interest of protection against environmental hazards. These social "costs" must be weighed and evaluated carefully as to the extent of benefit gained (protection against disease) for the imposition of certain values and beliefs and loss of certain freedoms.

As mentioned earlier, there are areas where two of the factors overlap (Fig. 8-14). These fall within the realm of specific protection within primary intervention, yet the character of interventions are different in that a high degree of susceptibility exists and if not reduced, disease is highly likely. This is known as the prepathogenic stage in the natural history of the disease. All that is needed is the presence of the third factor and disease results. It is this combination of environmental and agent factors that predispose a situation for malaria. The interaction of a "susceptible type" of child and the conducive environment predisposes lead poisoning. Poor refrigeration and the type of food susceptible to salmonella growth results in food poisoning in a high percentage of cases, once the host factor is added.

Heredity, socioeconomic factors, and the physical environment may be creating a disease state long before the disease is manifest or can be detected. The situation has such a high probability for developing into disease, that all that needs to be added is the third factor, whether it be agent, environment, or host. In these situations, the prevention activities are directed toward target groups with high risk potential for developing the disease. Case finding and routine screening become important to detect the point at which a high degree susceptibility becomes disease.

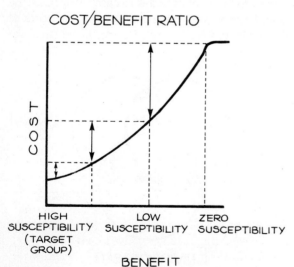

COST/BENEFIT RATIO

FIGURE 8-13. Hypothetical cost/benefit analysis for preventive measures based on degree of susceptibility.

Many situations persist in this chronic high risk or susceptible state. Some never develop into clinically manifest disease. There is confusion whether this is actually primary or secondary prevention. The level of knowledge and technology may be such that the disease is present, but we are unable to detect it at this stage. Or the situation may be that an individual host is actually a carrier of the disease yet will not manifest detectable symptoms.

Secondary Prevention

Once interactions take place between all three factors—the individual host, the disease agent, and conducive environmental conditions—the disease process begins (Fig. 8-15). The *pathogenic* process begins with a subclinical stage then progresses to the clinical stage, resulting in infirmity and death if no interventions are made. The nature of the progression and the rate depends on the disease's particular natural history and the continuing forces in the host, agent, and environment.

Subclinical pathogenesis of chronic disease is usually more difficult to detect than for acute diseases because of the subtlety of symptoms. Early signs and symptoms of malnutrition, mental illness, or arthritis are frequently missed or confused with other problems. Because of this, any deviation from "normal" is suspect for disease. But "normal" is not an absolute condition, and often complex interactions influence "normal" states in unknown ways. Therefore, clues for secondary prevention are sometimes obvious and at other times, indistinct, depending entirely on the individual, the observer, the settings, the time (day, month, or year), prior events, and concurrent events.

Because of these subtleties in early disease detection, this stage in secondary prevention relies heavily on the nurse to do initial screening based on her knowledge of "normal" states for various situations and growth and development levels. The school nurse and the industrial nurse can be instrumental in case finding at this level. Mass screening done by health departments contribute to the identification of subclinical states. The community health nurse and office or clinic nurse may identify clues about family members of the client under care. These suspect cases then are encouraged to follow-up on diagnostic screenings. The nurse's ability to educate clients about the signs and symp-

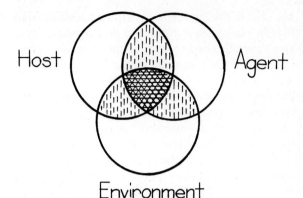

FIGURE 8-15. Secondary prevention focuses attention on the area of interaction of all three factors, that is, the disease process.

toms present and how those relate to the disease process are crucial in motivating individuals to initiate care. The nurse may also play a vital role in facilitating access to care, once the individual is motivated to initiate care. The health care system can be mystifying, bureaucratic, and frustrating in attempts to procure adequate care. As a client advocate, the nurse can make a crucial difference in the individual actually getting the appropriate care as well as influencing the quality of that care received.

If intervention at this early pathogenic stage is not made, the progression of the disease is influenced by several factors: length and intensity of exposure, the natural history of the particular condition, the resistance elements in the host, and the precipitative factors in the environment. The latter elements have a unique influence on the disease process. If all three factors are conducive to development of the disease, then only minimum exposure is needed. If each element is highly resistant or has a high tolerance level, then the likelihood of clinical manifestation is low.

The pathogenic course is (1) subclinical to (2) clinical without felt need to (3) clinical with felt need. Subclinical is defined as positive laboratory findings of abnormal tissue or other early measurement of deficiencies or deviations from "normal." Clinical abnormalities may be manifest but not perceived by the individual or others around him without routine or periodic examinations. Usually, however, clinical findings are not detected unless the individual has felt interference with normal activities, that is, feeling mildly ill or uncomfortable; unable to participate in normal routine activities for a short period; need to change the normal routine because of the chronicity of the condition; or directly effected in the individual's degree of independence in mobility and activities of daily living. At each of these stages, the disease process may be interrupted and stabilized, at which point convalescence begins. The degree of success in the pathogenic course of the condition depends on: (1) the completeness of knowledge regarding the natural history of the disease; (2) the opportunities to apply that knowledge; and (3) the actual application of that knowledge. Diagnosis is one part of application, and treatment is another in the effort to halt the disease process.

The nurse collaborates with others on the health care team in secondary prevention measures. The physician is trained in diagnostic skills and in determination of appropriate treatment. However, the success of that diagnosis and therapy depends on the client's initial motivation to seek care and subsequently to follow through with interventions. It is in these areas that nursing can play a crucial role. The nurse in the community may be influential in discovering a condition which is "non-normal" and in encouraging the individual to seek care. Whether the individual perceives a problem or not, the school nurse or industrial nurse may detect subtle clues that arouse suspicion, indicating that further evaluation is necessary. For example, a child falling on the playground may not be seen as having a problem, but an astute school nurse may put this situation together with other incidents and suspect signs of epilepsy. The detective skills of picking out bits and pieces of information about deviations from normal behavior are something in which the nurse is trained—that is, observation and assessment skills. Thus, the initial activities in secondary prevention—screening and diagnosis—are facilitated by a nurse's assessment and health teaching skills in getting the client initially involved in the health care activities.

Actual application of medical treatment is usually done by the nurse under the direction or initiation of a physician. The success of a therapeutic measure often depends on the exactness and completeness with which it is implemented, which is a primary responsibility of the nurse. Also, client cooperation and follow-through are influenced by

the client teaching done by the nurse. Interpretation of the rationale for treatment and explanation of the techniques and possible complications are important areas that the nurse shares with the client in an attempt to intervene in the disease process.

Nurses are also involved in another aspect of secondary prevention—that is, the contribution to the body of knowledge about the disease processes. Research is one mode of contribution, but perhaps more important is the reporting and documentation of observations of signs and symptoms and the changes observed after interventions are made. The documentation of these observations is often crucial in determining the nature of the continuous treatment and in influencing the course of rehabilitation—the third level of prevention.

In summary, secondary prevention includes detection and treatment once the disease process has begun. The ability to limit progression of the disease process depends on adequate and appropriate treatment to arrest the progression of the condition and to prevent further complications and sequelae. The medical diagnosis and interventions are directed at the disease agent. Changes in the environment and alterations in the individual host should accompany treatment of the organism. If only one factor is changed, the client remains susceptible and recurrence or relapse of the condition is likely. Nurses have the opportunity to intervene in these other factors so that movement back to "health" can be achieved. Treatment of the "whole person" rather than just the disease takes the individual host into account. Continuity of care in discharge planning anticipates needed alterations in the environmental factors. If a client becomes ill due to a high risk situation with a highly susceptible combination of two factors (host, agent, or environment) and is treated and allowed to return to the same situation, then secondary prevention efforts have been worthless.

There is a breakdown in the health care system if the condition has been allowed to progress to this acute state. The solution to this problem is complex, and perhaps not even achievable. However, nursing can make some differences by client education and nursing research. Educating the consumer to identify and detect early signs and symptoms is important. The role of the nursing profession in health screening is crucial. Facilitating the client in receiving appropriate care helps prevent the client from falling through the gaps in the health care system caused by specialization of both doctors and nurses. Further research needs to be done to identify early signs, symptoms, and causal factors of disease conditions. The nurse's identification of physical and psychosocial aspects of the client's situation contributes to the identification of precipitating factors contributing to the development of disease.

Tertiary Prevention

Tertiary prevention is intervention after an illness or injury has taken place with the purpose of preventing further complications due to the disease condition. An altered state of the individual exists, for example, limitations in movement or activities of daily living. Appropriate adjustments must be made so that altered levels of resistance can be established to avoid further complications in progression of disease and to reduce susceptibility to other conditions. For example, the paralyzed person is susceptible to decubiti as a result of the paralysis and to respiratory infections because of indirect complications of immobility. The client is exposed to problems that would not normally be difficult. If the condition is chronic, then permanent alterations need to be considered. If the situation is temporary, for example, as in postsurgery recuperation, then short-term tertiary prevention measures are considered.

Education of the client and those around him is needed in order to develop new levels of awareness to situations that perhaps were not even problems prior to the disability or illness. Because the client's ability to cope independently is altered, the nurse needs to work with the individual and the family in identifying the new levels of abilities and weaknesses. Rehabilitation training helps the development of new skills in activity management and in helping the individual develop new strengths in coping with his altered health status. Resistance and normal levels of functioning that are often taken for granted are not always present in the chronically ill or injured client. This additional susceptibility requires constant attention to early signs and symptoms.

The process of primary and secondary prevention begins all over again at this altered state. The framework of host, agent, and environment is the same, but the characteristics within each are altered, and the nature of the overlapping circles indicates even higher susceptibility. Thus, tertiary prevention is actually primary and secondary preventive measures applied to the individual with an altered health status. Retraining and counseling are essential to implementing the adjusted preventive measures.

Facilities with specially trained personnel are needed to implement education and counseling at this tertiary level. Occupational therapy in hospitals helps clients to readjust their skills to minimize the effect of their handicap, whether the problem be permanent or temporary. A sheltered environment allows a client to try out new behaviors and skills, thus minimizing the effect of failing. As rehabilitation progresses, changes must be made in the environment. Education of the client's family and friends is important to avoid unnecessary stress. Education of the public and the employment market to utilize this individual as a productive member of society is crucial. In this way the cost of the illness or injury to society and to the individual is minimized and the benefits of his skills and knowledge are put to use.

Again, the role of the nursing profession at this level of prevention is significant. Rehabilitation begins in the hospital as soon as the acute or chronic progression of the disease is altered. Measures to enable readjustment to the altered physical or psychosocial status are implemented by the health care team: doctor, nurse, social worker, dietician, physical therapist, and occupational therapist. Each member has a role, as well as reinforcing the activities of the other team members toward the goal of rehabilitation. Specific activities to prevent or minimize complications are carried out together with retraining and counseling about ability to cope with this altered state. Even though a condition may only be temporary, such as postsurgical appendectomy or hysterectomy, the same concepts of tertiary prevention should apply until the individual is independent and returned to his prior activity state.

The client may be transferred to another health care setting or discharged to his home for continued rehabilitation. If the individual returns home, a visiting nurse is available through referral to work with the client and family in the readjustment phase and to help with needed alterations in the environment for the new level of health status. Nurses contribute to community education and can influence legislation in society's utilization of the handicapped person.

Tertiary prevention is part of any illness or condition. The more common conditions which are thought of are those which inhibit mobility, sensory abilities, or independent achievement of everyday tasks. Examples are cerebral vascular accident paralysis, injuries due to accidents, alterations in sight, hearing, speech, or burns. Every "nonhealth" condition has a rehabilitative aspect; therefore tertiary prevention measures should be implemented. Usually physical alterations in status are considered, but the nurse should also be aware of psychological (emotional) and social alterations in health status. For example, tertiary prevention for substance abuse is essential if the individual is to be successful in rehabilitation. This applies to the overeater and the smoker as well as the alcoholic or drug addict. If the individual returns to the unaltered original situation that precipitated the problem, then the chances for relapse are very high. Alterations in the environment, host, and agent will help reduce this risk.

In summary, prevention is viewed in three levels: primary, secondary, and tertiary. Each level is related to the natural history of disease and its level of pathogenesis. Primary preventive measures are designed to alter the causal factors in the disease process by interventions in the environment, the individual host, or the disease agent. Secondary prevention measures are instituted after the pathogenic course has begun in an effort to detect the process at as early a stage as possible. Once the disease is identified, therapeutic efforts to halt or minimize the progress are implemented. Tertiary prevention measures are intertwined with therapeutic measures to prevent complications and facilitate adjustment to an altered state of health. Rehabilitation is continued until the individual is able to cope independently with the adjusted status. The process becomes cyclic in that primary and secondary prevention measures are again indicated and readjusted to this altered level of health status.

SCREENING

The concept of screening is presented in this chapter because of its importance in primary and secondary prevention. A nurse's activities in primary and early secondary prevention entail either health education or screening. A discussion of health education will be presented later in this chapter. In this section, the concept of screening will be defined. Tables of recommended screening procedures per age group are presented to give the reader a sense of the scope of the topic. The tables should not be used as a recipe for preventive services for particular age groups. Rather, they should be reviewed within the perspective of the breadth of the specialty of preventive health care and to gain insight into the application of the concepts that have been presented thus far.

To understand screening one needs to review the definition of disease. Three assumptions are held in order to define screening. First, disease is a process with *multiple causes*. Second, disease follows a *natural history* of development and progression. Third, disease process *can be altered* through appropriate interventions. Screening also implies that the disease process can be *detected*. Through a variety of tests, certain conditions begin to show deviations from normal. The definition of subclinical disease indicates the nature of screening tests. There are indications, laboratory or otherwise, of abnormalities under stress, then as the condition progresses, abnormalities appear at rest.

The nature of the abnormality and the type of test are interrelated. Laboratory tests detect tissue abnormalities. X-rays allow for observation of structural abnormalities or abnormal tissue masses. Growth and development screening tests detect problems in motor coordination, sensory, and speech development. Because diseases have multiple causes, there may be more than one screening test appropriate for detection of a problem. As disease progresses, more gross abnormalities are present, and the fineness of the screening instrument is less necessary. Once clinical symptoms are manifest, less precise means are needed to identify abnormalities.

A distinction needs to be made between screening and diagnosis. Diagnosis is the process of identification of a particular disease agent. It is a combination of positive identification and ruling out of exceptions. This is an important part in secondary prevention in order to apply appropriate interventions to alter the disease process. Screening is the identification of a "non-normal" element. It does not diagnose a particular disease, but rather identifies the *likelihood* of its presence or absence. A positive Venereal Disease Research Laboratories (VDRL) test does not mean that the individual has syphilis, for there are other conditions which trigger a positive test; however, the likelihood of syphilis is greater and further diagnostic tests are then indicated. A screening test may be an even less sensitive test, merely indicating "something is wrong," such as a positive stage I Pap test.

Nursing assessment skills are screening procedures. Given an understanding of normal ranges for physiological, psychological, and social behaviors, the nurse should be alert to deviations from expected observations. As discussed previously, the nurse then refers clients for appropriate diagnosis and therapeutic intervention or continues to monitor the client until a defined problem appears.

The role of the nurse in the screening process is similar. The actual procedures may be carried out by a nurse or technician depending on the nature of the test and the resources available. However, interpretation of the results, while often done by the nurses, usually follows protocol defined by nurses or physicians. Comparison of test results to normal parameter measurements is done. Knowledge of the false-positive and false-negative rates of the particular test in light of other testing circumstances as well as client characteristics influence the decision regarding referral. Choices for follow-up range from a return screening visit, a second screening procedure, to referral for specific diagnostic workup. The decision for follow-up at this phase is crucial as it may prevent any clinical manifestation of the disease. On the other hand, the nurse cannot refer every suspected abnormality because the resources in the health care system for adequate follow-up are limited. Judgment based on knowledge of the client, the screening procedure, and the disease process must be used.

Table 8-1 illustrates the variety of procedures available for screening. The table is divided by age groupings in which certain growth and development stages have higher susceptibilities to particular diseases. The column labeled "Procedure" lists testing procedures or specific laboratory techniques. Others are more general such as health assessment ("history") of clinical signs and symptoms or "counseling" for assessment of psychosocial problems. The "Condition" column lists the conditions for which the test is designed. The "Type

of Prevention" indicates two levels of prevention with which the test is concerned. A "1" identifies primary prevention where activities are directed at the disease agent, individual host's resistance characteristics, or toward the environmental realm. The primary prevention level includes intervention when two of these factors overlap and susceptibility to disease is suspected. A "2" is listed when the screening test is a secondary prevention measure. The disease is already present, either on a subclinical or early clinical level. The screening procedure is aimed at detection of specific characteristics that indicate the particular condition. Positive findings on these tests are more likely to need follow-up for definitive diagnosis.

The column labeled "Intervention" is an abbreviated list of recommended follow-up procedures if positive results are found. Again, discretion must be used in determining the accuracy of the test results and the appropriateness for follow-up in each situation. This list is given, not as a cookbook to screening techniques, but to demonstrate the variety of screening procedures available.

HEALTH EDUCATION

Health education is an integral part of every level of preventive health care. Alterations in the disease agent and environment can be carried out in mechanical ways. Alterations in the host, because it involves the individual within his personal realm, is most often accomplished by health education. Through education the individual gains an understanding of the condition and is usually motivated to alter his situation to intervene in the disease process. The responsibility for health teaching falls on each health care professional who is involved with the client. Nurses, however, are in the unique position of having the most frequent immediate contact with the client and thus should take the opportunity for maximizing client education. Objectives for health education can be stated as follows:

1. To improve the health of the people . . . by:
   (a) providing them the necessary information to help prevent illness and disability insofar as possible and to maintain the highest possible level of well-being even when ill or disabled; and (b) helping them to make the necessary modifications in individual life style or behavior when necessary.

TABLE 8-1. Procedures Available for Screening (Age Groupings According to Growth and Development Stages)

Procedure	Condition	Type of Prevention	Intervention
A. Mother and Fetus*			
History of menarche	Unplanned pregnancy (before pregnancy)	1	Contraception
Serological exam	Lack of rubella antibody (before pregnancy)	1	Immunization
Pregnancy test	Unwanted pregnancy	2	Abortion
History of pregnancy	Unsuccessful prior pregnancy	2	Counseling
History and counseling	Inadequate preparation for pregnancy	1	Counseling
History and counseling	Inadequate preparation for delivery	1	Counseling
History and counseling	Inadequate preparation for parenthood	1	Counseling
History and counseling	Smoking and other risks to developing fetus	1, 2	Counseling
History and counseling	Inadequate recognition of signs and symptoms of abnormalities	1	Counseling
Anthropometric examination and counseling	Nutritional abnormality	2	Counseling and diet
Hemoglobin/hematocrit	Anemia	2	Diagnosis and therapy
Urine albumin	Toxemia	2	Diagnosis and therapy
Pap smear	Genital tract malignancy	2	Diagnosis and therapy
VDRL	Syphilis	2	Diagnosis and therapy Counseling and contact finding
G.C. culture	Gonorrhea	2	Penicillin, counseling and contact finding
Blood grouping and Rh determination	Rh iso-immunization and other blood abnormalities	1	Antibody
Casual blood sugar	Abnormal glucose tolerance	2	Diagnosis and therapy
Blood pressure measurement	Hypertension	2	Diagnosis and therapy
Examination	Organic heart disease	2	Diagnosis and therapy
Physical exam	Pelvic inadequacy	2	Diagnosis and therapy
Physical exam	Reproductive organ abnormality	2	Diagnosis and therapy
Urine culture	Bacteriuria (after third pregnancy)	2	Diagnosis and therapy
Amniocentesis	Genetic disorders (women over 40)	2	Diagnosis and therapy
Blood test	Sickle cell trait (high risk groups only)	2	Diagnosis and therapy
B. Infant†			
History and counseling	Inadequate preparation for infant care (newborn)	1	Parent counseling
PKU	Metabolic disorders (newborn)	2	Diagnosis and therapy
Silver nitrate prophylaxis	Gonorrheal ophthalmia (newborn)	1	Prophylaxis
Observation and measurement	Congenital malformations (newborn)	2	Diagnosis and therapy
Vaccinations	Diphtheria, tetanus, and pertussis	1	Immunization
TOPV	Poliomyelitis	1	Immunization
Vitamin K	Hemorrhagic disease	1	Prophylaxis
Hematocrit	Anemia	2	Diagnosis and therapy
Developmental assessment including height and weight	Growth and development disorders	2	Diagnosis and therapy
Counseling	Accidents	1	Parent counseling

TABLE 8-1. Continued

Procedure	Condition	Type of Prevention	Intervention
	C. Ages 1–6 Years‡		
Observation and assessments	Growth and development abnormalities	2	Diagnosis and therapy
Observation and assessments	Neurologic disorders	2	Diagnosis and therapy
Anthropometric measurements	Malnutrition and obesity	1, 2	Counseling and diet
Hematocrit	Anemia	2	Diagnosis and therapy
Hearing and vision testing	Hearing, vision, and eye deficiencies	2	Diagnosis and therapy
Speech testing	Communication disorders	2	Diagnosis and therapy
Vaccination	Diphtheria, tetanus, and pertussis	1	Immunization
History and vaccination if indicated	Measles, mumps, and rubella	1	Immunization
History and TOPV if indicated	Poliomyelitis	1	Immunization
Dental exam	Dental defects	1, 2	Diagnosis and therapy
Counseling	Accidents	1	Parent counseling
Counseling	Poisoning	1	Parent counseling
	D. Ages 6–16 Years§		
Observation and assessment	Behavioral, intellectual, or communicative maladjustments	2	Counseling Diagnosis and therapy
History and counseling	Smoking	1, 2	Counseling
Examination and prophylaxis	Dental caries, malocclusions, and periodontal disease	1, 2	Prophylaxis
Hearing and vision testing	Visual and hearing defects	2	Diagnosis and therapy
Anthropometric examination	Musculoskeletal disorders	2	Diagnosis and therapy
Anthropometric examination	Malnutrition including underweight or overweight	1, 2	Counseling and diet
Skin examination	Acne	2	Diagnosis and treatment
History and examination	Sexual immaturity or disorders (2nd visit only)	1, 2	Counseling, diagnosis, and therapy
Counseling	Accidents	1	Counseling
Vaccination	Diphtheria and tetanus (2nd visit only)	1	Immunization boosters
History	Drug abuse and alcohol (2nd visit only)	1, 2	Counseling
Hematocrit	Anemia (2nd visit only)	2	Diagnosis and treatment
Blood pressure	Cardiovascular problems (2nd visit only)	2	Diagnosis and treatment
History	Unwanted pregnancy (2nd visit for high risk groups only)	1	Contraception
VDRL	Syphilis (2nd visit for high risk groups only)	2	Diagnosis and treatment; counseling and contact finding
G.C. culture	Gonorrhea (2nd visit for high risk groups only)	2	Diagnosis and treatment; counseling and contact finding

Preventive Health Care **125**

TABLE 8-1. Continued

Procedure	Condition	Type of Prevention	Intervention
	E. Ages 17—34 Years ‖		
History of completed immunization or booster in past 10 years	Tetanus and diphtheria	1	Td vaccine
Rubella HI	Congenital and rubella syndrome (females only)	1	Rubella vaccine
VDRL	Syphilis	2	Diagnosis and treatment
Culture of female	Gonorrhea	2	Diagnosis and treatment; contact; investigation
Height and weight	Malnutrition and obesity	1, 2	Counseling and diet; diagnosis-treatment
Blood pressure	Hypertension and associated conditions and complications	1, 2	Diagnosis and treatment
Cholesterol	Coronary artery disease	1	Counseling and diet
Hematocrit	Anemia	2	Diagnosis and treatment
Casual blood sugar	Abnormal glucose tolerance and diabetes	1, 2	Diagnosis and treatment
Cervical cytology	Cancer of cervix	2	Diagnosis and treatment
Breast exam (self)	Breast cancer	2	Diagnosis and treatment
Hearing and vision testing	Hearing and visual acuity disorders	2	Diagnosis and treatment
History/life style	Heart and lung diseases	1, 2	Counseling
History and counseling	Alcoholism and drugs	1, 2	Counseling
Counseling	Accidents	2	Counseling
History and counseling	Smoking	1, 2	Counseling
PPD	Tuberculosis	2	Diagnosis and treatment
	F. Ages 35—64 Years #		
History of completed immunization or booster in past 10 years	Tetanus	1	Td vaccine
VDRL	Syphilis	2	Diagnosis and treatment
Height and weight	Malnutrition and obesity	1, 2	Counseling and diet; diagnosis-treatment
Blood pressure	Hypertension and associated conditions and complications	1, 2	Diagnosis and treatment
Cholesterol	Coronary artery disease	1	Counseling and diet
Hematocrit	Anemia	2	Diagnosis and treatment
Stool for blood	Occult malignancy	2	Diagnosis and treatment
Glucose tolerance test	Diabetes	2	Diagnosis and treatment

TABLE 8-1. Continued

Procedure	Condition	Type of Prevention	Intervention
Breast exam	Breast cancer	2	Diagnosis and treatment
Mammography or xerography in all over age 50, and high risk less than age 50	Breast cancer (more frequent than every 5 years)	2	Diagnosis and treatment
History/life style	Heart and lung disease	1, 2	Counseling
Hearing and vision testing	Hearing and vision disorders	2	Diagnosis and treatment
History and counseling	Alcoholism and drugs	1, 2	Counseling
History and counseling	Smoking	1, 2	Counseling
Counseling	Accidents	1	Counseling
Cervical smear	Cervix cancer	2	Diagnosis and treatment
PPD	Tuberculosis (high risk groups only)	2	Diagnosis and treatment
	G. Age 65 and Over**		
History of completed immunization or booster in past 10 years	Tetanus and diphtheria	1	Td vaccine
Influenza immunization	Influenza and complications	1	Influenza vaccine
Height and weight	Malnutrition and obesity	1, 2	Counseling and diet; diagnosis-treatment
Blood pressure	Hypertension and associated conditions and complications	1, 2	Diagnosis and treatment
EKG	Arrhythmia	2	Diagnosis and treatment
Hearing and vision testing	Hearing and vision deficiencies	2	Diagnosis and treatment
Glucose tolerance test	Diabetes	2	Diagnosis and treatment
Hematocrit	Anemia	2	Diagnosis and treatment
Stool for blood	Occult GI disease	2	Diagnosis and treatment
Breast exam and mammography or xerography	Breast cancer	2	Diagnosis and treatment
History/life style	Heart and lung disease	1, 2	Counseling
History and counseling	Alcoholism and drugs	1, 2	Counseling
History and counseling	Depression and suicide	1, 2	Counseling
Counseling	Accidents	1	Counseling

*Reprinted with permission from: Task Force Reports: *Preventive Medicine, USA*. New York, PRODIST, 1976, p. 296.
†*Ibid.*, p. 297.
‡*Ibid.*, p. 298.
§*Ibid.*, p. 300.
‖*Ibid.*, p. 301.
#*Ibid.*, p. 302.
**Ibid.*, p. 303.

2. To help restrain inflation in health care costs by relieving some of the preventable demand on health services.
3. To involve the consumer-client positively and constructively in his own health maintenance and in responsible effective use of the health care delivery system.[3]

These are broad objectives, yet achievable within the domain of the nurse-client relationship. A large portion of client education is done on an informal one-to-one basis. These instances usually are under time constraints and often cannot provide the in-depth coverage of the topic needed. The quality and quantity of this type of client education varies widely. Yet if these contacts were planned and documented with the same attention and precision as wound care or postoperative monitoring, the contribution of the nursing profession to client education would gain in credibility and its effectiveness in movement toward health could be measured.

Organized classes and courses are another method for client education. These are usually for clients referred by their doctor or nurse for specific problems. These groups are organized around a particular topic, and the information and procedures are usually well established. Often, the instructor has greater experience in the area. Help may be needed for teaching methodology or group management skills, but the instructor has expertise in the content area. Usually these classes are one of three general areas: (1) classes for diabetics, cardiac clients or others with severe chronic disease or disability; (2) classes for expectant parents; and (3) preoperative instruction. Because of the nature of the topics, it is fairly easy to develop standardized teaching plans which can then be shared and adapted to other groups with similar needs. The nurse could also use these standardized outlines for individual client education.

Health education within the school setting is ideal for sharing knowledge about prevention of disease and needs for health care. However, there exists three major constraints typically in a school setting: (1) "A traditional low visibility and low priority for health education, (2) a narrow definition of the appropriate content and jurisdiction of health education efforts, and (3) a shortage of adequately trained health educators."[4]

The traditional perspective toward health education in the schools is to tuck it into physical ed-

ucation, biology, or home economics. This "integration" into the curricula would be ideal; however, the administrative structure of the school system frequently undermines serious attempts to make these sections relevant for the students. The qualifications of teachers do not depend on their skills in managing health related topics, such as sexuality and family planning, substance use and abuse, or hygiene as it relates to communicable diseases.

These topics solicit value conflict between the students, teachers, school administrators, school board, and parents. So, instead of facing the conflict and making the content relevant, the health related topics are avoided or watered down to the extent that there is no substantive content. The school nurse's role could be crucial in bringing attention to this deficit of the system. However, time and political constraints frequently frustrate any attempts at change. Also, the school nurse is usually alone and lacks the support of other health professionals in pushing for change within the educational system. It is unfortunate when one sees the attention given to driver's education as compared to the collective time and money given to relevant health education for the population between 5 and 18-years-old.

Occupational health is another area that could benefit from health education. Progress has been made to protect the workers against health hazards within the work environment. The enactment of the Occupational Safety and Health Act (OSHA) in 1970 was a milestone in preventive industrial health. Yet the majority of the working population remains ignorant of potential environmental safety and health hazards. Worker's compliance with wearing safety gear is low, which highlights the lack of understanding at this level of prevention. Unions and the federal government continue their efforts in identifying hazards and pressing for industrial reform and worker education.

The opportunities are vast in the occupational setting for identification of physical, mental, or emotional problems; screening for diseases; and counseling for substance abuse. Well-planned poster campaigns could have an immense effect on primary and secondary prevention. Lunchtime sessions could stimulate great changes in adult health practices.

Such efforts, as successful as they have proved to be in individual situations, have scarcely made a dent in the health problems of American workers. The blame, however, cannot be attributed primarily either to management or to the unions. The major culprits are the same four factors that hamper other forms of health education; namely, individual ignorance, public apathy, commercial pressures, and lack of any strong positive leadership on the part of either the government or the health professionals.[5]

Health education on a local community level is usually aimed at specific groups either by geographic location, age, socioeconomic status, ethnic characteristics, or other factors. Typical programs include screening for such diseases as hypertension, tuberculosis, breast cancer, sickle cell anemia, and lead poisoning. Health fairs help to disseminate information to large numbers of people. "Hot lines" are another community education method to deal with specific needs and to provide general information.

On the national level, some 70 health related agencies and organizations are affiliated with the National Health Council. Most of these organizations are involved with some sort of health education directed toward their specific area of concern. They are not particularly concerned with the individual but rather provide information for a larger segment of the population. A few examples of these national organizations are the National Cancer Society, the American Heart Association, the National Arthritis Foundation, Planned Parenthood Federation, the National Safety Council, Red Cross, Weight Watchers, and Alcoholics Anonymous. The National Health Council, acting as the umbrella organization for these major nongovernmental agencies, is currently trying to establish the framework for a national center for health education.[6] A major contribution of these nonprofit agencies is their involvement of consumers on all levels. Also, successful fund raising promotes further research and training for professionals in addition to the health education provided for the public.

The media is a major factor in health education. It influences a greater proportion of the values, mores, and health-related behavior of the American population than do our laws, schools, health, or religious institutions. The impact of the media is not known, but recent studies have tried to determine its influence. The Blue Cross Association, who commissioned a 1971 Harris Poll, found the following statistics: "29% of the American people get most of their medical information from TV advertising; 28% from newspaper medical columns; 26% from magazines; 25% from TV medical news. These were exceeded only by information from doctors, and doctors were named only by 51%."[7] Another study done by other researchers concluded: "If, however, 70% of all messages on television are not true, and 70% of these messages are believed by children, then television viewing, as presently programmed, might be labeled as hazardous to the health of future adults."[8]

However, the potential use for the media for special purposes is virtually limitless. If health professionals utilized marketing strategies as well as the drug industry, the cereal industry, or the auto industry, the demand for health care services could be made more appropriate and meaningful. The health education information that could be conveyed via the media is exciting to postulate. Time and energy spent condemning current media could be redirected toward competing with the marketing messages. Try to imagine attention redirected from toothpaste advertisements to preventive dental hygiene practices.

The involvement of the nursing profession in health education is probably greater than any other group involved in the health care field. Even though many of the nurses working in hospitals and nursing homes have extensive technical responsibilities and limited time to give to client education, it is generally assumed that client teaching is an explicit part of the job responsibilities. The nurse could be considered negligent if client education is not part of the delivery of professional client care. Out of 815,000 active registered nurses in 1973, the 54,800 in public health and school nursing, and the 20,000 in occupational health nursing have health education as a major component of their job.[9] The Nursing Practice Acts reinforce this responsibility for health education. Client education is a component of all state licensing examinations. Unlike the physician, the nurse is not primarily focused on the disease agent but rather on the client as a whole person. Time spent in client education activities should be viewed as a responsibility and challenge for effective health care rather than a resort for failure in diagnosis or treatment. Appropriate health education may be more effective, in certain cases, than surgical or pharmacological treatment. Nurses need to continue and step up their efforts in client teaching, or the vacuum will be filled by others more interested or more qualified.

The topic of prevention is enormous and difficult to contain within a single chapter. The fundamental theories and concepts of preventive health care have been given. It is now the responsibility of the reader to synthesize and apply these concepts into the care of *your* clients.

REFERENCES

1. Hanlon, J.: *Principles of Public Health Administration*, 5th ed. St. Louis, C. V. Mosby Co., 1969, p. 5.
2. Donabedian, A.: *Aspects of Medical Care Administration: Specifying Requirements for Health Care*. Cambridge, Mass., Harvard University Press, 1973, p. 73.
3. College of Medicine & Dentistry of New Jersey, Office of Consumer Health Education. *The CMDNJ-OCHE Program in Consumer Health Education*. Jan., 1975.
4. Task Force Reports: *Preventive Medicine, USA*. New York, PRODIST, 1976, 29.
5. *Ibid*, p. 34.
6. Van Ness, E. H.: Federal focus on health education. Proceedings of the Health Education Conference. Presented at the Communicable Disease Center, Atlanta, Georgia, June, 1974, pp. 9–11.
7. Blue Cross Association: Press release. Chicago, Dec. 29, 1971, p. 16.
8. Lewis, C. E., and Lewis, M. A.: The impact of television commercials on health-related beliefs and behaviors of children. *Pediatrics* 53:35, 1974.
9. U.S.D.H.E.W. National Center for Health Statistics, *Health Resources Statistics*, 1974, p. 245.

BIBLIOGRAPHY

Benenson, A. (ed): *Control of CD in Man*, 11th ed. Washington, D.C., *APHA*, 1970.
Clark, D., and MacMahon, B. (eds.): *Preventive Medicine*. Boston, Little, Brown, and Co., 1967.
Collen, M. (ed.): *Multiphasic Health Testing Service*. New York, John Wiley and Sons, 1978.
Dubos, R.: *Mirage of Health*. New York, Anchor Books, 1959.
Dubos, R.: *Man, Medicine and Environment*. New York, Mentor Books, 1968.
Frankenburg, W., and North, F.: *A Guide to Screening for Early and Periodic Screening, Diagnosis and Treatment Program CEBO under Medicaid*. Washington, D.C. USDHEW, Social and Rehabilitation Service in Cooperation with the American Academy of Pediatrics, 1974.
Goerke, L., and Stebbins, E.: *Mustard's Introduction to Public Health*, 5th ed. New York, Macmillan Co., 1968.
Hilleboe, H.,, and Larimore, G. (eds.): *Preventive Medicine: Principles of Prevention in the Occurrence and Progression of Disease*, 2nd ed. Philadelphia, W. B. Saunders Co., 1965.
Leavell, H., and Clark, E. G.: *Preventive Medicine for the Doctor in His Community: An Epidemiologic Approach*, 3rd ed. New York, McGraw-Hill Book Co., 1965.
Murray, R., and Zenter, J.: *Nursing Assessment and Health Promotion through the Life Span*. Englewood Cliffs, N.J., Prentice-Hall, Inc., 1975.
Murray, R., and Zenter, J.: *Nursing's Concepts for Health Promotion*. Englewood Cliffs, N.J., Prentice-Hall, Inc., 1975.
Nuffield Provincial Hospitals Trust: *Screenings in Medical Care: Reviewing the Evidence, A Collection of Essays*. London, Oxford University Press, 1968.
Roueche, B.: *Annals of Epidemiology*. Boston, Little, Brown, and Co., 1967.
Sartwell, P. (ed.): *Maxcy-Rosenau Preventive Medicine and Public Health*, 9th ed. New York, Appleton-Century-Crofts, 1965.
Smillie, W., and Kilbourne, E.: *Preventive Medicine and Public Health*, 3rd ed. New York, Macmillan Co., 1963.
Tinkham, C., and Voorhies, E.: *Community Health Nursing: Evaluation and Process*. New York, Appleton-Century-Crofts, 1972.
Tinkham, C., and Voorhies, E.: *Early Disease Detection: Health Screening in Private Practice*, vol. 2. Mount Kisco, N.Y., Futura Publishing Co., Inc., 1971.

CHAPTER 9

This chapter will speak to some issues relating to the process of the restoration of health. Restoration means simply, "bringing back to, or putting back into, a former position or condition."[1] The process may present relatively few problems in application to objects, but with human beings, it frequently has significant limitations which must be assessed on a progressive basis by the client, the family, and members of the health team. The inherent difficulty, however, is that the client cannot always return to the predisease state. Physical, psychological, and social factors must be considered as interrelating processes, not in isolation. They are not static events, but ongoing processes, in which previous events from the individual's history influence the present and future episodes of health.

In this chapter the restoration of health will be examined with reference to: (1) the individual, (2) the family, and (3) the community. These frameworks should not be differentiated into levels of importance but should be viewed as basic features

CONSIDERATIONS IN RESTORATION OF HEALTH

Linda G. Dumas, M.S., M.A., R.N.

or elements of the process of restoration. All significantly influence the return of health to the individual. The nurse has a major role in the planning and implementation of goals with the client and his family.

Return for a moment to the concept of restoration. Each person is unique, as are his relationships to the family and community. Two people may have the same illness, but the factors that affect their recovery will necessarily be different. Even under optimum conditions, not all individuals will be able to regain their health. Levels of health are relative; thus in establishing goals with the client and his family, health professionals must evaluate the health status on a continuum, choosing goals that are unique to each individual. For the purpose of this discussion, restoration can be seen as the process by which the individual, the family, and the health team move toward maximizing a mutually evaluated potential; for the individual, this will mean the realization of independence and productivity.

THE INDIVIDUAL

In the following paragraphs we will focus on two major influences on the client: the acuteness or the chronicity of the event which caused the disruption and the anticipated role changes which relate to the restoration process. Initial assessments of the acuteness or chronicity of the illness are made during the hospitalization. Evaluation of individual needs for treatment and rehabilitation are discussed by the physician, nurses, and members of the continuing health care team, prior to discharge. It should be emphasized that evaluation is ongoing throughout the entire process of restoration of health. There are many factors which are held in abeyance during the person's hospitalization; however, these will re-emerge when normal activities are resumed outside the confines of the hospital. These extenuating factors are influenced by the severity of the illness, specifically the residual effects, which can range from weakness, fatigue, or the healing of a wound, to long-term or perhaps permanent disability due to loss of function of a systemic or focal nature.

Any illness which disrupts an individual's normal routine is a potential threat, particularly an illness requiring hospitalization. Even with illnesses of a nonacute nature, there will be adjustments when the patient is discharged. Examples might be time lost from work, dietary restrictions, dressing changes, and the necessary rest required to return to the premorbid state. With more serious illnesses, long-term recovery phases may be indicated. The individual may be bedridden and in pain, requiring time-consuming care by family members or the utilization of outside support systems, which will be examined in more detail later.

Related to the acuteness-chronicity continuum are the changes in role. No matter how adequately the individual and his family are prepared by the hospital staff for anticipated alterations in role, the reality of events may indeed be devastating. Because we live in an age where medical technology is continually surpassing previous expectations, people are living longer, and those with illnesses, which at one time meant certain death, are now returning to the community. Many of the illnesses relate to losses in perception and coordination which accompany chronic and terminal disease processes. Think for a moment of the implications. Clients with chronic motor or sensory deficits are often depressed, frustrated, or angry. The daily activities which we take for granted, such as lifting an arm, feeding ourselves, dressing, walking, getting in and out of bed, and communicating, are no longer possible for many people. These are tasks which may require arduous effort, even with assistance. They are no longer independent. Often it takes months, or even years, to regain a semblance of the function which they had prior to illness. In caring and assisting individuals with motor or sensory disorders in the process of their restoration, it is important to empathize with their sense of loss.

Loss encompasses many areas, including loss of independent function which results in changes in work patterns, often with subsequent social and economic effects. These effects may lead to significant alterations in life style. Coping mechanisms vary, and with seemingly never-ending crises, adaptation is necessarily more difficult. Encouragement and patience are necessary for proper nursing care. Frequently, nurses are required to give sup-

port while the individual works toward goals which will maximize his potential for independent function. Technology, while often indispensable, is no substitute for the balance between reality and hope which the nurse and the client will realize through shared communication.

THE FAMILY

. . . For most people, however, the issue is not whether the family has a future, but *what* that future will look like. For after all the questions are asked and the speculations are done, the unshakable reality remains: most Americans of all classes still live in families and will continue to do so for the foreseeable future at least. And it is there—in those families—that the stresses and strains of everyday life are played out; that children are born and brought to adulthood; that women and men love and hate; that major interpersonal and intrapersonal conflicts are generated and stilled; and that men, women, and children struggle with the demands from the changing world outside their doors.[2] (Italics added.)

No individual enters the world in isolation from a reference group. Social changes in the eighteenth century reflected a decline in the extended family and in the influence of the collective.[3] The emergence of the nuclear family has necessarily made the members more dependent on fewer people; it may be that this dependence has made the family more fragile. Protective mechanisms manifested by deception and denial, despite the well-meant intentions, have placed family members on different levels of awareness. Relationships are thus more vulnerable to the strains imposed by crises or losses relating to illness and death.

Different contexts of awareness can be seen in the dynamics which often occur when a member is terminally ill. How many lies take place in the sickroom, and who lies? It would appear that the dying person and his family are engaged in mutual deceptions; for the family who masks truth and for the client who perpetuates their illusions. As Aries wrote, ". . . discretion is the modern form of dignity."[4] Group solidarity does not necessarily equate with group strength, and an important part of making accurate assessments relates to the paradox of appearances and their realities. Situations are often not what they seem to be, and as you develop your interpersonal skills and become more comfortable in your roles, you will begin to question the superficialities with tact and perception.

As nurses, you must understand the impact of role reversals and the concomitant social adjustments on the family members. Despite the changes in the male and female roles, particularly in relation to working women, our society continues to socialize men and women in the traditional patterns. Working men are socialized into their roles as providers, and if this ability to work is disrupted by serious illness or a loss, the sequelae can be extremely traumatic. The disruptions caused by illness and hospitalization place a burden on the individual and his family, the extent of which is often not realized until the sick person returns home.

Although this discussion has thus far centered on traditional family patterns, it must be remembered that there are many single parent families. If the single parent becomes ill, the family may be forced to seek alternative means of financial support. If there is only one caretaker, the maintenance of everyday activities becomes a serious problem. Also, mention must be made of those persons who are alone. The elderly comprise the majority of people in this category. It is estimated that 16 percent of the elderly population still live below the poverty level.[5] Their economic and social isolation is due, in part, to the emergence of the nuclear family. Families are small, and their aging members are often excluded from their center, and in this technological age, society caters to its most productive members.

The process of restoration is necessarily complex and difficult as the effects of multiple illnesses are combined with social isolation and depression.

> . . . There is only one solution if old age is not to be an absurd parody of our former life, and that is to go on pursuing ends that give our existence to a meaning—devotion to individuals, to groups or to causes, social, political, intellectual, or creative work. In spite of the moralist opinion to the contrary, in old age we should wish still to have *passions strong enough to prevent us turning in upon ourselves.*[6] (Italics added.)

de Beauvoir states the problem cogently. Yet in one form or another, the issue has been voiced before.

Social isolation, depression, poverty, and growing old more often than not add up to chronic illness. It is critical, therefore, that you see through the societal rhetoric and actively attempt to effect change. In assisting the elderly in the process of restoration, emphasis should be placed on restoring their sense of being a part of things. This is an important factor in a plan of care for anyone, young and old alike; however, for the latter group, it can mean the difference between life and existence; there is a distinct difference in the quality of the two forms.

The nurse's assessment of the individual and the family should include the demographic, economic, cultural, and social influences which have an impact on their life and health. When you make your initial assessment, remember that concrete, objective factors, such as housing, sanitation, plumbing, and heat, will influence the process of restoration.[7] Subjective assessments are accomplished by direct and indirect interactions. These take time and often cannot be completed in an interview. You will be using many of your senses, including sight, hearing, speech, and above all, good judgment. Remember, other ways of life may not necessarily be like your own, and there is no reason to expect they should be. Be attuned to the possibility of value imposition, and try to accept people for what they are. Nothing is accomplished when you negate the things which are important to someone else. A nurse has an important role in assisting people toward adjustments in situations which may seem irresolvable. Emphasize the positive factors in the situation and help the individual and his family to work through or around the realities of everyday life. While there is relatively little you can do to ameliorate most everyday realities, such as poverty and its effects, you can be supportive and encouraging and offer viable alternatives. Health is a multifaceted phenomenon, and you cannot restore it in isolation from the environmental variables which play a paramount role in its recovery or loss.

THE COMMUNITY

We have briefly considered the individual and the family, focusing on the variables affecting the restoration of health. Now we will look within a larger frame of reference—the community. A community is a spatially defined area where a majority of the members live, sometimes work, but usually share similar norms and values. A community may be large or small, and membership in a class is often a common bond for its members. You may see variations of the lower, middle, and upper classes which are frequently delineated by economic factors; however, economic influences encompass political, ideological, cultural, and social realms. None of these should be looked at in isolation, and nurses should make a point of being familiar with the extent to which these influence the individual and family ways of life. All affect restoration in that they significantly influence reactions and subsequent attempts at readjustment.

Many communities continue to reflect a strong collective sentiment. This may be observed in extended kinship systems or social relations based on ethnic or religious affinities. Often such groups are stable resources from which to draw support during crises. However, religious and ethnic factors may also exert constraints on the plan of care for the individual and his family. If possible such constraints should be evaluated prior to discharge. Nutrition is an area which reflects cultural, ethnic, or religious preferences, and special diets should be written with such influences in mind.

Demographic factors are important, especially those relating to the accessibility of the clinics and hospitals. Community transportation services and availability of support services in the area should be assessed. Health service agencies are of no value to the client if they are inaccessible.

Availability of Support Services

Support services with which health professionals should be familiar will now be addressed in more detail.

VISITING NURSES. The Visiting Nurses' Association is one of the most valuable supports in a community. This is an independent nonprofit organization which is financed by insurance, welfare, fee-for-service, and The United Way. Special arrangements are made when the client cannot afford to pay; some visits may even be free. It is an excellent resource and serves as a liaison to the hospitals, clinics, and other health services in the community. The organization is comprised of nurses who visit people in their homes. Each agency has

a nutritionist, physical therapist, and social worker available on a consultative basis. These people have a sound knowledge of the community characteristics, the referral services available, and the priorities of health problems in the area. The nurses are skilled in family assessment, and their interventions are of critical significance for individuals and families in trouble.

HOME SERVICES. Homemakers and home health aides are other important resources. They may be a part of a visiting nurses agency, or they may work out of private agencies. One of the primary assets of these people is that they are frequently members of the community in which they work; thus, they share similar values, norms, and ways of life with their clients. Homemakers do housecleaning, cooking, food shopping, and related tasks, while home health aides are trained to give personal care such as bed baths in addition to light housework and cooking. The services of these groups are being increasingly utilized, and the presence of a homemaker or home health aide may make the difference in the feasibility of restoring a person at home, as opposed to residence in a skilled care facility.

Meals-on-Wheels. Meals-on-Wheels is another service available in most communities. Hot meals are brought to the home once or twice a day for a minimal price, depending on the need. This is an important service for the elderly clients who live alone.

TRANSPORTATION. Transportation services are an important resource in the community. Most communities have such services as Medicab, federated vans, chair cars, and senior shuttle cars to provide transportation to clinics and hospitals. Criteria for the use of such services are based on the individual's capacity for ambulation. Persons who are able to walk are usually ineligible for Medicab; however, the federated vans will transport them. The vans transport the elderly and those who have difficulty getting to clinics. Use of all transportation services should be arranged well in advance of the clinic visit for the person to be brought to the facility and returned to the home. Clients should be informed of the services available to them.

ASSOCIATIONS. There are numerous resources in each community. Local divisions of the American Cancer Society, the Multiple Sclerosis Association, and the myriad of related support groups are available for assistance. It is impossible to be familiar with all of them, but when caring for an individual with a problem, the assessment of *relevant* resources is an important part of the care plan. Some persons derive much benefit from the groups in which members help each other by sharing similar problems. Others do not wish to be faced with persons who, like themselves, reflect illness and loss. It is a matter of personal choice for the individual, but the options should be offered.

In a previous section of this discussion, we mentioned the paradox of appearance and reality. It is again relevant in this context, for in your assessment of health services, you should maintain a critical stance, directing your attention to the objectives, goals, and effectiveness of such organizations. There are many health services, but their existence does not necessarily mandate their effectiveness in meeting client needs.

SUMMARY

Some physical, psychological, and social factors relevant to the process of restoration, viewing them as dynamic forces in the interrelationship of the individual, the family, and the community, have been discussed. These areas have been separated for the purpose of clarity; however, they should not be viewed in isolation. A nurse's overall goal should be to provide integrated nursing care to the client and his family. Because there are many ways of meeting common goals, do not expect *your* way to be the only way, or the best way. You will be attempting to formulate a holistic approach, through the assessment of physical problems, diagnoses, and interventions, along with the practical applications which are unique to the individual and his family environment. It should be emphasized that in restoration, the client is not cared for in isolation; your care, your rationale, and your judgments will involve the individual, his interactions with his family (or the people with whom he lives) and the community in which they all live. The characteristic which distinguishes the restoration process is the assessment of the client outside of the health care

setting, within the framework of the community. Health attitudes are often shared by members of a common group; therefore, interventions should be directed toward goals realistically related to interaction of members, coping mechanisms, and the health problems existent within a family and the community. You will become more adept in this area as you acquire experience, but it is important to remember that even with experience, one may make errors in judgment. Reflection on such errors results in growth of a personal and professional nature. There will be a continuity to your plans of care, and you should be consistent in their re-evaluation. Try to anticipate problems, for it is much easier to cope with their effects if you plan ahead.

Nurses have many support systems. Your colleagues on the health team are perhaps the most important, and sharing your problems with them often brings to light different ideas and perspectives on an issue. Such support systems are *intradisciplinary* and *interdisciplinary*. Limiting yourself to sharing only with the members of your discipline will narrow your perspectives and as a consequence, your assessments. As pointed out earlier, the process of restoration is complex, and it involves the expertise of members in other disciplines. Intelligent informed decision-making emanates from a broad base of information.

As restoration progresses, you will be critically reassessing your plans and re-establishing goals along with the means which will be utilized to meet them. Restoration is not a static event; it is a dynamic and ongoing process. To develop the ability to incorporate a "total picture," you will need to have a sound understanding of the rationale for drugs and treatment, an understanding of the family dynamics, and an ability to use teaching as an ongoing rather than episodic tool. You will be able then, to relate the larger environment of the community to the problems of the individual and his family.

There is no unique methodology which is applicable to all persons. You should be able to assess the reality and the feasibility of your plans of care in this respect. Be aware of the ways in which the problems in a community limit the individual and his family. Similarly, be aware of the positive factors which can be drawn on for support. Overall, you should be able to provide a sound rationale for your actions. Goals which are realistic for the client and his family, as well as for you, are critical. You may not always accomplish everything you set out to do, but you can certainly make inroads by the initiation of thoughtful plans of care for someone else to implement or modify.

Clients and their families are unique individuals. They have their own ways of conducting their lives, so they may not always be receptive to your plans for their well-being. Nursing implies mediation; however, as mediator, you must consult the person and the family with your intentions. You cannot do it alone, and your role is one of many roles in the restoration of an individual to health or to a realistic level of function. You are a member of a group, and this group is comprised of the client, his family, and the health team. You have a responsibility for assisting in the process of restoration, but the ultimate responsibility for decision-making rests with the client.

REFERENCES

1. ———: *Webster's New International Dictionary,* 2nd ed. Springfield, Mass., G. and C. Merriam Co., 1957, p. 2125.
2. Rubin, L. B.: *Worlds of Pain,* New York, Basic Books, 1976. p. 5.
3. Aries, P.: *Centuries of Childhood,* New York, Vintage Books, 1962.
4. Aries, P.: *Western Attitudes Towards Death.* Baltimore, Johns Hopkins University Press, 1974. p. 6.
5. Schulz, J. H.: *The Economics of Aging,* Belmont, Calif., Wadsworth Publishers, Inc., 1976.
6. de Beauvoir, S.: *The Coming of Age.* New York, Warner Books, 1970, p. 802—803.
7. Tinkham, C. W., and Voorhies, E. F.: *Community Health Nursing—Evolution and Process,* 2nd ed. New York, Appleton-Century-Crofts, 1977.

PART 3: ASPECTS OF THE HEALTH CARE SYSTEM

Having introduced in Parts 1 and 2 concepts relating to the client and his health/illness status, it is now appropriate to address the system with which the client interacts to achieve the maximum level of health possible for that particular individual.

Part 3 focuses on the various components that comprise the health care network—that is, the system itself and its political and economic influences, issues, and constraints; the expectations of the consumer; the demands the system places on the consumer; and the personnel who provide the various aspects of his care (Chapters 10–12).

An introduction to the process by which the menbers of all groups interact will help the student understand how the various (and often numerous) providers keep communications open among themselves. Ideally there will be continuity of care for all clients within this vast and often complicated system (Chapters 13 and 14).

Finally, the roles and functions of the registered nurse and the ethical and legal implications of being a humanistic licensed professional worker are discussed (Chapters 15–17).

CHAPTER 10

The study of the organization and delivery of health care services in the United States is a complex and bewildering task. The present system creates many problems for consumers and health professionals. This chapter broadly examines how health care is delivered in this country and suggests future trends that could affect nursing practice. It should be noted that each country has its own specific mechanisms for provision of health care services. Political, social, and economic factors affect the philosophy, planning, and implementation of these services. Examination of differing national modes of health care delivery, however, is beyond the scope of this chapter.

It is important that nurses understand health care delivery mechanisms, so that their clients receive the best health care available. Since nurses often have the initial contact with a client, they are responsible for introducing and guiding him through the network of available resources. Also, if the nurse is to act as an agent of change to improve the system, she must possess a thorough knowl-

THE DELIVERY OF HEALTH CARE

Mary Beth Hanner, M.P.H., R.N.

edge of the existing structure and how it functions.

Nurses not only provide care to individuals and families but also to neighborhoods and communities. The nursing process can be utilized to provide actions that will promote the optimal functioning of the community as a whole. Therefore, a second major focus of this chapter will be the application of the epidemiological approach in the community setting to improve the health status of groups of people.

To provide comprehensive care to clients, it is necessary to understand how the environment affects their health. Control or total elimination of disease can be best accomplished through a modification of the environment. Diagnosis and treatment of individuals do not significantly help to reduce the prevalence of disease or health problems; thus, a community approach is essential. Nurses are becoming more active in providing this type of care at the community level. They often work as members of a multidisciplinary team, so that each professional can contribute unique knowledge and

skills needed to deal with many complex community health problems.

HEALTH, MEDICAL, AND ILLNESS CARE SERVICES

The "health care delivery system" is a term used to describe the provision of all health, medical, and illness care services in this country. Although it is a frequently used phrase, it really does not appropriately describe the current state of health care services. Unfortunately, health care is not the primary focus in the provision of services to the public. Most services are designed to provide crisis-oriented illness and medical care. Too little emphasis is placed on keeping healthy people well. Most clients do not seek or receive services until they develop a health problem. To examine this issue more fully, it is necessary to differentiate between health, medical, and illness care. Clarification of these terms will also help in evaluating the effectiveness of current services.

Health care is the provision of services which are aimed at maintaining or improving the quality of the client's total internal and external environment to attain his optimal level of functioning. Health is a dynamic state that is constantly evolving toward a higher level of adaptation and self-actualization. The goal of this service is to keep the client on the positive side of the health-illness continuum. *Medical care* services are those which relate to the diagnosis and treatment of specific illnesses. The primary providers of medical care are physicians. *Illness care* refers to services provided to assist individuals and families to cope with the impact of a health problem and if possible, to regain a more positive state of health and prevent further disability. Illness care also involves assisting clients and families to cope with a terminal illness and helping clients face death with a sense of peace and dignity.

Many different kinds of health professionals are needed to provide comprehensive health and illness services. Although "health care" will be used in this chapter to describe health, medical, and illness care as a whole, it is very important to recognize that each type of service must be available to provide comprehensive care to individuals, groups, and communities.

The failure of the present system to deliver and promote health care services is an issue that is being discussed at all levels of government. The health care industry is the third largest business in this country. Spending for medical and illness care totals over 100 billion dollars annually. However, most health care dollars are spent almost entirely on diagnosing and treating illnesses, while only a very small amount is directed toward the prevention of illness and the promotion of health.

HEALTH CARE DELIVERY "SYSTEM": FACT OR FICTION

Banathy defines a system as: "deliberately designed synthetic organisms, comprised of interrelated and interracting components which are employed to function in an integrated fashion to attain predetermined purposes."[1] If we look at this definition in relation to health care delivery in the United States, it is easy to question if care is delivered in any systematic manner. Health related programs have sprung up independently, usually as stopgap measures directed toward existing health problems or illnesses. There is no overall plan from which specific programs are designed. Some of the many problems that have been identified within our present structure are:

1. Emphasis on crisis and illness, not on prevention.
2. Poor distribution of facilities and manpower.
3. Extremely high costs.
4. Lack of consumer participation.
5. Lack of coordination of services (i.e., fragmentation, overlaps, and gaps).

Services are fragmented. It is almost impossible to obtain comprehensive care from one service provider. There are multiple programs, providers, and agencies but little coordination of efforts or communication between groups. Each service has its own specific goals, seeks to meet its own interests, and provides care in whatever manner deemed best by the individuals who are in control. These services are not deliberately designed components that provide integrated, comprehensive care to clients.

Overlap of services within a community is demonstrated in numerous ways. For example, there are often several hospitals within a small geographic area that provide obstetric services. In recent years, with the declining birthrate, the need for beds in an obstetric unit has decreased. Yet, these units continue to be maintained, even though there is no indication of a present or future need. The logical solution would be to consolidate some of the obstetric units so that services are provided to local residents in some, but not all, of the area hospitals.

An example of a gap in necessary services would be the lack of extended care facilities and home nursing services for the elderly. Our population is changing; the percentage of people over age 65 is increasing. Since the majority of people in this age group have one or more chronic illnesses, the need for services has greatly increased. More money needs to be directed toward provision of comprehensive health, medical, and illness services to older citizens.

The unequal distribution of facilities and manpower is another significant problem. Many rural and poor areas are extremely underserved. Vital services are often lacking, and the few that are available are usually crowded and poorly staffed.

A system, according to the previous definition, should be designed with "predetermined purposes." Unfortunately, there is little agreement on what health is, how to stay healthy, or how to become healthier. The United States has not formulated a national health care policy with specific goals and objectives that can be measured and evaluated. Obviously, the ultimate goal of a health care system should be to improve the total well-being of all the people; however, there seems to be a lack of concensus on the best means to achieve that goal. A system needs to have components that complement each other and work *together* to achieve specific goals. One of the biggest challenges facing government today is the necessity of redesigning the present health care structure into a systematic network of services. Since nurses are the largest group of health care professionals, they have a tremendous responsibility to promote movements toward an effective system of health care delivery.

Present Structure

The present structure for delivery of health, medical, and illness services is divided into the public and the private sectors. The public sector includes the official agencies at the federal, state, and local levels of government. As the costs of health care escalate, more responsibility is being placed on the government for financing services. Therefore, governmental involvement is greatly influencing the organization and delivery of all three kinds of care.

PUBLIC SECTOR

FEDERAL GOVERNMENT. The federal government has some responsibility for the provision of direct services to special population groups. The Veteran's Administration, the Indian Health Service, the Public Health Service, and hospitals for military personnel are examples of such services. Most of the federal government's responsibility, however, does not relate to direct care services. Federal agencies propose legislation affecting health care, set standards for many state and local health agencies, and monitor the compliance of agencies with laws and standards. The federal health agencies usually communicate directly with state health departments, rather than local official agencies. The number of federal agencies involved in health related matters is large, and this has created some of the problems with delivery of services. The Department of Health, Education, and Welfare has the major federal responsibility for research, policy-making, planning, and funding related to health care.

STATE GOVERNMENT. The state health department was designed as a link between federal and local agencies. The main goal is to assist local areas in meeting health needs.[2] Therefore, many functions at the state level relate to advising community agencies and coordinating activities and programs within the state. Many state health departments provide state residents with direct services, such as massive screening and immunization programs, state hospitals, or institutions for the mentally ill or mentally retarded.

LOCAL GOVERNMENT. At the community level, the city or county health department is usually the largest official agency. The major responsibilities are provision of direct services to the population; identification of health needs specific to the area; and planning, implementation, and evaluation of programs to reduce or eliminate identified health problems. Some specific activities that should be basic to *every* local health agency are:

1. Collection of vital statistics.
2. Control of sanitary conditions.
3. Control of communicable disease.
4. Provision of special services to protect the health of mothers and infants.
5. Provision for some laboratory services.
6. Provision for public education on health matters.[3]

Many communities provide other resources, such as county or city hospitals, clinics, and community health nursing services. Community health nurses make home visits for health guidance and for illness care. They also work in clinics, provide health teaching to groups, and often provide service to schools, day-care centers, low income and senior citizen housing projects, and many other institutions. The role of the community health nurse in the provision of direct services to communities will be discussed in more detail later in this chapter.

PRIVATE SECTOR

One of the major advantages of our present health care structure is that we can choose physicians, hospitals, and other health care facilities. The private sector offers us a variety of services. Most service institutions, such as hospitals and nursing homes, are within the private sector of health care delivery. A major category of services within this sector is the voluntary agency. These agencies have more freedom and flexibility because they are not as restricted by governmental regulations. Voluntary agencies include such organizations as the American Cancer Society, Muscular Dystrophy Association, March of Dimes, and American Heart Association. Visiting nurse associations are also considered to be voluntary agencies.

Evaluation of Services within a Community

Health professionals must be able to examine and evaluate services within their own communities to determine their effectiveness. The three "A's" of health care services—availability, accessibility, and acceptability—can be used as a framework for evaluation. The stated objectives of the service and the levels of preventive care available should be considered within this framework. The following sections consider questions that should be asked when assessing community resources. The questions are not exhaustive but rather represent several factors that need to be considered in examining facilities that deliver health care within a community.

AVAILABILITY

Are there enough resources to provide adequate care for everyone in the community? Are services provided for each segment of the community's population? Do facilities provide health services as well as medical and illness services?

The nurse can facilitate the client's entrance into the network of services, as well as his progress through it. Therefore, it is important that the nurse be aware of community resources that are appropriate for her clients. It is equally important to identify services that are lacking but needed by community members. For example, a community health nurse who is working with an elderly, blind

client should have a thorough knowledge of available and needed resources within the area. Some appropriate referrals for this client might include:

1. Association for the Blind.
2. Friendly visitor service.
3. Senior citizen center.
4. Voluntary transportation service.
5. Meals-on-Wheels—hot meals delivered to home-bound clients.
6. Homemaker or home-health aide service.
7. Social service department—in order to determine eligibility for financial assistance.

Obviously, all of these resources might not be available nor appropriate for an individual client. A thorough nursing assessment will help to determine specific needs and problems for each person. The nurse and client should define problems and set goals mutually during the referral process.

ACCESSIBILITY

Do all community residents have equal access to care? If not, what barriers prevent access? Can each segment of the population get to the health care facilities? Are there transportation services available for the poor, the elderly, and the handicapped? Are there babysitting services or other arrangements for clients with children? Can people afford to pay for services?

Figure 10-1 illustrates some potential barriers that block access to services. Clients should be aware of resources that are available to them. Often they do not obtain help for a particular health problem simply because they are unaware that help is available. Emphasis on community education programs can greatly increase public awareness and result in better utilization of facilities.

Fear about the seriousness of the health problem is often a major deterrent to seeking health, medical, or illness services. The nurse can allow the client to verbalize fears, then present correct information, and stress the importance of early detection and treatment of health problems. Scare tactics or threats usually only increase fear of the unknown and tend to discourage people from seeking help.

Health professionals can do a lot to make service more accessible to clients. Ease of entry into the agency is a major consideration. How inconvenient

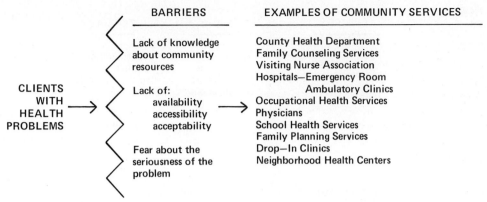

BARRIERS	EXAMPLES OF COMMUNITY SERVICES

CLIENTS WITH HEALTH PROBLEMS →

Lack of knowledge about community resources

Lack of:
availability
accessibility
acceptability

Fear about the seriousness of the problem

→

County Health Department
Family Counseling Services
Visiting Nurse Association
Hospitals—Emergency Room
           Ambulatory Clinics
Occupational Health Services
Physicians
School Health Services
Family Planning Services
Drop—In Clinics
Neighborhood Health Centers

FIGURE 10-1. Barriers to health, medical, and illness services and examples of community services. How can nurses help clients to break these barriers?

is it to make contact with the providers of care? Are appointments or referrals always needed? Is there ever a "drop-in" time for people who have problems that need immediate attention? Look at the hours that the center is open. Are the times for service convenient for the staff rather than the group who require care? Many services are open only from 8 or 9 am to 5 pm. These times may not be good for working families, and they may not fit into the life style and patterns of the community served. Ideally, working hours should be flexible to meet the changing needs of the community.

ACCEPTABILITY

Are services designed in accordance with community residents' values, life styles, and environment? Do clients utilize these services? If not, why not? Do the people served and the providers of care see the service as being appropriate, efficient, and effective? Do clients feel relatively comfortable in the setting? Is information presented in a manner that clients can comprehend?

OBJECTIVES AND OUTCOMES

Another area for consideration would be examination of the stated objectives of an agency. What is the purpose for its existence, and what do the staff expect to achieve? Compare the answers to the above questions with the actual services that are provided to consumers. Are the outcomes of care consistent with the goals of the agency?

LEVELS OF PREVENTION

Services within a community should also be evaluated in relation to the kinds of preventive care offered. All three levels of prevention—primary, secondary, and tertiary—should be offered to the consumer.

Primary preventive activities are aimed at promoting health and preventing the incidence of disease. Such activities would include immunizations and counseling on topics such as nutrition, exercise, smoking, sexuality, genetics, and mental health. *Secondary prevention* should detect health problems early and provide immediate intervention so that serious consequences can be prevented. Some examples would be developmental assessment of children, physical examination, and the Pap smear to detect cervical cancer. *Tertiary prevention* focuses on rehabilitation after an episode of illness to prevent further disability or complications. Teaching clients with chronic illnesses to monitor themselves to detect further problems is a preventive measure at the tertiary level.

Figure 10-2 illustrates a health-illness continuum. The left side of the continuum represents a positive state of health. The person who is well needs health services that include primary prevention. Nursing activities would include health promotion and maintenance. Medical and illness care is directed at people who have potential or actual disease conditions. Secondary and tertiary preventive nursing activities must then be considered in the assessment, planning, and evaluation of client care.

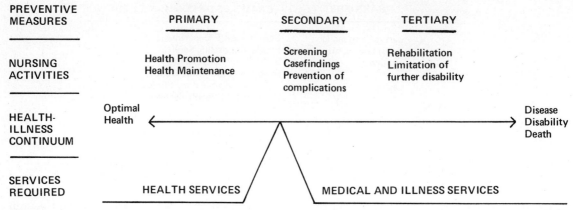

PREVENTIVE MEASURES		PRIMARY	SECONDARY	TERTIARY
NURSING ACTIVITIES		Health Promotion Health Maintenance	Screening Casefindings Prevention of complications	Rehabilitation Limitation of further disability

FIGURE 10-2. Services needed to provide primary, secondary, and tertiary care to clients.

Examination of the three "A's," objectives and outcomes, and the levels of preventive care will help to point out strengths and weaknesses of the services within a particular region. Increased availability, accessibility, and acceptability will promote better utilization of health resources and, hopefully, will improve the health status of consumers of these services.

THE RIGHT TO HEALTH

The belief that health care is a right and not a privilege is a philosophy that has been espoused for many years. However, it is a concept that is not a reality for many people, especially the poor. In 1966, the President's Commission on Human Rights developed four goals relating to the right to health for every citizen:

1. Every person should have maximum protection against diseases that need not happen and against illness and injury resulting from the hazards of the modern environment.
2. Every person should have ready access to basic medical care, despite social, economic, geographic, or other barriers, and should have the assurance of continuity of quality service through diagnosis, treatment, and rehabilitation.
3. Every person should have maximum opportunity for developing his capabilities in an environment that is not merely safe, but conducive to productive living.
4. All activities conducted in pursuit of health

should be carried out with full attention to the dignity and integrity of the individual.[4]

These four goals are based on the philosophy that quality health care is a basic right of all people. Health care legislation has been designed in an attempt to improve the delivery of service and to promote more equal access for everyone. The National Health Planning and Resources Development Act, enacted on January 4, 1975, authorized the development of new agencies at the local, state, and national levels. Congress, recognizing that many problems existed within the structure of health care delivery, proposed this legislation to provide a single network of authority for health planning and development. The act also mandates that guidelines be established for the development of a national health planning policy.[5] Specific information on this legislation is contained in Chapter 11 entitled "The Consumer of Health Care Services."

Another legislative proposal reflecting the right to health philosophy is the national health insurance plan. The enactment of this plan by Congress is predicted in the very near future. Many plans have been proposed, and there is widespread agreement on the need for national health insurance. Debate continues on methods of financing and administering the program. Basically, the purpose of all the proposals is to provide accessibility to health services for every citizen, regardless of their ability to pay.

The American Nurses' Association has issued a statement of their principles and positions in relation to national health insurance. The ANA is supporting a program that will do the following:

1. Guarantee coverage of all people for the full range of comprehensive health services.
2. Define the benefits clearly so that they can be understood by beneficiaries and providers alike.
3. Recognize the distinctions between health care and medical care, and provide options in utilization of health care services that are not necessarily dependent on the physician.
4. Provide for nursing care services as a benefit.
5. Recognize nurses as providers to be reimbursed for their services.
6. Provide that the data systems necessary for effective management of the program protect the rights and privacy of individuals.
6. Include provisions for peer review of services that will protect the right and responsibility of each health care discipline to monitor the practice of its own practitioners.
7. Provide for consumer participation in evaluation of the insurance program.
8. Provide for financing of the program through payroll taxes or payment of premiums by the self-employed, with coverage for the poor and unemployed paid for from general tax revenues.[6]

These two proposals, along with many others, are attempts to restructure services so that they are provided in a systematic, comprehensive, and effective manner. The development of a system that will remain open and responsive to the changing needs of our society and our environment is the desired outcome and the hope for the future. Tinkham and Voorhies[7] state their concern for the future of health care delivery in the following:

> To bring order out of chaos is a major task of all who are concerned with health. Americans have the knowledge and the resources, but have not been able or willing to implement a flexible, economically feasible plan of health organization through which quality service can be made available to all who need it. Our heritage of democracy and individualism, coupled with the complexity of an urban society, makes the task of planning quality care a herculean one. Whether

this can be done depends more on our wisdom and intelligence than on money or words.[7]

THE COMMUNITY AS A CLIENT: PROVISION OF NURSING SERVICES

The dilemma we face is how to improve the delivery of health care, but the solutions to this problem are not simple. More hospitals, nurses, doctors, and other health workers might help to increase the availability of services, but we now recognize other approaches are required to solve our major health problems. Man's total well-being is far more affected by his heredity, environment, and behavior than by the type of medical care services received. Research is presently being conducted on how to motivate people toward more health promotive behaviors and life styles. Future goals will be directed toward attempts to modify our genetic makeup in order to decrease our predisposition to specific diseases. The effect of the environment on health is a major concern of public health workers today. They recognize that health professionals must be prepared to go beyond treating individuals and families; they must have the ability to treat the community as a client. Knowledge and skills must be applied to the diagnosis and treatment of entire groups of people within defined community areas.

Evolution of a Community Approach

The history of medicine and health care demonstrates an evolution from a focus on treating client symptoms and diseases to one of comprehensive care and treatment of individuals, families, and communities. McGavran[8] states that changes in the health field since 1850 can be divided into four eras. Up until 1850, providers of care focused on the treatment of *symptoms* only. Most specific disease entities were unknown, and little could be done except to alleviate the presenting symptoms. Discovery of the germ theory led into a new era of scientific diagnosis and treatment of specific diseases. However, it was soon recognized that successful treatment of disease often did not improve the total well-being of the client. "The operation was a success, but the patient died" is a popular phrase used to describe this kind of care.

In the early 1900s it became evident that a more comprehensive approach to client care was required. The emphasis moved toward the needs of the *total* individual. A more holistic assessment was done in order to identify social, psychological, sexual, spiritual, and economic needs in addition to physical concerns.

The present era, which began around 1950, has an even broader focus, that is, on the scientific diagnosis and treatment of the total community. It has become clear that we must look at our entire environment to find solutions to health problems that plague the latter part of the twentieth century. Individual diagnosis and treatment of disease may help or cure one client, but only through a community approach can disease be controlled or eliminated. For example, advances such as improved sanitation, control of disease-carrying insects, immunizations, and pasteurization of milk have dramatically reduced the incidence of communicable diseases. Modification of man's internal and external environment brought about significant improvements in the health status of entire groups of people. The most effective methods to reduce the incidence and prevalence of disease are: (1) modification of the environment, (2) a change in the immunity status of groups of people (immunization or exposure to disease), and (3) quarantine. This fact has brought us to the present focus on provision of service to the entire community.

Epidemiological Approach

The epidemiological approach can be utilized to diagnose and treat health problems that affect groups of people within the community. Many health professionals use this framework to plan and implement primary preventive services to defined populations. Figure 10-3 depicts the basic steps of the epidemiological approach to the provision of primary prevention. The health worker must first define the target area for intervention. At what population is the program aimed? Service might be directed toward a specific group, neighborhood, geographic area, or perhaps a school or work setting. Once the target population has been determined, an assessment should be done to define the most prevalent health problems in that group. It is important to identify which of those problems could be prevented. Priorities for intervention can then

be determined by examining the degree of threat to the life and security of the group. Also, identify the problems that are considered as top priorities by community residents.

After selection of the priority health problem, examine factors that contribute to the development of the disease or health condition. These are called high-risk factors because they affect each person's vulnerability to illness. For example, such things as age, sex, weight, smoking, eating, drinking habits, and family history of disease can all affect an individual's susceptibility to disease.

The next step involves assessment of the people who have the health problem and of those people who have several high-risk factors that increase their chance of developing the health problem or condition. Planning and implementation of measures to modify or eliminate high-risk factors would then be carried out to decrease the vulnerability of the target group. Evaluation efforts should center on collection of data to analyze the results of efforts to control or reduce the health problem. Statistics should be kept to monitor the incidence (number of new cases) and prevalence (total number of cases) of the condition.

APPLICATIONS TO COMMUNITY HEALTH NURSING

The goals of nursing relate to the provision of service to individuals, families, groups, and communities. However, it is often difficult to understand the concept of the community as the nurse's client. How can an entire community be diagnosed and treated? How can health professionals prevent potential problems from developing in population groups? These are questions that often overwhelm the nurse who is working in a community setting.

The epidemiological approach to the provision of primary preventive services is a framework within which the nurse can operate. For example, a community health nurse who is assigned to a small, rural, moderate to low-income community may make many health guidance visits to parents with newborn infants. Her caseload may also include some families who have been referred from the local child protective agency for potential or actual child abuse or neglect. While very competent nursing intervention may be provided to each of these families, additional efforts are needed to pre-

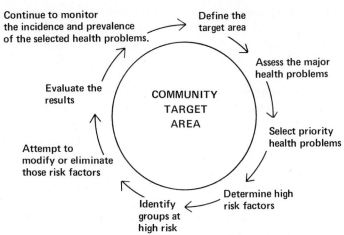

FIGURE 10-3. An epidemiological model for provision of primary prevention to communities.

vent child abuse before it occurs. Therefore, the nurse should investigate the extent of the problem in the area to determine if it is a serious health threat to a significant number of children. She should also determine what characteristics are common to abusive parents to identify families who would be in a high-risk category. High-risk factors for child abuse would include: social isolation, single parent families, parents who were abused when they were children, people with a low tolerance for frustration, and those parents who have unrealistic expectations of their children. The nurse would then assess which families in her caseload had several high-risk factors to provide an effective plan of primary prevention. In this situation, one alternative the nurse might consider is the formulation of a local parents' group with a babysitting service. This group could provide increased social support to decrease the feelings of isolation among the parents. Discussion of common parental concerns, problems, and frustrations might help group members to gain more insights about themselves and the needs of their children. Hopefully, this kind of approach would lead to a decreased incidence of child abuse and neglect cases in the target group.

Another example of the need for an epidemiological perspective can be demonstrated by cancer, which is the second leading cause of death in the United States. Many health professionals feel that cancer is a modern epidemic. This disease has been approached on an individual basis for many years. Activities were aimed at early case-finding (secondary prevention) to diagnose and treat cancer in its

early stages. Therefore, people were taught the seven warning signals of cancer and were advised to visit their physicians for frequent checkups. However, even after several years of frequent urging, the incidence of cancer is still increasing. Another approach must be utilized in addition to the methods described.

Cancer can also be examined from an epidemiological viewpoint. It is estimated that as much as 85 percent of all cancers are caused by environmental factors such as chemicals and other environmental pollutants. It is an established fact that highly industrialized states have the highest rates of cancer. Workers who are exposed to certain chemicals (e.g., vinyl chloride) develop cancer at much higher rates than the rest of the population. Therefore, employees who are working with these carcinogens (cancer-producing substances) are in a high-risk group. Thus, their working conditions must be modified to decrease their exposure to these substances. This should help to prevent future cases of cancer in the employee group by decreasing their vulnerability.

Not only are certain workers at risk for developing cancer, but food consumers are exposed to many known and suspected carcinogens. Since we all are consumers of food, we increase our risk of developing cancer by eating food additives. The Food and Drug Administration has the primary responsibility for determining which agents are carcinogenic so that they can be eliminated from the market. This is a very slow process, however, and the public is often not protected from potentially dangerous substances. Since it is not presently possible to alter our genetic make-up if we are predisposed to cancer, it is important to modify our environment by reducing the number of carcinogens to which we are exposed.

Examination of the entire group at risk utilizing the epidemiological method is not only appropriate for the problems of child abuse and cancer, but for most of our current health problems. As the era of community diagnosis and treatment continues to emerge, even greater emphasis will be placed on environmental factors, community health, and epidemiology. Nurses are also changing their focus to a more comprehensive examination of health and illness producing factors. Hopefully, this movement will help to create positive changes for both the nursing profession and for the consumer of health, medical, and illness services.

SUMMARY

The health care delivery system is, in reality, a tangled network of services that provides unequal distribution and quality of care throughout the United States. The focus today is one of disease orientation rather than one of health promotion and maintenance. Services are geared toward medical and illness care, but little emphasis is placed on providing health promotive services. Problems of health care delivery are numerous and relate to the poor distribution of services, inflation, and lack of coordination and consumer input. Services must be redesigned and organized so that they are available, accessible, and acceptable to all community residents.

Attempts to improve the present structure are being proposed by government. Legislative reforms may help to provide a better quality of care, but our focus of intervention must also broaden. A community approach to solving health problems will hopefully reduce or control the problems in a significant number of people within the community target area. The ideal outcome of changing the present structure would be the creation of a working *system* of health care delivery that is flexible, open, and responsive to the changing needs of the health care consumer.

REFERENCES

1. Banathy, B. H.: *Instructional Systems.* Palo Alto, Calif., Fearon Publishers, 1968, pp. 2–3.
2. Wigley, R., and Cook, J. R.: *Community Health: Concepts and Issues.* New York, D. Van Nostrand Co., 1975, p. 149.
3. *Ibid.,* p. 152.
4. U.S. Department of State: *For Free Men in a Free World: A Survey of Human Rights in the United States.* Washington D.C., U.S. Government Printing Office, (Publication #8434,) 1969, pp. 166–168.
5. Novello, D. J.: The national health planning and resources development act: what it is and how it works. *Nurs. Outlook* 24(6):354–355, 1976.
6. American Nurses' Association: *A National Policy for Health Care: Principles and Positions.* American Nurses' Association, December 1977, p. 3.
7. Tinkham, C. W., and Voorhies, E. F.: *Community Health Nursing: Evolution and Process,* 2nd ed. New York, Appleton-Century-Crofts, 1977, p. 194.
8. McGavran, E. G.: What is public health? *Can. J. Public Health* 44:441, 1953.

CHAPTER 11

A consumer is generally defined as the purchaser of a particular good or service. The definition of the consumer of health services is usually expanded to include the user of services as well and is interchangeable with client or patient. In a very broad sense, all taxpayers perform two consumer roles with regard to health services. (1) They pay for their own health care through insurance plans and out-of-pocket monies for the costs not covered by insurance. (2) Through taxes (city, state, and federal), the aggregate needs of citizens (emergency medical services) are supported and care is provided to those unable to pay for their own health care, primarily the aged and the sick poor. The use of public funds for any purpose is legislated by elected officials and is presumably responsive to the desires of the majority of the electorate.

The cost of all health care services has spiraled astronomically in the past 20 years. Figure 11-1 illustrates the rapid rise in health care since the enactment of Medicaid and Medicare in 1965. Although private payment, either for insurance cov-

THE CONSUMER OF HEALTH CARE SERVICES

Marion Isaacs, M.S., R.N.

erage or for those services which are not insured, is still slightly more expensive, the public expenditures for health services are formidable and likely to surpass private outlays even without national health insurance (Fig. 11-2). Programs such as Medicare, Medicaid, Veterans' services, CHAMPUS, CHAMP-VA, and the Federal Employees Insurance Benefits taken collectively account for most of the federal government financing for health care.

In a capitalist economy, such as the United States, the role of the consumer is crucial in maintaining a balance between the concerns of the producer-seller and the concerns of the consumer-purchaser. This balance results in profits for the seller which can either contribute to his personal wealth or be used for expansion and as a consequence, make a contribution to the wealth of the society by increasing production and employment. For the buyer, the balance results in prices which are within grasp and variety in the quality of goods and services. However, this ideal balance of market forces is difficult to maintain, and often the consumer feels that the goods and services received have been falsely advertised or are of inferior quality. The famous, old Latin quote, *caveat emptor* or "let the buyer beware," suggests the long felt attitude of impotence in combating the situation. In recent years with the impact of the consumer movement, attitudes are changing. The dictum, *populous lamdudum defutatus est*, hung on the door of the offices of the Health Research Group, the health arm of Ralph Nader's consumer oriented organization. It roughly translates to "the consumer has been screwed long enough."

Many consumer groups have sought political solutions to these economic problems. Senior citizens groups such as the Grey Panthers and special interest groups such as the Veterans of Foreign Wars have lobbied the federal government for programs to resolve their own or other constituent problems. Requests run the gamut of federal power from disbursement of general revenues through regulatory protection. In general, federal solutions are sought to resolve local problems when the problem (1) is

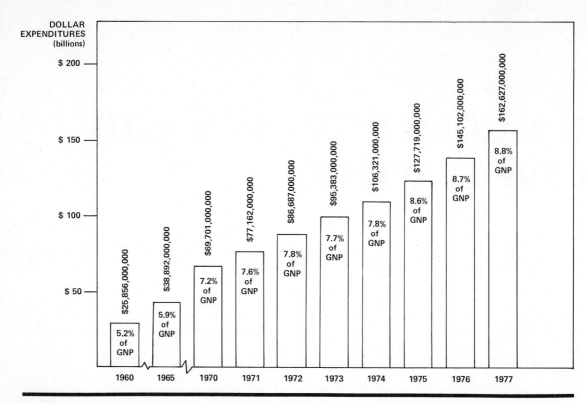

FIGURE 11-1. U.S. national health expenditures in dollars and as a percentage of the gross national product (GNP). (Source: U.S. Department of Health, Education, and Welfare, Social Security Bulletin, vol. 47, no. 7, 1978. Prepared by the Health Planning Council for Greater Boston.)

widespread affecting citizens throughout the country, (2) is too expensive to be paid for through state and local taxes, and (3) has an inherent social good which requires a fundamental change in public policy. The federal share of personal health care expenditures has increased, in part, as a function of expansion of services and programs. The expenditures of the Department of Health, Education, and Welfare exceed all other government budgets, including the Defense Department, and excluding only the budget of the government of the United States and the Soviet Union. Because the word health does not appear in the Constitution, it is often difficult to initiate federal regulatory programs. The argument of impingement on states rights is frequently raised by business groups to deter federal regulations which might provide protection to the consumer in the marketplace. The government is often left with the option of using dollars rather than regulation to address local problems and inequities. However, when the government or even the insurance industry purchases service for individuals, the direct bite of the consumer is lost in the transaction. This will be explored in more detail when the role of third-party payers in health care financing is discussed.

According to Rhodes,[1] the Republican Party has traditionally identified itself with the position that the consumer can fare well in the marketplace if the pure roles of consumer and seller are unfettered by government intervention. Consumer refusal to purchase inferior or overpriced goods creates the necessary incentive for industry to respond or go out of business. Liberal Democrats, on the other hand, believe essentially that there are basic necessities that should be provided to the American people which cannot be left to the market as an ultimate protection of the public good. On the federal level, the Food and Drug Administration is a regulatory agency; since its creation by law in 1906, it has been seen as the protector of the public's health with regard to foods, drugs, and cosmetics.

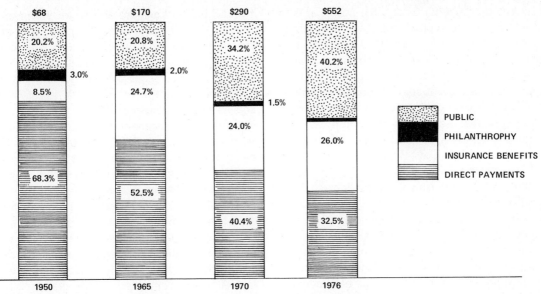

FIGURE 11-2. Percentage distribution of personal health care expenditures by source funds for fiscal years 1950, 1965, 1970, and 1976. (Source: U.S. Department of Health, Education, and Welfare, in a 1976 presentation to the House Interstate and Foreign Commerce Committee.)

Likewise, the Environmental Protection Agency was legislated to protect the public from environmental pollution (air, water, etc.). Laws determine the extent to which these regulatory agencies can influence industry, and statutes are periodically amended to reflect desired changes.

THE HEALTH MARKETPLACE

In the usual marketplace transaction, whether a good such as a rug is to be purchased, or a service such as auto repair, or a combination of these, such as occurs in dining out, the consumer responds to needs and desires by shopping for the quality article he desires, basing his decision on the variations in price. Other variables may enter into the transaction, such as the availability of alternatives or the pre-established relationships with specific merchants. The merchant's role is to try to make the sale, either by accommodating consumer needs regarding price and quality or with convenience factors such as hours open, delivery services, attractive advertising, or ambience. The consumer generally has an idea about whether he has been well served on the basis of his past experience with the product or his knowledge of what to expect from it. Generally, the merchant is aware that there are other

merchants with similar desires, services, and products and to make the sale, he must compete on several levels with them.

How then does the consumer-client differ from the consumer of other goods and services? Why is the health marketplace different from the general marketplace? Many factors influence the consumers and providers in the marketplace of health services delivery which have been proposed as constraints against the balancing forces of supply and demand. Without detailing each of these, several of the most important are presented here.

1. The view that health care is a right and the growth of third-party payers as a means of paying for it.
2. The unreliability of supply and distribution of providers as an influence on cost.
3. The mystical aspects of medical or nursing care (lack of advertising and the difficulty in evaluating the quality of the service provided).

Health Care as a Basic Right

The problem with viewing health as a basic right is that it requires collective decision-making on what constitutes quality services and the cost that is to be paid for them. The proliferation and general use of third-party payers has protected the consumer against many medical expenses but has curtailed his usual influence on cost and supply. The Blue Cross/Blue Shield plans started during the depression when so many people were unable to pay for hospital costs that they simply stayed at home. The providers (physicians) realized that a collective insurance plan such as the ''Blues'' was a means of continuing their services for the client and getting the bills paid. Simply stated, by pooling relatively small individual contributions, the group accumulates the resources to pay out large sums of money to individuals who need it. Unions, organizations, and other groups have seen the value of insuring against the cost of illness with this method, and the growth of private insurance coverage has been significant. In order for these plans to be successful, the premium cost is determined on the basis of the sickness liability of the particular group, considering age, occupation, and the illness experiences of the enrollees. Some individuals, such as those with sickle-cell anemia and other congenital problems, are often uninsurable. There are currently about 12 million Americans who have no private insurance and who are also ineligible for government health insurance.

In all instances, the presence of a third-party payer has removed to a certain extent, the client's role as consumer or purchaser of health and medical services. The policy-making process employed by most insurance companies, until very recently, excluded consumer input. Basic plans often stress coverage of expensive inpatient care while most ambulatory services (except emergency room care) are absent. This presence of money for acute hospital care has encouraged capacity expansion and use thereby discouraging less expensive preventive and other ambulatory services.

Presently when the federal and state governments pay for health coverage, they do so on the basis of the money available from tax revenues and by setting eligibility requirements based on income, physical disability, or age. The Medicare program, which is financed totally through federal funds, is a standardized package of benefits, regardless of the health status or employment of the individual, based on the individual's age. Almost all American women over 62 years of age and almost all men over 65 years of age are eligible for this insurance, after paying the initial deductibles and coinsurance requirements which are set at the federal level. Renal dialysis is the only specified disease category which is covered regardless of age.

Medicaid, on the other hand, is an expense shared by the state and the federal government. The federal government is responsible for a minimum of 50 percent of the costs of care (for special categories of recipients, a higher percentage may be paid). The state must comply with certain minimum regulations to receive the federal shares, but essentially Medicaid is a state-run program and covered services and eligibility criteria above a minimum are decided on the state level. In spite of this, some states still feel that federal regulations require too much in terms of administration and service. In fact, Arizona has no Medicaid program at all.

In addition to indirect decisions regarding benefits, there are several other problems created by third-party payment. They diminish the client's need for making a conscious decision against the costs of covered services; that is, once the plan has been paid for (often by deductions from the paycheck before it is even felt as actual income) the client, especially if there are no copayments or deductibles, has the incentive to get his money's worth rather than choose other alternatives to expensive hospitals or emergency room care.

The physician or provider is relatively unchallenged and unconcerned about choosing the most high-styled level of care because most of the cost will be paid. Therefore, a procedure may be chosen which has marginal necessity or requires a more frequent follow-up protocol than either the provider or the client would have chosen if the need to pay for the service was a factor. Thus, Elwood and McClure[2] suggest that in the contemporary provider-client relationship, it is actually the provider who is the purchaser of goods and services in that the provider decides the quality, method, and frequency of treatment, provided interest is not usually pecuniary. High-styled care and use of costly technology in even hopeless situations have become characteristic of hospital and outpatient health care, although there appears to be a rebellious trend.

In recent years, the historically provider-oriented insurance plans have responded to consumer pressure to assist in representing them more effectively.

(Although the cost of overutilization of marginally necessary services is not felt directly by the individual, he does pay for these services in the form of rate increases or tax increases.) In addition, industries which negotiate with union groups regarding the extent of health benefits have also taken steps to try to control the cost of health care. The Kaiser Corporation is best known for its early attempts to control the cost of care through the use of a prepaid group practice or health maintenance organizations (HMO). The HMO concept varies from other insurance plans in that the client chooses and identifies with the providers (because of the extensive preventive and informational programs offered) during times of wellness. The provider has the incentive of staying within cost limits to keep the plan solvent and has no incentive to overutilize services because he is either salaried or shares in the profits if there are savings. Nurse practitioners are used extensively as an adjunct to, and sometimes even a cost-effective, quality substitute for, physician services. The results indicate that most HMOs (organized on the Kaiser model) have fewer surgical procedures, shorter hospital stays, and broader preventive services than the traditional fee-for-service system, at a cost savings of between 10 and 30 percent.[3] There are currently approximately six million Americans enrolled in prepaid group practices. These plans have had varying support in their development by the federal government in the past, although the 95th Congress and the Carter administration have taken steps to improve this situation through the passage of the Health Maintenance Organization Act Amendments of 1978.

As a major purchaser of services, several unions have sought to have their insurance companies take a more active role in containing costs by refusing to pay providers for marginally necessary or outdated procedures and by requiring a second surgical opinion prior to surgery, leaving the ultimate choice of surgery to the client.

Perhaps in response to this pressure, the National Blue Shield Association in May 1977, recommended that its individual plans stop routine reimbursement for 28 surgical and diagnostic procedures considered outmoded or unnecessary, which at the time of this writing cost members $27.4 million a year.[4] Several Medicaid plans have adopted similar practices.

Other suggestions for revamping the third-party system, if it is to be perpetuated under national health insurance, are the inclusion of more extensive preventive services, more comprehensive ambulatory services, third-party review of all hospital and nursing home admissions for the rationale for admission and length of stay, on a concurrent rather than retrospective basis, prospective hospital budgeting, and more extensive denial of payment to providers[5] for inappropriate care (with no penalty to the client).

Supply as a Factor in Reducing Cost

In the usual scheme of market forces, oversupply should result in a decrease in the cost or value of goods or services. While this may be a relevant factor to nursing manpower, because of our status as employees, it has not been true of physicians still primarily engaged in private fee-for-service practice.

During the past two decades, the federal government has attempted to engage in manipulation of supply and distribution of nursing and medical personnel. The first major attempt was made in 1963 in the Health Professions Educational Assistance Act (HPEA) in which schools received federal assistance for their teaching activities. In subsequent years, health manpower subsidies were expanded and direct capitation grants were made to schools on the basis of enrollment in addition to the provision of loans and scholarships for medical, nursing, osteopathy, dental, and veterinary students. Nursing was removed from the general HPEA manpower legislation in 1964 and through the 1970s continued to receive separate authorization and appropriation through the Nurse Training Act. The principle rationale for government intervention centered around the following four major perceptions:

1. Unfettered market forces would continue to result in the exclusion of low or moderate income people and minorities from medical, nursing, and other health professions.
2. A 1970 prediction by the Carnegie Commission[5] and others that a shortage of physicians and nurses would have a deleterious effect on the health of the American people.
3. The mix of medical manpower was improper; specialists and surgeons being overrepresented and primary care providers seriously

underrepresented. (In 1977, only 45 percent of American physicians provided primary care compared to 75 percent of Britain's medical manpower.)[6]

4. There is a geographic maldistribution of nurses and physicians; rural areas have far fewer nurses and physicians per population than urban and suburban areas.

The effect of health manpower legislation on supply is impressive. From 1963–1973, the number of active, registered nurses increased by an overall 43 percent, and practical nurses increased by an overall 83 percent. However, Reinhardt[7] suggested that without a change in this manpower policy the supply of active registered nurses will increase faster than the population to be served. The

Table 11-1. Supply and Distribution of Active Registered Nurses and Doctors

Geographic division and state	1966		1972			1968		1973		
	Registered nurses employed in nursing	Population/ nurse ratio	Registered nurses employed in nursing	Population/ nurse ratio	Percent increase in employed nurses 1966-72	M.D.s	Population/ physician ratio	M.D.s	Population/ physician ratio	Percent increase in physicians 1968-73
United States	613,188	319	794,979	262	29.6	264,287	754	308,543	680	16.7
New England										
Maine	4,051	247	4,810	213	18.7	932	1,067	1,144	908	22.7
New Hampshire	3,521	193	4,445	174	26.2	846	838	1,068	743	26.2
Vermont	1,836	225	2,854	161	55.4	700	614	825	565	17.9
Massachusetts	28,743	193	37,620	154	30.9	10,536	533	12,183	476	15.6
Rhode Island	3,673	245	4,712	206	28.3	1,277	722	1,549	624	21.3
Connecticut	15,438	188	17,887	172	15.9	5,117	579	6,005	313	17.4
Middle Atlantic										
New York	74,280	240	89,375	206	20.3	38,902	464	42,156	432	8.4
New Jersey	24,942	275	31,943	230	28.1	9,015	777	10,930	670	21.2
Pennsylvania	45,809	255	61,927	192	35.2	16,356	718	17,889	663	9.4
East North Central										
Ohio	32,649	316	42,032	255	28.7	13,003	809	14,173	758	9.0
Indiana	72,829	390	15,841	334	23.5	4,753	1,072	5,422	978	14.1
Illinois	35,552	305	44,783	251	26.0	13,954	788	15,993	699	14.6
Michigan	23,441	363	30,546	295	30.3	10,049	865	11,543	785	18.7
Wisconsin	14,084	303	18,887	240	34.1	4,702	924	5,548	818	18.0
West North Central										
Minnesota	14,441	250	19,169	202	32.7	5,174	716	5,934	656	14.7
Iowa	9,981	277	11,959	241	19.8	2,696	1,040	2,865	999	6.3
Missouri	11,291	401	14,982	317	32.7	5,495	831	6,274	760	14.2
North Dakota	2,114	306	2,885	202	36.5	542	1,146	581	1,093	7.2
South Dakota	2,089	327	3,140	217	50.3	501	1,335	508	1,343	1.4
Nebraska	4,730	308	6,802	225	43.8	1,503	976	1,773	865	18.0
Kansas	6,895	319	9,098	249	32.0	2,324	954	2,621	864	12.8
South Atlantic										
Delaware	2,098	191	2,935	195	39.9	652	819	762	752	16.9
Maryland	10,005	369	14,847	273	48.4	6,170	618	7,748	526	25.6
District of Columbia	3,662	216	5,020	150	37.1	2,773	281	3,046	241	9.8
Virginia	11,511	387	16,647	286	44.6	4,853	939	6,072	798	25.1
West Virginia	4,707	377	6,255	287	32.9	1,655	1,065	1,868	957	12.9
North Carolina	12,126	404	16,649	314	37.3	4,947	1,012	5,984	886	21.0
South Carolina	5,625	448	7,916	340	40.7	2,004	1,277	2,589	1,052	29.2
Georgia	6,956	630	12,492	379	79.6	4,361	1,028	5,368	898	23.1
Florida	21,760	281	26,202	280	20.4	7,558	851	10,809	717	43.0
East South Central										
Kentucky	6,297	500	8,487	390	34.8	3,033	1,053	3,511	948	15.8
Tennessee	6,755	566	9,446	431	39.8	4,231	917	5,001	819	18.2
Alabama	5,912	586	7,847	449	32.7	2,754	1,251	3,194	1,110	16.0
Mississippi	3,670	612	5,129	440	39.8	1,653	1,342	1,889	1,227	14.3
West South Central										
Arkansas	2,609	728	3,776	532	44.7	1,560	1,219	1,794	1,134	15.0
Louisiana	6,758	525	9,133	409	35.1	4,015	897	4,466	839	11.2
Oklahoma	4,650	528	6,514	404	40.1	2,361	1,060	2,647	1,008	12.1
Texas	20,167	520	28,213	411	39.9	11,463	944	13,885	852	21.1
Mountain										
Montana	2,483	285	3,261	220	31.3	641	1,092	730	1,000	13.9
Idaho	1,954	353	2,518	300	28.9	596	1,166	710	1,093	19.1
Wyoming	1,209	267	1,480	234	22.4	286	1,133	332	1,063	16.1
Colorado	8,312	241	11,780	218	41.7	3,340	635	4,068	607	21.8
New Mexico	2,511	401	2,778	387	10.6	918	1,083	1,228	895	33.8
Arizona	5,862	275	8,513	231	45.2	1,902	884	2,994	692	57.4
Utah	2,347	430	3,260	346	38.9	1,298	793	1,631	705	25.7
Nevada	1,060	421	1,732	308	63.4	446	1,040	591	932	32.5
Pacific										
Washington	11,361	269	14,476	236	27.4	4,318	757	5,110	671	18.3
Oregon	6,814	289	8,790	249	29.0	2,643	758	3,266	679	23.6
California	58,694	321	68,668	297	17.0	32,334	600	38,749	533	19.8
Alaska	590	459	1,399	232	37.1	180	1,583	281	1,174	56.1
Hawaii	2,334	304	3,110	262	33.2	965	761	1,236	680	28.1

SOURCE: AMA Center for Health Services Research and Development: Distribution of Physicians in the U.S., 1973. G. A. Roback. Chicago. American Medical Association 1974. Table 9; AMA Center for Health Services Research and Development: Reclassification of Physicians, 1968, Chicago. American Medical Association. 1971. Appendix Table 1; U.S. Bureau of the Census: Population Estimates: Current Population Reports, Series P-25, No. 460, June 1971, and No. 533, October 1974. (Adapted from U.S. Department of Health, Education and Welfare, Public Health Service, Health Resources Administration: Health United States 1975, Tables B.1.13, P120 and Table B.1.19, P126, DHEW Publication No. (HRA) 76-1232.)

Department of Labor also says that "if trends in the number of persons enrolling in schools of nursing continue, some competition for more desirable, higher paying jobs may develop by the 1980s."

Likewise, the medical manpower supply has increased significantly in the past 10 years (Table 11-1). The Department of Health, Education, and Welfare claims that National Health Insurance will expand the user market and the demands on supply of medical (12 percent more needed) and nursing personnel (5 percent more) needed. However, they anticipate that the pool of inactive nurses can fill any short-term shortages.

Marc Lalonde,[8] Minister of National Health and Welfare in Canada, discussed the overall supply of doctors and nurses in selected countries (Table 11-2) in that country's working document on health issues. It is noteworthy that the United Kingdom, Sweden, and Denmark have fewer doctors per 10,000 population than the United States, and all three offer almost 100 percent health insurance coverage. Likewise, there are fewer nurses per 10,000 population in Sweden and the United Kingdom. The ratio of nurses to doctors is approximately the same in Canada, Denmark, and Sweden. The United Kingdom has fewest, and Australia has the most with a 5.6:1 nurse-doctor ratio. Reliable yet contradictory data and an apparent need prompted the 95th Congress to vote, by a wide majority, to extend for 2 additional years, federal support for nursing education through the passage of the Nurse Training Act of 1978. Congress and the nursing community were shocked by President Carter's pocket-veto of the legislation. The President's veto message contended that there was no longer a supply problem in nursing personnel. The only exception cited was the need for nurse practitioners who are viewed by many as necessary to shore up the current undersupply of primary care physicians. Reliable predictions on the need for supply levels are difficult to make. Many factors, such as population mobility, changes in practice, changes in role, and changes in demand for service as well as disease morbidity and mortality are important and often elusive variables. The most tenacious argument against increasing the numbers of health professionals, physicians or nurses, is the lack of improvement of health status. For example both the north central and southern states have low ratios of physicians and nurses to the population, but the life expectancy is high in the central midwest and low in the south. Factors such as sanitation, standard of living, housing, education and life style are often more deleterious to health than the absence of physicians and nurses.

The increase in supply did not result in corresponding decrease in cost. Cost incurred by the private and public sector for physicians' services in 1960 totaled $5,648,000; by 1973, this cost rose to $18,200,000.[9] In 1975, medical care prices on the whole, increased at nearly twice the rate of the consumer price average with prices for physicians leading the increase.[10] Reinhardt[7] suggested that the annual income of physicians, particularly specialists, has propelled them into the highest strata of the nation's income distribution. Likewise, though not comparable to the increase in income enjoyed by physicians, nurses have also enjoyed economic gains, perhaps as a result of prowess in collective bargaining and the repeal of an 18-year-old "no-strike" policy by the American Nurses' Association in 1968.[11] The historically low salary

TABLE 11-2. Health Insurance Coverage, Nurse and Physician Supply (1971)*

Country	Percent Covered by Medical and Hospital Insurance	No. Physicians per 10,000 Population	No. Nurses per 10,000 Population	Nurse/Physician Ratio
Australia	79% (hosp.) 75% (med.)	11.8	66.6	5.6/1
Canada	Almost 100%	15.7	57.3	3.6/1
Denmark	96.7%	14.5	53.4	3.6/1
Sweden	Almost 100%	12.4	43.7	3.5/1
United Kingdom	Almost 100%	12.5	35.1	2.8/1
United States	85% (hosp.) 65% (reg. med.) 35% (maj. med.)	15.3	49.2	3.2/1

*Adapted from Lalonde, Marc: *A New Perspective on the Health of Canadians,* Ottawa, Tri-Graphic Printing, 1975, p. 27.

ranges have also been a factor influencing the trend toward increases in the late 1960s when money was available and hospital and health workers were recognized as needing reparations. (See Table 11-3 for a comparison of nurses' and public school teachers' salaries.)

Increase in the supply of workers has also probably resulted in an increase in costs of care exclusive of wages or fees. Again looking at market forces, the increased supply of goods or services is especially affected by the interplay with demand for those services. In health care, the demand for service, as discussed in the section on third-party payers, is often provider-induced. While the larger cost increases can be attributed to physicians' behavior,[12] nurse behavior also contributes to increases in the total cost of health care. For example, one of the major functions of community health nurses is to case-find, that is, seek ill or potentially ill people and introduce them to the health delivery arena. The increase in supply is, in its simplest terms, met by the increase in demand before it can ever have a downward effect on costs. It is believed that interventions such as these or increasing the frequency of follow-up, the membership of the health team, or the time spent with clients is a priori

TABLE 11-3. Comparison of Earnings of Registered Nurses in Nonfederal Hospitals and Public School Teachers, 1960–1973

Year	Earnings of General Duty Nurses	Earnings of Public School Teachers*
1960–1961	$4,001†	$ 5,275
1963–1964	4,498‡	5,995
1966–1967	5,382‡	6,830
1969–1970	7,514‡	8,635
1972–1973	9,216§	10,305

*Computed from information presented in *Digest of Educational Statistics*, p. 48.

†The 1963 general duty nurse earnings data (3, 1970–71, p. 131) was adjusted back to 1960 using the 1960–63 change in general duty nurses in 13 cities (1, p. 80), (4,498) (4,193)/4,714 = 4,001.

‡Computed from Bureau of Labor Statistics information presented in *Facts About Nursing*, (3, 1970–71, pp. 131–135).

§The 1969 general duty nurse earnings data (3, 1970–71, p. 131) was adjusted forward to 1972 using the 1969–72 change in general duty nurses in 13 cities (3, 1972–73, p. 135, and 1970–71, p. 135) or 7.514 × 9,312/7,592 = 9,216.

Adapted from: Division of Nursing: *Trends in RN Supply*, United States Department of Health, Education and Welfare, Health Resources Administration (DHEW Pub. No. (HRA) 76-15), 1976, p. 74.

increasing the quality. Eventually, data will have to be accumulated to support these beliefs in terms of proven advantages for the client which justify the continued costs to individuals and society.

THE MEDICAL MYSTIQUE

Much has been written about the need for demystification of medical care, patients' rights, informed consent, client participation in decision-making, self-care, and other methods of making public the protected knowledge domain of health professionals. There is also concern about fraudulent and abusive practices by some providers (individual and institutional), and legislative and investigative efforts have attempted to uncover, prevent, and control these practices when they occur.

However, the average American believes in medicine, in the provider, in the hospital, in medical science, and in technology when he is sick. Most individuals look to the health delivery system for the treatment of disease, for the alleviation of pain, for comfort and reassurance, and for beneficial intervention. Although it may be that faith in the medical solution to so many problems is unwarranted or overestimated, and that, in general, medicine can do much less than the public believes, each client hopes it will succeed in his particular case.[13] This attitude and the fact that most people, especially those in the middle and upper classes (whose dealings with the less adequate aspects of the health care delivery system are less extensive than that of the poor) have mitigated any outside intervention into the system beyond the concern for rising costs.

Although a constant purchaser, the consumer is generally not a user until he becomes a patient. He does not actually become involved in the problems that others experience with the system except as a sympathetic friend or outraged reader until he or a family member becomes ill. This sporadic input by the well consumer, therefore, has had little impact on the provider and does not threaten the expert role the provider experiences once illness and need for services have been demonstrated. Clients are often afraid to question the busy provider and are often intimidated by the aura of hospital equipment and practices. Once in it they feel like captives of this system. They are loathe to do anything but go along with things "as they are" and then try to forget about it once it is over. It is for this reason that those most constantly involved with the system—providers and third-party payers—need to be held responsible for making positive system-wide changes. While it is true that the consumer of private pediatric care can rebel against the price, manner, or availability of the care, he is not likely to get a refund and may have considerable trouble finding an alternative which he is more certain to like and trust. This is perpetuated by distribution problems and by the lack of advertisement of fees, services, and qualification by providers.

Advertisement of Fees and Services

The important role that advertising plays in maintaining market balances has been discussed previously. Why then do health providers and other professionals disdain such practices? As with many practices which we look upon suspiciously with today's eyes, the historical development of the prohibition in advertising physicians' services was quite innocent. According to the American Medical News,[14] the American Medical Association in 1847, adopting Percival's Medical Ethics, developed from English common law the following position:

> It is derogatory to the dignity of the profession, to resort to public advertisements or private cards or handbills, inviting the attention of individuals affected with particular diseases, publicly offering advice and medicine to the poor gratis, or promising radical cures; or to publish cases and operations in the daily prints, or suffer such publications to be made; . . . to invite laymen to be present at operations; . . . to boast of cures and remedies; . . . to adduce certificates of skill and success, or to perform any other similar acts.
>
> These are the ordinary practices of empirics, and are highly reprehensible in a regular physician.[14]

The tone and portent of this "code" taken in its historical perspective is a natural reaction to the poor educational preparation and control of medical practice at that time. Physicians were thus dissuaded by peer professional ethics from acting like snake oil salesmen or medicine showmen.

Over the years, education for physicians has become more standardized and local and state governments now control and regulate health care providers through licensing. Similarly, professionals staked out their domain further by defining exclusive scope of practice and educational qualifications so that today, the early admonitions in the American Medical Association's stand on medical ethics seems less in the public interest and more useful as a protection of the private domain of physicians' qualifications, fees, services, and practices. On the other hand, advertising would have to be controlled to the extent that it does not mislead, seduce, or indirectly raise care costs.

The Health Research Group, in 1974, published what was probably the first consumer guide to physicians' fees. Attempting a survey of the physicians in Prince Georges County, Maryland, the Health Research Group was thwarted by the Maryland County Medical Society which sent notices to its members warning them to the effect that publication of information on fees or prescriptions is unethical and could be construed as advertising, which is illegal for physicians practicing in Maryland. The consumer group responded through litigation claiming that the medical society's warning to its members prevented it from publishing a complete directory and that the state law against professional advertising was unconstitutional. A three judge panel of the U.S. District Court abstained from hearing the case referring the Health Research Group to the Commission on Medical Discipline, an agency of the Maryland state government. The commission ruled in favor of the County Medical Society saying that participation in the directory did constitute advertising which would violate the state's medical practice act. Most controversial in this particular publication was the introduction which suggested that university affiliated, group practice, or staff appointed physicians could provide better service than physicians in practice alone.

This particular claim was the basis of the accusation that participation by physicians was tantamount to advertising. The Health Research Group responded by appealing the District Court's action to the U.S. Circuit Court of Appeals asking them to make the District Court decide on whether the state medical law against advertising was constitutional. While the outcome of this decision is still pending at the time of this writing, a similar suit by several lawyers concerning legal fees and services has been won and is already beginning to show signs of clearing up the murkiness of legal services and costs for the public.

Throughout the country, other consumer groups have followed the lead of the Health Research Group and begun publishing physician directories. In Evanston, Illinois, a suburb of Chicago, the Consumers' Health Group published a directory with a listing of physicians' routine charges and lab fees. That state's medical society did not feel this publication by the consumer group represented advertising. Similarly, in Tucson, Arizona, a physicians' union, the Professional Guild of Arizona, published fees in its Doctors Directory for Pima County. There have been no problems to date with either of these consumer-oriented activities.[15]

On the federal level in 1976, the Federal Trade Commission (FTC) filed a complaint against the American Medical Association (AMA) charging that their anti-advertising attitude was a restraint of trade. The FTC position is that the AMA "has been acting like a business, and its members have been acting like businessmen. They do compete with each other. People pay money for their services, and people should get the benefit of competition between them so far as these principles of ethics and competition restrict competition and hurt the public, then the antitrust laws should do something about them."[16] In December 1978, Commission administrative law Judge E. Barnes handed down the first ruling which found the AMA, the Connecticut State Medical Society, and the New Haven County Medical Association in violation of the FTC act by restricting physician advertising. The AMA plans to appeal the decision.

A. F. Dougherty, Jr., Deputy Director of the FTCs Bureau of Competition, was reported to have said, the commission was notifying "all professions—not just doctors—that there can be no dallying in their compliance with antitrust laws, which prohibit any form of price-fixing."[16] Nursing is not without its problems in this area either. The Attorney General of the State of Massachusetts recently charged the Massachusetts Nurses' Association with price-fixing with reference to its setting rates for private duty nurses.

In summary, it can be seen that the traditional influence of the consumer on the quality and cost of goods and services is somewhat altered in the health care delivery system. Several factors have been identified which contribute to this difference, such as the extensive use of third-party payers, the unreliability of supply as an influence on the cost, and the mystical aspects of health care.

CONSUMER MOVEMENT IN HEALTH DELIVERY SERVICE

There continues to be a growing recognition that consumer involvement in controlling delivery, public involvement in assuring quality and controlling cost, and the advances of the consumer movement toward the representation of consumers in government decisions may have far-reaching potential for improving the consumer influence and maintaining the desired balance of forces in the marketplace. Several major interventions have been suggested as public policy in behalf of consumers where health marketplace idiosyncracies or traditions have failed in assuring responsiveness to them. The remainder of this chapter will deal with three movements illustrative of these:

1. The inclusion of consumer-users in public policy decisions.
2. The patients' rights movement.
3. The movement for a federal agency to protect consumers' interests.

Consumer-users in Public Policy Decisions

Several legislative attempts have been made to increase the involvement of consumer-users in public policy decisions. A discussion of the two major laws—the Community Health Centers Act and the National Health Planning and Resources Development Act—will follow.

COMMUNITY HEALTH CENTERS ACT

The drive for social equity highlighted by the civil rights movement set the stage for the development of the Office of Economic Opportunity (OEO) and the plethora of programs it established for the poor and elderly during the years of John Kennedy's "War on Poverty" and Lyndon Johnson's "Great Society." The desire for consumer-user participation on community boards, formerly composed of upper class citizens or providers, was encouraged by legislative language requiring "maximum feasible participation" of the poor or of the residents of the area served and backed by withdrawal of funds for noncompliance. Gradually these consumers and sympathetic providers and policy makers began recognizing the extent of the outrages in the system and created needed changes. There was articulation of the general dissatisfaction and frustration the poor felt regarding long lines, lack of continuity, and general unresponsiveness of the public facilities and charity services. Reported also was the denial of services by many private and voluntary institutions.

Numerous examples of the plight of the poor to receive dignified care were cited as rationale for the need for a change in the power structure: Silver cited this example of what a Mexican-American indigent client had to do to obtain care in Monterey, California, in 1965:

> ... Most of the hospitals' clinics opened at 8 a.m. ... the patient would ... have to start his journey at 1 a.m. (from King City) boarding a Greyhound bus for the one hour trip to Salinas. He would then have to sit up the balance of the night, waiting for the clinic to open. Even if he were seen early in the morning, he still had to wait for a bus back, as the first bus for King City did not leave until afternoon. The status degradation and "mortification process" of county hospital care was perhaps the most significant hardship. Being classified as a second-class citizen, submitting to uncomfortable tests of financial means, suffering liens on property, and enduring long waits before appointments are implemented are all parts of the invidious class categorizations of the indigent and denigrate self image.[17]

Horror stories of similar circumstances prevailing in county and city-run facilities throughout the country were revealed. The poor began to denounce their exploitation, accusing the health care system for using them as "teaching material" for medical students and "research material" for scientists. In addition, they wanted the jobs which a health center could provide, because this meant real socioeconomic opportunity for them. Poor consumers were demanding and receiving a share in policy decision-making for the first time.

Although several authors[18-22] have reported problems in the early years, possibly a result of growing pains, most also felt that consumer participation in decision-making was an idea whose time had come. While there was no certainty that consumer participation would guarantee success, there was ample evidence that a professional design for ghetto health care without consumer input did not. One of the main functions of community participation was then seen as a means of obtaining a new kind of accountability of professionals to the client-consumer. Additionally, the involvement of the client in the decision-making of neighborhood health centers, schools, and other community programs was seen by community organizers and social scientists as a means of providing the poor with a greater stake in society which might reduce their alienation.

To assure that there is indeed the desired community participation, the federal regulations[23] which govern the granting of federal dollars for neighborhood or community health centers specify the size, composition, selection, functions, and responsibilities of center governing boards. Briefly, these boards are to consist of between 9 and 25 members, a majority of whom are clients of the center and can represent the individuals being served in terms of race, ethnic background, and sex. No more than half of the other members may be health professionals, and the remainder must be representatives of the community in which the centers catchment area is located. They are to be selected for their expertise in community affairs, local government, finance and banking, legal affairs, trade unions, and other commercial and industrial concerns or social service agencies within the community. The exact selection of members and the method for member selection is not specified but it is required that the method be written into the board's bylaws. The functions of the board include selection of the project director or chief executive officer of the center, establishment of personnel policies and procedures, financial policy activities evaluation, including client advocacy when complaints are raised, and service policies such as scope and availability of services, location, hours, and quality of care audits.

One of the major difficulties health professionals, especially those employed in centers which serviced the more outspoken, sometimes even militant, communities, was the sudden necessity for the accountability to lay persons of decidedly different, often disadvantaged educational and financial situations. Many professionals found it difficult and burdensome to explain, justify, and share with others in the decision-making process. The resistance to participation with consumers in either the client/provider role or in the consumer/administrative relationship had probably been less arduous for nurses than for physicians and hospital administrators. This in fact may be due to the perceived powerlessness felt by nurses that Davis[24] examines and therefore the greater identification nurses feel with the powerlessness of the client. In addition, nurses have long advocated a position in support of consumer satisfaction, client rights and client education which enables a sharing relationship to develop. Although the method and boundaries of consumer participation still remain cloudy, the mandate is clear.

As mentioned previously, the major conflicts which arise in the determination of role and function of the citizen or consumer participant in health planning or service delivery are those in which it is unclear whether the decision-making should be professional or public.

Nurses, particularly those engaged in community health nursing, are likely to become staff members, organizers or participants on a board or in a community planning agency where membership may include large numbers of consumers or community residents. In addition, it is possible that such a board can have an effect on the nurses' role and goals as employees in a service setting.[25]

Methods of Citizen Participation

In his analysis of citizen participation in health and welfare planning and service delivery, Burke[26] identified the more common methods of citizen participation, indicating the assumptions, conditions, and organization requirements for each. He identifies these strategies as: education-therapy, behavioral change, staff supplement, cooptation, and community power.

EDUCATION THERAPY. As the name implies, the major focus in this strategy is the education and therapy of the participant. The goal is the process of citizen involvement rather than the outcome of

the solution of a specific problem or performance of a specific task. This process of developing group cohesion, self-confidence, and self-reliance in decision-making was an underlying goal in many of the urban renewal and poverty programs of the 1960s. (The Office of Economic Opportunity hoped this would help the disenfranchised to turn away from the self-defeating and despairing culture of poverty.) This strategy was also utilized by the black power movement. Frustrating the use of this strategy in community planning is its inability to accommodate to organizational or institutional demands. When the aim is to build self-reliance, the outcome of decision-making, right or wrong, cannot be thwarted without causing a reinforcement of feelings of inadequacy or alienation. Public officials and budget managers often feel the price of failure, from poorly designed programs which are often too expensive, especially when compared to the unquantifiable success of community or citizen development. Therefore, without an independent financial resource, it is difficult to sustain such a project.

BEHAVIORAL CHANGE STRATEGY. Utilizing the assumptions that first, groups are a major force in changing individual behavior, and second, that individuals and groups resist decisions that are imposed upon them, the objective of this strategy is to induce change in the individual or subsystem by changing the behavior of either the system members or influencial representatives of the system. Here, there is specific task orientation, and it is felt that participation in the decision-making process will create a commitment to new objectives and will enhance the ability of members to support or carry out determined plans. Several conditions have been suggested as important for this to occur: the participants must have a strong sense of identification with the group and the feeling that their contributions and activities are meaningful, both to themselves and to the group. Gains or satisfactions, either through personal and group accomplishments or from association with the members, must also be felt. There needs to be an awareness of the need for change, and the consequent pressure for change must come from within the group as a shared perception. This strategy is often applied to health problems such as weight or smoking control groups as well as planning agencies. Planning agencies, however, find it more difficult to fulfill these conditions. The complexity of planning projects and the need to meet deadlines often subvert the attention of the professional from fostering group deliberation and initiative. To be successful in making change in a community, the consumer representative must be permitted opportunity to develop, commit himself to the course of action, and be in a position to gain the support and commitment of those he represents. This last is often cited as a major difficulty by opponents of community participation who challenge the representation and accountability of consumers to the aggregate. On the other hand, when only the wealthy and politically influential were chosen for positions, such as hospital trustees, their lack of accountability or contact with the aggregate was rarely challenged.

STAFF SUPPLEMENT STRATEGY. The staff supplement strategy is identified as the simple principle of voluntaryism. The major purpose of it is, as the title implies, the utilization of citizens to carry out work for an organization which does not have the staff resources to carry on the function itself. Hospitals, social welfare organizations, religious organizations, and educational institutions are examples of facilities which depend on voluntaryism for several important service functions. Few citizen volunteers are actually involved in policy-making roles. Cooperation with organizational goals is assumed when the volunteer is recruited. However, sometimes input into decision-making is desirable, and the voluntary expertise of citizens is solicited. In the realm of community planning, which at this embryonic stage of development, is not completely based on valid data or unanimity of direction, a situation may be created in which bargaining, negotiation, and compromise are methods most often involved in the decision-making, and even the expert volunteer is simply another opinion that must be considered.

COOPTATION. Burke[26] defines cooptation as the process of absorbing new elements into the leadership or policy-making structure as a means of avoiding threats to its stability and existence. Taking two forms, cooptation can be employed first, in response to specific power forces, where certain individuals are considered to have sufficient resources or influence (financial, legislative, or constituent) to vitally affect the operation of the orga-

nization and where capturing of the individual is a means of at least neutralizing or at most, encouraging their support for the organization's policies. Such identification with the organization may actually deter beneficial change where the more aggressive, uncoopted can serve as watchdogs outside the policy-making structure. The second form cooptation takes is more often used by health and social welfare organizations. Here leadership from the community is formally coopted because of the credibility they have that the organization needs in order to promote its goals. As Rosenstock[27] points out in his work on community health education, the clergy were extremely important in gaining participation by blacks in government-sponsored immunization programs against polio during the 1950s. Formal cooptation such as this does not have the same negative connotation of the informal cooptation described first. Health, social welfare, and educational institutions need to establish reliable and readily accessible channels of communication through which information and requests may be transmitted. Since the public is solicited by the organization for this specific purpose, its organizational power is not threatened, community participation, and sharing is encouraged especially in that it provides the participant with an opportunity to learn about the struggles and needs of the organization, increasing support and identification. It is not intended, however, to impede or redress organization goals and as such, like staff voluntaryism, may be a source of frustration to consumer representatives with behavioral change goals.

COMMUNITY POWER STRUGGLES. Power here is defined as the ability to exercise one's will over the opposition of others. Power is usually associated with wealth or the control of institutions. Community power gains its strength by virtue of the exertion of sheer numbers on the existing forces. The goal is change oriented, either social or economic. Few organizations can resist changing policies and procedures when consumers boycott, picket, or demonstrate against them. Likewise, legislators fear the power of a cohesive outspoken electorate. Success in developing community power depends on the presence of a charismatic leader who can mobilize the numbers required to have impact and who can maintain the level of emotional involvement this strategy necessitates if it is to have any duration. Martin Luther King, Jr., and Malcolm X were two leaders of this sort who had tremendous impact in developing cohesive group support and promoting change. Ralph Nader is another who is able to gather consumer support and obtain organizational impact.

In conclusion, community or consumer participation can take several forms. These strategies have been enumerated for the benefit of the nurse who is a staff member, or provider participant on a board or committee which also involves consumer participation. The success of any of these strategies, whether they be clear-cut or transitional, depends to a large degree on the knowledge, skill, and support of the professionals involved. Staff members should be sensitive to the individual differences of participants and enable them to contribute to the process. The goal is to work with the community representatives. Limitations in the organizational structure, the funding mechanism, and the effective cooperation by consumers must also be acknowledged so that strategies and goals can be set realistically.

NATIONAL HEALTH PLANNING AND RESOURCES DEVELOPMENT ACT

Another major legislative attempt to reorder the health delivery system which also creates a formal mechanism for consumer input is the National Health Planning and Resources Development Act of 1974 (PL 93-641). According to the Health Resources Administration[28] which administers this act, it combines and expands the mandates of several older laws: the Hill-Burton Act of 1946, the Comprehensive Health Planning and Public Health Service Amendments of 1960, and the Regional Medical Programs of 1965.

Updating Older Legislation

The *Hill-Burton Act of 1946* promoted the rehabilitation and construction of health care facilities. Appropriating $4.3 billion from 1947 to 1973 for the construction of 11,255 projects including 5,986 general hospitals, 1,795 long-term care facilities, 4,000 mental hospitals, tuberculosis centers, and outpatient departments.[29] In 1964, the Hill-Burton Act was amended to increase the number and the responsibility of planning agencies to determine the need for new construction and to encourage ren-

ovation and special services alternative to hospitals, such as nursing homes.

The *Comprehensive Health Planning and Public Health Service Amendments of 1960* authorized the establishment of area-wide comprehensive health planning agencies (CHP). At the local level, these were called 314B agencies, and at the state level, a consolidating 314A agency was designated. These agencies were authorized to plan for the needs of their regions; assume the responsibilities of the phased out Hill-Burton planning agencies; and participate in Section 1122 of the Social Security Amendments which was a precursor to the current certificate-of-need program. Section 1122 asked for, but did not require, the review of proposed hospital construction above the cost of $100,000 and the issuance of a certificate-of-need for approved projects. Unneeded facilities could be denied federal third-party payment and other Public Health Service monies. The CHP agencies involved communities and consumers in a decision-making capacity.

The *Regional Medical Programs of 1965* (*RMP*) promoted cooperative arrangements between health services organizations, research institutions, and medical schools to facilitate access to advances in diagnosis and treatment of special medical problems, namely, heart disease, stroke, and cancer. Manpower training in these areas were also provided for, as was the development of sophisticated emergency medical services such as cardiac care ambulances.

One of the problems with these last two programs was the overlapping of mandated planning responsibilities. Jurisdictional rivalry developed within several states. The development of the National Health Planning and Resources Development Act was seen as a means of capturing and retaining the best features of the comprehensive health planning legislation and the regional medical programs through their consolidation and expansion of responsibility.

Accessibility and Cost-Effectiveness of the Health System through PL 93-641

The National Health Planning and Resources Development Act (PL 93-641) created a multitiered, interdependent group of entities responsible for making the health system more accessible and cost-effective. There are three organizational structures within the system: (1) the Health Systems Agency (HSA), (2) the State Health Planning and Development Agency (SHPDA), and (3) the State Health Coordinating Council (SHCC).

Briefly, the Health Systems Agency replaces the local 314B agencies in the comprehensive health planning legislation. Comprised of a consumer majority governing board and supported by a staff paid for by the Department of Health, Education, and Welfare (DHEW), the HSA has the responsibility of preparing and implementing plans for the improvement of the health of the residents in its area, increasing accessibility, continuity, and quality of health services, controlling costs, and prevention of unnecessary duplication of services. A specific health plan is called for which includes long-term goals for the community. An Annual Implementation Plan is also required. Consistent with the concern for medical care cost containment, the HSAs are mandated to review and approve or disapprove applications for federal funds for health programs within the area. The first step in the certificate-of-need process, which will be described later, HSAs can also assist states in reviewing the appropriateness of existing services, although as yet the definition of "appropriate" and the mechanism for dealing with "inappropriate" facilities is so vague as to have resulted in inaction by most HSAs on this particular responsibility.

The *State Health Planning and Development Agency (SHPDA)*, a governor-appointed agency usually called the State Agency, replaced the 314A agencies in the CHP legislation. It has the responsibility to conduct health planning activities and implement parts of the state plans of the HSAs which relate to the government of the state. It integrates the health plans of the HSA into a preliminary State Health Plan and administers the state certificate-of-need program (which is a revision of the 1122 mandate in the CHP legislation). The certificate-of-need legislation followed the initiative of more than 30 states which had set up similar programs on their own to control costs by controlling expansion of hospital facilities. Under PL 93-641, all states must set up certificate-of-need programs to continue receiving DHEW monies, Medicaid, Medicare, and Maternal Child Health. DHEW set minimum standards for the process to be used in certificate-of-need programs but leaves penalties to the states. Generally, an agency wishing to start, expand, or modify health services, is required to submit a proposal to the HSA for approval. Disapproved programs can be favored by the SHPDA, but appeal of HSA decisions can only be obtained through the Secretary of DHEW or the courts.

The *State Health Coordinating Council (SHCC)* is composed of 16 members appointed by the governor. (Sixty percent of its members must be HSA members also, and 50 percent must be consumers.) The SHCC has the responsibility of approving the State Health Plan, reviewing the budget applications for assistance of HSAs, advising the State Agency on the performance of its functions, and setting criteria for determining the need for facilities and modernization of equipment. This legislation also calls for a 15 member National Advisory Council which consults with the Secretary of DHEW on the development of national goals, the implementation of the new law, and the evaluation of new technology for organizing, delivering, and equitably distributing health services.

Since the designation of the HSAs in all areas around the country has taken several years, as has the appointment of the National Advisory Council, a thorough evaluation of the success or failure of this relatively recent legislation is precipitous. However, several criticisms have been made regarding the consumer role in HSAs as now structured. It is generally agreed that it is desirable to have consumer involvement in the determination of resource allocation and the planning for establishment of health care which they pay for. Difficulty can arise in trying to get consumers who indeed represent a constituency of "consumer thought" and in assuring that they will take every opportunity to articulate it.

There are several differences in the consumer and provider roles which are seen to put the consumer at a disadvantage to the provider, for which even the majority position on governing boards may not compensate. Essentially, providers receive status as well as organizational support in terms of their salaries and staff to assist in information gathering and analysis. Consumers have to rely on the staff of the HSA for most if not all of their information. If the staff identifies more with the providers (as may be likely given professional ties and the prestige most providers enjoy), the consumer may not get the assistance necessary to fully understand the issues being decided. In addition, the out-of-pocket expenses that some consumers bear in terms of babysitting and transportation can be a hardship since their service on these boards is voluntary even though they provide a service to the community.

Another difficulty occurs in making sure that the consumer actually sees his role in insuring that the consumer-community gets the most and best for the money, rather than just the most. For example, if it is the perception of the consumer representative that new hospital construction can create additional jobs for a community, the goal of cost containment and comprehensive health planning may be thwarted by this self-interest.

Labor union representatives are often seen as especially valuable consumer representatives because they are knowledgeable about the cost of care and have resources with respect to policy analysis. Under our current system of third-party payments, it is often difficult to get a constituency for cost containment because the actual cost of care is collectively borne—that is, the individual is frequently not confronted with the actual expense. Labor union members, on the other hand, have to negotiate their benefits periodically as contracts with employers come up for renewal. When labor is presented with the information that the cost of the health care benefits have trebled in a 2 year period, diminishing the capital available for pay increases, there is immediate and real acknowledgement of the effects of inflated health care costs on the individual.

Public Citizen's Health Research Group published a handbook for consumers interested in having meaningful participation as HSA board members or as citizen watchdogs. Nurses may be interested in the suggestions offered as they are meaningful to the provider as well as to the consumer groups. Bogue's suggestions for consumer involvement in Health System Agencies are quoted in their entirety:

1. Identify and maintain constant contact with an HSA staff person or persons who are responsible for, or at least sympathetic to consumer involvement.
2. Obtain and familiarize yourself with copies of all documents governing the operation, structure, and procedures of the HSA.
3. Make certain the consumer representatives on the HSA Board and other HSA committees actually have no conflicts of interest, accurately reflect the demographic composition of the health service area, and are willing to be active and aggressive in confronting proposals by providers.
4. Get your group on the mailing list for all notices and information sent out by the HSA.
5. Make certain consumers from your group are represented and prepared at all meetings and hearings.
6. Adopt a data policy which requires reporting to the HSA of all relevant information by individual providers and guarantees that all information, documents, internal reports, etc., are disseminated or readily available to the public.
7. Be actively involved from the earliest stages in the initial development of the Health Systems Plan (HSP), the Annual Implementation Plan (AIP), and the procedures and criteria for certificate-of-need review. *No* proposals for new inpatient hospital construction or major capital equipment should be granted a certificate-of-need until these three documents are completed and approved.
8. During the HSA's period of conditional designation, be sure to document and complain about—informally, in written comments, and at public hearings—all instances of unresponsiveness to consumer interests. Copies of your complaints should be sent to the HSA Board, the Governor, the Statewide Health Coordinating Council (SHCC), your Congressperson(s), and Public Citizen's Health Research Group.[30]

As more nurses become provider-members of HSA governing boards or staff planners, it will be important for them to become fully informed of the issues involved in local health planning and assist the consumer membership as much as possible with obtaining and understanding the issues at hand.

PROFESSIONAL STANDARD REVIEW ORGANIZATION (PSRO)

Another important piece of health legislation will be mentioned here briefly, because although it has tremendous potential bearing on the cost and quality of health care provided to the majority of hospitalized patients, it has virtually no consumer involvement and absolutely no authoritative nursing involvement. The Professional Standards Review Organization Act (PL 92-603) was passed in 1972 as an amendment to the Social Security Act. According to Long,[31] this legislation was designed to provide for the peer review of hospital and nursing home care paid for by any of the provisions included in the Social Security Act (Medicaid, Medicare, Maternal Child Health); the objectives are the evaluation of the necessity for admission, the length of stay, the appropriateness of care, and the adequacy and quality of the service provided. Review is to be carried out by a local nonprofit professional organization composed of licensed physicians or osteopaths. Emphasis is placed on reduction in the cost of hospital care by controlling inappropriate utilization. This is also seen as a quality objective.

Audits of patient charts are most often performed by nurses who usually indicate the predetermined discharge date of a patient based on the PSROs established criteria for diagnosis and age of patient. Physicians generally handle problems with respect to physician compliance with these protocols and may alter treatment regimen if they deem it necessary. At the present time, PSRO of ambulatory and nursing home patients is not mandatory, although it is anticipated for the future. With respect to requirements for consumer participation on PSROs, the opportunity is minimal.

The State Professional Standard Review Council has the primary function of developing uniform data gathering procedures, evaluating the performance of local PSROs, and replacement of poorly performing PSROs. Its membership is legislated to include four doctors recommended by the State Medical Society and the State Hospital Association and one representative from each local PSRO (local PSROs have exclusive physician membership). In addition, four persons knowledgeable in health care can be selected, two by the governor. This group has an advisory council to assist it in its role. Membership of the advisory council is to include between 7 and 11 representatives of health care practitioners other than physicians. The National Professional Standards Review Council, an 11 member physician group, has the following responsibilities:

1. Advising the Secretary of DHEW in administration of the act.
2. Developing and distributing information to state and local PSROs.

3. Reviewing the operation of the councils and the organizations.
4. Reporting its findings annually to Congress.

It is fairly obvious that in addition to not promoting access to consumers in PSROs, nurses are also excluded under the current legislation. The American Nurses' Association (ANA) has expressed great concern over this, proposing full membership in PSRO for registered nurses and other licensed health care practitioners.

In as much as providers educated and practicing in professions other than nursing do not have the experience or educational background to effectively evaluate the necessity, appropriateness and quality of nursing care, it follows that members of the nursing profession should be involved in decisions as to the quality of professional care/service, rendered by nurses. . . . The need for nursing is one valid criterion for admission, assigning length of stay, and for continued stay review. Professional nurses should develop nursing criterion relative to admission and continued stay where interdisciplinary review is possible, they should participate in the development of such criteria.[32]

Logic and experience in other countries supports the claim by organized nursing that membership on PSRO evaluation teams and policy groups should be expanded.

The concept of exclusive review by peers, though laudable, is impractical in that it puts a great deal of pressure on the individuals involved to confront and redress each other. These are behaviors which are no easier for physicians to perform with respect to one another than they are for any other human being. Having consumer input and the input and involvement of the rest of the health care team, who have judgment responsibilities for client care, might increase the accountability of all these individuals.

Dyck[33] reported that the Canadian College of Physicians and Surgeons included consumers on a committee it organized (at the request of the Minister of Health) to study the rising rate of hysterectomies in the province of Saskatchewan. Similar to PSROs this group determined legitimate medical indications for hysterectomy, published them, and monitored the behavior of physicians. The effort resulted in a 30 percent decline in the rate of hysterectomy in the province between 1970 and 1974. At the time of the publication of the Canadian study, hysterectomies continue as the leading major surgical procedure in the United States.

Patients' Rights

In response to consumer demands and as an outcome of court cases finding in favor of consumers/ patients against hospitals (regarding such issues as human experimentation, surgical and medical treatment without informed consent, and incarceration in mental institutions without treatment) several attempts have been made to enumerate the specific rights of the hospitalized person. The American Hospital Association[34] (AHA) Board of Trustees with input from four consumers, put together one of the earliest of these model Patients' Bill of Rights. In distributing copies to its 7,000 member organization, it urged (but with no power to mandate) adoption of it. However, several hospitals have voluntarily adopted this model or a version of it as official hospital policy. Once a hospital adopts and publishes a Patients' Bill of Rights for its institution, it serves an important function to the patients who are informed, often for the first time, that they can have some specific expectations of the hospital experience. It also informs providers and staff that certain behaviors are expected of them vis-a-vis the patient. If such a policy is violated, and satisfaction cannot be gotten in the hospital, the patient can take legal action.

The State of Minnesota has enacted a Bill of Rights[34] for all hospitalized patients, which it requires to be posted in all hospitals and distributed to all patients. While this Bill is less inclusive than the AHA and the National League for Nursing (NLN) prototype (to follow), abusers of the declared patients' rights can be fined up to $1,000 and up to 1 year in prison.

The American Civil Liberties Union,[34] also produced a model Patients' Bill of Rights which is included in Table 11-4 with the AHA and Minnesota versions for comparison. In the same table is the NLN list of rights of patients. In suggesting these rights, the NLN[35] states "while regard for patients' rights can be taught and made part of institutional programs, the burden for upholding those rights falls inevitably on the individual provider of care. Wherever they work, nurses should not only dem-

onstrate their personal commitment to patients' rights through their actions, but should insist on institutional policies that respect the rights of patients, and should play an active role in teaching patients about their rights and in encouraging other health professionals to be knowledgeable about and to respect those rights."

SPECIAL INTEREST LOBBYISTS

In addition to addressing the generalized rights of hospitalized patients, other health advocacy groups have emerged for the protection of or support of specific client constituencies. The Grey Panthers, mentioned previously, formed in the 1960s to express the needs of the elderly to state and federal legislators. The Right to Life Organization, in addition to its yearly visit with congressional staff in Washington, is active on the state and local level in advocating antiabortion policies. The Candlelighters seek federal monies for research and treatment for cancer victims. These groups, making a commitment to the particular problem or disease that they wish to find support for, are generally founded and sustained because of some personal involvement with the issue. For example, the Committee to Fight Huntington's Chorea was founded by the widow of Woody Guthrie, after her husband died of that disease. Obviously the value of these groups in providing mutual support for one another or in channeling their political clout through cohesive organization is great. However, when such organizations lobby extensively for their own needs, they often do so at the expense of other problems equally justifiable in need but politically disadvantaged. The poor for example, are often not acknowledged politically because they have fewer representatives cognizant and sympathetic to their needs, and because they are disenfranchised politically.

It has been suggested by Ball[36] that any federally financed National Health Insurance must incorporate the poor in the same benefits and administrative programs as the middle class to prevent the recurrence of problems of cuts in services, benefits, and eligibility evidenced in the Medicaid programs. It is argued that lacking the technical and financial expertise of the middle class, programs exclusively designed for the poor are easily subverted, cut, or severely curtailed.

Federal Protection of Consumer Interests

The notion of including consumer input in public policy decisions is not a new one. Several attempts have been tried in the last decade to pass legislation which would create a Federal Agency for Consumer Advocacy. The purpose of this section is to briefly discuss the major historical precedents and the current congressional climate.

In response to the need for support of consumer interest caused by the depression, Congress proposed that a Consumer Council be established in 1929. That bill did not get to floor discussion until 1932, when it was attached, as an amendment to a larger, more promising bill. It passed Congress but was vetoed by President Hoover, tabling, for another year at least, any substantive legislation for consumers. Then, under the momentum for which Franklin D. Roosevelt was famous, four major consumer organizations were created within the federal structure. These were reported to have failed because there was "ambiguity in the definition of consumer and a "lack of formal policy for consumer protection."[37]

By 1937, an F.D.R. committee on federal reorganization recommended a plan which included a Department of Social Welfare, defining in its responsibility, an area of protection for the consumer. The plan was not adopted. Also during this period, Consumers' Research Inc., an organization with the stated purpose of determining or articulating consumer needs recommended a cabinet level consumer department. It was not until 1959, however, that a bill was introduced reflecting this recommendation. It was introduced by Senator Estes Kefauver (D-Tenn.) with 21 cosponsors, hardly sufficient to get off the ground. Kefauver proposed the creation of a Consumer Secretary in the Cabinet, attempting to construct permanent Presidential ties to the issue. The major alternative idea at the time (which remains so today) was for the creation of an independent agency for consumer protection, headed by an administrator who is not on the level of a Secretary. The Environmental Protection Agency (EPA) is organized on this model.

In 1962, John Kennedy issued the first Presidential message to Congress addressing consumer interests. He set up a consumer advisory council within the Council of Economic Advisors. How-

ever, this folded after 18 months and one written report.

In 1964, Lyndon Johnson issued an executive order creating the first President's Commission on Consumer Interest. Their first report in 1966 recommended a joint congressional committee on consumer interests like the joint economic committee. This was never implemented. Johnson did, however, create a part-time post of Special Assistant to the President for Consumer Affairs and named Esther Peterson (then Secretary of Labor) to the position. In 1967, Betty Furness was appointed, and in 1969 President Nixon appointed Virginia Nauer to fill this position on a full time basis. During one of the early appointments of the Carter Administration, Esther Peterson was renamed to fill the post.

From 1969 to 1970, five different prototypical consumer-related bills were introduced in Congress. One was for the creation of a permanent office of consumer affairs in the White House. Others were for a permanent Bureau of Consumer Protection, a permanent position of Consumer Special Assistant to the President, a consumer representative in the Department of Justice, and an independent Consumer Council, a nongovernmental organization. The alternative most sought after by consumer advocates is for the creation of an independent consumer advocacy agency. Authority would include the responsibility to serve as a consumer's advocate by monitoring and intervening in actions taken by other federal agencies; to initiate or participate in judicial appeals of agency actions which are perceived to be inimical to the interests of consumers; to receive and act upon complaints by individuals or groups of consumers; and to question private business in search of information related to consumer problems.[38]

Essentially, arguments for such a consumer agency say that the various existing federal agencies, particularly the regulatory ones (FDA, Consumer Product Safety Commission [CPSC], EPA), do not operate in the best interest of consumers. Opponents say the only way to protect the consumer is to improve the existing institutions of the government, not to add more government. The major argument for a Consumer Protection Agency is that regulatory agencies are bound by many conflicts: (1) The industries they try to regulate are often wealthier and more powerful, having thus a

TABLE 11-4. Four Prototypical Patients' Rights Positions

American Hospital Association Bill of Rights*	State of Minnesota Legislation†	American Civil Liberties Union Model Patient's Bill of Rights‡	National League for Nursing "Nursing's Role in Patient Rights"§
(1) The patient has the right to considerate and respectful care.	(1) Every patient and resident shall have the right to considerate and respectful care.	(1) The patient has a legal right to prompt attention especially in an emergency situation.	(1) Patients have the right to courteous and individualized health care that is equitable, humane, and given without discrimination as to race, color, creed, sex, national origin, source of payment, or ethical or political beliefs.
(2) The patient has the right to obtain from his physician complete current information concerning his diagnosis, treatment, and prognosis in terms he can be reasonably expected to understand. When it is not medically advisable to give such information to the patient, the information should be made available to an appropriate person in his behalf. He has the right to know, by name, the physician responsible for his care.	(2) Every patient can reasonably expect to obtain from his physician or the resident physician of the facility complete and current information concerning his diagnosis, treatment and prognosis in terms and language the patient can reasonably be expected to understand. In such cases that it is not medically advisable to give such information to the patient, the information may be made available to the appropriate person in his behalf.	(2) The patient has a legal right to a clear, concise explanation of all procedures in layman's terms, including the possibilities of any risk of mortality or serious side effects, problems related to recuperation, and probability of success, and will not be subjected to any procedure without his voluntary competent, and understanding consent. The specifics of such consent shall be set out in a written consent form, signed by the patient.	(2) Patients have the right to information about their diagnosis, prognosis, and treatment—including alternatives to care and risks involved—in terms they and their families can readily understand, so that they can give their informed consent.
(3) The patient has the right to receive from his physician information necessary to give informed consent prior to the start of any procedure and/or treatment, the medically significant risks involved, and the probable duration of incapacitation. Where medically significant alternatives for care of treatment exist, or when the patient requests information concerning medical alternatives the patient has the right to such information. The patient also has the right to know the name of the person responsible for the procedures and/or treatment.	(3) Every patient and resident shall have the right to respectfulness and privacy as it relates to his medical care program. Case discussion, consultation, examination, and treatment are confidential and should be conducted discreetly.	(3) The patient has a legal right to a clear, complete, and accurate evaluation of his condition and prognosis without treatment before he is asked to consent to any test of procedure.	(3) Patients have the legal right to informed participation in all decisions concerning their health care.
(4) The patient has the right to be advised if the hospital proposes to engage in or perform human experimentation affecting his care or treatment. The patient has the right to refuse to participate in such research projects.	(4) Every patient and resident shall have the right to expect the facility to make a reasonable response to the requests of the patient.	(4) The patient has a legal right not to have any test or procedures, designed for educational purposes rather than his direct personal benefit, performed on him.	(4) Patients have the right to refuse treatments, medications, or participation in research and experimentation, without punitive action being taken against them.
(5) The patient has the right to every consideration of his privacy concerning his own medical care program. Case discussion, consultation, examination, and treatment are confidential and should be conducted discreetly. Those not directly involved in his care must have the permission of the patient to be present.	(5) Every patient and resident shall have the right to obtain information as to any relationship of the facility to other health care and related institutions insofar as his care is concerned.	(5) We recognize the right of the patient to know the identity and professional status of all those providing service. All personnel have been instructed to observe themselves, state their status and explain their role in the health care of the patient. Part of this is the right of the patient to know the physician responsible for his care.	(5) Patients have the right to privacy during interview, examination, and treatment.
(6) The patient has the right to expect that all communications and records pertaining to his care should be treated as confidential.	(6) Every patient and resident shall have the right to every consideration of his privacy and individuality as it relates to his social, religious, and psychological well being.	(6) No patient may be transferred to another facility unless he has received a complete explanation of the desirability and need for the transfer, the other facility has accepted the patient for transfer, and the patient has agreed to transfer. If the patient does not agree to transfer, the patient has the right to a consultant's opinion on the desirability of transfer.	(6) Patients have the right to confidentiality of all records (except as otherwise provided for by law or third-party payer contracts) and all communications, written or oral, between patients and health care providers.
(7) The patient has the right to expect that within its capacity a hospital must make reasonable response to the request of a patient for services. The hospital must provide evaluation service, and/or referral as indicated by the urgency of the case. When medically permissible, a patient may be transferred to another facility only after he has received complete information and explanation concerning the needs for and alternatives to such a transfer. The institution to which the patient is to be transferred must have accepted the patient for transfer.	(7) The patient and resident have the right to expect reasonable continuity of care which shall include but not be limited to what appointment times and physicians are available.	(7) We recognize the right of all potential patients to know what research and experimental protocols are being used in our facility and what alternatives are available in the community.	(7) People have the right to health care that is accessible and that meets professional standards, regardless of the setting.
(8) The patient has the right to obtain information as to any relationship of his hospital to other health care and educational institutions insofar as his care is concerned. The patient has the right to obtain information as to the existence of any professional relationships among individuals, by name, who are treating him.	(8) Every patient and resident shall have the right to know by name and specialty, if any, the physician responsible for coordination of his care.	(8) The patient has a right, regardless of source of payment, to examine and receive an itemized and detailed explanation of his total bill for services rendered in the facility.	(8) Patients have the right to information about the qualifications, names, and titles of personnel responsible for providing their health care.
		(9) The patient has a legal right to refuse any particular drug, test, procedure or treatment.	(9) Patients have the right to information on the charges for services, including the right to challenge these.
		(10) The patient has a legal right to all the information contained in his medical record while in the health-care facility and to examine the record upon request.	(10) Patients have the right to coordination and continuity of health care.
		(11) We recognize the patient's right of access to people outside the health care facility by means of visitors and the telephone. Parents may stay with their children and relatives with terminally ill patients 24 hours a day.	(11) patients have the right of access to all health records pertaining to them, the right to challenge and to have their records corrected for accuracy, and the right to transfer of all such records in the case of continuing care.
		(12) The patient has a legal right to informed participation in all decisions involving his health care program.	(12) Patients have the right to refuse observation by those not directly involved in their care.
		(13) We recognize the right of a potential patient	(13) Patients have the right to privacy in communicating and visiting with persons of their choice.
			(14) Patients have the right to appropriate instruction or education from health care personnel so that they can achieve an optimal level of wellness and an understanding of their basic health needs.
			(15) Above all, patients have the right to be fully informed as to all their rights in all health care settings.

TABLE 11-4. Continued

American Hospital Association Bill of Rights*	State of Minnesota Legislation†	American Civil Liberties Union Model Patient's Bill of Rights‡	National League for Nursing "Nursing's Role in Patient Rights"§
(9) The patient has the right to examine and receive an explanation of his bill regardless of source of payment. (10) The patient has the right to refuse treatment to the extent permitted by law and to be informed of the medical consequences of his action. (11) The patient has the right to expect reasonable continuity of care. He has the right to know in advance what appointment times and physicians are available and where. The patient has the right to expect that the hospital will provide a mechanism whereby he is informed by his physician of the following discharge. (12) The patient has the right to know what hospital rules and regulations apply to his conduct as a patient.		to complete and accurate information concerning medical care and procedures. (14) The patient has a legal right to both personal and informational privacy with respect to: the hospital staff, other doctors, residents, interns and medical students, researchers, nurses, other hospital personnel, and other patients. (15) We recognize the right of a patient to discuss his condition with a consultant specialist at his own request and his own expense. (16) The patient has a legal right to privacy respecting the source of payment for treatment and care. This right includes access to the highest degree of care without regard to the source of payment for that treatment and care. (17) The patient has a legal right to leave the health care facility regardless of physical condition or financial status, although he may be requested to sign a release stating that he is leaving against the medical judgment of his doctor or the hospital. (18) A patient has a right to be notified of discharge at least one day before it is accomplished, to demand a consultation by an expert on the desirability of discharge, and to have a person of the patient's choice so notified. (19) The patient has a right to competent counseling from the facility to help him obtain financial assistance from public or private sources to meet the expense of services received in the institution. (20) The patient has a right to timely prior notice of the termination of his eligibility for reimbursement for the expense of his care by any third-party payer. (21) At the termination of his stay at the health care facility we recognize the right of a patient to a complete copy of the information contained in his medical record. (22) We recognize the right of all patients to have 24 hours a day access to a patient's right advocate who may act on behalf of the patient to assert or protect the rights set out in this document. (23) We recognize the right of any patient who does not speak English to have access to an interpreter.	

*Source: American Hospital Association, A Patient Bill of Rights, (A.H.A. Cat. No. 5009 45M-3754333) Chicago, 1975. (Reprinted with the permission of the American Hospital Association.)
†Source: Annas, G.: The Rights of Hospital Patients. New York, Avon, 1975.
‡Ibid.
§Source: National League for Nursing. Nursing's Role in Patient Rights, National League for Nursing, New York (Pub: No. 11-1671), 1977.

greater influence on some legislators than is desirable. (2) Federal political appointees have a short shelf-life and rely on industry for future employment. Former Federal Communications Commissioner Nicholas Johnson supported the need for additional consumer support in the bureaucracy:

To look to the Federal government for any real hope that regulatory agencies will serve the public interest is becoming, more and more, an incredible act of faith. The evidence to the contrary is overwhelming. You can just write off the Federal government, because the agencies are owned lock, stock, and barrel by the large corporations and industries they are supposed to regulate. It's not that government officials are corrupt; in most cases, they are simply responding to social pressures, to power, to people with whom they associate and who can influence their careers.[37]

Joan Claybrook, appointed in 1977 as administrator of the National Highway Traffic Safety Administration, said that that agency was supposed to have informed consumers about which automobiles were the most crashworthy by law in 1972. While $2.7 million has been spent on studies, to date, there have been "no useful results passed on to consumers."[39]

Opponents to a new central agency for the representation of consumers argue that in addition to the Office of Consumer Affairs, currently headed by a Special Assistant to the President, numerous consumer representatives can be found functioning throughout the government. The Federal Trade Commission, which is the largest federal agency concerned primarily with consumer protection, is one of 253 consumer protection and advancement activities in 33 federal agencies and departments. A more recent survey, published in Congressional Quarterly 1969, found that the number of agencies and departments involved had increased to 39, and in 1969 Virginia Nauer stated that a study for the President "found that 413 units of the Federal government were administering 938 consumer-related activities."[37]

Based on this information and massive lobbying against an independent consumer advocacy agency by organized business, particularly the Chamber of Commerce,[38] the idea is again the subject of furious debate. Ralph Nader published a series of reports which dramatically confirmed what earlier studies had shown, essentially that governmental agencies established to regulate an industry to protect consumers typically ended up as instruments of the industry they were supposed to regulate, thus, enabling industry to protect monopoly positions and to exploit consumers more effectively. Although Nader's analysis of the problem is consistent with opponents of the establishment of yet another bureaucracy, he believes that there is nothing innately wrong with the political process that produces this result; what he sees lacking is a well-defined, well-organized, explicitly-instructed agency to protect consumers and supervision by consumers to insure that this is done.

It would seem that the Carter administration was expressing accord on the issue of the present lack of responsiveness of the Administration to consumer interests. In support of the legislation, Peterson, Special Assistant to the President for Consumer Affairs, said:

Experience has shown that the consumers' voice simply is not heard in most regulatory arenas and that this imbalance in advocacy, time and time again results in decisions which fail to take full account of the impact on consumers. The job of the Consumer Agency would be to help balance the record upon which governmental decisions are made and, in so doing, to give the consumer's viewpoint, as well as the producer's viewpoint, the weight it deserves. We do believe that government decision-makers will strike a fairer balance when determining what constitutes the "public interest" in a particular case when they do so on the basis of a full and balanced record.[40]

In its support, Congress Watch[41] suggested ways in which this new agency could positively affect government. For example, the Agency for Consumer Protection (ACP) can pressure for less government regulation by agencies like the Civil Aeronautics Board (CAB) and the Interstate Commerce Commission (ICC), which fix prices far above the competitive rates. Those troubled by bureaucracy should appreciate the savings and efficiency of replacing many ineffective consumer offices within government with one effective consumer advocate.

Further, it is argued that the proposed annual budget of $15 million or 10 cents per capita could produce considerable benefits in savings to consumers and balance out business oriented federal outlays. (The Commerce Department gets $1.7 billion to "foster, promote, and develop commerce and industry.") Also, in support of the legislation for a consumer agency, according to Green of Citizens' Watch,[41] are the President, the Speaker of the House, Tip O'Neil, and more than 150 consumer, farm, senior citizens, environment and labor groups, including Consumer Federation of America, American Association of Retired Persons, American Bar Association, the National Conference of Mayors, Consumers Union, Common Cause, the AFL-CIO, and Friends of the Earth. Opposed are the U.S. Chamber of Commerce, The Business Round Table, The National Association of Manufacturers, General Motors, and Proctor and Gamble.

The *Washington Post*[42] released results of a Harris Poll questioning the public's opinion on the matter. Harris is said to have called it "a landmark, documenting the phenomenal growth of the consumer movement, which he said is staggeringly larger than similar ones of the past, such as the Populist, Labor, or Equal Rights for Blacks movement. The consumer constituency dwarfs all of them . . . . consumers are disgusted with the whole range of problems they blame on business. Soaring prices, products of questionable safety, false advertising claims, woefully inadequate service, warranties, and guarantees that don't mean anything, lack of redress and extreme difficulties in receiving common justice in the marketplace." Approximately 1500 Americans were polled, 522 persons from leadership groups composed of consumer activists, senior business managers, business and government consumer affairs specialists, and insurance and noninsurance regulators.

Congress Watch provided several examples where an agency for consumer protection could save citizens' lives and dollars in the health area:

1. The FDA does not warn of dangers of vaginal cancer—the FDA routinely makes decisions affecting the public health and safety. Most of these decisions are made behind closed doors and with little or no opportunity for consumer participation. The FDA has approved the use of DES as a morning after birth control pill despite evidence linking DES to vaginal cancer in the offspring of women taking DES during pregnancy. FDA does not require that women be warned of this risk, even though the morning after pill is not 100% effective.

2. HEW permits waste in the health care system—our system of health care tolerates incredible amounts of wasteful costs. Unnecessary hospitalizations cost about $10 billion every year, and unnecessary surgeries cost over $4 billion a year. For years, HEW, with the power to reduce substantially some of this waste, did nothing to require second surgical opinions or other waste-trimming measures, such as preadmission testing, which has been shown to be effective in reducing costly overutilization without sacrificing quality of care.

3. The Consumer Product Safety Commission fails to protect consumers—four years ago, industry designed a new extension cord to keep children from being burned when they put cord receptacles in their mouths. It asked the CPSC for help in imposing the design on every extension cord still sold in America. The CPSC has taken no action, and cords still burn children.

4. Cockroaches, flies, and rodents in food-processing plants—the General Accounting Office (GAO) in 1972, found that about 40% of food manufacturing plants, which are regulated by the FDA under the Food and Drug Act, were operating under conditions that were unsanitary or worse. This report, and FDAs own inspecting practices, demonstrate why consumer expectations of clean food are so low.

5. HEW fails to enforce Fire Safety Standards for Nursing Homes—about 7,000 skilled nursing homes received HEW, Medicare, and Medicaid funds. A GAO audit of 32 of these homes, found that 23 or 72% had one or more deficiencies with respect to fire safety regulations.

6. Defective heart pacers in the FDA—the 1975 report by the Controller found that the FDA did not follow its own procedures in a "life-threatening situation" when it failed to investigate the cause of a recall of cardiac pace-

makers by manufacturers. The common defect in the pacemakers was a leakage of body fluids through the plastic seal of the pacemaker causing short circuiting and the sudden speeding up or slowing down of the electronic heart pacing. The FDA did not independently establish how many deaths or injuries have been caused by this defect.[41] Publicity and legal action against the government by organizations such as the Health Research Group and the Environmental Defense Fund have resulted in significant gains for consumers with these and other undesirable policies.

The National Consumer League in its support for an agency for consumer protection has stated "that consumer concerns are essential because the government must receive a balanced presentation of the issues in order to determine where the public interest truly lies. The public interest as they define it, is made up of the business, the labor, the farm, the international, and the consumers' interest. All of these interests overlap and interrelate—they all have a right to call upon their government to hear and protect them. At the present time, the decision-maker has ample opportunity to hear from business, labor, and the farm community who have been well represented in Washington for decades. But consumers have no institutionized representative in the halls of government. Too often decision-makers do not consider the impact of their actions on the consumers. They lack the incentive, since the consumer voice is not a full partner in the action and they lack the data."[43]

At the time of this writing, legislation for an agency for consumer protection died in the Ninety-fifth Congress. History suggests it will be reintroduced in future sessions of Congress.

REFERENCES

1. Rhodes, J.: *The Futile System*. New York, Hawthorne Books, 1976.
2. Elwood, P., and McClure, W.: Health Delivery Reform Memorandum. Interstudy. P.O. Box S, Excelsior, Minnesota, November 17, 1976.
3. McClure, W.: The Medical Care System under National Health Insurance: Four Models That Might Work and Their Prospects. Paper presented before the American Political Science Association, Interstudy, Minneapolis, Minn., Sept. 2, 1975.
4. Brody, J.: Blue Shield acts to curb payment on procedures of doubtful value. *New York Times*, May 19, 1977.
5. Carnegie Commission on Higher Education: *Higher Education and the Nation's Health*. New York, McGraw-Hill Book Co., 1970.
6. Starr, P.: Too many doctors. *Washington Post*, March 13, 1977.
7. Reinhardt, U.: Health Manpower Policy in the United States. Issues for Inquiry in the Next Decade. Paper presented to the Bicentennial Conference on Health Policy, University of Pennsylvania, Nov. 11–12, 1976.
8. Lalonde, M.: *A New Perspective on the Health of Canadians*. Ottawa, Trigraphic Printing, 1975.
9. Executive Office of the President: *Compendium of National Health Expenditures Data*. Washington, D.C., U.S. Department of Health, Education and Welfare (DHEW 70, SSA 76-11927), 1976.
10. Health Resources Administration: *Health United States 1975*. Washington, D.C., U.S. Department of Health, Education, and Welfare (DHEW Pub. No. (HRA) 76-1237), 1976.
11. Miller, M.: Nurse's right to strike. *Nurs. Digest* 4:47–51, 1976.
12. Executive Office of the President—Council on Wage and Price Stability: *The Complex Puzzle of Rising Health Care Costs: Can the Private Sector Fit it Together*. Washington, D.C., U.S. Government Printing Office, 1977, p. 241.
13. National Commission for Manpower Policy: *Employment Impacts on Health Policy Developments*. Washington, D.C., Special Report No. 11, October 1976.
14. Rolands, M.: MDs, Madison Avenue don't mix, ethnicist says. *American Medical News*, January 12, 1977.
15. Lewis, R.: MD directories popular with patients, but physicians' reactions are mixed. *American Medical News*, June 20, 1977.
16. Nicholson, T.: Advertising: doctor's dilemma. *Newsweek*, pp. 63–64, January 5, 1976.
17. Silver, G.: Community participation and health resource allocation. *Int. J. Health Ser.* 3:117–131, 1973.
18. Dans, P., and Johnson, S.: Politics in the development of a migrant health center. *N. Engl. J. Med.* 292:890, 1975.
19. Kane, T.: Citizen participation in decision-making: myth or strategy. *Admin. Men. Health,* (Spring) 1975, p. 29.
20. Milio, N.: Dimensions of consumer participation and national health legislation. *Am. J. Pub. Health* 60:6, 1970.
21. Notkins, H.: Community participation in health services: a review article. *Am. J. Pub. Health* 27:11, 1970.
22. Sparer, G., et al.: Consumer participation in O.E.O. assisted neighborhood health centers. *Am. J. Pub. Health* 60:6, 1970.

23. Grants For Community Health Services: Title 42 Public Health, Federal Register, 41:23−1(Part 51C), 1976.
24. Davis, A. J., and Underwood, P.: Role, function and decision-making in community mental health. *Nurs. Res.* 25:256−258, 1976.
25. Bernal, H.: Power and interorganizational health care projects. *Nurs. Outlook* 24(7):418−421, 1976.
26. Burke, E.: Community participation strategies. *Am. Ins. Planners* 34:287, 1968.
27. Rosenstock, I., et al.: Why people fail to seek poliomyelitis vaccination. *Public Health Rep.* 74(2):98, 1959.
28. Health Resources Administration: *Health Planning and Resources Development Act of 1974*. Washington D.C., Bureau of Planning and Resources Development (DHEW Pub. No. (HRA) 75-14015), 1974.
29. Rogers, P., and Hyde, L.: Planning for quality health care, in *Public Health in America 1776−1976*, Washington, D.C., U.S. Department of Health, Education, and Welfare, 1977.
30. Bogue, T. and Wolfe, S.: *Trimming the Fat Off Health Care Costs: A Consumer's Guide to Taking Over Health Planning*. Washington, D.C., Public Citizen's Health Research Group, 1976 ($2.00 a copy, $1.00 for three or more).
31. Long, R.: *Background Material Relating to PSRO's*. Washington, D.C., Committee on Finance, United States Senate, U.S. Govt. Printing Office (32-7680), 1974.
32. Kaplan, A. (ed.): *A Report from Washington on Professional Standards Review Organizations*. PSRO Letter, No. 52, October 1, 1975.
33. Dyck, F. J., et al.: Effect of surveillance on the number of hysterectomies in the Province of Saskatchewan. *N. Engl. J. Med.* 296:1326−1328, 1977.
34. Annas, G.: *The Rights of Hospital Patients*. New York, Avon Books, 1975.
35. National League for Nursing: *Nursing's Role in Patient Rights*. New York, National League for Nursing, (Pub. No. 11-1671), 1977.
36. Ball, R.: What are the prospects for national health insurance? *Am. Lung Assoc. Bull.* 62(6):7, 1976.
37. Legislative Analyses: *Consumer Protection Legislation*. American Enterprise Institute for Public Policy Research, Washington, D.C., 1977.
38. Keefe, M., et al.: *Consumer Protection Agency*. Washington, D. C., Congressional Reference Service, Library of Congress Issue Brief (#1B 74083), 1977.
39. Associated Press: New head of agency says it failed to fulfill law. *New York Times*, p. 18, May 10, 1977.
40. Peterson, E.: The Agency for Consumer Protection. Memorandum to Congressman James J. Florio, The White House, June 2, 1977.
41. Green, M.: The Agency for Consumer Protection. Memorandum to Congress, Public Citizen, May 31, 1977.
42. Burrus, M.: Consumer unrest staggering. *Washington Post*, May 17, 1977.
43. Willet, S.: The Agency for Consumer Protection. Memorandum to Congress, National Consumers' League, May 1977.

CHAPTER 12

EXPANSION OF THE PROVIDER GROUP

Supporting Factors

The client's search for an entry point into the health care system and for guidelines explaining its utilization is a dilemma recognized by consumers and providers in the system. Another dilemma is the health care industry's apparent inability to reconcile the political, economic, professional, and social forces which could come together to produce effective organization and ultimately utilization of services. The consumer's search for care and the system's state of disorganization are closely linked to the proliferation of health care providers, their preparation, utilization, and productivity.

In the last two decades, government and private resources have stimulated the growth, diversity, and stratification of groups of health care providers. Traditional care agencies and newly created facilities have tried to accommodate clients' needs for

PROVIDERS OF HEALTH CARE

Diane O. McGivern, Ph.D., R.N.

services and the varigated responses from professionals. The proliferation of provider groups has resulted from a number of factors: (1) federal support, (2) identified lack of services, (3) recognition of health as a right, (4) emphasis on health promotion, (5) technological expansion, and (6) experimentation.

The *flow of federal funds* into the training of practitioners within the traditional disciplines has had a significant influence on the growth of provider groups. In addition, there has been federal support for training programs which provide access to career ladders, thus moving community residents into the first level of health service related positions. While this has created a new strata of providers, there is a limited appreciation at all levels of how to use these providers effectively.

Identification of major gaps in health care services, which are correlated with consumers' geographic and socioeconomic characteristics has supported the expanded scope of practice for some practitioners. It has also contributed to the creation of new classifications of providers in an effort to place more services at the disposal of poorly served consumers.

The emphasis through the 1950s and 1960s on individual and civil rights changed the concept of health; it is now thought of as *an individual right* which should be available to everyone. This, combined with subsequent legislation, produced a concept of health as a valued, available commodity. It also resulted in a significant increase in demand for services, which could not be met by the number of traditional providers available or by the scope of their practices. The recent appreciation of *health promotion and health maintenance* activities has also influenced the proliferation of provider groups. Health promotion and maintenance services are also seen as potentially cost-effective.

The fifth factor, the *technological sophistication,* which has created an array of diagnostic and therapeutic equipment and procedures, requires a new group of highly trained specialists and technicians, each trained in an increasingly narrow field. This need for highly trained personnel coincides with the overall emphasis on specialization in the health care field and the resultant loss of the generalist at entry points in the health care delivery system.

The last factor which has contributed to the profusion of providers is the movement within the traditional disciplines associated with their mutual examinations of scope of practice. There is the conflict associated with (1) determining the degree of cooperation and overlay between practice areas, (2) the major issue of reimbursement, and (3) the development of new or expanded models of practice.

As health care issues become more complex, comprised of community, social, legal, nutritional, and environmental components, individual providers are being supplemented with provider *teams*. Practitioner teams, formed in response to a more complicated and multifactored focus, often incorporate members from the newer provider groups.

These factors and others are responsible for the alterations in the traditional provider groupings and the additions of new and sometimes controversial provider groups to the health care delivery system.

Effects

The delivery system has been visibly affected by the impact of the provider explosion. Professional journals, care agencies, and educational programs reflect this rapid change. One result has been the strain experienced within the traditional professions where professional and technical practices overlap, forcing disciplines to share functions and responsibilities which had been separate until recently. The expansion and realignment of responsibility for new and more common health care services among traditional and newly created providers has produced a second effect; that is, confusion on the part of the consumers, the general public, and providers, regarding the jurisdiction and responsibility of various practitioners.

Accurately or not, the expansion of the provider group and the increased numbers of direct and indirect health care providers have been associated with the rise in health care costs. Predictions of future cost escalations are frequently cited when nontraditional practice models are proposed. The traditional hierarchy of professional and occupational groups has always influenced the operations of the health care delivery system. The effect of the realignment of positions and relationships within the provider sector on the final form of national health insurance and alternate forms of reimbursement is not clear but certainly anticipated. Also, the changing provider picture intensifies the competition among professional and occupational health care groups for public and private support of basic education, specialized training, and research. Practitioners anticipate that competition will change the economic base of their present practices.

Advantages and Disadvantages

The addition of new health care specialists and redefinition of the established disciplines must have some advantages for users of the health care system. The most obvious advantage is the potential ease of access to the system and an extensive array of services. Access to the system and services may be greatly enhanced as nurses, social workers, dentists, and others gain the necessary sanctions to bring clients into the system and health care facilities, and are eligible for reimbursement for services. Physicians who have been the traditional gatekeepers of the system are freed for better utilization of their time in keeping with their educational and clinical preparation for acute illness care.

The emergence of new providers and the upgrading of traditional roles allows for testing new models of practice which may in fact be more economical, more humane, and produce better health. The development of new health care workers and new delivery models may prove disadvantageous, however, if each professional practice area is defended on the basis of precedent and not re-negotiated on the basis of effectiveness.

Structure and Distribution

The organization and utilization of health professionals within a setting, agency, or geographic area will be determined by a variety of factors, including purpose or focus of the institution, characteristics of the potential client population, indigenous health problems, and availability of community resources. Within a health care setting, the ways in which the health care provider group is structured and provides services to clients depend on the purpose of the institution or setting. Agencies that serve clients whose needs are acute, pathology-oriented, and short-term require a proportionately greater number of prepared practitioners to provide these services. Health care agencies which aim to provide health maintenance care to a population on a long-term basis, need a cadre of professionals prepared to function in this way.

The characteristics of the client population should determine the number, distribution, and utilization of the provider groups. A resident population in a geriatric facility might require more attention from providers who focus on long-term health promotion and health maintenance activities. An emergency room in a high trauma area will utilize more providers geared for acute short-term services. Frequently, the traditional professionals, physicians, nurses, or social workers have been utilized in the traditional ways without a clear understanding of the incongruence of professional services to the needs of the population being serviced. The demographics of the community help to anticipate the prevailing health problems and consequently identify the types of professionals who will be most useful.

HEALTH CARE PROVIDERS

Who are the health care providers that have traditionally and more recently provided health promotion, health maintenance, and sick care to client populations in institutions and in communities? Arbitrarily, health care providers can be divided into professional, paraprofessional, nonprofessionals and indirect provider groups. The specific characteristics which distinguish professions and professionals include service orientation, autonomy, specialized knowledge, protected areas of function, system of professional values, relevance to basic societal values, training periods which are lengthy, specialized, and abstract, and commitment to life-long pursuit.[1]

Professional Services

Within this definition, professional groups include medicine, dentistry, pharmacology, dietetics, social work, nursing, and therapies, including speech, physical, occupational, and recreational. In line with the characteristics of professions, each group is identified by an educational preparation, licensure or certification, and degrees of specialization.

Physicians' educational preparation has traditionally included completion of 4 years of undergraduate education and 4 years of a professional curriculum; however, one or both curricula may be time compressed. Other variations of educational-professional preparation include medical school and graduate school, leading to a M.D.-Ph.D. Medical school curricula have focused on basic science education and clinical apprenticeship. State licensure is mandatory for practice and achieved through passing the Federation Licensing Examination.[2] Examples of specialization include radiology, anesthesiology, and surgery. Medicine provides access to many roles, including direct care provider, researcher, and academician. While these roles are not mutually exclusive, we are concerned primarily with the provider role in this discussion.

Dentistry parallels medicine in a variety of ways. Education includes 4 years of undergraduate education and 4 years in a professional school program. Dental school curricula also incorporate basic science education and clinical practice. While most postgraduate training has been basic to specialization, more recently postgraduate training has also become preparatory to general practice. State licensure is mandatory for practice. An example of additional certification or recognition includes Board certification. Dentistry also gives professionals access to a number of roles, including care provider, researcher, and academician.

Pharmacology bases its professional preparation on the traditional structure of undergraduate and graduate education. Basic preparation in a school of pharmacy and subsequent licensure allows the graduate to dispense medications prescribed by physicians and dentists. The pharmacist also advises health professionals on various aspects of therapeutics and provides information to consumers regarding appropriate drug usage. Graduate education prepares professionals in areas such as toxicology and clinical pharmacology.

Preparation for professional *nursing* practice is through baccalaureate education and state licensure. Nurses are prepared to provide a wide range of services which promote health, prevent illness, and are supportive and restorative. Clients may be individuals, groups, or communities. Clinical specialization is studied at the master's level. Doctoral education prepares practitioners for advanced practice, research, teaching, and administration. Certification recognizing clinical practice is a relatively recent development.

Physical therapy is concerned with the preservation of functional capabilities, restoration of function, and prevention of disability due to acute or chronic illness or accident. Physical therapists evaluate the presence and extent of physical disability by identifying and interpreting data which describe degrees of impairment. Preparation for practice may be within a baccalaureate program or a specialized postbaccalaureate certificate program. Licensure is required for practice.

Occupational therapy focuses on the provision of selected activities to promote and maintain health and prevent further disability. Therapists evaluate behaviors and treat clients with physical or psychosocial dysfunction through the use of creative acts, activities basic to daily living, and pre- and avocational skills. Basic preparation is through undergraduate education, but licensure by examination is not required by all states. Examination by the American Occupational Therapy Association is required for admission to the Registry of Occupational Therapists.

Preparation for a career in *social work* is achieved through a baccalaureate program or through master's level education. Social workers are prepared to assist clients through the development of a relationship by which the client is helped to achieve a better adjustment with his life situation. Social work is not exclusively a health care discipline. Medical and psychiatric social work are more directly involved with the health care delivery system.

Dietitians are prepared to take responsibility for the nutritional care of individuals and groups. Education for this area of practice is a bachelor's degree with specialization in foods and nutrition. A 1 year internship is recommended to qualify for recognition by the American Dietetic Association. Dietitians counsel and teach patients and families about how to apply the principles of nutrition to the selection of foods necessary for health or therapeutic regimens.

Paraprofessionals, Nonprofessionals, and Indirect Providers

The paraprofessionals who supply a significant portion of the health care services currently available include such groups as physician's assistants, inhalation therapists, practical nurses, emergency medical technicians, and medical laboratory technicians. These groups require variable lengths of academic preparation, focus on technical components, and are under the direct supervision of appropriate professionals.

Physician's assistants are one of the newer provider groups, beginning in the early 1960s.[3] The scope of the physician's assistant's practice is a defined set of activities delegated by the employing physician. The assistant is specifically trained to carry out many of the tasks formerly done by the physician. Training for this career takes place in 1 to 2 year programs. Assistants may be employed to work for physicians in hospitals, rural health clinics, specialty clinics, or in private practices. National certification for physician's assistants began in 1973.[4]

Inhalation therapy technicians must complete a 2 year training course approved by the American Medical Association. This technician administers and instructs clients in the use of inhalation equipment, aerosol inhalants, and breathing exercises.

Practical nurses work under the direction and supervision of professional nurses in hospitals, clinics, nursing homes, and other health care settings. Practical nurse programs vary in length, but licensure is necessary for practice.

A wide variety of *technicians* provide services to and for consumers of health care. Preparations for these occupations vary but are usually not beyond the associate degree level; however, specialized training is required. Technicians work under the direct supervision of physicians or technologists.

The *nonprofessional provider* class is characterized by limited training which is primarily employment-institution based. Health care services are supported in this category by such workers as nursing assistants and laboratory assistants.

A wealth of other disciplines (*indirect providers*) supply health related information, contribute to the organization and administration of the group or facility providing direct health care services, and plan on a community, state, or regional level for the services and facilities that will be available to the total population.

INTERDISCIPLINARY HEALTH CARE TEAM APPROACH

The concept of interdisciplinary provider teams was developed and written about as early as the 1940s.[5] Since then, hospital-community projects have utilized the model of team practice. In the 1960s, the Office of Economic Opportunity guidelines for Neighborhood Health Centers included the team approach, and this prompted its popularization. Therefore, in direct response to funding requirements and perceived health system inefficiencies, the interdisciplinary team model became a new solution built into the delivery system despite the lack of supporting evidence.

The team concept has generated a number of variations on the model and a variety of definitions. The definitions in the literature, despite their diversity, incorporate the following commonalties; they are characterized by a common purpose, differential professional contributions, and a system of communication. The team model has developed a variety of categories as well. A team may be single or multidisciplinary. An interdisciplinary team may be basic or nuclear—that is, the minimal team required to carry out the essential functions of a specific service. A team may be extended or second level, including professionals who contribute to the diversity of service provided by the basic team, or a team may be consultative or third level—that is, an extended team joined by specialists for a limited period of time.

Multidisciplinary teams may function in several ways. Observation of the pattern of team behavior may indicate that decisions are not really made by team concensus but by the designated leader of the group and that the members function independently. Another behavioral pattern for team functioning would include no designated group leader, decisions made through group concensus, a significant blurring of roles, and interdependent functioning. The multidisciplinary team approach reflects many of the problems that all professions are grappling with individually. For all the reasons enumerated earlier, professions and therefore teams, are confronting the problems of defining appropriate roles, utilizing and integrating paraprofessionals, maintaining flexibility in the interprofessional situation, and developing balance between the specialized and generalized skills within and between the professions.

The interdisciplinary team approach has several advantages for the clients and professionals in the health care delivery system. Because clients have multiple problems with multiple causations and because both problems and causes cross the traditional disciplinary lines of knowledge and skills, a team approach to such complex foci would be broader. The second advantage would stem from this; the client would receive improved services with a minimum of duplication.

The multiprofessional approach makes health care teams one way to control and appropriately apply the rapidly expanding body of technical and treatment information. Teams, as either the cause or effect, are viewed by some, as an organizational solution for the proliferation and diversification of health care workers. Several advantages associated with the multidisciplinary approach accrue for the team members. Multidisciplinary teams provide and enhance mutual support and professional growth. Also, the team format provides a way to begin to equalize the status of the professions.

The disadvantages or unresolved aspects of the multidisciplinary team approach cited by participants and observers may seem to equal or outweigh the advantages. Team health care delivery is described as cumbersome and damaging to the traditional one to one provider-client relationship. Also, it contributes to a loss of final responsibility through the concept of shared responsibility. A critical factor, which may be viewed as a disadvantage, is the length of time it takes for the group to develop as an operating team; time to develop trust, clarify vocabulary, goals and roles, and time for decision-making and problem-solving.

From the point of view of the health care provider, team members complain about the isolation from one's own profession associated with the blurring of traditional professional boundaries and the limited representation of each discipline. There has been the expressed concern that credentials and professional status may continue to affect team member behavior. A related question is whether the factors of personality and background of people who select various professions affect team interaction and consequently team care.

Several critical questions need to be studied to determine whether the multidisciplinary approach to care is a valid, efficient model:

1. What is the appropriate measure of efficiency?
2. What is the best educational preparation for this model of practice and can the differences in educational preparation be resolved?
3. Can systems of remuneration be developed to adequately cover team care?
4. What will be the real impact of the multidisciplinary team approach to health care costs?

The problem of establishing appropriate parameters for measuring the effectiveness of care is not as superficial as it might seem. It requires a change of values about health and the human aspects. The prized concepts of health must incorporate humaneness, maximum health through promotion and maintenance activities, and utilization of all health care professionals who incorporate caring as well as curing.

REFERENCES

1. Kane, R. A. S.: The interprofessional team (with special reference to the role and education of the social worker). Paper presented to the Graduate School of Social Work, University of Utah, Salt Lake City, June, 1975, p. 30.
2. Riddle, J. W.: Education and medical licensure. *J. Am. Med. Assoc.* 236(26):3042–3043, 1976.
3. Jewett, R. E.: Characteristics of physician's assistant program. *J. Med. Educ.* 50:95, 1975.
4. Sadler, A. M., Jr.: New health practitioner education: problems and issues. *J. Med. Educ.* 50:69, 1975.
5. Kindig, D. A.: Interdisciplinary education for primary health care team delivery. *J. Med. Educ.* 50:97, 1975.

BIBLIOGRAPHY

Aradine, C. R., and Hansen, M. F.: Interdisciplinary teamwork in family health care. *Nurs. Clin. North Am.* 5:211, 1970.
Beloff, J. S., and Karper, M.: The health team model and medical care utilization. *J. Am. Med. Assoc.* 219:359, 1972.
Beloff, J. S., and Willet, M.: Yale studies in family health care. III. The health care team. *J. Am. Med. Assoc.* 205:73, 1968.
Bergman, R.: Typology for teamwork. *Am. J. Nurs.* 74:1618, 1974.
Bullough, B.: Nurse practice acts. *Nurs. '77* 7(2):73, 1977.
Chapoorian, T., and Craig, M. M.: PL 93-641, Nursing and health care delivery. *Am. J. Nurs.* 76:1988, 1976.
Cohen, R.: New careers a decade later. *NY Univ. Educ. Q.* 8:2, 1976.
Hoekelman, R.: Nurse physician relationships. *Am. J. Nurs.* 75:1150, 1975.
Kane, R. L.: Sounding board: primary care, contradictions and questions. *N. Engl. J. Med.* 296:1410, 1977.
Keyes, J. A., Wilson, M. P., and Becker, J.: The future of medical education: forecast of the council of deans. *J. Med. Educ.* 50:319, 1975.
Levinson, D.: Sounding board: roles, tasks, and practitioners. *N. Engl. J. Med.* 296:1291, 1977.
Rothberg, J. A.: Nurse and physician's assistant: issues and relationships. *Nurs. Outlook* 21:154, 1973.
Somers, A. R.: *Health Care in Transition: Directions for the Future.* Chicago, Hospital Research and Educational Trust, 1971.
Szasz, C.: Education for the health team. *Can. J. Public Health* 61:386, 1970.

CHAPTER 13

A group refers to associations between two or more persons who are in some kind of *interdependent* relationship. Interdependence is one of the key properties that defines groups as opposed to mere collectivities or aggregates of people. The concept of interdependence calls our attention to the ways in which people *organize* together; it refers to situations in which one person's actions affect another person's behavior or perceptions. If people interact and communicate, taking one another into account, modifying their own behavior in light of the behavior of others, then we would say for all practical purposes they belong to a group.

Group process is a way of looking at groups. A group process perspective directs attention to certain aspects of reality; it helps organize our experience and provides us with the tools we need for better understanding. When we speak about group

---

*From Sampson, Edward and Marthas, Marya: *Group Process for Health Professions*. John Wiley and Sons, Inc., New York, 1977, reprinted by permission John Wiley and Sons, Inc.

GROUP PROCESS*

Marya Sampson Marthas, Ed.D., R.N.

process, we are adopting a perspective that emphasizes the following: (1) how structures and relationships emerge within a group; (2) how they grow and develop over time; (3) how they are maintained at a relatively steady or stable state; and (4) how they are transformed or changed. The process perspective directs attention to the ways in which groups deal with their task and maintenance problems, the ways in which members are recruited and socialized into their particular roles, how decisions are made, how conflicts and disagreements are handled, how leadership and authority are exercised, and how relationships develop and evolve over time.

The understanding of this process and the ability to facilitate it requires knowledge and skill. The recognition of the necessity for such skills is relatively new. Holistic and comprehensive nursing care demand a knowledge of the self and the other in relation to groups. We all have a group character which has become an integral part of nursing practice.

GROUP CHARACTER

We are many kinds of beings. We are biological organisms possessing qualities that we share with all living systems and with others of our species. We are psychological beings with distinctly human capabilities for thought, feeling, and reason. But more than that, we are social, group beings with a complex web of interconnections that link us to others. These links help define our group character and play a major role in our daily lives as well as our professional practice. It is difficult to imagine an activity in which our group character is not involved. The range is broad, extending from simple conversations with clients and colleagues, to meetings, rounds, conferences, training, and sessions.

Nothing mysterious is intended when we speak about a person's group character. The concept directs our attention to two important issues. First, we usually conduct our practice within the actual presence of one or more other persons. And second, in light of this fact, we typically take them into account, adjusting our behavior to theirs, even as they adjust to ours, thereby becoming participants in a group process. Our group character, therefore, refers to the bonds that connect us with others, a figurative line between persons representing the give-and-take adjustments each makes in the presence of the other.

Direct Connections

At times, these links are direct and relatively obvious:

> Nurse Allen is obtaining intake information on her client. She is preoccupied with asking questions and carefully recording the answers in their proper place on the many forms she must complete. The client is anxious about this procedure. The more questions that nurse Allen asks, the greater the client's anxiety becomes; soon, the anxiety interferes with her ability to hear the questions and even to think clearly enough to provide coherent answers. Nurse Allen has many other clients to deal with and so responds with growing annoyance to the client's halting replies. She becomes more abrupt and demanding. The client responds with even greater anxiety and difficulty in providing answers.

What might appear to be a routine matter, obtaining intake information, involves a group process. The nurse's behavior is one element in that process; the client's behavior, the other. Nurse Allen is not simply doing an interview to assess a client on intake as a technician might assess a blood sample. Rather, she is involved as a participant in a process in which her behavior in conducting the interview affects the client's response; in turn, the client's responses affect the nurse's own behavior. Each is involved in adjusting her behavior to the behavior of the other; this is the link that joins them.

In speaking of nurse Allen's group character, we call attention to the idea that who she is is affected by who the other person is in the intake interview. Her character is someone who is annoyed and impatient. This is not a comment on her personality as much as on her manner of adjusting her behavior to her client. The client likewise has a group character. Anxiety is not necessarily a quality she possesses separately from her reaction to nurse

Allen and the intake procedure. Each participant not only evokes a particular kind of response from the other but also responds to the other.

Subtle Connections

The links that relate us with others may also be subtle. We may participate in a group process with little awareness of the group character we are portraying.

> The client and her husband are about to leave the hospital; in her desire to reassure them that all is well, Dr. Welch tells the wife not to worry, nothing really is wrong with her husband, just some indigestion. The couple begins to argue vehemently as they leave. Dr. Welch turns around and continues with her other work, not realizing that her simple reassurance played a part in their family drama. Her assurance as a medical professional undercut the legitimacy of the husband's illness. Dr. Welch had defined him as not sick, never realizing that he had been using sickness as a way of avoiding responsibilities at home.

This is not to suggest that Dr. Welch should not have offered reassurance; this example is presented to illustrate how the health professional may become a part of a group process without being aware that this has even happened. In this case, Dr. Welch's behavior had a greater effect on others than their behavior affected her; nevertheless, she became a member of that family's group process, if only for a brief moment. Obviously, knowledge of group process would have helped her in this type of intervention.

GROUP PROCESS IN LIFE AND IN PRACTICE

Listed here are several reasons why it is important to begin to understand group process and to develop as keen a sensitivity to our group character as we have of our biological character.

1. Our life and our professional practice involve other persons.
2. Our group character emerges as we interact with these others.

3. We rarely, if ever, practice without taking others into account, just as they must act in the context we provide for them.
4. We participate in a group process even when we are unaware of our participation and even when "the group" includes only the nurse and the client or the nurse and one other person.

Many of us do not think of a group or of group process as involving the cases cited above. We have an intuitively larger context or longer-term relationship in mind. The examples focus on small groups of two or three persons; likewise, they examine relatively brief encounters. The study of group process includes both of these cases and those we more typically understand when referring to groups—that is, relationships that have a relatively greater permanence in time and thus permit the development of relationships and structures and relationships that include larger numbers of persons, encompassing both clients as well as other persons (e.g., colleagues and community groups).

It will be helpful in the understanding of group process in the health professions to examine the wide variety of contexts, settings, and groups within which nursing practice tends to occur. Figure 13-1 outlines some of the major areas of group participation of relevance to the health professional.

Human Growth and Development

The life history of human beings can be written in terms of the nature and types of groups in which they have been reared and in which they are presently involved. We are all born helpless and unable to function without support provided by other members of our species. Unlike many animals who achieve independence within a relatively brief period after birth, the story of the human infant is one of continued dependence on others for a substantial period of life. Even as adults, the true hermit who can function independently of others is more myth than reality.

PRIMARY GROUPS

Research has suggested some of the serious consequences that face developing children who do not receive their due amount of human interaction

and contact. The sociologist, Cooley,[1] early recognized the critical role that these *primary group* contacts played in the emergence of social feelings and civilized persons. For Cooley, a primary group involved a close, face-to-face association of the sort one finds in the family, in play groups, and in many neighborhood and informal work groups. Such groups are characterized by their sense of "we" and "our" rather than the more individualistic "I" and "mine." These primary groups are the source of the person's emerging human social qualities; and for adults, they remain an important source of support and nurturance.

Although it has become fashionable to speculate on the breakdown of primary groups (e.g., neighborhood and friendship groups) in our modern society, much research suggests the continuing importance and role of these groups in the life of the individual. Litwak and Szelenyi,[2] for example, determined where people would turn for help if they had a 1-day stomach ache, a 2-week appendectomy, or a 3-month broken leg. Their data suggested the importance of friendship and neighborhood groups for dealing with these and related types of health problems. In other words, even in our modern, urban, and often impersonal society, persons in trouble turn to primary groups for help and support.

The role of the primary group, especially the family, in health care has become increasingly relevant in the management of heart and cancer clients. The psychological impact of cancer, for example, has led health professionals to see the need to extend their treatment plans beyond the medical. The initial diagnosis of cancer sets up a process that has a wide ranging impact on clients and their families. Often, the initial shock gives way to anger, followed by guilt and blame. The client is angry but so too is the family, now threatened by the loss of one of their own. Clients and their families will often blame themselves for their illness: "perhaps we should have urged you to seek medical attention earlier; it's our fault." Fear is also a part of this process: "If my father has cancer, will I have a better chance of getting it myself?"

The process which we have briefly outlined is one that implicates the clients and their primary group; the management of the client, therefore, must take that primary group network into account. When the course of the disease is long-term, as it so often is with cancer, the center of treatment must include the family. The health professional must recognize the clients' need for a continuing connection to and support from their families at a time when the families' fears and worries could lead them to withdraw, thereby failing to provide the mutual support and comfort that is so necessary. Our need for our primary group relationships does not fade once we reach adulthood; the need remains and is implicated in many areas of our lives that fall within the purview of the health professional.

HOSPITALISM

While much criticism has been leveled at the work of Spitz on what he called *hospitalism*, it stands as further testimony to the critical role that early group experiences play in our lives.[3] Spitz observed children in institutions; although they did not lack physical comforts, they lacked the vital social stimulation of other human beings. According to Spitz, these children not only developed lesser intelligence, but also were later unresponsive to and disinterested in people.

The research of Bowlby among others further illustrates this finding.[4,5] The child who is not provided with a strong mothering relationship tends to have difficulty forming attachments to others. It would seem, then, that one function of our early group experiences is to help us develop intellectually and socially; that is, to help us become capable of later forming those kinds of attachments with others that make the entire fabric of social life and human culture possible. Although Harlow[6] worked with monkeys, he reached the same conclusion as Bowlby that both mothering and play with peers are essential to normal adult heterosexual relationships and competency in the tasks of adulthood (e.g., in later being a mother or mothering figure one's self). Our peer group forms one of the key primary groups necessary to our development.

In addition to these effects on the developing child, the reduction and stimulation, including both sensory (e.g., sight, sound, and touch) and social (e.g., interaction and contact with other persons) also has serious consequences for adults. Early research[7,8] has demonstrated a decrement in intellectual functioning and in problem-solving ability

when normal sensory input is reduced for a period of time. Such persons also become more open to believing fantastic things (e.g., in ghosts) toward which they otherwise would take a more critical attitude.

Sensory or social isolation, while not usually introduced into adult lives by intention, nevertheless can result from some medical procedures in which the person is isolated for a period of time (e.g., during radiation therapy). A similar pattern of *hospitalism* in adults has been described by Sommer and Osmond[9] among others. It is said to involve such symptoms as the following:

1. Deindividuation or a reduced ability to think and act independently; almost an increased passivity and dependence and loss of a distinct self.
2. Disculturation or an adoption of institutional attitudes and values, and a correspondent loss of one's earlier attitudes and values.
3. Isolation and estrangement or a loss of one's contacts and commitments to things in the outside world.
4. Stimulus deprivation or a tendency to adapt to a world within the institution that has a tempo that differs dramatically from that on the outside.

These symptoms are said to occur both within clients and staff who are under extensive institutional care. The implications of this pattern for both client care and staff development within institutional settings are clear; use of groups to oppose these symptoms might well become a central aspect of hospital programs.

THE THERAPEUTIC MILIEU

The concept of the therapeutic milieu is a relatively recent one; its origins lay primarily in psychiatric settings but has recently been extended to a consideration of the hospital ward or unit as a therapeutic milieu. Basically, to avoid the effects of hospitalism and sensory limitation, the health professional, especially the nurse who has greatest hour-by-hour contact with the client, must attend carefully to creating a total therapeutic context for client care. The seemingly little attentions and human concerns shown for clients can play an important role in their recovery. An attitude of extreme clinical detachment, for example, helps contribute to hospitalism and sensory limitation; the client's milieu, therefore, becomes one that hinders recovery rather than one which facilitates it. The quality of the milieu is only as good as the people working in it; they must function as a unit. This requires that they deal with some of their own feelings and concerns and with the host of interpersonal issues that develop within any functioning unit. Knowledge and use of group process is essential at two points: (1) in helping develop and maintain a therapeutic milieu for the clients; (2) in dealing with the professional staff and their interpersonal issues as they function together in creating a healthful milieu.

We grow and develop emotionally and intellectually by virtue of contacts with other people; we remain relatively intact and functioning, as long as such contacts persist. Without our group memberships and belongingness, therefore, we soon experience various symptoms of deficit. Group processes are critical to all human growth and development and to the maintenance of healthful functioning.

Behavior Maintenance and Change

The social psychologist, Lewin, formulated the issue for us in his analysis of the way in which persons change their attitudes and habits.[10] Although his initial efforts were concerned with changing eating habits by getting people during wartime to serve less well-known cuts of meat (e.g., kidneys and brains), the issue remains the same, whether it is eating behavior, smoking behavior, or other health-related attitudes and behaviors that we need to understand or to change. Lewin's analysis can be stated in terms of several key ideas.

1. Our individual attitudes and habits do not exist in isolation but rather are related to the attitudes and habits of significant groups to which we belong or to which we aspire. The teenager, for example, may take up smoking as a habit because a peer group he or she belongs to or would like to join values smoking.
2. We tend to be rewarded with acceptance and a sense of sharing a common view of things when our behavior generally fits within the norms and guidelines of the groups to which we belong; we meet rejection, hostility, or pressure to change, when our behavior strays too much from our groups' standards. A nurse, working in a setting in which everyone is known on a first-name basis, is accepted as long as this policy is adhered to. Pressure to be like the others is brought to bear if this person breaks this implicit group understanding by using the more formal type of address (Dr. Jones).
3. Lewin suggested that since behaviors are frozen within supportive group settings, to change those behaviors it is necessary to *unfreeze* them from their settings. This means that the individual's support in the group in which the behavior is frozen must be reduced or the group's own standards (i.e., norms, guidelines, and implicit or explicit understandings) for the particular behavior must be altered. For example, the smoking teenager's habit may be frozen in a particular group of friends. That behavior can be changed if the teenager's dependence on the group is lessened or if the entire group's evaluation of smoking is changed.
4. To retain the new behavior, the person must be within a group context that will support rather than undermine it. This involves a process that Lewin calls *refreezing*—that is, locating the new behavior in a supportive group, a group whose standards enforce conformity to the new behavior. These ideas of Lewin have obvious relevance to such treatment programs as Alcoholic's Anonymous; the member of AA both deattaches himself from his former "drinking buddies" and simultaneously becomes a member of a group that opposes drinking.

Let us take another example that will help to clarify these points. Suppose that the issue involves helping a person to stop smoking or at minimum to cut down significantly. First, we must recognize that smoking is a habit that not only developed within a group context but is maintained as a habit within a group context. Thus, to change the individual's smoking behavior, we must work upon the groups that support that habit. For example, it should be easier to get clients to stop smoking if the smokers could be brought together in a group that discusses and examines smoking and that collectively agrees to reduce it, than by trying to deal with the individual in isolation. To deal with habits in isolation from the groups to which they are related is not likely to change those habits; the person returns to his old ways too easily. Most self-help groups work along these lines. To understand or to change poor health habits or to reinforce positive habits, therefore, we must work on the level of the group or groups to which persons belong rather than on the individual in isolation. And to work on the level of groups requires that we learn group process skills.

It is not stretching the point to suggest that understanding this key function of group process in the change and in the maintenance of individual attitudes and behaviors makes our understanding of such processes indispensable to our practice. The promotion and maintenance of health means that the health professional must become sensitive to these processes and capable of working with them effectively.

Health Promotion and Maintenance

The preceding discussion emphasized the important functions that groups play in behavior maintenance, and no area is more critical in this regard than that of health promotion. The interesting research study of Cohen and his coworkers[11] from the psychiatric literature focuses more clearly on this point.

The problem facing this particular psychiatric team involved the treatment of a group of aggressive male and female outpatients through the use of tranquilizing drugs. To provide a proper test of the usefulness of the drugs, a drug group was compared with a matched placebo group over a period of some 3 months. Measures of the client's aggressive behavior at home were obtained both before and after drug or placebo treatment. Additional measures were obtained of the client's home environment. Data from the study are reported in Table 13-1. The measures are discrepancies in reported aggressiveness before treatment and after treatment. The negative values indicate that *all* clients showed reductions in their aggressiveness after the 3 months of treatment. In comparing the data for drug vs. placebo treatment, the most striking finding was that there appeared to be no apparent difference. A closer examination of the data, however, showed that the one instance in which the drug was significantly better than the placebo occurred in the low-conflict family environment. Only when the client's family setting is low in conflict did the use of a tranquilizing drug prove to be more effective than a placebo. But why?

This research highlights the important function that groups play in health maintenance. The authors suggested several parts to the process. (1) The behavior of the person in the high-conflict family setting begins to change as a function of the drug. (2) They are in a group in which conflict is the norm and standard, that is, a group in which aggression and hostility are expected and approved forms of behavior. (3) Any deviation from that normative

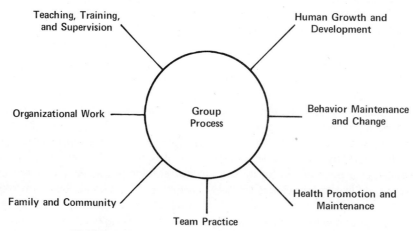

FIGURE 13-1. Group process in life and in practice.

TABLE 13-1   Average Change in Aggressiveness

FAMILY SETTING	TRANQUILIZING DRUG	PLACEBO
High conflict	− 5.67	−6.50
Low conflict	−15.13	−5.36

pattern, as happens with the tranquilizing drug, is met with increased pressure to shape up and remain a good group member. (4) In the case of a high conflict family, being a good group member requires being hostile and aggressive. (5) Thus, the group process conflicts with the drug treatment program, resulting in the overall ineffectiveness of the drug as compared with the placebo.

Basically, only when the group process reinforces the drug treatment, as in the low-conflict setting, is the treatment program more effective than the placebo. The lesson to be learned is very clear. Anyone involved in the treatment of illness, whether this be psychiatric as in the research example or nonpsychiatric, must carefully evaluate the group factors involved in the success or failure of the treatment program *and* how to intervene in the group process in the service of health. To ignore the group processes that are involved, therefore, is to engage in what might prove to be questionable client care.

As was previously noted, heart disease or cancer offer us other clear instances in which the medical treatment must be expanded to take cognizance of the group factors that are either supportive or undermining the medical treatment program. At minimum, there must be a sensitivity to such group processes. For example, what is the meaning to the family's existing interaction patterns or the meaning to the man's business associates of a change in his activity after myocardial infarction? The health professional must become increasingly aware of the role of group processes in such cases. The health professional must also develop skills in working with relevant processes as part of client care. Acknowledging group effects is the first step; doing something about them is the next. The importance of group and social processes in the health continuum cannot be overly emphasized. The material that follows provides a convenient summary of some of these important relationships.

1. *Causes different states of health:* the stress of certain kinds of occupations or of certain types of roles within groups, such as positions with executive responsibility.

2. *Affects the reporting of symptoms and of disease:* ethnic groups vary in their reporting of symptoms.[12,57]

3. *Affects the sick role:* persons and groups vary in their willingness to take on the role of the sick person.[14] Some evidence suggests the importance of training clients in the role of patients so they may better participate in their own recovery.[15]

4. *Influences the course of a disease:* the effectiveness of medical treatment varies as a function of the client's role in the family; persons in dependent family roles adapt better to long-term illness at home than persons whose family roles are a more active and independent one. The latter have more difficulty in home adaptation and seem to benefit more from other care arrangements or from interventions designed to help them adapt better at home.[16]

5. *In treatment and in client management:* sensitivity to the group and social factors involved in maintaining a state of illness when joined with skills in the use of group process for healthful intervention can be a vital part of the health professional's client care plan.

Team Practice

We are living in an era of specialization and often narrow areas of expertise. It is an era of comprehensive health care in which the *team* is the key treatment unit.[17] For most aspects of our daily practice, therefore, we find ourselves as one person among several who have different kinds of responsibility for managing the health care of clients. Our skills as a team member or organizer are important to the effectiveness of practice. A team working with heart clients, for example, may consist of the physician, cardiac nurse, occupational and physical therapists, social service workers, dieticians, and perhaps other specialists as well. Or, a team working with colostomy clients may consist of a nurse specialist (helps the client tend to her colostomy so that it would not be a nuisance to her or her family), a nutritionist (helps the client learn about proper foods), a physical therapist (helps client rebuild strength and recover basic functions), a psychologist or psychiatric nurse (helps client and family deal with the emotional aspects of the surgery), and perhaps even a client-advocate or social worker (to help deal with the variety of questions and problems that arise in connection with social services). We each have different functions to carry out, but we all share the same concern with the client's well-being. Busying ourselves within our own specialized focus and forgetting how the team works can have serious implications for the client; it is easy to forget holistic care. The following is an example in which poor or questionable team practice produced serious consequences for the client.

Ms. Munroe is a clinical nurse specialist on a medical-surgery unit at a city hospital. She is just beginning her practice and still sees herself as a neophyte with much to learn. In the context of that hospital, however, she is expected to take on increasing responsibility for her patients. Many of the staff turn to her as an expert. Some of the nursing staff, many of whom have much greater expertise than she, nevertheless occupy positions in the hospital's hierarchy that lead them to hesitate to express their judgment especially when it varies from hers or the doctors'. One of Ms. Munroe's patients, that she and the others see as a part of their daily rounds, has developed a severe and disabling back pain. The private physician brings in an orthopedic consultant; both recommend immediate surgical treatment. Though inexperienced and unsure of herself in such matters, Ms. Munroe feels that a more conservative treatment program would be preferred at least initially. Two of the nurses on the daily rounds share her assessment but hesitate to support her in the discussions with the private physician and the consultant. They feel it is best to let the physicians argue it out on their own. Because she is unsure of her own competencies, Ms. Munroe hesitates to press her own view of the proper treatment. She makes a few abortive attempts, but these are met with barely disguised hostility and abrasiveness on the part of the private physician: "Who does this nurse specialist think she is!" Ms. Munroe senses that to question the doctors too closely is to engage in a battle of egos with them; they would feel threatened and resentful. She decides not to take them on and press her views, but rather just to sit back, and like the rest of the nursing staff, let them decide on surgery.

This case illustrates many different points, not the least of which involves the implications of the power and status relationships between various health professionals for client care. It illustrates how a group of persons, all of whom have the care of the client in mind and all of whom ostensibly function as a team, hesitate to openly discuss and evaluate the case. The client's care is given over to the decision of one physician who is never really introduced to the good arguments for an alternative treatment program, or to the hour-by-hour assessments of the persons involved in the intimate on-going care of the client.

The point is important. It is not being argued that someone other than the physician in charge of the case should be responsible for the client's overall management. What is being noted, however, is that how team members' inability to work effectively together as a team prevents their providing the client with the kind of care that might otherwise be received. Viable alternatives are never fully introduced or explored. It can be said that this team's group process resulted in what might turn out to be poor practice.

Family and Community Work

Except in some rare instances, it is not an exaggeration to suggest that the various states of health are not simply attributes of the individual as such but can be seen to be attributes of the family and the community as well. This is a conclusion consistent with Lewin's position.[10] It is also a position increasingly adopted among health professionals who see illness as a total physical, social, and psychological disturbance that affects the complex network of group relationships of the client. The health professional does not simply confront the disease entity that the client presents, but, in addition, confronts a person who was, is, and will again be a member of a family, a community, or of some group network.

As we have seen, the cancer client, for example, is much more than one with a specific set of symptoms. Their symptoms are not only individual characteristics with their own history and course of development; they have meaning and consequences for the person's daily living within social groups. Insofar as we relate only to the symptoms as properties of the client, we lose sight of their broader contexts of meaning. To attend solely to the disease entity as such, is to extract it from its group context and thereby to miss what are critical elements in the course and treatment of the disease as well as the client's overall health status. Clients typically have many anxieties about their physical condition as well as issues involving their family, their occupation, and their financial situation. They need to communicate these anxieties and their doubts and uncertainties to the health professionals in whose care they are placed.[18]

The less specialized the health professionals' role, the greater their responsibility for the broad, daily-living aspects of the client, the more important are group processes for client care. One does not confront a disease, but rather a small cast of human characters tied together into group networks. Treatment and care, therefore, require that the health professional be able to comprehend this expanded focus and be able to operate effectively in that group context. Although working with families differs in some respect from working with other kinds of groups, there are sufficient similarities in the nature of the group processes involved to permit the professional who can learn about groups to make significant headway in family work.

For example, Hospice, a group of seven nurses, two physicians, and two social workers was formed in Connecticut to deal with 35 clients and their families as a unit rather than the client in isolation. The clients are all terminally ill but plan to remain at home throughout this difficult period. The health professional staff works with the family at home to help everyone participate in the client's care; all deal with the terminal illness as a matter for family involvement and concern, not just as something happening to the client or as a matter between the client and the health professional. The health professionals, in this case, must not only be skilled in their technical specialty, but must also be sensitive to group process as it develops within the family. Their unit of treatment is the entire family; their skills must therefore be broadened to encompass this larger concept of "client."

Health professionals are often called upon to participate in groups within the community as well—for example, client groups, teacher groups, and groups formed specifically around particular kinds of health problems (e.g., obesity, sexual dysfunction, and cardiac care). A nurse's function in such groups may vary, though in the typical case, the health professional is called on to provide expertise as a consultant; in other instances, the professional may be instrumental in organizing the group.

Several noteworthy examples of the use of client groups as part of health care have recently been developed. One program, for example, called Leukemia Society Outreach Program, is chaired by two health professionals; one is an administrative assistant in pediatric oncology, and the other is a clinical oncology nurse. The goals of the program can perhaps be best captured through some comments of parents and clients: "My husband and I have never had a chance to sit down and talk with the parents of another child with leukemia . . . I have never looked another such parent in the eye, and I would very much like to." Through the organization of parents into a group, it is possible to share experiences and provide mutual support; in addition, it is also possible to provide parents and clients with information regarding community services and support facilities that are available to them.

An adult leukemia patient noted why he needed this type of organization. ". . . There has been one element missing [in my life]. While I had my own thoughts, the love of friends and relatives and the care of concerned medical staff, I was always aware that I had no other patients to share my thoughts and feelings." This patient addresses himself to the need for others with a similar illness to come together to discuss their experience, to universalize what would otherwise appear to be peculiar individualistic feelings, and to share problems and possible solutions.

The issue facing the health professional involves the best ways of organizing client groups or of working with groups that are already formed and functioning. Skills in group process and in leadership are clearly essential to effective practice of this sort. These are all areas in which definite skills can be learned and must be learned; we are not all intuitively capable of working effectively with groups. Our medical and nursing expertise does not make us experts in group, family, or community work. We cannot simply appear on the scene and practice our specialty without an adjunct ability to work effectively in and with groups.

Teaching, Training, and Supervision

Health professionals' practice does not only involve them with clients, client groups, families, or community groups; most are also involved as educators or supervisors, either formally or informally. In formal educational settings, the health professional may organize a small discussion or seminar presentation, or the health professional may be in a supervisory position in which skills of effective leadership are critical parts of the role. In less formal settings, the professional may be in the role of teacher or supervisor, helping to provide training or supervision to others who are less experienced.

In all cases, the professional must teach, train, or supervise others, individually and in small group settings. As with any similar endeavor, teaching, and supervision do not simply involve transmitting one's own knowledge and skills to another. Rather, an interchange between persons takes place; the effectiveness of the learning depends in great measure on both the skills and expertise of the teacher in his or her field of specialization and the skills and expertise of the teacher in group process. Learning to work with a group in training is vital to any health professional who will participate in teaching or supervisory functions. This type of role is especially important in the health professions; much of the training is based on an in-service or supervisory model.

Organizational Work

Another area within which a knowledge of group process is important for effective functioning involves organizational structures and informal groups. Most health professionals either center their work in some kind of organizational (i.e., institutional) setting or at various points in their practice must work within the structures and with the informal groups of some organization. Organizations include hospitals, clinics, mental health agencies, and educational institutions. And, significant issues in most institutional settings, but especially hospitals, involve the *coordination* of diverse persons and the effective exercise of authority and leadership. Group process skills are relevant to both of these issues—that is, to issues of coordination of specialized professionals and to issues of authority and leadership.

A considerable amount of work in sociology and psychology has demonstrated the important role that small groups play within even the most highly structured and seemingly rigid organization.[19-22]

These tend to be the more informal groups of the sort that Cooley termed primary groups; they crisscross throughout organizations and provide an often complex network of human relations that any practitioner interested in organizational change or effective work within the organization must get to know, to understand, and be able to work with.

The health professional may wish to introduce a new practice, for example, to develop a sexuality advising program for clients; they are likely to run into the problems involved in working within organizations to institute any change. These problems stem not only from the administrative level, but are very much rooted in the practices and functioning of the network of informal groups that compose the organization; many see any change to be a threat or disturbance to their own status and well-being.

The health professional may realize that the existing structure of the organization itself thwarts their practice; under such circumstances, the professional must consider ways to change those organizational elements that work to their disadvantage.

Ms. Robinson, during her nursing education, was quick to note how the structure of the family planning clinic at which she was interning interfered with her effectively working with her clients. She was expected to provide intake interviews with women coming in for a pelvic examination and for follow-up family planning information and advice. Many of the women were shy and embarrassed about the procedures; they were hesitant to discuss their own needs; they were reluctant to examine the type of family planning they wanted and their feelings about the complex social and psychological issues that were involved. Ms. Robinson sought to help them explore these matters prior to meeting the physician for the actual examination. She knew that the doctors were busy and took little time to do more than agree to whatever ideas the client might have. Thus they might recommend an abortion to a young girl who says that is what she would like without ever fully exploring her real feelings on this matter. The clinic itself was located in the hospital's emergency room; thus, the interview rooms that Ms. Robinson used could be taken from her, even during an interview, by the needs of the emergency room. In addition, the doctors were on call upstairs and would often come down for a few quick examinations when their own schedule permitted; this would interrupt the intake interviewing often at a very sensitive point. As though this were not enough, doctors frequently had to return to a case upstairs, leaving clients waiting for their return.

This case is illustrative of an organizational arrangement that made Ms. Robinson's work difficult to carry out effectively. Her initial feelings were to blame herself for her poor practice. She lost self-confidence in her ability to interview and to counsel and thought several times of leaving nursing entirely; after all, she seemed unable to do her job well. As she came to a better understanding of the organizational structures within which she was carrying out her work, however, she became less prone to blame herself for the problems of practice. At the same time, she was better able to find ways to work more effectively within this arrangement. Her understanding could also have been put to use in attempting to change the clinic's arrangements. Of course, not all organizational features are readily changeable; but there is usually much more flexibility and leeway than may initially appear. One must be able to develop an understanding of how organizations and groups within organizations work so that one's own practice can be developed to its fullest potential.

The scope of the practice of the professional nurse ranges from direct client care to working in training and supervisory roles with colleagues and others. This scope makes it apparent that group processes are implicated in one way or another at some of the most significant points of practice. It therefore is not a luxury but a necessity for the health professional to develop skills and knowledges about group process for effective practice.

Effective group leadership and participation require four fundamental elements: (1) genuine care and concern for the group, its members, and its functioning together; (2) the development of the perceptual and interpersonal skills needed to intervene in a group's ongoing process; (3) the knowledge of group process concepts and theories; and (4) sensitivity to oneself and one's impact on group process as a participant-observer. These four factors are like the legs of a table; any one that is missing causes wobbling, uncertainty, and insecurity.

Genuine care and concern, while not as readily taught, often derives from the sense of self-confidence that the other three elements provide. As individuals develop a solid foundation in group process concepts and theory, the perceptual and interpersonal skills required to intervene in a group and awareness of themselves as participants in the process of the group, they can acquire a greater interest in and concern for the group they lead or in which they are members. It is difficult not to develop this genuine concern once we know something about how groups function and about the ways we can intervene to facilitate the improvement of that functioning.

REFERENCES

1. Cooley, C. H.: *Social Organization: A Study of the Larger Mind*. New York, Charles Scribner's Sons, 1909.
2. Litwak, E., and Szelenyi, I.: Primary group structures and their functions: kin, neighbors, and friends. *Am. Sociol. Rev.* 34:465–481, 1969.
3. Spitz, R.: Hospitalism: an inquiry into the genesis of psychiatric conditions in early childhood. *Psychoanal. Study Child.* 1:53–74, 1945.
4. Bowlby, J.: *Attachment and Loss, vol. 1: Attachment*. New York, Basic Books, 1969.
5. Bowlby, J.: *Attachment and Loss, vol. 2: Separation*. New York, Basic Books, 1973.
6. Harlow, H.: The heterosexual affectional system in monkeys. *Am. Psychol.* 17:1–9, 1962.
7. Bexton, W. H., et al.: Effects of decreased variation in the sensory environment. *Can. J. Psychol.* 8:70–76, 1954.
8. Scott, T. H., et al.: Cognitive effects of perceptual isolation. *Can. J. Psychol.* 13:200–209, 1959.
9. Sommer, R., and Osmond, H.: Symptoms of institution care. *Soc. Probl.* 8:345–362, 1960.
10. Lewin, K.: *Field Theory in Social Science: Selected Theoretical Papers*, edited by Cartwright, D., New York, Harper and Row, 1951.
11. Cohen, M.: Family interaction patterns, drug treatment, and change in social aggression. *Arch. Gen. Psychiatry* 19:50–56, 1958.
12. Clausen, J. A.: Social factors in disease. *Ann. Am. Acad. Polit. Soc. Sci.* 346:138–148, 1963.
13. Croog, S. H.: Ethnic origins, educational levels, and responses to a health questionnaire. *Hum. Organ.* 20:65–70, 1961.
14. Mechanic, D., and Volkhart, E. H.: Illness behavior and medical diagnosis. *J. Health Hum. Behav.* 1:86–93, 1960.
15. Harm, C. S., and Golden, J.: Group worker role in guiding social progress in medical care institutions. *Soc. Work* 6:44–51, 1961.
16. Deutsch, C. P.: Family factors in home adjustment

of the severely disabled. *Marr. Fam. Liv.* 22: 312–316, 1960.

17. Steiger, W. A., et al.: A definition of comprehensive medicine. *J. Health Hum. Behav.* 1:83–85, 1960.
18. Brown, E. L.: Meeting patients psychosocial needs in the general hospital. *Ann. Am. Acad. Polit. Soc. Sci.* 346:117–125, 1963.
19. Coch, L., and French, J. R. P., Jr.: Overcoming resistance to change. *Hum. Rel.* 1:512–532, 1948.
20. Homans, G. C.: *The Human Group.* New York, Harcourt, 1950.
21. Homans, G. C.: *Social Behavior: Its Elementary Forms.* New York, Harcourt, Brace, and World, 1961.
22. Roethlisberger, F. J., et al.: *Management and the Worker: An Account of a Research Program Conducted by the Western Electric Company, Hawthorne Works, Chicago.* Cambridge, Mass., Harvard University Press, 1939.

BIBLIOGRAPHY

Argyris, C.: Theories of action that inhibit individual learning. *Am. Psychol.* 31:638, 1976.

Bales, R. F.: *Interaction Process Analysis: A Method for the Study of Small Groups.* Cambridge, Mass., Addison-Wesley, 1950.

Bales, R. F.: *Personality and Interpersonal Behavior.* New York, Holt, Rinehart, and Winston, 1970.

Benne, K. D., and Sheats, P.: Functional roles of group members. *J. Soc. Issues* Vol. 4, 1948.

Bennis, W. B., and Shepard, H. A.: A theory of group development. *Hum. Rel.* 9:415, 1956.

Bion, W. R.: *Experiences in groups.* New York, Basic Books, 1959.

Buck, R., et al.: Sex, personality, and physiological variables in the communication of affect via facial expression. *J. Pers. Soc. Psychol.* 30:587, 1974.

Cartwright, D., and Zander, A.: *Group Dynamics*, 3rd ed. New York, Harper and Row, 1968.

Gibb, C. A.: Leadership, in *Handbook of Social Psychology*, 2nd ed., vol. 4, edited by Lindzey, G. and Aronson, E. Reading, Mass., Addison-Wesley, 1968.

Hare, A. P.: *Handbook of Small Group Research.* Glencoe, Ill., Free Press, 1962.

Jourard, S. M.: *Disclosing Man to Himself.* Princeton, N.J., Van Nostrand, 1968.

Kelman, H. C.: Compliance, identification, and internatization; three processes of attitude change. *J. Confl. Resolu.* 2:51, 1958.

Lippitt, G. L.: How to get results from a group, in *Group Development*, edited by Bradford, L. P., Washington, D.C.: National Training Laboratories, National Education Association, 1961.

Lippitt, R., and White, R. K.: An experimental study of leadership and group life, in *Readings in Social Psychology*, 3rd ed., edited by Maccoby, E. E., et al., New York, Holt, Rinehart, and Winston, 1958.

Raven, B. H., and Rubin, J. Z.: *Social Psychology: People in Groups.* New York, John Wiley, 1976.

Sampson, E. E.: *Social Psychology and Contemporary Society.* New York, John Wiley, 1976.

Storms, M. D.: Videotape and the attribution process: Reversing actor's and observers' points of view. *J. Pers. Soc. Psychol.* 27:165, 1973.

Thibaut, J. W., and Kelley, H. H.: *The Social Psychology of Groups.* New York, John Wiley, 1959.

Watzalwick, P., et al.: *Pragmatics of Human Communication.* New York, Norton, 1967.

Yalom, I. D.: *The Theory and Practice of Group Psychotherapy.* New York, Basic Books, 1975.

CHAPTER 14

DEFINING CONTINUITY OF CARE

The concept of comprehensive, continuous health care is as old as organized community health. However, the existence of a concept does not guarantee its accomplishment in the real world of health care delivery. Continuity of care implies the long-term, ongoing care of individuals or families as a unit, regardless of their status on the health-illness continuum, beginning before birth and lasting throughout their lifetimes. Such ongoing care further suggests what French described as an organized "system of personal and family-centered services, rendered by a well-balanced, well-organized core of professional, technical, and vocational personnel who, by using facilities and equipment that are physically and functionally related, can deliver effective care at a cost that is economically compatible with individual, family, community, and national resources."[1]

From this definition, it can be concluded that continuity of care is influenced by: (1) where care

CONTINUITY OF CARE

Jo Joyce Tackett, M.P.H., R.N.

is given—that is, health service resources; (2) who the care-giver is—that is, health manpower resources; and (3) the cooperation that exists within and between the health service resources and the manpower resources—that is, teamwork capabilities. In this chapter, these three components are examined as they have been modified through time in an attempt to achieve continuity of care in our evolving health care delivery system.

COORDINATING HEALTH SERVICE RESOURCES

Comprehensive Health Care

Providing comprehensive, continuing care at an affordable cost requires a unified network of health services in which timing of intervention and setting are significant factors. Logic tells us that primary preventive services (sustaining health)—that is, staying well—saves a great deal in terms of personal, social, and health costs. Secondary preven-

tive services (early detection and treatment of disease), though more costly, are nonetheless essential and have, until recently, more comfortably met social demand. Tertiary services (chronic disease control, restorative and rehabilitative care, curative research) are very costly but are also necessary as our society becomes increasingly committed to valuing the potential of every human being.

Setting is just as important as affordable, continuous care. Institutional care, especially long-term institutional care, has involved steadily increasing social and health costs, until the costs are almost exhaustive. Consequently, society is now rediscovering what was once done from necessity, that "the most therapeutic and least costly method of health care delivery is to treat the client where he is, where he lives, so that health care becomes a national element of life style."[2] Various studies, including those producing stress-adaptation theories, have shown that treating the client "where he lives" decreases his recovery time, diminishes the amount of psychological-social disruption he experiences, affords a quicker return to his usual social roles, increases the incentive for healthful living, and promotes more economical use of health manpower.[2]

The specific health services required in a community vary as local needs, preferences, customs, and capacities differ, but a full range of services from primary to tertiary levels, available to all age groups, should be the goal of every community, including the related social and environmental services necessary to healthful living.

Many communities already have a good beginning toward the provision of comprehensive, continuous health services. What is still cardinal to coordinated care is a melding of the various existing service systems into one community-wide program. Such an endeavor should preclude any new construction or expansion of services which, history shows, usually only fosters further fragmentation or duplication of services.[3]

Evolutionary Development

Traditionally, coordination of health care services was not particularly difficult as the number of facilities was limited to a general community hospital or dispensary and one (or a handful if a community was large enough) family physician. Care that was not complicated enough to require hospitalization was provided in the home by family members or neighbors under the direction of the family physician. For many years, this simple health care delivery system was sufficient, but as community populations grew, advancements in technology abounded, knowledge of health and disease expanded, and social expectations (health as a right) and consumer demands (bill of rights) changed, and more health care facilities, providing a multitude of diverse services, came into existence. Suddenly there was a drastic change in the health care delivery system, but no corresponding coordination of the increasing number of services occurred.

As a result, the current picture of our health care delivery system is one of fragmentation, duplication, service gaps, poor distribution, and only minor efforts at coordination. The consequences have been exorbitant health care costs, inappropriate use of existing health resources, and great problems of access into the system for many potential consumers.

As both providers and users in the health care system have become unsettled by this so-called "nonsystem," some alterations in the situation are occurring, not only at the community level, but nationally. On the local level many physicians have merged to form group practices.[4] Some have even combined with various other health facilities to structure health maintenance organizations (HMO). Early HMOs were initiated at the urging and financial persuasion of industry (e.g., Kaiser-Permanente).[5] Eventually, the federal government produced guidelines and financial inducements for their development (1974). As the character of the population changed (e.g., more aged and more chronic diseases), progressive care facilities were created, of which many were attached to acute care hospital facilities.[6] Neighborhood health centers were supposed to coordinate the delivery of health care, making it accessible to underserved neighborhoods.[7]

In recent years, studies have been conducted nationally to devise ways to provide for continuity of care in fields such as infant and maternity care.[3] A likely enticement for these studies was our declining status internationally with regard to neonatal, infant, and maternal mortality rates.

Perhaps the largest scale effort taken by government and health service facilities at all levels in recent years was initiated by the Comprehensive Health Planning Act, a "Partnership for Health" program (P.L. 89-749, 1966).[8] The aim of this act was to develop an organized way to coordinate health service resources so that comprehensive, continuous care could be accomplished. Attainment of the goals of this act had built-in failure incentives, however, because it did not consider the milieu in which health service delivery must occur or the significant relationships health services have with the economic and social systems.

Following the general failure of that act, another was introduced with the same objective of comprehensive, coordinated health services in mind. The National Health Planning and Resources Development Act (P.L. 93-641)[9] established federal, state, and regional health coordinating councils. These coordinating groups are to give direction for coordination of existing agencies and limit needless duplication of the various health, social, and welfare agencies necessary to comprehensive and continuous health care.[10] It remains to be seen whether this approach will produce a means for continuity in health care.

National health insurance bills continue to be introduced before Congress, making the eventual passage of one extremely likely. All bills under consideration incorporate arrangements for the coordination of health service resources; most of these tend to simulate an HMO structure. Many hospitals and agencies in local communities are already planning for such a structure, with the hospital as a possible central agency around which all other health agencies would be coordinated.[6,11] Other innovative delivery system proposals which deserve attention include those described by Garfield[12] and Leininger.[13]

Garfield[12] proposes a delivery system that separates the sick from the well. Clients would enter through a health testing service. After health testing the client would be referred to facilities for sick care, health care, or preventive maintenance as required and would be transferred among services as his condition changed. A computer center would coordinate this system.

Leininger's[13] model is similar to Garfield's proposal, but more emphasis is placed on preserving cultural and neighborhood involvement by placing health testing centers in satellite clinics and neighborhood health centers. No computerized coordination is mentioned in her proposal.

Dynamics for Teamwork

The small scale coordination that has been achieved has already revealed the advantages of interagency coordination.[14,15] The political and social pressures from special interest groups upon individual agencies are more relaxed, thereby reducing competition between agencies and reassuring smaller agencies. The health service offerings to the consumer become much broader and more affordable. An increase in the availability of scarce resources to *all* consumers is made possible, and the health delivery industry is able to make more efficient use of its health care dollars and its provider resources.

Comprehensive services can be realized by numerous methods and varying degrees. Arnold[8] categorizes these methods into three types of endeavors: (1) A *cooperative endeavor*, which involves some mode for information exchange, often in the form of a referral arrangement, is an informal partnership between participating agencies that is not binding upon any of the participants. (2) In a *coordination endeavor*, which involves some mu-

tual adjustments, usually in program objectives, service provisions, and hours, participating agencies formally agree to conjoin parts of their programs according to each other's needs without diminishing the independent function of each. (3) An *integration endeavor*, which involves a merging of services, is a coordination endeavor in which an agency subsumes the services of another agency(ies). Whatever approach to comprehensive services is employed, each health service agency must recognize the individual contributions to total health care and be willing to work collaboratively with each if quality health care services are going to be available on a continuing basis. The success of any approach will depend upon long-range planning, flexibility of all agencies to adapt to the changing health care climate, earnest joint effort, and regular evaluation.

COORDINATING HEALTH MANPOWER RESOURCES

The Multidisciplinary Team

The concept of the health care team has existed for years, and it is generally accepted by health providers that teams with various types of manpower are beneficial to the delivery of health care. Yet, the transition of the health team from concept to reality continues to have a slow and agonizing growth and development. It has not evolved because of the efforts of the various health professions, but despite the organizational, political, ethical and legal problems that have denied or discouraged any cooperative efforts.[16] While there appear to be many advantages and disadvantages to the multidisciplinary team approach as outlined in Chapter 12, "Providers of Health Care," it should be examined in depth as one possible means of improving health care delivery.

Probably the largest motivation to make interdisciplinary health teams a reality has been the multicausal crisis in health care delivery. Due to the change in emphasis from "sick care" to "health care," the older health professions, especially nursing, have taken on new roles and reshaped old ones.[17,18] Additionally, the health care business has seen a rapid influx of many new health personnel. Specialization, a necessity of the rapid increase in knowledge and advancement of technology, has added confusion to what the consumer already perceived as disjointed health care; clients now often feel that there is no one they can approach who is responsible for them as a total person. The result has been concisely summed up by French[1] who said that "every profession is to some degree surrounded by a zone of ambiguity. The trouble with this zone of ambiguity is not that it is a 'no man's land,' but that it seems to be 'every man's land.' And often this leads to undeclared war between the adjacent occupations."

The need for teamwork among health personnel is obvious simply because there are now so many people who need to know what each is doing. True, there is an overlapping of roles, but a sharing of roles, information, and ideas is imperative when the critical need of the client is frequently shifting. The appropriate allocation of therapeutic roles at any one time in the client's life depends on coordination by a cooperating team of health manpower. Each specialist's unique contribution is necessary for the achievement of health team goals; therefore, each specialist's individual differences must be used constructively (not competed against) so that the specialist's contributions blend with the contributions of other members in a functional manner to accomplish the purposes of comprehensive, ongoing health care.

Experiments with student health teams have revealed much misunderstanding among the health professions about educational preparation and roles,[19-21] presenting a serious barrier to effective teamwork. However, if comprehensive health care for more consumers is to be a reality, the multidisciplinary team may provide a means by which the skills of all available manpower may be tapped.

The use of teamwork to manage health care provides for a system of checks and balances which aids in the elimination of subjective biases by individual team members and enables a more reasoned treatment plan to emerge. Some of the additional benefits of the multidisciplinary team have been summarized by Rubenstein and Levin:[15]

1. The team provides a forum for the exchange and cross-fertilization of divergent views.
2. Individual members can use the rest of the team as a consultative resource.
3. The team provides an arena for the mutual exploration and evaluation of innovative techniques and procedures.

4. Teamwork assists in deleting lengthy delays between client referral, need identification, and therapeutic intervention.

Some cooperation between health providers evolves from the natural association of the staff(s) working with the same clients, and cooperation is essential to teamwork. Marwell and Schmidt[22] investigated the cooperation phenomenon. Looking at some of the descriptions of cooperation they presented gives insights into what teamwork involves.

1. Behavior directed toward the same . . . end by at least two individuals.
2. A situation in which a goal . . . can be reached by one individual . . . only if all individuals [involved] . . . also have the same goal.
3. The meshing of activities or contributions in such a way that the outcome is a unit.
4. A situation in which the combined behavior of two or more organisms is needed to produce positive, or remove negative, reinforcement for either.
5. Cooperation occurs when . . . by emitting activities in concert, at least two [individuals] achieve a greater total reward than either could have achieved by working alone.
6. Cooperation is a joint or collaborative behavior that is directed toward some goal in which there is common interest or hope of reward.[22]

Collectively these descriptions of cooperation spell out five important components of teamwork. These components are: (1) goal-directed behavior; (2) positive reinforcement for each member; (3) distributed responsibilities; (4) coordination of effort through open communication; and (5) social respect for other participants.

The client is the central core of the health care team because his needs mandate the initial and continuous existence and operation of the team. Other health team members include the physician, nurses, and other specialized or allied health professionals. Each member contributes according to his educational preparation, his clinical experience, his personal capabilities, and his functional usefulness (i.e., the range of roles he can perform) to the overall care of the client. Each team member may also supervise an intradisciplinary team (e.g., nursing team) which is also involved, usually through direct care, with the client.

Interdisciplinary teams of three types may exist in a health system, interacting with each other, to provide continuity of care for the client. Any one individual professional may serve on more than one type of team. (1) The primary care team consists of a group of health professionals and allied health personnel who together provide the essential services that involve direct contact with the client. The physician and nurse are usually the main members, with the involvement of others dependent on the client's needs and problems. (2) The medical care team is a group who provides essential backup services to the primary care team (e.g., pharmacists and lab technicians). (3) The members of the health care team are less involved in direct client care and relate more to the entire community. Their concern is with the delivery of all services and factors relevant to continuity of care.

The regular interaction within and among these three types of health teams makes it possible for the client to have easier access to comprehensive health care on a continuous basis from coordinated health service facilities. However, the client should have a central point of entry into the system which should be responsible for the integration and continuity of all health related services. The health professional who is that central figure should have a continuing relationship with the client, and all pertinent health related information should be channeled through that professional, regardless of what institution, agency, or individual provider renders the service. That central figure should have access to all health related resources of the community and must possess the ability to mobilize those resources for the client.[3]

Professional nurses, particularly community health nurses who have had previous experience in both hospital nursing and a community based health agency, are key resources at the central point of entry to the primary care team. The community health nurse has a familiarity and working relationship with all health related community resources, holds a family-centered orientation to health care delivery, meets the client "where he lives," and has highly developed primary prevention and crisis intervention skills.[17,23]

The primary care team has several responsibilities to which all members should make contributions.[24] First is the intake process. Though the individual or family enters into the team's care through one central figure, all those disciplines that are going to be necessary to the team's membership will need to make an initial contact with the client. During this initial contact the team member(s) from each discipline gather data and make assessments relevant to their realm of practice. The information gathered by each team member is shared at the team intake conference so that the team can set need priorities and construct a comprehensive plan of care. A part of this plan will include decisions by the team as to which member(s) will carry primary responsibility for each client need identified. The team will then collaboratively implement the plan, including client-family participation. Maintenance of continuity requires formal or informal team conferences on a regular basis to: (1) continually update care plan priorities; (2) supply additional data from the ongoing assessments of each member; (3) evaluate member contributions, client progress, success of client-family involvement, and (4) determine need for referral to other health resources. Any member should feel free to intercede to provide support or apply crisis intervention skills as the need arises or when it seems appropriate to take on those roles. Other team responsibilities may accrue in any particular set of circumstances, but the aforementioned responsibilities should consistently be managed by the multidisciplinary primary care team.

The medical care team should, of course, act upon the directions of the primary care team, but medical care team members may, at times, participate in the primary care team.

The health care team also has mutual member responsibilities. Those ongoing responsibilities for maintenance of continuous, comprehensive health care to the citizenry served include: (1) program planning and program evaluation; (2) identification of the need for planning, development, and coordination of community resources; (3) consultation with the various health manpower groups; (4) interpretation of health care services and their coordination to consumer and health manpower groups; (5) ongoing research necessary to identify and solve community health care problems; and (6) proper implementation of the comprehensive community health care plan.[24]

Evolutionary Development

The traditional pattern has been that health disciplines tended to function in relative isolation, and are often unaware of the educational preparation or range of roles of other disciplines. Whatever collaboration did occur was usually initiated and controlled by the physician, and because nursing perceived itself to have, and was perceived by others to have, basically a handmaiden role, catering to the physician's needs, the physician's authoritative, omniscient control was not challenged. Even after nursing began to emerge and recognize itself as something more than a handmaiden, being a female-dominated profession and not yet stirred up by any women's liberation movement, there was a lack of self-confidence in the nurse's ability to make a creative contribution to any health team and a general feeling of powerlessness to question the authority of the "greater medical profession."[25,26] These same conditions, along with the proliferation of nursing into several educational programs, have also hindered intraprofessional colleagueship among practicing nurses.[25] Until recently, nursing grand rounds and nursing care conferences, long a part of medical practice, have been unheard of as a part of nursing practice.

Thus one major problem hindering continuity in health care was, and continues to be, in many areas, a status schism which forbids a coalition or partnership among nurses or between nursing and medicine.[27] A simple example of that schism was the existence of separate dining rooms and lounges for various disciplines—a practice which is not altogether extinct. Even today peer group solidarity persists as these disciplines refuse to combine some common aspects of their academic training programs into core courses and interdisciplinary clinical experiences. Most interdisciplinary academic efforts that do exist are classified as "experiments."[21,28,29] Yet, those "experiments" have shown that student teams with core courses and common clinical experiences learn to share problems, with intergroup feelings emerging then submerging as commonalties of purpose are realized by these student team members.

The reality of the health team has traditionally existed largely as a figure of speech. In many regions of the United States today, health manpower is arranged in more of a hierarchy than a team.

Nonetheless, the goal of teamwork is worthwhile and essential to comprehensive, continuous care and should not be pushed aside as too consuming a task to attempt. Current efforts at teamwork should bolster the sagging morale of nursing and other health disciplines. The transition of nursing and nursing education into the realm of professionalism, supported by changes in society in which women are more often placed on an equal plateau with men, has energized nursing's efforts for equal recognition and power in this business of health care delivery. Examples include the construction of joint practices (referred to as group practice attachments in Europe and Britain) in which physicians, nurses, and, at times, other health related professions, form corporations which then contract with hospitals and other health service facilities to provide medical, nursing, or other types of services. Nurse practitioners are leading this movement.[27,30] Typical consequences of joint practices have been: (1) Nurses and physicians rendering the same service are charging the same fees. (2) There has been a reduction in malpractice suits. (3) There has been an increase in the number of consumers served, accompanied by increases in the quality of care provided. (4) Overlaps in roles and functions are productively resolved. (5) Client waiting time is reduced, and there is a substantial elevation in client satisfaction toward services rendered. (6) Joint planning and decision-making exists, allowing additional time for counseling and health education during client contacts.[4]

The changing emphasis toward home-community care has seen greater cooperation by various disciplines with the community health nurse, accompanied by greater respect for the coordinator role the community-home based nurse can play in the management of continuous health care of clients. Also, the problem oriented medical record (POMR), has facilitated teamwork and care continuity. In fact, the whole objective of POMR is to facilitate health team communication and practices toward establishment of common goals and coordinated resolution of client needs.[16] POMR also provides a mechanism by which the health team can audit care.[31]

Some futuristic approaches to teamwork are also in various stages of discussion, planning, and experimentation. One such endeavor is the co-care team at Veteran's Hospital in Palo Alto, California.[20] The team consists of the client's primary physician, a nurse coordinator who represents the nurses rendering direct care, a community health nurse, a social worker, and other discipline representatives that the client's needs dictate. Their job consists of all the basic responsibilities of a primary care team as discussed earlier in this chapter.

A generalist team is proposed and described by Golden and his coworkers[32] with curricula already in various stages of development for preparation of this team. The team's objectives are threefold: (1) to deliver comprehensive primary care of quality on a family basis; (2) to provide continuous primary care to families at a lower cost through nonphysician teams that work conjointly with a group of physicians and health specialists, rather than through traditional physician-nurse teams; and (3) to deliver 80 percent of the primary care the community requires. Figure 14-1 illustrates the relation-

ships of these teams. Depending on the population unit to be served, the generalist team would have two to four family health advocates, one or two family health assistants, and one family health associate. Table 14-1 describes the responsibilities and roles of each team member, including educational requirements.

A venture a few nurses have already taken and which others are sure to follow in the future to provide continuity of care for clients is the complemental nurse in independent nursing practice.[33,34] The nurse is directly employed by the client, similar to the physician-client contract. The independent nurse practitioner then follows the client throughout the length of the contract, coordinating his health care, helping him meet his health needs, collaborating with other disciplines who are involved in his care at any given time, and giving direct care during "critical incidents." This role requires a registered

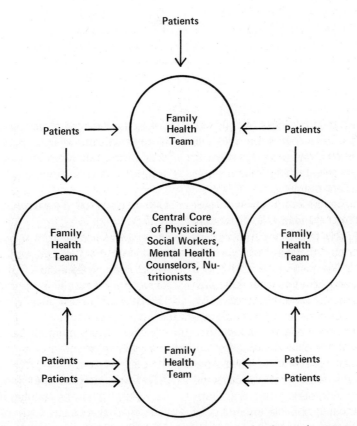

FIGURE 14-1. Family health teams give continuous primary care to families and patients and are supported by a core staff of physicians and other health specialists. (Reprinted with permission from: Golden, A., Carlson, D., and Harris, B.: Non-physician family health teams for H.M.O.'s. *Am. J. Public Health* 63:733, 1973.)

TABLE 14-1. Roles and Educational Preparation of the Generalist Team's Members[32]

Team Member	Roles and Responsibilities	Education Requirements and Preparation
Family health advocate	1. First contact client has with team in home or clinic. 2. Social ombudsman. 3. Provides continuity of concern. 4. Collects assessment data, majority of history information. 5. Does some of physical exam and lab tests. 6. Home visits to assess home life. 7. Health educator. 8. Catalyst for client utilization of needed community resources.	1. High school graduation not required, but must be literate, articulate, and establish rapport easily. 2. Preferably from geographical area of their team assignment. 3. Receive 6 months special training.
Family health assistant	1. All the above as listed for family health advocate. 2. Do more complicated aspects of health assessment, physical exam, lab diagnosis, and health maintenance aspects. 3. Process health checkups. 4. Manage chronic disease clients. 5. Work at all levels (individual, family to total community) on health related problems.	1. Six months practice in a health setting prior to this training. 2. Six months of theory with clinical practice. 3. Six months internship.
Family health associate	1. Coordinator of team. Also the above. 2. Responsible for day-to-day operation of team. Plans well person care. 3. Makes health diagnosis and Rx plans for moderate to mild health problems. Refers other problems.	1. Must be a registered nurse or a military corpsman who had independent duty. 2. Six months theory and clinical practice. 3. Six months internship.

nurse who has had advanced training beyond the basic degree and who is able to work on a flexible schedule. This practitioner has mobility, moving from health agency to private health services to home, wherever the client requires care.

Technological advances in communication systems will also increasingly aid team efforts for care continuity.[26] Not only will televisions, monitoring devices, and remote controls have increasing effect, but computers will provide immediate access to a multitude of information, including treatment protocols and referral resources. Data banks will make health information about consumers instantly accessible, even after they have changed location.

Peer review, an intradisciplinary procedure in most health delivery settings currently, should become a health team undertaking that evaluates the whole team, thereby reinforcing the team approach. To the fullest extent possible, members of the health team should receive not only their basic education jointly, but also their continuing education should be available as a multidisciplinary en-

terprise so that there can be an initial and continuing growth in the appreciation of the goals and skills of the other professions and ongoing development in the job of working together productively.

Dynamics of Teamwork

One can conclude from recent research and past experience that there are certain rules by which the health team must abide if their collaborative endeavor for continuity in care is to be fully realized. The rules of success seem to be these:

1. Each team member has knowledge of group dynamics and a clear image of what a team is.
2. Each member has knowledge and understanding of the training and functional range of roles of each other professional member.
3. Common goals for the team have been defined and each member feels a commitment to help achieve those goals.

4. Equity exists in that each member has equal voice and influence and is equally valued. This is important as a sense of inequity is the greatest factor influencing member dissatisfaction with the team relationship.[22]
5. Mutual respect reigns, including a readiness to learn from other members and to positively reinforce the efforts of other members.
6. Members are able to communicate using a common language. This helps to eliminate misunderstandings and misinterpretations between members, facilitates communication generally, and reduces role misconceptions.
7. Interdependence exists. So that members can collaborate, not compete, flexibility of leadership and role exchange is maintained. In this way roles can pass from one member to another as individual expertise is needed, depending on the client's current needs and his responsiveness to particular members. Lysaught[35] stressed that it is important for roles that interact (as do those of most health professionals) to be defined in context, rather than unilaterally.

Not only do health teams have rules to abide by, they can also anticipate moving through several phases during their development into a mature multidisciplinary team.[21,22] Initially a sense of competition prevails, until each member learns to yield some autonomy and peer identity to fulfill team goals. As these feelings are ventilated within the group, a state of compromise emerges and with it a growing rapport among team members. Cooperation is achieved next as members realize that different members' skills will be in demand at different times in the client's life. Collaboration is accomplished when team members can finally allow for fluidity of roles. When each member begins to feel he is an intricate part of the team, with valuable, unique skills to offer that team, full maturity of teamwork has arrived and comprehensive, continuing health care can be a reality. To quote Booker T. Washington, the health team will be "separate as the fingers, but united as the hand."

SUMMARY

Continuity of care has yet to achieve a full reality, though it has long been a concept of health care delivery. Continuous health care means care of the total client, throughout his life span, regardless of his health status. Such continuous care is possible only if a qualified, coordinated system of health services and manpower exists.

Both timing of intervention and the setting in which intervention occurs are important if care is to be both continuous and affordable. Primary preventive services are least costly, and tertiary services are most costly, but all are essential to a community's health care system. Likewise, home care offers the least expensive setting alternative, while long-term institutional care can be exorbitant. How many and which kinds of health services will vary from community to community, but all communities need coordinated services that cover the needs of all age groups contained by the community.

Coordinating health services was traditionally a simple matter because of the few health services and health manpower resources in existence. But as technology, knowledge, and consumer character have changed, a multitude of autonomous health services and manpower groups were created, without any planned means of coordination for care continuity, resulting in the "nonsystem" of today. Legislative action and efforts by both consumer and manpower groups are bringing about some experimental attempts for planned, coordinated, continuous health care delivery.

Achieving comprehensive health services can be done through cooperation endeavors, coordination endeavors, or integration endeavors. Coordination efforts already attempted have realized many positive consequences.

The health care team is not a new vision to health care delivery, but it is a concept whose full contribution to comprehensive, continuous health care has not yet been realized. The current health care crisis testifies to an emphasis on interdisciplinary teamwork. Teamwork has proved profitable in other occupations and the small scale efforts in the health business have revealed teamwork to be productive and practical. Five basic components of cooperative teamwork are: (1) goal directed behavior; (2) positive reinforcement for members; (3) distributed responsibilities; (4) coordinated effort through open communication; (5) social respect of and for other members. The client is the central focus of the team, with health manpower membership varying with the client's altering needs. Primary care teams, medical care teams, and health care teams make up the interdisciplinary team network. The client's central point of entry into this network is through a member of the primary care team. The nature and character of the nursing profession, especially community health nursing, lends itself nicely to being that central point of entry. Each of these teams has specific responsibilities that are consistently theirs to perform.

Traditionally, health professionals functioned in relative isolation, with little understanding of the functional potential or common goals of other professions. Currently, however, nursing and other related health professions are beginning to feel confident of the contribution they can offer health delivery as equitable team members. Several approaches to collaborative teamwork are in various stages of planning, development, and experimentation, and still others are being conceived. Perhaps the most fully developed futuristic approach is the generalist team created by Golden and coworkers.[32] Nurse practitioners are surging ahead to open communication channels between nursing and other manpower resources.

Several team rules have emerged out of successful team efforts. Teams can also anticipate movement through several phases before reaching a mature level of functioning in which they will be "separate as the fingers, but united as the hand."

REFERENCES

1. French, R. M.: *The Dynamics of Health Care.* New York, McGraw-Hill Book Co., 1968, pp. 7–10, 67–82, 105–114.
2. Wilson, R.: *The Sociology of Health: An Introduction.* New York, Random House, 1970, pp. 33–68.
3. National Commission on Community Health Service: *Health Is a Community Affair: Report.* Cambridge, Mass., Harvard University Press, 1967.
4. National Joint Practice Commission: *Together: A Casebook of Joint Practice in Primary Care.* Chicago, National Joint Practice Commission, 1976.
5. Collen, F., et al.: Kaiser permanent experiment in ambulatory care. *Am. J. Nurs.* 71:1078, 1971.
6. Lane, D., and Mazzola, G.: The community hospital as a focus for health planning. *Am. J. Public Health* 66:465, 1976.
7. Fry, R. E., and Lech, B. A.: *An Organized Developmental Approach to Improving the Effectiveness of Neighborhood Health Care Teams.* Cambridge, Mass., Alfred P. Sloan School of Management, Massachusetts Institute of Technology, 1971.
8. Arnold, M. F.: Basic concepts and crucial issues in health planning. *Am. J. Public Health* 59:1686, 1969.
9. Matek, S., and Hiscock, W. (eds.): Policy statements offered for APHA. *The Nation's Health,* September 1976, pp. 5–7.
10. Osborn, B.: *Introduction to Community Health.* Boston, Allyn and Bacon, Inc., 1967.
11. Alford, R. R.: *Health Care Politics.* Chicago, University of Chicago Press, 1975, pp. 110–137.
12. Garfield, S.: The delivery of medical care. *Sci. Am.* 222:15, 1970.
13. Leininger, M.: An open health care system model. *Nurs. Outlook* 21:714, 1973.
14. Morris, R.: Basic factors in planning for the coordination of health services. Part II. *Am. J. Public Health* 53:462, 1963.
15. Rubenstein, J., and Levin, S.: A model for interagency cooperation in provision of mental health services to youths. *Hosp. Community Psychiatry* 27:404, 1976.
16. Providing a climate for the utilization of nursing personnel. Paper presented at joint programs of the National League for Nursing and the American Hospital Association, Publication No. 20, New York, 1975, p. 1566.
17. Notter, L., and Spalding, E.: *Professional Nursing: Foundations, Perspectives and Relationships,* Philadelphia, J. B. Lippincott Co., 1976, pp. 35–36, 90–98.
18. Somers, A.: *Health Care in Transition: Directions for the Future.* Chicago, Hospital Research and Education Trust, 1971, pp. 87–100.
19. Jacobson, S.: A study of interprofessional collaboration. *Nurs. Outlook* 22:751, 1974.
20. Riley, M., and Moses, J.: Coordinated care: making it a reality. *J. Nurs. Admin.* 7:21, 1977.
21. Schmidt, C.: Five become a team in Appalachia. *Am. J. Nurs.* 75:1314, 1975.
22. Marwell, J., and Schmitt, D.: *Cooperation: An Experimental Analysis.* New York, Academic Press, 1975, pp. 183–188.
23. Freeman, R. B.: *Community Health Nursing Practice.* Philadelphia, W. B. Saunders Co., 1970, pp. 74–108.
24. George, M., Ide, K., and Vambery, C.: The comprehensive health team: a conceptual model. *J. Nurs. Admin.* 1:7, 1971.
25. Nolan, M. G.: Wanted: colleagueship in nursing. *J. Nurs. Admin.* 7:41–43, 1976.
26. Sutterloy, D., and Donnelly, G.: *Perspectives in Human Development: Nursing throughout the Life Cycle.* Philadelphia, J. B. Lippincott Co., 1973, pp. 303–314.
27. Sills, G.: Nursing, medicine, and hospital administration. *Am. J. Nurs.* 76:1432, 1976.
28. Davis, A.: Undergraduate interdisciplinary educators in the health sciences: innovative education. *J. Nurs. Educ.* 15:22, 1976.

29. Tanner, L., and Soulary, E.: Interprofessional student health teams. *Nurs. Outlook* 20:111, 1972.
30. Peterson, G.: *Working with Others for Patient Care.* Dubuque, Iowa, Wm. C. Brown Co., 1969, pp. 45–56.
31. Robinson, A.: Problem-oriented record: uniting the team for total care. *RN* 38:23, 1975.
32. Golden, A., Carlson, D., and Harris, B.: Non-physician family health teams for health maintenance organizations. *Am. J. Public Health* 63:732, 1973.
33. Walford, H.: Complemental nursing care project. *Nurs. Forum* 3:9, 1974.
34. Wolford, H., Whitson, B., and Hartley, L.: Complemental nursing: originator's viewpoint. *Am. J. Nurs.* 77:984, 1977.
35. Lysaught, J.: *An Abstract For Action.* New York, McGraw-Hill Book Co., 1970, p. 88.

BIBLIOGRAPHY

McHugh, J. and Chughtai, M.: The importance of teamwork in geriatric care. *Nurs. Times* 70:140, 1975.
McIntosh, J.: Communication in teamwork. *Nurs. Times.* 71:85, 1974.

CHAPTER 15

CONTEMPORARY ROLE OF THE REGISTERED NURSE

Practice roles for registered nurses are rapidly changing in response to a continually expanding knowledge base, consumer health care needs, government, and numerous other societal forces. New approaches to health care delivery are reflected in nursing roles which can best be described as innovative, challenging, and rewarding. No other health professional has a role which is as broad in scope and as dynamic as that of the registered nurse.

The three major elements of the nursing profession—practice, education, and research—find expression in all aspects of the nurse's role in health care delivery. The contemporary role of the registered nurse is truly a multifaceted one. While the requirements of a nurse's specific position and practice setting may require emphasis on particular components of the role, all of the components dis-

THE REGISTERED NURSE

Sarah B. Pasternack, M.A., R.N.

cussed below are inherent in the contemporary role of the registered nurse.

Health Care Provider

Nursing exists to serve people; therefore, the most important role of the registered nurse is that of health care provider. Nurses practice in schools, community health agencies, mobile health units, homes, industry, private practice (solo or joint practice with nurse colleagues or other health professionals), and hospitals. While the basic educational preparation allows the registered nurse to assume a beginning role as a nursing care provider, usually as a *staff nurse* in a hospital or ambulatory care agency, advanced preparation and experience enable the nurse to assume more specialized roles.

PRIMARY NURSING

Hospital-based nursing care may be provided through either *primary nursing* or *team nursing*.

Developed during the late 1960s, *primary nursing* has received wide acceptance by clients, nurses, and health care agencies. (Primary nursing should not be confused with primary health care which will be discussed shortly.) In primary nursing, the nurse assumes responsibility for using the nursing process in planning and implementing care for a given number of clients. The nurse is responsible for the coordination and provision of the client's care, on a 24-hour basis, from the time of admission to discharge from the hospital. Clients with chronic illnesses, which necessitate repeated hospital admissions, are usually assigned to the same primary nurse during subsequent admissions. In many agencies, the primary nurse also makes home visits following the client's discharge from the hospital. The primary nurse works in a collaborative relationship with the physician and other health professionals who may be involved in care of the client.

Primary nursing allows the nurse to practice in a truly professional manner; it also facilitates development of a therapeutic nurse-client relationship. The primary nurse bears responsibility for initiating and implementing the nursing process in each nurse-client relationship and is directly accountable to the client for the care rendered. Because of the responsibility the nurse must assume under a system of primary nursing, most agencies assign only registered nurses to this role. Since it is impossible for the nurse to be present 24 hours a day, an "associate nurse" assumes responsibility for carrying out the plan of care devised by the client's primary nurse when she is off duty. The role of the associate nurse is usually assumed by either a registered nurse (who is usually also a primary nurse for a group of clients) or a licensed practical nurse. A caseload of between four and eight clients is considered optimum.

In addition to the advantages for the client and the nurse, primary nursing offers a significant financial advantage for the hospital. As compared with the older mode of care—team nursing, primary nursing is indeed cost-effective for the employing institution;[1] it allows the nurse to focus on client care while other less costly personnel are utilized to perform non-nursing tasks. The benefits derived from implementation of primary nursing have allowed consumers, nurses, and hospital administrators to view nursing's contribution to health care in a new light. Consequently, many hospitals are in the process of employing all registered nurses. Selected references on primary nursing have been included in the bibliography.

TEAM NURSING

Although primary nursing has become the favored modality in nursing care, there are numerous hospitals that continue to employ team nursing. Team nursing was developed in the late 1940s and 1950s in response to a steadily increasing population with significant health care needs and a shortage of registered nurses. A "team" composed of at least one registered nurse and several nonprofessional staff members (i.e., practical nurses and nursing assistants) is responsible for providing care to a group of clients. Although a team may vary in size, there are generally three to eight members. Likewise, the number of clients for whom the team must provide care may vary. In some hospitals the client group is as small as 10 or 12 while in others it may exceed 30 clients.

Since the team leader should be the person who possesses the most knowledge and skill, this role is assumed by a registered nurse. The team leader makes the daily client care assignment for team members and is also responsible for supervising care provided by members of the team. In some instances, the team leader assumes direct client care responsibilities; at other times, the team leader assumes more of a managerial role in coordination of care. Also, the team leader is usually responsible for developing nursing care plans for clients assigned to the team and for conducting client care conferences.

When contrasted to primary nursing, the shortcomings of team nursing become quite evident. The most obvious disadvantages are the lack of individualized care for the client and the relatively infrequent interactions between the registered nurse and client. Indeed, the person with the least amount of skill is actually closest to the client.

PRIMARY HEALTH CARE PROVIDER

One of the newer roles for the registered nurse is that of primary health care provider. The terms "primary care" and "primary health care" refer to the client's point of entry into the health care system. Nurses are assuming the role of primary health care provider in ambulatory care settings where the ongoing health care of clients is the nurse's responsibility. The primary care nurse (nurse practitioner) must have highly developed health assessment skills (i.e., the health history and physical assessment techniques are discussed in another section of this book) to perform effectively in this role. The primary care nurse must be an astute observer, a skilled interviewer, and be able to draw on theoretical knowledge to make decisions about client care. However, it is important that the primary care nurse not exceed the legal boundaries of nursing practice; hence, she must be able to communicate and collaborate easily with other health professionals and disciplines; she must also be able to recognize the proper times to refer clients to these other professionals.

The nurse's role as a primary health care provider is rather new (less than 15-years-old), and it is still a controversial one within the profession, among other health professions, in legislatures (i.e., in relation to nurse practice acts and third-party reimbursement for health care services), and among the general public. Those who support the concept of the nurse as a primary care provider believe that direct access to the nurse by the consumer will permit the nurse to make a significant contribution to health care. Proponents of this emerging role view the nurse as especially well prepared to provide *health* care—care which is more than and different from *medical* care—through such activities as health promotion and maintenance, health teaching, and counseling.

Some have questioned whether the nurse is actually an appropriate primary health care provider.[2] Nurse-physician roles in primary care often overlap, and professional practice boundaries are often in flux when primary care is provided in an interdisciplinary fashion. Those who oppose the role of the nurse as a nurse practitioner believe that the nurse is actually taking on the physician's role and neglecting the nurse's role.[2,3] Resolution of this issue is one of the most perplexing dilemmas currently facing the nursing profession.

Teacher

Client teaching and health are important components of the registered nurse's role. Among all health professionals, the nurse is perhaps the best prepared to assume responsibility for planning and implementing health education. It is important that the nurse view health teaching as *integral* to the nurse's role in providing care. The nurse should strive to make *every* nurse-client interaction a learning experience for the client.

The most important teaching role of the nurse is most often an informal one. Correct utilization of the nursing process requires the nurse to assess the client's knowledge about his health status and formulate a teaching plan which is incorporated into the overall nursing care plan. It is important for the nurse to incorporate the family and significant others into the teaching plan when appropriate.

The nurse is also well prepared to assume a formal role in *consumer health education*. The nurse's knowledge of health, human behavior, pathophysiology, and teaching definitely qualify the nurse to assume a leadership role in health education for consumers of all ages. The possibilities for nurse involvement in consumer health education are extensive. Some examples of the registered nurse's role in health education follow.

1. Providing specialized instruction to individuals with identified health problems, such as diabetes or hypertension.
2. Teaching cardiopulmonary resuscitation in the community.
3. Teaching senior citizens how to select nutritious but economical foods in the supermarket.
4. Teaching first aid measures to school teachers, cafeteria personnel, and maintenance staff.
5. Teaching day-care providers about child health, safety, and accident prevention.
6. Teaching techniques of breast self-examination to women in the community.
7. Teaching the families of handicapped persons how to adapt the home environment to meet the needs of the handicapped individual.
8. Providing formal health education within a school system.
9. Providing childbirth preparation classes for expectant parents.
10. Teaching parents how to provide sex education for their children.

Client Advocate

As a client advocate, the nurse is responsible for defending and promoting the rights of the client. An episode of illness frequently places an individual and family in a state of crisis. It is important, therefore, that the nurse take the initiative for providing the client and family with thorough explanations regarding the client's status and impending treatment procedures. The nurse should never assume that the physician has given the client an adequate explanation *in terms that the client can comprehend* nor should the nurse assume that the client does not have any questions, concerns, or fears merely because he does not verbalize them.

Clients are often fearful of medical procedures, hospitals, and health care providers, and usually unaware of their rights in health care matters. It is important then that the nurse not only make sure the client is fully informed about his rights but also that the client's rights are properly upheld. The nurse's role as a client advocate takes on even greater significance when the client is incapable of understanding his rights and acting in his own behalf. Infants, children, the aged, the handicapped, the mentally ill, and the imprisoned are especially in need of the nurse's advocacy role. The nurse should be aware that defending a client's rights can be a risky, lonesome venture. Frequently, the nurse finds that colleagues are unwilling to back up their verbal promises of support or that the nurse has placed her job or, even worse, her license in jeopardy. There are times when the nurse *must* take a risk on behalf of the client, but it is also important for the nurse to be informed of the possible legal consequences of the nurse's advocacy role. In addition to reading the selected references on client's rights listed in the bibliography, the student is urged to read the sections of this book which discuss client's rights and legal aspects of the nurse's role.

Counselor

Providing a relaxed, therapeutic environment and establishing rapport with the client, family, and significant others is essential if the nurse expects to achieve success in the role of counselor. Most individuals who enter the health care system are somewhat anxious about their health, but each reaction to encounters with illness or the health care setting is unique. Many individuals actually feel quite comfortable in sharing their feelings with a nurse, but frequently the *nurse* must take the initiative in the counseling situation.[4]

Counseling clients and families is, perhaps, one of the most demanding and exhausting aspects of the registered nurse's role. Counseling requires the nurse to become "involved," to make therapeutic use of the self, to *care*. It is never easy, and frequently there are no "answers" for the client's concerns nor are there "solutions" to the client's problems. The nurse must be willing to give the client time to develop trust in her. Most importantly, the nurse must be willing to *listen* and be able to use communication skills to assist the client in exploring his concerns and in weighing alternatives when such exist. The nurse's goal must always be to facilitate the *client's ability* to deal with his problems; hence, she must never give the client "advice" or direction in the counseling relationship.

Coordinator

It is essential that the nurse work collaboratively with other disciplines to provide the client with the care and resources which will assist the client and family in reaching the established goals. The nurse is responsible for initiating referrals to other health care providers to insure continuity of care after discharge from the hospital or between visits to the health care agency. Planning for a client's recovery and eventual discharge is a professional nursing responsibility which should begin shortly after the client is admitted.

In addition to coordinating the health services, the nurse must also place high priority on coordinating the client's daily activities. It has been estimated that as many as 30 different individuals enter a hospitalized client's room each day. Hospitalization imposes numerous stresses on a client; the most frequent are the exhausting daily care, treatment, and diagnostic testing routines which are compounded by sleepless nights. Frequently, it is necessary for the nurse to intervene to provide the client with a schedule which includes adequate rest and privacy.

Researcher

A steadily growing nucleus of nurse researchers is continually adding to the evolving body of nursing science knowledge. Technical knowledge of the present day will be short-lived; new knowledge provides nurses with fresh insights which can be utilized to provide better care to clients. Nursing research is far from being dull, sterile, or isolated in a remote laboratory. Rather, nursing research is a creative, disciplined endeavor which seeks answers to questions about variables which affect the nature of the life process in people during health and illness. Nursing research is generally directed toward the development of a *theoretical* body of knowledge rather than testing of new nursing care *techniques*. However, the knowledge generated by nursing research findings provides the practicing nurse with a theoretical rationale upon which direct nursing care can be based. It is imperative that there be a close alignment between nursing research and clinical nursing practices. As one noted nurse researcher states: ". . . knowledge production in nursing depends on a flowing kind of interaction—a movement back and forth between the concrete realities of nursing work and the abstract world of those interrelated propositions known as theories."[5] Although many nurses do not choose to conduct nursing research, *all* practicing nurses have a responsibility of keeping abreast of findings generated by nursing research, critically reviewing the validity of the findings, and incorporating relevant findings into daily practice.

Change Agent

The registered nurse must be a leader in establishing and maintaining high standards of nursing care in the practice setting. In addition to implementation of the American Nurses' Association *Standards of Nursing Care*[6] (see section on Quality Assurance), the registered nurse must assume a leadership role in promoting creative approaches to client care.

The nurse must develop skills in clinical judgment and decision-making in addition to expertise in clinical nursing care to influence and, thus, promote change in the quality of care provided by the health care system. Change is always a difficult process for human beings, and health care professionals and health care institutions are often *most* resistant to change. Students and beginning practitioners are frequently frustrated and discouraged as they desperately attempt to implement their innovative, and quite often valuable, ideas. Surely, *all* nurses, including administrators and educators, must learn to be more receptive to the new ideas proposed by students and beginning registered nurses. In the meantime, however, "developing" change agents might find the information provided in the following list to be of some assistance in their quest for creativity and change. In addition some helpful references related to the change process have been included in the bibliography.

1. The assumption that change agents are creative individuals is often *true*.
2. It is *true* that the ideas of creative people are often regarded as somewhere between slightly odd and wildly outlandish.
3. It is *true* that most successful change agents usually cultivate strong, loyal, reliable *allies* before attempting to introduce change.
4. The popular belief that change is a *very slow* process is *very true*.
5. The belief that creative persons generally possess strong commitment to their endeavors is generally *true*; also, it is *true* that they often succeed in reaching their goals.
6. The popularly held belief that change agents should learn to be satisfied with *very small, widely-spaced* rewards is generally *true*.
7. The popular notion that change agents must be courageous is *true*.
8. It is generally *true* that recognized *leaders* and *authorities* on a given subject are more likely to be successful in introducing change than other individuals.
9. The assumption that a positive correlation exists between the traits of creativity and intelligence is often *true*.
10. It is *true* that change agents suffer from a malady known as chronic frustration.
11. The belief that change agents are usually resourceful enough to learn how to handle their frustrations appropriately is generally *true*.
12. The popularly held belief that knowledge of "change theory" is invaluable for any aspiring or practicing change agent is *true*.
13. The assumption that nursing students and new graduate nurses "don't know anything about nursing" is *most definitely false*. (It is also nothing more than ancient mythology.)

Case-finder

The nurse is quite frequently in a position to identify health problems which were not previously identified. Some of these discoveries may be inadvertent, but quite often they are detected because of the nurse's keen observational and communication skills. For example, a nurse caring for an individual may identify an equally significant, but untreated, problem in a family member. Referral to the most appropriate health care professional is, of course, the next logical step after case-finding. Case-finding should extend beyond the individual level. Identifying a community's needs for nursing care, health education, or health screening are all within the scope of case-finding.

Consultant

The role of consultant (formal or informal) is a rather new one for nurses. The expertise of nurses is often sought by groups and organizations within the nursing profession as well as by groups and organizations outside the profession. For example, a pediatric nurse might serve as a consultant for a day-care agency, or a well-known nurse educator might be requested to conduct a curriculum evaluation workshop for a nursing faculty in another part of the country. Some health care agencies employ nurses with advanced educational and practice skills as consultants for their own nursing staff. For example, a nurse with a master's degree in psychiatric nursing might provide nurses on general medical-surgical units with assistance in identifying and responding to client's psychosocial needs. Except where the nurse is employed by the agency, nurse consultants usually provide consultation on a fee-for-service basis. Many nurses, however, waive consultation fees for agencies and groups in their own communities.

While relatively few nurses engage in formal consultation, *most* registered nurses (and nursing students) participate in the informal type of consultation. Ironically, they do so quite frequently, despite the fact that very few nurses recognize the process as consultation. For example, a nursing student who is engaged in an independent study of nursing audit might seek guidance from a faculty member who has a special interest and familiarity with nursing audit. Also, the student might seek an appointment with chairpersons of the nursing audit committees in various hospitals and community agencies. A primary nurse who is having difficulty in implementing a nursing care plan might seek out a nurse colleague to identify and explore alternative approaches.

Informal consultation in the practice or education setting is the only component of the contemporary role of the registered nurse which does not directly involve the client. However, it is a most important and necessary part of the registered nurse's role. Nurses are no different from other people; each nurse possesses special skills which may be quite different from the expertise of another individual. Nurses can and should serve as consultants to each other more frequently and on a more conscious level. *No* nurse can be knowledgeable and skilled in *all* aspects of nursing. In professional nursing, seeking out one's peers for consultation or validation does *not* signify lack of knowledge or incompetence; rather, it signifies a deep concern for quality client care and a sincere desire to improve one's practice.

EDUCATIONAL PREPARATION OF REGISTERED NURSES

The system of formal nursing education in the United States is just over 100-years-old. To say that nursing education has been beset by confusion, controversy, and conflict would be an understatement. Some changes in the nursing education system have been accomplished with amazing rapidity and ease, whereas others continue to evolve in an almost *painfully slow* manner. Nevertheless, the history of nursing education in the United States and abroad is most fascinating. It is an aspect of the profession with which every nurse should be acquainted. Since a detailed account of this development is not within the scope of this chapter, the student is referred to the readings on the history of the profession which have been incorporated into the bibliography.

Early Beginnings

The system of "modern" nursing education was initiated by Florence Nightingale in England, circa 1860. At a time when "nice ladies" did not work outside the home, Florence Nightingale proposed the following radical (for the times) ideas:

1. Care of the ill is a worthy endeavor.
2. Nursing should be viewed as a profession.
3. There should be formal educational preparation for nurses which should be provided in schools that are *independent of hospitals* in order to emphasize education, not service to the institution.
4. Nursing should be concerned with *health*, not just "sickness."
5. Nursing is a career which is quite distinct from medicine.
6. Nurses should be highly paid.
7. Individuals seeking admission to nursing schools should be qualified to pursue the course of study.
8. Individuals who are admitted to schools of nursing must be carefully selected.

The founder of modern nursing was a most remarkable individual. One nursing historian describes her as "a brilliant thinker, an intrepid fighter for the causes she believed in, and an outspoken advocate for progress in the nursing, hospital, and home care of the sick."[7]

Diploma Nursing Schools

News of Florence Nightingale's nursing school spread to the United States, and by 1873, three "Nightingale" schools were established: the Bellevue Training School (Bellevue Hospital, New York City), the Connecticut Training School for Nurses (New Haven Hospital, New Haven), and the Boston Training School for Nurses (Massachusetts General Hospital, Boston). Actually, the placement of "Nightingale" schools under hospital control, which was contrary to the beliefs of Florence Nightingale, has been termed an "historical accident."[8] Nevertheless, the hospital-based school was widely accepted, and diploma schools proliferated. By 1900, there were 40 diploma schools, and by the 1950s, there were well over 1,000.[9] However, the rapid escalation of operating costs and the implication of the American Nurses' Association's 1965 "First Position on Education for Nursing"[10] have been responsible for the steady decline in the number of diploma nursing schools since the mid-1960s. As of 1976, 390 diploma schools of nursing remained open.[11] Nurses who graduated from diploma schools accounted for 25.5 percent of all graduating nurses in 1975–1976.[11]

Collegiate Nursing Education

BACCALAUREATE PROGRAMS

Although collegiate education for nurses developed slowly, it is not a recent innovation. The very first baccalaureate nursing programs were established in 1877 at Howard University (Washington, D.C.) and in 1910 at the University of Minnesota (Minneapolis). The early 1900s was a time of educational reform for many professions in this country. As a result of Flexner's extensive study,[12] the medical profession rapidly moved from an apprentice-style educational system to collegiate education for physicians. A similar movement occurred in the teaching profession, when minimal education for teachers was removed from "normal schools" and transferred to 4-year colleges.

Numerous reputable studies of the nursing profession and nursing education have been conducted since the beginning of the twentieth century. Beginning with the 1923 publication of the Goldmark report,[13] study after study recommended that basic education for nurses should take place within a baccalaureate program. Despite the general reluctance to endorse baccalaureate nursing education, collegiate nursing programs slowly but steadily increased in number. By 1950, there were about 195, and by 1976, the number of baccalaureate programs had increased to 341.[11] The 1975–1976 graduates of baccalaureate programs accounted for 29 percent of all graduating nurses.[11]

Most of these programs admit diploma school and associate degree program graduates who wish to earn a baccalaureate degree. A number of baccalaureate nursing schools have recognized the unique needs of the registered nurse student. Therefore, some baccalaureate programs now offer students the option of "self-paced" and independent study, transfer credit for courses completed in other accredited colleges, and exemption or "challenge" examinations.

ASSOCIATE DEGREE PROGRAMS

Research conducted by the noted nursing educator, Montag,[14] provided the blueprint for modern associate degree (A.D.) nursing education. Montag proposed that there was a need for a "nursing technician" whose preparation should be less extensive than that of the professional nurse but more than that of the practical nurse. She envisioned the nursing technician as being able to assume responsibility for client care and for making some nursing judgments. The nursing technician was expected to perform under the supervision of the professional nurse, but was not prepared to assume administrative responsibilities. Also, the associate degree program outlined by Montag was intended to be a "terminal degree" program; that is, it was not designed to be the first 2 years of a baccalaureate program.

Not only were the first graduates of the A.D. program able to assume the expected clinical practice role, they were also able to pass State Board Examinations which led to licensure as a registered nurse. Easy access to A.D. programs in local community colleges, low tuition, and in many programs, an "open-admissions" policy have made A.D. programs highly attractive to students of all ages. The growth of A.D. programs has been quite rapid. In 1976, less than 30 years after they were established, A.D. nursing programs numbered 642, and accounted for 47 percent of all programs leading to registered nurse licensure.[11] Associate degree graduates accounted for 45 percent of all graduating nurses.[11]

New Trends in Collegiate Preparation

The nursing profession is steadily attracting large numbers of individuals of all ages and both sexes. Also, many individuals who have earned degrees in other fields are seeking entry into nursing education programs. At the same time, the cost of a college education continues to rise. As a result of the diverse educational backgrounds and needs of individuals seeking entry into programs which prepare the student for practice as a registered nurse, some innovative programs have recently emerged.

NEW YORK STATE REGENTS EXTERNAL DEGREE PROGRAMS

The External Degree Program enables individuals to earn a college degree without requiring the student to either enroll in a school or attend a class. This program uses a combination of transfer credit, proficiency examinations, and other special evaluation techniques to assess the learner's knowledge. Currently, it is possible for individuals to earn either an associate degree or a Bachelor of Science degree. Candidates must demonstrate both theoretical nursing knowledge and clinical proficiency. Both programs have been carefully developed to insure that their standards are comparable to traditional nursing education programs. It is not necessary for candidates in either program to reside in New York State to complete the program as *most* (but not all) states consider graduates of the Regents External Degree Program eligible to take the State Board Examination. Upon written request, the External Degree Program will provide interested individuals with further information about the program. The address of the program has been listed at the end of the book.

GENERIC MASTER'S DEGREE AND DOCTORATE

A small number of colleges and universities have developed generic (basic) master's degree nursing education programs which are designed expressly for individuals who already hold a bachelor's degree in another discipline. The course of study generally ranges from 2 to 3 years in length. Graduates of these programs are eligible to take the State Board Examination for licensure as a registered nurse. Upon successful completion, graduates of the generic master's degree program are prepared to assume beginning level positions in nursing. Generic master's degree programs are quite different from the traditional master's degree programs which prepare nurses who already hold a bachelor's degree in nursing to assume specialized roles in nursing.

The most recently developed nursing education program which prepares graduates to seek a license as a registered nurse is the Doctor of Nursing program.[15] Developed by the nursing faculty at Case Western Reserve University, this program will be approximately 3 years in length. Candidates for admission must have either a baccalaureate degree in a non-nursing discipline or they must have completed at least 3 years of college. (This latter group will complete their fourth year of college during the course of the nursing program.) The program, which, as of this writing, was scheduled to admit its first class in the fall of 1979, is designed to place the graduates on the same academic level as that of physicians and other health professionals.[15,16] The Nursing Doctorate (N.D.) should not be confused with doctoral nursing programs which lead to either the Ph.D. or D.N.Sc. degree. These doctoral programs prepare candidates (who must hold a master's degree in nursing) to conduct scholarly research in nursing and to assume leadership roles in nursing education and nursing administration.

Minimum Preparation for Nursing Practice

The *four* types of nursing education programs through which individuals can become eligible to take the State Board Examination leading to licensure as a registered nurse are: the diploma, associate degree, baccalaureate, and generic master's degree programs. As of 1982, graduates of the new Doctor of Nursing program will also be eligible to take the licensure examination. Even to the uninformed observer, pure logic suggests that such widely diverse educational programs *cannot possibly* produce the same type of practitioner.

Although there has always been a nucleus of nurses who support collegiate nursing education, recommendations to move nursing into higher education generally went unheeded until 1965 when the American Nurses' Association issued its "First Position on Education for Nursing,"[10] commonly referred to as "The ANA Position Paper." This paper explored significant factors in education, society, and health care which influenced both the education of nurses and the practice of nursing. It recommended that (1) education for *all* licensed to practice professional nursing should take place within the system of higher education;[10] (2) minimum education preparation for *professional nursing should be a baccalaureate degree in nursing*; and (3) minimum preparation for technical nursing practice should be an *associate degree in nursing*.

As one might expect, the "Position Paper" touched off heated debate among nurses who were prepared in the various educational programs. However, it also provided the impetus for the closing of numerous diploma schools; each year, the number of diploma schools continues to dwindle. Concomitantly, the "Position Paper" facilitated growth of both baccalaureate and associate degree programs.

Unfortunately, the "Position Paper" did not go as far as to recommend that nurses who practice on different levels should *also* be licensed accordingly (i.e., there should be different state board examinations). Although the terms "professional" and "technical" generate endless disputes, most nurses are beginning to recognize that lack of definitive licensure, according to the type or level of practice, will continue to generate difficulty for nurses, consumers, other health professionals and employers.

Various individuals and nursing groups now strongly advocate licensure of the nurse who holds a minimum of a baccalaureate degree in nursing as a registered professional nurse and licensing of individuals who hold a diploma or associate degree under a different category. (Terminology for this category is uncertain at the present time.) At the 1978 Biennial Convention of the American Nurses' Association, the House of Delegates resolved that the baccalaureate degree should be the minimum preparation for entry into professional nursing practice by 1985. Also, the delegates resolved that national guidelines for implementing the two categories be developed for presentation to the 1980 House. The concept of "grandfathering" was also endorsed by the group. Therefore, diploma and associate degree program graduates who are licensed to practice as registered professional nurses prior to 1985 will not be affected.[17]

STANDARDS OF NURSING PRACTICE

Accountability, authority, and autonomy are interdependent qualities which are essential to professional nursing practice (see Fig. 15-1). Although these concepts may seem abstract, they are qualities which influence every aspect of the registered nurse's practice. In fact, accountability, authority, and autonomy are no less important to nursing practice than are the visible components, such as technical and interpersonal skills.

Accountability

Accountability may be defined as the quality of professional practice which holds the professional person answerable for the extent to which actions taken were consistent with his responsibility.[18] Accountability carries with it the *responsibility* to perform the activity for which one is held accountable.[18] The source of professional nursing accountability is the registered nurse's license to practice. Not only does the license *permit* the practice of nursing within the given state, it also allows the nurse to use the designation, R.N.

Licensure signifies that the nurse is qualified to practice the profession, and it also establishes direct accountability *to the consumer*. The nurse is, therefore, responsible for the *outcome* of all actions and decisions carried out in relation to the care of the client. To be accountable to the client, the nurse must always assign the highest priority to the client's safety and well-being. The registered nurse's accountability to the client is evaluated by

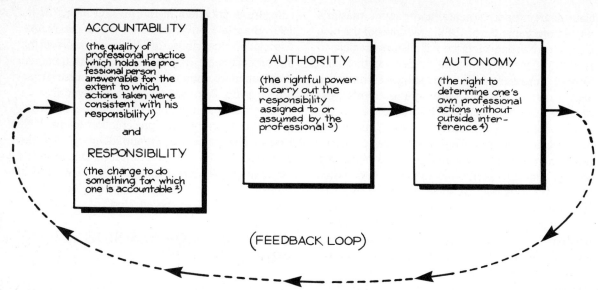

FIGURE 15-1. Accountability, authority, and autonomy are interdependent qualities which are essential to professional nursing practice. [1]Adapted from Peplau, H.: Responsibility, authority, evaluation, and accountability of nursing inpatient care. *Mich. Nurse* 44:5–8 and 20–23, 1971. [2]Ibid., p. 7. [3]Adapted from Passos, J. Y.: Accountability: myth or mandate? *J. Nurs. Admin.* 3:19–22, 1973. [4]Adapted from Maas, M., Specht, J., and Jacox, A.: Nurse autonomy: reality not rhetoric. *Am. J. Nurs.* 75:2201, 1975.

examining the nurse's *actual performance* in relation to the expected performance.

Quality assurance is a term used to denote structure and process involved in assuring that the client receives the type of care which is most advantageous to his recovery, health, and well-being. Quality assurance programs are used to determine whether an individual nurse, or a group of nurses, actually meets the expected standard of practice. In other words, quality assurance programs evaluate whether nurses demonstrate accountability in practice. Quality assurance involves: (1) evaluating the excellence of results derived from care rendered; and (2) taking action to make improvements that are likely to effect a higher quality of care in the future.[19] Because extensive discussion of quality assurance is not within the scope of this chapter, only selected methods of evaluating quality of care will be discussed here. The student will find additional references on quality assurance in the bibliography.

Standards are definitive criteria against which a nurse's performance can be compared. The American Nurses' Association's *Standards of Nursing Practice* are frequently used to evaluate nurses'

performance. The standards, which are listed below, are correlated to specific criteria which can be used for evaluation.

Standard I: The collection of data about the health status of the client/patient is systematic and continuous. The data are accessible, communicated, and recorded.

Standard II: Nursing diagnoses are derived from the health status data.

Standard III: The plan of nursing care includes goals derived from the nursing diagnoses.

Standard IV: The plan of nursing care includes priorities and the prescribed nursing approaches or measures to achieve the goals derived from the nursing diagnoses.

Standard V: Nursing actions provide for client/patient participation in health promotion, maintenance and restoration.

Standard VI: Nursing actions assist the client/patient to maximize his health capabilities.

Standard VII: The client's/patient's progress or lack of progress toward goal achievement is determined by the client/patient and the nurse.

Standard VIII: The client's/patient's progress or lack

of progress toward goal achievement directs reassessment, reordering of priorities, new goal setting, and revision of the plan of nursing care.[6]*

In addition to the generic *Standards of Nursing Practice* listed here, there are Standards of Practice for Medical-Surgical, Maternal-Child, Geriatric, Psychiatric, and Community Health Nursing. Each practicing nurse should be thoroughly familiar with these *Standards of Practice*, copies of which may be obtained from the American Nurses' Association for a nominal fee.

Peer review is a mechanism whereby a professional submits evidence of his practice to his peers for purposes of evaluation. Peer review is gradually replacing the older, more structural tools used by head nurses and supervisors to evaluate clinical performance of staff nurses. In a peer review evaluation, evidence of professional practice may consist of written care plans, client evaluations of the nurse's performance, evaluation completed by professional coworkers and evidence of continuing education.

Nursing audit is a system which evaluates whether the desirable level of client health or recovery was secured by the nurse's goal-directed activities. To conduct a nursing audit, the nursing staff of an agency develops the expected client outcome condition/behavior for a given problem and then reviews client records to determine whether the outcome was achieved. For example, if the expected client behavior for a newly diagnosed diabetic is: "client can state the signs and symptoms of insulin shock," records of newly diagnosed diabetics would be reviewed for documented evidence that the client achieved the desired outcome. An alternative audit method consists of evaluating the nurse *at the time care is being given*.

Authority

Authority may be defined as the rightful *power* to carry out the responsibility *assigned to* or assumed by the professional.[20] Authority—that is, the *power* to act—allows the nurse to establish a direct rela-

tionship with the client to render highly specialized care through use of the nursing process. Authority, then, is a necessary condition for the achievement of nurse-client accountability (see Fig. 15-1). There are two main sources of the nurse's authority in professional practice. The first of these is the definition of professional nursing in the state's Nurse Practice Act. In each state there is a statutory law called the Nurse Practice Act. Each Nurse Practice Act contains a definition which delineates the boundaries of the nurse's practice. The second source of authority is the specialized knowledge, skill, and judgment which is necessary in order to qualify for licensure. The nurse must engage in continuing education to maintain the knowledge and skill necessary to exercise professional authority.

Autonomy

The accountability established between the nurse and client and the authority to carry out care enable the nurse to initiate and implement the nursing process *autonomously*. Both accountability and authority are therefore necessary prerequisites to autonomy (see Fig. 15-1). Autonomy in professional nursing practice may be defined as the right to determine one's own acts without outside interference.[21]

The autonomy of the professional nurse arises from three main sources. The first is the specialized knowledge required to practice the profession. The second is the "service ideal" possessed by members of the profession—that is, the primary goal of the profession is to provide a specialized service which is necessary and valuable to the well-being of the consumer. The third source of autonomy in nursing practice actually comes from the consumers *served* by the profession. Consumers grant a profession autonomy on the basis of a *trust* that the practitioners of the profession place concern for the well-being of the client above *self* concern. The consumer also grants a profession autonomy when there is sufficient evidence that the members of the profession possess a special knowledge and skill. However, the *regulation* of practice also comes from the consumer through the Nurse Practice Act; hence, the consumer requires the registered nurse to demonstrate accountability. It is, therefore, not possible to separate accountability, authority, and autonomy (see Fig. 15-1).

---

*Reprinted with permission from American Nurses' Association: *Standards of Nursing Practice.* Kansas City, Mo., The American Nurses' Association, 1973.

It is important for the nurse to recognize that the autonomy which characterizes nursing practice is related to the nurse's expertise in applying the nursing process in clinical practice. In other words, the registered nurse does not require "permission" from another discipline, such as medicine, to practice nursing, nor does the nurse require direction from another discipline to carry out the nursing process. The nurse is *the* authority on nursing care. However, it is *essential* that the nurse know the boundaries of nursing practice. The autonomy of the registered nurse does *not* permit the nurse to make a *medical* diagnosis or to institute *medical* treatment. Also, the nurse must clearly understand that autonomy in practice does *not* mean that the nurse practices in *isolation* of other professionals. Rather, the complex nature of health care delivery requires that *all* professions collaborate in providing the highest possible quality of care to clients. The

American Nurses' Association and the International Council of Nurses have developed codes of ethics (Tables 15-1 and 15-2) which provide the nurse with a framework for integrating the qualities of accountability, authority, and autonomy into nursing practice.

PROFESSIONAL NURSING ORGANIZATIONS

Membership in a professional nursing organization is a voluntary undertaking. Frequently, an individual *seeks* membership in a particular organization or group because he values the purposes, goals, and functions of that group. There are numerous professional nursing organizations. Many nurses find that membership in just one organization does not adequately satisfy their professional, intellectual, and educational needs. Hence, it is not unusual to find that many nurses hold membership in both a multipurpose organization, such as the American Nurses' Association, and in an organization related to their area of clinical practice, such as the American Association of Critical Care Nurses. Only the major nursing organizations will be discussed in this chapter. A listing of some of the clinically oriented nursing specialty organizations may be found at the end of this chapter.

The American Nurses' Association (ANA) is the one officially recognized professional organization for registered nurses. Only registered nurses and new graduates of nursing education programs which prepare individuals for registered nurse licensure are eligible to belong to the ANA. The purposes and functions of the ANA may be found in Table 15-3.

Many nurses do not readily perceive the benefits one derives from membership in the ANA because they are often intangible. It is important for ANA members and nonmembers alike to recognize that the ANA's positions on health and nursing issues largely determine the future growth and survival of the nursing profession. Because the ANA is the official professional organization, the consequences of decisions and actions taken (or *not* taken) by the ANA will *substantially* affect *every* registered nurse and the practice of nursing. A nurse's decision to join the ANA is often an expression of the individual

---

TABLE 15-1. Code for Nurses

1. The nurse provides services with respect for human dignity and the uniqueness of the client unrestricted by considerations of social or economic status, personal attributes, or the nature of health problems.
2. The nurse safeguards the client's right to privacy by judiciously protecting information of a confidential nature.
3. The nurse acts to safeguard the client and the public when health care and safety are affected by the incompetent, unethical, or illegal practice of any person.
4. The nurse assumes responsibility and accountability for individual nursing judgments and actions.
5. The nurse maintains competence in nursing.
6. The nurse exercises informed judgment and uses individual competence and qualifications as criteria in seeking consultation, accepting responsibilities, and delegating nursing activities to others.
7. The nurse participates in activities that contribute to the ongoing development of the profession's body of knowledge.
8. The nurse participates in the profession's efforts to implement and improve standards of nursing.
9. The nurse participates in the profession's efforts to establish and maintain conditions of employment conducive to high quality nursing care.
10. The nurse participates in the profession's effort to protect the public from misinformation and misrepresentation and to maintain the integrity of nursing.
11. The nurse collaborates with members of the health professions and other citizens in promoting community and national efforts to meet the health needs of the public.

Reprinted with permission from American Nurses' Association: *Code for Nurses with Interpretive Statements.* The American Nurses' Association, Kansas City, Mo., 1976, p. 3.

TABLE 15-2. 1973 Code for Nurses: Ethical Concepts Applied to Nursing

Code for Nurses

The fundamental responsibility of the nurse is fourfold: to promote health, to prevent illness, to restore health and to alleviate suffering.

The need for nursing is universal, inherent in nursing is respect for life, dignity and rights of man. It is unrestricted by considerations of nationality, race, creed, colour, age, sex, politics or social status. Nurses render health services to the individual, the family, and the community and coordinate their services with those of related groups.

Nurses and People

The nurse's primary responsibility is to those people who require nursing care.

The nurse, in providing care, respects the beliefs, values and customs of the individual.

The nurse holds in confidence personal information and uses judgment in sharing this information.

Nurses and Practice

The nurse carries personal responsibility for nursing practice and for maintaining competence by continual learning.

The nurse maintains the highest standards of nursing care possible within the reality of a specific situation.

The nurse uses judgment in relation to individual competence when accepting and delegating responsibilities.

The nurse when acting in a professional capacity should at all times maintain standards of personal conduct that would reflect credit upon the profession.

Nurses and Society

The nurse shares with other citizens the responsibility for initiating and supporting action to meet the health and social needs of the public.

Nurses and Co-Workers

The nurse sustains a cooperative relationship with co-workers in nursing and other fields.

The nurse takes appropriate action to safeguard the individual when his care is endangered by a co-worker or any other person.

Nurses and the Profession

The nurse plays the major role in determining and implementing desirable standards of nursing practice and nursing education.

The nurse is active in developing a core of professional knowledge. The nurse, acting through the professional organization, participates in establishing and maintaining equitable social and economic working conditions in nursing.

Reprinted with permission from International Council of Nurses, Geneva, Switzerland, 1973.

---

nurse's values about the profession and its role in health care delivery.

Nurses' Coalition for Action in Politics (N-CAP) is the political action arm of the ANA, officially organized in 1974 as the outgrowth of NPA (Nurses for Political Action) to promote the improvement of health care of the people by:

1. Encouraging and stimulating nurses and others to take a more active and effective part in governmental affairs.
2. Educating nurses and others to become aware of government, the important political issues, and the records of office holders and candidates.
3. Assisting nurses and others in organizing themselves for effective political action.
4. Raising funds for the aforementioned purposes, and from such funds making contributions to assist persons in political work without regard to party affiliation, who by their acts have demonstrated their interest in the health of the nation.

5. Taking any actions necessary or desirable for attainment of the purpose stated above.

Membership is open to *all* interested persons, including students.

Membership in the *National League for Nursing (NLN)* is open to anyone (nurses and non-nurses) who is interested in furthering the association's overall goal, "meeting the nursing needs of the people." The major programs of the NLN are:

I. *Nursing Education:* Through its four councils—the Council of Baccalaureate and Higher Degree Programs, Council of Associate Degree Programs, Council of Diploma Programs, and the Council of Practical Nursing Programs—the NLN fosters the development of nursing education.
A. Special Services
1. Accreditation of basic, graduate, and continuing education programs.
2. Consultation services.
3. Continuing education programs.

TABLE 15-3. Purposes and Functions of the American Nurses' Association

I. Purposes of the ANA. (These purposes shall be unrestricted by considerations of nationality, race, creed, life style, color, sex, or age.)

A. Work for the improvement of health standards and the availability of health care services for all people.

B. Foster high standards of nursing.

C. Stimulate and promote the professional development of nurses and advance their economic and general welfare.

II. Functions of the ANA.

A. Establish and enunciate standards of nursing practice, nursing education and nursing service and to implement them through appropriate channels.

B. Establish a code of ethical conduct for nurses.

C. Stimulate and promote research in nursing, disseminate research findings and encourage the utilization of new knowledge as a basis for nursing.

D. Provide for continuing education for nurses.

E. Promote and protect the economic and general welfare of nurses.

F. Assume an active role as consumer advocate in health.

G. Analyze, predict and influence new dimensions of health practices and the delivery of health care.

H. Act and speak for the nursing profession in regard to legislation, governmental programs and national health policy.

I. Represent and speak for the nursing profession with allied health, national and international organizations, governmental bodies and the public.

J. Serve as the official representative of the United States nurses as a member of the International Council of Nurses.

K. Promote relationships and collaboration with the National Student Nurses' Association.

L. Ensure a national archive for the collection and preservation of documents and other materials which have contributed and continue to contribute to the historical and cultural development of nursing.

Adapted with permission from the American Nurses' Association: *By-Laws* (As Amended, June 1976). American Nurses' Association, Kansas City, Mo., 1976, pp. 5–6.

4. The Division of Measurement offers Achievement Tests in Nursing, a nursing pre-admission test. The Division is also the test service agency for the State Board Test Pool Examinations for R.N. and P.N. licensure.

5. Research on educational trends and practices.

II. *Nursing Service*

A. Council of Hospital and Related Institutional Nursing Services.

B. Council of Home Health Agencies and Community Health Services.

III. *Community Planning for Nursing Care:* Through its 44 constituent leagues, NLN participates in local and state health programs.

IV. *American Lung Association Department at NLN:* A joint venture between the two organizations for the purposes of promoting the practice and education of nurses involved in the care of patients with actual or potential respiratory problems.

V. *Publications:* Directories of accredited basic and graduate nursing education programs and practical nursing programs.

VI. *Interorganization Committees:* With ANA, AMA, American Dietetic Association and others.

Membership in the *National Student Nurses' Association (NSNA)* is open to all students in diploma, associate degree, baccalaureate and generic master's degree programs. The NSNA is sponsored by the ANA and the NLN. Therefore, its goals are similar to those of the parent organizations. Membership in the NSNA affords nursing students with an excellent opportunity to participate in making important decisions which affect the nursing profession. Chapters are organized on state and local levels. *Imprint* is the official publication of NSNA.

Sigma Theta Tau, the National Honor Society of Nursing, was founded in 1922 by six students at the Indiana University Training School for Nurses. Membership is extended, by invitation, to individuals who have earned a minimum of a bachelor's degree in nursing and to selected students enrolled in baccalaureate or higher degree programs. The purposes of Sigma Theta Tau are to:

1. Recognize the achievement of scholarship of superior quality.
2. Recognize the development of leadership qualities.
3. Foster high professional standards.

4. Encourage creative work.
5. Strengthen commitment on the part of individuals to the ideals and purposes of the profession of nursing.

Nursing Literature

Nursing students should become familiar with the nursing literature resources early in their career. Students who make a habit of reading the current professional literature will be rewarded by the acquisition of knowledge which may be applied in clinical practice, nursing science course work, and in writing research papers. Every practicing nurse has a responsibility to keep abreast of the current literature. Reading current nursing journals is one of the most effective means of keeping one's practice up to date. Reading nursing journals is also important to the registered nurse because the current nursing literature is the primary medium through which members of a profession communicate with one another. A list of the most frequently used nursing journals appears in Table 15.4.

TABLE 15-4. Major Nursing Journals

A. Journals which focus on the profession in general:
1. *American Journal of Nursing*—the professional journal of the American Nurses' Association.
2. *Nursing Outlook*
3. *Nursing Research*—the primary journal of nurse researchers.
4. *Nursing '79*—(previous years: *Nursing '78, Nursing '77*).
5. *Nursing Forum*.
6. *Nursing Clinics of North America*—quarterly.
7. *Image*—official publication of Sigma Theta Tau, National Honor Society of Nursing.
8. *Imprint*—official publication of the National Student Nurses' Association.
9. *Canadian Nurse*
10. *R.N.*

B. Journals which focus on selected aspects of nursing practice:
1. *American Journal of Maternal Child Nursing*—bimonthly.
2. *American Journal of Public Health*—published by the American Public Health Association.
3. *AAORN Journal*—published by the American Association of Operating Room Nurses.
4. *Bulletin of the American Academy of Nurse Midwives*.
5. *Issues in Comprehensive Pediatric Nursing*—Bimonthly.
6. *Issues in Health Care of Women*—Bimonthly.
7. *Issues in Mental Health Nursing*—Quarterly.
8. *Journal of Continuing Education in Nursing*.
9. *Journal of Nursing Administration*.
10. *Journal of Nursing Education*.
11. *Journal of Obstetric and Gynecological Nursing (JOGN)*—published by the Nurses' Association of the American College of Obstetricians and Gynecologists.
12. *Journal of Psychiatric Nursing and Mental Health Services*.
13. *Maternal Child Nursing Journal*—published quarterly by the Graduate Faculties of the Departments of Obstetrical and Pediatric Nursing, University of Pittsburgh.
14. *Nurse Educator*.
15. *Perspectives in Psychiatric Care*.
16. *Supervisor Nurse*.

REFERENCES

1. Marram, G.: *Cost-Effectiveness of Primary and Team Nursing*. Wakefield, Mass., Contemporary Publishing, Inc., 1976.
2. Rogers, M. E.: Nursing: to be or not to be? *Nurs. Outlook* 20:42−45, 1972.
3. Aiken, L. H.: Primary care: the challenge to nursing. *Am. J. Nurs.* 77:1830, 1977.
4. Walke, M. A. K.: When a patient needs to unburden his feelings. *Am. J. Nurs.* 77:1164−1166, 1977.
5. Benoliel, J. Q.: The interaction between theory and research. *Nurs. Outlook* 25:112, 1977.
6. American Nurses' Association: *Standards of Nursing Practice*. Kansas City, Mo., The American Nurses' Association, 1973.
7. Kelly, L. Y.: *Dimensions of Professional Nursing*, 3rd ed. New York, Macmillan Publishing Co., Inc., 1975, p. 34.
8. Rogers, M. E.: *An Introduction to the Theoretical Basis of Nursing*. Philadelphia, F. A. Davis Co., 1970, p. xi.
9. Kalish, P. A., and Kalish, B. J.: *The Advance of American Nursing*. Boston, Little, Brown and Co., Inc., 1978, p. 508.
10. American Nurses' Association: First position on education for nursing. *Am. J. Nurs.* 65:106−111, 1965.
11. Johnson, W. L.: Educational preparation for nursing, *Nurs. Outlook* 25:589, 1977.
12. Flexner, A.: *Medical Education in the United States and Canada*. New York, Carnegie Foundation, 1910.
13. Goldmark, J., et al.: *Nursing and Nursing Education in the United States*. New York, Macmillan Publishing Co., 1923.
14. Montag, M.: *The Education of Nursing Technicians*. New York, G. P. Putnam's Sons, 1951.
15. Schlodtfeldt, R. M.: The professional doctorate: rationale and characteristics. *Nurs. Outlook* 26:302, 1978.
16. Case Western Reserve doctoral program for nurses. *Chronicle of Higher Education*, June 26, 1978, p. 15.

17. American Nurses' Association Convention '78. *Am. J. Nurs.* 78:1232, 1978.
18. Peplau, H.: Responsibility, authority, evaluation and accountability of nursing in patient care. *Mich. Nurse* 44:5–8 and 20–23, 1971.
19. Zimmer, M. J.: Quality assurance for outcomes of patient care. *Nurs. Clin. North Am.* 9(2):307, 1974.
20. Passos, J.: Accountability: myth or mandate? *J. Nurs. Admin.* 3:19–22, 1973.
21. Maas, M., Specht, J., and Jacox, A.: Nurse autonomy: reality not rhetoric. *Am. J. Nurs.* 75:2201, 1975.

BIBLIOGRAPHY

Perspectives on the Registered Nurse and the Nursing Profession

Books

American Nurses' Association: *Facts About Nursing, '76–77.* Kansas City, Mo., American Nurses' Association, 1977.
Chaska, N. (ed.): *The Nursing Profession: Views through the Mist.* New York, McGraw-Hill Book Co., 1978.
Fundamental Issues in Nursing, edited by the Staff of the *Journal of Nursing Administration,* Wakefield, Mass., Contemporary Publishing Co., 1975.
Grissum, M., and Spengler, C.: *Woman Power and Health Care.* Boston, Little, Brown and Co., 1977.
Kelly, L. Y.: *Dimensions of Professional Nursing,* 3rd ed. New York, Macmillan Publishing Co., 1975.

Articles

Ashley, J.: This I believe: about power in nursing. *Nurs. Outlook* 21:637, 1973.
Beletz, E. E.: Is nursing's public image up to date? *Nurs. Outlook* 22:432, 1974.
Cleland, V. S.: To end sex discrimination. *Nurs. Clin. North Am.* 9:563, 1974.
Diers, D.: A different kind of energy: nurse power. *Nurs. Outlook* 26:51, 1978.
Elmore, J. A.: Black nurses: their service and their struggle. *Am. J. Nurs.* 76:435, 1976.
Hassenplug, I. W.: Nursing *can* move from here to there. *Nurs. Outlook* 25:432, 1977.
Hiede, W. S.: Nursing and women's liberation—a parallel. *Am. J. Nurs.* 73:824, 1973.
Jacox, A.: Address to the next generation. *Nurs. Outlook* 26:38, 1978.
Kalisch, B. J.: The promise of power. *Nurs. Outlook* 26:42, 1978.
Kelly, L. Y.: Our nursing heritage: have we renounced it? *Image* 8:43, 1976.
Kritek, P., and Glass, L.: Nursing: a feminist perspective. *Nurs. Outlook* 26:182, 1978.

Mayo, R. P.: A nurse can be a man or a woman. *Am. J. Nurs.* 76:1318, 1976.
Mullane, M. K.: Nursing care and the political arena. *Nurs. Outlook* 23:699, 1975.
Nurses and nursing issues: a round table discussion. *Am. J. Nurs.* 75:1848, 1975.
Partridge, K. B.: Nursing values in a changing society. *Nurs. Outlook* 26:356, 1978.
Schlotfeldt, R. M.: Nursing is health care. *Nurs. Outlook* 20:245, 1972.
Sheahan, D.: Scanning the seventies. *Nurs. Outlook* 26:33, 1978.
Stanton, M.: Political action and nursing. *Nurs. Clin. North Am.* 9:579, 1974.
Styles, M. M.: Dialogue across the decades. *Nurs. Outlook* 26:28, 1978.
Winstead-Fry, P.: The need to differentiate a nursing self. *Am. J. Nurs.* 77:1452, 1977.

The Registered Nurse and Patient Advocacy

American Hospital Association: Patient's bill of rights (1972). *Nurs. Outlook* 24:29, 1976.
Bandman, E., and Bandman, B.: There is nothing automatic about rights. *Am. J. Nurs.* 77:867, 1977.
Fay, P.: In support of patient advocacy as a nursing role. *Nurs. Outlook* 26:252, 1978.
Kelly, L. Y.: The patient's right to know. *Nurs. Outlook* 24:26, 1976.
Nelson, L. J.: The nurse as an advocate: for whom? *Am. J. Nurs.* 77:851, 1977.
Ohio Nurses' Association: The patient's rights to nursing care. *Am. J. Nurs.* 75:1112, 1975.

Accountability, Authority and Autonomy in Nursing Practice

American Nurses' Association: *Code for Nurses with Interpretive Statements.* Kansas City, Mo., American Nurses' Association, 1976.
American Nurses' Association: *Perspectives on the Code for Nurses.* Kansas City, Mo., American Nurses' Association, 1978.
Bandman, B.: Do nurses have rights? . . . no! *Am. J. Nurs.* 78:84, 1978.
Bandman, E.: Do nurses have rights? . . . yes! *Am. J. Nurs.* 78:84, 1978.
Christman, L.: Accountability and autonomy are more than rhetoric. *Nurse Educ.* 3(4):3, 1978.
Driscoll, V.: Liberating nursing practice. *Nurs. Outlook* 20:24, 1972.
Fagin, C. M.: Nurses' rights. *Am. J. Nurs.* 75:82, 1975.
Guy, J. S.: Institutional licensure: a dilemma for nurses. *Nurs. Clin. North Am.* 9:497, 1974.
Kellams, S. E.: Ideals of a profession: the case of nursing. *Image* 9:30, 1977.
Kelly, L. Y.: Credentialing of health care personnel. *Nurs. Outlook* 25:562, 1977.

Kelly, L. Y.: Nursing practice acts. *Am. J. Nurs.* 74:1310, 1974.

Lewis, E. P.: The right to inform (editorial). *Nurs. Outlook* 25:561, 1977.

Maas, M., Specht, J., and Jacox, A.: Nurse autonomy: reality not rhetoric. *Am. J. Nurs.* 75:2201, 1975.

McClure, M.: The long road to accountability. *Nurs. Outlook* 26:47, 1978.

Nurses attaining stronger professional identity (editorial). *Am. Nurse* 8(10):4, 1976.

Ozimek, D., and Yura, H.: *Students Have Responsibilities as Well as Rights.* New York, National League for Nursing, 1977. (NLN Pub. No. 15-1666)

Quality Assurance

Books

American Nurses' Association: *A Plan for Implementation of the Standards of Nursing Practice.* Kansas City, Mo., American Nurses' Association, 1975.

American Nurses' Association: *Guidelines for Review of Nursing Care at the Local Level.* Kansas City, Mo., American Nurses' Association, 1976.

American Nurses' Association: *Standards of Community Health Nursing Practice.* Kansas City, Mo., American Nurses' Association, 1973.

American Nurses' Association: *Standards of Geriatric Nursing Practice.* Kansas City, Mo., American Nurses' Association, 1973.

American Nurses' Association: *Standards of Maternal and Child Health Nursing Practice.* Kansas City, Mo., American Nurses' Association, 1973.

American Nurses' Association: *Standards of Medical-Surgical Nursing Practice.* Kansas City, Mo., American Nurses' Association, 1974.

American Nurses' Association: *Standards of Psychiatric and Mental Health Nursing Practice.* Kansas City, Mo., American Nurses' Association, 1973.

American Nurses' Association: *Standards of Rehabilitation Nursing Practice.* Kansas City, Mo., American Nurses' Association, 1978.

American Nurses' Association: *Quality Assurance Workbook.* Kansas City, Mo., American Nurses' Association, 1976.

Mayers, M., Norby, R. B., and Watson, A. B.: *Quality Assurance for Patient Care: Nursing Perspectives.* New York, Appleton-Century-Crofts, 1977.

Phaneuf, M. C.: *The Nursing Audit: Profile for Excellence.* New York, Appleton-Century-Crofts, 1972.

Articles

Hauser, M. A.: Initiation into peer review. *Am. J. Nurs.* 75:2204, 1975.

Hover, J., and Zimmer, M.: Nursing quality assurance system. *Nurs. Outlook* 26:242, 1978.

Lamberton, M., Keen, M., and Adomanis, A.: Peer re-

view in a family nurse clinician program. *Nurs. Outlook* 25:47, 1977.

Lang, N. M.: Quality assurance review in nursing. *MCN: Am. J. Mat. Child Nurs.* 1:75, 1976.

Ramphal, M.: Peer review. *Am. J. Nurs.* 74:63, 1974.

Zimmer, M. J. (ed.): Symposium on quality assurance. *Nurs. Clin. North Am.* 9:303, 1974.

Creativity and Change in Nursing

Gortner, S. R.: Strategies for survival in the practice world. *Am. J. Nurs.* 77:618, 1977.

Gunderson, K., et al.: How to control professional frustration. *Am. J. Nurs.* 77:1180, 1977.

Harty, M. B.: Goal-oriented creativity. *Image* 5(3):7, 1973.

Klug, C. A.: Judgment and creative thinking. *Image* 5(3):10, 1973.

Levine, M. E.: On creativity in nursing. *Image* 5(3):15, 1973.

McGriff, E. P.: The courage for effective leadership in nursing. *Image* 8:56, 1976.

Mullaly, L. M., and Kervin, M. C.: Changing the status quo. *MCN: Am. J. Mat. Child Nurs.* 3:75, 1978.

Peplau, H. E.: Creativity and commitment in nursing. *Image* 6(3):13, 1974.

Primary Nursing

Dahlen, A. L.: With primary nursing we have it all together. *Am. J. Nurs.* 78:426, 1978.

Hegyvary, S. T.: Symposium on primary nursing. *Nurs. Clin. North Am.* 12:185, 1977.

Lewis, E. P.: Everybody's patient is nobody's patient (editorial). *Nurs. Outlook* 23:551, 1975.

Marram, G. D., and Schlegel, M. W.: *Primary Nursing.* St. Louis, Mo., C. V. Mosby Co., 1974.

Marram, C. D., et al.: *Cost-Effectiveness of Primary and Team Nursing.* Wakefield, Mass., Contemporary Publishing Co., 1976.

Team Nursing

Douglass, L. M.: *Review of Team Nursing.* St. Louis, Mo., C. V. Mosby Co., 1973.

Kron, T.: *The Management of Patient Care*, 4th, ed. Philadelphia, W. B. Saunders Co., 1976.

Lamberton, E.: *Nursing Team Organization and Functioning.* New York, Bureau of Publications, Teachers' College, Columbia University, 1953.

Primary Health Care: The "Nurse Practitioner," and Changing Nurses' Roles

Aiken, L. H.: Primary care: the challenge for nursing. *Am. J. Nurs.* 77:1828, 1977.

American Nurses' Association: Nurses in the extended

role are not physician's assistants. Kansas City, Mo., American Nurses' Association, July 1973. (Mimeographed)

Anderson, M. De C.: Our expanding role: notes on not nursing. *Nurs. '77* 7:16, 1977.

Bullough, B.: Influences on role expansion. *Am. J. Nurs.* 76:1476, 1976.

Levine, E.: What do we know about nurse practitioners? *Am. J. Nurs.* 77:1799, 1977.

Mauksch, I. G., and Rogers, M. E.: Nursing is coming of age through the practitioner movement: pro (I. Mauksch) and con (M. E. Rogers). *Am. J. Nurs.* 75:1834, 1975.

Nursing at the crossroads (symposium on "expanded" roles). *Nurs. Outlook* 20(1):21, 1972.

Schorr, T. M.: Is that name necessary? (editorial) *Am. J. Nurs.* 74:235, 1974.

The nurse practitioner question. *Am. J. Nurs.* 74:2188, 1974.

The nurse practitioner: research and evaluation (entire issue). *Nurs. Outlook* 23(10):622, 1975.

Nursing Education and Entry into Practice

American Nurses' Association: First position on education for nursing. *Am. J. Nurs.* 65:106, 1965.

Fagin, C., McClure, M., and Schlotfeldt, R. M.: Can we bring order out of the chaos of nursing education? *Am. J. Nurs.* 76:98, 1976.

Graduate education in nursing (entire issue). *Nurs. Outlook* 23(10):622, 1975.

Leininger, M.: Doctoral programs for nurses: trends, questions, and projected plans. *Nurs. Res.* 25:201, 1976.

Lenburg, C. B.: The external degree in nursing: the promise fulfilled. *Nurs. Outlook* 24:422, 1976.

Lewis, E. P.: One nurse or two (editorial)? *Nurs. Outlook* 26:237, 1978.

McGriff, E. P., and Simms, L. L.: Two New York nurses debate the NYSNA 1985 proposal. *Am. J. Nurs.* 76:930, 1976.

National League for Nursing: Competencies of the associate degree nurse on entry into practice. *Nurs. Outlook* 26:457, 1978.

Rines, A. R.: Associate degree education: history, development and rationale. *Nurs. Outlook* 25:496, 1977.

Sorensen, G.: In support of the generic baccalaureate degree program. *Nurs. Outlook* 24:384, 1976.

Continuing Education in Nursing

Cooper, S.: Continuing education: yesterday and tomorrow. *Nurse Educator* 3(1):25, 1978.

Cooper, S.: Continuing education: how? *MCN: Am. J. Mat. Child Nurs.* 3:242, 1978.

Dake, M. A.: CEU: a means to an end? *Am. J. Nurs.* 74:103, 1974.

O'Connor, A. B.: Diagnosing your needs for continuing education. *Am. J. Nurs.* 78:465, 1978.

Whitaker, J. S.: The issue of mandatory continuing education. *Nurs. Clin. North Am.* 9:475, 1974.

Nursing Research and the Practicing Nurse

Benoliel, J. Q.: The interaction between theory and research. *Nurs. Outlook* 25:108, 1977.

Jacox, A.: Nursing research and the clinician. *Nurs. Outlook* 22:382, 1974.

Kalisch, B.: Creativity and nursing research. *Nurs. Outlook* 23:314, 1975.

Lindemann, C. A.: Priorities in clinical research. *Nurs. Outlook* 23:693, 1975.

Notter, L.: The case for nursing research. *Nurs. Outlook* 23:760, 1975.

Smoyak, S. A.: Is practice responding to research? *Am. J. Nurs.* 76:1146, 1976.

Historical Perspectives on the Nursing Profession

Books

Ashley, J.: *Hospitals, Paternalism, and the Role of the Nurse.* New York, Teachers' College, Columbia University, 1976.

Ehrenreich, B., and English, D.: *Witches, Midwives, and Nurses: A History of Women Healers.* Oyster Bay, N.Y., Glass Mountain Pamphlets, 1972.

Kalisch, P. A. and Kalisch, B. J.: *The Advance of American Nursing.* Boston, Little, Brown and Co., 1978.

Articles

Ashley, J.: Nursing and early feminism. *Am. J. Nurs.* 75:1465, 1975.

Austin, A. L.: Nurses in American history: wartime volunteers—1861–1865. *Am. J. Nurs.* 75:816, 1975.

Bullough, B.: Lasting impact of World War II on nursing. *Am. J. Nurs.* 76:118, 1976.

Dolan, J.: Nurses in American history: three schools—1873. *Am. J. Nurs.* 75:989, 1975.

Rawnsley, M. M.: The Goldmark report: midpoint in nursing history. *Nurs. Outlook* 21:380, 1973.

Selaven, I. C.: Nurses in American history: the Revolution. *Am. J. Nurs.* 75:592, 1975.

Smith, G. R.: From invisibility to blackness: the story of the National Black Nurses' Association. *Nurs. Outlook* 23:225, 1975.

Professional Nursing Organizations

ANA convention '78: Tomorrow's health/today's challenge. Proceedings of the biennial convention of the American Nurses' Association, Honolulu, Hawaii, 1978. *Am. J. Nurs.* 78:1231, 1978.

ICN '77: Proceedings of the quadrennial Congress of the

International Council of Nurses, Tokyo, Japan, 1977. *Am. J. Nurs.* 77:1303, 1977.

Minor, I., and Shaw, E.: ANA and affirmative action. *Am. J. Nurs.* 73:1738, 1973.

NLN convention report, 1977: Proceedings of the biennial convention of the National League for Nursing, Anaheim, California, 1977. *Nurs. Outlook* 25:378, 1977.

NSNA today (National Student Nurses' Association). *Am. J. Nurs.* 77:624, 1977.

Zimmerman, A.: ANA: its record on social issues. *Am. J. Nurs.* 76:588, 1976.

APPENDIX: SELECTED NURSING ORGANIZATIONS AND GROUPS

American Association of Critical Care Nurses
P.O. Box C-19528
Irvine, Calif.

American Association of Industrial Nurses
79 Madison Ave.
New York, N.Y.   10016

American Association of Nurse Anesthetists
Suite 929
111 East Wacker Drive
Chicago, Ill.   60601

American College of Nurse Midwives
Suite 500
1000 Vermont Ave., N.W.
Washington, D.C.   20005

American Indian Nurses' Association (AINA)
Suite 502
2241 W. Lindsey
Norman, Okla.   73069

American Nurses' Association (ANA)
2420 Pershing Road
Kansas City, Mo.   64108

ANA Washington Office
1030 15th Street, N.W.
Washington, D.C.   20005

Association of Operating Room Nurses
10170 East Mississippi Ave.
Denver, Colo.   80231

Association of Pediatric Oncology Nurses
c/o Lorraine Bivalec
Children's Oncology Program
Children's Hospital of Stanford

520 Willow Road
Palo Alto, Calif.   94304

Association of Rehabilitation Nurses
1132 Waukegen Road
Glenview, Ill.   60025

Emergency Department Nurses' Association
P.O. Box 1566
East Lansing, Mich.   48823

International Council of Nurses
Box 42
1211 Geneva 20
Switzerland

National Association of Spanish-speaking and Spanish-surnamed Nurses
300 West 108th Street
New York, N.Y.   10025

National Black Nurses' Association (NBNA)
P.O. Box 8295
Canton, Ohio   44711

National League for Nursing (NLN)
10 Columbus Circle
New York, N.Y.   10019

National Student Nurses' Association (NSNA)
10 Columbus Circle
New York, N.Y.   10019

Nurses' Association of the American College of Obstetricians and Gynecologists
Suite 2700
1 East Wacker Drive
Chicago, Ill.   60601

Nurses Coalition for Action in Politics (N-CAP)
Suite 408
1030 15th Street, N.W.
Washington, D.C.   20005

Orthopedic Nurses' Association
Suite 501
1938 Peachtree Road, N.W.
Atlanta, Ga.   30309

Sigma Theta Tau—National Honor Society of Nursing
P.O. Box 1445
Indianapolis, Ind.   46206

New York Regents External Degree Program
Cultural Education Center
Albany, N.Y.   12230

CHAPTER 16

Look at me. Please see me
Not my hospital gown
Or my white uniform.
Open your heart, so you can see mine.
I do not ask you to agree with
Or understand all you see
For I don't even do that.
Just look at what is really me
And allow it to be.[1]*

The above verse captures the essence of the invitation inherent in a dialogical encounter to exercise the most basic human right—the right to creatively define self within a shared relationship. This invitation emanates from both client and nurse and is addressed to each "other" in their respective roles. It is an invitation characterized by spirited encouragement to take the rough clay of the moment's experience and to toss it back and forth in a series

---

*Based on the poem, "Look at Me, Please See Me," in reference 1.

THE NURSE AS A HUMANISTIC ARTIST

Patricia Chehy Pilette, Ed.D., M.S., R.N.

of dialogical exchanges until it has formed into a definition of each participant—a definition created from the boundaries stretched by deliberate choices of the individuals.

Anyone who participates in genuine dialogue participates in a process of discovery and creation of self, experiencing the meaning of the existential phrase "to be." The setting in which this self-realization may be experienced is the nurse-client encounter. The nurse-client relationship is the cornerstone of the art of humanistic nursing. The dialogical encounter is the creative arena within the nurse-client relationship, wherein the humanistic challenge to find the "real" self can be accepted. To the extent that the nurse professes and practices this nursing art form, she is a humanistic artist drawing upon her own humanness in order to humanize more effectively her nursing interactions. To the degree that she lacks this art form in her practice, she is merely another technician, for it is through the interaction characteristic of the dialogical encounter that the nurse's fundamental observational

capabilities and ultimately her critical reflective skills are realized.

The concept of the nurse as a humanistic artist, the major concern of this chapter, is viewed from the perspective of existential philosophy. In assuming such a perspective, an effort is made to distinguish the differences among the crucial elements of the nurse's artistry (i.e., art per se, dialogue, and the interrelationship of the two concepts). Through conceptual analysis of these elements, the meaning of the phrase, "The nurse as a humanistic artist," will hopefully be made clear to the reader.

EVOLUTION OF THE ART OF NURSING

The well-worn aphorism, "Nursing is an art and a science," has a long history in nursing literature, but the art of nursing predates the science of nursing. Art, our most basic birthright, can be traced to the biblical character Phoebe and her charitable manner of ministering to the Romans. This early intuitive art meant no more or less than comforting and caring for another human being.

As nursing struggled toward its professional identity, it more clearly defined the skills and techniques it possessed. Consequently, the art of nursing became more restricted, designating the skillful manner in which nursing techniques were performed. Technical competence and speed were crucial components of a "skillful manner."

A further evolution of art's definition occurred in the early 1900s, during the Scientific Revolution, when the first attempts were made to wed the art of nursing with an embryonic science of nursing. The effect of such efforts resulted unfortunately in a tug of war over the primacy of art and science in nursing, instead of the hoped for partnership. Within nursing, as well as outside the profession, fears of scientific dominance were expressed, followed by pleas to maintain the primal importance of art: "For, important as is the underlying science, the art must always predominate."[2] Such warnings failed, and the much-feared de-emphasis of art became a reality. Over the past 60 years, the professional pendulum has gradually swung toward the scientific domain. This has led to refinement of the definition of art; now nursing skills are performed "in accordance with scientific principles."

Today's nursing demands further expansion of the old definition of art. It requires an art that is as sophisticated and effective as the science it meets and weds. In this humanistic era, it is fitting that nursing has reclaimed and updated its birthright. The art of the nurse today lies in the creative management of the human dimension of the nursing role, which is realized in interrelationships with others. The art of nursing has its deepest roots in the human care transaction and is confirmed in the dialogical process or "I-Thou" relationship (Fig. 16-1).[3]

DIALOGICAL ENCOUNTER

The "I-Thou" relationship describes an intense interaction between the self (the "I") and another human being (the "Thou" or "Other"). It is a "meeting" of two human beings who, while recognizing their differences, can still enter into an accepting and subsequently growth-promoting encounter.

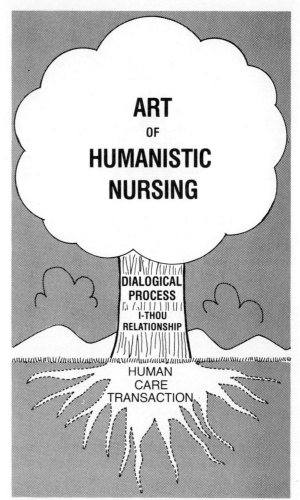

FIGURE 16-1. The dialogical process or the "I-Thou" relationship.

The heart of the "I-Thou" or dialogical relationship is the invitation "to be." The idiom "to be" means "to exist." Since existence is always in relation to the surrounding world, the key to understanding the human self is found in the social nature of man. Relationship is a fundamental reality of life.

The etymological roots of the phrase "to be" denote the reality of existence. Inherent in this reality is the implication of change and "becoming." In other words, there is potential within each person that has not yet been realized. "To be" involves process, a process which is experiential and subjective in nature. "To be," therefore, is rooted in human experience, possessing the basic qualities of the life process—change and growth.

Personal growth is a transactional process. The self has been described by some psychologists as a fluid or changing whole. The self emerges during human interaction; the quality of interaction determines the quality of self. Wholeness is a defining characteristic of humanity. A whole person should be seen as a feeling, thinking, and willing organism. Wholeness is unique, like fingerprints, illustrating the diverse possibilities for expressing experience of the world. Uniqueness, however, is a mixed blessing since it is an affirmation of our separation from others and guarantees some degree of isolation.

Dialogue is a bridge from the isolation of the individual to the discovery of common humanity. In dialogue there remains a genuine regard for the "other's" unique humanness while each reaches beyond it to that special sphere which Buber[4] called "the between" (Fig. 16-2). The origin of the term dialogue is the Greek "dia-logos," that is, "between meanings." The "between" is a special dimension of experience. It is the interhuman—intersubjective-free-space—in which mutual growth occurs. This growth comes about as new meanings for existence are created, and old meanings are expanded or refined. Man is the only animal capable of creating these meanings. The dialogical interrelationship is an amorphous reality which harnesses man's creative powers to shape life's meanings.

Meaning can be conceptualized as a pattern—that is, a design born of experiences that man gives to his world. Because individuals are unique, so too are their meanings. Some meaningful experiences occur like an explosion of insight, while others come gradually like the dawn. Today's meaning will undergo change and further clarification when it meets future, significant experiences. It is important to understand that man is concerned with meanings. The existential psychologist, Frankl, maintains that "man's concern about a meaning of life is the truest expression of being human."[5]

Perhaps at no other time in life is the concern for meaning so acute as when confronted with such ontological life experiences as death, illness, psychological trauma, and birth. These events are what Kenniston refers to as "developmental separations."[6] They are normal occurrences of life to be sure, but for the individual they are crises, connoting an acute sense of separation and isolation from the rest of humanity. In such crises, the deepest significance of the meaning "to be" becomes apparent.

The Chinese character for crisis is a pictograph composed of the symbols for danger and opportunity. This synthesis conveniently conveys both the inherent danger of continued separation and the opportunity for personal growth. In dialogue, the separation and isolation of the individual in crisis can be transcended. Thus, the dialogical interaction of the nurse and the client can dissolve the bonds of separateness. The nurse encounters the humanness of the client in ontological crisis through her own humanity—a humanity that is her major resource.

Genuine dialogue requires the courage to go beyond role facades and to risk the "real" self (Fig. 16-3). Risk, in this case, is vulnerability; as vulnerability increases so does the possibility that self will be rejected and then so does the potential for deep hurt. As a protection against vulnerability, some nurses perfect the art of pretending rather than the art of nursing. Seeming to be invested in the moments' events, they display a plastic friendliness and cordiality that shields them from the suffering they risk with change or growth. Pretending is, therefore, a more secure posture to assume in nursing life.

When examined, however, pretending is clearly seen as an evasion of responsibility. This responsibility is to be responsive, and responsiveness

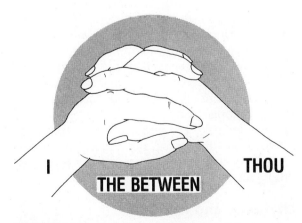

FIGURE 16-2. In dialogue, "the between" is a genuine regard for the other's unique humanness.

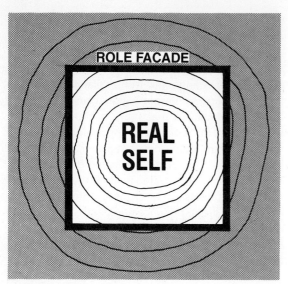

FIGURE 16-3. Genuine dialogue requires the "real" self.

means simply the ability to respond to another. The response in dialogue is to fully attend to the "other," focusing him in the "I" 's consciousness, intensifying his presence in the experience of the moment. This expanded awareness of the "other" is accompanied by a deep sense of empathy. The "I" sees the "Thou" as the "Thou" sees himself. This process is reciprocal and the "Thou" (client) also responds empathetically to the nurse.

The dialogical encounter is an experience in which the nurse works on her identity as a person and affirms that of the "other." She interacts in a "meeting" process, yet observes from within the human dimensions disclosed, and creates new meanings for her own existence. She is both the flower in bloom and the gardener in this human process.

Dialogue is only one level of human communication. Anyone engaged in a dialogue shows a marked increase in his energy level, appearing wholly committed to listening and responding, to being attentive to the "other." Dialogue is draining yet, paradoxically, refreshing. Emotionally, it is difficult to maintain the energy level necessary for dialogue. Sometimes it is less taxing to involve only a part of the self in an interaction. For example, the nurse may engage in a technical level of communication. In these moments, she functions to convey information, not insight. With objective under-

standing as her goal, only the cognitive part of her person is involved. Alternatively if she focuses on performing a specific task or procedure, the psychomotor as well as the cognitive may be the domains she utilizes. This is not to say that she is devoid of feeling when she provides information or performs a task. The choice of this technical mode of communication reflects the decision of some nurses to remain more emotionally distant and formal in their presentation of self. While this last mode of communication produces less growth, the individual nurse ultimately chooses to function within the confines of her current stage of social development.

Another level of communication sometimes appears to be a dialogue but is really a monologue. The nurse and client appear to establish a relationship but each speaks only to himself; the conversation is only superficially communication. Nothing is learned; there is very little exchange and no real concern for the "other." Everyone is familiar with moments filled by this "empty talk" of everyday life.

All of these levels of communication, apart from dialogue, are characteristic of an "I-It" relationship,[3] or subject-object relationship in which "I" treats the "other" as an object. A classic example is the nurse who refers to a client by his disease (e.g., "the gallbladder in room 303"). The "I-It" relationship is what one might call a "test-tube" relationship; the "I" observes the "other" without entering into a responsive relationship. Guardedness is the hallmark of an "I-It" relationship.

Dialogue, on the other hand, is characterized by spontaneity. This spontaneity is not to be confused with impulsiveness; the former is goal-directed, whereas the latter is oriented to immediate gratification. Dialogue is a spontaneous turning toward the "other" in search of a mutual self-realization. Because dialogue is spontaneous, communicants should be open and receptive to its possibilities, responding freely. The response can be spoken or silent, where the nurse and the client "meet" through glance, gesture, tone of voice, or just "being there."

Dialogue and Art

As elusive as is a precise definition of the structure-less reality of a dialogical encounter, in experience this type of relationship is easily recognized. This chapter has attempted to express the essential aspects of a relationship between a client and a nurse that meet the criterion of this self-affirming experience. If the art of nursing—the human dimension of nursing—is expressed through a dialogical encounter, the relationship that forms should be open and spontaneous, conveying a full, deep, authentic commitment of self and displaying an empathetic responsiveness to the "other" with the shared intent of creating new personal meanings for life. The verse at the beginning of this chapter suggests that discovery of the real meaning of "being" requires casting off pretentious role stereotypes; it pleads for a chance for the "real self" to evolve within the context of the nurse-client relationship.

The dialogical encounter and the nurse-client relationship are as closely bound together as the lungs and the heart and are equally important to the art of humanistic nursing. It is the dialogical encounter that gives an enlivened humanness to the nurse-client relationship, much as the human spirit enlivens the body.

Dialogue does not require special techniques. The whole being aids in answering the dialogical invitation. Just be! Remember that you can choose "to be" whatever you wish. If that choice is to engage in an intensive unfolding of humanness through a dialogical encounter, then you are *becoming* a humanistic artist. You are accountable for the humanity which is, after all, the medium and message of your nursing practice.

REFERENCES

1. Hoddinott, P.: Look at me, please see me, quoted in *Finding Yourself, Finding Others,* by Moustakas, C., Englewood Cliffs, N.J., Prentice-Hall, Inc., 1974, p. 6.
2. Worcester, A.: Is nursing really a profession? *Am. J. Nurs.* 2(2):908, 1902.
3. Buber, M.: *I and Thou.* New York, Charles Scribner's Sons, 1970.
4. Buber, M.: Between man and man: the realms, in *The Human Dialogue: Perspectives on Communication,* edited by Matson, F. W., and Montagu, A., New York, Free Press, 1967.
5. Frankl, V.: Quoted in *The Encapsulated Man,* by Royce, J., Princeton, N.J., Van Nostrand Co., Inc., 1964, p. 84.
6. Kenniston, K.: *The Uncommitted: Alienated Youth in American Society.* New York, Dell Publishing Co., Inc., 1965, p. 456.

BIBLIOGRAPHY

Beland, I.: *Clinical Nursing: Pathophysiological and Psychosocial Approaches 2.* London, Macmillan Co., 1970.
Brown, E.: *Nursing for the Future.* New York, Russell Sage Foundation, 1948.
Gale, R.: *Who Are You?* Englewood Cliffs, N.J., Prentice-Hall, Inc., 1974.
Howard, J., and Strauss, A.: *Humanizing Health Care.* New York, John Wiley, 1975.
Price, A.: *The Art, Science and Spirit of Nursing 2.* Philadelphia, W. B. Saunders Co., 1962.
Robb, I. H.: *Nursing Ethics: For Hospitals and Private Use.* Cleveland, E. C. Koechert Publisher, 1928.
Wiedenbach, E.: *Clinical Nursing: A Helping Art.* New York: Springer-Verlag, 1964.

CHAPTER 17

GLOSSARY

agency. The relationship in which one person acts for or represents another, either as employer and employee or master and servant.

assault. An intentional act designed to make the victim fearful and which produces reasonable apprehension of harm.

battery. The touching of one person by another without permission.

civil law. That part of American law which does not deal with crimes.

common law. Legal traditions of England and the U.S. where part of the law is developed by means of court decisions.

crime. An unlawful act committed against society as a whole in violation of the criminal law. Crimes are prosecuted by and in the name of the state.

defendant. The person denying the allegation; the party against whom relief or recovery is sought in a cause of action.

defamation. The injury to a person's reputation or character by willful and malicious statements

LEGAL ASPECTS OF NURSING

Maureen Cushing, J.D., R.N.

made to a third person. Inclusive of both *libel* (written word) and *slander* (spoken word).

essential elements of a negligence cause of action. Duty, breach (dereliction), proximate cause (direct causation), and damages.

guardian ad litem. A guardian appointed by a court of justice to stand in the shoes of the incompetent person to represent him.

malpractice. Professional misconduct, improper discharge of professional duties or failure to meet the standard of care of a professional which results in harm to another.

malpractice insurance. A contractual agreement to have someone else pay for any liability or loss resulting from negligent professional practice, in return for the payment of premiums.

negligence. Carelessness, failing to act as an ordinary prudent person or acting in a way contrary to what a reasonable person would have done.

plaintiff. Party to a civil suit who brings the cause of action (suit) seeking damages or other legal relief.

proximate. Direct or immediate. In a negligence case the careless act must be the proximate cause of the injury.

res ipsa loquiter. Literally translated meaning "the thing speaks for itself." The doctrine is applied in cases where some foreign object, as a sponge, drain, or clamp has been left in the patient's body.

respondeat superior. "Let the master answer." Under agency law the employer is responsible for the legal consequences of the acts of the servant/employee while he acts within the scope of his employment.

standard of care. Those acts performed or omitted that an ordinary prudent person would have done or not have done. A measure against which the defendant's malpractice conduct is compared.

statutory law. A declaration of the legislative branch of government having the force of law (i.e., child abuse statute in Massachusetts is found in Massachusetts General Laws, chapter 119, section 51-A).

statute of limitations. A legal limit on the time one has to file a suit in civil matters, usually measured from the time of the wrong or from the time that a reasonable person would have discovered the wrong.

tort. A civil wrong or injury.

There are many legal implications for all categories of nursing practitioners. This chapter identifies for the nursing student the essential legal principles which delineate the current and emerging responsibilities which affect their nursing practice. The force of the law on the health care delivery system is profound and the implication for nursing firmly established.

Case cites are included to illustrate a legal principle and identify the duty of the nurse to conform to standards which are mandated by professional nursing organizations and the very nature of their service oriented profession. It is the author's fervent hope that the nurse will be motivated to think in terms of rendering the highest quality client care rather than giving these materials a malpractice prevention focus. It should be clear from the case illustrations that the legal decisions do not give rise to the standards, but more readily serve to reinforce the knowledge, judgments, and activities upon which the profession is based.

Nursing, like the law, has had a remarkable evolution, and it is a profession that continues to develop and accommodate itself to the ever changing needs of society. For example, in the *Darling* case (1965), an 18-year-old student broke his leg in a football game. Shortly after a leg cast was applied, it was noted that the observable limb parts were discolored and swollen. Nursing records showed that the client received considerable pain controlling drugs with no relief over a period of several days. There was courtroom testimony that bloody drainage was seen when the cast was bivalved, and one witness testified that the stench at that time was the worst he had experienced since World War II. Two weeks after the injury, the client was transferred to another health care facility, and in spite of intensive therapeutic management, the leg had to be amputated. While many precedents were set in the case, the nursing implications were that the nurses failed to properly observe the toes for changes of color, sensation, and movement. Evidence established that these essential nursing activities were performed only a few times a day, and that was inadequate.

The court said that the hospital owed more than a duty to exercise reasonable care in selecting competent nurses. It extended the hospital's responsibility to see that proper procedure was followed by the nursing staff and that nurses had a further duty to inform the attending physician of the circulatory impairment. If the physician failed to act upon the nursing assessment, they were bound to advise the hospital authorities so that appropriate action might be taken.

The impact of the *Darling* case on the quality of health care provided by both the nursing and medical professions was substantial. In addition, it charged the hospital, previously not held accountable, with the responsibility of having a system which assures that the medical and nursing staff were carrying out their activities in a competent manner. The case also set precedent when it allowed the plaintiff to introduce licensing regulations, hospital bylaws, and the Joint Commission on Accreditation of Hospitals' standards to show noncompliance by the hospital.[1]

LEGAL BASIS FOR NURSING

Every professional nurse should understand the influence that the three branches of the Federal Government have on the practice of nursing, particularly the legislative and judicial components. That is not to say that the executive branch of government does not have a tremendous impact on the profession as well, and predictably, it will continue to exert its influence. It is imperative that the profession continue to be accountable for policing its membership performance to retain as much control over the professional activities as the nature of the profession demands. The reader must understand the process by which the governmental branches are empowered to act and the constraints placed upon them.

Legislative Law

Each state must assume the responsibility to protect its citizenry in matters of public well-being. This is accomplished by creating statutes. *Black's Law Dictionary* distinguishes statutory law from common law by defining it as an act of the legislature which declares, commands, or prohibits something and represents a written will of the legislature.[2] When interpreting statutes, it is important to read each word carefully to determine such factors as: the class of persons coming under the protection of the statute; the circumstances under which it becomes operative; the penalty, if any, for failure to comply with it; and the legal interpretation of terminology used in the statute. It is not infrequent that a statute is challenged on a constitutional issue (e.g., a state's abortion statute).

In recent years, nursing has recognized an urgency to redefine Nurse Practice Acts to give viability to the expanded role of the nurse. All nursing organizations strongly support the individual licensure system in contrast to the institutional licensure movement which in recent years has been proposed by some nonnursing groups.

The California Nurse Practice Act passed in 1974 begins on a very promising and unique note. It represents a departure from the more traditional nurse practice act format. It begins with a preamble which sets forth the intent of the legislature. This is important as it gives some indication as to how the statutory provision should be interpreted in light of legislative design. The statutory provision recognizes that "nursing is a dynamic field, the practice of which is continually evolving to include more sophisticated patient care activities." This section appears to support the contention that the identification and listing of distinct nursing functions, other than in broad terms, should not be specifically identified within the framework of the statute. Such specific identification does not allow for the growth and evolution of activities inherent in the profession and would necessitate statutory amendments each time a unique nursing function expanded.

The most important concept identified in the preamble is the recognition by the legislature of the existence of overlapping functions existing between physicians and professional nurses.[3] This gives status to the independent function of the nurse practitioner, as well as distinguishes it from the more traditional dependent, assistant role. The very essence of the concept of the extended role of the nurse is embodied in that statement.

The New York Nurse Practice Act, passed in 1972, represents an example of a totally rewritten definition of nursing practice. The distinctions which in the past have existed between the nurse practice act and the medical practice act are no longer as discernible, and this has led nurses to become more assertive in maintaining control of their profession. The new definition of nursing roles incorporates the concept that within the practice of nursing there must be a differentiation of the levels of practice. Three sections of New York's Nurse Practice Act are set forth here. (Laws of New York State Revision of Title VIII, "The Professions"; Article 139, Nursing, as amended and signed into law March 15, 1972.)

I. Section 6910.
   Definitions: as used in Section 6902:
   1. "Diagnosing" in the context of nursing practice means that identification of and discrimination between physical and psychosocial signs and symptoms essential to effective execution and management of the nursing regimen. Such diagnostic privilege is distinct from a medical diagnosis.
   2. "Treating" means selection and performance of those therapeutic measures essential to the effective execution and management of the nursing regimen, and execution of the prescribed medical regimen.
   3. "Human Response" means those signs, symptoms, and processes which denote the individual's interaction with an actual or potential health problem.

II. Section 6902.
   Definition of the practice of nursing:
   1. The practice of the profession of nursing as a registered professional nurse is defined as diagnosing and treating human responses to actual or potential health problems through such services as casefinding, health teaching, health counseling, and provision of care supportive to or restorative of life and well-being, and executing medical regimens as prescribed by a licensed or otherwise legally authorized physician or dentist. A nursing regimen shall be consistent with and shall not vary any existing medical regimen.
   2. The practice of nursing as a licensed practical nurse is defined as performing tasks

and responsibilities within the framework of casefinding, health teaching, health counseling, and provision of supportive and restorative care under the direction of a registered professional nurse or licensed or otherwise legally authorized physician or dentist.

III. Section 6909.
    2. Nothing in this article shall be construed to confer the authority to practice medicine or dentistry.[4]

While at first glance, it would seem that the failure to define nursing regimen was an oversight by the drafters of the act; on further perusal, it would appear that this approach was intentional and preserved the trend of "opening up" nursing functions. It is clear the redefining of nurse practice acts does not create a new licensing group, rather it expands the professional nurse's activities. Nurses have begun to meet the challenge of making the profession relevant to their clients and are assuming a prominent role in making health services available. Nursing is no longer confined to an assister role in therapeutic intervention; it is now responsible for health education, health maintenance, preventive measures, and restorative services.

Boards of registration in nursing must assume the responsibility for maintaining the regulatory controls which govern this new practice. An example of a regulation is a joint statement concerning the handling of drugs by professional nurses. One such statement establishes "dispensing" as a pharmacy act consisting of a pharmacist removing one or more doses from a bulk drug container and placing them in another properly labeled container for subsequent use.[5] Reference should be made to other state laws governing the health care professions to assure that their provisions do not restrict nursing activities or place nurses in a position of practicing another profession without a license.

The nurse practitioner movement has largely been brought about as a result of the crises in medical care which failed to make quality health care accessible. Independent functioning is an integral part of the nurse practitioner. Some revised or amended practice acts remove the restriction on medical diagnosis and treatment, whereas other states prohibit these extended functions under all circumstances.[6] Almost all acts expanding the nurse's function stipulate that policies and protocols will be jointly promulgated by boards of medicine and nursing.

Dr. F. Abdellah, Chief Nurse Officer, believes that as nurse practitioners become recognized and accepted for their vital contribution to the health care delivery system, Americans will be the beneficiary group.[7] It is anticipated that in the future judicial interpretation of nurse practice acts will expand the professional nurse's role, especially with respect to the nurse practitioner.

Brown reports of the creation of joint private practices by health practitioners of varied disciplines as a result of the dissatisfaction with current health care agencies. Such groups may include a psychiatric social worker and nurse, a physical therapist and orthopedist, or a variety of team groupings.[8]

One classification of paramedical personnel should be identified before the discussion of the legislative branch of government is concluded. Bullough, commenting on the psychological barriers to expanding the nursing role, states, "when the need for some type of middle medical worker emerged, many physicians simply did not think of nurses as being capable of independent or cooperative decision-making, turning instead to physician's assistants."[9] It should be well understood that physician's assistants are not licensed professionals; that is, they function in a dependent role. New York recently proposed legislation which would have prohibited the physician's assistant from writing medical orders and prescriptions. The bill was withdrawn by the drafter after public hearings determined that they work and prescribe medications under the supervision of physicians. The hearings identified a need to provide uniformity for training physician's assistants, and a future bill will be introduced to address this lack of standards and may also require that they pass a competency test in pharmacology.

The physician's assistant functions under the legal authority of the physician's license to practice. There is a need for uniformity with regard to the extent to which physicians can delegate activities to the physician's assistant. The professional nurse needs to understand that activities which are carried out illegally by the physician's assistant may place the nurse's license in jeopardy if he carries out any illegal therapeutic orders. One state advisory opinion stated that physician's assistants may not practice nursing without being licensed.[10] Nursing organizations frequently request the Attorney General of a state to render an advisory opinion on questions submitted to his office, for example, Attorneys General have been asked to determine whether intravenous puncture was within the realm of a nurse's function.

Judicial Law

There are several legal definitions which are an integral part of the remaining materials. The common law is that body of law derived from the early traditions of England as well as from the judgments and decrees of the courts. Once the court has created a principle of law based upon a given statement of facts, it will apply that principle to all future cases where the facts are essentially the same. This doctrine is known as *stare decisis.*

There is built into the legal system a time limit as to the viability of a civil suit. Each state via statute establishes a time period within which actions may be brought upon certain claims. Some states have built into the statute that the tolling of the statute of limitations begins at the time of the wrong in contrast to the time of discovery of the wrong. Failure to bring the cause of action within the time period results in a dismissal of it. The time period as it relates to minors extends beyond the normal limit.

Once a cause of action has been adjudicated in a proper court and upon its merits it is said to have *res judicata.* The same issue(s) and parties are precluded from a second cause of action. The court proceeding may be tried before a judge and jury or a judge alone. The right to decide this belongs to the party bringing the cause of action. The law is clear when it delineates the role of the jury as triers of fact and the role of the judge as that of maintaining procedure and applying the law to the facts. There exists a right to appeal a lower court's decision so long as this right has been reserved at the trial level. Generally the appellate proceeding considers infringement of procedure or improper application of the law by the judge.

LEGAL RELATIONSHIPS

Duty to Employer

Within the primary care setting, many legal relationships exist. Some of these are based upon agency law principles. For example, a private duty nurse, physician, or medical consultant, so long as they are not employed by the hospital, function within an employer-independent contractor relationship; that is, they are held individually liable for their own acts of negligence because the contractual relationship is between the client and the respective provider of care.

The relationship which exists between the nurse and the hospital, if employed by the hospital, is that of employer and employee. The nurse acts for or represents the hospital and thus is bound to function within the policies and protocols of the employing hospital. This is based on the concept that the health care facility has a right to establish and implement policy which most effectively achieves its philosophical beliefs. As long as nurses perform within the scope of the authority under which the hospital has determined they function, the hospital will be liable for negligent acts committed by them. This legal relationship creates a doctrine known as *respondeat superior.* Succinctly stated it means, "Let the master answer." However, this does not mean that the nurse may not be sued individually. In the case, *Martin v. Perth Amboy Hospital*, the court decided that the hospital was not liable. When a surgeon ordered the metal detection rings removed from the laparotomy pads during surgery, the court held that at that time, the surgeon became the surgical nurse's employer and was, therefore, responsible for the nurse's actions when the sponge count was incorrect.[11] When the physician exerted such control over the nurse's activity the court applied the doctrine of the borrowed servant and held the surgeon and the nurse liable. Control helps determine the relationship or lack of it between the employer and employee.

Professional nurses are responsible and owe a duty to their employer, the client, and other personnel. The hospital has an obligation to advise new employees regarding the scope and parameters of their professional duties. Nurses should request this information regarding the philosophy of nursing service, a relevant job description, and policies affecting the position if it is not offered. This will enable them to practice their profession with the greatest degree of professional contentment as well as afford protection of their licenses.

Duty to Client

TORTS AND CRIMES

As we have seen the law speaks in terms of an obligation or a duty created by a legal relationship. A *tort,* as defined in a malpractice context, is a civil wrong or injury. It must always be a violation of a duty owed to the client by the provider of care. The duty generally is created by operation of law rather than a mere agreement of the client and provider of care. Such a cause of action is brought in the names of the parties such as, *Jones v. Clark.* A criminal cause of action differs from a tort cause of action in that the latter is an unlawful act committed against society as a whole in violation of the criminal law and is brought in the name of the state, such as *The State of New York v. Smith.*

NEGLIGENCE AND MALPRACTICE

The distinction between negligence and malpractice is best illustrated by comparing their definitions. Negligence is carelessness; that is, failing to act as an ordinary prudent person or acting in a way contrary to what a reasonable person would have done. It does not necessarily require a legal relationship. A person who intentionally drives through a stop sign and causes injury to a person or property is said to be negligent. Malpractice is professional misconduct, improper discharge of professional duties, or a failure to meet the standard of care of a professional which results in harm to another. It requires a legal relationship. A student nurse was negligent when she caused permanent damage to an infant's leg when she injected medication meant to be administered intravenously into the muscles of the infant's buttocks. In this case she failed to read the warning on the ampule that it was for intravenous use only.[12]

Inherent in both definitions are acts of omission and acts of commission. Thus, failing to observe for circulatory impairment and initiate action to reverse the finding in the *Darling* case was a negligent ac-

tion as a result of omitting to do what the ordinary prudent nurse in the same or similar circumstances would have done. A client received a substantial award for permanent disability in a case where the nurse negligently instilled sodium hydroxide instead of a saline solution while assisting in a gastric analysis.[13] This case illustrates the principle that no nurse should undertake to make a nursing diagnosis, institute a plan of care, or perform a procedure that is beyond her qualifications.

Establishing the standard of care is not as difficult as it first appears. It is actually a measure against which the defendant-nurse's action is compared. In a courtroom proceeding, it would be established by the plaintiff-client's attorney bringing in an expert witness nurse, introducing into evidence the relevant criteria set forth by the professional nursing organizations and professional writings. The American Nurses' Association and the Association of Operating Room Nurses are examples of professional organizations whose published standards of care would help prove the plaintiff's case. All state boards of nursing formulate rules and regulations to guide nursing professionals, and while these regulations are not law, they have the force of law.

In every negligent or malpractice cause of action, certain legal elements must be established to sustain the suit. They include duty, breach, causation, and damages. Consider application of these elements in the following case involving a wrongful death cause of action against a defendant hospital.[14] A patient was admitted to the hospital for emergency surgery. Due to her restlessness and respiratory distress, she was transferred from the recovery room to a private room. When the nurses attempted to connect the oxygen outlets to the wall, the gauges did not fit, whereupon a nurse ran for the portable oxygen. There was a delay of 5 minutes in getting the portable unit to the bedside. In spite of cardiopulmonary resuscitation, the patient died, and the next of kin brought suit. The court held that a legal *duty* to provide functioning emergency equipment was owed the patient by the hospital and that it *breached* that duty by not having an adequate emergency oxygen supply available when faced by a functional defect in the normal supply. This latter was the *proximate cause* of the patient's death. The *damages* included pain and suffering and wrongful death.

This case should draw attention to the necessity

of having written protocol for the maintenance of equipment. This is one reason why job descriptions should be frequently revised and made available to all hospital personnel so that each person is aware of his responsibility in the scheme of keeping the environment safe. Most hospitals delegate the responsibility for daily checking of the emergency cart to the professional nurse. Consider the nurse's liability when the endotracheal tube is malfunctioning or when there is only one Bristojet of sodium bicarbonate available when a cardiac arrest occurs on the unit. Generally, the nurses who check the contents of the emergency cart sign and date the check sheet attached to the cart. Carrying liability one step further, consider the hospital's duty to institute a viable cardiac arrest procedure and periodically evaluate it for effectiveness.

Examination of Specific Duties

ABANDONMENT

While the law imposes legal duties on the nurse in carrying out the activities and responsibilities of her profession, it is most important to provide the highest quality client care according to the standards of the profession. Consider this 1972 case which dealt with *abandonment* of the client.[15] A 53-year-old bank guard was shot at close range and critically wounded. He was classified as expectant care upon his arrival at the emergency room and survived for an hour and a half during which time his family members observed his care. The family alleged that the hospital breached the duty owed him by failing to render critical care during the 90 minutes he was under its care. Evidence determined that while many physicians, including a neurosurgeon, visited him no supportive care in the form of blood, intravenous fluids, or shock intervention was carried out. The hospital defended by stating that the physicians had placed him in the expectant care category and that his chances for recovery were hopeless. The autopsy showed extensive brain damage. The court held for the next of kin saying that the physicians could not rely on autopsy data to justify a previous clinical decision not to treat.

The concept of abandonment or failure to treat which emerges from this case has considerable applications for nursing activities. A nurse could be liable for failure to render cardiopulmonary resus-

citation to a client who has had a sudden cardiac arrest when the nurse's inaction was based upon a physician's verbal order not to resuscitate. Proper hospital and nursing protocol require that a physician communicate such an order via the doctor's order sheet so that there is a written record of the order.

DUTY TO REMAIN COMPETENT

An important legal conclusion to bear in mind is that clients have the right to expect that the persons caring for them have the competency to meet their needs. The courts have said that as laudable as nurses' intentions are in helping out on a unit which is short staffed, they must not undertake functions with which they are unfamiliar. For example, an incorrect medication dose resulted in an infant's death when a nursing supervisor, who was not familiar with pediatric doses, gave an adult dose of digitalis. She had gone to the unit to give assistance in a staffing shortage.[16]

The competency issue frequently places nurses in a moral dilemma when asked to "float" to another unit. Under these circumstances, nurses should alert the person requesting the reassignment to their educational or experiential limitations. The hospital nursing service department has the responsibility not to rely excessively on a reassignment policy as it would be evidence of a continuing lack of staff pattern.

One of the findings and recommendations of the Secretary's Commission on Medical Malpractice was that an increase in the number of professional nurses in health care facilities would substantially decrease the numbers of malpractice causes of action.[17] Many professions are weighing the question of how best to prepare their membership with the competency to meet the needs of the group they serve. Nursing has become the vanguard of the movement.

PROVISION OF SAFETY IN CLIENT CARE

Nurses need to continually examine and evaluate client care activities in order to bring about safe practices in addition to a safe environment. Poor nursing judgment is a prime factor in many of the hospital mishaps which occur. The nurse must be vigilant in applying the steps of the nursing process to all client situations. While the courts have not directly taken notice of these components, they have a long history of referring to them in terms of lack of judgment and failure to act upon client findings.

RESTRAINTS

In the past it was not considered within the scope of nursing practice to apply restraints independent of a physician's order. That limitation would probably still hold true with respect to the rigid leather wrist restraints used so frequently a decade or two ago. It is common nursing knowledge that these restraints frequently yielded a nerve compression injury. There are many factors within an episodic health care delivery system which increase the responsibility of nurses to provide for the client's well-being or to intervene in an adverse client finding. Some examples of situations which require nursing intervention include psychological adverse drug response from medications and anesthesia, disorientation to the physical environment, and pathological changes which impair judgment.

Once the nursing decision to apply restraints to protect the client from causing harm to himself or others has been made it must be coupled with reasonableness. The nurse must determine if the situation would have been best dealt with by having someone sit with the client, administering medication to sedate him, or changing the client's room facilitating more frequent checking by the staff. It should be clear that nursing judgment is not confined to a single option, and the situation requires careful evaluation. A sudden emergency greatly influences the examination and selection of options, and this would be taken into account in the event that a cause of action arose.

An equally important factor in the use of client restraints needs to be identified, that is, the duty to observe for the possible adverse effects resulting from the use of restraints. There is an increased duty for the nurse to inspect the area of the body restrained to assure that the restraint is not impairing circulation or harming the tissues. The most frequently employed restraining methods are hand wraps or a Posey belt. In one client situation, it may be deemed adequate to inspect once per shift,

whereas in another, the history of diabetes or arm edema after a mastectomy may require more frequent supervision. These variable factors in client status should influence the selection of restraint or supervision determined best for the client. It should be clear that the transfer of scientific theory to the client situation is an integral component of the nursing process. Determination that the method of restraint was adequate is frequently a jury question.

FALLS

It is not difficult to understand why falls are a frequent suit area. The reasons for the high incidence of client injury from falls are too numerous to cite here, but some of the more unusual factors include: sensory deprivation, especially visual; faulty design or use of bed rails; and poor assignment of clients necessitating prolonged stretches or lack of observation and care. One recent court decision held that a client may be expected to administer to her own need when the hospital staff failed to respond to her call light. In that case the client fell while attempting to get out of bed when there was no response to her call for a bed pan.[18]

The nurse need not foresee harm for liability to exist nor is she held negligent for every fall which happens to her client. The determinant is: Where is the negligence? Where does this nurse stand in relationship to the reasonable and prudent nurse?

CLIENT IDENTIFICATION

Client identification represents a special problem when caring for young children and unconscious clients. Most hospitals have instituted the system whereby the client's *wrist band* and not the bed or room is the means of identifying him. Akin to client identification problem is the need to make providers of care aware of *client allergies*. This is most frequently accomplished by putting an *allergy bracelet* on the client on admission. The breakdown of the system occurs when the bracelet becomes wet and thus illegible or when the client remembers a forgotten allergy several days after admission. There is the likelihood that this essential client data does not find its way to the allergy bracelet which is potentially dangerous for the client's welfare.

BURNS

Because the use of direct heat in treatments and diagnostic procedures is a frequent occurrence in a hospital setting, it is not uncommon for burns to occur. Chemicals, when not properly diluted are also a source of heat injuries. Consider the issues in the following two cases. An operating room circulating nurse was held negligent when she failed to redrape a patient after dripping excessive amounts of a flammable solution she was using in preping the client. The client was severely burned when a Bovie machine ignited the drapes.[19] A client who had been receiving hot pack treatments for several days fell asleep and was burned. The court allowed the nurse to introduce evidence to show that the client was competent to assume responsibility for the treatment and that he had been doing so for several days. At that time contributory negligence was an absolute defense, and the court held that the nurse was not negligent.[20] Change the facts a little to involve a perineal lamp positioned a foot from the bed and the fact that the client had received a maximum dose of narcotic for pain just before the heat treatment. The reasonable, prudent nurse would assume responsibility to remove the lamp when the exposure time had expired as well as supervise the treatment throughout.

FOREIGN BODIES

The operating room is particularly vulnerable for negligence suits involving foreign bodies. Lost sponges, needles, and instruments comprise the bulk of the suits. The trend in recent years is away from the "Captain of the Ship Doctrine" which stated that the surgeon is in complete charge of all that goes on in the operating room. The concept has been replaced by considering the sponge count as an administrative function of the hospital which holds the circulating and scrub nurses accountable for the correct count. As employees of the hospital, they have a responsibility to inform the surgeon if the count is incorrect, and he is bound to take measures to determine if the lost material is in the wound. As employees of the hospital, the nurses are under the control of the hospital; however, it is possible that the surgeon can exert so much control over the nurses that they become his employ-

ees. Consider the situation where the surgeon's own scrub nurse is responsible for the sponge loss.

Ordinarily the plaintiff-client has the burden to show that the defendant was negligent. However, there is an exception to this procedure and that is when the doctrine of *res ipsa loquitor* ("the thing speaks for itself") applies. The doctrine shifts the burden to the defendant to show that he was not negligent. In order for the concept to apply, it must be shown that the instrument was under the exclusive control of the defendant, the plaintiff was not contributively negligent, and that the occurrence causing the injury would not have occurred if reasonable care had been used. Sponges left in the patient during surgery frequently bring into question the application of this doctrine.

TEACHING

While client teaching has always been an important component of health care it has risen to new dimensions as a result of the client's desire to be involved in the decision-making aspect of his health care. It has become essential that documentation of client teaching be included in the patient's hospital record to assure continuity of care. It is just as important to explain the hospital environment and routine to the client as it is to teach the limitations on activity after a femoral angiogram. Harm to the client is foreseeable in both situations, albeit, it may be a more predictable life threat if the client gets out of bed 2 hours after returning from the angiography laboratory.

A male client suffered genitourinary injury when he voided directly into the collection jug rather than into his urinary receptacle. According to proper laboratory methods, the jug contained a preservative which splashed on the genital area burning it. The physician had ordered the urine collected for a 24 hour examination. It was unclear whether the nurse had properly taught the client the procedure for collecting the urine. The hospital argued that the client was contributively negligent, and it operated as a complete defense in the state where the cause of action was brought.[21]

A bus driver, who had earlier in the day taken his first dose of Pyribenzamine, lost consciousness while driving and injured one of the passengers. The drug had been prescribed by his private physician who did not teach him any of the side effects of the drug. The policy of the bus company was that an employee was to inform the company health office of any medication prescription ordered by a noncompany physician, and the employee had not done this. The suit against the bus company was not successful as the proximate cause of the injury was determined to be failure on the part of the physician to do essential health counseling.[22]

ADMINISTRATION OF MEDICATION

The administration of medications requires concentration and compliance with procedure. Needless to say, there is considerable case law to support the contention that this aspect of nursing activity is frought with potential liability. Too frequently nursing judgment is not stressed as great a factor in medication errors as it should be. Many errors associated with medications occur as a result of omitting them or in transcribing them. The duty of a nurse differs considerably when she administers 2 mg of Valium three or four times a day to provide sedation than when she administers 20 mg of the same drug three or four times a day to relieve the severe spasms associated with low back pain. The latter dose requires that the nursing care plan include assistance in walking and constant elevation of bedside rails.

A Department of Health, Education, and Welfare news release in October 1977 reported that the Food and Drug Administration would require brochures explaining the benefits and risks of drugs containing the female sex hormone. The brochure is written in lay language, and the purpose of the prescription insert is to inform the users what to expect. Dr. D. Kennedy, Commissioner of Food and Drugs, supported the concept that people have the right to know what drugs they are taking, why they are taking them, and the beneficial and adverse results.[23]

For the nurse to safely administer medications, she should be aware of the therapeutic goal of the drug and the essential nursing observations and activities associated with its administration. It is essential to understand the desired effect of the drug to make an intelligent nursing decision. What should be the response by the nurse when the client vomits the 10 grains of aspirin? If the therapeutic goal was to relieve a headache or fever, then the nurse must determine if the client still has the symptom. If, however, the dose represents the method the physician has selected to control the client's clotting mechanism after hip surgery to prevent the complication of emboli, the nurse would have to communicate the incident to the primary physician at the time of its occurrence. One situation would be within the nurse's scope to determine an appropriate action, whereas the other would not be within the scope of nursing practice to decide how to dispose of the problem. Nurses must remember that they must practice within the framework of their own license; they can not carry out an activity or order which is questionable. They must comply with the drug literature and make nursing judgments supported by scientific knowledge.

It is important for nurses to know that they have the prerogative of refusing to carry out a questionable order. The nurse is bound to use nursing judgment to assess the clinical accuracy of the order. The nurse can not escape liability by saying that the order was incorrectly written by the physician. Take, for example, the case *Barnes* v. *St. Francis Hospital.* A physician ordered via the telephone that Dramamine be given "hypodermically." The literature stated that it could only be given intramuscularly, but the nurse gave it subcutaneously in the hip. The court ruled that the nurse should have known to give it intramuscularly, even though the doctor's order was not specific. The court also found that due to the client's girth, the nurse used poor judgment in using a needle which was not long enough.[24]

Compare the results of the next two court decisions. In the case, *Wilmington General Hospital* v. *Nichols,* a client sustained an irreversible footdrop as a result of a nurse's negligence in injecting a proper medication dose in the wrong area of the buttock. The client recovered damages.[25] In the case *Southwest Texas Methodist Hospital* v. *Mills,* a client complained of a stinging sensation in her left leg after receiving her preoperative medication intramuscularly in the left buttock. She was taken to surgery and placed in lithotomy position throughout the procedure. Several buttock intramuscular injections were given in the recovery room, and that same day she complained of left leg numbness. The patient did not recover damages due to the fact that she was unable to prove that the sciatic nerve injury was due to the negligence of the nurse. The defense introduced multiple possible causes of the injury, including inadequate blood and oxygen supply to the area during the operation as well as continuous pressure on the nerve during the procedure.[26]

This latter case illustrates the point that injections are a calculated risk. Infections and other adverse reactions might result from injections by nurses and in and of itself, it does not imply negligence. The plaintiff-client must show negligence. The nurse must show that she executed precise and clinically safe orders, that protocol was adhered to, and the injection was carried out in a skilled manner.

COMMUNICATION AND DOCUMENTATION

Failure to report a change in client status to the physician is a frequent reason for clients bringing negligence causes of action. Akin to this suit-prone activity is a delay in communicating client findings. It would be prudent procedure for the nurse to make a specific notation of the time the physician was called and the implementation of his orders or directions.

A recent Maryland case ruled against the hospital under the *respondeat superior* doctrine when the emergency room nurse failed to inform the physician that a mother had removed ticks from the head and chest of one of her two children. She brought both children to the hospital for emergency services when they developed a rash on their scalp and chest and conveyed these facts to the nurse. The court held that the failure of the nurse to give an accurate history was a violation of a duty owed and that this negligence resulted in the death of one of the boys. The physician was not held liable when he treated the children for measles as this failure was not negligence based upon the history given to him by the nurse.[27] This case illustrates that the assessment process, nursing or medical, is a basis for planning care.

The physician removed a "T-tube" the day before discharging a client. A short time later the client complained of pain, and upon being notified, the physician ordered pain medication. Although the nurses responded to the client's call light, there was no further record of contacting the physician in the presence of increasing pain with bloody vomiting.

Twelve hours after the onset of symptoms, the client was diagnosed as having an acutely dilated stomach which required an additional 3 weeks in the hospital. The court held that the length of delay was unreasonable.[28]

Significant quotes of the client should be included in the nursing notes. In the *Darling* case the plaintiff's attorney used the nurses' notes to establish the fact that he was in an unusual amount of pain over a continuous period which should have alerted the staff of the need to intervene. Moans of a client can be used to establish pain and suffering which can be an aspect of the damages award.

While most states have legislative provision to keep nurses' notes as part of the hospital record after the client has been discharged, some states do not. That is unfortunate, as it may be the most valuable weapon in a court proceeding to rebut the plaintiff's contention of negligence. Most hospitals have a written policy identifying the purpose and situations in which documentation of care must be done. While the nursing process is easily identifiable in a problem-oriented system of recording, it is essential that it be clear and concise in a source-oriented system as well. All documentation of care should reflect nursing judgment, nursing evaluation, and nursing action.

It is a discredit to the profession that many attorneys representing the plaintiff find that the nurses' notes, which lack exactness, help their cause. No event should be recorded without some professional nursing interpretation and appropriate nursing action. Nurses should keep in mind that the suit is frequently years removed from the point in time of rendering the nursing care. It is not that the courts will not allow oral testimony, but there is a greater tendency of a judge or jury to give more weight to documentation of care done at the time it was given. This is because the potential of a pending suit is not anticipated. Courts will sometimes accept verbal testimony of nurses on the rationale that many of the routine activities need not be charted. However, other courts will exclude testimony contrary to or inconsistent with charted observations by nurses.

Professional nursing is based upon a scientific body of knowledge and in the situation of the client who had a femoral angiogram done earlier in the day and who got out of bed, the documentation of that event must reflect the nursing process. Nursing judgment requires affirmative action by the nurse, and documentation of care should include that the client was returned to bed, the dressing checked, vital signs taken, and the physician notified. Observing, reporting, and recording go hand in hand.

NONNEGLIGENT TORTS

Invasion of Privacy. This is an appropriate cause of action when unauthorized persons are permitted to see a client's operative procedure. The law is protective of a person's right to be left alone and not be subjected to publicity. Public figures do not have the extent of protection as do nonpublic persons. A recent court determination held that publishing a story which included photographs and names of students in a public school's special education program was an invasion of privacy. The students were identified as mentally retarded, and the court regarded that designation as delicate and private in nature.[43]

A New York Health Law section was struck down as an undue invasion of privacy when it required the reporting to state authorities of the names and addresses of clients receiving prescriptions for "Schedule II" drugs. Recognizing the state's right to curtail drug abuse, the court still considered the client's right not to have his name published a greater right.[44]

Assault and Battery. Assault is an intentional act designed to make the victim *fearful* of pending harm. Battery, as previously defined, is the *carrying out* of an assault. The two terms are viewed together, and the most common nursing situations considered as assault and battery are giving an injection or medication against the known wishes of the client.

Incident Reports

At one time accidents or injuries would be reported on an "accident report," but the trend today is to refer to them as incident reports. Every situation which requires completion of an incident report warrants informing the physician. In most reports, this requirement is built into the wording of the tool. It is not an uncommon practice to see an incident report lying on top of the desk at the nurses' station

the day after the incident awaiting the physician's signature. There are times when a telephone call to him is sufficient to inform him of the incident and get direction if needed. In this event, the client's record should state specifically the time that the physician was called.

The purpose of incident reports is to give hospital administration notice of situations which may require procedure or policy change. It is this aspect which generally categorizes them as being inadmissible in a court proceeding due to their status as committee reports or business records. The rationale is that hospitals would not require these reports if the threat existed that they could be introduced in evidence and used against them. As a result an opportunity to improve client care or to correct a problem would fail to materialize. Because the hospital record may be introduced as evidence, the report should not be included in the medical record as it would lose that protection. It should be pointed out that the incident report is not absolutely protected as it may be subpoenaed in court, partially or as completed. Many incident reports include a question, "How could this incident have been prevented," which necessitates citing a specific statement as to why it occurred and what should be done to prevent it occurring again. The incident report is reviewed by a designated hospital committee, and if it is written up in factual terms, the opportunity for the nurse to confer with the committee will provide specific information as well as measures to prevent similar mishaps. Because of the possibility, albeit remote, that the incident report may find its way into the court, statements specifically identifying liability should not be included in the writing up of such a report.

CLIENTS' RIGHTS

In 1973 the American Hospital Association proposed a 12 point "Patients' Bill of Rights." These rights are included in Table 11-4 in Chapter 11; however, it is appropriate to expand on the issues affecting health care as they have evolved from case law and statutory provisions. There have been no suits thus far based upon enforcement of the Patients' Bill of Rights, although it can be introduced into evidence to establish a standard of care. This is probably so, even if a respective hospital or state has not adopted it.

Currently, all 50 states allow the clients access to their medical records, although some states require the filing of a cause of action. The Report of the Secretary's Commission on Medical Malpractice cites the unavailability of the hospital record, except by instituting a suit, as one of the causes of unnecessary malpractice actions.[29] Massachusetts allows clients direct access to their hospital or clinic records.[30] Records of a hospital or clinic under the control of the department of mental health may be available when there is a proper judicial order or when the client requests that his attorney be allowed to inspect the record.[31]

A government agency report urged that a Federal policy toward computer systems in hospitals, which store and retrieve client records, be created to prevent abuse of confidential information.[32] Better monitoring of the quality, quantity, and cost of health services delivered is one of the benefits of computerized medical records.

The Right to Emergency Care

The right to emergency care was established by the *Manlove* case in 1961. The issue involved in the case was whether a private hospital had a right to refuse emergency treatment in its emergency room. Parents of a 4-month-old infant took the child on two successive days to a physician who prescribed medications and other treatment. Due to the child's temperature, and because the physician did not have office hours that day, the mother took the infant to the defendant's hospital where a nurse on duty did not examine the child. The child at that time was not coughing or crying, and the nurse explained that the policy of the hospital prohibited treatment as the child was already under a physician's care. She did make attempts to contact the treating physician but failed to reach him. The nurse then suggested that the mother bring the child into the pediatric clinic the next morning. Upon returning home the mother made an appointment for later in the evening with the physician who had been treating the infant, but the infant expired before being seen.

The court held that the hospital owed a duty to render emergency care. The court's reasoning was that the public relies upon the fact that the hospital can provide emergency services even if the hospital does not have an emergency room. The court also said there was no duty to establish an emergency room or admit the client to the hospital facility, merely a duty to treat until the client was out of danger.[33] Subsequent cases have held that emergency care is independent of the ability to pay, and the hospital can transfer the client to another facility in a safe manner once the client is out of danger.

Rights of Psychiatric Clients

The courts have given particular attention in the last decade to the rights of psychiatric clients. A landmark case was decided regarding psychosurgery when the court ruled, that:

1. Clients involuntarily committed in state institutions are legally incapable of giving competent, voluntary, knowledgeable consent to experimental psychosurgical operations which will irreversibly destroy brain tissue.
2. The first amendment freedoms of speech and expression presuppose a right to generate ideas which could be destroyed or impaired by psychosurgery.
3. The constitutional right to privacy would be frustrated by unwarranted medical intrusion into a client's brain.[34]

The due process rights of psychiatric clients seeking voluntary admission to a mental health facility have been protected by requiring a hearing with legal counsel unless the client waives it.[35] By statutory and case law, minors have a procedural due process right in commitment proceedings. Any commitment deprives a person of his liberty and such proceedings should have safeguards.

Informed Consent

The doctrine and case law involving informed consent are evolving rapidly. It would appear that an essential principle of health care, that of involving the client in the decision-making aspect of his diagnosis and treatment, is finally being complied with. The current trend is that the risk disclosure is not that which the reasonable client would comprehend, but of such a nature that the particular client in question would understand. While there is considerable debate within the medical community regarding the concept of informed consent, it should be acknowledged that care based solely upon trust and expectation (sometimes, not realistic) is not an alternative to the client's own reasoned judgment based upon all the considerations. The idea of a second opinion yields considerable benefit to both the client and the physician. A frequent issue for the jury to decide is whether the client would have withdrawn the consent if he had the facts presented to him prior to the procedure.

Blanket consent forms are not recommended by attorneys involved in health care because there has been difficulty circumventing their ambiguity and lack of specificity. Sometimes nurses are requested to obtain a client's signature prior to going to the operating room or x-ray for a diagnostic test; however, they should not do so if the client appears unaware of the procedure or has questions surrounding it. It would be essential that the nurse communicate the information to an immediate superior. Under these circumstances, regardless of the legal significance of the signature, it would be unwise to go forward with the procedure. It would expose the nurse and the hospital to liability, but most importantly, it would deprive the client of his right to be involved in the decisions surrounding his care.

A physician can not delegate the obtaining of an informed consent to a nurse where the disclosure of the *risks, benefits,* and *alternatives* to medical treatment are an integral component of that signature. Clearly, nurses do not possess the degree of medical knowledge necessary to assist the client in making a decision. The nurse may expose herself to peril if the client were to allege that he decided upon a course of treatment in reliance on inaccurate or incomplete information given by the nurse.

The following two cases based upon similar facts illustrate the necessity for and emergence of the *informed consent doctrine,* which is distinct from a negligence cause of action. In the case, *DeFillipo v. Preston,* decided in 1961, a client was unable to speak above a whisper after a surgeon performed a thyroidectomy. Expert testimony established that the statistics showed a 2 percent incidence of permanent damage to the laryngeal nerve, even in the absence of negligence. The woman "consented" to the procedure; however, the surgeon failed to inform her of any surgical risks. The court decided it on a negligence cause of action, and the surgeon was not liable.[36] In a case decided in 1973 (*Con-* *grove* v. *Holmes*) based upon similar facts and again involving a thyroidectomy, the surgeon was held liable, not for lack of his surgical skill, but rather, for failure to obtain an informed consent.[37]

Lack of consent is traditionally a battery against the person. *Battery* is generally defined as an intentional touching of another person. The key element is the absence of consent to the touching by the plaintiff.[38] Consent is invalid if it was obtained (1) when the client was awakened from sleep in the middle of the night to sign an "operative permit," (2) after the client received preoperative medication but before being removed to the operating room, and (3) when the explanation is given in medical terminology to a lay person. There are two court sanctioned reasons for proceeding without obtaining an informed consent: when the risk-disclosure element would be so intimidating that it becomes unfeasible from a medical point of view to give the information and where a delay in beginning treatment may place the client in peril.[39]

The client's right to refuse medical intervention is well established. However, the courts have made a clear determination to intervene in cases where the involved party is pregnant, in his minority, or does not possess intellectual capacity to decide upon a course of therapy. Health care providers should be aware of the factors in a hospital setting which may bring into question the validity of a client's refusing medical care. Advanced pathology which affects intellectual capacity and the influence of intellectual altering drugs are examples of factors which could render a supposed refusal invalid. Hospitals would be well advised to petition the court for instructions in such cases. Documentation of findings by the nurse of activities of the client indicating that he was lucid at a given point of time may be important in a cause of action where the state of his mind is in issue.

The Right to Die

The "right to die with dignity" controversy is complex. It appears to the lay person, as well as those in the medical community, that instead of nearing resolution it is becoming more complex. Recent court decisions, beginning with the *Quinlan* case, have addressed some of the complicated issues surrounding the use of medical technology in caring for terminal clients. While there are many unanswered questions, the court decisions have helped to identify some guidelines. The Euthanasia Educational Council first published a document referred to as "a living will" in 1961. It was vague in wording and lent itself to be interpreted several ways. Medical technology has moved so swiftly that the ethical, moral, and legal aspects were left behind and the issues associated with the possibility of sustaining terminally ill clients indefinitely still confronts the health care profession.

While the competent terminally ill client has the right to refuse treatment, the incompetent client is unable to convey his wishes to those caring for him. California, in 1976, was the first state to pass legislation on a "Natural Death Act." Since then several states have enacted similar legislation, and more states are in the process of proposing similar statutes. Some California physicians have complied with the statutory provision in caring for their clients who have signed such a document. The concept of a living will has its critics who maintain that no matter how specific the wording there will still be abuses. Some critics caution that a client can not know at the time the document is signed how he will feel about dying some time in the future of an unpredictable cause. Clearly, a state that has not enacted legislation creating a living will will not recognize a document created in another state; however, the living will gives evidence as to the state of mind of the person at the time of the signing.

Another controversy which surrounds the "right to die" issue is who should make the decision not to treat the person and when withdrawal of life support equipment may be done. In August 1977, the Massachusetts Supreme Judicial Court became the highest state appellate court in the country to adopt the Harvard Ad Hoc Criteria for "brain death."[40] However, the court sought to negate any misunderstanding that its decision would affect the numerous other situations in which the question might arise when death occurs. The court considered the issue of "brain death" only as it related to a criminal conviction. That same court, when ruling on another case, said that the courts rather than an ethics committee should make the right to die decision for terminally ill clients who are incompetent to decide for themselves.[41] The court adopted a procedure to be followed in similar cases which will arise in the future. It requires that a judge appoint a guardian ad litem who is charged with the responsibility to make a complete investigation with the best interests of the incompetent client kept paramount. The court will then consider the recommendation of the guardian ad litem in rendering its judicial decision whether affirmative treatment of the client must be continued or not.

In May 1978, the Massachusetts Appeals Court took under advisement a case involving an elderly widow dying from an incurable brain disease with concomitant condition of arteriosclerosis. The client was unable to speak in her own behalf due to her brain pathology, and her physician anticipated that she would have a sudden cardiac arrest sometime in the near future. The court said that based on the facts, the decision not to do cardiac resuscitation was for the physician to determine as it would be in keeping with the highest medical profession tradition. In essence, the court said that the decision not to resuscitate was not dependent upon judicial approval. The children of the client agreed with the physician that she be allowed to die peacefully when the arrest occurred.[42]

The Making of a Will

Because nurses are in close contact with persons who are critically ill they may be involved in the activities surrounding the making of a will. The law of the various states differs with respect to the number of witnesses it requires, and the procedure is not as simple as merely signing your name. It is not unknown for a person's will to be successfully contested after his death due to invalid witnessing procedures. For this and other reasons, most hospitals have a policy which only allows certain members of the staff to perform this function. Many large hospitals have a notary public on their staff who is competent to direct the activities surrounding the witnessing of a will. While many hospitals do not allow nurses to act as witnesses, the nurse may be requested to give testimony in a court of law regarding the state of mind of the person making the will if the will is being contested due to alleged intellectual incapacity at the time it was made.

Good Samaritan Laws

Good Samaritan Laws were created to protect the public when they became injured. There is considerable variance in the wording of different states' statutes; therefore, it is important to read the statutory provision with care to determine the groups protected by it and in what circumstances. Some states require that assistance be given by all citizenry, whereas others apply the law to specified categories of health care professionals.[45] Most require that the aid be rendered in good faith and without negligence.

The reason for the law is that those most able to help an injured person will do so without fear of a future law suit. It is important to note that there are few cases involving judicial consideration of the Good Samaritan Laws.[46] Because the rendering of care is not done within a health care setting, the standard of care is not expected to be the same as that which would be given in an emergency room. In essence, the standard is not as high as it would be in the controlled setting where experience, equipment and readiness would be a factor. However, the emergency care provided must be done in a reasonable manner. An example of care rendered in a grossly negligent manner would be where a nurse attempts to manually reduce a compound fracture before immobilizing it. This is so because no reasonable, prudent nurse would have cared for a compound fracture in this manner.

REFERENCES

1. *Darling* v. *Charleston Community Memorial Hospital,* 211 N.E. 2nd 253 (1965), 383 U.S. 946 (cert. denied, 1966).
2. *Black's Law Dictionary*, 4th ed. St. Paul, Minn., West Publishing Co., 1951.
3. California Code, Business and Professions, sec. 2725.
4. New York Education Law, sections 6910, 6902, 6909.
5. Massachusetts Nurses' Association: *Guidelines to Ethical and Professional Nursing Practice.* Joint statement concerning the handling of drugs by professional registered nurses, 1971.
6. Bullough, B.: The law and the expanding nursing role. *Am. J. Public Health* 66(3):249-253, 1976.
7. Abdellah, F.: Nurse practitioners and nursing practice (Editorial). *Am. J. Public Health* 66(3):245-246, 1976.
8. Brown, K.: Nature and scope of services: joint practice. *J. Nurs. Admin.* 7(10):13-15, 1977.
9. Bullough, *op. cit.* p. 249.
10. Woodahl, R.: Opinion of the Attorney General, Helena, Mont. August 28, 1975.
11. *Martin* v. *Perth Amboy Hospital*, 250 A. 2nd 40 (N.J., 1969).
12. *O'Neil* v. *Glens Falls Indemnity Co.*, 310 Fed 2nd 165, (1962).
13. *Gault* v. *Poor Sisters and St. Joseph's Hospital*, 1967 CCH Neg. Cases 1223.
14. *Berraire Hospital* v. *Campbell*, 510 So. West 2nd 94, (1974).
15. *Bubry* v. *Gardena Medical Center*, California, 1972.
16. *Norton* v. *Argonaut Insurance Co.*, 144 So. 2nd 249, (1962).
17. *Report of the Secretary's Commission on Medical Malpractice.* (DHEW Publication No. (OS) 73-88) Washington, D.C., U.S. Government Printing Office, 1973.
18. *Newhall* v. *Central Vermont Hospital*, 349 A. 2nd 890.
19. *Bing* v. *Thunig,* 143 N.E. 2nd 3 (1957).
20. *Dittert* v. *Fisher*, 36 P. 2nd 592 (1934).
21. *Chamberlain* v. *Deaconess Hospital*, 324 N.E. 2nd 172, (1974).
22. *Kaiser* v. *Suburban Transportation System*, 401 P. 2nd 350, (1965).
23. Kennedy, D.: *HEW NEWS* (P77-39, DHEW) Washington, D.C., U.S. Government Printing Office, October 17, 1977.
24. *Barnes* v. *St. Francis Hospital*, 507 P. 2nd 288 (1967).
25. *Wilmington General Hospital* v. *Nichols*, 210 A. 2nd 861, (1965).
26. *Southwest Texas Methodist Hospital* v. *Mills*, 535 S.W. 2nd 127.
27. *Ramsey* v. *Physicians Memorial Hospital et al.*, 373 A. 2nd 26 (1977).
28. *Karrigan* v. *Nazareth Convent & Academy, Inc.*, 510 P. 2nd 190 (1973).
29. *Report of the Secretary's Commission on Medical Malpractice*, p. 212.
30. M.G.L. c. 111, sec. 70.
31. *Ibid.*
32. Office of Technology Assessment: *Study on Policy Implications of Medical Information Systems.* Washington, D.C., Congressional Report, 1977.
33. *Wilmington General Hospital* v. *Manlove*, 174 A. 2nd 135, (1961).
34. *Kaimowitz* v. *Department of Mental Health*, Civil No. 73-19434-AW, Circuit Court, Wayne County, Michigan, 1973.
35. M.G.L. ch 123, sec. 6.
36. *DeFillipo* v. *Preston*, 173 A. 2nd 333, (1961).
37. *Congrove* v. *Holmes*, 308 N.E. 2nd 765, (1973).
38. Prosser, W.: *Law of Torts*, 4th ed., p. 143, sec. 30, St. Paul, Minn., West Publishing Co., 1971.
39. *Canterbury* v. *Spence et al.*, 464 F. 2nd 772, (1972).
40. *Commonwealth* v. *Golston*, 377 N.E. 2nd 744, (1977).
41. *Superintendent of Belchertown* v. *Saikewicz*, 370 N.E. 2nd 417, (1977).
42. *Boston Globe*, June 30, 1978, p. 1.
43. *Deaton* v. *Delta Democrat Publishing Co.*, 326 So. 2nd 471, (1976).

44. *Roe* v. *Ingraham*, 403 F. Supp. 931, (1976).
45. M.G.L. ch. 112, sec. 12B.
46. Zaremski, M., "Good Samaritan" statutes: do they protect the emergency care provider?, *Medicolegal News* 7(1):5-7, Spring 1979.

BIBLIOGRAPHY

Annas, G.: *The Rights of Hospital Patients.* New York, Avon, 1975.

Bernstein, A.: Contemporary consent cases *Hosp., J. Am. Hosp. Assoc.* 49:101, 1975.

Bok, S.: *The Dilemmas of Euthanasia.* New York, Doubleday, 1975.

Carpenter, W.: The nurse's role in informed consent. *Nurs. Times* 71(27):1049, 1975.

Creighton, H.: *Law Every Nurse Should Know,* 3rd ed. Philadelphia, W. B. Saunders Co., 1975.

Hall, R.: Hospital committee proceeding and reports: their legal status. *Am. J. Law Med.* 1(2):245, 1975.

Hayt, E., and Hayt, E.: *Law of Hospital, Physician and Patient,* 3rd ed. Chicago, Ill, Physician's Record Co., 1972.

Imbus, S.: Autonomy for burned patients when survival is unprecedented. *N. Engl. J. Med.* 29(6):308, 1977.

Kaplan, R.: Euthanasia legislation—a Survey and a Model act. *Am. J. Law Med.* 2(1):41, 1976.

Law, S.: The patient's right to refuse treatment. *Hosp. Med. Staff* 5(10):1-7, 1976.

Pontoppidan, H.: Optimum care for hopelessly ill patients. *N. Engl. J. Med.* 295(7):362-364, 1976.

Rabkin, M.: Orders not to resuscitate. *N. Engl. J. Med.* 295(7):364-366, 1976.

Regan, W.: Nursing service problem: incident reports. *Regan Report on Nursing Law,* July 1974.

Secretary's Committee: Extending the scope of nursing practice. A report of the Secretary's Committee to study extended roles for nurses, Washington, D.C., Department of Health, Education, and Welfare, November, 1971.

Springer, E.: The *Darling* case: ten years later. *Hosp. Med. Staff* 4(6):1, 1975.

Williams, B.: Malpractice: how good is your insurance protection? *Nurs. '76* 6:81, 1976.

PART 4: INDIVIDUALIZING HEALTH CARE NEEDS

The delivery of health care is not a haphazard process. It is carefully evaluated, organized, and implemented. The nurse, in conjunction with the client and the various members of the health team, utilizes critical thinking in orchestrating the care of her clients. For care to be effectively administered and received, it is first necessary for the nurse to *assess* the situation. The collection of *subjective* and *objective* data about the client, his past and present health history, and his socioeconomic as well as sociocultural familial background are included in the assessment.

Viewing the information collected in light of the knowledge available to the health professional enables the nurse to draw some conclusions about the client's *problems* that need resolution. Once these problems have been identified or diagnosed (therefore being called *nursing* diagnoses), the nurse can formulate *objectives* or *goals* with the client and significant others and then initiate a *plan of care.* This plan reflects the client's strengths and weaknesses, the environment from which he comes and to which he will return, and considers how these factors enhance or detract from the suggested interventions. After *implementation* of the plan, *evaluation, modification* and *revision* will be necessary to determine if care has been successful or if further action must be planned.

Chapters 18 to 21 introduce the student to goal-directed assessment of clients, their families, or significant others when appropriate. Chapter 18, "Introduction to Goal-Directed Assessment: Observation of Nonverbal Behavior," examines the language of the body—the messages or clues that everyone, including the nurse, send out to the world. The nurse skilled in assessment possesses a valuable tool—a sharpened power of observation—and uses this much as she would any other instrument, such as a stethoscope or a thermometer.

Chapter 19, "Interviewing: A Tool for Data Collection," carries the observation skills discussed in Chapter 18 a step further. The student is introduced to the goal-directed verbal exchange between the client and nurse. Purposeful conversation and communication to gather data is the second most important skill in the assessment process.

Chapters 20–22 look specifically at the major tools of assessment—the health history and the physical examination. Chapter 21 is limited to adolescents and adults, while Chapter 22 explores the differences in assessing infants and preadolescents. Chapters 22 to 26 focus on the remaining steps in the nursing process as described above.

CHAPTER 18

1920s: On the screen the dark and handsome
  sheik, Valentino, gazed into the young
  woman's eyes; he picked her up and carried
  her off into his tent. Women in the audience
  literally swooned. During that same era of the
  silent screen, Charlie Chaplin and the Keystone Cops had audiences roaring with laughter at their antics.

1960s: The table was laden with food. A man
  and a woman sat across from one another and
  had one of the most memorable meals in
  movie history. The audience watching the couple consume the food slowly realized that they
  were watching a very erotic seduction scene.
  If asked today about the movie, *Tom Jones*,
  many people remember that scene more readily than others.

1970s: The ultimate exchange of nonverbal
  communication in cinematic history occurred
  in the movie *Close Encounters of the Third
  Kind*. In the final scene depicting man's face-
  to-face encounter with extraterrestrial beings,

INTRODUCTION TO GOAL-DIRECTED ASSESSMENT: OBSERVATION OF NONVERBAL BEHAVIOR

Elise D. Navratil-Kline, M.S., R.N., and
Arlyne B. Saperstein, M.N., R.N.

no spoken words were used between humans and aliens. Extremely sophisticated photographic techniques made this exchange seem realistic and believable. Many observers were moved by the feelings of gentleness and tenderness they felt the aliens conveyed with their eyes alone.

The examples above were taken from motion pictures, a predominantly visual medium of communication. In each example, whether from 50 years ago in the dawning years of films or currently, no conversation was necessary to convey a point or make an impact on the audience. It is obvious from examples such as these and other visual forms of entertainment, such as Marcel Marceau and mime troops or charades, a game which most of us have seen or played, that a message can be transmitted and received without any accompanying verbal emphasis or explanation. Nonverbal communication has been a mode of sending out information since the first creatures walked the earth. In the

animal kingdom, there are specific gestures and behaviors which have special significance to other members of the species. Although man has added language to his means of communication, he still incorporates nonverbal signals into verbal exchanges.

Nonverbal behavior has been described by Barnlund as "an elaborate code that is written nowhere, known by none, and understood by all."[1] Blondis and Jackson describe nonverbal behavior as that which fills in the gaps that are left when messages are verbally transmitted, making the message complete.[2] While words can be fairly well controlled with accuracy, nonverbal behavior cannot. Therefore, this may be why behavior is more believable and trusted than the words themselves. The significance of this is that "words are often not what they seem and are sometimes used to camouflage what is actually felt."[2]

Why is it so important that the nurse be familiar with nonverbal behavior? Just as all physical complaints or disorders are accompanied by an emotional component and vice versa, all communication between individuals has a nonverbal component whether or not a verbal exchange occurs. If the nurse overlooks this aspect of communication, she will always receive incomplete, messages; a holistic picture of the client and what he is projecting will never emerge.

Before we can observe the behaviors and feelings of others, we must first become aware of our own. Autodiagnosis, according to Burgess and Lazare,[3] is a process in which the observer (in this case, the nurse) examines her own feelings and reactions to a situation in order to understand it. Awareness of these feelings makes them not only less intimidating but also more easily controlled. This is important, especially if the nurse is feeling anxious. Robinson[4] stated that the feelings of discomfort experienced with anxiety are basically the same in everyone, whether the individual is a nurse, a physician, or a client. However, the constructive use of anxiety is possible if the person feeling it can identify and then alter its nature and source (conflict). Conversely, to experience the anxiety and act involuntarily to dispel uncomfortable feelings rather than coming to terms with the problem can be counterproductive. When nursing students begin to interact with clients they may experience a great deal of anxiety. While much of this may be due to their own feelings of insecurity and inexperience, observing behavior that is unexpected or difficult to accept may produce anxiety. An example might be seeing an adult lose bladder or bowel control, thereby soiling the bed. While the student may not yet be sophisticated or knowledgeable enough to uncover all of the reasons why she feels nauseated, angry, or frustrated, she can identify the fact that she is feeling one or more of these emotions. This is the first step in learning to deal with our own and then our clients' behavior constructively.

THE SENSES

Perception

In learning and practicing the skill of observation, it is important to remember that being human, we can never be totally objective and impartial. Everything we see is colored by our previous experiences and our sociological, ethnic, and economic backgrounds, as well as how we are feeling at that particular moment. Therefore, it is important that we sharpen our perceptive skill as much as possible. To do this requires that we become conscious of all our senses and expand our knowledge base (i.e., social and behavioral sciences as well as physical sciences). Hein has stated that, "Without knowledge, we see without understanding the subtleties and nuances of each patient with whom we interact. The use of observation implies skill in knowing what to look for and the relationship and significance it has to the patient, his family, and his community."[5]

In order for interpersonal communication to occur, we use both motor and sensory skills.[6] Most people are not aware of the functioning of all of our senses until something brings one to our attention. For example, our sense of smell usually goes unnoticed until the odor of something overpowering reminds us of its presence. Although the senses work together, they will be discussed separately for ease of presentation.

Sight

According to *Psychology Today,*

The problems encountered in studying vision are similar to many of the problems found in other areas of psychology. We observe many forms of behavior in response to visual stimuli, ranging from something as simple as stopping at a traffic light . . . to the complex reactions that may result from seeing a beautiful painting or the judgments we may make about another person by observing the way he dresses or his facial expressions. . . . The visual system responds differently to the environment by enhancing certain features of the physical changes taking place and by de-emphasizing others. It has no alternative. The total amount of information contained in all the physical changes taking place in our environment is far beyond the capacity of any living organism to register much less analyze. . . . In order to interpret stimuli properly we have to use contextual information; we have to combine our expectations of what we think should be occurring with what actually does occur. This fact means, of course, that the message we get from a physical signal may depend as much on what we expected the stimulus to be as on what it actually was. In fact, we often see what we expect to see rather than what actually occurred. . . . This important aspect of human functioning appears to operate by a process of internal synthesis, in which an image of the world is created and matched against the sensory input.[7]

According to Hein, "Seeing is believing or so the saying goes. Seeing is not believing, however, because observation has an inherent selectivity based on our experiences, our senses, our present frames of reference. . . . Since each of us has different experiences and interests, our ability to see also differs even when we are all looking at the same thing."[8] For these reasons, it is important that in nurse-client interactions we verify our observations by discussion with others who have observed the client or with the client himself. In that way, we may validate that what we saw was actually taking place. Even then there may be times that the client will be unaware of certain behaviors and will be unable to acknowledge your perceptions.

Hearing

Just as with sight, selective hearing can also take place. People often hear what they want to hear rather than what is actually said. This frequently occurs when one is overly anxious about the topic of conversation, as the client who is discussing his diagnosis with the physician and cannot accept what it is he is hearing. He may later ask the nurse what his diagnosis is even though he already "heard" it. With a great deal of practice, the nurse who learns to listen well, will hear and later be able to fairly accurately reconstruct conversations between clients or other individuals and herself.

When dealing with the senses, perhaps it is even more important to be aware of other aspects of conversation than just the words. "Paralanguage," according to Blondis and Jackson, "deals with how something is said, rather than what is said. A whole range of nonverbal cues are involved, such as voice quality, pitch, tone, and tempo—and vocal characteristics, including coughing, whining, clearing of the throat, and so on."[9]

It is a unique experience to hear a recording of our own voice since we do not hear ourselves as others hear us. It is important to know what you sound like to others. Is your voice well-modulated, high, shrill, grating, calm, musical, difficult to hear or understand? Knowing how you sound may make it possible to improve or correct certain characteristics that might be irritating or impede communication.

Smell

What does the sense of smell have to do with observation? When we are in an enclosed space or in close proximity to another individual, our sense of smell may tell us certain things about him. Hein claims that:

These clues relate various aspects of culture, personal preferences, impending trouble, and moods. . . . Within intimate and personal distance, we can determine through our olfactory receptors the various perfumes or after-shave lotions preferred by those we encounter. These scents often communicate the presence of a person before we actually see him. . . . These aromas become as familiar as the person to us. Odors derived from smoking, drinking, eating highly seasoned foods . . . also are discernible within these zones. Body odor, halitosis, and odors connected with excretory functions and infectious processes can also be detected.

Fear or anxiety are also detectable through our olfactory receptors. Some patients who are diaphoretic under stress exude odors different from those evidenced through perspiration due to intense heat or work.[9]

Not only should the nurse use her sense of smell as one of her assessment tools, but she should not forget that she, too, will give olfactory clues to those in her immediate vicinity. Good physical hygiene is mandatory when close contact with clients is demanded. It should be noted that when a client is ill, certain odors, especially strong or overpowering ones, may be unpleasant or even nauseating; this would indicate to the nurse that heavy perfumes or scented lotions, powders, and sprays need to be used in moderation, if at all.

Taste

The importance of our sense of taste was also described by Hein:

The organs of taste and smell are connected physiologically by a web of nerve receptors located near each other—adjacent to the nasal passages along the base and surface of the tongue. The organs rely on each other and provide concurrent experiences. . . . Of the two senses, taste seems to have less impact upon communication between ourselves and patients. It does, however, add to our knowledge from a sociocultural and a socioeconomic point of view. The offering of a cup of coffee is a cultural ritual often as important as the content of the interview, because in this exchange we can discover clues to a person's social conduct, economic status, and abilities to prepare food. . . .

We must become aware of the economic and cultural significance of food to each individual and family, particularly if their behavior suggests food is being used as a mode of communication. . . . The importance of sociocultural influences on dietary habits and preferences cannot be underestimated wherever nursing is practiced. These factors are often not considered in planning therapeutic diets in a hospital, but they may have an impact on patients, especially if they involve a restriction of certain types of foods or seasoning. . . .

The sense of taste (as it concerns food) can also be put to use in other ways within our relationships with patients. For example, it can become the medium through which definite therapeutic goals are realized. It can become a sensory tool—a neutral and socially acceptable way to elicit beneficial results that cannot be obtained through other methods. When used in situations that lend themselves to such an approach, it can promote self-esteem and ego-integrity and reactivate one's previous interests and roles.[11]

Touch

The last of the senses, touch, has been described by Blondis and Jackson as

. . . the most personal of our senses because it brings two human beings into close relationship. It is the most basic and primitive of the senses; the infant uses touch to explore its world, and while still a fetus, responds to the vibrations of the mother's heartbeat. Our first contact with life is through touch. The newborn feels the obstetrician's hands, reacts to the feel of touch during rocking, soothing, bathing, and feeding. The baby's first cry is usually silenced when he is placed on his mother's belly and experiences her warm comfort. Our first comfort in life comes from touch, and usually our last, since touch may communicate with the comatose, dying patient when words have no way of breaking through. . . .

Touch contacts are so vital to human development that children will fail to grow and to mature without them. A total deprivation of touching leads to cachexia in some children, which can cause death or retardation, while other children given a scant ration of physical affection grow into destructive, violent adults. . . .

Unfortunately, many adults have mixed feelings about touch. Some carry childhood taboos into adulthood, whereas others see tactile contact as an invasion of their privacy or are bothered by feelings of embarrassment and inferiority. Understanding our own feelings will help us empathize with our patient's responses to touch. . . . To be truly therapeutic, tactile communication must be used at the appropriate time and place. Each person considers a certain amount of space around him as private, and touch can be seen as an invasion of that privacy unless it is desired by each person. Touch must be used at the right time and in the right way; otherwise misinterpretation of the message will occur.

The use of touch by people is not limited to communication. It also is used as a means of becoming familiar with the environment. Children fondle a new toy, examine every inch of it with their fingers. . . . Adult patients exhibit the same kind of touch exploration when they pat the hospital bed or run their fingers up and down the raised safety bars. The patient's need to keep in touch with his environment is real, and the observant nurse will be aware that the patient's touch behavior has significance. A patient who is constantly touching a certain area of his body might be experiencing pain, unusual sensations, or fear that this part of his body is in danger.[12]

It is apparent that the utilization of touch as a therapeutic communication device must be accompanied by a great deal of discrimination on the part of the nurse. Later in this chapter a closely related topic, territorial rights (i.e., need for space), will be explored. This, too, will be a concern of the nurse in her interaction with clients.

From the information above it becomes clear that observation of the client for the purpose of assessment is far more involved than just looking at him. Many factors, some of them extremely complex, influence the nurse and the client as this process is implemented. The nurse's perceptual skill must be sharpened by continuous practice before it can be exercised in an appropriately critical manner. To do this she must become aware of not only what is happening externally, but what is occurring internally as she relates to her client. She then must be able to exercise some constructive control over the emotions she is feeling. This also includes a look at her own value systems and beliefs. Value systems not only include feelings about politics, religion, and race but also issues such as moral and ethical behavior, cleanliness, dress codes, and food preferences. When these are different or at odds with those of the client, then the possibility of friction, conflict, and mutual distrust increases. Naturally, as stated before, the identification of the feeling experienced by the nurse must take place before any controls or mastery can be achieved. Further, the nurse must have a basic knowledge of the forces affecting her perceptions and behaviors as well as those of her clients. It is for that reason that the student studies the behavioral and social sciences as well as the physical sciences. To understand behavior one must know how information is interpreted and how distortions can occur. While the student nurse certainly does not have the knowledge to analyze and interpret a client's behavior in depth, it is important for her to understand, in general, basic motivations and behavioral patterns. While the student will not have to expound upon the deep psychological significance of a specific behavior, she will be expected to describe what it was that she did observe, how it made her feel, and

how she responded to the situation or occurrence. In addition, a nurse may also be asked why a client has behaved in a certain manner and whether or not his behavior was merely a response to her behavior or actions.

APPEARANCE OF THE CLIENT

General Appearance

What is it that we note upon our first encounter with another individual? When we meet people we often get a certain sense or feeling about them, even before becoming acquainted. Have you ever spoken to someone on the telephone and later met them? They may not have looked at all the way you might have expected them to. Have you been to a party and at first glance "known" with which persons you wanted to socialize? What is the "chemistry" that draws us to one individual and makes us shrink from another? Once again *value systems* emerge. There are certain body prototypes that appeal to each of us—that is, height, weight, body build, musculature, coloring, facial features, scents, or odors—and others that we may find less attractive or even offensive. This is also true for manner of dress, styles, and colors. The pressure and influence of the family unit, community, and society cannot be minimized in the development of these predilections or prejudices. The initial impact that a person makes on us may tell us a lot about him. However, it is important, especially in professional situations, that generalizations not be made on the basis of a very limited glimpse of a client.

One of the first things that should be noted on meeting a client is the physical appearance. Clothing may tell us a lot about socioeconomic status, life style, and cultural background, and primarily, concept of self. The way in which we "put ourselves together" may have a purpose that is obvious or subtle. Some people dress to look like their peers, such as in adolescence, while others care nothing about expectations of friends and dress for their own psychological and physical comfort. Our clothing can be physically protective, as from the sun or the cold, or can conceal a "multitude of sins," or defects (real or imagined) such as birth marks, blemishes, fat, or bruises. Just as some feel the need to cover up and look less attractive, there are others who expose more in order to be seductive. While the information that is conveyed to you by the mode of dress may say a lot, it could also be very misleading. A stain on a dress could have been caused quite by accident just prior to the interview. In another case, it just might be that the person's habits of cleanliness are poor, and the stain has never been laundered. Clothing that is out of current style could indicate a lack of interest in trends or it also could be due to lack of funds to keep up with fashions. Other information must be collected to validate our initial assumptions. What standard of hygiene and grooming has been adhered to? Is the client's hair clean and combed or unkempt? (If the latter, is it very windy outdoors?) Is there a noticeable body odor or halitosis? Does the person wear perfume or cologne? Is the scent sweet, fresh, light, or very heavy? Has the client shaved, or if he has a beard is it neat? Are the nails clean or dirty, split, or broken? The list could go on and on. Remember that the whole picture of an individual must be studied before any conclusions can be formulated.

Not only should the client's appearance be looked at in terms of how he is groomed but also from the standpoint of appropriateness. Is the person's wearing apparel, accessories, or cosmetics in accordance with the person's position, the time of day, the season, or the occasion? A banker in a pair of tattered jeans may not be inappropriate in certain instances, but if he has just come from the bank, it may not be at all appropriate. A long-sleeved wool dress worn on a hot summer day or a halter top and shorts in midwinter would be inappropriate. Again, there may be circumstantial reasons for deviance from the norm or what might be expected.

In addition to the above characteristics, the interviewer should also note the body movement of the client—that is, his *kinetic behavior*. Just as a person may say something about themselves to us by choosing a specific cologne or type of clothing, so they may also communicate with their gestures and the motion of their whole body. The nurse should be aware of how the client reacts to her. What is his behavior while they are together? Does he move around during the exchange or does he appear to be relaxed? Does he convey anxiety, fear, or shyness? Is he open and cooperative or rigid and noncompliant? Does his behavior, both physical and emotional, change after being with the nurse for a period of time? The remainder of this chapter examines specific aspects of the client's nonverbal behavior that we observe in making an assessment, such as postures, limb movements, facial expressions, affect, and stereotyped behaviors.

Posture

Posture—the way we carry ourselves when standing, walking, or sitting—is a way of communicating information about ourselves. Factors affecting posture include physical limitations due to past or present illnesses, injuries or occupations, body image, self-esteem, and affective (emotional) disturbances.[13] If a person is in pain he may bend over and "protect" his abdomen with his arms. A person with curvature of the spine or severe arthritis may also appear stooped, while someone who has had a spinal fusion may sit rigidly upright. An individual who has spent 8 hours a day, every day for years bent over a piece of equipment at his job will often continue to use this posture even when not working. The person who is slumped over may be depressed, unhappy, sad, or just tired, while the one who remains erect could be happy, relaxed, alert, or rigid. Care must be taken so that generalizations about posture are not made. A stooped position does not necessarily mean that a tall woman desires to be shorter and less conspicuous, nor does it always indicate a depressed state. As stated, it could be exhaustion or a past illness. It should be noted that shifts in postures may indicate that something is occurring; these shifts should be looked at in relation to the situation as a whole. If a person is seen on only one occasion, posture may be an insignificant clue to their behavior. Observing a person on many occasions, with knowledge of his occupation and past health history, is a more valid means of drawing tentative conclusions.

Gestures

The various gestures that are used by individuals can be thought of as punctuation marks in communication. Much of what we do not express verbally is done with the head, arms, hands, and occasionally the legs. Kicking or swinging the legs and feet while seated could possibly indicate anxiety or restlessness. On the other hand, after being seated for quite a while, this could be a means of increasing circulation to the parts, consciously or unconsciously.

The head may nod in order to tell a speaker to continue talking and that we agree with him. Shaking the head could say, "stop," or indicate disagreement. When offering sympathy or expressing feelings of hopeless acknowledgment, some individuals will be seen shaking their head, adding still another significance to the traditional way of saying "no."

Most gesturing is done with the arms and hands. People from various cultures tend to use gestures in different fashions. Latin Americans, for instance, often use arms and hands in sweeping motions with every statement. People from the Mediterranean countries, such as the Italians, also gesticulate in conversations. Western Europeans and North Americans tend to be more controlled and use less hand illustrating. It should be remembered that while hand gesturing is not standard and usually varies from person to person, it most often emphasizes or reinforces what is being said. Hand gestures, however, can be a language in themselves with a very specific translation into words. The sign language used by the deaf is an example of this type of gesturing.

Facies and Affect

Facies refers to how the face appears to the observer, while affect denotes emotional tone that is a reaction to an experience. When observing facies, one looks at the general appearance of the face, such as the shape; the condition, color, and tone of the skin; the individual features, including eyes, nose, mouth, chin and jaw; distinctive markings; distribution of hair; and the condition of the teeth. Equally important is the expression on the face. When observing expression or affect, the major consideration is whether it is appropriate to or in context with the situation. For instance, one would not expect a client to smile brightly when he is discussing the recent death of a loved one. Of equal significance would be the lack of affect on a client's face.

The nurse in observing affect looks for relaxation or tension; a calm, peaceful countenance or a pained, angry, hostile, or tormented expression;

fear or worry; apathy or happiness; radiance and joy. Blushing, blanching, winking, blinking, tics, tears, crying, sniffling, coughing, smiling, laughing, giggling, and the quality, pitch, and tone of the voice are other indicators of feelings or emotions that can be observed by the nurse.

While the saying that "the eyes are the windows of the soul" may be overstating the case, there is an element of truth in it. Very often the client's eyes are very revealing and tell us much more about what the client is experiencing than any other body part can. Eyes not only reflect emotions but also certain physical conditions such as neurological disturbances or drug usage and withdrawal.

Eye contact is an important mode of communication. We tell each other with our eyes whether we agree or disagree with what they are saying, whether we want an answer or are not willing to be interrupted at a particular moment, whether we are self-assured or uncertain about what we are saying, and whether we are interested or disinterested with the other person's conversation. In addition, our eyes may reveal feelings of embarrassment, fear, guilt, and domination, or subordination.

Space and Territory

Most of us are aware that animals stake out a specific circumscribed area or territory that they will defend against penetration even to the death. Man, too, marks off certain spaces including that area immediately surrounding him as his personal territory. He also may exhibit defensive behavior if he suspects that his space is about to be or has been invaded. Space is a very individualized matter. For some people, their personal space may be a very small area, while for others, a much larger area is needed around them to maintain their psychological comfort. Culture and ethnicity as well as socioeconomic factors play a large part in how much space a person may need without feeling uneasy. Americans, especially males, usually do not stand very close together when speaking, whereas Latins and Arabs will stand very close to one another. The American talking to the Arab would probably pull his head back as the Arab moves into his intimate (immediate) space. If the invasion of his space continues, he would probably back away. While each culture has its own attitude toward space and territory, conditions of poverty and overcrowding can become a stronger force influencing territoriality than the original background.[14]

An illustration of typical behavior regarding personal territory can be seen in crowded elevators. As the car stops at each floor people rearrange themselves to make more room for each additional person. Usually nobody touches one another in the elevator until it is absolutely mandatory. If you are *alone* in an elevator and someone enters and stands next to you, touching you slightly, would you move away from them or continue to stand there in such close proximity? Would you feel uncomfortable? Would you consider this person's behavior inappropriate? If so, your personal space would have been violated.

The nurse when caring for clients must perform procedures within a very close range. Some clients will feel this to be an invasion of their territory. While little can be done to alter the distance, an explanation of the care to be given prior to initiation of the procedure, as well as an attempt to convey respect for the client's feelings may be of assistance in allaying some of the discomfort. As little touching as possible may also decrease anxiety in clients who dislike having strangers in close proximity, for these people feel very threatened when their personal space is invaded. Eventually as communication and trust increase, touching may be less intimidating. However, this usually takes a great deal of time; the client should not be pressured to accept the nurse's touching behavior before his readiness is ascertained.

CONCLUSIONS

We have all been using our powers of observation throughout our lifetime, but for most of us it has not been a goal-directed tool. This chapter is merely an introduction to the observation of a client. It by no means encompasses all of the characteristics and behaviors of which a skilled practitioner should be aware. While a number of observable areas have been cited, it will be very difficult, if not impossible, for the beginning student to focus on all at one time. Therefore, a great deal of practice time will be necessary to attempt to observe each area individually. Eventually, the student's strengthened powers of observation and recall will allow her to synthesize more than one point at a time. The following exercise is recommended in order to assist the student to develop this skill: with a partner, seat yourself in a place, such as a park bench, laundromat, or restaurant, and as unobtrusively as possible observe an individual for 10 minutes. Focus at first on only one area, such as posture, gestures, or facies. At the end of this time, and without discussion, write down all of the observations you have made. Then discuss them with your partner for similarities and differences. Alter the exercise by looking at different areas and eventually focus on several at a time.

The skill of observation is an absolute necessity to assess a client and his family. The nurse, in fulfilling most of her functions is in a position to utilize this skill frequently. She has more exposure to client's behaviors than the physician or other members of the multidisciplinary team. It is for this reason that she is the one who is called upon to set up a plan of care based on observation, assessment and conclusions drawn about the client's strengths, weaknesses, problems, and needs.

REFERENCES

1. Barnlund, D. C.: *Interpersonal Communication—Survey and Studies,* 2nd ed. New York, W. W. Norton and Company, 1963.
2. Blondis, M. N., and Jackson, B. E.: *Nonverbal Communication with Patients: Back to the Human Touch.* New York, John Wiley and Sons, 1977, p. 20.
3. Burgess, A. W., and Lazare, A.: *Psychiatric Nursing in the Hospital and the Community,* 2nd ed. Englewood Cliffs, N.J., Prentice-Hall Inc., 1976, pp. 14–15.
4. Robinson, L.: *Psychiatric Nursing as a Human Experience,* 2nd ed. Philadelphia, W. B. Saunders Company, 1977, p. 115.
5. Hein, E.: *Communication in Nursing Practice.* Boston, Little, Brown and Company, 1973, p. 155.
6. *Ibid.:* p. 151.
7. *Psychology Today: An Introduction.* Del Mar, Calif., Communications/Research/Machines, Inc., 1970, pp. 314–315, 344–345.
8. Hein, *op. cit.,* p. 152.
9. Blondis and Jackson, *op. cit.,* p. 5.
10. Hein, *op. cit.,* p. 201.
11. *Ibid.,* pp. 198–200.
12. Blondis and Jackson, *op. cit.,* pp. 6–8.
13. Francis, G. M., and Munjas, B. A.: *Manual of Socialpsychologic Assessment.* New York, Appleton-Century-Crofts, 1976, p. 158.
14. Fast, J.: *Body Language.* New York, Pocket Books Inc., 1970, p. 177.

CHAPTER 19

This chapter focuses on interviewing as one of the tools used in the collection of data. Before discussing interviewing, a brief look at the factors affecting communication is helpful to understand the process that occurs when two people have a meaningful or directed conversation or exchange of information.

FACTORS AFFECTING COMMUNICATION

Communication is a process in which information is sent out by one source and received by another. In order for this process to occur successfully, the sender's meaning must be clearly understood by the receiver. Feedback from the receiver must then be returned to the sender to verify not only that the message came through, but that its intended meaning remained intact. Interviewing is based on the full cycle of this process and cannot be successful if any of its elements or steps are lacking.

Chapter 18 dealt with observation and assessment of verbal and nonverbal behavior. All of the

INTERVIEWING: A TOOL FOR DATA COLLECTION

Maureen O'Brien Modesty, M.S., R.N., and
Arlyne B. Saperstein, M.N., R.N.

information in that chapter should be considered when interacting with or interviewing a client. The client's verbal responses cannot be isolated from the nonverbal; communication takes place on both levels, and words and actions combine to form a whole. Nonverbal behavior can verify a verbal response; take for example the question, "What did you think of the chemistry exam today?" If the answer, "Oh, I thought it was pretty simple. I was prepared for it," was accompanied by a smile, a look of confidence, and a relaxed body stance, the behavior appears to complement the answer. In other instances, the verbal and nonverbal responses may appear mismatched or at odds with one another. Consider the same question and answer, but this time the response is accompanied by tapping fingers, knitted brows, and a frown on the face. In this case, the impression is that the answer did not reflect the individual's true sentiments. In cases where there are inconsistencies between verbal and nonverbal responses, communication can break down or present problems. In addition to this

problem, the following list presents *factors which can positively or negatively affect the communication process* and should be considered when interacting with clients or other individuals. It should be noted that these factors affect both the client and the interviewer.

1. The environment in which communication takes place.
   a. Is the setting appropriate, comfortable, pleasant, and private?
   b. What are the distractions—noises, hectic activity, or other people?
2. The physiological status of both individuals involved.
   a. Is either person ill or experiencing any sensations or conditions which could be distracting—that is, pain, discomfort, headache, nausea, chills, or exhaustion?
   b. Are all senses functioning adequately, (e.g., hearing and sight)?
   c. Is there any alteration in functioning (e.g.,

decreased consciousness due to illness or medications, or an inability to stand, sit, or walk)?

3. The psychological status and personality traits of both individuals.

   a. Is there any problem with or alteration in perception or cognitive functioning? Do distortions occur? Are there delusions, hallucinations, or faulty logic?

   b. Are there specific behavioral patterns or characteristics—for example, withdrawal, dependence, anxiety, hostility, combative behavior, or insecurity?

   c. Is either individual concerned with personal, economic, or emotional problems other than those being discussed?

4. The intellectual, social or cultural characteristics of both individuals.

   a. Is a common language used? Are there differences in speech patterns, grammar, slang, use of technical terms, or jargon?

   b. Are there educational or intellectual differences that affect the communication and understanding of ideas or thoughts?

   c. Are messages decoded in the same manner? Do they have the same meaning for both individuals or can a second meaning exist?

   d. What are the individuals' personal philosophies, beliefs, and ethical and moral values as related to the material discussed?

   e. What cultural traits are apparent (e.g., gesturing with hands, short, clipped statements, stoicism, or aversion to discussing "personal" information (need for privacy)?

5. The circumstances involved in the current relationship between the individuals.

   a. What are the preconceived ideas that the individuals may have about one another? Has a client had an uncomfortable or negative experience with a nurse before which makes him now wary of this individual simply because she is a nurse? Is the person seen as an authority and, therefore, to be respected and accepted?

   b. Does the other individual appear to be considerate, warm, interested, "safe" or "trustworthy," or rude, cold, uninterested,

"threatening" or "untrustworthy"?

   c. Are the individuals strangers? How do they deal with personalities unknown to them?

   d. Is the topic of discussion perceived by both individuals as pleasant or unpleasant, meaningful or meaningless, relevant or irrelevant, important or trivial?

While the factors listed above can give the student a beginning understanding of the various things that interfere with or enhance communication, it is by no means complete. Communication is an intricate process; the variables are endless; any two people who interact bring to the situation different backgrounds, experiences, expectations, and feelings. For the nursing student who is facing her first interviewing experience, however, the information listed above should supplement a review of her studies in other areas to provide a comprehensive understanding of the basic concepts and principles of communication. English and language arts teach communication, both verbal (speech) and nonverbal (writing and reading). Psychology courses introduce the concepts of perception and cognition which influence the manner in which we communicate with and understand one another. Sociology and anthropology provide information on how social and cultural differences alter or affect communication between individuals or groups.

INTERVIEWING

There are innumerable reasons for conducting an interview; among these, the most prevalent is the collection of data to:

1. assess the client's past and present health status;
2. determine the client's health needs;
3. plan for his care; and
4. evaluate the effectiveness of care given.

Interviews are also utilized for health teaching, therapeutic purposes, and counseling.

This chapter focuses on the type of interview that is meant for assessment—the gathering of information or data. The principles discussed here, however, can be applied to all meaningful exchanges among the nurse, the client, and his family.

Interviewing is a process that is learned and refined through experience. A comfortable style for one individual may be quite different from that of another; there is no right or wrong way to interview a client. Therefore, rather than listing the specific steps to be used in interviewing, this chapter examines the issues and concerns that students universally experience when first confronted with the interviewing process. Instructors can be invaluable in helping students explore various "techniques" that may be useful in developing individual styles.

Being a professional person has many built in *responsibilities* to clients. The development of skill in interviewing is necessary for the nurse to meet the client's needs. Interviewing is a fairly easy task, yet a responsible one. Taking a position of responsibility as an interviewer is important to elicit information; determine needs; assist in carrying out the nursing process; and give the client a sense of dignity, importance, and individuality. This sense of responsibility is necessary whether the interview session is initiated by the client or the nurse. To achieve success in interviewing, it is necessary to remember what one is doing, the questions one is asking, the information one is eliciting, and the importance of this to the client and his health.

Beginning the Interview

An interview session does not necessarily take place in an office; most interviews conducted by nurses are in waiting rooms, examining rooms, or clients' rooms. Wherever they are conducted, it is important that both persons are comfortable. Many students in initial interviews may conduct the session by standing next to the seated client or they may even squat down next to the client, which is an uncomfortable position to conduct any meaningful exchange. This can convey to the client a need to keep the session superficial—that there is little time available for the session, although in fact there may be a great deal of available time.

In addition to *comfort,* the *surroundings* should be quiet. If the client is accompanied by others, it is necessary to provide *privacy* to allow the client to speak freely. This, except in rare situations, necessitates a place where the client and interviewer are alone. At some point in the session, it may be necessary to interview the accompanying relative

or significant other either with or without the client present; however, this should always be done with the permission of the client and with his awareness of the purpose of the exchange with the relative.

An appropriate opening statement or *introduction* is often neglected by new practitioners. An example of a suitable introduction is, "Good morning Mrs. Jones, I am Miss Smith, the nurse practitioner. I have some time to talk with you about how the clinic may be helpful to you." Since names are easily forgotten, a name tag is most helpful. In addition, if a time constraint exists, the client should be told of the limitations of the session at the onset.

The *purpose of the interview* should also be introduced at the beginning of the session with statements such as: (1) "How can we be helpful to you?" (2) "What brings you in?" or (3) "It would be helpful to your therapy if you could begin to share with me some of the concerns and thoughts you've had about your illness (or situation)." Each of these are *open-ended statements* that allow the client to begin anywhere. Some clients will respond, "Where shall I begin?" A useful answer might be, "How about at the beginning." Although in an interview situation most of the nurse's comments should be open-ended, this takes practice; the new interviewer will often ask questions that are more specific or *closed*. These will be examined later in this chapter. Questions which are leading such as, "You feel better today, don't you?" must be avoided as they actually set the client up for an expected or stereotyped response. This can drastically reduce the possibility of eliciting a spontaneous, informative answer since the client will usually fall into the trap of following "the script" or saying what he thinks he is supposed to say.

Additionally, asking more than one question at a time can be both confusing and self-defeating. To ask, "Have you been experiencing any other symptoms besides nausea during this pregnancy and how has the nausea affected your work in the restaurant?" splits the focus. The client can only respond to one aspect of the question, leaving the remaining question unanswered, lost, or forgotten as the client progresses with an attempt at answering the portion on which she focused. Dealing with the issues separately will assure that the questions are both addressed. Thus, one way to measure the nurse's interviewing skill is through her ability to phrase clear, open-ended questions which encourage the client to express himself.

Note Taking

It is possible to remember the information obtained in the interview without taking *copious* notes during the session if the interviewer listens carefully and allows time immediately following the interview to write notes. Note taking during the interview should be kept to a minimum, as many clients become self-conscious or concerned when they feel that everything they say is being recorded. Watching the nurse writing profusely may make the client feel that the interview is quite impersonal since eye contact and facial expressions are diminished, and pauses may be needed to allow the interviewer to complete her notes. Generally, the collection of demographic data necessary for forms and workings of the institution can be accomplished within the first several minutes of the session (i.e., name, address, age, type of work, ages of children, and telephone number). After this basic information is collected, the interviewer should put down the pencil and proceed with the interview. If necessary, she can then write down a few key words that will assist in reconstructing the interview after its termination. While seemingly difficult at first, this skill becomes easier with time, practice, and self-assurance.

Confidentiality

An extremely important issue which should be addressed at some point in *every* interview session is confidentiality. Although this can be discussed at any time during the interview, it is generally done either in the beginning or at the end of the session. Clients, when they seek professional help assume automatically that the data they share about themselves will be handled in a discreet and helpful way; that is, only those who need to know what they have shared about themselves will be allowed access to the information.

At the onset of the interview a general statement such as, "The things we discuss here will be confidential," is inadequate as it is lacking in scope as to the handling of the data gathered. The client should be told if material will be shared in a conference or an oral report to other health care personnel. When the limits of confidentiality are dis-

cussed early in the session, the client knows the system in which he is operating and can then make a judgment as to whether to continue in the session or to alter the terms. This discussion on the utilization of the material generally requires only two or three statements from the interviewer. For example, "I did want to say something about the way in which we operate here. What we talk about today will be discussed in a small staff conference in an attempt to determine how we may best assist you. Do you have any questions regarding this?"

What is discussed regarding confidentiality at the end of the session is generally a restatement of earlier comments as to the operating policies of the setting. It is useful to make a comment at the conclusion of the interview that lets the client know what will be done with the information that he has given. For instance, "It has been helpful to understand the difficulty you had in taking your medication. I will share this problem with the staff here at the clinic so that we can find a way to help you."

On occasion when the session is initiated by the client, for example, in a hospital unit or in a clinic, the client may approach the nurse and immediately begin to discuss a problem with which he is concerned. It is at the end of the interaction that the nurse makes a statement regarding confidentiality if the material is to be shared with others. However, it is not necessary for the nurse to make a comment regarding confidentiality in *every* client situation, but as a rule in formal nurse-client interviews, an explanation of how data will be handled is usually necessary.

Often a client will say or will wish to say something personal about himself and will ask the nurse not to share this information with others. It is important for the interviewer not to promise anything, such as *secrecy,* which may ultimately have to be rescinded. It is necessary for the practitioner to keep in mind that the reason for a nurse-client interaction is to provide help and assistance. What the nurse needs to convey to the client at this point is a desire to be of assistance, and if that help requires sharing information with others, she would, of course, let him know before doing so. If the nurse promises not to share something, then as a helping person she may be preventing assistance to a client who may be in great need of that help. Often when clients ask for a pledge of secrecy, they are really trying to ascertain whether they can *trust* that whatever they have just shared or are about to disclose to the interviewer will be handled discreetly—in a way which will help them yet not harm others. If the nurse perceives this to be the situation, then it is necessary to respond with a statement validating this awareness. The following is an example of this kind of interchange.

Client: If I tell you something will you promise not to tell anyone?

Nurse: Are you asking me if it is all right to talk with me about matters which are important to you and whether I will handle these things with respect and discretion?

Superficiality

It appears that the hesitancy of many new practitioners to take a responsible position in an interview session is related to their wondering, "What will I do if a client turns to me and requests things that I cannot deliver?" To minimize or avoid this terrifying situation (as perceived by the student), the total interview session is structured in a way that prevents the client from turning to the nurse and expecting more of her than she believes she can deliver. For this reason, the student needs considerable supervision with her interviewing skills to overcome her inclination toward keeping the interview on a superficial level. For clarification of situations in which students are asked a question to which they cannot respond, the following example is offered. A client turns to the student and asks, "What can I do to help me sleep better as I have not been sleeping well lately?" The student immediately forgets that the task in this session is to collect data and believes she must respond immediately in a supposedly helpful way by telling the client what to do to sleep more easily. However, she begins to have some concern because she has not yet attended "the class" on how to encourage sleep in insomniacs. She frets inwardly about the need to be responsible to clients and recalls in years past her grandmother drinking warm milk to help her with sleep. She then shares with the client the benefits of warm milk prior to retiring. This is a situation repeated constantly on the part of new practitioners—that is, being faced with a question by a client, believing any responsible and experienced practitioner would be able to respond to any

question, and trying to find an answer, sometimes from the reading but most often from their past experiences and observations.

The key to being a skilled interviewer is *not to feel a need to implement* at any time without adequate data. Since the goal of an interview is to know more about the person, the task is to collect data. This often requires that either the client's questions or his responses (or both) may need further exploration and clarification. In this way the nurse should make no assumptions about his intent or meaning but get as much information as possible before proceeding further. Most often implementation is easy once adequate data are collected. In the situation of the client who asks how he might sleep better, the interviewer needs to ask specific questions to gauge the degree of difficulty with sleep. Examples of questions that might be asked are:

1. What exactly has your sleep pattern been recently?
2. What time do you go to bed? How long before you fall asleep? How long before awakening?
3. How has the sleep pattern changed from that in the past?
4. What have you done to help increase sleep?
5. What has helped? What has not helped?
6. Have you received suggestions from others? If so, have they been helpful?

Then the most important question that the interviewer can ask the client is, "In thinking about your sleeplessness, why do you think there has been a change in your sleep pattern?" The interviewer must remember that clients most often think about the why of their behavior, and although they may not be able to identify the exact cause of difficulty, they may provide a number of interesting and important clues which provide valuable insight as to what they are like.

A second way in which superficiality is manifested is exemplified by the interviewer who says just what *she* thinks the client wants to hear; for example, "Don't worry about a thing, we will have you better in no time." In essence, this cuts the client off; it does not allow him to state his concerns and express his anxiety. It immediately suppresses the necessary exploration of material which may be painful and difficult. There is no gain here (other than avoidance of issues) for either the interviewer or the client.

Superficiality is also evident in the nurse's failure to pursue to any degree meaningful content mentioned or alluded to by the client. The following example is one in which the interviewer might not pursue content offered freely by the client:

A client talks about her husband's sudden and massive illness which has resulted in his hospitalization for open heart surgery. The student gains information about his present state, his concerns about recurrent heart problems, and a view of his life previous to the sudden onset of his difficulties—all important information, but lacking in data related to the effects on the family. As the wife describes the extraordinary measures taken to keep this man alive, an issue which one immediately might wonder about is the toll this situation has taken on the family. Very often these problems may take the form of a financial crisis, yet the new interviewer often believes that she is intruding if she asks about money. An appropriate and simple question might be, "Did insurance cover all the expenses?" (Obviously many other questions would also be appropriate.)

It is important to collect data on issues related to the one being discussed, with some degree of completeness, to develop a total picture of the situation. As in the above example, cost of the hospitalization, changes in the family's life style, changes in the sex life of the couple, and effects on the children are just a few areas that might be pursued. The appropriate time at which to ask questions about finances or sex can only be gauged with experience; however, if a wife and husband are discussing their marriage in detail and fail to bring up either subject, it is perfectly legitimate and necessary for the interviewer to then ask directly, "Are there any difficulties with finances?" or "Have there been any problems or changes in your sexual relationship?" Clients, when asked these questions, often respond in a candid way, frequently thankful that a subject of concern to them has been opened by the interviewer, an accepting neutral person with whom to talk about these issues. A frequent problem on the part of the new practitioner is the belief that asking personal questions of the client is an *intrusion* into his personal affairs. This belief hampers the nurse in following up issues and concerns of the client and almost invariably causes the session to be a waste of time, with neither the client nor the nurse gaining much from the session.

The ability to ask relevant questions about an area of difficulty helps the client turn to the nurse as someone with whom he can talk and who shows an interest in him. The goal in an interview session (i.e., to collect data) needs to be remembered continually by the practitioner in order to discover how clients maintain their health, what are the pitfalls in maintaining health, and what are issues they face in their attempts to increase or maintain their health status. To enhance the interview session so that the clients find the interviewer a helpful, caring person, someone who is easy to talk with, the interviewer needs to *focus* in and collect comprehensive data on any issue that has been identified as a problem. At this point when collecting data, there is no need on the part of the practitioner to believe any implementation needs to take place.

A way of gauging a successful interview is in the collection of relevant data which are helpful both to the client and the nurse for clarification and planning. A favorable attribute for an interviewer is the development of the belief that "I am someone to whom people can open up." As the nurse improves her ability to conduct a meaningful or helpful interview, clients will frequently comment, "It is so nice to have someone to talk to about these concerns," or "You are the first one I have been able to share these things with." These verbalizations of the client help the nurse to improve her interviewing skills.

Value Judgments

As the student learns the ways of interviewing, she will often identify those persons or individuals with whom she is most successful. New practitioners often have no way of gauging a successful interview and instead tend to make judgments as to how nice the person was; that is, the client has not told them anything which new practitioners deem as unacceptable in relationship to their own values. Making value judgments on the data collected is one of the first items which must be discarded by the new practitioner; for example, "This client is terrible because he beats his wife and children," or "This woman is bad because she has had innumerable affairs throughout her marriage." Instead, the student should feel delighted that the client can share these problems with her, that she can create an environment in which the client can speak about his personal life without fear of criticism and with a feeling of acceptance of him as a person.

The gauge of being a successful interviewer is not to be able to list all those behaviors that people deem as the least acceptable, but to derive a more complete picture of the person being interviewed. Equally important is having a sense of *the client's successes.* A partial list of some successes people might have includes: (1) being able to maintain a marriage or relationship with a significant other; (2) to hold a job for more than a brief time; (3) to give to and care about people; (4) to maintain family ties; and (5) to achieve success in their play.

Erikson has defined health as the ability to work, to love, and to play.[6] As interviewers nurses should be interested in how people maintain their health, what things have they done in each of the areas identified by Erikson to strive for health, and what have been the pitfalls in the maintenance of health.

Behavioral Changes in the Interviewer

To develop skills in interviewing, the student should make certain changes in her behavior. It is necessary for the interviewer to avoid any *distracting behaviors* such as toying with objects, such as pencils or paper clips, tapping fingers, or swinging feet while seated. The time available for the session is the client's time, not the interviewer's. Knowing this, any behaviors which put the focus on the practitioner need to be put aside. The most important way in which to accomplish this is *being quiet about oneself.* The need to interject personal feelings and experiences about similar events in the client's dialogue should be suppressed; this seems to be one of the most difficult skills for the practitioner to incorporate. Examples of the dialogue between students and clients showing the interviewer's tendency to do this are frequently evident. An illustration of this would be:

Client: I have recently moved to the city.
Student: Me too—what an adjustment—especially being afraid to go about the city.

Client: Oh yes, someone tried to steal my pocketbook this past week, but I just pulled it away. When I lived in Meadowbrook that never happened; I could even leave the door unlocked when I went out for the day.
Student: Oh, you were from Meadowbrook? I am from Shady Grove, the next town away.

What happened in this dialogue was the failure to collect data about the client's situation—that is, a *lack of focus on the client.* Instead the new practitioner easily assumed her own way of relating to someone as if this was strictly a *social exchange.* Having had this recent experience, the student probably was in a most favorable situation to elicit data from the client on the adjustments and difficulties in moving to the city. The student failed to use her own insight to enhance the data collected in this session. The following two statements would have helped the interviewer to focus on the client and her situation rather than on the similarities between the client and herself: "Have you found it an adjustment moving into the city?" and "What brought you to the city?" To be able to focus on someone outside oneself and to put aside the need to share similar experiences with the client are mandatory. In most cases, it is not necessary or helpful for the client to hear that you attended the same high school or that you also had a close relative die of cancer.

Learning how to interview is like learning a part in a play; initially it may seem mechanical and stilted. Frequently the new interviewer will fight being cast into some strange role that seems to be preventing her real self from coming forth and that appears to treat the client as less than unique. Learning this skill requires some change in the new interviewer, but after a short time in this new role her comfort and satisfaction with her ability to focus in on another person is a delightful experience.

To be a skilled interviewer, the nurse needs experience with life; an excitement and joy at looking at human behavior; and an appreciation, sensitivity, and acceptance of the many ways in which people behave. At times the interviewer may be caught up with her own values, but these, like the need to share some of her similar experiences with the client, must be discarded. The student in developing her interviewing skills should focus on all of the behaviors she sees about her and on her knowledge of human behavior and its landmarks in development. This knowledge of human life is important as it helps the nurse to formulate *relevant questions* in the interview. Two examples of questions which are relevant follow. Naturally many other questions could be relevant.

1. A woman is pregnant with her first child. *Interviewer:* "What do you foresee as changes that will come about in your marriage with the birth of the baby?"
2. A woman talks about her present life and some of the increased responsibilities she has: her 90-year-old mother who is living with her is becoming increasingly frail; her retarded adult child needs more of her supervision because of the frailness of the client's mother; her husband has been hospitalized most of the past year with some vague physical and emotional symptoms necessitating increased responsibility on her part in maintaining the family business. *Interviewer:* "How are you coping with all of this increased stress?"

Perceptions of the Interviewer

To be a successful interviewer, the nurse must recognize her own perceptions—that is, she should have an awareness of personal feelings and reactions throughout the session. This can only come about after the student ceases to interject her own experiences, has minimized her need to judge a client's behavior as either acceptable or unacceptable and has developed the ability to focus on the client. Sharing perceptions with the client for validation helps to enhance this focus and adds immeasurably toward the goal of interviewing for data collection. When sharing perceptions, it may be useful to say, "It seems as if," or "I wonder if," or "It sounds as if." Generally the perceptions are shared in the form of a statement with a question mark, rather than a direct question. The ability to recognize, use, and validate our perceptions in terms of what the client is talking about is perhaps the most useful and exciting skill to develop. The following are examples of the sharing of perceptions:

1. An elderly woman is talking about living on social security, having just received a 5 per-

cent increase in her check to keep up with the cost of living. She then adds that Medicare payments went up $1.70 a month; her rent is going up $7.00 next month and she has learned that it is questionable whether she remains eligible for food stamps with her social security increase. *Interviewer:* "It sounds like it is pretty difficult making a go of things financially?"
2. A client lives alone, hampered with limited mobility due to severe arthritis, and seldom leaves her apartment. She states, "Oh, I have been waiting for you all day. I was hoping you would not forget." *Interviewer:* "It gets lonely for you at times?"

The reader may or may not have the same perceptions in the above examples, but it is not important that our perceptions are identical or similar. What is important is that we are recognizing our perceptions and validating them with the client.

Validation of perceptions allows the interviewer to develop her own style, but this occurs only after she has developed a beginning ability to focus first on the client. Validation occurs only after one begins to *listen and hear* what clients are saying. Perceptions are inner feelings, an awareness within the interviewer as to the struggles and issues that are confronting the client being interviewed. Often the new practitioner is hesitant to share her perceptions with the client because she is fearful that she may not be accurate. This is just the point. Perceptions are shared to validate our inner feelings and awareness of the issues confronting the individual. Generally, whether our perceptions are accurate or not they enhance the collection of data, and they most often create in the client an awareness of someone who is listening and interested in them, and help the client with the articulation of those matters they wish to discuss.

The Issue of Age

An issue that seems to be of concern to many new interviewers is that of the client's age in comparison to their own, particularly when students are in their late teens or early twenties. Frequently the student is confronted with a client who might reflect on how young she is, and the student often feels young, inexperienced, and awkward when interviewing someone the same age as her parents. The issue of age is almost a universal concern for the student. However, age is generally irrelevant to the interviewing process, and the student must keep in mind that many helping professionals are younger than the clients, a fact to which clients must become accustomed. With this awareness on the part of the interviewer, the issue of the young practitioner generally requires little attention in the interview. If there is need for comment, the practitioner can take the issue of being young as a compliment or wonder with the client if they are finding many health or other professionals as younger than themselves. Most often there is no need for comment unless further pursued by the client.

Hesitancy

Another issue that arises in an interview session is the hesitancy of clients to talk about issues and concerns with which they are presently faced. This is almost a universal difficulty when interviewing adolescents whether the interviewer is the same age as the adolescent or older. Hesitancy or lack of an adequate response may be observed in the interview session when clients respond to specific questions on the subject asked without any further elaboration. For example:

Interviewer: How many children do you have?
Client: Three.
Interviewer: Boys and girls?
Client: No, all boys.
Interviewer: What are their ages?
Client: 9, 11, and 15.

Questions such as these are examples of *closed questions*; they demand a direct answer or statement—most often a "yes" or "no"—and do not leave the client an opening for discussion or exploration. This type of question is often appropriate when very specific information is needed (e.g., "What is the name of the medication you are currently taking for your diabetes?"). In the situation presented above, the client responds to the direct question without offering any further information. Here the interviewer must use some specific techniques to aid in the dialogue of the client. If a new subject is raised by the interviewer, as in this example with the issue of children, the interviewer needs to preface her question with an explanation of why the subject is being introduced. For example, "One of the things I am interested in hearing about is your everyday life; for example, what about children?" This presents an area for the client to talk about because he has been informed of the direction the interview is to take. It may be necessary to add a comment about how important it is for an interviewer to understand the client's present life style in order to thoroughly comprehend the health related issue for which he initially sought help. For instance, "It is helpful to my understanding of what can be done for your headaches if I know what your everyday life is like. For example, do you work? Do you have children?"

Often the new practitioner is unwilling to accept hesitancy or *silence* at all in the interview session, and she finds herself asking any question that comes to mind in order to seem as if she is in perfect control of the session. Students should remember that it is perfectly legitimate to *pause and reflect* on what the client has just stated. The pause and reflection may be done silently by the interviewer or one can *recap* verbally with the client the essence of the recent exchange. An interviewer might say "Let's see. You have two sons who are 4 years apart, 4 and 8, and you have been married 12 years. You returned to work 1 year ago for the first time in your marriage. Was there any particular reason for your returning to work a year ago?" Also, the interviewer should allow the client time to pause without immediately asking another question. It is much easier to collect data if the interviewer's questions are few. To do this, it is necessary to create an expectation that this is the client's time to talk. Use statements such as, "Could you tell me about that?" or "Go on," or "What other things do you do," or "When that happens, tell me what goes through your mind." Each of the above statements are open-ended, do not introduce a new topic, and most often create within the client the feeling that his role in this interview is to talk about himself. Generally, avoiding direct questions and having the client initiate the discussion is more helpful in the collection of data, as the client most often will bring up issues and concerns which are relevant to himself. When the interviewer takes the role of initiating discussions on most topics during the session, it can generally be assumed that items of concern for the client have been overlooked. It is important then to realize that during the session, it will most often be necessary for both the client and interviewer to pause and to allow moments for silence, where each participant has time to reflect on what has been discussed, and for the interviewer to form questions that may be more open-ended.

When the client seems reluctant or hesitant to talk about an issue or even talk at all, it is necessary for the interviewer to validate this perception with the client: "You seem hesitant to talk about your marriage (your physical complaints or your earlier life, etc.)." It is important to remember that although the interviewer may initiate an area of discussion, validation of the client's desire not to talk about an issue needs to occur. It is then useful to make the statement, "Fine, we do not have to discuss this, but I was wondering about your hesitancy." Initiate the discussion of the hesitancy rather than the subject itself. The above statement is most helpful in obtaining a more complete awareness of the client. It is generally a good rule to question or to look into all behaviors that may be seen; for example, in the waiting room the interviewer sees the client accompanied by a man. She may check her perceptions during the interview by, "Was the person in the waiting room your husband?" but only when it fits into the discussion. If the person is carrying a book, awareness of what he is reading may be helpful in creating a more complete picture of the client.

Hesitancy is often reflected in the client's comments, "I do not want to bore you," or "You are too busy to have time to listen to all this," or "I have told people all of this before." In some situations you may need to reassure the client of your willingness to listen and state that in fact this is exactly what you want to hear from him. In other situations, the client may need some further clarification as to what is to be done with the data that are being collected, how it will be helpful to him, and specifically with whom the information will be shared. If none of the suggestions above are successful, the client can be asked if there is someone else with whom he wishes to speak. There is no way, after all, that he can be forced to participate.

Termination of the Interview

At what point does an interview end? How is it concluded? Termination is usually individualized and unique. When the nurse's or the client's time constraints have been identified at the onset of the interview, then the point at which the session ends is rather clear. When this distinction has not been made, then it may be up to the nurse to determine what constitutes "the end." Ideally both participants will feel that their goals have been achieved and that further discussion is not needed at this time. A natural break is usually quite apparent in this case. Clues such as restlessness, distraction, or a tired expression may indicate that the client wants to conclude. It is quite appropriate to ask, "Are you feeling weary?" or "Would you prefer to continue this discussion at another time?"

When the interviewer is aware that time is running out, it is often very effective to make a statement such as, "It appears that time is getting short (or the hour is getting late), so perhaps we should stop at this time. I would be happy to answer any questions that may remain before you leave." Of course it should be reiterated that the collection of data is an ongoing process. Although an interview ends, quite likely there will be some form of follow-up by either the same individual or another member of the health care team.

CONCLUSION

What then does the client gain from an interview session? Most clients have operated for some time within the health care system and are aware that there usually are no easy answers to questions they may have. However, the ability of practitioners to focus on any problems or issues identified by the client helps the client sense their concern; verbalizations are important and worthy of focus and exploration. Any recognition by the health care professional of what it is that the client considers relevant and important creates an immediate feeling within the client that there is someone who cares and is paying attention to him. In society, in the everyday world of exchange between people, most individuals are not particularly interested in how people feel and what their health concerns might be. This is easily seen in the mechanical expression often used by people in greeting each other, "How are you?" "Fine, thank you," whether that is the case or not. So what we automatically give clients in an interview situation is permission to talk about their health and themselves for a given period of time without fear or concern that the focus on themselves and their health is unacceptable. Acceptance, a forum to talk about oneself and one's health, is not to be negated by the practitioner; it is all important in beginning any exchange between the client and the nurse. "But is this all we can give clients?" is often the concern of the student without remembering that an interview is only one of the many skills available to the nurse in assisting clients. The interview does not accomplish all that we wish to do for and with clients, nor should it ever be thought of as more than a beginning exchange between client and nurse. If the nurse has too many goals for an interview, she negates its importance.

The ability to learn how to interview can be taught fairly easily to most students, although at present too little time is given to the teaching and development of this skill. The art of interviewing cannot be learned in a 2 hour class or after reading a chapter. Although both may be helpful, this skill is most often developed in school and with on-the-job supervision. It should be remembered that skill in interviewing takes years of practice and that the ideas and thoughts presented here will not be incorporated by the student nurse immediately.

REFERENCES

1. Becknell, E., and Smith, D. M.: *System of Nursing Practice.* Philadelphia, F. A. Davis Co., 1975.
2. Bernstein, L., Bernstein, R., and Dana, R.: *Interviewing: A Guide for Health Professionals,* 2nd ed. New York, Appleton-Century-Crofts, 1974.
3. Bird, B.: *Talking with Patients,* 2nd ed. Philadelphia, J. B. Lippincott, 1973.
4. Bolozoni, N., and Beach, B.: Premature reassurance: a distancing maneuver. *Nurs. Outlook* 23:49–51, 1975.
5. Engel, G., and Morgan, W.: *Interviewing the Patient.* Philadelphia, W. B. Saunders Co., 1973.
6. Erikson, E.: *Childhood and Society.* New York, W. W. Norton Co., 1963, p. 266.
7. Fowkes, W. Jr., and Hunn, B.: *Clinical Assessment for the Nurse Practitioner.* St. Louis, C. V. Mosby Co., 1973.
8. Gillies, D., and Alyn, I.: *Patient Assessment and Management by the Nurse Practitioner.* Philadelphia, W. B. Saunders Co., 1976.
9. Hardiman, M. A.: Interviewing? or social chit-chat? *Am. J. Nurs.* 71(7):1379–1381, 1971.
10. Loesch, L., and Loesch, N.: What do you say after you say mm-hmm? *Am. J. Nurs.* 75:807–809, 1975.
11. Marshall, J. C., and Feeney, S.: Structured versus intuitive intake interview. *Nurs. Res.* 21:272, 1972.
12. Rogers, C.: *On Becoming a Person.* Boston, Houghton-Mifflin Co., 1961.
13. Sundeen, S., et al.: *Nurse-Client Interaction.* St. Louis, C. V. Mosby Co., 1976.

CHAPTER 20

The health history is a comprehensive record of the client's health background, his manner of living, present and past health problems, and family health perspective. The accumulated health data base determines the direction for exploring the client's problem. Accuracy facilitates a relevant physical examination and permits correlation of physical findings with the information acquired.

The objective of the health history is to gather information about the client and his problem which is not available from other sources. Recording the history establishes a relationship between a member of the health care team and the client that facilitates the process of diagnosis and treatment and affords the client a better understanding of his problem.

The quality of the health history depends upon the skills of the interviewer. The interview should be a formal oral exchange of information and feelings for the purpose of eliciting meaningful data. (See Chapter 19 on interviewing.) To elicit information fundamental to evaluation of a client's con-

THE HEALTH HISTORY

Pearl P. Rosendahl, Ed.D., R.N., and
Arlyne B. Saperstein, M.N., R.N.

dition, a good working relationship must be established. The interviewer should radiate warmth and caring and exhibit a nonjudgmental attitude.

The interview is opened with a courteous greeting and an introduction which includes the interviewer's name and title. The interviewer must listen carefully to the client's story. It is important to use open-ended statements that provide the client opportunities to express his concerns. Questions are asked to clarify data and direct attention to the specific area under investigation. If the client is encouraged to speak freely, greater insight will be gained into the client's personality and mental status. In addition, it is necessary to observe and interpret nonverbal communication or body language, comparing statements with facial expressions, postures, and gestures that convey feelings. This examination begins when the interview opens and continues until the history is complete.

As data are collected, evaluated, and synthesized, a nursing diagnosis can be contemplated, and appropriate plans can be constructed. An or-

ganized and logical health history should be obtained from the client. The following health history-taking format logically considers the components of an effective health history:

1. Basic data.
2. Informant.
3. Chief complaint—that is, the reason for visit.
4. Personal and social history.
5. History of present problem.
6. History of past problems.
7. Review of systems.
8. Family history.

ANALYSIS OF COMPONENTS OF HEALTH HISTORY

Basic Data

Basic data should include the client's name, nationality, age, sex, race, date and place of birth, and occupation.

Informant

Initially, the source and reliability of the information obtained should be listed. The client is usually the informant. However, if the client is a child, or is confused, unconscious, or incapable of speech, other sources are used, for example, family members, old records, or social workers.

Chief Complaint

The chief complaint will be divulged as the interviewer requests, "Tell me about your problem." Once identified, this should be recorded verbatim with quotation marks; it should not be translated into a diagnosis. Also the duration of the complaint should be ascertained.

Personal and Social History

The *personal and social history* aid in evaluating the client holistically. To determine the client's marital status, education, military service, economic status, living environment, dietary habits, and use of tobacco, alcohol, and medications the following questions should be asked: "Are you or have you ever been married?" If so, the number and duration of marriages, and the age, status, and health of spouses and children should be elicited. "What is the extent of your education?" will provide a clue to the client's level of comprehension. "What is your present occupation?" may help with planning when the client is discharged from care. In addition, prior jobs and military service that may have a causal relationship to the present illness should be analyzed. Certain occupations are considered hazardous since they entail exposure to toxins or physical and emotional stresses. Questions such as "What is your combined yearly family income, including all sources?" and "Do you have health insurance?" may identify financial concerns that can interfere with the client's treatment regimen. Referrals to other members of the health team, such as social workers, should be effected when necessary. Environmental factors may impinge upon the client's health; pertinent questions might be: "Do you live in an apartment or a house? How many rooms are in your home? How many bathrooms? Are there stairs? How many members are in your household? What are their ages? What are their

relationships to you?" The client's responses will assist in the design of a meaningful home rehabilitative care plan. "What are your favorite foods? What is your typical breakfast? Lunch? Supper? Snacks?" Probing questions enable assessment of the nutritional adequacy of the client's diet. Inquiries about the client's use of drugs, alcohol, and medications should include quantities, frequencies, and intolerances. As most people tend to minimize consumption, always ask the client for an *exact* estimate of quantity. "*How many* bottles of beer (or hard liquor) do you drink each day?" "*How many* packages of cigarettes do you smoke each day?" "What specific medications do you take during the course of the day?" These include oral contraceptives, aspirin, aspirin-like compounds, antacids, and other patent medicines.

History of Present Problem

The history of the present problem is a narrative description of the problem of primary importance to the client. All symptoms relating to the chief complaint are described chronologically, both subjectively and objectively, beginning when the complaint first arose and continuing to the present, being sure to sequentially date events and symptoms and include all hospitals, medications, physicians, special studies, and surgical procedures involved. Each symptom requires the following: (1) date and mode of onset; (2) character of the complaint; (3) course and duration; (4) location; (5) a review of the specific organ systems likely to be involved; (6) relationship to other symptoms, bodily functions, and activities; and (7) effect of measures taken to relieve or improve the client's condition.

Suggested questions to obtain this information include: "Tell me about your problem from the time it began until now." "Describe your symptoms." If the client has difficulty describing a symptom, for example, pain, descriptive terms can be provided typically in a question to assist him. "Is it gnawing, shooting, or throbbing?" The client should also be asked the duration of a single attack as well as the frequency of the problem. "Point to where you are uncomfortable" is a reliable way to pin down the troubled site, since the client's perception of location may be quite different from the interviewer's. A complete review of the organ systems which seem to be implicated should be done. A complaint of "chest pain" for example, should include all questions pertinent to the cardiovascular system; however, it is important to remember that disorders of other systems could also cause chest pain. (See Review of Systems.) Questions such as, "Was your discomfort aggravated when you ingested food or climbed stairs?" and "What relieved your discomfort?" aid in the identification of symptoms. Significant findings should also be recorded. It is important to learn what clusters of symptoms tend to reflect changes in tissues, organs, or functions.

History of Past Problems

The history of past problems should contain a review of health maintenance practices, childhood diseases, allergies, serious medical illnesses, surgical procedures, injuries, mental illnesses, obstetrical history, and systems review. Each category should include the dates of occurrence, complications, if any, and sequelae. Health maintenance data should include the results of the last complete physical examination and the dates of all immunizations and any reactions (mumps, measles, German measles (rubella), whooping cough, tetanus, smallpox, poliomyelitis, tuberculosis, and diphtheria). The client should be asked if and when he contracted chickenpox, diphtheria, measles, rubella, rheumatic fever, scarlet fever, or whooping cough. Females should be asked for the date and results of the last Papanicolaou test. Allergies and drug sensitivities are determined by: "What allergies do you have?" "Do you get reactions from any drugs?" "Are you allergic to any foods, insect stings, or other phenomena?" "Are you susceptible to asthma, hay fever, hives, or eczema?" "Tell me about other illnesses you have had." The client is asked about specific symptoms, causes, course of illness, treatment, complications, and any residual disability. "Have you ever been hospitalized?" If so, information about the institution, diagnosis, treatment, and recurrence should be obtained. "Tell me about your operations." If any, ask when and where the surgery was performed, what the procedure was, and who was the surgeon. "Have you ever had a severe injury or accident?" Inquire about stitches, broken bones, or a loss of consciousness. "Have you ever had a nervous breakdown or other emo-

tional problems?" If there has been trauma, determine what precipitated the occurrence. Symptoms, treatment, and persistent emotional disturbances must be detailed. Obstetrical history should include the client's age at menarche; the type, frequency, duration, and volume of blood flow; the number of pregnancies and live births, including any complications of pregnancy and delivery; age at menopause; and the quality of sexual relationships.

Review of Systems

The *review of systems* is a set of questions about common symptoms involving every organ system progressing from the head towards the feet. This review enables the interviewer to ask the client about the past and present status of every organ system and to search for symptoms that may be relevant to the present problem. Grouping of symptoms helps to identify relationships. Initially, questioning should be general; for example, "Have you had any difficulty with your skin?" If the response is positive, specific questions requiring explanations and details are asked. The absence, as well as the presence, of symptoms should be recorded to avoid later confusion about their existence. If the symptoms have previously been recorded in the data collection of the *history of present problem,* a referencing notation is made in the appropriate section of *review of systems.* The divisions of the review of systems are listed in Table 20-1.

GENERAL STATE OF HEALTH. The client should be asked about his general well-being, including recent changes in weight, fatigue, fever, chills, and weakness.

TABLE 20-1. Systems to Review during the Health History

General state of health	Respiratory system
Skin	Cardiovascular system
Neurological system	Gastrointestinal system
Head	Urinary system
Ears	Genitalia
Eyes	Musculoskeletal system
Nose and sinuses	(including extremities)
Mouth and throat	Endocrine system
Neck	Hematopoietic system
Breasts	

SKIN. Ask about past dermatological problems and current changes in the texture, temperature, and color of the skin, hair, and nails; also inquire about allergies, infections, lesions that are slow to heal, nevi, pain, and trauma.

NEUROLOGICAL SYSTEM. The client should be questioned about susceptibility to seizure disorders, syncope (dizziness or fainting), and loss of consciousness. Questions are introduced relating to mental status if the client does not think clearly, forgets easily, evidences disturbed interpersonal relationships, or appears to be disoriented, nervous, or depressed. Any history of psychiatric therapy should be noted. Psychiatric questions would concern nervousness, depression, insomnia, and nightmares. Questions related to motor disturbances would be proper if the client has diminished strength in his arms or legs, weakness on one side of his body, paralysis, or a loss of balance or coordination. Sensory changes of significance include numbness, tingling, or burning sensations anywhere in the body.

HEAD. Ask if there is any history of head injuries or persistent headaches. The source of most headaches is either vascular (migraine) or muscular (tension headaches), but headaches may also arise from eyestrain, infections, tumors, fatigue, allergies, and alcohol.

EYES. The client should be asked when his eyes were last examined and if he wears corrective lenses. Has he any history of glaucoma or cataracts? Visual problems may stem from hyperopia (farsightedness), myopia (nearsightedness), astigmatism (change in curvature of the cornea or lens), strabismus (both eyes do not focus in same direction), nystagmus (constant movement of eyeball), color blindness, glaucoma, or cataracts. Other problems which should be unraveled are pain, inflammation, infection, discharge, diplopia (double vision) and excessive or decreased tearing.

EARS. Ask about a hearing aid and the results of any hearing tests. Determine exposure to unusually loud noises, taking particular note of duration. Current problems requiring investigation are infections, earaches, hearing problems, tinnitus (ringing in the ear), and vertigo (dizziness or a feeling of moving in space).

NOSE AND SINUSES. Question the client about the annual frequency of colds, nasal discharge, recurrent epistaxis (nosebleeds), polyps, allergies, sinusitis, sneezing, or any change in the sense of smell.

MOUTH AND THROAT. Ask about the last dental examination; dentures; pain; sore throats; hoarseness; lesions of the tongue, gums, teeth, or throat; and difficulty in chewing, tasting, or swallowing.

NECK. Investigate any limitation of movement, pain, swelling of the lymph glands, or enlargement of the thyroid gland.

BREASTS. Ask the age of onset of breast development and lactation. Ascertain if the client has any history of breast lumps, mammography (x-rays of breast), surgery, or trauma. Males and females alike should be questioned concerning discharge, other changes in the nipples, dimpling or tenderness; men should be asked about gynecomastia (abnormally large breasts). Is the client taking oral contraceptives or hormonal replacements? Does she examine her own breasts regularly? Any findings of breast self-examination should be recorded.

RESPIRATORY SYSTEM. Take a history of chest colds, pneumonia, tuberculosis, and other lung diseases. If the client smokes, ask how many packages per day and for how many years. Record the date and results of the last chest x-ray. Current problems to be investigated include coughing; dyspnea (difficult respirations); hemoptysis (bloody sputum); pain associated with breathing; sputum production; and wheezing. Coughs should be described as dry or productive; dyspnea by its time of occurrence, degree, and type; hemoptysis by amount and time of occurrence; pain associated with breathing by location, character, and duration; sputum by its consistency, volume, and odor; and wheezing by its timing and severity.

CARDIOVASCULAR SYSTEM. The client should be asked if he has a history of rheumatic fever, hypertension, heart attack, heart murmur, enlarged heart, edema, abnormal chest x-ray or electrocardiogram, elevated blood lipids (i.e., cholesterol or triglycerides), other special tests, such as cardiac catheterization, or circulatory disorders, such as varicose veins, and thrombophlebitis. Pain should be characterized by location, radiation, quality, severity, duration, time of occurrence, and manner of aggravation or relief; associated symptoms, such as dyspnea on exertion (e.g., walking a few blocks or up a flight of stairs), palpitations (e.g., rapid beating, forceful beating, or irregular beating), and syncope (related to vascular or central nervous system conditions) should also be noted.

GASTROINTESTINAL SYSTEM. Ask about any history of hernias; hepatitis; jaundice; ulcers; and surgery or trauma to the appendix, gallbladder, liver, or spleen. Does the client wear a prosthesis or a colostomy appliance? If the client reports anorexia (loss of appetite), then severity, duration and associated nausea and vomiting are noted. Is there pain that may be associated with certain anatomical areas within the gastrointestinal tract: for example, esophageal pain appears in the midsubsternal area; gastric pain in the midepigastrium; biliary and hepatic pain in the right upper quadrant with radiation to the right infrascapular region; colonic pain in the midline and slightly to the side of the affected colon; and splenic pain through radiation, to left chest and shoulder. (These will be described further in the following chapter.) Nausea and vomiting, pyrosis (heartburn), and flatulence may be associated with biliary tract disease or peptic ulcers. Note also any changes in bowel habits, frequency or stool color (particularly clay-colored or black, tarry stools), and the presence of hemorrhoids. The client should identify the character, color, and frequency of all excretions (e.g., drainage, bleeding, stool, or vomitus). Any abdominal pain should be characterized by location, quality, onset, manner of aggravation and relief, and other associated symptoms. Ask the client about his use of antacids and laxatives.

URINARY SYSTEM. Take histories of urinary infections or protein (albumin) or sugar in the urine. Current problems of frequency and urgency may be associated with infection of the urinary tract; hesitancy and nocturia (excessive urination at night) may indicate benign prostatic hypertrophy (enlarged prostate gland) or nocturia alone, diabetes, or congestive heart failure. Changes in urine are manifested by hematuria (blood in the urine),

pyuria (pus in the urine), and sediment; these arise not only as a result of disease but also from diagnostic tests and medications. Incontinence should be characterized according to frequency, time and relation to activity.

GENITALIA. Male. Ask about surgery (e.g., circumcision, hernia repair, hemorrhoids, prostate gland), venereal disease, carcinoma, testicular pain or swelling, problems with the prostate gland, sexual problems, (e.g., impotence, altered sexual drive, and sterility) burning, lesions, or discharge, (which may be related to venereal diseases or herpes genitalis).

Female. Ask about venereal disease, blood clots, abnormal bleeding, (characterized by amount and time of occurrence), leukorrhea (white or yellow vaginal discharge), pruritus (itching), burning, pain, lesions, changes in temperament or mood, sexual habits and method of contraception.

MUSCULOSKELETAL SYSTEM. Ask for a past history of trauma, surgery, arthritis, gout, or the use of back braces. Conceivable current problems are swelling of varicose veins; intermittent claudication (pain and lameness in the calf muscles); extremity pain during walking; continuously cold hands and feet; joint pain, swelling, heat, redness, stiffness, and deformity; bursitis; muscle weakness (sometimes associated with neurologic or muscular disease); myalgia (muscle pain); backache (sometimes caused by a herniated intervertebral disc); and abnormal gait. Determine if there is any limitation of normal daily activities caused by malfunctions of the musculoskeletal system.

ENDOCRINE SYSTEM. Ask about histories of goiter, exophthalmos (protrusion of the eyeball), unusual growth pattern, changes in skin pigmentation, unusual weight gain, and any special tests (e.g., basal metabolism or urine tested for sugar and acetone). Check for current heat or cold intolerance; changes in skin texture, pigmentation, dryness, or perspiration; changes in hair distribution; and polyuria (increased urine production); polydipsia (increased thirst); or polyphagia (increased hunger).

HEMATOPOIETIC SYSTEM. Ascertain whether the client has had anemia, bleeding tendencies, lymphadenopathy (swelling of lymph nodes), blood dyscrasia, exposure to toxic agents, and transfusions or transfusion reactions. Document the client's latest blood count. Check for current fatigue, easy bruising, and tender or suppurative (pus producing) nodes. The client's blood type should be recorded.

Family History

The family history is helpful in resolving the client's problem. Assess the health status of the client's family (mother, father, siblings, and children), recording ages and health status of those still living and the ages and causes of death of the deceased. Ask if any other family member has a similar complaint. Use a history form or the list of diseases in Table 20-2 to determine the prevalence of specific diseases among family members; care should be taken to list affected family members.

After complete information has been collected, a brief summary of each category of the health history is formulated and recorded.

EXAMPLE OF A HEALTH HISTORY

Basic Data

Miss Nancy Adams
80 Storrow Drive
Boston, Massachusetts 02215

Date of birth: 9/16/1938, Boston, Massachusetts

Age: 42

Informant

Client, herself, who appears reliable.

Chief Complaint

Intermittent "chest pains" during the prior week.

Personal and Social History

Miss Adams is single, never married, a college graduate, a grammar school teacher, and is financially responsible. She consumes a high protein diet, mainly chicken and fish, supplemented

TABLE 20-2. Diseases for which Prevalence Must Be Determined in a Health History

Heart disease	Tuberculosis
Hypertension	Renal disease
Obesity	Mental disease
Diabetes	Migraine
Cancer	Alcoholism
Arthritis	Venereal disease
Gout	Stroke
Ulcers	Seizures
Allergy	Rheumatic fever
Asthma	

amply with vegetables and fruit, with minute utilization of salt and sugar. She has smoked one and a half to two packages of cigarettes daily for the past 25 years, and consumes several cocktails a week. In addition to medicines noted under the History of Present Problem, she has taken two aspirins regularly at the onset of her menstrual period to relieve headaches.

History of Present Problem

Miss Adams first experienced episodic chest pains 2 years ago (December 1978). In conjunction with heavy exertion, eating, or cold weather, severe pain was felt as a substernal pressure sensation which radiated to her left arm. Duration was several minutes; pain stopped when activity ceased. Her physician informed her that she had angina. Nitroglycerine tablets were prescribed as needed for similar pain.

One year ago (March 1979), she was awakened at night with a prolonged episode of severe, substernal pain. Nitroglycerine tablets did not relieve her suffering. University Hospital admitted her to the coronary care unit. After tests, she was informed by Dr. William White that she had had a heart attack. After 3 weeks observation and treatment, she was discharged with a daily prescription of warfarin, 7.5 mg., and requested to obtain a prothrombin time monthly.

This week, she again experienced chest pain associated with exertion and shortness of breath. She has been awakened twice with episodes of paroxysmal nocturnal dyspnea. She denies ever having had rheumatic fever, hypertension, or murmurs. She has not experienced palpitations, cyanosis, edema, cough, or syncope.

History of Past Problems

Health maintenance: Her last complete physical examination was 6 months ago. Her condition was good. A Papanicolaou test was graded class I (normal). She received Sabin vaccine in 1968, tetanus in October 1972, and a tuberculin test (negative) in 1976.

Childhood diseases: Measles at age seven, chickenpox at age eight.

Allergies: No known allergy.

Medical illnesses: No major diseases other than illnesses under History of Present Problem.

Surgical procedures: Hospitalized at age 12 for tonsillectomy.

Injuries: None recalled.

Mental illnesses: No known mental disorder.

Obstetrical history: Onset of menses at about 13-years-old. Her cycle is 29 days; menses 4 days with moderate flow. She has never had sexual intercourse and has not experienced any signs of menopause.

Review of Systems

General state of health: Declared fair for the past 2 years. She has experienced a weight loss of 20 pounds during the past 6 months and has felt increasing fatigue.

Skin: There have been no changes in texture, temperature, or color of the skin, nor in the appearance of the hair and nails. She denies any rashes, infections, lesions, or pain.

Neurological system: Expresses anxiety since the onset of her illness. She denies seizures, syncope, loss of consciousness, paresis, paralysis, balance problems, paresthesia, or psychiatric therapy.

Head: Usually experiences a headache monthly associated with her menstrual cycle. She denies dizziness or trauma.

Eyes: Wears glasses for reading and had her eyes re-examined last year. Denies cataracts, glaucoma, hyperopia, myopia, astigmatism, strabismus, nystagmus, color blindness, pain, inflammation, infection, discharge, or diplopia.

Ears: Denies infections, earaches, hearing problems, tinnitus, and vertigo.

Nose and sinuses: States that she has several colds yearly. Denies nasal discharge, recurrent epistaxis, polyps, allergies, sinusitis, or any change in her ability to smell.

Mouth and throat: Has multiple dental fillings, does not wear dentures, and has semiannual dental examinations. Has an occasional sore throat not requiring treatment. Denies pain, hoarseness, lesions of the tongue, gums, or throat, and difficulty in chewing, tasting, or swallowing of fluid or food.

Neck: Denies any limitation of movement, pain, swelling of lymph glands, or enlargement of the thyroid gland.

Breasts: Breast development at "12- or 13-years-old." She denies breast lumps, dimpling, discharge, any change in nipples, tenderness, mammography, surgery, or trauma. She examines her breasts "after each period."

Respiratory system: Her latest chest study was performed in 1979. Denies a history of chest colds, pneumonia, exposure to tuberculosis, asthma, cyanosis, cough, hemoptysis, wheezing, sputum, or operations.

Cardiovascular system: See History of Present Problem.

Gastrointestinal system: Has normal stools and bowel habits. Denies anorexia, nausea, vomiting, dysphagia, hematemesis, abdominal pain, pyrosis, flatulence, jaundice, diarrhea, constipation, rectal bleeding, melena, or hemorrhoids.

Urinary system: States no dysuria, urgency, hesitancy, hematuria, incontinence, or renal calculi. Has had nocturia several times a night for the past 6 months.

Genitalia: Does not use any method of contraception. Denies venereal disease, abnormal bleeding, leukorrhea, pruritus, pain, burning, lesions, or masturbation.

Musculoskeletal system: States no varicose veins, intermittent claudication, bursitis, joint pain or swelling, muscle tenderness or weakness, backaches, or skeletal deformities.

Endocrine system: Volunteers no history of goiter, intolerance to weather change, polyuria, polydipsia, or polyphagia.

Hematopoietic system: Denies ever having anemia, abnormal bleeding, lymphadenopathy, excessive bruising, or exposure to toxic agents. Has never had a transfusion, nor does she know her blood type.

Family History

Her maternal grandmother died of a cerebral vascular accident in 1960 at the age of 84. Her maternal grandfather died from a heart attack in 1950 at age 78. Her father died of a heart attack in 1953 at age 56. Her mother is 78-years-old and in fairly good health except for osteoarthritis. Her brother, age 46, is in good health. There is no evidence of alcoholism, allergies, asthma, cancer, epilepsy, diabetes mellitus, gout, hypertension, mental illness, migraine, obesity, blood disorders, renal disease, rheumatic fever, seizures, tuberculosis, ulcers, or venereal disease in the family.

Sonya Hawkins, R.N.

BIBLIOGRAPHY

Brownie, J., and Boucher, R.: *Primary Care, Readings-Guidelines.* Xerox, 1975.

DeGowin, E., and DeGowin, R.: *Bedside Diagnostic Examination.* New York, Macmillan Co., 1976.

Fowkes, W., and Hunn, V.: *Clinical Assessment for the Nurse Practitioner.* St. Louis, C. V. Mosby Co., 1973.

Froelich, R., and Bishop, M.: *Clinical Interviewing Skills: A Programmed Manual for Data Gathering, Evaluation, and Patient Management.* St. Louis, C. V. Mosby Co., 1977.

Gebbie, K., and Lavin, M. (eds.): *Classification of Nursing Diagnoses.* St. Louis, C. V. Mosby Co., 1975.

Gillies, D., and Alyn. I.: *Patient Assessment and Management by the Nurse Practitioner.* Philadelphia, W. B. Saunders, 1976.

Mahoney, E., Verdisco, L., and Shortridge, L.: *How to Collect and Record a Health History.* Philadelphia, J. B. Lippincott, 1976.

Prior, J., and Silberstein, J.: *Physical Diagnosis: The History and Examination of the Patient.* St. Louis, C. V. Mosby Co., 1977.

CHAPTER 21

GLOSSARY

anasarca. Severe generalized edema.

anesthesia. Partial or total loss of sensation. Consciousness may or may not be present.

aphasia. The loss of ability to verbalize and comprehend spoken words.

apices. Plural of apex. (The maximum point or summit; for example, the apex of the heart is the point of maximum impulse.)

bruit. One of a variety of sounds, originating in veins or arteries, heard on auscultation.

cachexia. A pronounced state of malnutrition and wasting.

consolidation. A solidified state usually referring to a condition of the lungs as in pneumonia.

crepitus (crepitation). A crackling or grating sound or sensation associated with certain diseases or bone fractures.

dysesthesia. A prickling or crawling sensation or impaired sensitivity to touch.

PHYSICAL EXAMINATION OF THE ADULT

Pearl P. Rosendahl, Ed.D., R.N., and
Arlyne B. Saperstein, M.N., R.N.

edema. An excessive amount of fluid in the tissue.

fremitus. Tremors caused by vibrations (such as vibrations of the voice) felt through the chest.

hypesthesia (hypoesthesia). A dulled or diminished sensibility to touch.

murmur. A soft blowing sound produced by vibrations of blood moving within the heart and adjacent vessels.

nicking. A constriction of the blood vessels of the retina.

paresthesia. Increased sensitivity or the experiencing of abnormal sensations seemingly without cause.

plethora. Blood vessel distention causing a reddened skin tone.

pneumothorax. The entrance of air or gas into the pleural cavity causing the lung to collapse.

polycythemia. An increase in the amount of red blood cells.

rales. An abnormal sound caused by air passage through constricted or mucus filled bronchi heard on auscultation.

thrill. An abnormal tremor accompanying a cardiac murmur.

torpid. Sluggishness or reduction in normal vigor.

The process of physical assessment requires that the client be considered in his entirety. There are various strategies employed in examining the client. Some nurses will learn to examine from the head and move downward to the toes. Others will assess the client by systems. No one method is correct or incorrect provided that the information (data) presented by the client is collected, and the examiner is comfortable, consistent, and thorough in the examination.

The beginning student will not be expected to do a complete physical examination but will become aware of the necessity of constant, ongoing, goal-directed assessment. As the student progresses in her education, she will add more and more of the knowledge and skills needed for examination of the client until she is able to assess the client as a whole. While she will not be expected to make a medical diagnosis, she will be able to differentiate normal from abnormal characteristics and report (as well as record) them appropriately.

The physical examination is broken down into the following components: methods and tools of assessment, general impression, the integument, the neurological system, head and neck, breast and axilla, thorax and lungs, heart, abdomen, genitourinary and rectal examination, and the extremities and vertebral column. Finally, an example of a recorded physical examination is presented. Many examples of medical conditions are included to illustrate abnormalities. They are not meant to teach the student to make a diagnosis but to clarify what symptoms may be found when assessing the client.

As stated above, the physical examination plays a very important role in the collection of a data base. It is essentially a set of observations utilizing the senses of *sight, smell, touch,* and *hearing.* Four classic techniques, or cardinal skills—*inspection, palpation, percussion,* and *auscultation*—correlate with these senses in doing a physical assessment.

From the study of anatomy, physiology, pathophysiology, and repetitive experiences in assessing or examining clients, the student learns to recognize what is a normal or abnormal finding. Repetition is essential not only in the learning process but also in maintaining proficiency in the performance of these skills.

METHODS OF ASSESSMENT

The four cardinal skills mentioned above are used in the following sequence to examine each section of the body: (1) inspection, (2) palpation, (3) percussion, and (4) auscultation.

Inspection

Inspection is the careful and comprehensive observation of the client for meaningful physical attributes. When this skill is developed, its application will automatically include awareness of the client's posture, movements, gait, stature, nutrition, skin, speech, and behavior.

POSTURE. The client's posture often gives the examiner invaluable clues. As stated in Chapter 18 on observation of nonverbal behavior, posturing may tell us much about how the client feels about himself. It can also indicate to the observer what physical as well as emotional feelings or symptoms are present. For instance, a client with heart disease is often more comfortable lying on his right side or leaning his body over or against tables. A client suffering from pain may assume unusual positions to obtain relief.

MOVEMENT. Movement may be noted in one specific area or may be so generalized that the entire body is involved. Often, you may notice involuntary movements of eye muscles and muscles of the face and neck, commonly known as *tics* or *spasms.* The client with chorea makes sudden, unexpected, and purposeless movements of the arms and legs or the entire body. Another example of movement which can be either localized or general is convulsions which can occur with, or without, a loss of consciousness.

GAIT. While each of us has our own characteristic manner of walking and carrying ourselves, certain gaits may be symptomatic of disease. An example would include the client with *hemiplegia* who usually drags the affected leg around in a semicircle when walking. A *spastic gait* is a choppy and stiff style of walking. (This can be seen in neurological diseases involving lesions of the upper motor neuron, e.g., multiple sclerosis.)

STATURE. Stature, or body build and size, varies from one individual to another; however, in most cases it is found within an expected though fairly wide range that we consider to be normal. Abnormal stature is classified as dwarfs or giants. Ateliotic dwarfs are well proportioned but small in their various parts; achondroplastic dwarfs usually have abnormally short legs, and cretins are less than 3 feet tall. Their extremities are short with the spine deviated to either side. Giants result from hyperactivity of the anterior lobe of the pituitary gland. When the pituitary hyperactivity begins during adolescence, gigantism develops; and when the hyperactivity begins in adulthood, acromegaly occurs.

NUTRITION. The client's nutritional status can be assessed in a variety of ways, but his weight is often the most important clue. This state is usually perceived as within normal limits, underweight or overweight. Underweight can result from a loss of weight consistent with increased metabolism as in hyperthyroidism. It can also be due to excessive destruction of tissue (e.g., cachexia caused by a cancerous condition). Overweight is usually caused by overeating. Edema, or anasarca, may result in a rapid increase in weight (e.g., in kidney or heart disease).

SKIN. When inspecting a client, the skin is one of the first characteristics we notice. Assessment of the skin will be discussed in detail later in this chapter.

SPEECH. The characteristics of the voice or speech are resonance, tone, pitch, volume, and articulation. In listening to the client speak, voice changes may be noted. These changes, which can be readily noted or can be quite subtle, may have an affinity with a disease process. For instance, diseases of the larynx may cause the voice to be weakened, hoarse, and rough. A client with motor aphasia has a loss or defect in the power of expression of speech.

BEHAVIOR. Note how the client acts. Is he alert, competent, nervous, or is he dull, confused, or depressed? Behavior may be symptomatic of emotional and physical problems. For example, clients with hyperthyroidism are generally nervous and unusually alert and agile. Clients are dull, apathetic and torpid with hypothyroidism. Clients with Korsakoff's syndrome describe imaginary people whom they have just met or imaginary travels they have just completed.

Palpation

Palpation is the feeling or touching of a part of the body in order to learn someting about its structure or function. It is also employed to confirm the findings of an inspection. The finger tips are used, as they are highly sensitive, for tactile discrimination. The dorsa of the hands or fingers are used, as the skin is much thinner, for temperature sensing. Use the palmar aspects of the metacarpophalangeal joints to experience vibrations and the grasping fingers to feel sensations from the joints and muscles.

With practice, thrills and murmurs over the heart area, vocal fremitus over the thorax, tenderness in tissues, crepitus in bones, tendon sheaths, and masses can be palpated. Masses are assessed for location, size, shape, consistency, adherence to other organs, tenderness, mobility, pulsation, and any changes of the overlying skin. Palpation is subdivided into *light palpation, deep palpation,* and *ballottement.*

LIGHT PALPATION. In light palpation, the palm of the hand is laid lightly but firmly upon that part of the body you are palpating. Fingers are gently pressed into that part to a depth of about 1 cm. Light palpation would be used on the abdomen to assess tenderness and resistance from muscle spasm.

DEEP PALPATION. Use the entire palmar surface of the hand with the fingers pressed into that part of the body to a depth of 4 or 5 cm. The tactile sensations are felt with the finger pads. Another method is the using of both hands for deep palpation. The right hand is placed on the part to be palpated, and the fingers of the left hand are pressed upon the terminal interphalangeal joints of the right hand. The left hand produces the pressure while the right hand receives the sensations. This is a good method for assessing deep-lying organs, such as the kidney and liver.

BALLOTTEMENT. Ballottement is a type of palpation used to detect large amounts of fluid in a body cavity, for example, for the detection of ascites (fluid) in the peritoneal (abdominal) cavity. One flank is tapped sharply with the hand. The other hand receives the impulse when placed against the other flank. Since fat in the mesentery will cause a similar impulse, the client or another person, exerts firm pressure on the midline of his abdomen with the edge of his hand. A wave passing this block and felt by your receiving hand is usually caused by fluid.

Percussion

The surface of the body is tapped to produce sounds that will vary in quality in accordance with the density of the underlying tissues. The purpose is to ascertain the density of tissue by the sound produced when it is struck. The source of every sound is a vibrating body which produces a series of waves in the surrounding medium. These waves, which vibrate at the same rate as the vibrating body, reach the ear causing a vibration of the ear drums and middle ear producing a sound.

Percussion sounds will enable the examiner to locate normal structures and to be able to detect abnormalities. To elicit percussion sounds, hyper-extend the middle finger of the left hand (the plex-imeter finger) and place it flatly and firmly upon the chest wall. (Otherwise, the note can be altered.) Strike the base of the first phalanx of the left middle finger of that hand with the flexed finger of the right hand. A much clearer note can be obtained if the hand, at the moment of striking, is moved at the wrist while the forearm is kept fixed. The percussion stroke must be sharp, clear, and decisive, and the percussing finger, after striking the blow, must be immediately raised.

Various densities produce sounds which have been given names such as *hyperresonance, reso-nance, tympany, dullness,* and *flatness.* These notes are distinguished by differences in *pitch, in-tensity,* and *duration.*

PITCH. When speaking of the high or low quality of a sound, one is referring to pitch. Pitch depends upon the number of vibrations produced. When the vibrations are rapid, the pitch is higher than when they are slower.

INTENSITY. The intensity of a tone depends upon the amplitude of the vibrations. A loud tone has a wider amplitude of vibrations than a soft tone. The tone over a lung is louder than over the liver since lungs have more elastic tissue and vibrate more readily when struck.

DURATION. Duration is another characteristic assisting in analysis of the percussion note. A res-onant note is well sustained, whereas a note over a solid organ is abbreviated.

Auscultation

Auscultation is the art of hearing sounds that are produced by pertinent organs of the body to as-certain physical signs. You can hear by applying an ear directly to the body's surface, but a stethoscope will amplify body sounds. The beginning examiner initially may hear too much. The ability to distin-guish between important and unimportant sounds is acquired by practice. The ideal environment for auscultation is a soundproofed room that is devoid of all extraneous noises. Realistically, you must learn not to be distracted and to concentrate com-pletely on the sounds delivered by your stetho-scope. You must identify the sounds you hear as being from interior parts of the body. Erroneous assumptions can be made when hearing certain sounds, including *sounds produced by friction of the stethoscope on hair.* Body hair under the steth-oscope may produce crackling sounds which may be confused with rales. If the client has a hairy chest, wet the chest with water to press the hairs down. If absolutely necessary the skin may have to be shaved.

The scope of auscultation is varied. It can be used to examine: the vessels of the neck for mur-murs (bruits); the lungs for breath sounds, voice and whisper sounds, rales, and friction rubs; the heart for valve sounds, for splitting, murmurs, and rhythm disturbances; the abdomen for bowel sounds and murmurs from aneurysms; and the joints, tendon sheaths, and bones for crepitus.

Auscultation, as with observation, palpation, and percussion, should follow a prescribed routine to thoroughly examine each part of the body.

MUSCLE, TENDON, AND JOINT SOUNDS. Clients who are chilled, nervous, or hold their mus-cles tensely may produce soft sounds in their mus-cles. Muscular sounds are crumpling, muffled, and indistinct and are not affected by coughing. Sounds produced by joints and fasciae usually disappear when the client relaxes.

ASSESSMENT TOOLS

A number of tools assist in various aspects of phys-ical examination and assessment. For the *general examination* a sphygmomanometer (blood pres-sure cuff; see Chapter 29, "Vital Signs"), a ruler marked in centimeters, a penlight, tongue depres-sors, and an oto-ophthalmoscope are used. The otoscope and ophthalmoscope are adjuncts oper-ating from the same power source. The otoscopic portion of the instrument is used to visualize the external ear canal and tympanic membrane with magnification. There are several speculum tips that fit this instrument. The largest size speculum that will fit into the ear canal is used. There is usually a short, wide, speculum available for the nostrils. The ophthalmoscopic portion of the instrument includes a series of neutralizing lenses together with a light source and filters to enable the examiner to look directly at the fundus of the eye with magnification. The image is erect without reversal or inversion. These lenses, which are numbered, are called diopters. A diopter is used as a unit of measurement in refraction. Numbers range to a high of 40 diopters. The zero setting indicates no lens, the plus numbers (usually in black) indicate convex lenses, and the negative numbers (usually in red) indicate concave lenses. Lenses are adjustable by rotating the wheel in the ophthalmoscopic head. Positive numbers bring the focal point closer to the examiner, and negative lenses move the focal point away. Therefore, the hyperopic (or farsighted) eye requires more of the plus sphere for clear focus, and the myopic (or nearsighted) eye requires more of the minus sphere for clear focus. An additional attachment provides a light source for use as a sinus transilluminator.

The stethoscope is also used in the assessment of the client for auscultation. Many stethoscopes come with variously sized ear tips and diaphragms. The ear tips must fit comfortably and snugly to prevent sound leakage. The tubing is double and thick-walled, about 25 to 30 cm in length and 3 mm in internal diameter. Most stethoscopes have combination heads consisting of a diaphragm and a bell. The diaphragm is used for detecting low frequency sounds, diastolic and third heart sounds, and is appropriate for identifying first and second heart sounds as well as high-pitched murmurs. The bell is best suited for sensing low and medium pitched sounds and murmurs.

For *rectal and vaginal examinations*, gloves, lubricant, and a vaginal bivalve speculum (available in three standard sizes) are needed.

Equipment used for the *neurological examination* includes a reflex hammer (which comes in various shapes and sizes) and a tuning fork (which varies in frequency). A 512 cycle per second fork is employed to test hearing. A 128 cycle per second fork is utilized for testing vibratory sense and is too low pitched for hearing. However, a 250 cycle per second fork is usually adequate for testing both hearing and vibratory sensations. In addition, cotton (for testing light-touch sensations), safety pins (for testing superficial pain sensations), and several test tubes (for testing temperature sensations) are needed.

EXAMINATION OF THE CLIENT

For the examination of a client, the examining room should be comfortably warm, free of drafts, well lighted, and quiet. All equipment must be accessible, clean, and in good working order.

If possible, have the client walk to the examining table, so that stature, gait, posture, movements, and any visible abnormalities can be observed. See that the client is completely undressed but draped protectively at all times. Wash your hands in front of the client before and after the examination. The client should be addressed slowly; each action should be explained. Seat the client and examine his head, neck, chest, and back. Then, place the client in a recumbent position and examine the axilla, breasts, lungs, heart, abdomen, genitalia, and extremities. Compare the findings on one side with the other side, as the body is bilaterally symmetrical. The techniques of inspection, palpation, percussion, and auscultation are employed for each section of the body as applicable. All clients should be treated with respect, consideration, and gentleness.

General Impression

A general impression of the client includes appearance, health status, height, weight, and vital signs. (See Chapter 29, "Vital Signs.")

GENERAL APPEARANCE. Initially, record demographic data on the client including his age, sex, and race. Scrutinize the client's posture, movements, stature, physical development, nutrition, skin, behavior, and any gross visible abnormalities.

STATUS OF HEALTH. The client's apparent status of health is assessed. Is he ambulatory or confined to a bed? Is he well or chronically ill? Are there any signs of distress, such as dyspnea (difficulty in breathing), orthopnea (respiratory difficulty in any but the sitting or standing position), or coughing? Is the client using oxygen or other life-supporting apparatus? Does he appear younger or older than his stated age?

MEASUREMENTS. Height and weight are measured; the client's measurements are compared with a chart on desirable factors. This will indicate then, whether or not he is malnourished or obese. If the client is obese, observe the distribution of fat. This will help in differentiating between simple obesity and an abnormality such as truncal fat seen in Cushing's syndrome. *Vital signs* include temperature, pulse, respirations, and blood pressure which are more thoroughly described in Chapter 29. All physical findings are recorded to interpret the functional efficiency of each part of the body.

Integument

SKIN

The skin supports the peripheral nerve endings and contributes to temperature regulation by radiation, conduction, and convection of heat and the emission of sweat. The underlying tissue is protected by the skin from injury, infection, and dehydration. Since the skin covers the entire body, diseases of the other organ systems are often reflected in it. Differences between various sections of the body are seen and signs of abnormalities may be noted. Many skin conditions can be derived from general systemic disease or diseases of the skin. Examination of the skin also includes the nails and the hair. Skills utilized in the physical examination of the skin, nails, and hair are inspection, aided by palpation. These are interrelated and utilized synchronously.

Certain skin diseases are confined to different regions of the body. Examples are: (1) acne which is found on the face, shoulders, and upper trunk;

(2) lupus erythematosus which spreads across the nose and face in a butterfly pattern; (3) cutaneous moniliasis which appears in moist folds, such as under the breasts, in the axillae, inguinal, and perianal regions and gluteal folds; and (4) stasis dermatitis which is found on the legs.

All the integument is examined, observing the *state of skin,* the *color,* and the *presence of any lesions.*

STATE OF SKIN. The state or condition of the skin is noted by assessing for elasticity, turgor, swelling, moistness (or lack of moisture), texture, thickness, and temperature. Very loose skin may indicate that the client has lost weight. Edema of the skin might indicate a condition such as nephritis or heart disease. Moist skin may denote hyperthyroidism, whereas dry skin is frequently associated with myxedema (hypofunction of the thyroid). A marked thickening and harshness of the skin is characteristic of the skin disease scleroderma. Skin temperature depends on the volume of blood circulation permeating the dermis. A localized area of hyperthermia (excessive heat) results from increased blood flow (e.g., a localized skin infection). A localized area of hypothermia (lower temperature) is symptomatic of decreased blood flow, which results in cooling of an area, as seen in peripheral arteriosclerosis.

COLOR. The four known groups of pigmented substances of normal skin are: carotene, oxyhemoglobin, reduced hemoglobin, and melanin (Table 21-1).

The skin is observed for jaundice, flushing, and cyanosis. *Jaundice* may be caused by carotenemia (excessive ingestion of carotene). Noncarotene yellow skin changes occur in hepatitis, xanthomatoses (deposits of lipids in the tissues), and ecchymoses

TABLE 21-1. Skin Pigmentation

Compounds	Hue	Location in Skin
Carotene	Yellow	Melanocytes of epidermis and hair matrix, melanosomes, and dermal macrophages.
Oxyhemoglobin	Bright red	In red blood cells—arterial.
Reduced hemoglobin	Bluish red	In red blood cells—venous.
		Both are found in various quantities at various depths in dermis, subcutaneous fat, and underlying muscle masses.
Melanin	Brown	Melanocytes of epidermis and hair matrix, melanosomes, and dermal macrophages.

(hemorrhagic spots) from breakdown of hemoglobin products. *Flush* is caused by a disturbance in hemoglobin pigmentation. There is an increase in oxygen and a change in hemoglobin. This condition evidences plethora or polycythemia. *Cyanosis* is a distinctive deep purplish-blue color. This is caused when reduced hemoglobin reaches 5 g/dl. Examples of conditions in which cyanosis may be present are pneumonia and congenital heart disease with right and left shunts.

LESIONS. Skin eruptions are divided into primary and secondary lesions. *Primary lesions* appear immediately after a stimulus (e.g., macule, papule, nodule, vesicle, bullae, pustule, and wheal). *Secondary lesions* result from alterations in the underlying primary lesions (e.g., scales, lichenification, fissure, excoriation, and scars). Attributes of these lesions are: *macule*—flat nonpalpable spot; *papule*—palpable spot less than 5 mm; *nodule*—palpable spot greater than 5 mm; *vesicle*—blister smaller than 5 mm; *bulla*—blister larger than 5 mm; *pustule*—vesicle filled with pus; *wheal*—hive; *scaly* or *squamous*—loose outer cornified layer; *fissure*—crack through the epidermis; *lichenification*—thickening of the skin with accentuation of normal skin lines; and *scar*—replacement of injured tissue by connective tissue (Fig. 21-1). The skin is observed for any cutaneous abnormalities (e.g., lesions). If any are present, they are identified by type, grouping, and distribution. Lesions discovered should be palpated to distinguish morphology and infiltration. Some lesions are grouped in distinctive patterns: *annular*—circles, (e.g., psoriasis and urticaria); *linear*—lines (e.g., lymphangitis and poison ivy); and *zosteriform*—broad bands, usually following area of nerve distribution, (e.g., herpes zoster).

NAILS

The nail organ consists of the nail plate and supportive surrounding tissues. The nail plate is made of horny material that grows until cut or worn away by usage. Nail differs from hair in that its growth is continuous rather than cyclic. Fingernails extend at a rate of approximately 0.1 mm a day while toenails grow less quickly.

Diseases of the nails are seldom diagnosed without reference to the rest of the cutaneous system.

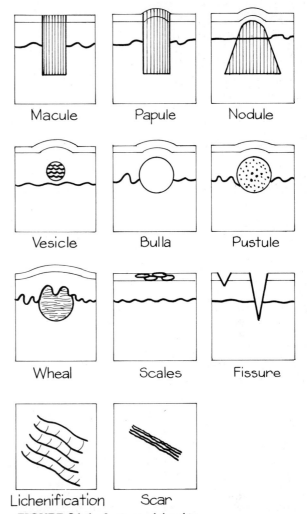

FIGURE 21-1. Lesions of the skin.

Since the nail is capable of only a limited number of reaction patterns, a particular alteration may have many causes. The fingernails and toenails are observed for *shape* and *color*.

SHAPE. *Ridges* and *furrows* in the nails, either longitudinal or transverse, are often identified with systemic disease but may also be caused by direct injury to the matrix, or the source of new nail. *Beau's lines* are transverse furrows in nails usually appearing after a severe illness and disappearing gradually over several months. (Fig. 21-2). *Clubbing* of the tips of the fingers and toes is associated with many serious systemic diseases. Hypoxia (decreased oxygen supply) may be a causal factor. Attributes of clubbing of the tips of fingers and toes

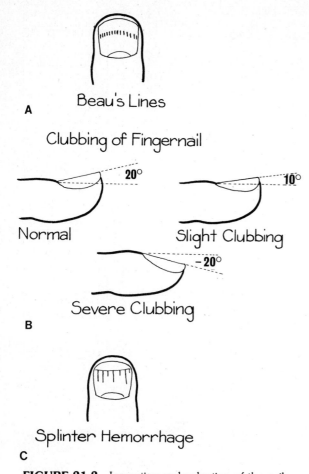

A

Beau's Lines

Clubbing of Fingernail

Normal 20°   Slight Clubbing 10°

Severe Clubbing −20°

B

Splinter Hemorrhage

C

FIGURE 21-2. Inspection and palpation of the nails.

are thickening, widening, terminal phalanges, glossy skin at the roots of the nail, obliteration of the normal angle between nail and skin fold, and exaggerated longitudinal convexity of the nail (Fig. 21-2).

COLOR. The nail plates are transparent. Changes in the underlying vascular system can be seen in the nail beds, as in anemia or cyanosis. Another abnormality is splinter hemorrhages. They are red or brown linear streaks in the nail bed, running from the free margin for approximately several centimeters. They are commonly associated with subacute bacterial endocarditis (Fig. 21-2).

HAIR

The hair is inspected for distribution, amount, and texture.

DISTRIBUTION. The human body is covered with hair except on the palms, the dorsa of the distal phalanges, the soles, the inner surface of the prepuce, the labia minora, and the glans penis. There are distinctive sexual hair patterns appearing after puberty. Any change in the normal developmental pattern identified with the opposite sex suggests an endocrine problem.

AMOUNT. Hair loss may occur in a disease process, such as syphilis. In some clients with a pituitary insufficiency, the hair may be extremely sparse. With alopecia areata, the client suddenly loses patches of hair, leaving spots of baldness.

TEXTURE. The texture of the hair can feel coarse or fine, dry or oily. In some individuals hair may be dry and brittle because of physical or chemical injury, or due to a condition such as myxedema. In hyperthyroidism, the hair exhibits a very fine texture.

Neurological System

The purpose of a systematic neurological examination is to discover any and all motor, sensory, and coordinative defects. The examination is based on both the client's history and a series of observations of spontaneous behavior, movement, posture, coordinated, and reflex actions. When the history is obtained from the client, consideration should be given as to how well the client speaks, and comprehends, if he has a thought disorder, and whether or not he is confused or appears to have a behavioral disorder.

Observation of the client may detect symptoms such as homonymous hemianopsia (which causes the client to turn his head to see directly ahead), the ptosis and crossed-eyes encountered with oculomotor weakness, or the masklike face and tremor-at-rest of Parkinson's disease. Observe the client's gait. He may have an absence of arm-swinging, an ataxic gait from loss of position sense, hemiplegic posturing, or the shuffling gait of Parkinson's disease. The client's *mental status, cranial nerves, motor system, reflexes, sensory* and *coordinative functions* should be tested systematically to assure a complete assessment.

MENTAL STATUS

Content and flow of the client's thought while the history is taken can provide data relevant to the client's mental status. Assessment of mental status includes consideration of states of consciousness, general behavior and appearance, mood, verbal function, memory, manipulation of knowledge, and mental content.

STATES OF CONSCIOUSNESS.
Consciousness is a state in which the client is aware of his environment and himself and is responsive to stimuli. Terms such as alertness, confusion, stupor, semicomatose, and coma have been given many meanings. You must describe the stimulus given to the client and the response to that stimulus. Consciousness should be identified in terms of *awareness* as in the following examples:

1. Alert, oriented, responds to time, place and person.
2. Slightly drowsy, responds to spoken name; responds to name but not to time or place.
3. Light coma, responds to shouted name, drifts off immediately afterward.
4. Deeper coma, responds to painful stimuli rather than verbal stimuli. Pain may include pinching of the skin, shaking, or pricking with a pin. The client, once aroused, is able to carry out some simple commands.
5. Can still be aroused with painful stimulation rather than verbal. However, the client does not follow simple commands.
6. Client is unresponsive. Responds to stimulated deep pain by withdrawal of that portion of the body stimulated.
7. In profound coma, there is no response to deep pain. Corneal, pupillary, pharyngeal, swallowing, and cough reflexes are abolished. The client is incontinent of urine and feces.

GENERAL BEHAVIOR AND APPEARANCE.
The client's behavior is ascertained as to whether he is cooperative, hostile, aggressive, or negative. There can be subtle changes to indicate a lowering of consciousness—for instance, a client who cannot feed himself, or one who is incontinent. Appearance may be described as neat or messy, or appropriately (or inappropriately) dressed for age and situation.

MOOD.
The appropriateness of mood is noted. Inappropriateness would be exemplified if the client is experiencing severe pain but is smiling. Quick mood shifts from laughter to weeping or happiness to sadness should also be noted as this may indicate diffuse brain disease.

VERBAL FUNCTION.
Speech, reading, and writing should be evaluated to ascertain the level of cerebral functioning. During the health history, the examiner should note articulation, word choice, sentence structure, and comprehension of dialogue. Cerebral dysfunction may result in aphasia which can be either expressive (unable to communicate), receptive (unable to comprehend communication), or global (loss of all speech function).

MEMORY.
There are three separate functions—immediate recall, recent memory (the ability to learn), and remote memory (retrieval of previously learned material). A good test for immediate recall is to utter a series of numbers and have the client repeat them forward and backward. Recent memory can be assessed by showing three objects and asking the client to remember them 5 minutes later. Remote memory can be tested by referring to events in the distant past (i.e., naming past presidents, birthdays, or anniversaries).

MANIPULATION OF KNOWLEDGE.
Inability to calculate is an index of cerebral disease and dominant parietal lesions. Simple calculations, for instance, serial sevens (i.e., subtracting seven from 100 and successive sevens from previous results) is a test for this evaluation. The ability to perform generalizations constitutes the highest functioning of the brain. This is tested by requiring the client to produce abstract generalizations from concrete examples. He can be given a proverb or fable and asked for its meaning (e.g., "a stitch in time saves nine"). A client with abstract reasoning would respond that an effort to resolve a problem now would avert difficulty later. A client without abstract reasoning would respond with the number of stitches needed to mend a garment.

MENTAL CONTENT. The presence of hallucinations, delusions, obsessions, phobias, and lack of insight and judgment indicates impairment of mental function or severe emotional conflicts. Questions should be asked to clarify the problem. Questions such as "Have you had any strange experiences lately?" to ascertain hallucinations or delusions, and "Do you perceive yourself differently than you were several months ago?" to ascertain insight.

CRANIAL NERVES

This portion of the neurological examination is a mixed motor and sensory examination of the structures of the head and neck.

Cranial Nerve I (Olfactory)

To evaluate the sense of smell the client is asked to close his eyes and one nostril. Each nostril should be tested separately, using distinctive but not irritating or overpowering odors (e.g., coffee, tobacco, or peppermint).

Cranial Nerve II (Optic)

Visual acuity (*central vision*) is tested with a Snellen chart. Using the Snellen notation, acuity is expressed first by recording the test distance, commonly 20 feet, and then recording the distance at which the smallest letter seen should be read by an average normal eye. Thus, if the client, at 20 feet, reads letters of a size that the average person could see, the Snellen notation is 20/20. If at a test distance of 20 feet, the client can only see the letter that should be seen at 30 feet, his Snellen notation is 20/30. Newspaper print is approximately 20/50 at usual reading distance and can be used if a Snellen chart is not available.

In conducting the test (confrontation perimetry) for visual fields (peripheral vision), the client covers one eye and looks at a designated eye of the examiner. (The examiner covers his opposite eye in order to compare field of vision with the client.) The examiner starts at the periphery of each quadrant of vision and moves his finger or a cotton-tipped applicator, in front of and toward the center of the client's vision. The client is asked to indicate when he initially sees the finger or the applicator. Each quadrant and each eye is tested separately.

Cranial Nerves III, IV, VI (Oculomotor, Trochlear, and Abducens)

The functions of the third, fourth, and sixth cranial nerves, which command eye movement and pupil function, are tested together because all three supply muscles for eye movement. The *oculomotor nerve* innervates the superior rectus, inferior oblique, the medial rectus, and the inferior rectus muscles. This nerve also innervates the muscles which constrict the pupils and those which elevate the eyelids. The *trochlear nerve* innervates the superior oblique muscle, and the *abducens nerve* innervates the lateral rectus muscle.

The position of the eyes at rest and in movements in all directions is appraised. Are the eyes symmetrical at rest? Do they move conjugatively? Does each eye move fully in all directions? Eye movements and pupil functioning can be tested by having the client hold his head erect and by following the examiner's fingers. The movements for testing these muscles are shown in Figure 21-4.

As the client is following the finger in the upward and lateral gaze, the examiner should pause and watch for *nystagmus*. Nystagmus should be critiqued during examination of eye movements; it is a sudden jerking motion of the eyeballs usually associated with visual fatigue, refractive error, or certain diseases of the central nervous system.

The examination of pupils should be done in a darkened room. The pupils are examined for size, shape, and regularity. The pupillary light reflex is evaluated by shining a light into one eye, and then the other, while the client fixes on a distant object. Both direct and consensual (occurring on the opposite side from the stimulation) pupillary reflexes should be observed.

To evaluate the *accommodation reflex,* ask the client to focus on a distant object, and then to focus on an object held close to the face. Normally, the *pupils constrict* when the client focuses on this object. With involvement of the oculomotor nerve, the client will not be able to look up medially or down with the affected eye. There will be dilatation of the pupil and ptosis of the lid. If the trochlear nerve is involved, the client will not be able to look downward and laterally. If the abducens nerve is involved, the client will not be able to look laterally.

Cranial Nerve V (Trigeminal)

To evaluate facial sensation, the client is tested for perception of pain, temperature, and touch in each of the three divisions: *ophthalmic* (first), *maxillary* (second), and *mandibular* (third). Power and bulk of the temporal, masseter, and pterygoid muscles are assessed. The corneal reflex which is mediated through the ophthalmic division is then tested. The ophthalmic branch provides sensation to the skin of the anterior scalp, forehead, and to the cornea; the maxillary branch provides sensation to the upper teeth and jaw, the cheeks, and oral, pharyngeal, and nasal mucosa; and the mandibular branch provides sensation to the tongue, lower teeth, and buccal surface. The motor fibers innervate the masseter, temporalis, and pterygoid muscles, which are involved in mastication.

For testing the sensory divisions of the nerve the client closes his eyes. Pain and temperature have similar pathways; therefore, only pain needs to be tested. Pain is tested by pricking the client's forehead and the area over the mandible in the infraorbital region with a pin, or these areas are touched lightly with a wisp of cotton. This nerve can also be tested for the corneal reflex. The client is asked to look upward, while the cornea is briefly stroked from the side and from below.

To test the motor portion of this nerve, the client is asked to open his mouth and move his chin from one side to the other while the movement is opposed with manual pressure against the ramus of the jaw.

Cranial Nerve VII (Facial)

This nerve has a large motor and a small sensory component (on the anterior 70 percent of the tongue). Facial nerve motor functioning is measured by noting symmetry of the face at rest, especially the nasolabial folds. Voluntary movement of the facial muscles is observed as the client is asked to smile, show his teeth, frown, raise his eyebrows, and as his eyes are forcibly closed.

Sensory function can be evaluated by testing the accuracy of the taste sensation. The client is asked to identify sugar or salt on the anterior aspect of each side of the protruded tongue.

Cranial Nerve VIII (Vestibulocochlear)

This nerve is evaluated for hearing and postural and equilibratory function. Auditory acuity (*cochlear nerve*) is tested in each ear separately. The client is asked to attempt to detect the ticking of a watch, a whisper, or other faint sound. If tuning forks are available, the Rinne and Weber tests (see below) are helpful in determining if there is a hearing loss. Normally, air conduction is better than bone conduction.

The vestibular nerve is tested by observing for spontaneous nystagmus (usually observed during examination of eye movements), disorders of gait, and muscular control.

RINNE'S TEST. One ear is tested at a time. The handle of a vibrating fork is pressed against the mastoid process. The client is asked to signal when he can no longer hear the sound. At that signal the fork is removed, and the still vibrant tines are placed in front of, but not touching, the client's ear. Normally, air conduction is longer than bone conduction; this is said to be "Rinne positive." When bone conduction is longer, the test is said to be "Rinne negative."

WEBER TEST. The base of the vibrating fork is placed on top of the client's skull. The client is asked in which ear the sound is louder. With normal perceptive hearing, and no conductive loss, the sounds will be heard equally in both ears. If the perceptive hearing is normal but there is conductive loss, the sound will lateralize to the side of the conductive loss (which shuts out room noises). Perceptive loss on one side causes sound to lateralize on the other side. Therefore, lateralization of sound to the left ear is caused by a conductive loss of the left ear or a perceptive hearing loss of the right ear.

ROMBERG TEST. This can be used to test the function of the vestibular portion of the eighth nerve. The client stands with his feet close together and his eyes closed. He must be assured that he will not fall as you will keep your arms around him without touching him. If the client has damage to the vestibular portion, he will be unable to stand erect and will sway and fall if not supported, particularly when his eyes are closed.

Cranial Nerves IX and X (Glossopharyngeal and Vagus)

The motor and sensory function of the palate, pharynx, and larynx are evaluated together. Motor fibers of the glossopharyngeal nerve innervate the muscles of the pharynx. Sensory fibers transmit sensations of touch and temperature from the pharynx and taste sensation from the posterior tongue.

Motor fibers of the vagus nerve innervate the soft palate, pharynx, and larynx. The sensory fibers carry impulses from many of the thoracic and abdominal viscera.

In testing the glossopharyngeal nerve, swallowing is observed. The gag reflex is tested bilaterally by touching both sides of the posterior pharyngeal wall with a tongue blade. The client is asked to swallow some water. If paralysis is present there will be regurgitation. Tasting sensation is assessed by having the client mouth small amounts of sugar, salt, or vinegar with closed eyes. To test the vagus nerve the client is asked to open his mouth and say "ah" while the examiner notes whether or not the uvula elevates and is in midline. Hoarseness of the voice may indicate involvement of both ninth and tenth cranial nerves.

Cranial Nerve XI (Accessory)

For the evaluation of function of the sternomastoid and trapezius (upper portion) muscles, the client is asked to turn his chin to each side against the examiner's resisting hand. To test for trapezius muscles, the client keeps his shoulders shrugged while the examiner attempts to push them down. Impairment of this nerve will be characterized by the client's weakness in these tests.

Cranial Nerve XII (Hypoglossal)

This nerve innervates the muscle of the tongue. The client is asked to protrude his tongue. Voluntary movements of the tongue are observed. Any abnormal involuntary movements are noted. Muscle bulk is evaluated. Involvement of this nerve may cause weakness on one side as manifested by deviation of the protruded tongue towards the side

with the lesion. One can observe atrophy and increased coating on the paralyzed side.

MOTOR FUNCTION

This examination includes assessment of muscle size, tone, strength, and movements. Examination for the routine evaluation of the following muscle actions would be sufficient: elbow and wrist flexion and extension; hand grip (finger abduction and adduction), and knee and ankle flexion and extension. The examiner needs to note skeletal muscle mass and the shape of each body part, always comparing muscles of similar parts of the body for symmetry.

Whenever possible, the circumferences of two counterparts (arms, thighs, and legs) are compared at the same level with a measuring tape. Atrophy (loss of muscle bulk) or hypertrophy (enlarged, abnormal muscle bulk) are noted. The muscles are felt to palpate their bulk for tenderness, lumps, and tone. Resistance to passive range of motion is noted as is any rigidity, spasticity, or flaccidity. Strength is assessed on a scale of 0 to 4, muscle group actions, and individual muscular functions; grade strength normal = 4; plegia (paralysis) = 0.

Movement is assessed by observation: the client at rest for involuntary movements; volitional movements, performed upon request; smoothness, jerkiness, or slowness of movements; or lack of movement. A slight limp, awkwardness in turning, and loss of associated arm-swinging are examples of important findings.

If possible, the client's spontaneous movements and activities in bed should be observed. One may discover one side is not moved as much as the other, indicating hemiparesis (one-sided paralysis).

While the client is seated, he is asked to hold his arms outstretched in front of him with elbows fully extended, wrists dorsiflexed, fingers extended, and eyes closed while the examiner observes for "drift." Usually, a normal person can hold this posture without any change. Weakness on one side leads to gradual relaxation of the finger extensors, the wrist and elbow extensors, and the flexors of the shoulder. A similar test can be done with the legs. While the client lies prone, ask him to flex his knees at a 45 degree angle and strongly dorsiflex his ankles. If both limbs on the same side show "drift," there may be a contralateral cerebral lesion.

The purpose of assessing motor and sensory functioning are to determine if any pathways are affected and if so, to localize the lesion to either the peripheral nerves, nerve roots, spinal cord, brain stem, cerebellum, basal ganglia, or the cerebral hemispheres. Two general principles in motor function testing are:

1. Upper motor neuron lesions are characteristic of hypertonicity of muscles, hyperactive deep tendon reflexes, and pathological reflexes.
2. Lower motor neuron lesions are characteristic of hypotonicity of muscles, atrophy, hypoactive deep tendon reflexes, and no pathological reflexes.

REFLEXES

The most commonly tested reflexes are stretch, or the deep tendon reflexes, and superficial or cutaneous reflexes. All reflexes require the participation of sensory receptors, afferent neurons, central synapses, and sometimes interneurons, efferent neurons, and effectors.

Reflexes are usually graded from 0 to 4, depending upon the response. Gradings are as follows: 0 = no response; 1 = low normal; 2 = normal; 3 = brisk, may not be indicative of pathology; and 4 = hyperactive, usually indicative of pathology. The biceps, triceps, brachioradialis, patellar, achilles, and plantar reflexes are included in the examination.

STRETCH, DEEP TENDON, REFLEXES. Stretch or deep tendon reflexes are tested by tapping a tendon close to the body surface with a reflex hammer. This action stimulates a stretch receptor which elicits a reflex contraction of the attached muscle. Reflexes of one side are compared with similar reflexes on the opposite side.

BICEPS REFLEX. The client's elbow is supported in your hand while placing your thumb over his biceps tendon. The reflex hammer is struck so that the blow is aimed directly through your thumb at the biceps tendon. The contraction of the biceps muscle under your thumb is observed or felt.

TRICEPS REFLEX. The client's arm is flexed at the elbow and pulled across his chest. The triceps tendon is struck just above the elbow and quick extension of the forearm is watched for.

BRACHIORADIALIS REFLEX. The forearm is pronated, and the radius is struck about 2 to 5 cm above the wrist. Observation is for flexion of the forearm and the fingers.

PATELLAR REFLEX. The client is asked to sit or lie down. The knee is supported in slight flexion. The reflex hammer is tapped lightly at the patellar tendon just below the patella; this should cause a quick extension of the knee.

ACHILLES REFLEX. The client is asked to sit or lie down with the leg somewhat flexed at the knee; the ankle is dorsiflexed. The reflex hammer is tapped lightly just above the os calcis with the expected result of quick plantar flexion of the foot.

PLANTAR REFLEX. The client's ankle is grasped by the examiner. A blunt point, either the dull end of a reflex hammer, a wooden applicator tip, or the end of a split wooden tongue blade is used to stroke with moderate pressure the lateral border of the sole from the heel toward the ball of the foot, curving medially to follow the bases of the toes. The normal movement will be flexion of the toes. In the presence of upper motorneuron lesions, the stretch or deep reflexes will be exaggerated.

SUPERFICIAL REFLEXES. The superficial reflexes are tested by scratching the skin with an object such as a pin or the end of a split wooden tongue blade. The reflexes usually tested are the abdominal and cremasteric reflexes. To test the *abdominal reflex,* the skin of the abdomen is lightly stroked from the periphery to the umbilicus in four quadrants. The normal reaction will be contraction of the abdominal muscles and deviation of the umbilicus toward the stimulus. The *cremasteric reflex* is tested in males by lightly stroking the skin of the medial aspect of the thigh. The normal reaction will be elevation of the testicle on that side. In the presence of upper motor neuron lesions, the superficial abdominal and cremasteric reflexes are attenuated.

ABNORMAL REFLEXES. Other reflexes that indicate pathologic motor involvement are the Hoffman, Babinski and Chaddock's reflexes. To test the

Hoffman reflex, the client's hand is held with his fingers extended and relaxed. His extended middle finger is supported and his fingertip flicked up or down. In the presence of pyramidal tract disease, there will be flexion and adduction of the thumb. The *Babinski reflex* is tested with a blunt instrument, which is used to stroke the lateral aspect of the sole of the foot from the heel toward the ball of the foot, curving medially to follow the bases of the toes. Normally, this would elicit the plantar flexion of the great and small toes. In the presence of pyramidal tract disease, Babinski's reflex results. Manifestations are dorsiflexion of the big toe, fanning of the toes, dorsiflexion of the ankle, and flexion of the knee and thigh. There may be partial responses to the stimuli; these partial responses relate to the different degrees of pathology of the pyramidal tract. If discomfort or ticklishness occurs and interferes with the testing, the *Chaddock reflex* may be tested instead. In this test, the lateral aspect of the foot is stroked beneath the lateral malleolus of the ankle. In the presence of pyramidal tract disease, the same extensor response as is seen in the Babinski reflex will be noted.

SENSORY FUNCTION

The examination of sensation is difficult as tests may be inadequate and responses to sensory stimuli may not be readily evaluated objectively. Generally, it must be determined if sensory findings are the same in symmetrical parts of the body. If the client is alert and cooperative, the examination would include testing his perceptions of *pain, temperature, light touch, position, vibration,* and *stereognosis.* The client is asked to close his eyes during tests. For more detailed testing, the client's eyes are screened from the part being examined.

Superficial pain is tested clinically by pricking the skin with a pin. Different parts of the body are touched with either the sharp or dull end of the pin. The client is asked to respond properly to sharp and dull sensations. Deep pain is elicited by applying pressure on deep structures, such as squeezing the Achilles tendon.

Sensation to *temperature* is not usually tested because the pathways for temperature perception are close to those for pain. Therefore, temperature perception needs to be tested only when there is a questionable response to pinprick. Temperature sensation is then assessed by applying test tubes filled with hot and cold water to various body parts. The client answers "hot" or "cold" each time that particular test tube touches his skin.

Wisps of cotton are used to *lightly touch* different areas on both sides of the body simultaneously. Then concentration is on separate sides. The client is asked to describe perceived sensations. Numbness is a word used sometimes by stroke clients to describe their symptoms. It may mean dysesthesia, paresthesia, anesthesia, hypesthesia, or even weakness or paralysis without sensory symptoms.

To test a sense of *position* the terminal phalanx of each digit is grasped by its sides and each digit moved up or down. The client is asked to identify that direction.

Vibration sense combines touch and rapid alterations of deep pressure sense. To test this a tuning fork is placed over the bony prominences of the body. The client responds primarily to vibration, and not to the pressure of the tuning fork. The client is asked to indicate when he no longer feels the vibrations. At that time you can apply it to your own body, comparing the client's threshold for vibrations with your own body's reaction. Advancing age may diminish this sense, particularly, at the toes and ankles.

Stereognosis is the ability to recognize shapes and identify objects by means of touch alone. This is a cerebral cortical function, but the tactile elements of information travel through the dorsal columns of the spinal cord and the medial lemniscus in the brain stem. Articles (e.g., pins, nails, or apples) are placed in the client's hands, and he is asked to identify the articles by touch. The lack of recognition of shape and form is frequently found with cortical lesions.

COORDINATION

The usual tests for coordination, *finger-to-nose, heel-to-shin,* and *rapid, repeated alternating movements* are commonly classified as "cerebellar" tests. Skillful performance of these tests requires, however, that other parts of the motor apparatus are in good order. The perfect execution of acts is called *eupraxia* and loss of this ability in performance is *apraxia.* Slowness in the performance of these tests can be the only abnormality, and while that slowness is consistent with a cerebellar disorder, it is not enough for identification as a disorder. Finger-to-nose and heel-to-shin tests can often be made to bring out the highly significant, side-to-side tremor. The client should be made to do the tests accurately and precisely. Rapid, repeated alternating movements are particularly helpful when seeking cerebellar incoordination in the legs.

The client is evaluated for general coordination of movement (e.g., arm-swinging) and smoothness of actions. A test for coordination is the Romberg test. (See Romberg test in preceding pages.) A client with lack of balance resulting from motor disorders will sway more if his visual cues are removed (i.e., truncal ataxia).

FINGER-TO-NOSE TEST. Muscle coordination of the upper extremities is assessed by this test. The client brings his arms from an outstretched position to touch his nose with one index finger and then with his other index finger first with eyes open, and then, closed. With a cerebellum disorder, the client will undershoot or overshoot his nose.

HEEL-TO-SHIN TEST. Muscular coordination of the lower extremities can be tested by having the client place his left heel on his right shin, run his heel down the full length of the shin, then repeat using the other leg. With a cerebellum disorder, the client's heel will slip from one side to the other side of the shin.

ALTERNATING MOVEMENTS. The client holds his forearms vertically and alternately pronates and supinates in rapid succession. With a cerebellum disorder, the movements will be incomplete or slowed.

Head and Neck

HEAD

Inspection and palpation are the principal means for examination of the head. Percussion and auscultation are minor contributing factors. Examination of the head will focus on its size, shape, and movement; the skin, eyes, ears, nose, oral cavity, and neck are all included in the assessment.

The head is observed for symmetry. The hands are run over the cranium and felt for irregularities. An *abnormally small* head may connote mental re-

tardation. Hydrocephalus is typified by a large head with a bulging forehead. Unusual movements of the head are noted as they may often suggest the presence of disease. For example, in Parkinson's disease, a slight tremor can be seen. Clients with tics or habitual spasms perform sudden, unexpected movements of the head. The movement of the head may be limited as in cervical osteoarthritis or torticollis. The scalp and skin are inspected for rashes and bulges. A tumor originating in the skin or the subcutaneous tissue of the forehead may produce a striking appearance as seen in lipoma of the forehead. Sebaceous cysts of the scalp are common. Using fairly deep pressure, palpate the cranium and face for tenderness. Marked tenderness of the forehead may be exhibited in frontal sinusitis.

FACE

Examination of the face should include attention to the skin, the symmetry, and the client's expression. The skin of the face may be markedly thin and tightened, such as in scleroderma. Moles and warts occur on the skin of the face; they should be examined carefully for signs of malignancy, such as darkened color or itching. The eyelids are examined and any evidence of edema noted. Symmetry and proportion of facial structures are assessed. Opposing sides of any body are never exactly alike, but marked differences may be indicative of an inflammatory process, neoplastic growth, or trauma. The nasolabial folds are noted in particular. One side of the face may sag as a result of paresis or paralysis of the facial muscles resulting from Bell's palsy or a cerebral vascular accident.

EYES

The components of the eye examination are: visual acuity and visual fields, which were discussed under the neurological examination, and assessment of the external eye.

Conjunctiva

The conjunctiva divides into the bulbar and the palpebral. The bulbar conjunctiva covers the eye up to the junction of cornea and sclera; the palpebral conjunctiva lines the posterior lid surface. The bulbar conjunctiva is readily examined by separating the lids widely and having the client look up, down, and to each side. Many small blood vessels are visible. Dilation of these vessels may produce redness caused by a variety of eye conditions.

The palpebral conjunctiva cannot be seen until the lids are everted. The upper lid is everted as follows: (1) The client looks down. (2) The upper eyelashes are grasped and pulled gently down and forward. (3) An applicator stick is placed across the lid and pushed downwards to evert the lid over the stick (this is used for inspection of the conjunctival surface). (4) The lid is returned to normal position by having the client look upwards.

The lower lid is everted as follows: The client looks upwards, and simultaneously the lid is slid downwards over the lower orbital rim. The conjunctiva is markedly reddened if conjunctivitis is present. It can be stained yellow in jaundice. A raised yellow plaque, a pinguecula, may occur in the bulbar conjunctiva on either side of the iris; its size increases with age (Fig. 21-3).

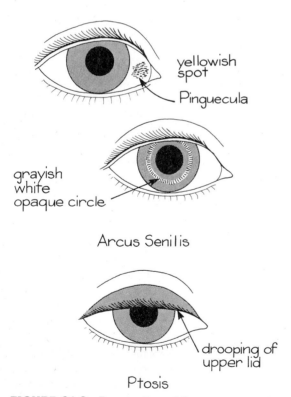

FIGURE 21-3. Examination of the eye: conjunctiva, cornea, and lid.

Sclera

The sclera is normally white. Exceptions may be pinguecula, some patches of pigment, or visible peripheral vessels in cases of tuberculosis of children and young adults.

Cornea

Normally, the cornea is perfectly smooth and transparent. The cornea is examined by obliquely moving illumination. Each cornea is compared. The corneal reflex was discussed previously with the neurological examination. The cornea may evidence opaque scars resulting from an old injury or a previous infection. Inflammation of the cornea, which can be caused by congenital syphilis, displays a clouding of the cornea. Arcus senilis is a thin grayish-white opaque circle, or a part of a circle, around the outer margin of the cornea (Fig. 21-3). When present in young people, it may suggest hypercholesterolemia. An annular, brownish-green ring of pigmentation (Kayser-Fleischer ring) on the posterior corneal surface near the limbus may be seen in Wilson's disease.

Eyelids

The eyelids serve a protective function. When the eyes are opened, the space between the opened upper and lower eyelids is called the palpebral fissure. The two angles of the eye slit are the external and the internal canthi. When the eye is opened, the lower lid is just under the junction of the cornea and sclera (the limbus).

It should be determined whether or not the palpebral fissures are equal in size. The eyelids are inspected and palpated for *position, infection, edema, entropion,* and *ectropion.* Pressure on the eyes when trying to separate the lids should be avoided. The lower lid can be retracted by pulling the skin downward over the cheek bone. The upper lid is lifted by pressing upwards over the brow. Ptosis of the upper lids results from paralysis of the third cranial nerve (Fig. 21-3). Weakness of the upper lids may be caused by myasthenia gravis. Distention of a meibomian gland with secretion may result in a cyst identified as a *chalazion* (Fig. 21-4). An infection of the hair follicles may produce a *hordeolum* (sty). Edema of the eyelids may be caused by allergies, nephritis, or hyperthyroidism. *Entropion* is an introversion, whereas *ectropion* is an eversion of the eyelids. Both processes are usually caused by trauma or inflammation.

Pupils

Normal pupils are equal in size, perfectly round, and constrict to light and accommodation. Direct reaction to light ensues whenever the pupil constricts by receiving increased light. Consensual pupil reaction occurs whenever the opposite eye constricts, although that pupil did not receive extra light.

The pupils are examined for equality in size and regularity. Inequality in the size of the two pupils is called *anisocoria,* which is often associated with many types of central nervous system diseases (Fig. 21-4). Constriction of the pupil, or *miosis,* is seen in inflammation of the iris and after the use of certain drugs such as morphine. Dilatation, or *mydriasis,* occurs in localized use of drops, in ocular trauma, or in acute glaucoma. Constriction or dilatation is most significant when it is unilateral (on one side only). Irregularity of pupil contour may occur from adhesions of the iris. This characteristic is visible in syphilis of the central nervous system or in trauma. The pupillary light reflex is tested by having the client fix on a distant object. A light is shined into each eye while observing for constriction of the pupils from the light stimulus. Simultaneously, inspection for consensual pupil reaction is done. The pupils of elderly persons may react sluggishly to light. However, reactions are hastened after several stimulations.

If there is monocular blindness, the pupil of the affected eye will not respond directly but will react consensually whenever the opposite eye is stimulated. However, stimulation to the affected eye will not produce a consensual reaction to the opposite eye. To test for the accommodation reflex, the client focuses initially on a distant object, and then, at a finger held 5 to 10 cm from his nose. Normally, the pupils constrict whenever the client focuses on the nearer object. Pupils that react actively to accommodation but not to light are called *Argyll Robertson pupils.* They are often related to syphilis of the central nervous system.

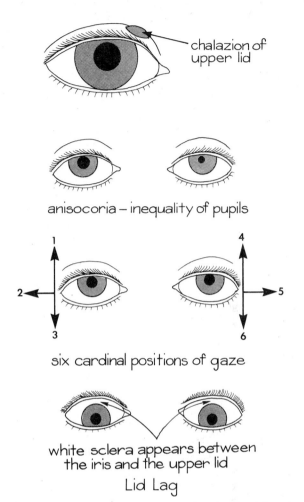

chalazion of upper lid

anisocoria – inequality of pupils

six cardinal positions of gaze

white sclera appears between the iris and the upper lid
Lid Lag

FIGURE 21-4. Examination of the eye: eyelid and pupils. Six cardinal positions of gaze.

Extraocular Muscles

Of the six muscles that control eye movements, four are innervated by the oculomotor nerve. The remaining two muscles are innervated by the trochlear and abducens cranial nerves. Extraocular movements are best tested by moving the eyes into six cardinal positions of gaze (Fig. 21-4).

To assess extraocular movements the examiner stands in front of the client. The client's head is immobilized by having his chin held. He is directed to focus on the examiner's finger through the six cardinal positions of gaze (Table 21-2). Inability to turn one's eyes to a given position indicates that the muscle is weakened or paralyzed.

TABLE 21-2. Normal Extraocular Movements

Extraocular Muscle	Position
Superior rectus (third nerve)	Up and temporal
Inferior rectus (third nerve)	Down and temporal
Lateral rectus (sixth nerve)	Straight temporal
Medial rectus (third nerve)	Straight nasal
Superior oblique (fourth nerve)	Down and nasal
Inferior oblique (third nerve)	Up and nasal

Other abnormalities in extraoculomotor movements are strabismus, lid lag, and nystagmus which can be observed through the six cardinal positions of gaze. Disparity between the movement of the eyes is manifested in *strabismus*. *Lid lag* is tested by holding a finger above the client's eye level; as the finger moves downwards, the client's upper lids are observed. Normally, the eyelid will overlap the iris in its downward movement. Whenever there is some white sclera exposed during the downward movement, the lid appears to lag behind the globe. This is typified in Graves' disease. To test for *nystagmus,* a pause is made during the upward and lateral positions of the six cardinal fields of gaze. Nystagmus is a rapid and jerky motion of the eyeballs as the client looks up and down and from side to side. It may be the result of visual fatigue, refractive error, or associated with central nervous system diseases. To test for convergence of the eyes, the capacity of the eyes to turn inward whenever looking at a close object is observed. This can be assessed whenever testing the pupillary reaction to accommodation. The medial recti muscles contract to move the eyes into alignment to focus images on the same part of the retina. Otherwise, the two images will not fuse, and *diplopia* (double vision) will result.

Funduscopic Examination

During the funduscopic examination, the appearance of the optic disc, the macula, the blood vessels, and the remaining retina are observed.

The room is darkened and the seated client looks 20° upward and temporally at a distant object. The client is instructed to hold his eyes perfectly still. The ophthalmoscope is set at +8 or +10 lens (identified by the black numbers). The examiner's left eye examines the client's left eye, and the right eye is employed for examination of the client's right eye. The examiner's nose is parallel to the client's right eye and his cheek. The left forefinger is utilized to change the lens while the right hand rests upon the head of the client. The right thumb can retract and hold the client's upper lid gently to prevent blinking. Starting 12 inches (30 cm) from the client's eye, the light is shined through the pupil and a golden-red reflex should be seen. Any black spots showing against the red aura should be noted. These are opacities interrupting the red reflex. Holding the ophthalmoscope, the examiner starts moving closer to the client until it is about 3 inches (8 cm) from the client's eye and at a 15 degree angle; then the lens disc is rotated in the sight hole from +10 diopters (indicated by the black numbers), to −5 diopters (indicated by the red numbers). This exercise will aid in finding the optimal magnification for a distinct view of the retina. When a cataract has been extracted, approximately +10 is needed for correction. If both the client and the examiner have normal vision, then the best view is obtained whenever the lens disc is turned to zero.

When the correct setting for the ophthalmoscope is found, the examiner moves in closer to the client until the forehead rests firmly against the right thumb that is over the client's forehead. The fundus should now be seen in the vicinity of the optic disc. The following characteristics of the optic disc are noted: (1) the shape is round or oval; (2) the color is primarily light red; (3) the margin should be sharp and clear; (4) the physiologic cup is a pale (normally yellowish-white) area in the temporal side of the disc devoid of nerve fibers and forms a slight depression. The size and shape of the cup will vary in normal eyes. Blood vessels may be distinguished as follows. (1) Arterioles are bright red with a central white reflex stripe. (The width of the reflex stripe is noted). Arterioles do not pulsate in the retina. They are about two-thirds to four-fifths the diameter of veins. (2) Veins are a darker red and lack a central white reflex stripe. They normally pulsate. Their size is normally one-quarter wider than the arterioles. Normally the arterioles and veins interweave into the retinal periphery without sharp changes in direction. Therefore, veins at the arteriovenous crossings are observed for nicking, humping, tapering, and banking which is suggestive of retinal arteriolar sclerosis (Fig. 21-5). The background of the retina is red-orange. There may be

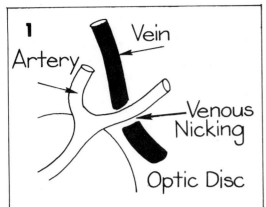
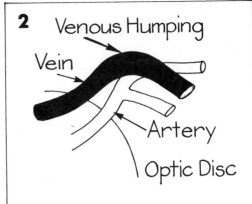
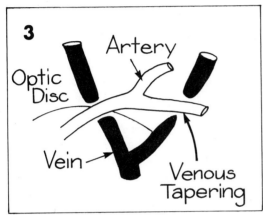
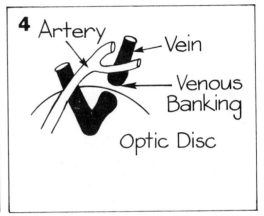

FIGURE 21-5. Ophthalmoscopic examination of the fundus of the eye: venous nicking, humping, tapering and banking.

varied amounts of black pigments as influenced by complexion and race. White areas caused by scarring, hemorrhages, and exudates are scanned for. These are usually attributed to retinal hypertension or diabetic retinopathy (Fig. 21-6). To examine the macula, the client is asked to look directly into the light, and the macula can then be visualized. It is about two to three disc diameters to the temporal side of the disc margin and appears as a small red disc area with a central white or shining dot, called the fovea centralis.

Intraocular Pressure

The measurement of intraocular pressure is achieved by palpation (digital tonometry) and the use of a tonometer.

Digital tonometry or palpation, can only discern *extremes* of intraocular pressure. Place the tips of both forefingers on the closed upper lid. Apply gentle alternating pressure. Press the eyeball gently with one forefinger, and assess the amount (large or small) of pressure needed to move the other forefinger outwardly.

The most accurate measurement of intraocular pressure is determined with the tonometer. After the eye is anesthetized with drops, the tonometer is placed on the cornea. The midportion of the cornea is displaced inwardly by pressure applied by a plunger. Intraocular pressure is the amount of this displacement. The normal intraocular pressure is usually from 10 to 30 mm of mercury with 15 mm Hg, the average. The principal usages of tonometry are inquiry for open angle glaucoma and for an increase in pressure after the pupils have been dilated. This test should be included in every routine physical examination of all clients over the age of 40, unless the eye is infected.

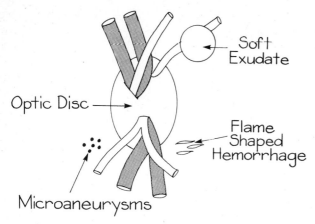

FIGURE 21-6. Ophthalmoscopic examination of the retina.

EAR

The three divisions of the ear are the external, middle, and inner ear. The auricle and external canal comprise the external ear; the tympanic membrane (which is pearly-gray in color and translucent), the tympanic cavity with the three ossicles, and the eustachian tube comprise the middle ear, and the labyrinth comprises the inner ear (Fig. 21-7).

The pinna or auricular and mastoid processes are inspected first. Then the otoscope using the largest speculum that fits the canal comfortably is selected. The pinna is pulled upwards and backwards in an adult to straighten the external canal bringing the tympanic membrane or the drum into position where it can be viewed. The speculum is inserted and the external canal examined for foreign bodies, discharge, lesions, or edema. Redness, excoriation and inflammation of the external canal may be due to infection or external otitis (known as swimmer's ear) (Fig. 21-8). The speculum is adjusted in the canal until the eardrum is visualized. Debris or cerumen (wax) may have to be carefully removed with a cotton tipped applicator in order to visualize the eardrum. The eardrum is inspected and the landmarks identified (pars flaccida, short process and handle of the malleus, umbo, light reflex, and pars tensa). Color, perforations, scars, position of the handle of the malleus, inflammation and bulging of the eardrum are noted (Fig. 21-9). The color of the eardrum is pearly-gray; areas of transparency (healed perforations) or white-chalky opacity (calcification) should be noted. An amber or red color would be a notable contrast to the normal color. The handle of the malleus stands out as a ridge

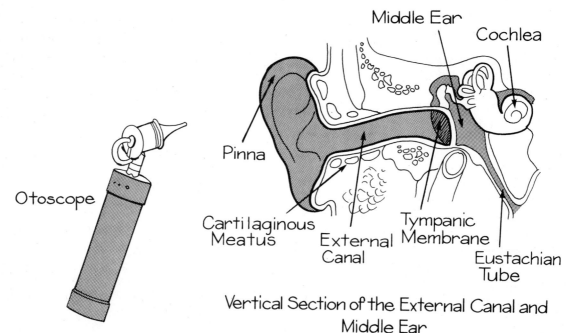

FIGURE 21-7. Examination of the structures of the ear.

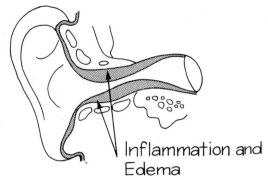

Inflammation and Edema

FIGURE 21-8. Examination of the ear: external otitis.

running downwards and backwards across the upper half of the eardrum. Occasionally, a few dilated vessels are seen along the bone. In the anteroinferior portion of the eardrum, there is a triangular, glistening area in which the light reflex can be seen. These landmarks may be obscured when there is bulging of the eardrum.

The client is instructed to perform the Valsalva's maneuver by occluding the nostrils and attempting to breathe forcefully through the nose. This applies pressure through the eustachian tube to the middle ear. If the eustachian tube is patent, an outward motion of the eardrum is observed by a change in the configuration of the light reflex. The function of the middle ear mechanism is dependent upon the patency of the eustachian tube; if the tube does not open intermittently to replenish the air in the middle ear space, a partical vacuum results causing a transudation of fluid into the middle ear with resultant hearing loss.

HEARING TESTS. The client's hearing ability is ascertained by the following tests: identifying the ticking of a watch, the Weber test, and the Rinne test (See previous discussion of Weber and Rinne tests in preceding pages.) Hearing losses are of two types: *perceptive* (nerve deafness) and *conductive* losses. Perceptive losses may occur from congenital deafness, hereditary deafness, drug toxicity, infections, or trauma. Conductive losses may occur from disorders of the eardrum, or middle ear, or otosclerosis.

LABYRINTHINE TEST. The inner ear has a function in controlling balance or equilibrium. This is assessed by performing the labyrinthine test for

falling (Romberg's sign) (See previous discussion under neurological examination.)

NOSE

The lining of the nose is a mucous membrane that enables material to go into solution and stimulate the olfactory nerves. The mucus also provides a source of water from which the inspired air is humidified. The lining epithelium is ciliated so that the mucus is carried along with inhaled particulate matter into the pharynx. The blood supply of the nose is particularly generous in the region of the anterior end of the inferior turbinates. The sinuses arise as diverticula from off the nasal cavities and assume their full size as the face finally reaches adult dimensions. The sinus is equipped with cilia to enable mucus to be carried through the ostium to join the nasal stream (Fig. 21-10). The external nose should be inspected for its symmetry, any deformity, and for any loss of structure. Deviation of the nose may be caused by an old fracture of nasal cartilage (Fig. 21-11). The syphilitic nose may resemble a "saddle nose" caused by erosion of the nasal bones (Fig. 21-11). The bulbous and discolored nose may be caused by chronic acne rosacea (Fig. 21-11).

Using the short wide nasal speculum, the otoscope is gently inserted and the lower portions of the nose are examined. The client's head is tilted slightly backwards to inspect the roof of the cavity. Care must be taken not to touch the very sensitive nasal septum. The mucous membrane is assessed; its normal color is pink. The mucosa is reddened in viral rhinitis and bogged in allergic rhinitis. The inferior and middle turbinates and meatus lying lateral to the middle turbinate are inspected. Any

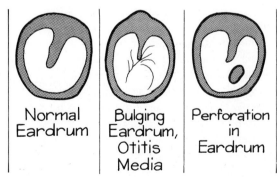

| Normal Eardrum | Bulging Eardrum, Otitis Media | Perforation in Eardrum |

FIGURE 21-9. Examination of the ear: eardrum.

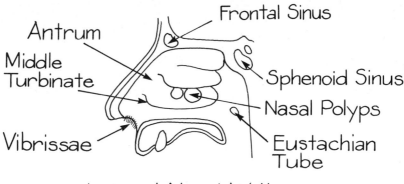

FIGURE 21-10. Examination of the nose: internal structures.

swelling, increased redness, pallor, or polyps should be noted. Clients with chronic rhinitis may develop nasal polyps, which physically are soft, pale, spherical masses of mucosa. Pressure exerted over the bony ridge just below and behind the eyebrow will detect any frontal sinus tenderness. Pressure exerted over the malar eminence will uncover any maxillary sinus tenderness.

ORAL CAVITY

In the oral cavity, where food is broken into small fragments, saliva is provided by the major and minor salivary glands to prepare the food for passage through the esophagus. The pharynx is equipped with lymphoid tissue. The larynx has powerful adductor muscles to perform as an efficient sphincter.

The breath should be noted as certain odors are characteristic of conditions. In oral sepsis, there is halitosis. The breath in diabetes mellitus has a sweetish, fruity odor. In uremia, the breath may have a urinous odor. The breath of a client with severe parenchymal liver disease may have an amine odor.

When examining the oral cavity, a tongue depressor is used to retract the lips and cheeks for visualization. The lips are checked for color, fissures, lesions, and structure. They show a marked cyanosis in pneumonia, congenital heart disease, and in polycythemia vera. Fissures in the corner of the mouth are called angular stomatitis or *cheilosis.* One of the common lesions of the lips is herpes simplex. The lips may be deformed from birth, such as cleft lip. The state or repair of the teeth and the condition of the gums should be noted. If the client has dentures, they should be removed and checked for fit. Gingivitis is usually caused by poor dental hygiene and occurs in deficiency diseases such as blood dyscrasias or metallic poisoning. Hyperplasia (excessive proliferation) of the gums may be caused by monocytic leukemia or the anticonvulsant drug, Dilantin.

The mucosa should be inspected for color, hydration, lesions, and nodules. Particular attention is paid to the floor of the mouth. Palpation of suspicious areas is essential. Any white areas of thickened epithelium (leukoplakia) should be noted. Leukoplakia resembles dried white paint. Any part of the oral mucosa plus the tongue may be involved. Leukoplakia may be a precancerous lesion.

The parotid and submaxillary glands should be identified. The openings of the parotid glands are located in the oral mucosa opposite the second upper molar and the submaxillary glands at the base of the tongue. Swelling behind the mandibular ramus (which is always present in parotid enlargement) should be palpated with the fingers. Free flowage of saliva is ensured by compressing these glands. Absence of clear saliva may indicate the presence of a calculus in the duct.

The client should be asked to show his tongue. Both surfaces of the tongue are inspected for color, markings, movement, ulcers, and symmetry. There may be pallor of the tongue as well as smoothness and glossiness in conditions such as pernicious anemia and sprue. The papillae on the upper surface and sides of the tongue will be diminished or absent. Marked furrowing of the tongue may be

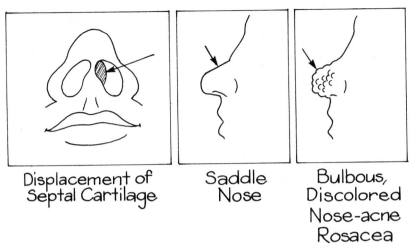

Displacement of Septal Cartilage   Saddle Nose   Bulbous, Discolored Nose-acne Rosacea

FIGURE 21-11. Examination of the nose: deviations from normal.

characteristic of syphilis. In lesions of the hypoglossal nerve, the tongue will not protrude in the midline but will deviate towards the side on which the lesion is located. The tongue may be atrophied on the side of the lesion. Ulcers of the tongue may be caused by carcinoma, syphilis, or tuberculosis. Normally, the hard palate is whitish in color and has rugae running transversely, whereas the soft palate is pink and has fine vessels under the mucosa. The color and condition of the palates is noted. The mobility of the soft palate is checked by having the client say "ah." The soft palate rises on phonation. During the examination of the soft palate, any limitation of opening of the mouth (trismus) should be noted. The presence or absence of the tonsils should be noted, and the adjacent retromolar area inspected. The nasopharynx can only be examined with a small mirror, and frequently, the examination is difficult; the choana and the eustachian tube orifices should be observed. With a laryngeal mirror, one should be able to see the base of the tongue with its normal lymphoid tissue, the epiglottis, and the color and movements of the vocal cords.

NECK

The following structures are carefully identified and palpated; lymph nodes, cervical muscles and vertebrae, jugular veins, carotids, thyroid gland, and the trachea. The carotid arteries and the thyroid gland are then auscultated. The client should be seated and the neck inspected for masses, scars, and symmetry.

LYMPH NODES. The client is asked to flex his neck slightly forward. The neck is palpated with the pads of the index and middle fingers by moving the skin over the underlying tissue in each area in a rotating motion. Consistency, location, moveability, size, and tenderness of any palpable nodes are noted. The various groups of lymph nodes to palpate are: (1) the posterior cervical which are found at the anterior edge of the trapezius; (2) the anterior cervical which are located along the side of the sternocleidomastoid muscles and along either side of the trachea; (3) the submandibular which are under the ridge of the mandible; (4) the preauricular found in front of the ear; (5) the postauricular which are anterior to the mastoid process; (6) the occipital at the base of the scalp; and (7) the supraclavicular in the supraclavicular fossae (Fig. 21-12). Slow, gentle sliding or rotary motions with the palpating fingers should more easily reveal slightly enlarged nodes. The lymph nodes in the neck may be enlarged (lymphadenopathy) in many diseases. Lymphadenopathy may be caused by extension of infection or cancer of the mouth or throat, or in Hodgkin's disease, leukemia, measles, or infectious mononucleosis.

CERVICAL MUSCLES AND VERTEBRAE. It should be noted if the neck is supple, or if there are any deformities of the cervical spine. The client is

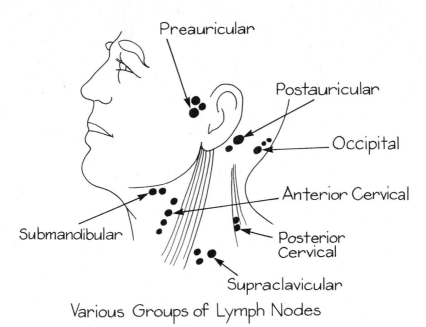

Various Groups of Lymph Nodes

FIGURE 21-12. Examination of the neck: lymph nodes.

asked to touch his chin to his chest, extend his neck posteriorly, and to turn his neck to either side. Limitation of head and neck movements may result from cervical muscle spasms, cervical arthritis, or meningeal irritation. A torticollis or wryneck causes deviation of the head toward the affected side as sternocleidomastoid muscles are shortened. Torticollis can be congenital, or a dislocation of the upper cervical vertebrae may produce the condition.

JUGULAR VEINS. Examination of the external and internal jugular veins enables accurate estimation of venous pressure and aids in determining the presence of disease. Normally, they are not distended when the client is sitting. When the client is in a recumbent position, the veins fill. It should be noted if the client's jugular veins are distended when his head is elevated to 45 degrees. Normally, they do not fill more than 1 or 2 cm above the clavicles at 45 degrees. Venous pressure can be estimated by measuring the height of the veins from the sternal angle. Venous pressure more than 4 cm H_2O above the sternal angle is considered elevated. In congestive heart failure, pulmonary hypertension, or constrictive pericarditis, the veins of the neck are usually engorged.

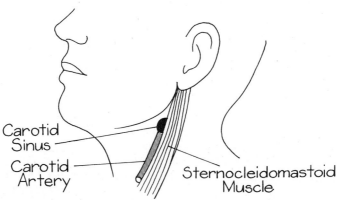

FIGURE 21-13. Palpation of carotid artery.

CAROTID ARTERIES. The common carotid is deep in the neck near the anterior border of the sternocleidomastoid muscle (Fig. 21-13). In thin clients, it may be possible to observe the carotid artery through the tissues of the neck. In aortic disease of the heart, the carotid arteries often beat with unusual force. Gently press the carotid artery in the lower part of the neck by rolling the fingertips over the medial border of the sternocleidomastoid muscle. Pressuring the artery in the upper half of the neck should be avoided as it is the site of the carotid sinus. The force of impulse is noted, and the carotid pulsations on one side should be compared with that of the other side. During auscultation the client is asked to hold his breath briefly. The carotid artery is lightly auscultated in the lower half of the neck. A carotid artery that is narrowed by arteriosclerosis will often evidence a bruit, which is a sound resulting from turbulent blood flow through the stenosed area.

THYROID GLAND. The thyroid gland is butterfly-shaped and lies just below the thyroid cartilage (Fig. 21-14). The normal thyroid is usually not palpable, or is just slightly palpable. In a thin neck, the isthmus of the thyroid may be palpable at the level of the third or fourth tracheal ring. By simple extension and lateral deviation of the neck, any enlargement of the thyroid in the lower half of the neck in the anterior triangles can be observed. If the normal thyroid gland is palpable, a firm, smooth mass, which moves upwards with swallowing will be felt. The examiner stands behind the seated client and places the thumbs in back of the client's neck and positions the fingertips of both hands firmly over the thyroid gland. The thyroid isthmus just below the cricoid cartilage is felt for first. Then each lateral lobe is palpated. Whenever necessary, the client is asked to swallow; thyroid tissue rises with swallowing. The thyroid gland slips between the fingers permitting evaluation of each lateral lobe for size, contour, firmness, and for any nodules (Fig. 21-15). Palpation can also be done while the examiner is seated in front of the client. With one thumb the trachea is pushed toward the right side. The other thumb and forefinger are pressed deeply behind the sternocleidomastoid muscle. The underlying lateral thyroid lobe is palpated with these two fingers. The procedure is reversed for the other side (Fig. 21-15). Auscultation over an enlarged thyroid may reveal a systolic bruit, resulting from increased blood flow through the tissue. Enlargement of the thyroid gland may be suggestive of carcinoma (Fig. 21-15).

TRACHEA. The trachea normally lies in the midline of the neck. The trachea is checked for deviation by placing the index finger into the sternal notch to palpate the trachea. Then the finger is rolled off the trachea first on one side and then on

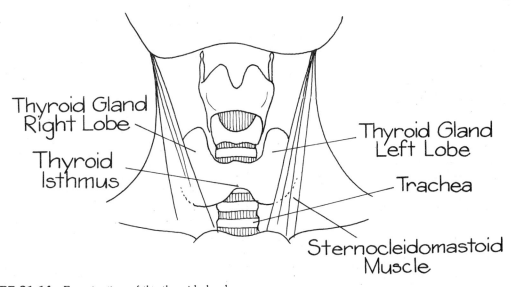

FIGURE 21-14. Examination of the thyroid gland.

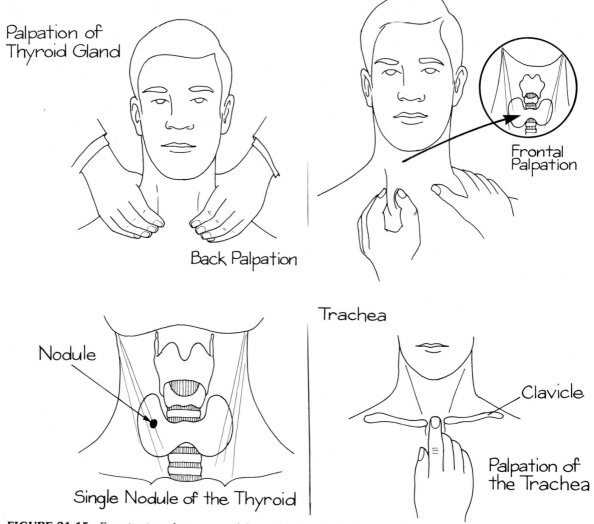

Palpation of Thyroid Gland

Back Palpation

Frontal Palpation

Trachea

Nodule

Single Nodule of the Thyroid

Clavicle

Palpation of the Trachea

FIGURE 21-15. Examination of structures of the neck: thyroid gland and trachea.

the other side. The distance on both sides between the trachea and the manubrium is measured. Deviation of the trachea may be caused by a mass in the upper neck (Fig. 21-15). The trachea and mediastinum may deviate to the opposite side with spontaneous pneumothorax. Deviation to the ipsilateral side occurs in pulmonary atelectasis.

Breast and Axilla

FEMALE BREAST

The breast functions as an integral part of the reproductive system. Glandular tissue forms 15 to 20 lobes arranged radially about the nipple, and adipose tissue envelops the stroma between and around the lobes. The central portion is primarily glandular while the peripheral area is mostly fat. Breast tissue forms a circular area and from this circle the axillary tail of gland tissue extends laterally along the axillae fascia. Lymph drainage from the breasts flows into the internal mammary and axillary lymph nodes. The skin of the nipple, which is pigmented and wrinkled, extends outwardly on the surface of the breast to form the areola. Color of the areola and nipple in nulliparae (never having been pregnant) ranges from pink to brown. Pregnancy and oral contraceptive medications increase areolar pigmentation. It should be noted that the physical assessment of the breasts should be implemented in the postmenstrual cycle since the menses may mask or confuse findings, and the breasts may be sensitive just prior to menstruation. Tenderness may indicate an underlying inflammatory process or widespread chronic cystic mastitis.

The client should disrobe to the waist. The breasts are inspected for symmetry. Breast inspection should initially be performed with the client sitting erect with her arms at her sides and then with her arms raised. This technique frequently will outline asymmetry, fixation of the nipple, or fixed masses under or adjacent to the areola. The size and shape of each breast is compared as small differences may exist. Although asymmetry is usually a difference in development, enlargement of one of the breasts may be caused by a cyst, inflammation, or a tumor (Fig. 21-16).

Areolar Nodes and Nipples

The areolar nodes and the nipples should be compressed. Colostrum, normally, may be expressed from the nipples of parous (having been pregnant) women many years after pregnancy.

The nipples should be inspected for retraction, shape, appearance, ulcers, and discharge. If there is evidence of recent retraction of the nipple, there may be disease (e.g., carcinoma) in progress (Fig. 21-16). Dry scaling, excoriation, and fissures are noted. Breaks in the nipples are inspected for ulcers. Ulceration of both nipples usually indicates a dermatological disease; ulceration of one nipple may indicate a malignant process (e.g., Paget's disease, see Fig. 21-16). A discharge of any kind may identify disease along the ductal system; if present, consistency and color are noted. About 1 percent of clients with carcinoma of the breast will experience sanguineous discharge. Greenish, yellowish, or bluish secretion may indicate chronic cystic mastitis.

Skin

Retraction is characterized by a dimpling of a part of the skin of the breast. Because of the proximity of the breast tissue to the skin, any infiltration that

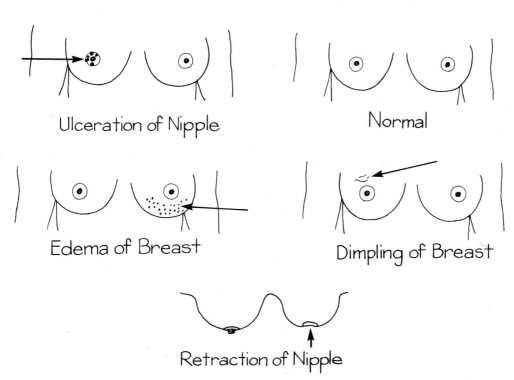

Ulceration of Nipple

Normal

Edema of Breast

Dimpling of Breast

Retraction of Nipple

FIGURE 21-16. Examination (inspection) of the female breasts and axillae.

inhibits traction on some of the ligaments results in dimpling over the area of the lesion (Fig. 21-16). Any maneuver that causes contraction of the pectoral muscles may elicit retraction. For determination of the presence of retraction, the client raises her arms, or presses her hands against her hips. Very minor skin retraction may be the earliest sign of carcinoma. The breast is examined for peau d'orange, edema of the skin, characterized by a "pig-skin" or "orange-peel" appearance. It is caused by a tumorous cell blockage of the lymphatic glands, that is, lymphadema (Fig. 21-16).

Axillae and Supraclavicular Area

Inspection should include the axillary and supraclavicular regions as they are important constituents in the lymphatic drainage system. They are scrutinized for bulges, edema, infection, and retractions.

A systematic examination of the breasts is then performed while the client is alternately erect and supine. Mentally the breasts are divided vertically and horizontally, intersecting at the nipple, into quadrants. These quadrants are identified as the upper medial and lateral quadrants, with a protrusion called the axillary tail, and the lower medial and lateral quadrants (Fig. 21-17). The axillary tail, is breast tissue which approaches the axillae. Masses in the breast are best probed by palpation with the flat surface of the hand rather than by the tips of the fingers. A rotary motion is used to compress the breast tissue against the chest wall. Starting at an outer quadrant of the breast, movement is towards the nipple and then away until all tissue in all quadrants has been examined. Systematically, the entire breast is palpated for thickening and masses. Any thickening in the upper outer quadrant

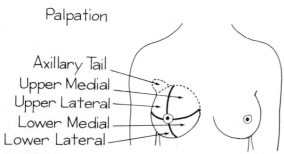

Palpation

Axillary Tail
Upper Medial
Upper Lateral
Lower Medial
Lower Lateral

FIGURE 21-17. Examination (palpation) of the female breasts and axillae.

of the breast should be noted. Observations should be repeated since about 65 percent of all cancers of the breast occur in this quadrant.

As the client sits, the left axilla is palpated with the right hand. The right hand is placed in the axilla with the fingers pointed towards the apex of the axilla and the palm towards the chest wall (Fig. 21-18). The fingers are brought downwards over the surface of the ribs. An attempt to feel the nodes as they are compressed against the chest wall should be made. The central group of nodes is located near the center of the thoracic wall of the axilla; the lateral axillary group is near the upper part of the humerus; the pectoral group is beneath the lateral edge of the pectoralis major muscle; the subscapular group is under the anterior edge of the latissimus dorsi muscle; and the area above the clavicle is palpated for the supraclavicular group (Fig. 21-18). Inflammatory process in the breast may be due to adenitis extending into the supraclavicular lymph nodes. The procedure is reversed in examining the opposite axilla.

MALE BREAST

The male breast consists of an areola and nipple above a thin disc of undeveloped breast tissue. The size of each breast is assessed. Then the male breast is examined for carcinoma, mastitis (inflammation of the breast), and gynecomastia (abnormally large mammary glands in the male). The areola and nipple are inspected and palpated for nodules, masses, and ulcerations.

Thorax and Lungs

Landmarks are necessary to identify the location of underlying structures and to describe the exact location of any abnormalities. All abnormalities should be described as so many centimeters medial or lateral to specific interspaces and vertical lines (see below).

A maximum amount of information may be gained during the examination of the thorax and lungs by following these suggestions: (1) Have the client undress completely to the waist. (A sleeveless paper gown for female clients prevents exposure while permitting examination.) (2) Tell the client to sit up straight or in a dorsal recumbent position. Alterations in expansion or symmetry may be vis-

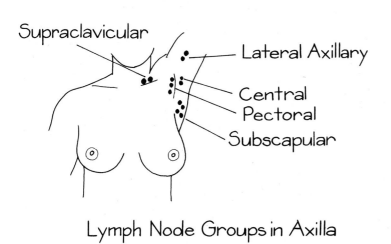

Lymph Node Groups in Axilla

Palpation of Left Axilla

FIGURE 21-18. Examination (palpation) of the axillae: lymph nodes.

ualized well in the recumbent position. (3) Oblique lighting is preferable. (4) Tell the client to breathe through the mouth more deeply than normal to increase the intensity of breath sounds. (5) Examine and compare one side of the thorax with the opposite side going from the apex to the base. (6) Relate a finding to the intercostal space and the distance from the vertical lines.

INSPECTION

Bony Landmarks

The manubriosternal junction or *angle of Louis* is a helpful landmark (Fig. 21-19). This is a visible bony ridge caused by the joining of the manubrium to the body of the sternum. This ridge corresponds to the second rib, and its costal cartilage serves as a starting point for counting ribs. The interspace immediately below it is the second interspace. The manubriosternal junction is also significant in the location of other structures in the thorax as it marks the location of the tracheal bifurcation, the body of the fourth thoracic vertebra, and the upper level of the aortic arch.

The most accurate way to count ribs and interspaces is to start from the second costal cartilage. The tip of the scapula is at the sixth and eighth rib depending on the degree of scapular elevation. The lowest rib palpable posteriorly is the eleventh or twelfth, depending on the individual.

The most prominent spinous process is called the vertebra prominens and is usually the seventh cervical vertebra.

Surface Markings and Vertical Lines

On the *anterior surface* of the chest the following vertical lines are used: (1) the midsternal line which

Sternum

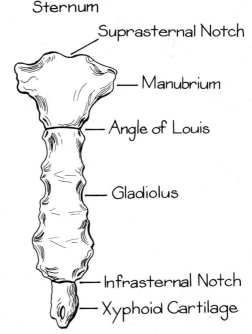

Suprasternal Notch

Manubrium

Angle of Louis

Gladiolus

Infrasternal Notch

Xyphoid Cartilage

FIGURE 21-19. Examination of the thorax: sternum.

Physical Examination of the Adult 319

is located in the middle of the sternum; and (2) the midclavicular line which runs directly downward from the midpoint of each clavicle (Fig. 21-20). On the *lateral surface* of the chest the vertical lines used are: (1) the anterior axillary line which runs downward from the origin of the anterior axillary fold along the anterolateral aspect of the chest; (2) the midaxillary line which runs downward from the apex of the axilla; and (3) the posterior axillary line which runs downward along the posterolateral wall of the thorax. On the *posterior surface* of the chest the vertical lines used are: (1) the midvertebral line which runs down the posterior spinous processes of the vertebrae; and (2) the scapular line which

goes through the inferior angle of the scapula when the client is erect and his arms are at his sides.

Apices of the lungs extend 3 to 4 cm above the clavicles. Lobes are separated by fissures so that location of these gives the location of the lobes. *Oblique fissures* separate the left lower lobe from the left upper lobe and the right upper and the right middle lobe from the right lower lobe. This extends from the thoracic vertebra downward and laterally to the junction of the fifth rib and the midaxillary line, thence anteriorly and medially to the sixth costochondral junction. *The horizontal fissure* is located anteriorly in the right hemithorax and separates the right upper lobe and the right middle lobe.

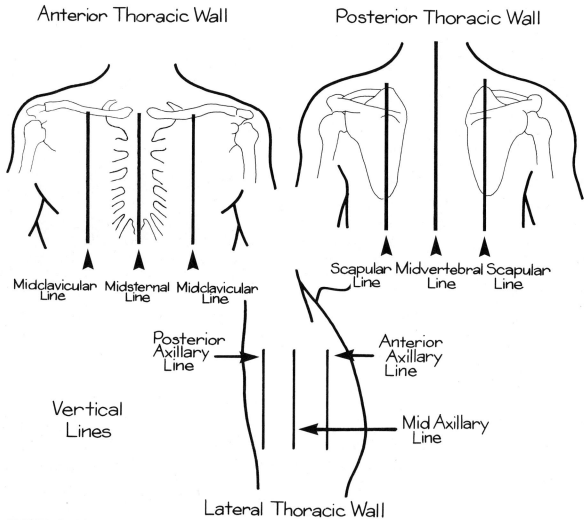

FIGURE 21-20. Examination of the thorax: surface markings.

This extends approximately from the midaxillary line at the level of the fifth rib horizontally to the third interspace at the right sternal border.

Knowledge of surface markings is important in making a correlation between physical findings and pathology. In auscultation of the chest it is often not possible to listen over every square centimeter of the chest, but one can at least listen over every segment.

Configuration of the Thorax and Integument

The symmetry is never perfect, but normally deviations are minor (Fig. 21-21). The sternum usually lies posterior to the midclavicular line. It is depressed behind the frontal plane of the thorax in the congenital defect known as pectus excavatum. The lower two-thirds of the sternum are primarily involved (Fig. 21-21). The xiphosternal junction may be drawn in posteriorly, and the upper end of the sternum may protrude anteriorly; this is known as pectus carinatum (Fig. 21-21).

In adults, the thorax is oval with a ratio of anteroposterior to lateral diameter ranging from 1:2 to 5:7. The ratio of anteroposterior to lateral diameter 1:1 or barrel chest, is present in some normal, short, stocky people or in the presence of thoracic

kyphosis. However, it is usually associated with emphysema (Fig. 21-21).

The skin of the thorax is normally smooth, supple and reflects the color of the skin elsewhere on the body. Skin is observed for cyanosis, excess veins, scars, seborrheic dermatitis, or spider nevi (angiomas) which are seen in cirrhosis of the liver. The adult male has a variable amount of hair on the thorax. Lack of hair may be a significant finding.

The musculature of the thorax consists of the pectoral and shoulder girdle; pectoral muscles may be larger on the side of the dominant hand. In neurological or muscular disease, wasting of the musculature or winging of the scapula may be observed. Interspaces are normally visible beneath the skin but may become greatly accentuated in cachexia or in neuromuscular disease causing wasting. Localized swellings may be due to lipomas or other skin tumors, tumors of the chest wall, or tumors of the rib.

The spine is observed for kyphosis or for scoliosis, with its attendant deformity of the ribs.

Respirations

Respirations are assessed as to their rate and character. Respiration in males tends to be diaphragmatic, whereas in females, it tends to be more cos-

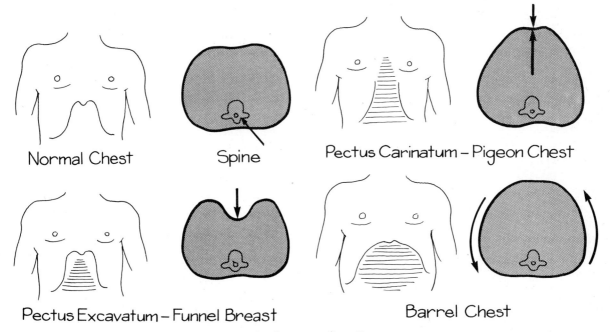

Normal Chest   Spine   Pectus Carinatum – Pigeon Chest

Pectus Excavatum – Funnel Breast   Barrel Chest

FIGURE 21-21. Examination (inspection) of the thorax: configuration.

tal. (See also Chapter 29, "The Assessment of Vital Signs" and Chapter 36, "Maintenance of Respiratory Status and Pulmonary Functioning.") *Quiet respirations* have a rate of 12 to 20 per minute, are regular, not very deep, use no accessory muscle, and are not accompanied by retraction of interspaces. In *deep breathing,* the normal chest wall moves symmetrically. Asymmetry indicates that chest wall or pleuropulmonary disease (e.g., acute pleurisy) with muscle splinting, pleural effusion, or pulmonary fibrosis may be present. The extent of excursion from full inspiration to full expiration is observed. The time for a complete forced expiration is normally less than 4 seconds. The following terms describe different types of respirations.

dyspnea. Discomfort or difficulty in breathing often associated with respiratory obstruction or abnormalities of rate and depth.

orthopnea. Dyspnea that is greatly worsened by recumbency.

bradypnea. Abnormally slowed respirations, such as that seen in opiate intoxication.

apnea. Cessation of respiration.

tachypnea. Increased rate of respirations.

hyperpnea. Increased depth of respirations.

hyperventilation. Increased minute ventilation seen in metabolic acidosis and emotional states.

periodic respiration. Regular alternation of periods of apnea and hyperpnea (Cheyne-Stokes asthma) seen in heart failure and brain disease and occasionally in infancy during sleep.

sighing respiration. Interspersed deep inspirations. (This is not due to organic disease.)

stertorous respiration. Noisy respiration due to the presence of secretions in the main airways. This may be seen in terminal or in any very weak or comatose client.

PALPATION

Palpation may validate the findings noted on inspection. The thorax is palpated for crepitations, masses, pulsations, and tenderness. To assess thoracic expansion, the examiner's hands are placed over the lower thorax anteriorly, with the thumbs pointing toward the xiphoid process and the fingers extended over the anterolateral wall. Symmetry of motion during quiet and deep breathing is assessed. Motion may be limited in one hemithorax, or both, as the result of fractured ribs, pleurisy,

pleural effusion, or trauma to the thorax (Fig. 21-22).

Fremitus is a term that means vibration. Fremitus is produced by phonation which sets in motion the thoracic wall. These vibrations can best be felt by the hand at the root of the neck, along the trachea, and at the major bronchi both anteriorly and posteriorly (Fig. 21-23). The client is asked to repeat a phrase ("ninety-nine") in a moderately loud voice. Symmetrical areas of the client's thorax are palpated to detect transmitted vibrations and compare them. Palpation is carried out with the ulnar border of the hand or the finger tips. Normal fremitus varies considerably in intensity over a single hemithorax; therefore, bilateral comparison is essential. The intensity of the vibration is determined by the following:

1. *Loudness of the voice*—vibrations are more intense with volume.
2. *Pitch of the voice*—the lower the pitch, the better the transmission of vibrations.
3. *Patency and proximity of the bronchi to the chest wall*—diminished vibrations are transmitted through a plugged bronchus.
4. *Thickness of the chest wall*—there is an increase of vibration in thin people and a decrease in obese people.
5. *State of the lung*—solidified lung tissue transmits vibration better than aerated tissue, such as in lobar pneumonia.
6. *Air-tissue interface*—seen in pneumothorax or air-fluid interface as seen in pleural effusion will damp out vibrations.

A *pleural friction rub* is a coarse grating sensation resulting from the rubbing of inflamed visceral and parietal pleura over one another. This can best be felt by using the flat of the entire hand.

PERCUSSION

When the chest is struck in a systematic way, the entire chest wall and underlying tissues will be set into motion, producing audible sounds. This enables the examiner to determine the relative amount of air and solid material in the underlying lung. It also helps to delineate the boundaries of organs or portions of the lung which differ in structural density. Percussion will locate only gross ab-

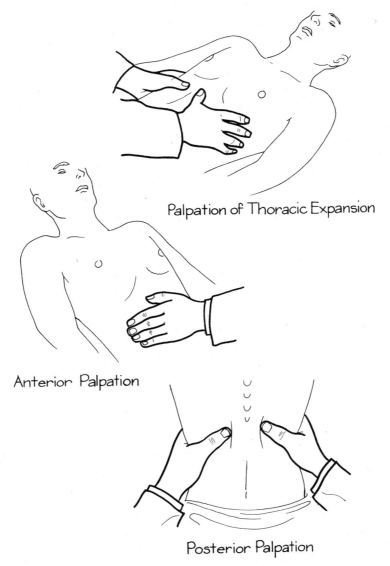

Palpation of Thoracic Expansion

Anterior Palpation

Posterior Palpation

FIGURE 21-22. Examination (palpation) of the thorax: anterior, posterior, and expansion.

normalities since it penetrates only about 5 to 7 cm into the chest, and lesions must be 2 to 3 cm in diameter to be detectable.

The client is positioned so that his head and shoulders are erect. Percussion proceeds downward from the apices to the bases, interspace by interspace, anteriorly and posteriorly. The client then raises his arm and each lateral wall is examined, beginning in the axilla and working down to the costal margin (Fig. 21-24). One side of the thorax must be compared with the opposite side. A careful analysis is made of the intensity, pitch, duration, and type of sound elicited by the percussion (Table 21-3).

Pitch of the sound depends upon the number of vibrations per second. When vibrations are rapid, the tone is high pitched, whereas when the vibrations are slow, the pitch is low.

Intensity of the sound depends upon the amplitude of the vibration. The loud tone has a greater amplitude of vibration than the soft tone. The porous lung is louder than the sound over the liver because the lung is more elastic, thereby vibrating with greater amplitude.

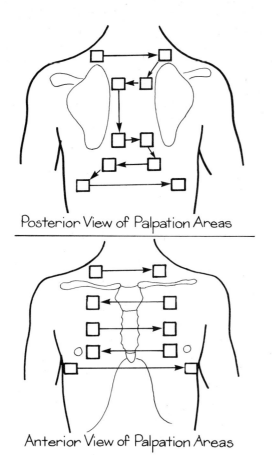

Posterior View of Palpation Areas

Anterior View of Palpation Areas

FIGURE 21-23. Examination (palpation) of the posterior and anterior thorax: fremitus.

Listening to *duration* of the sound helps to analyze the percussion note. The types of percussion sounds are classified as resonance, hyperresonance, dullness, flatness, and tympany. Resonance and hyperresonance are long in duration, whereas dullness and flatness are much briefer.

resonance. The percussion note that is emitted from the air-filled lung.

hyperresonance. A percussion note that has a deep, booming character. It is found normally in children; in the adult it is commonly the result of emphysema.

dullness. A note that sounds more like a thud. It is the opposite of resonance.

flatness. A note that sounds more like the sound emitted from striking a barrel filled with water. Flatness is considered as a more extreme manifestation of dullness.

tympany. A note that has a relatively musical sound. It results from air in an enclosed chamber.

Percussion sounds vary considerably from client to client depending on the amount of bone, muscle, or fat in each area. Comparison of symmetrical areas and a broad experience with the normal are essential. Percussion sounds vary with the intensity of the blow struck by the plexor (hammer or instrument of percussion). A lighter blow is often more helpful in determining the point of change from resonance to dullness.

Below the dome of the right diaphragm (fifth interspace in the midclavicular line) there is a flatness shading into dullness resulting from the liver. Below the fifth interspace in the midclavicular line on the left there is tympany resulting from the gas-filled stomach and colon. An enlarged spleen will encroach on this area; a left pleural effusion will obliterate it. There is dullness to the left of the sternum due to the presence of the underlying heart. In the left fifth interspace, this dullness normally extends

Percussion Sounds

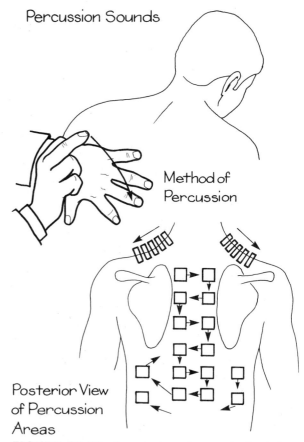

Method of Percussion

Posterior View of Percussion Areas

FIGURE 21-24. Examination (percussion) of the thorax and lungs.

TABLE 21-3. Characteristics and Nature of Structures of Percussion Sounds

Percussion Sound*	Pitch	Intensity	Duration	Nature of Structure
Resonance	3	3	4	Normal lung under chest wall.
Hyperresonance	2	5	5	Pneumothorax or pulmonary hyperinflation. Very thin chest wall over normal lung. Some musical quality.
Dullness	4	2	2	Solid organ, consolidated lung, thickened pleura or a thin layer of fluid under chest wall (rib or interspace).
Flatness	5	1	1	Solid organ, fluid or extensive scarring beneath chest wall.
Tympany	4	4	4	Musical note over a gas filled hollow viscus (e.g., stomach, colon).

*Graded on a 1–5 point scale of increasing pitch, intensity, and duration.

to a point 1 or 2 cm toward the midclavicular line (Fig. 21-25).

Diaphragmatic excursion (or the movement of the diaphragm), is usually determined posteriorly with the client in a sitting position. Diaphragmatic position is determined by the lower border of resonance. In midrespiration this is normally at about the ninth posterior interspace.

The client is instructed to exhale and hold his breath. The examiner percusses down and marks the point of transition from resonance to dullness. The client is then asked to inhale and hold his breath. The level of descent is percussed. The upper and lower borders can be marked during respiration by using the ring finger as a pleximeter to mark the upper border and the middle finger to

mark the lower border. The distance between these levels indicates the range of the diaphragm. This procedure is repeated for the opposite hemidiaphragm. The normal diaphragmatic excursion is about 3 to 5 cm (Fig. 21-26). Abdominal distention will cause elevation of the diaphragm such as that in hepatomegaly or ascites. Pulmonary overdistention will cause depression of the diaphragm.

AUSCULTATION

Auscultation of the lungs assesses the air movement of the bronchotracheal tree. This air movement produces vibrations that are perceived as *breath sounds*. These vibrations occur not only in normal breathing but from air moving in constricted or di-

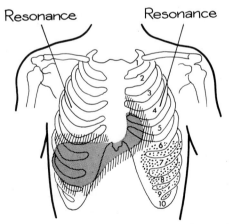

Dullness Surrounding Heart and Liver Area

Flatness Over Heart and Liver

Tympany Over Stomach

FIGURE 21-25. Examination (percussion) of the thorax and lungs: normal percussion sounds.

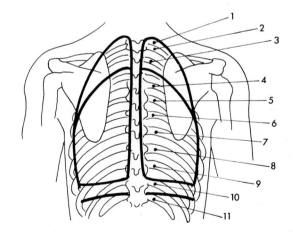

Normal Diaphragmatic Excursion Posterior Thorax

FIGURE 21-26. Examination of the posterior thorax and lungs: normal diaphragmatic excursion.

lated tubes, from fluid mucus, or from an obstruction moved by the air. The absence of breath sounds indicates blockage or an abnormal screening of breath sounds in the pleural cavity.

Breath Sounds

There are several types of breath sounds: bronchial, vesicular, and bronchovesicular. They are characterized by rising pitch during *inspiration* and falling pitch during *expiration* (Fig. 21-27). The duration of these two phases of respiration is the characteristic feature of the different breath sounds. The shorter the phase, the softer the sound in that phase; conversely, the longer the phase, the louder the sound in that phase (Table 21-4).

Voice Sounds

Spoken and whispered voice sounds are valuable in detecting pulmonary atelectasis, consolidation,

and infarction. Normally spoken and whispered words are faint and their syllables are not distinct, except over the main bronchi. When these words are loud and distinct, there is a pathological significance.

The sound heard with the stethoscope as the client phonates the word "ninety-nine" is known as *vocal resonance.* The vibrations produced in the larynx are transmitted to the chest wall, but in passage through the bronchi and alveolar tissue, they are decreased in intensity and are altered so that syllables are not distinguishable. When the vocal resonance is increased in intensity and clarity, *bronchophony* is said to be present. Intensity of vocal resonance is caused by: loudness of the voice; pitch of the voice—low pitched sounds are transmitted best; patency and proximity of the bronchi to the chest wall—vibrations are poorly transmitted through a plugged bronchus—vocal resonance is often greater over the right hemithorax posteriorly; thickness of the chest wall; an air tissue or air fluid interspace—this will damp out vibrations (as in

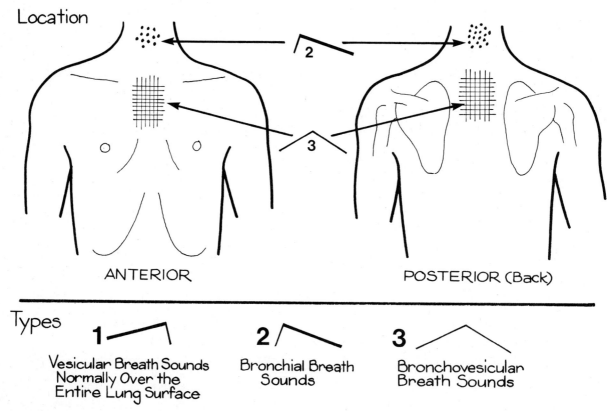

FIGURE 21-27. Types and location of breath sounds.

TABLE 21-4. Breath Sounds

Breath Sounds	Description	Significance
Bronchial or tubular	Harsh, blowing, "high-pitched sound with a blowing hollow character." The expiratory phase is usually longer than the inspiratory.	*Normally:* Heard over the trachea—never over lung parenchyma. *Disease:* Denotes partial or complete pulmonary consolidation with a patent bronchial tree. The solid lung tissue transmits centrally arising sound to the periphery with little modification.
Vesicular	Low-pitched, soft rustling sound. Inspiratory phase is louder and usually longer than expiratory.	*Normally:* Heard over most of the lungs. *Disease:* Vesicular breath sounds may be present but diminished in many disease states.
Bronchovesicular	Intermediate between vesicular and bronchial. The inspiratory phase is the same as vesicular. Expiratory phase is prolonged, higher pitched, harsher, and more blowing.	*Normally:* Heard over each side of sternum first and second interspace and upper interscapular area. Posteriorly bronchovesicular breath sounds are often more marked on right. *Disease:* In areas where vesicular breath sounds usually heard—indicates a mixture of aerated and consolidated parenchyma.

pneumothorax or pleural effusion); and solidified lung tissue with a patent bronchus (results in bronchophony).

Egophony is a modified form of bronchophony. There is not only an increase in intensity with the spoken word, but its character is altered. It is most readily elicited when the client says "eee." Over an area of consolidation or when there is fluid associated with pneumonic consolidation, the spoken "eee" will sound as "aaa" and will have a nasal character. This change from "e" which the client spoke to "a" during auscultation indicates the presence of egophony.

Pectoriloquy is the whispered voice. Auscultation of the whispered voice in the normal person yields a sound which is only faintly audible and in which syllables cannot be distinguished. It is essential that the words be whispered and not softly spoken. The client is asked to whisper "ninety-nine." Normally these whispered voice sounds are not heard or are diminished at the lung bases. However, when there is pulmonary consolidation, these sounds are transmitted with greater intensity and, therefore, the syllables will be clearly distinguished. This is one of the most reliable tests for the presence of pulmonary consolidation.

Adventitious Sounds

Adventitious sounds are "extra" sounds and are not normally heard over the chest. They are sounds that are superimposed upon the breath sounds, that may be normal or abnormal.

"Rale" means "rattling." These are bubbling or crackling sounds. They may vary from a single clicking sound to showers of short clicks. They may seem continuous, but actually are composed of many discrete sounds. Rales are the result of the passage of air through secretions in the respiratory tract. Therefore, they are produced by air flow and abnormal moisture. Dependent upon the size of the air chambers involved and the character of the exudate, rales will vary in size distribution, duration, and intensity. They are heard chiefly on inspiration, arise in the respiratory airways (e.g., respiratory bronchioles and alveoli), and indicate the presence of a parenchymal disease. However, they give no indication as to whether the disease is recent and active or long-standing and inactive. Rales may be described as fine, medium, or coarse.

Fine rales have a fine crackling quality. They are the result of moisture in the alveoli and are not cleared by coughing. They indicate inflammation or congestion involving the alveoli and can be heard in pneumonia, pulmonary congestion, and other diseases. *Medium rales* are a gradation between fine and coarse rales. They tend to occur earlier in respiration than do fine rales. They result from the passage of air through mucus in the bronchioles. *Coarse rales* originate in the larger bronchi and trachea. They gurgle and usually occur in a client who is too weak to clear fluid from his airways.

Rhonchi or wheezes are sounds which occur relatively continuously and are generally musical in character. They are sounds with a definite duration as heard by the human ear and may be heard on inspiration with an increase usually noted on expiration. They are best described as being low, medium, or high-pitched sounds and arise in the terminal bronchioles or larger airways. Low-pitched sounds arise in the trachea and main bronchi, the higher-pitched sounds arise distally. Wheezes are indicative of an obstructive process in the nonrespiratory airways. It is not possible to determine the nature of the obstructing process from the character of the sounds. Five basic principles follow: (1) Wheezes due to secretions tend to vary greatly from time to time, and are generally changed by coughing. (2) Inspiratory wheezes tend to be produced by the higher degrees of airway obstruction. (3) Wheezes may disappear altogether in very high grade obstruction because insufficient air is being moved to generate the sound. (4) In the presence of low grade obstruction, wheezes may be audible only on forced expiration or on the dependent side in lateral recumbency. (5) When the obstruction is structural (e.g., a tumor or fibrous stenosis), wheezes tend to be more constant.

Pleural friction rubs are produced by roughened visceral and parietal pleura rubbing over one another during respiration. Fibrinous exudate is the most common cause. The sound is a characteristic one and is usually heard during both phases of respiration. The rub may vary from breath to breath and may be heard only during a deep respiration. Pleural friction rubs are often accompanied by pleuritic pain. The rub is most often heard over the lower lateral and anterior thorax, the site of the greatest chest wall motion.

Adventitious sounds may also be of chest wall origin. *Crepitation*, which may be mistaken for rales, is due to hair between the skin and the stethoscope. Firmer application of the stethoscope gen-erally stops these sounds. They are close to the ear and are generally easily recognized with experience.

Muffled, distant, low-pitched, rumbling, sometimes roaring sounds are due to contraction of chest wall muscles. Variations can be produced by changing the client's position. They often occur in the chilled or nervous client and must be distinguished from rales which are usually louder, higher pitched, and more discrete sounds.

To summarize, auscultatory examination of the lungs begins as the client is instructed to breathe a little deeper with his mouth open. One side of the thorax is compared with the opposite side going from the top to the bottom, thus, anterior/posterior lung fields bilaterally:

(R) upper ———————→ (L) upper
(R) mid   ———————→ (L) mid
(R) base ———————→ (L) base

Normal breath sounds are listened for first, (that is, vesicular (⌃), bronchovesicular (⌒), and bronchial (⌄). They are noted and described in terms of *quality* (any distinctive feature), *intensity* (loud or soft), and *duration* (the relative duration of the expiratory and inspiratory phases). Abnormal sounds (e.g., rales and rhonchi) are then listened for. If consolidation or compression of lung tissue is suspected, abnormal voice sounds are listened for (e.g., bronchophony, egophony, and whispered pectoriloquy).

Heart

The clinical appraisal of the cardiovascular status of the client is based on conclusions made from auscultation of the heart. However, knowledge of the physiological correlation of auscultatory findings with normal and abnormal cardiac dynamics establishes a more educated approach to physical assessment. Normally, blood flow is the result of the precise anatomical and physiological nature of the heart. This organ, under normal circumstances, pumps blood effectively, 100,000 times a day. Whenever pathology develops, the valves, myocardium, and supporting structures frequently begin to function abnormally. Hemodynamic changes which originate with dysfunction result in clinical findings explainable within the framework of anatomical and physiological factors. The following areas of the heart must be recognized: right and left atrium, ventricles, mitral, tricuspid, pulmonary and aortic valves, aorta, pulmonary artery, vena cava, and pulmonary veins.

For a cardiovascular examination the client is examined seated, in a supine position, and in a left lateral side-lying position. Various positions are tried to elicit abnormalities. The examiner listens for the rate at the apex. Rhythm is determined. Is it regular or irregular? Are there extra beats? Each of the following areas are auscultated routinely starting either with the mitral valve and progressing to the aortic valve, or vice versa: (1) *the mitral (apical) area*: fifth left intercostal space, 1 or 2 cm medial to the midclavicular line; (2) *the tricuspid area*: fifth left intercostal space, close to the sternum; (3) *the epigastric area*; (4) *Erb's point*: third left interspace, where murmurs of aortic and pulmonic origin may often be audible; (5) *the pulmonic area*: second left intercostal space, lateral to the sternum; and (6) *the aortic area*: second right intercostal space, lateral to the sternum. These are areas on the chest in which valve sounds are transmitted with the greatest intensity and do not correspond to sequential anatomical locations.

CARDIAC CYCLE

One cardiac cycle is equivalent to one complete heart beat, lasts 0.8 second, and consists of two parts: the systolic and the diastolic.

Systole is the period of the cardiac cycle in which the ventricles are actively contracting and ejecting blood. The pulmonary and aortic valves are open, and the mitral and tricuspid valves are closed. Through the aorta during systole, oxygenated blood is pumped from the left ventricle to the tissues of the body. Through the pulmonary artery during systole, deoxygenated blood is pumped from the right ventricle to the lungs.

Diastole is the period in which the ventricles are not contracting and are filling with blood. The pulmonary and aortic valves are closed, and the mitral and tricuspid valves are open. Blood is returned to the heart by the vena cava and pulmonary veins.

PRECORDIUM

Parameters of the precordium that must be known are the apex; base; pulmonic area; aortic area; midclavicular line; anterior, mid, and posterior axillary lines; and interspaces. The anterior surface of the chest closest to the heart and aorta is called the precordium. Normally, the central area of the precordium is the projection of the right ventricle. The left border and apex are formed by the left ventricle, and the right atrium constitutes the right border. Examination of the cardiac system includes inspection, palpation, percussion, and auscultation.

With the client supine, the precordium is inspected for deformities. A protrusion of the bony thorax over the right ventricle may occur from cardiac enlargement associated with congenital heart disease. An apical pulse (also called PMI—point of maximal impulse) is obtained (Fig. 21-28). In about one-fifth of normal clients, an impulse, synchronous with the beginning of ventricular systole can be found. Normally, the impulse is a light tap that can be felt in an area of 1 to 2 cm in diameter. Its usual position is in the left fifth intercostal space, 7 to 9 cm from the midsternal line. When a left ventricle enlargement is caused by dilatation or hypertrophy, the apical pulse is shifted downward and to the left. The impulse may be shifted to the right by a left pneumothorax or right pleural adhesions. An increased impulse may result from heightened myocardial tone. Other abnormal visible pulsations are looked for. An impulse along the left sternal border may indicate an aneurysm. Visible pulses in the pulmonic or aortic areas are usually abnormal in clients over 25 years of age.

Findings made by inspection are generally apparent by palpation. Areas where pulsations were visible should be probed (Fig. 21-28). Palpation is done with the finger pads which are more sensitive to pulsations. The *apical pulse* may be felt, more definitively, with the client lying in the left lateral side-lying position. Its diameter, amplitude, and location are assessed. Thrills are palpated with the palmar surface of the hand (which is more sensitive to vibrations) [Fig. 21-28]. The entire precordium is felt starting with the apical area and then sequentially assessing the right ventricular area, the epigastric area, the third left interspace (Erb's point), the pulmonic area, and the aortic area. Any abnormality, forceful movements (*heaves*), palpable murmurs (*thrills*), or S_3 and S_4 gallop (see p. 331) are noted. *Thrills* are vibrations, resembling a cat's purr, felt over the precordium. They are usually associated with murmurs. Their location and sequence in the cardiac cycle should be described.

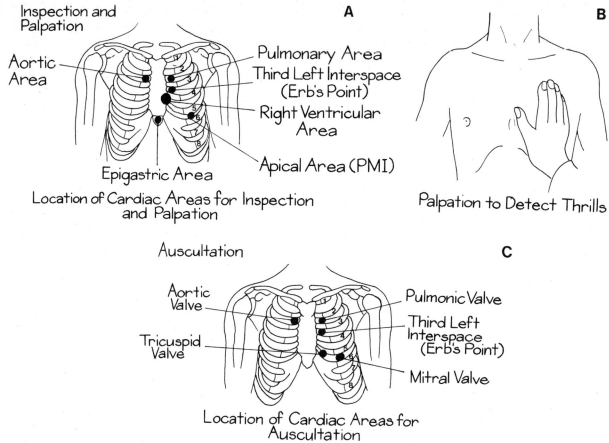

Inspection and Palpation

A

Aortic Area

Pulmonary Area
Third Left Interspace (Erb's Point)
Right Ventricular Area

Epigastric Area

Apical Area (PMI)

Location of Cardiac Areas for Inspection and Palpation

B

Palpation to Detect Thrills

Auscultation

C

Aortic Valve

Tricuspid Valve

Pulmonic Valve

Third Left Interspace (Erb's Point)

Mitral Valve

Location of Cardiac Areas for Auscultation

FIGURE 21-28. Examination (inspection, palpation, and auscultation) of the heart.

HEART SOUNDS

With abnormally rapid venticular filling (e.g., occurring into a ventricle composed of abnormal myocardium) discernible vibrations are produced by palpation and auscultation. When heard, they are identified as S_3 *gallop* and S_4 *gallop heart sounds*, which are discussed in more detail below. They are frequently palpable; sometimes, palpation of these sounds is easier than auscultation. Generally, these findings are manifestations of organic heart disease.

Although traditionally taught as a valid tool for appraising the cardiovascular system, *percussion* actually offers little input. Dullness extending beyond the sternal borders at the base of the heart may signify aneurysmal widening. Although not strongly advocated in examination of the heart, percussion is valuable in evaluating other organ systems.

Auscultation is performed to analyze the components of heart sounds. Sound is basically the sensation of vibrations as interpreted by the auditory apparatus. The quality of any sound is the product of several characteristics which are determined by the mechanical process creating the vibrations. Heart sounds are not pure tones but a combination of tones of varying frequency (Fig. 21-28). The pitch of the sound is determined by the frequency of the vibrations. Since heart sounds are not the result of pure tones, but a combination of a number of frequencies or overtones, the quality is imperfect. Since the mechanical energy related to heart sounds is limited, the duration of the sound is limited and variable. The intensity of heart sounds is determined by the amplitude of the vibrations. When auscultating the heart, the diaphragm of the stethoscope is used to hear high-pitched sounds and the bell portion to audit low-pitched sounds.

Progressively, the normal heart sounds, S_1 and

S_2 are listened for over all areas of the precordium. (These will be discussed in depth in the following pages.) The S_1 should be identified and evaluated for rate, rhythm, intensity, whether split and if so, the degree of splitting, and the relationship to inspiration and expiration. The S_2 is, likewise, analyzed systematically. Extra sounds in systole such as S_4 gallop, ejection sounds, systolic clicks, and sounds in diastole such as normal third sound, S_3 gallop, or opening snap are listened for (see following pages). Finally, murmurs, initially in systole and then, in diastole are listened for. Logically, each component of the cardiac cycle can be well analyzed. If murmurs are heard they should be characterized by location, quality, intensity, duration, and transmission. Whenever a murmur is heard, the surrounding chest surface is explored to determine transmission. The base of the neck and carotids are auscultated for transmission of a murmur in the aortic area; the axilla is auscultated for transmission of a murmur in the mitral area.

Normal Heart Sounds—S_1 and S_2

Under totally normal circumstances, only two sounds are produced during each cardiac contraction. The first heart sound (S_1) is the result of vibrations transmitted from the area of the mitral and tricuspid valves as they are shut at the onset of ventricular systole. These vibrations are transmitted through the various underlying tissues of the body to the surface. Similarly the second heart sound (S_2) is made up of vibrations originating in the closing of the semilunar aortic and pulmonic valves. Valve motion, closing and opening, is a result of a pressure gradient across the valve. During systole, the pressure in the contracting ventricle is considerably higher than in the corresponding atrium. The mitral and tricuspid valves are, therefore, forcibly closed, and blood is prevented from regurgitating into the atria. As long as the ventricular pressure is greater than that in the atrium, the valve will remain closed. During diastole, and particularly during atrial systole, the pressure in the atrium is greater than in the noncontracting ventricle; the atrioventricular valves (mitral and tricuspid) are forced open to allow filling of the ventricles. Closing of the atrioventricular valves is an audible event, while normally the opening process is clinically silent. Semilunar (aortic and pulmonary valves) opening occurs when during systole the pressure generated

in the ventricles reaches and exceeds the diastolic pressure in the aorta and pulmonary artery. This allows systolic ejection to take place and blood flows into the artery. As the descending limb of the ejection curve falls below the diastolic level in the aorta or pulmonary artery, the pressure gradient is such that the semilunar valves are forced shut. As with the atrioventricular closing, this event is audible, whereas the opening is normally silent. The valves on the left side of the heart always close with more force than the valves on the right side. Therefore, heart sounds are always dominated by the closure of the valves of the left side of the heart; for example, mitral and tricuspid valves, S_1, and the aortic and pulmonic valve, S_2 (Fig. 21-29).

Whenever the two valves close asynchronously, the ensuing sound is called *"splitting."* Physiological splitting of the aortic and pulmonic components of S_2 is commonly heard and has greater clinical usefulness. This splitting can be heard normally, varying with the phase of respiration. On inspiration, venous return to the right heart is increased. This provides a volume load to the right ventricle requiring a longer systolic period and delaying pulmonic closure (Fig. 21-29). The same effect is not seen on the left side of the heart since the increased blood volume is easily absorbed by the lungs. In certain pathophysiologic states, this splitting may be altered providing a clinical clue to an underlying abnormality. An example of pathological splitting may be seen in conditions of increased blood flow or increased pressure in the right ventricle. There may be fixed splitting of the second sound, that is, the two components of the second are audible throughout the entire respiratory cycle. It may occur in atrial septal defect or pulmonic stenosis (Fig. 21-29).

Third Heart Sounds—S_3

In healthy young persons, particularly if the heart rate is slow or low pitched, sound may be heard early in diastole and louder at the apical area. These vibrations are produced by rapid ventricular filling. Beyond the age of 30, this sound is usually abnormal (Fig. 21-29).

Gallop Sounds—S_3 and S_4

These sounds represent abnormal findings. They are so named because the rhythmic cadence pro-

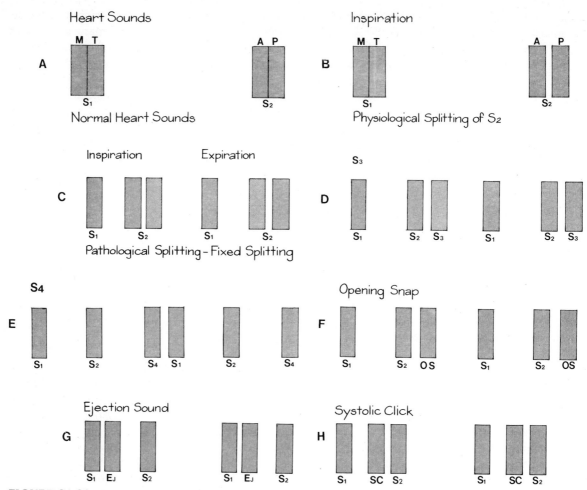

FIGURE 21-29. Examination (auscultation) of the heart: heart sounds.

duced is reminiscent of a galloping horse. These sounds identify hemodynamic abnormality and may originate from either ventricle. S_3 *gallop* can be distinguished from the normal third heart sound. The quality and timing of the sound is the same as the physiological third heart sound but is almost always associated with a tachycardia. The sound results from rapid filling of a relatively nondistensible dilated ventricle occuring in congestive heart failure and mitral insufficiency. In general, it represents volume overloading of the ventricle. S_4 *gallop* occurs in the presystolic period coinciding with atrial systole and represents filling of a nondistensible ventricle from increased pressure in the atrium. This is most commonly observed whenever there is a pressure load on the ventricle (e.g., hypertension and semilunar valvular stenosis) [Fig. 21-29].

Other Heart Sounds

VALVE OPENING SOUNDS. Normally the opening of both the atrioventricular and semilunar valves is a silent event clinically. The exact mechanism for the production of valve opening sounds (*opening snap*) is not known. The atrioventricular valve is stenosed requiring mobility of one leaflet. The opening snap (o.s.) occurs 0.08 seconds after the second heart sound, later than the split second sound, but earlier than the third heart sound (Fig. 21-29).

EJECTION SOUNDS. These are high-pitched sounds discernible early in systole at the point of maximum ejection. Since they are aortic or pulmonic events, they are heard most definitively at the base of the heart. Exercise can distinguish the ejection sound from a split first heart sound. They are present when the aorta or pulmonary artery is dilated, especially when arterial hypertension exists (Fig. 21-29).

SYSTOLIC CLICKS. Systolic clicks should not be confused with ejection sounds which are very similar in quality. They occur in mid or late systole. In most cases, this sound is not associated with any recognized pathology. A tensing of the pericardium is the probable cause in these situations. More recently, a late systolic click has been found in association with hemodynamically insignificant mitral regurgitation (Fig. 21-29).

PERICARDIAL FRICTION RUB. In pericarditis, the fibrinous pericardial surfaces rub together and produce grating sounds synchronous with the motion of the heart. Classically, a rub has three components: atrial systole, ventricular systole, and diastole. One, two, or all three factors may be present. A pericardial rub is notorious for appearing and disappearing mysteriously.

Heart Murmurs

Normally the passage of blood through the cardiac chambers and the vessels is not an audible event. However, whenever the flow becomes turbulent, the sound is interpreted as a murmur. Turbulence may be caused by an increase in the velocity of

flow through a normal vessel or tube, or by a deformity of the vessel or tube which causes a change in the flow (Fig. 21-30). Murmurs vary in their location, quality, intensity, and timing.

1. *Location*: Murmurs relating to valves are usually heard over the valvular areas. Murmurs relating to congenital septal defects and abnormalities may be heard near the sternum, base of the heart, and neck.
2. *Quality*: Murmurs may be described as blowing, rumbling, harsh, rasping, or musical. Murmurs can also be classified as crescendo (increasing), decrescendo (decreasing), or crescendo-decrescendo (diamond-shaped).
3. *Intensity*: Murmurs are graded from 1 to 6 in intensity: grade 1—very faint; grade 2—quiet and may be heard immediately upon listening with the stethoscope on the chest; grade 3—moderately loud; grade 4—loud and associated with a thrill; grade 5—very loud and associated with a thrill; and grade 6—may be heard without a stethoscope on the chest and associated with a thrill.
4. *Timing*: Murmurs are timed according to the phase of the cardiac cycle. They are classified as: systole—early, middle, late, and sometimes throughout the cycle (holosystolic or pansystolic), and diastole—early (protodiastole), middle, or late (presystole) [Fig. 21-31].

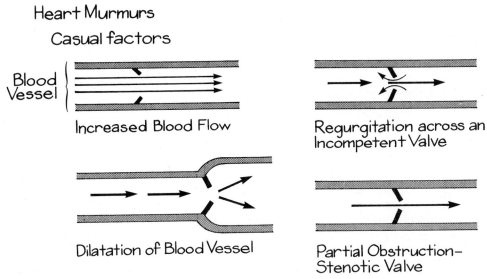

Heart Murmurs

Casual factors

Blood Vessel

Increased Blood Flow

Regurgitation across an Incompetent Valve

Dilatation of Blood Vessel

Partial Obstruction—Stenotic Valve

FIGURE 21-30. Examination (auscultation) of the heart: causes of heart murmurs.

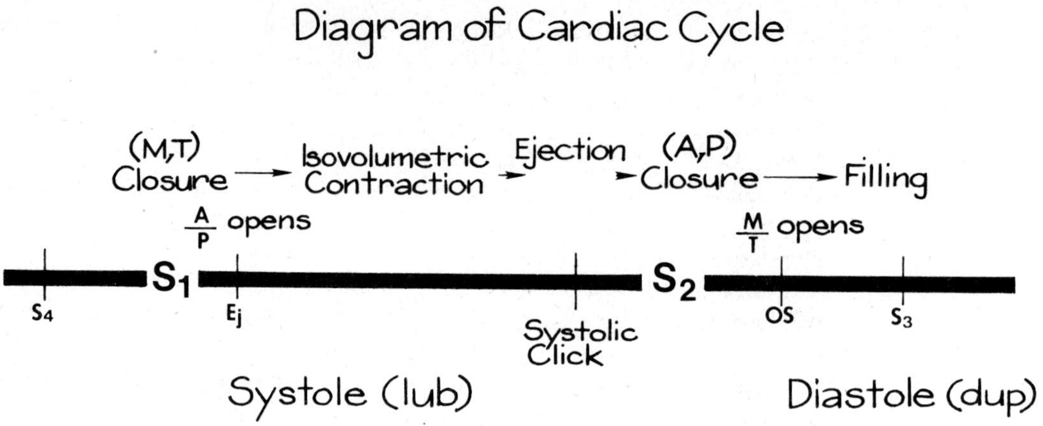

Diagram of Cardiac Cycle

(M,T) Closure → Isovolumetric Contraction → Ejection → (A,P) Closure → Filling

$\frac{A}{P}$ opens

$\frac{M}{T}$ opens

S₄ S₁ Ej Systolic Click S₂ OS S₃

Systole (lub) Diastole (dup)

FIGURE 21-31. The cardiac cycle.

SYSTOLIC MURMURS. This type of murmur originates between S_1 and S_2 and does not necessarily represent pathological abnormality. They occur, frequently, in normal people and are identified as *functional* or *benign* murmurs. They are caused by blood flow with a velocity sufficient to produce turbulence despite normal anatomical structure. Conditions which increase cardiac output—fever, exercise, or anemia—may exacerbate these murmurs.

SYSTOLIC EJECTION MURMURS. This type of murmur is caused by turbulent flow of blood during ventricular systole. The duration is the period during which the semilunar valves are open, usually following the crescendo-decrescendo pattern. Examples are the murmurs of aortic and pulmonic stenosis (Fig. 21-32).

PANSYSTOLIC MURMUR. This murmur begins with S_1 and extends to, and sometimes beyond S_2. Its production is based on flow inappropriately directed, as with shunting through a ventricular septal defect or mitral regurgitation (insufficiency). These murmurs are blowing in quality (Fig. 21-32).

Auscultation of Heart Murmurs

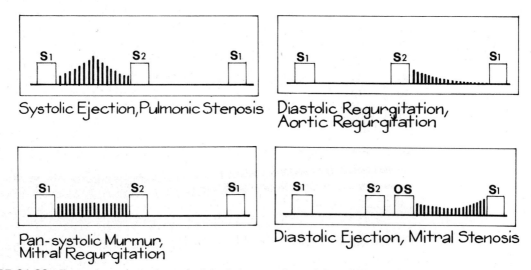

Systolic Ejection, Pulmonic Stenosis

Diastolic Regurgitation, Aortic Regurgitation

Pan-systolic Murmur, Mitral Regurgitation

Diastolic Ejection, Mitral Stenosis

FIGURE 21-32. Examination (auscultation) of the heart: systolic and diastolic murmurs.

DIASTOLIC MURMURS. This murmur occurs between S_2 and the subsequent S_1. They represent either valvular disease at the site of the murmur or a hemodynamic alteration. Two basic types exist (Fig. 21-32). Examples are murmurs produced by semilunar regurgitation or atrioventricular stenosis.

CONTINUOUS MURMURS. These occur when the pressure in one vessel exceeds the pressure in a vessel with which it has a pathological communication. An example is seen in patent ductus arteriosus since the aortic diastolic pressure never drops to the systolic pressure in the pulmonary artery.

Abdomen

The abdominal examination provides rewarding information when performed objectively. The abdomen is the site of many important organs that are susceptible to disease. In assessment of the abdomen, each constituent organ should be separately evaluated. Identifiable viscera are either hollow or solid. Hollow visera consist of the stomach, gallbladder, small intestines, colon, and urinary bladder, which is normally not palpable. They may

become distended from gas or fluid. Lesions, too, often may be felt. The contour of the abdomen is controlled by the stomach muscles and is modified by the accumulation of adipose tissue in the subcutaneous layers. The recti abdomini are two large muscles extending from the anterior costal margin near the midline to the symphysis pubis. The spleen, liver, adrenals, kidneys, and pancreas are solid viscera. Most of these organs retain their original shapes during enlargement; they may be palpable.

There are several differing systems describing the location of the abdominal organs. A simple system is to divide the abdomen into four quadrants by axial and transverse lines through the umbilicus:

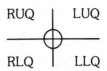

Utilizing this quadrant map, organ positions for either sex are as they appear in Table 21-5.

Another nonpreferred system divides the abdomen into nine smaller areas. However, the quadrant plan occasionally refers to several of these

TABLE 21-5. Organ Position within the Quadrant Map

Right Upper Quadrant	Left Upper Quadrant
Liver and gallbladder	Spleen
Pylorus	Stomach
Duodenum	Body of pancreas
Head of pancreas	Left adrenal gland
Right adrenal gland	Portion of left kidney
Portion of right kidney	Splenic flexure of colon
Hepatic flexure of colon	Portions of transverse
Portions of ascending	and descending colon
and transverse colon	
Right Lower Quadrant	**Left Lower Quadrant**
Cecum and appendix	Sigmoid colon
Portion of ascending colon	Portion of descending colon
Bladder (if distended)	Bladder (if distended)
Right ovary and salpinx	Left ovary and salpinx
Uterus (if enlarged)	Uterus (if enlarged)
Right spermatic cord	Left spermatic cord
Right ureter	Left ureter

Note.—Loops of small bowel are found in all quadrants.

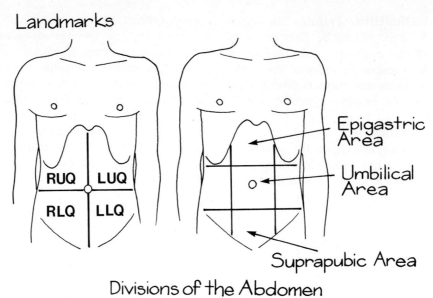

Landmarks

RUQ | LUQ
RLQ | LLQ

Epigastric Area
Umbilical Area
Suprapubic Area

Divisions of the Abdomen

FIGURE 21-33. Examination of the abdomen: landmarks.

areas, for example, epigastric, umbilical, suprapubic, and the flanks (Fig. 21-33). The logical abdominal examination sequence is usually inspection, auscultation, palpation, and percussion.

The undressed client is placed in supine position and draped to expose the abdomen completely from the xiphoid process of the sternum to the symphysis pubis. Since the client's abdominal musculature should be relaxed, provide a warm environment. The client's bladder should be emptied at the start. There should be good fields of vision from overhead and laterally towards the examiner.

INSPECTION

The abdomen is *inspected* for *contour, engorged veins, hernias, visible masses, pulsations, scars,* and *striae.*

CONTOUR. The contour of the abdomen can be described as flat, rounded, or scaphoid. A rounded abdomen is abnormal in adults and may be caused by excessive fat, lack of abdominal muscle tone, ascites, or distention. A scaphoid abdomen may be evidenced in thin, dehydrated, or malnourished clients (Fig. 21-34).

ENGORGED VEINS. Normally, veins of the abdominal wall are scarcely visible, whereas engorged

veins are commonly visible through the abdominal wall. Normal blood flow in the veins is upwards above the umbilicus and downwards below the umbilicus. To determine the direction of blood flow, a vein is compressed with both index fingers. A short segment of the vein is stripped of blood by moving one index finger away from the other for a few centimeters. One finger is removed and refilling time from that direction observed. The procedure is repeated, this time releasing the opposite finger, and refilling time from that direction compared. The rate of filling will be faster in the direction of blood flow. Whenever there is an obstruction of the superior vena cava, blood will flow downwards. An obstruction in the inferior vena cava causes blood to flow upwards, a reversal of normal venous blood flow.

HERNIAS. Hernias cannot be ruled out by inspection alone. Palpation is done to determine their presence. Whenever there is an operative scar exhibited, the client should be asked to perform the Valsalva maneuver. Bulging is checked for near the operative scar indicating a potential incisional hernia. The same analogy applies to an umbilical hernia. The navel may protrude, or increase, with the performance of the Valsalva maneuver. (Examination for inguinal and femoral hernias will be detailed in a subsequent unit on the genitalia.)

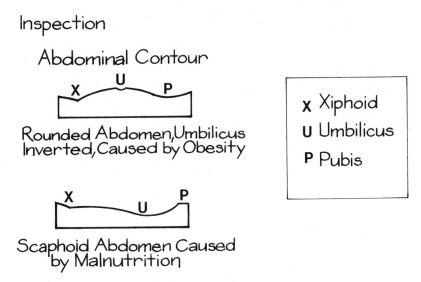

Inspection

Abdominal Contour

Rounded Abdomen, Umbilicus
Inverted, Caused by Obesity

X Xiphoid
U Umbilicus
P Pubis

Scaphoid Abdomen Caused
by Malnutrition

FIGURE 21-34. Examination (inspection) of the abdomen: contour.

VISIBLE PULSATIONS. A slight pulsation in the epigastrium caused by the abdominal aorta may be visible.

VISIBLE PERISTALSIS. In very thin people, peristalic waves may be seen in the upper abdomen. They usually begin near the left upper quadrant and gradually move downwards and to the right. If abnormally powerful waves are discernible beneath a normal wall, obstruction should be considered.

STRIAE. Striae are stretch marks running axially under the epidermis. If they have occurred recently, their color will be pink or blue, older scars will be white or silver. They are caused by distention of the abdomen from ascites, edema, obesity, pregnancy, or tumors.

AUSCULTATION

Auscultation is performed prior to palpation. Otherwise, the bowel wall may become irritated causing increased peristalsis.

Bowel Sounds

Bowel sounds relate to intestinal peristalsis and are relatively high-pitched, soft and gurgling. They are characterized by intensity, degree of activity, and pitch.

Intensity is an indication of the force and velocity of intestinal contraction. Many factors affect intensity, such as obesity and a muscular abdominal wall; loud bowel sounds are clinically useful only when changes are extreme.

Degree of activity of bowel sounds is intermittent, occurring usually every 2 to 10 seconds. The rate of bowel sounds varies according to the anatomical site. Peristalic waves traverse the gastric antrum approximately three times per minute. Jejunal contractions occur 11 times per minute, and ileal contractions occur eight times per minute. The colon is active approximately half of the time. Loud bursts of sound which reach an acme of intensity, and then regress, are called *peristalic rushes*.

Pitch of bowel sounds is derived from vibration of the intestinal wall caused by intestinal contractions. Pitch is a function of the tension and thickness of the intestinal wall and the air-fluid mix of the luminal contents. Increased pitch may signify intestinal distention.

All quadrants and the epigastrium are assessed with the diaphragm of the stethoscope (Fig. 21-35). To hear bowel sounds, the stethoscope is placed below and to the right of the umbilicus and gurgles are listened for. If they are not immediately audible, it is best to wait for 5 minutes. Bowel sounds are

Auscultation

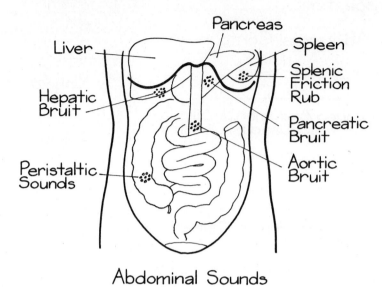

FIGURE 21-35. Examination (auscultation) of the abdomen: abdominal and bowel sounds.

hyperactive, high-pitched, and rushing if early intestinal obstruction or other disturbances, such as diarrhea, are present. Increased peristalsis produces increased frequency and intensity of bowel sounds (called borborygmi) which may be caused by enteritis or small bowel obstruction. A diminishing or absence of sounds may transpire if there is ileus from peritonitis, pneumonia, enterocolic ulceration, or advanced intestinal obstruction.

Bruits

All quadrants are auscultated with the bell of the stethoscope for bruits. A bruit over the epigastric area may result from an aneurysm of the abdominal aorta. A bruit in the flank or in the costovertebral angle may be caused by sclerotic narrowing of the renal artery.

Peritoneal Friction Rub

A peritoneal friction rub develops from the rubbing of the parietal peritoneum over an area of inflamed visceral peritoneum. The rub may be heard over the lower left costal margin in infarction of the spleen, or in the right upper quadrant, suggesting neoplastic involvement of the liver (see also discussion under Heart).

PALPATION

Palpation constitutes the most important part of the abdominal examination. It is executed with light and deep palpation and ballottement.

For *light palpation* the client must be relaxed since abdominal muscle tension will render palpation difficult. The client should be asked to breathe deeply through his mouth or flex his legs. He will need frequent reassurance. The examiner's hands should be warm. The entire abdomen is palpated lightly for discovery of areas of tenderness, increased resistance from muscle spasm, and solid masses. Tender areas should always be palpated last. The palm of the hand is laid lightly on the abdomen. The fingers are pressed in to a depth of 1 cm. A gentle, light dipping motion is used avoiding jabs (Fig. 21-36A). Superficial organs, tenderness, and any resistance should be ascertained. Tenderness may result from a localized inflammation. A solid organ is tender if its capsule is distended. Resistance to palpation is voluntary; maneuvering will be necessary for its elimination. Involuntary resistance may be caused by peritoneal infections or neoplastic irritation. Masses may increase resistance to palpation. If a mass is discovered, identification of whether it is in the cavity or the wall is attempted. An attempt to elicit rebound

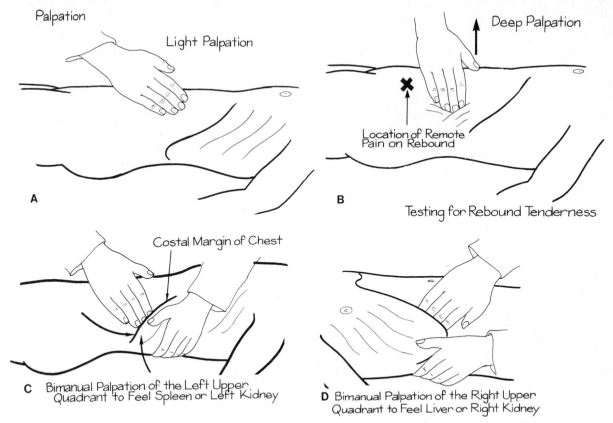

Palpation

Light Palpation

A

Deep Palpation

Location of Remote
Pain on Rebound

B Testing for Rebound Tenderness

Costal Margin of Chest

C Bimanual Palpation of the Left Upper
Quadrant to Feel Spleen or Left Kidney

D Bimanual Palpation of the Right Upper
Quadrant to Feel Liver or Right Kidney

FIGURE 21-36. Examination (palpation) of the abdomen.

tenderness (Blumberg's sign) in tender areas is made. The tips of the fingers are pressed gently into the abdominal wall, then suddenly withdrawn from contact (Fig. 21-36B). Transient pain, after withdrawal of pressure, is called *rebound tenderness*. If the site of tenderness has already been identified, a remote spot is pressed in deeply.

Deep palpation should occur with the client in supine position, the palmar surface of the fingers are used to feel all quadrants more deeply in a clockwise manner. Findings from inspection and light palpation should be elaborated. Most sensations should be received on the pads of the index and middle fingers. The finger pads should cause the abdominal wall to glide over the underlying structures forwards and backwards within a range of 4 or 5 cm. Again, another search for masses, tenderness, and the delineation of organs is made. Findings are identified according to their parameters. Organs that may be delineated are the liver, kidneys, spleen, and the abdominal aorta (Fig. 21-36C).

Ballottement is a type of palpation used for detection of large amounts of fluid in a body cavity and estimation of sizes of masses. One hand is pushed into the anterior abdominal wall. With the other hand, the flank is palpated to estimate the thickness of the mass.

Liver

A normal liver may be palpable just below the right costal margin on deep inspiration (Fig. 21-37). However, if the client has a low diaphragm as in emphysema, the liver's edge may be well below the costal margin.

Bimanually, the liver is palpated with the examiner at the client's right side; she should place the left hand under the client's right flank parallel to the eleventh and twelfth ribs. The liver is pushed toward the anterior abdominal wall. The right hand is placed under the right anterior lower thorax and the fingers curled under the lower ribs. The client is asked to breathe deeply and sustain it (Fig. 21-

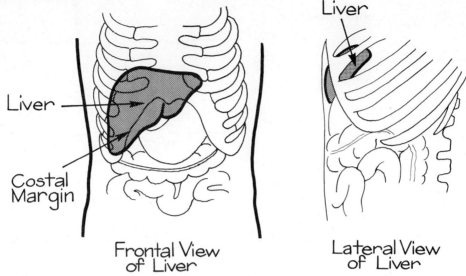

Liver

Costal
Margin

Liver

Frontal View
of Liver

Lateral View
of Liver

FIGURE 21-37. Examination (palpation) of the liver.

36D). On inspiration, the diaphragm descends to force the liver's edge downwards. If it is palpable, the liver will slip between the examining hands, deflecting them upwards. This maneuver is repeated several times. The positioning of the right hand is varied each time to feel as much of the liver as is possible. A normal liver's edge feels moderately firm and sharp. An inflamed liver will feel tender to the client. In portal cirrhosis, the liver will feel nodular.

Kidneys

The lower pole of a normal right kidney may be palpated (Fig. 21-38). The diaphragm, on inspiration, causes the kidneys to descend. The right kid-

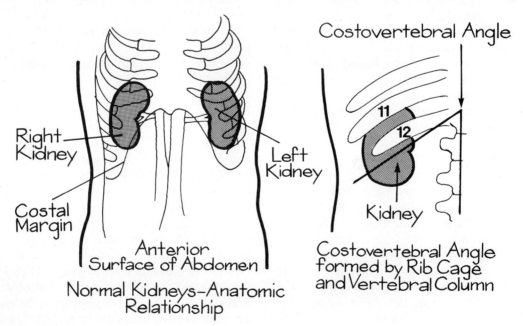

Costovertebral Angle

Right
Kidney

Left
Kidney

Costal
Margin

11

12

Kidney

Anterior
Surface of Abdomen

Normal Kidneys–Anatomic
Relationship

Costovertebral Angle
formed by Rib Cage
and Vertebral Column

FIGURE 21-38. The kidneys.

ney is more easily felt than the left kidney as it lies in front of the right twelfth rib. The left kidney lies primarily in front of the eleventh rib (Fig. 21-38).

Bimanual palpation is utilized with the left hand under the client's right flank and the right hand on the anterior abdominal wall in the midclavicular line at the level of the umbilicus. The client is asked to inhale. The anterior wall is pressed deeply at the height of inspiration. At exhalation, pressure is increased slightly on the anterior wall, and an attempt to feel the kidney as it slips upwards between the hands is made (Fig. 21-36D). If the right kidney is palpable, it is checked for contour, size, and tenderness. The same procedure is utilized to examine the left kidney (Fig. 21-36C). The right hand is reached across the abdomen and placed under the client's flank, and the left hand positioned on the anterior abdominal wall. A normal left kidney is not usually palpable.

To check for *costovertebral tenderness* the palm of the hand is placed over the soft tissues of the costovertebral angle between the spine and the twelfth rib. The left hand is struck with the right fist. Normally, the client should feel a jar. Tenderness in this area may indicate inflammation of the kidney.

Spleen

Normally, the spleen is not felt in an adult. It lies under the vault of the left diaphragm and has a spread of approximately 7 cm, from the ninth to the eleventh rib (Fig. 21-39). In diseases such as pernicious anemia, polycythemia, hepatitis, hemolytic disorder, the spleen may be enlarged and palpable. The procedure for palpating the spleen is similar to palpation of the liver. It is done at the left costal margin close to the anterior axillary line. The right hand is placed under the eleventh and twelfth ribs posteriorly, and lifted forward. The fingers of the left hand are pressed below the costal margin at the anterior axillary line (Fig. 21-36C). If a large firm mass in the left lower quadrant was felt on light palpation, the left hand is employed well below a suspected enlarged spleen (Fig. 21-39). Then the hand is moved higher towards the right side in an attempt to define the splenic border. The client is asked to inhale and hold his breath. If the spleen is palpable, on inspiration a firm mass will be felt when you tap your fingers. Acute infections may result in moderately enlarged soft spleens with blunted edges, whereas chronic disorders cause hard or firm spleens with sharp edges.

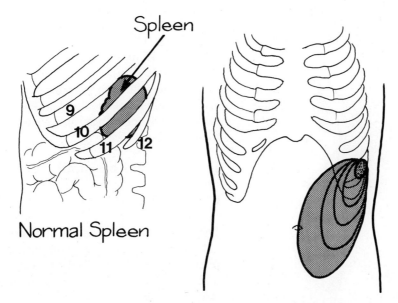

FIGURE 21-39. The spleen.

Abdominal Aorta

The abdominal aorta begins at the aortic hiatus of the diaphragm and descends ventrally to the vertebral column ending on the body of the fourth lumbar vertebra and dividing into the two common iliac arteries. Pulsations may be felt slightly to the left of the midline of the upper abdomen.

The client is instructed to breathe deeply, then the upper abdomen and slightly to the left of the midline are pressed into deeply. The thumb is placed on one side of the aorta and the fingers along the other side (Fig. 21-40). Once the aorta has been identified, it is noted whether the pulsations are transmitted forwards (normal) or laterally (suggesting an aortic aneurysm).

PERCUSSION

Percussion of each of the four quadrants for organ dullness is used to measure the size of the liver, the spleen, a distended bladder, or the presence of fluid.

To check the size of the liver, percuss in the right midclavicular line downwards from lung resonance to liver dullness (usually between the fifth and seventh intercostal spaces). Then, percussion in right midclavicular line from the level of tympany below the umbilicus upwards to liver dullness is performed. The vertical span of liver dullness, normally ranging between 6 and 12 cm in the right mid-

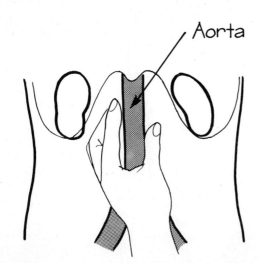

Identification of Aortic Pulsation
FIGURE 21-40. Palpation of abdominal aorta.

clavicular line is measured (Fig. 21-41A). Liver diameters in females are smaller than in males. A very enlarged liver may indicate presence of metastatic carcinoma.

Percussion of the area of splenic dullness is desirable. If the spleen has a normal diameter, splenomegaly (enlargement of the spleen) is almost always excluded. Its 7 cm width spreads from the ninth to the eleventh rib just posterior to the midaxillary line. A moderately enlarged spleen may be caused by hepatitis or lymphoma. A greatly enlarged spleen may be caused by myelocytic leukemia.

A distended bladder will also present dullness in the suprapubic area. Normally, the remaining abdomen is tympanitic to percussion as gas is present in the small and large intestine. Solid masses will be dull to percussion; and accumulations of peritoneal fluid will evidence shifting dullness on position.

To check for free fluid, the client is placed in supine position. The free fluid will migrate into the flanks. The midabdomen will present tympany caused by the underlying bowel. Percussion is performed toward each flank and a line drawn on the abdomen where the dullness begins in each flank (Fig. 21-41B). The client is turned on his side. Then, percussion is again done towards each flank. If ascites is present, the fluid will shift to the dependent flank. The new origin of fluid is marked (Fig. 21-41C). This is then repeated on the client's other side. By this procedure, an estimate can be made of free fluid from the distance of the old to the new line (although this procedure will not detect less than 500 ml of free fluid). The greater the shift, the greater the probability it is caused by fluid rather than by fat or feces.

Female Genitalia and Rectum

EXTERNAL GENITALIA

The female genitalia consists of external and internal groups. The external group includes the mons pubis, labia majora and minora, clitoris, vestibule, and the vestibular glands. The *mons pubis* is the fatty tissue underlying the integument in front of the pubic symphysis. Hair covers this area at puberty. The *labia majora* are rounded folds of adipose tissue which correspond to the scrotum of the

Percussion

Measurement of the Liver

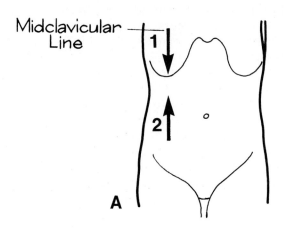

Midclavicular
Line

A

Ascitic Fluid

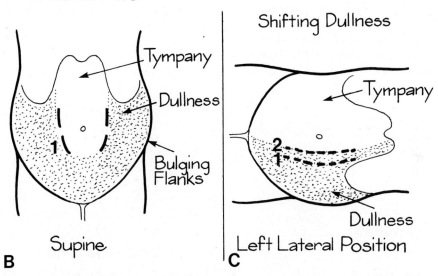

Tympany

Dullness

Bulging
Flanks

Supine

B

Shifting Dullness

Tympany

Dullness

Left Lateral Position

C

FIGURE 21-41. A, Measurement of liver size: (1) percuss from liver resonance down toward liver dullness; (2) percuss from tympany upward toward liver dullness. B, Level (1) of ascites (fluid) in supine position: tympany from gas-filled gut; dulness from ascitic fluid; bulging flank from dependent fluid. C, Previous level of ascitic fluid (1); new level of ascitic fluid in left lateral position (2).

male. The *labia minora* are the two folds which form the prepuce anteriorly covering the clitoris. The *clitoris* is the erectile tissue, which varies in size, that corresponds to the penis of the male. The *vestibule* is an almond-shaped space between the labia

minora. Four structures open into the vestibule: the urethra anteriorly, the vagina posteriorly, and the two ducts of the Bartholin's glands. The *urethral orifice* is about 2.5 cm dorsal to the clitoris and immediately ventral to the vagina. The *Skene's glands* are located around the urethral orifice. The *vaginal orifice*, or *introitus*, will vary in size inversely with that of the hymen. The *hymen* is a fold of mucous membrane normally partially covering the introitus. Once ruptured, the hymenal remnants heal as caruncles (small fleshy growths). The vestibular glands, or *Bartholin's glands*, are two small bodies situated on either side of the introitus (Fig. 21-42).

Inspection and Palpation

The external organs are superficial to the urogenital diaphragm and are below the pubic arch. The perineal area, labia minora, clitoris, vestibule, urethral opening, the vaginal introitus, and the support of the vaginal outlet should all be inspected.

The client should be asked to empty her bladder, disrobe, and assume the lithotomy position on the examination table. Clients who are unable to assume the lithotomy position should use the left lateral side-lying position. The client is draped well to avoid embarrassment. An attendant should be present to assist with the pelvic examination; this is especially helpful if the client needs additional support or feels more comfortable. The equipment, within reach, should include an examining lamp, head mirror or flashlight, an appropriately sized vaginal speculum, materials for making Papanicolaou smears (cancer screening test), lubricating jelly, gloves, and gauze. The examiner sits in front of the perineum within reach of the equipment.

The *perineal area* should be inspected for distribution of pubic hair, skin lesions, swelling of the labia, and discharge. Enlargement of the *clitoris* may suggest some form of masculinization. Redness and excoriation of the *vestibule* are characteristics of pruritus caused by monilial or trichomonas vaginitis. If there is any discharge from, or about the urethral orifice, the Skene's glands are inspected. A specimen is obtained by inserting the index finger into the vagina and milking the urethra gently outwards. Any discharge is cultured for the presence of gonorrhea. The presence or absence of the hymen is recorded. The Bartholin's glands are checked for labial swelling. The gloved index finger is inserted into the *vagina introitus* with the thumb on the outside near its posterior part. The tissue on each side is palpated. Any discharge is cultured. *Support of the vaginal outlet* is assessed by spreading the labia apart, and requesting the client to bear down as if to defecate. Bulging of the

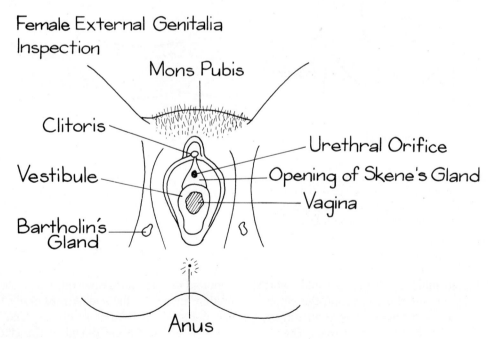

FIGURE 21-42. Examination (inspection) of the external female genitalia.

anterior vaginal wall may indicate a cystocele, and bulging of the posterior vaginal wall and rectum may evidence a rectocele. A *cystocele* is a portion of the bladder, covered by vaginal mucosa, which emerges from the introitus as a small, soft, spherical tumor. Pelvic laceration may have occurred during childbirth. A *rectocele* is a portion of the rectum, covered by vaginal mucosa, which emerges from the introitus. This condition may also have arisen at childbirth.

INTERNAL GENITALIA

The internal group consists of the vagina, uterus, fallopian tubes, and ovaries. The *vagina* is a hollow tube extending from the vestibule to the uterus. Its axis forms an angle of over 90 degrees with that of the uterus. The recess of the vagina behind the cervix is called the *posterior fornix*; recesses on either side of the cervix are called the *lateral for- nices*. The *uterus* is pear-shaped and flattened anteroposteriorly. It is normally inclined forward (anteflexed) 45 degrees from the horizontal plane of the erect body. It is supported in this position by two broad ligaments, the round ligaments, the utero- sacral ligaments, and ligaments attached to the bladder. There are three areas: (1) the body, or

fundus, is the expanded upper portion; (2) the isth- mus or constricted central area; and (3) the cervix or the lower portion of the uterus located in the upper part of the vagina. The *cervix* appears as a smooth button pierced by a small orifice, identified as the cervical os. The *fallopian* or *uterine tubes* extend from each side of the fundus terminating near the ovaries. Each tube is about 10 cm long and is not, normally, palpable. The *ovaries* corre- spond to the testes of the male. They are supported by ligaments near the uterine tubes, about 4 cm in length and 2 cm in width. The term, *adnexa*, refers to ovaries, uterine tubes, and ligaments. The chief methods for examination of the female genitalia are inspection and palpation. Application of these skills can reveal many disorders of the lower abdomen, reproductive organs, and the lower urinary tract. Some clinicians consider the pelvic examination an extension of abdominal palpation.

Speculum Examination

The internal organs, the vagina, uterus, and ad- nexa, are situated within the pelvis (Fig. 21-43). The pelvic examination per speculum is conducted with the client still in the lithotomy position, the buttocks extending just beyond the edge of the ta-

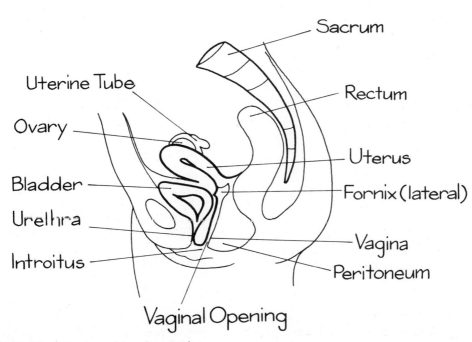

FIGURE 21-43. Side view of female genitalia.

ble. A speculum is selected that will cause the least amount of discomfort while permitting adequate examination of the vaginal structures. After selection of the proper speculum, it is checked for proper operating condition to ensure that the screws of both valves will loosen and tighten and that the lower blade will slide into the track on the handle. All items are placed closely within reach.

Clean surgical gloves are worn. The vaginal cavity is illuminated. The speculum is moistened with warm water for lubrication; both screws of the bi-

valve speculum are loosened. Holding the closed blades of the instrument between the index and second finger of one hand, the handle is gripped in the palm of the same hand. With the thumb and index finger of the other hand, the labia are spread wide at the lowest end of the introitus. Spreading the labia in this way prevents the speculum from dragging the pubic hairs and folds of the labia minora into the vagina. Stretching the introitus minimizes contraction of the vaginal sphincter and facilitates the entry of the speculum. The closed

Speculum Examination of the Vagina

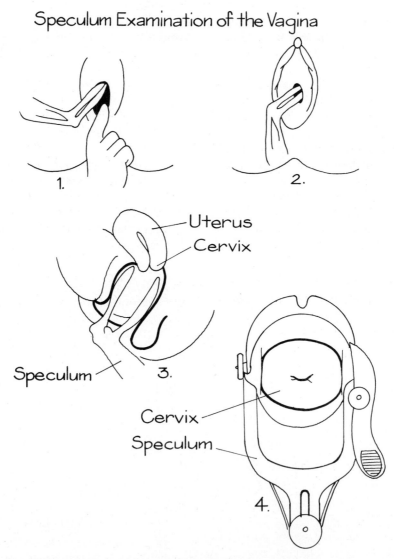

FIGURE 21-44. Speculum examination of the vagina: 1, introitus retracted by index finger, and speculum inserted vertically; 2, upon full insertion, speculum rotated to horizontal position; 3, blades of speculum opened to view cervix; and 4, exposure of cervix on the anterior vaginal wall.

speculum is inserted with the blades at a 45 degree angle over the fingers. The speculum is directed downwards to avoid the sensitive urethra. After the speculum has entered the vagina, the fingers are removed and the blades are turned into a horizontal position. While continuing to exert downward pressure, the blades are opened; they are locked open with the set screw. The speculum handle of the blade tips is moved to expose the cervix on the anterior vaginal wall (Fig. 21-44).

A slide preparation for the Papanicolaou test is made by rubbing the os of the cervix with the long end of a wooden scraper. It is smeared on a slide and ether-alcohol fixative applied immediately. Similarly, a sample from the vaginal pool is withdrawn. (Most cytologists require both samples for evaluation.)

The os of the cervix is inspected, and the color, position, nodules, masses, and any discharge determined. The cervical os before childbirth is small and round. After childbirth, the os evolves into a slit. The cervix is covered by smooth pink epithelium. During pregnancy, the color is a dusky blue. In cervicitis, the mucosa reddens. Normally, the uterus is anteflexed; the cervix is directed posteriorly. When the uterus is in retroversion, the cervix is directed anteriorly. Cervical erosion occurs whenever the cervical mucous glands, which occupy the endocervical canal, extend onto the surface of the cervix. If present, there will be a reddish area around the cervical os. Early cervical carcinoma

Variations of the Cervix

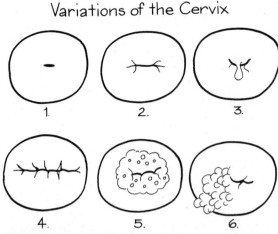

FIGURE 21-45. Variations of the cervix: 1, normal virginal cervix; 2, small laceration; 3, cervical polyp; 4, eversion; 5, erosion; and 6, carcinoma of cervix.

begins near the cervical os as a hard granular surface with an irregular margin. It is friable, bleeds easily, and may be difficult to distinguish from cervical erosion. Cervical polyps are bright red globular structures that protrude through the cervical os and bleed easily (Fig. 21-45).

To remove the speculum, the screws of both valves are loosened as much as possible without detaching them from the speculum. The speculum is drawn back off the cervix so that it is freed from the blades. The blades are closed by securing them between the index and second fingers. Finally, the closed speculum is drawn out of the vagina. As the speculum is slowly withdrawn, the vaginal mucosa is inspected. Normal vaginal mucosa is pinkish and smooth, exhibiting a bluish color before the onset of menstruation. White, curdlike exudate on the mucosa may indicate Candida albicans (moniliasis) infection. A thick, yellow, frothy discharge suggests Trichomonas vaginalis.

Digital Bimanual Examination

The purpose of the bimanual examination is to palpate the vagina, cervix, uterus, and adnexa between the fingers placed in the vagina and the other hand which lies flat on the lower abdomen. A water-soluble lubricant is used to lubricate the first two fingers of the gloved hand which enters the vagina. The thumb is kept abducted, and the other fingers flexed. The second finger of the gloved hand is inserted into the introitus. The introitus is stretched by putting pressure on the lower vaginal wall with a finger of the other hand. Next the index finger is inserted. With palm upwards, the fingers are advanced deeper into the vagina, sweeping the vaginal walls to detect any abnormalities.

The *cervix* is located and explored for size, consistency, and abnormalities. With the cervix between the two fingers, it is wiggled from side to side. If the client finds this maneuver painful, there may be infection present. A soft cervix identifying pregnancy, is called Hegar's sign. The gloved hand is opened and the thumb flattened against one side of the labia with the third finger against the other side of the labia. This position allows the fingers maximum penetration into the vagina. The hand on the abdomen is placed about midway between the client's umbilicus and symphysis pubis. The fingers are pressed downwards (Fig. 21-46). This ac-

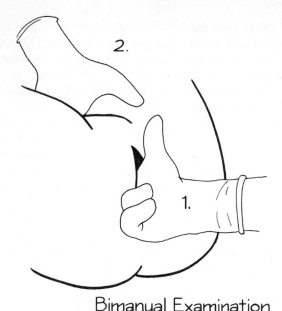

Bimanual Examination

FIGURE 21-46. Bimanual vaginal examination: 1, the index and middle fingers are inserted into the vagina; and 2, the hand on the abdomen pushes the uterus downward and forward.

tion will depress the pelvic organs to enable their outline to be identified by the fingers in the client's vagina. The fingers in the vagina are slid over the upper lip of the cervix.

Maintaining the fingers in contact with the cervix, the fingers are advanced deeper into the vagina until the body of the *uterus* beginning to curve is felt. The fingers are raised towards the hand on the abdomen that is pressing on the abdomen. The uterus is traced with the tips of the fingers. The fingers are separated in order to explore the uterus for its position, size, and the presence of masses. Displacement of the uterus is commonly posterior. Retroversion is the tilting backwards of the uterus with the cervix pointing forward towards the symphysis pubis. This condition is present in 25 percent of normal women. Retroflexion is the backward angulation of the body of the uterus with the cervix remaining in its normal axis (Fig. 21-47). Uterine enlargement is usually caused by pregnancy in a woman of fecund age. To differentiate enlargement by pregnancy from tumors, an attempt to assess for fetal parts and fetal heart sounds is made.

Very often benign growths, myomas or fibroids, develop in the uterine muscle. Frequently multiple, they are felt as hard but painless nodules attached to the fundus. Nodules and fundus will move readily together on palpation.

To examine the *adnexa*, the fingers in the vagina are brought closely together. They are moved to the left alongside the body of the uterus. The hand on the abdomen is moved to the left to depress the tissues between the fingers of both hands. An attempt to capture the ovary between the fingers of both hands is made. The adnexa are explored. The ovaries and the uterine tubes may be able to be palpated. If the ovaries can be palpated they are assessed for size, shape, mobility, tenderness, and masses. The normal ovary is somewhat tender. Generally, the uterine tubes cannot be palpated unless there has been a prior infection. Infection causes them to feel like fibrous bands. The fingers are withdrawn from the vagina, and the rectovaginal examination is begun.

Rectovaginal Examination

This examination permits the finger which is placed in the rectum to palpate behind the cervix and the posterior surface of the uterus. The objective is to confirm the findings of the pelvic examination, to check nodules and masses, and is done postpartum to check episiotomy repairs.

The rectal examination is uncomfortable. It is important to be gentle, supportive, and explain each step to the client. More lubricant is added to the second finger of the gloved hand. The client is

Retrodisplacement of the Uterus

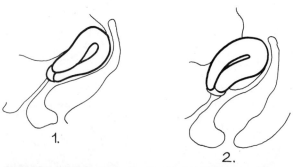

FIGURE 21-47. Retrodisplacement of the uterus: 1, first degree retroversion of uterus—uterus tipped slightly posteriorly; and 2, retroflexion of the uterus—backward angulation of the body of the uterus in relation to the cervix.

asked to bear down as if to defecate. The second finger is slipped slowly into the rectum. The index finger is inserted into the vagina. The rectovaginal wall is then between these two fingers. The thickness and security of the wall are checked. If a third or fourth degree laceration (rectal sphincter tear) occurred during childbirth, the presence of strictures of the sphincter are ascertained. With the index finger on the cervix, the second finger in the rectum is used to explore under the cervix and to either side. An attempt to detect whether the uterus is in a retroverted position should be made. The ovaries and tubes are explored for masses or unusual enlargement. With the second finger in the rectum, the cervix is touched through the rectovaginal wall. The pelvis is explored with the index finger in the vagina over the cervix. An attempt to outline the uterus in the antiverted or midline position is made.

RECTUM

The rectum can be assessed during the rectovaginal examination. The finger in the rectum palpates the rectum for masses, tenderness, and drainage. Both fingers are then withdrawn. The perineum is wiped downward and over the rectum with a tissue or softswipe. Any fecal material left on the glove should be tested for occult blood. Hemorrhoids are dilated veins, either external or internal. External hemorrhoids are located around the anal orifice, distal to the pectinate line. When inflamed they will cause pain and pruritus (itching). Internal hemorrhoids arise proximal to the pectinate line. On straining, they may prolapse into view as red masses covered with mucosa. They usually are manifested by painless bleeding. Anal fissures are linear ulcers on the margin of the anus. They may result in rectal bleeding and are palpated as defects that are quite tender to the client. Rectal abcesses and fistulas are connections between the lower bowel and the external skin. They usually cause drainage into the perianal tissue.

Male Genitalia and Rectum

EXTERNAL GENITALIA

The male external genitalia include the penis and the scrotum. The cone-shaped head of the penis,

glans penis, contains the urethral orifice. The covering foreskin (or prepuce) is frequently removed by circumcision. If present, a thin membrane (the frenulum) connects the foreskin with the glans. The shaft of the penis is formed by three columns: two lateral columns (the corpora cavernosa penis) and the third or median column (corpus spongiosum) which contains the urethra. The urethra is located ventrally in the shaft of the penis. The three columns are joined by fibrous tissue and are covered by skin (Fig. 21-48). The *scrotum* is the double pouch containing the testes and part of the *spermatic cord*. The *testis* is an ovoid body about 4.0 cm long and 2 to 2.5 cm in width. The testes are suspended by the spermatic cord, a structure extending from the inguinal ring to the testis. Normally, the left testis is somewhat lower than the right. The comma shaped epididymis is attached vertically to the posterior surface of the testis and leads to the *vas deferens*, becoming part of the spermatic cord. Other components of the spermatic cord are arteries, veins, nerves, and lymphatic vessels. From the testis, the cord extends upwards entering the external inguinal ring, moving through the inguinal canal to the abdominal inguinal ring, where the components diverge. The vas deferens continues behind the peritoneum joining the duct of the *seminal vesicle* to become the ejaculatory duct.

Inspection and Palpation

The penis and scrotum are examined. The presence of inguinal and femoral hernias are ascertained.

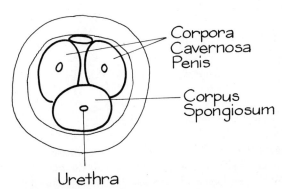

FIGURE 21-48. Cross-section of shaft of penis.

The natural state of the *penis* is inspected. If the prepuce is present, the client is asked to retract it to enable detection of any ulceration, tumor, or infection. The location of the urethral meatus is noted. The urethra is palpated with gloved hand, for evidence of scarring or stricture. Any discharge is noted and cultured.

The *scrotum* is examined by inspection and palpation (Fig. 21-49). The scrotum pouch and the perineum between the anus and the base of scrotum, are inspected and palpated to evidence that there are two testes present and whether or not swelling exists. Any mass should be transilluminated in a darkened room by shining a penlight from behind the scrotum to conclude whether the mass is translucent or opaque. Fluid-filled masses are translucent; most solid masses are opaque. *Hydrocele* of the testis (accumulation of serous fluid from infection or trauma) is translucent. The mass feels smooth and resilient. A *variocele* (originating from varicosities of the pampiniform plexus of veins) is opaque. It feels like a "bag of worms." This condition occurs predominantly on the left side. A scrotal inguinal hernia is opaque except

Scrotal Contents

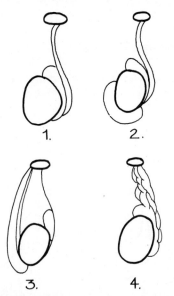

FIGURE 21-49. Scrotal contents: 1, normal contents—testis, epididymis, spermatic cord, and external inguinal ring; 2, hydrocele of the testis; 3, scrotal inguinal hernia; and 4, varicocele.

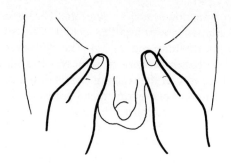

Palpation of Spermatic Cords

FIGURE 21-50. Palpation of spermatic cord.

when it contains translucent gas-filled gut. Since this hernia descends into the scrotum from the inguinal ring, the fingers used for the examination cannot get above it in the scrotum.

The *spermatic cord* is palpated (Fig. 21-50). The vas deferens, spermatic artery, and veins of the pampiniform plexus are identified. The presence of any lymphedema, induration, or tenderness of the spermatic cord are determined. The testis, epididymis, and portion of the cord adjacent to the epididymis are palpated; it should be noted if the epididymis is in normal position. Any areas of irregularity on the surface of the testis and epididymis are identified. Acute epididymitis emerges with direct spread of bacteria from urinary tract infections, or from prostatitis. The scrotal skin over the epididymis may be red and warm to the touch.

The inguinal and femoral areas are inspected for hernias. Inguinal hernias are classified as indirect or direct. An *indirect hernia* occurs whenever the peritoneal sac and possibly a loop of the bowel, penetrates the internal inguinal ring, travels the inguinal canal, and emerges through the external inguinal ring, possibly entering the scrotum. A *direct inguinal hernia* happens whenever the peritoneal sac and possibly a loop of the bowel, penetrates directly at the location of the external inguinal ring. The client is asked to stand with his ipsilateral (on the same side as the hernia) leg slightly flexed. The gloved index finger is inserted low into the scrotum, invaginating the scrotal skin; the spermatic cord is followed upwards to the triangular slitlike opening of the external inguinal ring. If possible, an attempt is made to advance the index finger 4 to 5 cm through the inguinal canal to the internal inguinal ring. The client is asked to bear down as if to defecate (Fig. 21-51). Any mass touching the finger is noted. If felt against the fingertips the hernia is indirect. If felt alongside the finger, the hernia is direct. A femoral hernia is a protrusion of a peritoneal sac through the femoral ring in the thigh. It can be palpated in the groin medial to the femoral artery (Fig. 21-52).

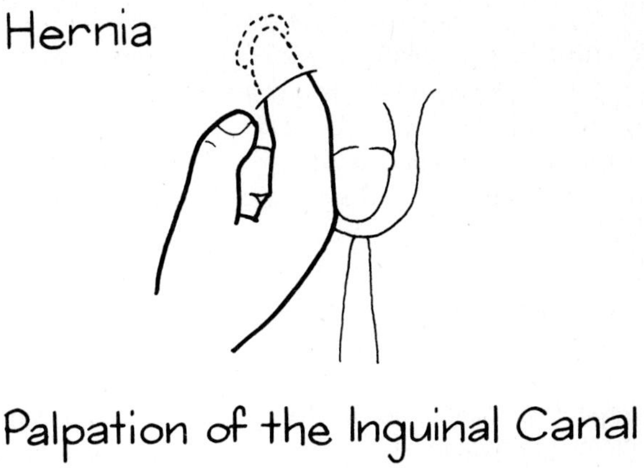

INTERNAL GENITALIA

The internal genitalia includes the prostate gland, seminal vesicles, and the bulbourethral glands. The *prostate gland*, a firm body consisting of gland and muscle, is situated in the pelvic cavity below the caudal part of the symphysis pubis, ventral to the rectum (through which it can be palpated). Measurements are 4 cm transversely at the base, 2 cm in anteroposterior diameter, and 3 cm in vertical diameter. Except for the upper portion, a shallow median furrow divides the posterior surface into right and left lateral lobes. The *seminal vesicles* are two lobular pouches between the fundus of the bladder and the rectum. Usually, they approximate 7.5 cm in length but may vary among males. Only

Hernia

Palpation of the Inguinal Canal

FIGURE 21-51. Palpation of the inguinal canal for hernia.

their lower portions may be palpated in the rectum. The bulbourethral glands (*Cowper's glands*) are two small, rounded, bodies about the size of peas. One gland lies on each side of the membranous urethra between the inferior edge of the prostate gland and the inner border of the anal canal. Primarily, inspection and palpation are used for physical examination of the external and internal genitalia.

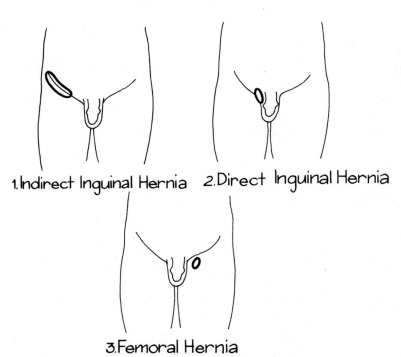

1. Indirect Inguinal Hernia   2. Direct Inguinal Hernia

3. Femoral Hernia

FIGURE 21-52 Inguinal and femoral hernias.

Rectal Examination

The internal genitalia (Fig. 21-53) are assessed with a rectal examination. The client should be examined while on his hands and knees or while bent over the examining table.

The anus is examined carefully for evidence of pruritus, dermatitis, fissure, or hemorrhoids. The glutei are held apart, and the client is asked to bear down as if to defecate. While he is bearing down, a well-lubricated index finger is inserted into the anus. Lateral and posterior surfaces of the anus are palpated for nodules or irregularities. While examining the anterior surface of the anus, the two lobes, and the median furrow of the prostate gland are identified; size, shape, and consistency are noted. The normal prostate gland is firm, small and rubbery. It should be noted whether the prostate gland is moveable or fixed. If the gland is soft and tender, it suggests prostatitis. If hard and irregular, a malignancy may be present (Fig. 21-54).

Superior to the prostate gland, the fingertips may reach the *seminal vesicles* on either side of the midline. Normally, they are not palpable. Only diseased seminal vesicles can be felt.

Normally, *bulbourethral glands* are not palpable. They can be felt only if they are enlarged or inflamed. One gland on each side of the midline just inferior to the caudal border of the prostate gland, and the inner border of the anal canal is palpated. In chronic inflammation, they enlarge to the size of a hazelnut and can be felt as rounded masses in the anterior rectal wall.

Extremities and Vertebral Column

General examinantion of the extremities includes assessment of peripheral pulses, veins, joints, muscles, bones, and the vertebral column. Cardiac action maintains blood pressure in arteries and veins. Left ventricular contractions produce pulses in accessible arteries, whereas right ventricular contractions produce venous pulses only in the upper torso. Therefore, pressure is highest in arteries, much less in capillaries, and almost nonexistent in veins. Visible arterial pulsations are palpable but not venous pulsations. Arterial blood pressure is altered by cardiac output via the left ventricle and the amount of peripheral resistance caused by the caliber of the arteries (e.g., blood pressure = peripheral resistance × cardiac output).

PERIPHERAL PULSES

Inspection and palpation are utilized for physical examination of peripheral pulses. Some of the palpable arteries are: brachial (which lies near the elbow in the biceps-triceps furrow), radial (medial to the outer border of the radius), femoral (at the inguinal ligament midway between the anterior-superior iliac spine and the symphysis pubis), popliteal (behind the knee), dorsal pedis (on the groove between two tendons on the medial side of the dorsum of the foot), and posterior tibial (behind the medial malleolus) [Fig. 21-55].

INSPECTION. Any visible pulsations are noted. The extremities are inspected for color, tempera-

Internal Male Genitalia

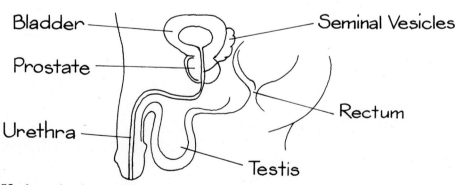

FIGURE 21-53. Internal male genitalia.

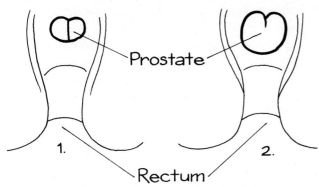

FIGURE 21-54. Prostate gland: 1, normal prostate; and 2, benign prostatic hypertrophy.

ture, lack of hair, shiny skin, and ulceration of the arms, legs, and feet.

PALPATION. Each arterial pulse is palpated bilaterally for related comparison. Condition, symmetry, pulse volume, and tissue effects are evaluated. The walls of the arteries are palpated for signs of arteriosclerosis or spasm. A spastic artery feels like a small cord. Arteries are palpated to determine if there is pulsation. Arteries can be partially or completely occluded. Complete occlusion suggests embolism or thrombosis. Arterial deficit causes dermal pallor, coldness, and malnutrition. If a thrill is felt over any major vessel, it is auscultated for a bruit.

VEINS

Veins from the upper torso drain into the superior vena cava while those of the lower part of the body drain into the inferior vena cava. The flow of venous blood in the lower extremities is, essentially, passive. Contraction of leg muscles (which causes a milking action), and the one way valvular system of the deep veins, force the flow of blood towards the heart. Good venous return flow of blood to the heart is accomplished by patent vessels, competent valves, and muscular contractions. These deep veins are well supported. Conversely, superficial veins are subcutaneous with little support from surrounding tissue. There are many communicating veins between the deep and superficial venous system (Fig. 21-56).

INSPECTION. The client is asked to assume the supine position. The presence of venous stasis and stasis pigmentation of the legs is checked. The client

is then asked to stand. Dilated veins and varicosities in the arms and the legs are assessed for their presence.

PALPATION. Palpation is done for pitting edema, thrombophlebitis, and valvular competency. The thumb is pressed firmly over the shin or dorsum of the foot for 5 seconds. It is then released and any pitting noted. Inadequate drainage of venous blood from the extremities is manifested by edema. Stasis pigmentation of the lower legs results from capillary damage. Ulceration may be attributed to malnutrition of the tissues. To test for deep thrombophlebitis, swelling is checked by measuring the circumference of the calves and the thighs of both legs and the respective size is compared. Another assessment is Homan's sign. Forceful dorsiflexion of the foot should produce pain in the calf muscles (Homan's sign) if there is deep thrombosis of the leg.

Peripheral Pulses

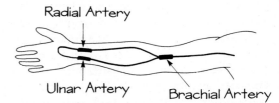

Palpable Arteries of the Upper Extremities

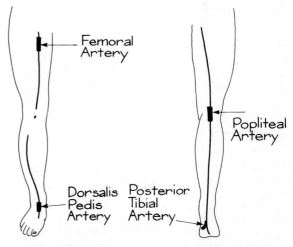

Palpable Arteries of the Lower Extremities

FIGURE 21-55. Palpable arteries of the upper and lower extremities.

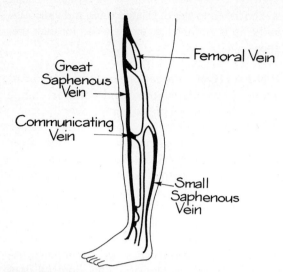

FIGURE 21-56. Large veins of the lower extremity: deep veins—femoral veins; superficial veins—the great and small saphenous veins; and deep and superficial veins are joined by communicating veins.

JOINTS

There are three main types of joints: synarthrosis (immovable articulations), amphiarthrosis (slightly movable articulations), and diarthrosis (freely moveable articulations). Diarthrodial joints outnumber the other types. They are lined by synovial membrane, enclosed in a capsule of connective tissue, and are supported by ligaments and muscles (Fig. 21-57).

Joints are examined, systematically, from the distal interphalangeals to the wrists, elbows, shoulders, acromioclaviculars, sternoclaviculars, dorsal spine, lumbar spine, sacroiliacs, hips, knees, ankles, and feet. Corresponding joints are compared systematically. Inspection and palpation supplement each other in evaluation of joints. Many clues are easily obtained as the client is observed. The client is asked to remove his clothes, get on and off the table, come to a sitting position, or turn on the table. The client's exposition of his functional skills can be correlated with what is he is able to demonstrate.

When focusing on a single joint for examination, it is inspected for color, presence of skin rash, nodules near the joint, joint swelling, deformity, and wasting of muscles proximal and distal to the joint. Joints are palpated for swelling, tenderness, nodules, range of motion, and crepitation. The face of the client should be watched when applying gentle pressure to the joints. Consistency and character of any nodules palpated is observed. Palpation for tenderness is done. Location and degree are noted when palpating joint enlargements to differentiate: bony swelling (hard surface at edges of joint); periarticular edema (involves tissues outside the joint in the subcutaneous tissue and usually "pits"); synovial effusion (test by ballottement); capsular thickening (periarticular and hard, does not pit, and is associated with a resistance to joint motion); and inflamed synovial swelling (feels doughy and velvety in consistency). Normally synovial membranes are not palpable. In osteoarthritis, small nodules, Heberden's nodes, may develop (Fig. 21-58). They are irregular bony enlargements at the dorsal surface of the distal interphalangeal joints. In rheumatoid arthritis, there are fusiform swellings (Haygarth's nodes) (Fig. 21-58) or muscular atrophy on the proximal interphalangeal joint. The periarticular tissue involved is inflamed in rheumatoid arthritis.

The joint is gently moved through a full range of motion (Fig. 21-59). Stability in the mediolateral, anteroposterior, and rotational directions is tested. The degree of pain and its location as range of

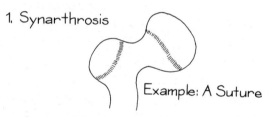

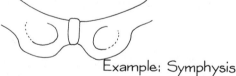

FIGURE 21-57. Types of joints.

motion is produced passively is assessed. Crepitations (crackling or rubbing sounds) should be heard and felt. If the range of motion is limited, the reason for its limitation is assessed. Joint motion limitations may stem from a tight capsule, pain and reflex guarding of muscles, actual bony ankylosis or bridging of the joint space with fibrous tissue, thickening and fibrosis of the joint capsule, shortening of muscles, shortening of tendons, and scarring of overlying skin and subcutaneous tissues.

MUSCLES

Muscles are inspected and palpated for atrophy, strength, tenderness, consistency, and abnormal movements. They are inspected for size and compared with corresponding muscles of the opposite side. Circumference measurements should be made at a definitely measured distance from a bony landmark for bilateral comparisons. Atrophy should be distinguished from congenital absence by palpation and tests for strength. Hypertrophy needs to be distinguished from pseudohypertrophy where a muscle is also enlarged, but less than normal strength is demonstrated as contrasted with the situation in true hypertrophy. Abnormal movements (e.g., fasciculations which are wormlike uncoordinated contractions) should be noted. *Fasciculations* are discharges of bundles of the muscle fibers and are not under voluntary control which may signify degenerating nerve fibers with foci of irritation. *Fibrillations* (spontaneous contractions of individual muscular fibers which signify denervation) are visible only when they occur in the tongue.

To test for muscular strength of the upper extremity, the client is asked to hold his elbows flexed with his arms close to his sides. He is instructed to hold this position firmly and to resist the examiner's attempts to change his position. Upward force is applied to the elbows and an outward force to the elbows. Then the hands of the client are grasped alternately applying force in all planes to test the flexors of the fingers, the flexors and extensors of the wrist, the pronators and supinators of the forearm, the flexors and extensors of the elbow, and the flexors and extensors of the shoulder. To test the muscles of the lower extremity, the client is asked to walk in his ordinary pattern, walk on heels, toes, stand or walk with hips and knees bent, squat and stand, stand on one foot, and raise his leg straight from the supine position.

Joints

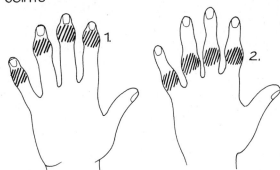

FIGURE 21-58. 1, Heberden's nodes; 2, Haygarth's nodes.

To test the muscles of the trunk, the client is asked to do a sit-up from a supine position and extend his neck, back, and hips from a prone position. Palpation for tenderness is done by gently squeezing the muscular masses of each extremity between the thumb and index finger. Consistency of muscle varies from the flabby feel in acute denervation or chronic conditions of the lower motor neuron, the doughy feel when there is an inflammatory exudate, the firm feel of fibrosis as in ischemic contracture, and the feel of spasticity and rigidity elicited mostly on movement resulting from lesions of the central nervous system.

BONES

The presence of bone pain and deformities are evaluated. Pain may be accompanied by swelling and tenderness and may be intensified by movement or weight-bearing. Bone pain may be caused by fractures, infections, osteosarcoma, osteoporosis, osteomyelitis, or Osgood-Schlatter disease. Fractures, dislocations and tumors of bones may result in deformities (Fig. 21-60). The shape of the legs may be altered by *genu varum* (bowlegs) or *genu valgum* (knock-kneed). *Talpes* (clubfoot) may be the equinus type (client walks on anterior portion of the foot) or the calcaneus type (client walks only on heel of the foot). In either type, the foot may be everted or inverted. In *pes planus* (flatfoot), the longitudinal arch of the foot is lost.

UPPER EXTREMITY

SHOULDER. The sternoclavicular joint, acromioclavicular joint, greater tuberosity, and bicipital

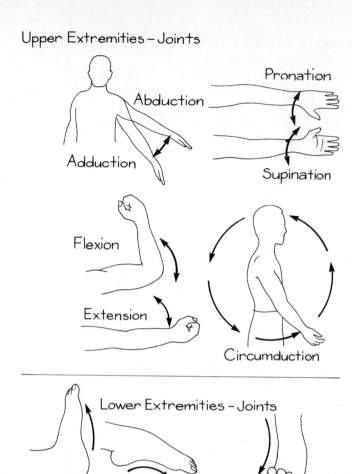

Upper Extremities – Joints

Abduction

Adduction

Pronation

Supination

Flexion

Extension

Circumduction

Lower Extremities – Joints

Dorsiflexion

Plantar Flexion

Inversion

Types of Movement by Diarthrodial Joints

FIGURE 21-59. Types of joint movement.

groove are palpated. The stability of the glenohumeral joint is tested by attempting relative anteroposterior and superinferior movements between the humerus and the scapula. Full abduction of the shoulder is a combination of 120° of glenohumeral motion and 60° of scapular rotation. Scapular winging may be produced by rhomboid, trapezius, or serratus muscle weakness.

ELBOW. The medial and lateral epicondyle of the ulna and olecranon fossa are palpated and an assessment of the stability of the head of the radius and its integrity in forearm pronation and supination is done.

WRIST. The key wrist joints are the radiocarpal,

the distal radioulnar, the transcarpal, and carpal metacarpal joints. These four joints together allow wrist dorsi and plantar flexion, radial and ulnar deviation, and forearm pronation and supination. The stability of the distal radioulnar articulation is tested.

HAND. The integrity of the metacarpal phalangeal joints are palpated for swelling, stability, and subluxation (partial dislocation). The ability of the hand to perform opposition of the thumb against the second and third digits (finger pinch) are observed and tested; the strength of full grasp (fist closed) is also tested. The thumb's capacity to oppose the pads of the remaining digits, and to flex across the palm are assessed.

The Upper Extremity

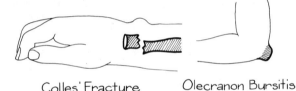

Colles' Fracture   Olecranon Bursitis

FIGURE 21-60. Causes of pain in upper extremity.

LOWER EXTREMITY

HIP. The area over the hip joint is palpated anteriorly and posteriorly. The greater trochanter and the ischial tuberosity are palpated. Hip motion is tested for flexion from the extended position, adduction, abduction, and medial and lateral rotation.

KNEE. Can the knee be fully extended and can the tibia be moved anteriorly or posteriorly relative to the femur and laterally with respect to the femur with the knee extended? Any crepitus on movement of the patella over the femur is noted.

ANKLE. Whether or not there is bulging of the synovium of the ankle joint is observed. Any tenderness over the medial deltoid ligament, the lateral ligament, or the distal tibial fibular articulation is noted. The ankle joint (tibiotalar) allows only dorsal and plantar flexion.

Spine

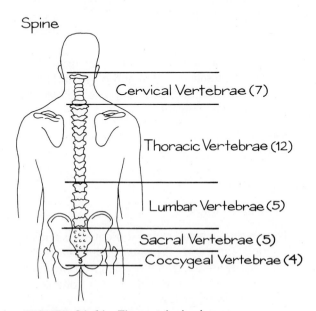

Cervical Vertebrae (7)

Thoracic Vertebrae (12)

Lumbar Vertebrae (5)

Sacral Vertebrae (5)

Coccygeal Vertebrae (4)

FIGURE 21-61. The vertebral column.

FOOT. Shoes are inspected for uneven wear. Whether the metatarsal phalangeal joints are subluxed, plantar fascia is contracted, metatarsal heads are tender, or if there is abnormal callous formation should be determined.

VERTEBRAL COLUMN

The entire vertebral column should be examined for deformities as well as for paravertebral and vertebral tenderness (Fig. 21-61).

The vertebral column is inspected for scoliosis, kyphosis, degree of lumbar lordosis, and whether these curves disappear or exaggerate on bending forward or lying down (Fig. 21-62).

The paravertebral muscles are palpated for spasm. Observation is made as to whether the spasm relaxes when weight is shifted from one leg to the other. Involuntary spasm does not relax whereas voluntary contraction relaxes. Palpation is done for tenderness. It should be assessed whether or not palpation produces radiating pain. The vertebral column is also percussed for radiating pain.

Vertebral column motions for the cervical and the thoracolumbar spine include forward flexion, extension, right lateral flexion, left lateral flexion, right rotation, and left rotation. The client is instructed to execute these motions and observed for limitation of range of movement and pain.

With the client supine and knees straight, the leg is gently flexed to extreme position. It is observed at what angle pain may be produced, and its location (straight leg raising test). With the leg supported in flexion and with the knee straight, the client's foot is dorsiflexed to put tension on the

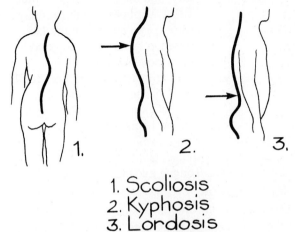

1. Scoliosis
2. Kyphosis
3. Lordosis

FIGURE 21-62. Curvature of the spine.

sciatic nerve. If pain is produced, this test is positive (Lasèque's sign).

A PHYSICAL EXAMINATION

General

Miss Adams is an alert, well-developed, thin, 41-year-old white woman appearing her age and evidencing no gross abnormalities or distress.

Measurements

Height: 167.6 cm (5'6")
Weight: 55.3 kg (122 lbs)
Temperature: 37°C (98.6°F)
Pulse: 88
Respiration: 16
Blood pressure: RA (right arm) 130/82 upright; LA (left arm) 126/78 upright; RA 126/80 supine; LA 126/78 supine.

Skin

Warm to the touch, good turgor, pink in color, no lesions.
Hair and nails appear normal.

Neurological System

Mental status: Tense, but alert and cooperative; orientation and memory intact; thought coherent; appropriate behavior and speech.

Cranial Nerves

I. Not tested.
II. Vision 20/20 both eyes; visual fields normal.
III, IV, VI. EOM (extraocular muscles) intact. PERRLA (pupils equal; round; reactive to light and accommodation).
V. Sensation intact, strength good.
VII. Facial movement good.
VIII. Hearing intact, Weber, no lateralization, Rinne air > bone.
IX, X. Gag reflex intact, swallowing normal, no hoarseness.
XI. Head movement and shrug of shoulders intact.
XII. Tongue midline, no tremor.

Motor System

Size, strength, and tone same bilaterally, no atrophy, weakness, or tremors.

Reflexes

	Biceps	Triceps	Brachio-radialis
RT.	2+	2+	2+
LT.	2+	2+	2+
	Patellar	Achilles	Plantar
RT.	2+	2+	↓
LT.	2+	2+	↓

Sensory: Screening for pain, light touch, position, vibration, stereognosis intact.
Coordination: Finger-to-nose, heel-to-shin, alternating movements—well done; Romberg negative.

Head and Neck

Head: Scalp and skull normal.
Face: Symmetrical, appropriate expression.
Eyes: Able to read fine print without difficulty. Lashes and brows present. Conjunctiva clear. Red reflex and fundi normal. Right eye and left eye discs flat and well delineated. No arteriolar narrowing, A-V nicking, hemorrhages or exudates.
Ears: No masses, lesions, of auricles or external canals. Wax partially obscuring the left tympanic membrane. Right tympanic membrane normal color, no perforations, light reflex present. Acuity good to watch ticking and whispered voice.
Nose: No septal deviation, patent bilaterally, mucosa pink and no sinus tenderness.
Oral cavity: Teeth in good repair. Mucosa pink. Tongue protrudes midline. Tonsils absent. Pharynx negative.
Neck: No lymphopathy. Veins not distended. Carotid pulsations equal and of good quality. Thyroid isthmus barely palpable. Lobes not felt. Trachea midline.

Breasts

Right breast slightly larger than left breast. No retraction or masses. Nipples erect and without discharge.

Thorax and Lungs

Thorax symmetrical, expansion equal bilaterally. Good excursion. Fremitus equal bilaterally. Lungs resonant. Diaphragmatic excursion 4 cm on inspiration. Breath sounds normal, no rales, rhonchi, or rubs.

Heart

Apical impulse palpable in the fifth interspace, 8 cm from the midsternal line. Physiologic splitting of S_2. A soft S_4 heard at the apex in the left lateral position. No murmurs or thrills are present.

Abdomen

Abdomen flat, no lesions, hernia, or pulsations. Bowel sounds normal. No masses or tenderness. Liver, spleen, and kidneys not felt. Liver span 8 cm in the right midclavicular line.

Genitalia and Rectum

External genitalia normal. Vaginal and cervical mucosa normal. Uterus in midposition, smooth, not enlarged. Ovaries normally palpable. No tumors, or masses evident. Rectovaginal examination confirms findings.

Rectal: No abnormalities, guaiac examination negative.

Extremities and Spine

Radial, brachial, femoral, dorsalis pedis and post tibial pulses palpable and equal. No venous dilation. No joint or bone disease. Full range of motion. Muscle strength intact. Normal curvature of spine. No paravertebral tenderness.

Sonya Hawkins, R.N.

BIBLIOGRAPHY

Alexander, M., and Brown, M.: Physical examination, part 12: chest and lungs. *Nurs. '75* 5(1), 1975.

Alexander, M., and Brown, M.: Physical examination, part 16: the musculoskeletal system. *Nurs. '76* 6(4), 1976.

Bates, B.: *A Guide to Physical Examination.* Philadelphia, J. B. Lippincott Co., 1979.

Beeson, P., and McDermott, W. (eds.): *Textbook of Medicine,* 14th ed. Philadelphia, W. B. Saunders, 1975.

Brown, M., and Alexander, M.: Physical examination, part 15: female genitalia. *Nurs. '76* 6(3), 1976.

Brown, M., and Alexander, M.: Physical examination: part 8: hearing acuity. *Nurs. '73* 3(4), 1973.

Browne, J., and Boucher, R.: *Primary Care Readings—Guidelines.* New York, Xerox, 1975.

DeGowin, E., and DeGowin, R.: *Bedside Diagnostic Examination,* 4th ed. New York, Macmillan Co., 1976.

Delaney, M.: Examining the chest, part I: the lungs. *Nurs. '75* 5(8), 1975.

Egan, R., et al.: A nursing guide to breast cancer prevention, *Nurs. Update* 6(11), 1975.

Fowkes, W., and Hunn, V.: *Clinical Assessment for the Nurse Practitioner,* St. Louis, C. V. Mosby Co., 1972.

G. I. Series—Physical Examination of the Abdomen. Parts 1–6. A. H. Robins Co., Richmond, Va.

Gillies, D., and Alyn, I.: *Patient Assessment and Management by the Nurse Practitioner.* Philadelphia, W. B. Saunders, 1976.

Gray, H.: *Gray's Anatomy of the Human Body.* Philadelphia, Lea and Febiger, 1974.

Guyton, A.: *Textbook of Medical Physiology,* 5th ed. Philadelphia, W. B. Saunders, 1976.

Hudak, C., et al.: *Clinical Protocols—A Guide for Nurses and Physicians.* Philadelphia, J. B. Lippincott, 1976.

Keough, G., and Nubel, N.: Oral cancer detection—a nursing responsibility. *Am. J. Nurs.* 73(4), 1973.

Malasanos, L., et al.: *Health Assessment.* St. Louis, C. V. Mosby Co., 1977.

Mansell, B., et al.: Patient assessment: examination of the abdomen. *Am. J. Nurs.* 74(9), 1974.

Mechner, F.: Patient assessment: examination of the ear. *Am. J. Nurs.* 74(3), 1974.

Mechner, F., et al.: Patient assessment: examination of the head and neck. (Programmed Instruction). *Am. J. Nurs.* 75(5), 1975.

Mechner, F.: Patient assessment: examination of the eye. Part I. *Am. J. Nurs.* 74(11), 1974. Part II. *Am. J. Nurs.* 75(1), 1975.

Mechner, F.: Patient Assessment: neurological examination. Part I. *Am. J. Nurs.* 75(9), 1975. Part II. *Am. J. Nurs.* 75(11), 1975. Part III. *Am. J. Nurs.* 76(4), 1976.

Megahed, M., and Rosendahl, P.: Brain tumors—an assessment for nurse practitioners. *The Nurse Practitioner,* July-August, 1977.

OMNI: Ortho Breast Examination, Raritan, N.J., Ortho Pharmaceutical Corp., 1974.

Prior, J., and Silberstein, J.: *Physical Diagnosis: The History and Examination of the Patient.* St. Louis, C. V. Mosby Co., 1977.

Roach, L.: Assessing skin changes: the subtle and the obvious. *Nurs. '74* 4(3):64, 1974.

Roach, L.: Color changes in dark skins. *Nurs. '72* 2(11): 19, 1972.

Sana, J., and Judge, R.: *Physical Appraisal Methods in Nursing Practice.* Boston, Little Brown and Co., 1975.

Sauve, M., and Pecherer, A.: *Concepts and Skills in Physical Assessment.* Philadelphia, W. B. Saunders, 1977.

Sherman, J., and Fields, S.: *guide to Patient Evaluation,* 2nd ed. Flushing, N.Y., Medical Examination Publishing Co., 1976.

Thorn, G. et al. (eds.): *Harrison's Principles of Internal Medicine,* 8th ed. New York, McGraw-Hill Book Co., 1977.

Traver, G.: Assessment of thorax and lungs. *Am. J. Nurs.* 73(3), 1973.

CHAPTER 22

GLOSSARY

acrocyanosis. Cyanosis (blue color) of the hands and feet.

apnea. Cessation of respirations.

caput succedaneum. Swelling (edema) of the scale of the newborn infant.

cephalhematoma. An area of swelling where blood has collected beneath the newborn's scalp.

coarctation. A stricture or compression of the walls of a blood vessel.

conjunctivitis. Inflammation of the conjunctiva of the eye.

ecchymosis. The escape of blood into the tissue beneath the skin causing it to appear "black and blue."

edema. An excessive amount of fluid in the tissue.

epispadias. A congenital anomaly in which the urethra opens on the posterior surface of the penis.

CHILD HEALTH ASSESSMENT

Dorothy De Maio, Ed.D., R.N., F.A.A.N.

epithelial pearls (Epstein's pearls). Small white elevations found on both sides of a newborn's hard palate.

erythema toxicum. A rash found on the newborn which disappears spontaneously. The cause is unknown.

fontanelles. The soft spaces found anteriorly and posteriorly between the bones of the infant's skull.

grunt. A sound heard during the expiratory phase of respiration when there is difficulty breathing. The closing of the glottis to prevent collapse of the alveoli in the lungs produces this sound.

hydrocele. An accumulation of serous fluid in a saclike cavity. In the male infant it may be seen associated with the testes.

hypertrophy. An increase in the size or bulk of a structure or organ.

hypospadias. A congenital abnormality in which the urethra opens on the undersurface of the penis.

jaundice. Yellow coloration of the skin due to de-

posits of bile pigment; a result of elevated bilirubin (yellow pigment) blood levels.

lanugo. Fine downy hair found on the body of the newborn.

metatarsus adductus. A deformity of the anterior foot in which supination and adduction are found.

milia. Tiny white nodules in the skin of the newborn caused by retained secretions of the sebaceous glands.

mongolian spot. Deposition of pigment causing a bluish area on the buttocks and/or lower back of infants. Usually associated with infants other than Caucasians.

Ortalani maneuver. A test utilized to detect congenital dislocation of the hip.

petechiae. Tiny pinpoint hemorrhagic spots found on the skin.

polydactyly. The presence of additional fingers or toes.

retraction. A state of drawing back. For example, with intercostal retractions (associated with respiratory distress), the tissue between the ribs is pulled inwards on inspiration.

sutures. The uniting lines between the bones of the skull.

syndactyly. The congenital fusion of two (or more) fingers or toes.

tachypnea. Abnormally rapid respirations.

talipes equinovalgus; talipes equinovarus. Forms of the congenital deformity clubfoot, in which there is deviation in the shape, position, and line of movement of the foot.

telangiectasis. A red spot on the skin caused by dilation of tiny blood vessels.

torsion. In a state of being twisted.

torticollis. Drawing of the head to one side with the chin pointing to the opposite side. Caused by contraction of the neck muscles.

vernix caseosa. Somewhat greasy, white coating on the skin of the newborn. Consists of sebaceous gland secretions and cells from the outer layer of skin.

virilization. Development of male sexual characteristics in the female.

Most health problems in children can be identified by effective interviewing and examination of the child and the parents. Data collection of this nature is an integral component of the nursing process when caring for clients during any phase of their life cycle. Historically, techniques of data collection were utilized by child health nurses, school nurses, community health nurses, and occupational health nurses who functioned in ambulatory care settings that required a total assessment of the client to maximize the nursing and medical care. Today, nurses have access to diagnostic tools that have been perfected by advanced technology, thereby increasing their competency in assessing the health status of children. The tools provide an extension of the nurse's eyes and ears. The interviewing and history taking process are also more comprehensive in scope and more systematically recorded. As a consequence of these advancements in technology and practice, nurses are now planning and managing care using a more accurate data base.

To examine and elicit a health history from a child and family, a prerequisite knowledge base should include a sound understanding of anatomy and physiology, the behavioral sciences, the techniques of communication, growth and develop-

ment, and the nursing process. This understanding is critical to the data collection process because it increases the potential for accurate identification of client problems and allows for a more accurate nursing diagnosis. An accurate nursing diagnosis is essential for the development of an effective nursing plan of care for the child. A nursing diagnosis differs from a medical diagnosis in that the focus is on health maintenance, education, hygiene, comfort, and safety, whereas a medical diagnosis is "the determination of what kind of a disease a patient is suffering from especially the art of distinguishing between several possibilities."[1] When the nurse's findings indicate that a medical problem may be present, referral to a physician is necessary.

A substantive part of the nursing care plan devised for children and their families should be directed toward communication, health education, and health supervision. The impact of age-appropriate health education for children will significantly enhance the parents' ability to meaningfully manage their physical and emotional health. Early preventive health education and counseling will have a lifelong effect on the child. The use of data collection techniques, such as history taking and the physical examination, as a vehicle for teaching parents and children has been effectively demonstrated by primary health care nurses. Inclusion of parents and children in health care transactions affords them their right of involvement in achieving their potential for a healthy family.

Nursing assessment of children has four primary goals:

1. Collection of a complete data base through interviewing, history taking, and physical examination.
2. Determination of a nursing diagnosis for a purposive independent nursing intervention.
3. Development of a plan of nursing care including the key components of child health care, such as concepts of child growth and development, health education, health prevention, comfort, safety, and mental hygiene.
4. Differentiation of deviations from normal and referral to the appropriate health care provider.

Assessment of the health status has long been one of the primary functions of nurses, particularly in child health and community health settings. Detailed information on the total concept of physical examination (Chapter 21) and history taking (Chapter 20) can be found elsewhere in this textbook. The purpose of this chapter is to highlight the differences that exist between the child and the adult of which nurses should be aware. The most significant difference can be found in the body systems, developmental age, and communication level. This will not be an extensive review nor will it include physical diagnosis. Those providing health care to infants and children are encouraged to seek other relevant resources and references.

CHILD'S HEALTH HISTORY

The goals of a health history of a child are similar to that of an adult, that is, to obtain information that, when combined with laboratory findings and physical examination, will permit a thorough health evaluation. In the case of the child, additional data are required from an informant (parent or child caretaker) to substantiate subjective and objective findings. Also, the nurse must be cognizant of parent-child interactions, verbal and nonverbal behavior, sibling and peer relationships, as well as the developmental level of the child, parent, and family unit. In addition, it is important to understand that the parents may not have total recall of all incidents and dates relevant to their child's health. Eliciting these kinds of data requires an accepting interviewing climate that is nonthreatening and nondirective. Open ended questions such as, "Tell me about Jimmy when he was a baby," can encourage healthy communication.

It is important, also, to include the child in the interviewing process; children from as early an age as 2 are capable of giving descriptive information. Involvement of the child assists in the establishment of a therapeutic relationship with the family unit. With the school age child, it is sometimes effective to interview the child alone initially and then with his parents. Whatever the circumstances, however, the individuality of the child and the family being served should be respected.

Data specific to child health that must be collected include prenatal and postnatal status, developmental milestones, nutrition and growth patterns, weight changes, learning and thought competencies, language development, social be-

havior, parental-sibling-peer relationships, and self-esteem. Progress in school, environmental conditions (e.g., housing and exposure to pollutants), and family life style are also important. Interviewing and history taking in the area of child health is a challenging task that requires considerable understanding and practice.

Developmental Assessment

An essential frame of reference for nurses performing a developmental assessment is the concept of the family. It is important to recognize that families, as well as the individuals that comprise them, are born, develop, mature, and age. At each sequential stage, there are new developmental tasks to achieve. The assessment of a child is best accomplished within the context of the family. Although developmental behaviors are highly individualistic, they often fall within a predictable frame of reference.

Developmental data specific to the individual child are required for a sound data base. Knowledge of a child's developmental status provides the clues for early detection of delays or advances in development. This in turn permits counseling of parents on methods of stimulating children to enhance their developmental potential, allowing for appropriate guidance on the acceptance of their strengths and weaknesses, thereby fostering healthy parent-child relationships. Data must be collected on key developmental components integral to child health (Table 22-1). These include prenatal and postnatal status, growth patterns, weight changes, gross and fine motor adaptation, language, and personal-social developmental milestones. In the older child, attention should be given to learning and thought competencies, parental and sibling relationships, progress in school (age-appropriate), peer relationships, and social development.

Appraisal of developmental levels can also be accomplished by utilizing widely available standardized screening tests. One of the best known is the Denver Developmental Screening Test (Fig. 22-1) which screens for developmental status of children from 1 month to 6 years of age. It is fairly simple to administer once the nurse is familiar with the theory and the techniques of administration. Other developmental tests found to be effective in developmental assessment are the Weschler Intelligence

TABLE 22-1. Child Development from 1 Month to 5 Years

1 Month

Motor
1. Moro reflex present.
2. Vigorous sucking reflex present.
3. Lying prone (face down): lifts head briefly so chin is off table.
4. Lying prone: makes crawling movements with legs.
5. Held in sitting position: back is rounded, head held up momentarily only.
6. Hands tightly fisted.
7. Reflex grasp of object with palm.

Language
8. Startled by sound; quieted by voice.
9. Small throaty noises or vocalizations.

Personal-social-adaptive
10. Ringing bell produces decrease of activity.
11. May follow dangling object with eyes to midline.
12. Lying on back: will briefly look at examiner or change his activity.
13. Reacts with generalized body movements when tissue paper is placed on face.

2 Months

Motor
1. Kicks vigorously.
2. Energetic arm movements.
3. Vigorous head turning.
4. Held in ventral suspension (prone): no head droop.
5. Lying prone: lifts head so face makes an approximate 45° angle with table.
6. Held in sitting position: head erect but bobs.
7. Hand goes to mouth.
8. Hands often open (not clenched).

Language
9. Is cooing.
10. Vocalizes single vowel sounds, such as: ah-eh-uh.

Personal-social-adaptive
11. Head and eyes search for sound.
12. Listens to bell ringing.
13. Follows dangling object past midline.
14. Alert expression.
15. Follows moving person with eyes.
16. Smiles back when talked to.

3 Months

Motor
1. Lying prone: lifts head to 90° angle.
2. Lifts head when lying on back (supine).
3. Moro reflex begins to disappear.
4. Grasp reflex nearly gone.
5. Rolls side to back (3-4 months).

Language
6. Chuckling, squealing, grunting, especially when talked to.
7. Listens to music.
8. Vocalizes with two different syllables, such as: a-a, la-la (not distinct), oo-oo.

Personal-social-adaptive
9. Reaches for but misses objects.
10. Holds toy with active grasp when put into hand.
11. Sucks and inspects fingers.
12. Pulls at clothes.
13. Follows object (toy) side to side (180°).
14. Looks predominately at examiner.
15. Glances at toy when put into hand.
16. Recognizes mother and bottle.
17. Smiles spontaneously.

4 Months

Motor
1. Sits when well supported.
2. No head lag when pulled to sitting position.
3. Turns head at sound of voice.
4. Lifts head (in supine position) in effort to sit.
5. Lifts head and chest when prone, using hands and forearms.
6. Held erect: pushes feet against table.

Language
7. Laughs aloud (4-5 months).
8. Uses sounds, such as: m-p-b.
9. Repeats series of same sounds.

Personal-social-adaptive
10. Grasps rattle.
11. Plays with own fingers.
12. Reaches for object in front of him with both hands.
13. Transfers object from hand to hand.
14. Pulls dress over face.
15. Smiles spontaneously at people.
16. Regards raisin (or pellet).

5 Months

Motor
1. Moro reflex gone.
2. Rolls side to side.
3. Rolls back to front.
4. Full head control when pulled to or held in sitting position.
5. Briefly supports most of his weight on his legs.
6. Scratches on table top.

Language
7. Squeals with high voice.
8. Recognizes familiar voices.
9. Coos and/or stops crying on hearing music.

Personal-social-adaptive
10. Grasps dangling object.
11. Reaches for toy with both hands.
12. Smiles at mirror image.
13. Turns head deliberately to bell.
14. Obviously enjoys being played with.

Table 22-1. Continued

6 Months

Motor
1. Supine: lifts head spontaneously.
2. Bounces on feet when held standing.
3. Sits briefly (tri-pod fashion).
4. Rolls front to back (6-7 months).
5. Grasps foot and plays with toes.
6. Grasps cube with palm.

Language
7. Vocalizes at mirror image.
8. Makes four or more different sounds.
9. Localizes source of sound (bell, voice).
10. Vague, formless babble (especially with family members).

Personal-social-adaptive
11. Holds one cube in each hand.
12. Puts cube into mouth.
13. Re-secures dropped cube.
14. Transfers cube from hand to hand.
15. Conscious of strange sights and persons.
16. Consistent regard of object or person (6-7 months).
17. Uses raking movement to secure raisin or pellet.
18. Resists having toy taken away from him.
19. Stretches out arms to be taken up (6-8 months)

8 Months

Motor
1. Sits alone (6-8 months).
2. Early stepping movements.
3. Tries to crawl.
4. Stands few seconds, holding on to object.
5. Leans forward to get an object.

Language
6. Two-syllable babble, such as: a-la, ba-ba, oo-goo, a-ma, mama, dada (8-10 months).
7. Listens to conversation (8-10 months).
8. "Shouts" for attention (8-10 months).

Personal-social-adaptive
9. Works to get toy out of reach.
10. Scoops pellet.
11. Rings bell purposely (8-10 months).
12. Drinks from cup.
13. Plays peek-a-boo.
14. Looks for dropped object.
15. Bites and chews toys.
16. Pats mirror image.
17. Bangs spoon on table.
18. Manipulates paper or string.
19. Secures ring by pulling on the string.
20. Feeds self crackers.

10 Months

Motor
1. Gets self into sitting position.
2. Sits steadily (long time).
3. Pulls self to standing position (on bed railing).
4. Crawls on hands and knees.
5. Walks when held or around furniture.
6. Turns around when left on floor.

Language
7. Imitates speech sounds.
8. Shakes head for "no."
9. Waves "bye-bye."
10. Responds to name.
11. Vocalizes in varied jargon-patterns (10-12 months).

Personal-social-adaptive
12. Plays "pat-a-cake."
13. Picks up pellet with finger and thumb.
14. Bangs toys together.
15. Extends toy to a person.
16. Holds own bottle.
17. Removes cube from cup.
18. Drops one cube to get another.
19. Uses handle to lift cup.
20. Initially shy with strangers.

1 Year

Motor
1. Walks with one hand held.
2. Stands alone (or with support).
3. Secures small object with good pincer grasp.
4. Pivots in sitting position.
5. Grasps two cubes in one hand.

Language
6. Uses "mama" or "dada" with specific meaning.
7. "Talks" to toys and people, using fairly long verbal patterns.
8. Has vocabulary of two words besides "mama" and "dada."
9. Babbles to self when alone.
10. Obeys simple requests, such as: "Give me the cup."
11. Reacts to music.

Personal-social-adaptive
12. Cooperates with dressing.
13. Plays with cup, spoon, saucer.
14. Points with index finger.
15. Pokes finger (into stethoscope) to explore.
16. Releases toy into your hand.
17. Tries to take cube out of box.
18. Unwraps a cube.
19. Holds cup to drink.
20. Holds crayon.
21. Tries to imitate scribble.
22. Imitates beating two cubes together.
23. Gives affection.

Table 22-1 Continued

15 Months

Motor
1. Stands alone.
2. Creeps upstairs.
3. Kneels on floor or chair.
4. Gets off floor and walks alone with good balance.
5. Bends over to pick up toy without holding on to furniture.

Language
6. May speak four to six words (15-18 months).
7. Uses jargon.
8. Indicates wants by vocalizing.
9. Knows own name.
10. Enjoys rhymes or jingles.

Personal-social-adaptive
11. Tilts cup to drink.
12. Uses spoon but spills.
13. Builds tower of two cubes.
14. Drops cubes into cup.
15. Helps turn page in book, pats picture.
16. Shows or offers toy.
17. Helps pull off clothes.
18. Puts pellet into bottle without demonstration.
19. Opens lid of box.
20. Likes to push wheeled toys.

18 Months

Motor
1. Runs (stiffly).
2. Walks upstairs—one hand held.
3. Walks backwards.
4. Climbs into chair.
5. Hurls ball.

Language
6. May say six to 10 words (18-21 months).
7. Points to at least one body part.
8. Can say "hello" and "thank you."
9. Carries out two directions (one at a time), for instance: "Get ball from table." "Give ball to mother."
10. Identifies two objects by pointing (or picking up) such as: cup, spoon, dog, car, chair.

Personal-social-adaptive
11. Turns pages.
12. Builds tower of three to four cubes.
13. Puts 10 cubes into cup.
14. Carries or hugs a doll.
15. Takes off shoes and socks.
16. Pulls string toy.
17. Scribbles spontaneously.
18. Dumps raisin from bottle after demonstration.
19. Uses spoon with little spilling.

21 Months

Motor
1. Runs well.
2. Walks downstairs—one hand held.
3. Walks upstairs alone or holding on to rail.
4. Kicks large ball (when demonstrated).

Language
5. May speak 15-20 words (21-24 months).
6. May combine two to three words.
7. Asks for food, drink.
8. Echoes two or more words.
9. Takes three directions (one at a time), for instance: "Take ball from table." "Give ball to Mommy." "Put ball on floor."
10. Points to three or more body parts.

Personal-social-adaptive
11. Builds tower of five to six cubes.
12. Folds paper once when shown.
13. Helps with simple household tasks (21-24 months).
14. Removes some clothing purposefully (besides hat or socks).
15. Pulls person to show something.

2 Years

Motor
1. Runs without falling.
2. Walks up and down stairs.
3. Kicks large ball (without demonstration).
4. Throws ball overhand.
5. Claps hands.
6. Opens door.
7. Turns pages in book, singly.

Language
8. Says simple phrases.
9. Says at least one sentence or phrase of four or more syllables.
10. Can repeat four to five syllables.
11. May reproduce about 5-6 consonant sounds. (Typically: m-p-b-h-w).
12. Points to four parts of body on command.
13. Asks for things at table by name.
14. Refers to self by name.
15. May use personal pronouns: I-me-you (2-2½ years).

Personal-social-adaptive
16. Builds five to seven cube tower.
17. May cut with scissors.
18. Spontaneously dumps raisin from bottle (without demonstration).
19. Throws ball into box.
20. Imitates drawing vertical line from demonstration.
21. Parallel play predominant.

2½ Years

Motor
1. Jumps in place with both feet.
2. Tries standing on one foot (may not be successful).

Personal-social-adaptive
9. Builds tower of eight cubes.
10. Pushes toy with good steering.

Table 22-1. Continued

3. Holds crayon by fingers.
4. Imitates walking on tiptoe.

Language
5. Refers to self by pronoun (rather than name).
6. Names common objects when asked (key, penny, shoe, box, book).
7. Repeats two digits (one of three trials).
8. Answers simple questions, such as: "What is this?" "What does the kitty say?"

11. Helps put things away.
12. Can carry breakable objects.
13. Puts on clothing.
14. Washes and dries hands.
15. Eats with fork.
16. Imitates drawing a horizontal line from demonstration.
17. May imitate drawing a circle from demonstration.

3 Years

Motor
1. Stands on one foot for at least one second.
2. Jumps from bottom stair.
3. Alternates feet going upstairs.
4. Pours from a pitcher.
5. Can undo two buttons.
6. Pedals a tricycle.

Language
7. Repeats six syllables, for instance: "I have a little dog."
8. Names three or more objects in a picture.
9. Gives sex. ("Are you a boy or a girl?")
10. Gives full name.
11. Repeats three digits (one of three trials).
12. Knows a few rhymes.
13. Gives appropriate answers to: "What: swims-flies-shoots-boils-bites-melts?"

14. Uses plurals.
15. Knows at least one color.
16. Can reply to questions in at least three word sentences.
17. May have vocabulary of 750 to 1,000 words (3-3½ years).

Personal-social-adaptive
18. Understands taking turns.
19. Copies a circle (from model, without demonstration).
20. Builds three-block pyramid (⌂).
21. Dresses with supervision.
22. Puts 10 pellets into bottle in 30 seconds.
23. Separates easily from mother.
24. Feeds self well.
25. Plays interactive games, such as "tag."

4 Years

Motor
1. Stands on one foot for at least five seconds (two of three trials).
2. Hops at least twice on one foot.
3. Can walk heel-to-toe for four or more steps (with heel one inch or less in front of toe).
4. Can button coat or dress; may lace shoes.

Language
5. Repeats ten-word sentences without errors.
6. Counts three objects, pointing correctly.
7. Repeats three to four digits (4-5 years).
8. Comprehends: "What do you do if: you are hungry, sleepy, cold?"
9. Spontaneous sentences, four to five words long.
10. Likes to ask questions.
11. Understands prepositions, such as: on-under-behind, etc. ("Put the block on the table.")

12. Can point to three out of four colors (red, blue, green, yellow).
13. Speech is now an effective communicative tool.

Personal-social-adaptive
14. Copies cross (+) without demonstration.
15. Imitates oblique cross (×).
16. Draws a man with four parts.
17. Cooperates with other children in play.
18. Dresses and undresses self (mostly without supervision).
19. Brushes teeth, washes face.
20. Compares lines: "Which is longer?"
21. Folds paper two to three times.
22. Can select heavier from lighter object.
23. Cares for self at toilet.

5 Years

Motor
1. Balances on one foot for eight to ten seconds.
2. Skips, using feet alternately.
3. May be able to tie a knot.
4. Catches bounced ball with hands (not arms) in two of three trials.

Language
5. Knows age ("How old are you?").
6. Performs three tasks (with one command), for instance: "Put pen on table—close door—bring me the ball."
7. Knows four colors.
8. Defines use for: fork-horse-key-pencil, etc.
9. Identifies by name: nickel-dime-penny.
10. Asks meaning of words.
11. Asks many "why" questions.

12. Relatively few speech errors remain—90% of consonant sounds are made correctly.
13. Counts number of fingers correctly.
14. Counts by rote to 10.
15. Comments on pictures (descriptions and interpretations).

Personal-social-adaptive
16. Copies a square.
17. Copies oblique cross (×) without demonstration.
18. May print a few letters (5-5½ years).
19. Draws man with at least six identifiable parts.
20. Builds a six-block pyramid from demonstration.
21. Transports things in a wagon.
22. Plays with coloring set, construction toys, puzzles.
23. Participates well in group play.

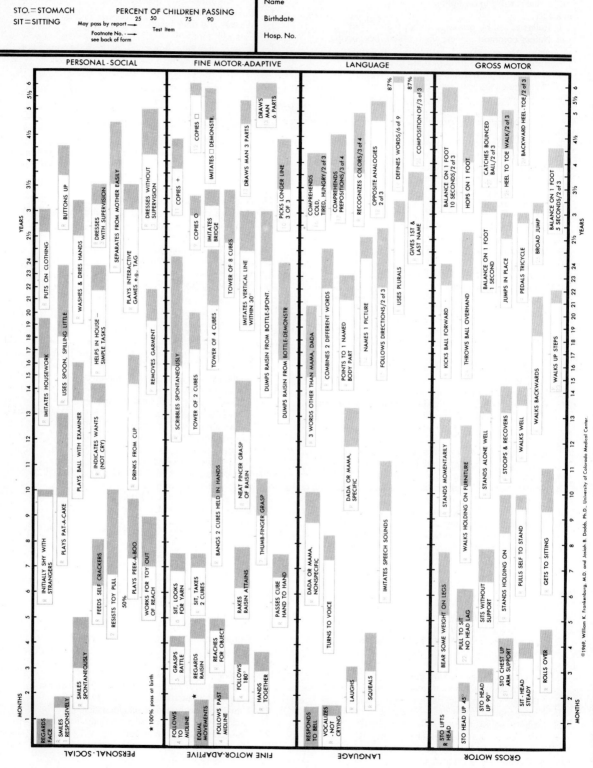

FIGURE 22-1. Denver Developmental Screening Test, Part 1. (Reprinted with permission from William K. Frankenburg, M.D., University of Colorado Medical Center, Denver, Colorado.)

1. Try to get child to smile by smiling, talking or waving to him. Do not touch him.
2. When child is playing with toy, pull it away from him. Pass if he resists.
3. Child does not have to be able to tie shoes or button in the back.
4. Move yarn slowly in an arc from one side to the other, about 6" above child's face. Pass if eyes follow 90° to midline. (Past midline; 180°)
5. Pass if child grasps rattle when it is touched to the backs or tips of fingers.
6. Pass if child continues to look where yarn disappeared or tries to see where it went. Yarn should be dropped quickly from sight from tester's hand without arm movement.
7. Pass if child picks up raisin with any part of thumb and a finger.
8. Pass if child picks up raisin with the ends of thumb and index finger using an over hand approach.

 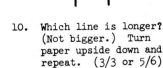 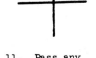 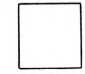

9. Pass any enclosed form. Fail continuous round motions.
10. Which line is longer? (Not bigger.) Turn paper upside down and repeat. (3/3 or 5/6)
11. Pass any crossing lines.
12. Have child copy first. If failed, demonstrate

When giving items 9, 11 and 12, do not name the forms. Do not demonstrate 9 and 11.

13. When scoring, each pair (2 arms, 2 legs, etc.) counts as one part.
14. Point to picture and have child name it. (No credit is given for sounds only.)

 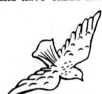 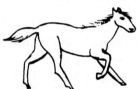 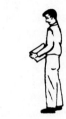

15. Tell child to: Give block to Mommie; put block on table; put block on floor. Pass 2 of 3. (Do not help child by pointing, moving head or eyes.)
16. Ask child: What do you do when you are cold? ..hungry? ..tired? Pass 2 of 3.
17. Tell child to: Put block on table; under table; in front of chair, behind chair. Pass 3 of 4. (Do not help child by pointing, moving head or eyes.)
18. Ask child: If fire is hot, ice is ?; Mother is a woman, Dad is a ?; a horse is big, a mouse is ?. Pass 2 of 3.
19. Ask child: What is a ball? ..lake? ..desk? ..house? ..banana? ..curtain? ..ceiling? ..hedge? ..pavement? Pass if defined in terms of use, shape, what it is made of or general category (such as banana is fruit, not just yellow). Pass 6 of 9.
20. Ask child: What is a spoon made of? ..a shoe made of? ..a door made of? (No other objects may be substituted.) Pass 3 of 3.
21. When placed on stomach, child lifts chest off table with support of forearms and/or hands.
22. When child is on back, grasp his hands and pull him to sitting. Pass if head does not hang back.
23. Child may use wall or rail only, not person. May not crawl.
24. Child must throw ball overhand 3 feet to within arm's reach of tester.
25. Child must perform standing broad jump over width of test sheet. (8-1/2 inches)
26. Tell child to walk forward, ⬠⬠⬠⬠→ heel within 1 inch of toe. Tester may demonstrate. Child must walk 4 consecutive steps, 2 out of 3 trials.
27. Bounce ball to child who should stand 3 feet away from tester. Child must catch ball with hands, not arms, 2 out of 3 trials.
28. Tell child to walk backward, ←⬠⬠⬠⬠ toe within 1 inch of heel. Tester may demonstrate. Child must walk 4 consecutive steps, 2 out of 3 trials.

DATE AND BEHAVIORAL OBSERVATIONS (how child feels at time of test, relation to tester, attention span, verbal behavior, self-confidence, etc,):

FIGURE 22.1 Denver Developmental Screening Test, Part 2.

369

Scale for Children (WISC), the Stanford Binet Intelligence Scale, the Peabody Picture Vocabulary Test (measures verbal intelligence), the Developmental Test of Visual-Motor Integration (the Beery Test, the Goodenough Draw-a-Man Test, and The Preschool Readiness Experimental Screening Scale). When administering developmental tests, the nurse must keep in mind that innumerable variables influence the results of the test. The child may be tired, irritable, uncomfortable in a strange environment, anxious, or not feeling well. Significant deviations from the norm should be retested and referred for further evaluation.

Newborn Assessment

Newborn assessment is a multifaceted, multistaged process. Physical and developmental evaluation of the newborn requires an understanding of the normative variations of the newborn. The total assessment encompasses evaluation of the interactional behaviors of the parents and infant as well as the family unit. The initial assessment of the newborn takes place in the delivery room. At birth, the universally accepted assessment tool, the Apgar scale, monitors the status of the newborn (Table 22-2). At 1 and 5 minutes postdelivery, the heart rate, respiratory effort, muscle tone, reflex irritability, and color of the infant are scored on a scale ranging from 0 to 2 in each category. A total score of 10, 2 in each category, reflects an infant in excellent physical condition. An infant scoring below 5 requires immediate medical intervention.

The normal newborn is a unique individual from the moment of birth. The assessment of the infant's state of health is not only essential for planning nursing, and medical interventions, but it will serve as a data base when assessing the health-illness status of the child in the future. Therefore, the as-

sessment should be comprehensive and recorded systematically, concisely, and accurately.

Physical and developmental evaluation of the newborn requires an understanding of the normative characteristics of the age as well as the numerous normal newborn variations. Differentiation of the extremes of normal from abnormal becomes fairly simple as the nurse gains greater expertise in clinical practice.

Assessment commences with observations on the general appearance of the newborn, followed by measurements of height, weight, chest, and head circumference. These measurements provide an index that is of critical importance in monitoring the child's health status during the first 2 years of extremely rapid growth. The average newborn is approximately 20 inches (50 cm) in height. Weight is more variable, but the average newborn weighs approximately 7½ pounds (3.4 kg). Head circumference, an important clinical measurement, averages between 33 to 35 cm (13–14 inches) from the occipital to the frontal bone. Head circumference should be taken with a tape measure (usually paper), which is placed in the middle of the forehead and encircled around the greatest circumference, the occipital protuberance. Chest circumference, which ranges from 30 to 33 cm (12–13 inches), is often the same as the head circumference. These indices of health status and physical growth must be evaluated and recorded longitudinally in early childhood. Ideally the measurements should be depicted graphically (Figs. 22-2, 22-3, 22-4, and 22-5). In addition to the parameters of height, weight, and chest and head circumferences, the following data should be obtained.

GENERAL APPEARANCE AND BEHAVIOR. Note color, nutritional state, muscle tone, reflexes (measures of neurologic status), and inter-

TABLE 22-2. Apgar Scoring Chart

Sign	0	1	2
Heart rate	Absent	Slow (below 100)	Over 100
Respiratory effort	Absent	Slow, irregular, weak cry, hypoventilation	Good strong cry
Muscle tone	Flaccid, limp	Some flexion of extremities	Well flexed, active motion
Reflex irritability	No response	Some motion, grimace	Cry, cough, or sneeze
Color	Blue/pale	Body pink, extremities blue or pale	Completely pink

action of mother and infant. The Brazelton assessment tool rates the interactive behaviors of the newborn, identifies behavioral assets as well as neurologic functioning, and is useful for counseling parents on the behavior of their child.

SKIN. Under good light examine the infant for jaundice, acrocyanosis, edema, ecchymosis, mongolian spots, texture, milia, dimples or sinuses, lanugo, erythema toxicum, petechiae, and telangiectasis.

HEAD. Examine cranial vault for overriding sutures, symmetry, anterior and posterior fontanelles (soft spots), edema of scalp (caput succedaneum), and cephalhematoma.

EYES. Note ability to follow and fix gaze on a bright moving object, red reflex, lens opacity (congenital cataracts), excessive tearing (lacrimal duct obstruction), conjunctivitis, and subconjunctival hemorrhages (commonly result from delivery).

EARS. Note whether the ears are normal in configuration, low set (suspect renal or chromosomal anomalies), or have preauricular sinuses or tabs, anomalies and infections of the canals and drums. (This is not always feasible in the newborn because of the presence of vernix caseosa in the canal.)

NOSE. Observe for patency of nasal passages, milia.

MOUTH. Note color of the mucous membrane, tooth buds, erupted teeth, and size of tongue; visualize and palpate hard and soft palate for defects; check for adequacy of frenulum linguae, and the presence of epithelial pearls (Epstein's). Assessment should also include the characteristics of the infant's cry for pitch, intensity, quality, and effort.

NECK. Inspect for webbing, torticollis, position of trachea, and masses.

THORAX. Note symmetry, presence of supernumerary nipples, possible fractured clavicle, complete Moro reflex (see Reflexes), and hypertrophy of the breasts. *Respiratory assessment* should include rate, (30–60 per minute increased immediately after birth and with increased activity), periods of apnea, transient tachypnea, auscultatory findings, respiratory grunt, and retractions. Normal variations include short periods of apnea, irregularity, and shallow respirations.

HEART. The techniques of observation, inspection, palpation, and percussion are used to examine the heart. Inspect chest wall, and note pulsation and point of maximal intensity (PMI) which is normally in the midclavicular line between the fourth and fifth intercostal space. Record murmurs and deviations from normal of the first and second sound. (Significant murmurs persist after the first 6 months of life.) Note heart rate variations—below 100 and above 180 are abnormal at birth. After 30 minutes the heart rate will usually range between 120 and 150. Brachial and femoral pulses, which should both be examined at the same time, will provide clues to coarctation or aortic insufficiency.

ABDOMEN. Note status of umbilicus, contour of the abdomen, possible enlarged kidneys (difficult to palpate in newborn), gross abnormalities such as absence of abdominal musculature, and distortion of the abdomen (possible diaphragmatic hernia). Auscultation for bowel sounds should precede palpation. Palpate liver and spleen when possible.

GENITALIA. Note ambiguity of genitalia, virilization, distance between introitus and anus (should be one finger tip in length on female). A white vaginal discharge which may be tinged with blood is sometimes noted. In the male, note prepuce, size and position of urethral meatus (epispadias and hypospadias) and testes. Examine for presence of inguinal hernia and hydrocele. First voiding should be recorded and urinary stream of male observed.

ANUS. Note patency, fissures, or abnormal location. Digital examination for imperforate anus or rectal atresia may be done.

EXTREMITIES. Note orthopedic deviations such as talipes equinovarus and equinovalgus, metatarsus adductus, webbed fingers and toes, polydactyly and syndactyly. With the infant in supine position note flexion and abduction (Ortalani maneuver) of the hips. Also note the length of the legs and skin folds, and observe normal variations such as tibial torsion and bowing.

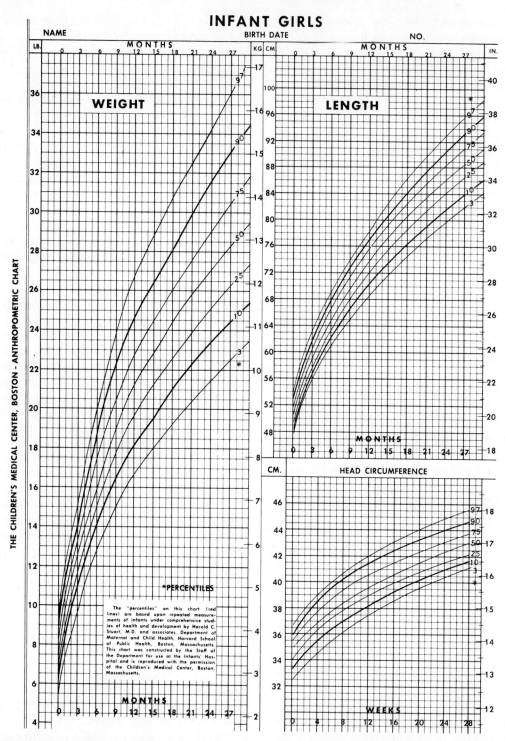

FIGURE 22-2. Percentile chart for measurements of infant girls. (Reprinted with permission from the Children's Hospital Medical Center, Boston, Mass.)

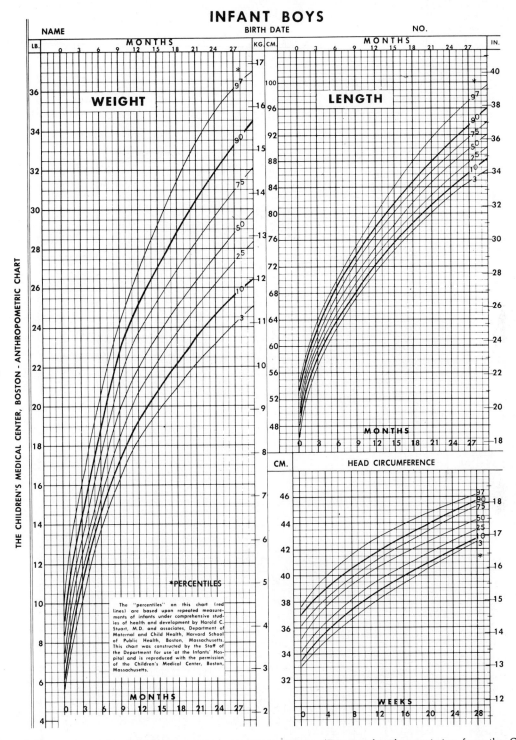

FIGURE 22-3. Percentile chart for measurements of infant boys. (Reprinted with permission from the Children's Hospital Medical Center, Boston, Mass.)

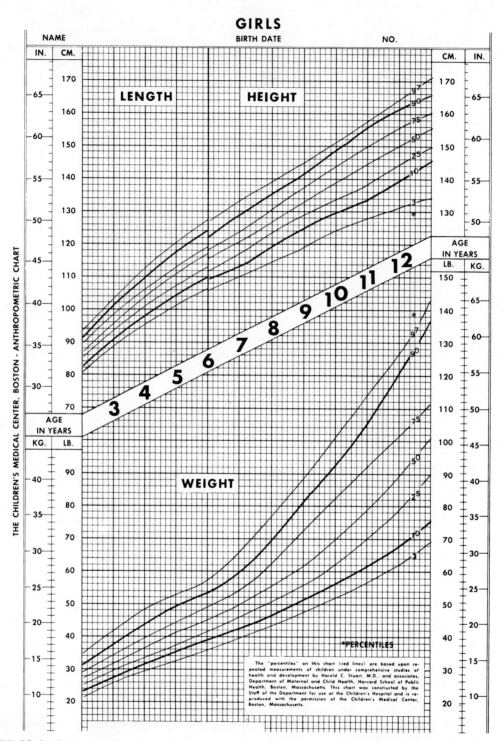

FIGURE 22-4. Percentile chart for measurement of girls. (Reprinted with permission from the Children's Hospital Medical Center, Boston, Mass.)

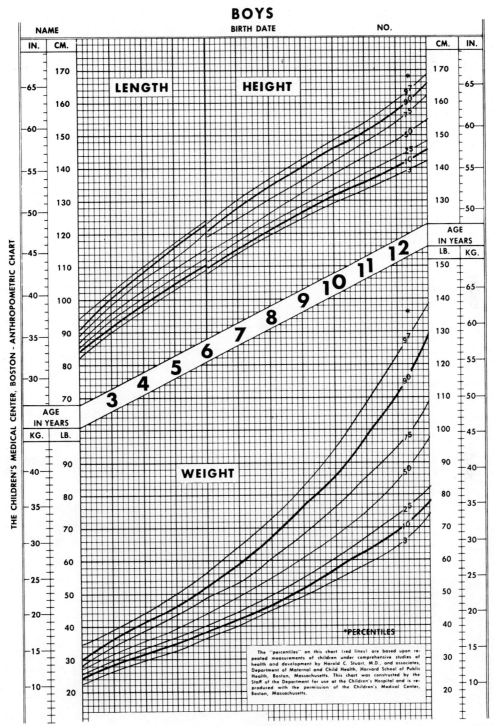

FIGURE 22-5. Percentile chart for measurements of boys. (Reprinted with permission from the Children's Hospital Medical Center, Boston, Mass.)

SENSORIMOTOR REFLEXES. Elicit and note the following reflexes:

Rooting. Touch infant's cheek; infant opens mouth and moves head toward source of stimulation (Fig. 22-6).

Sucking. This occurs in response to anything placed in the mouth, when the infant is hungry, and when there are stimuli to other parts of the body (Fig. 22-6).

Grasp. Press finger of examiner into infant's palm; infant will grasp finger (palmar). By pressing a finger against the ball of the foot, toes will flex (plantar).

Placing. Hold infant upright and allow dorsal side of foot to come in contact with edge of table. The foot will rise and place on the table (Fig. 22-7).

Moro. Sudden movement of the crib or the table will elicit abduction and extension of the arms followed adduction of the arms, as in an embrace (Fig. 22-8).

Tonic neck. Observe this reflex while the child is in a supine position and not crying. This is often referred to as the fencing position; the arm and leg are extended in the direction that the head is turned to; the opposite arm and leg are flexed at the same time.

Blink. Shine a light suddenly in the infant's eyes; infant will blink.

Babinski. The toes flex in response to the stroking of the lateral aspect of the infant's sole.

LOW BIRTH WEIGHT INFANTS

The infant weighing less than 2500 g is considered at risk for adapting to extrauterine life. Low birth weight may result from premature delivery or the infant being small-for-date, more commonly known as small for gestational age (SGA). These infants require a more specific assessment of their physiologic and neurologic status. Early identification of these infants allows for anticipatory preparation to treat a number of complications that may arise, such as hypoglycemia, changes in temperature, or frequent apneic spells.

Low birth weight infants have a high mortality rate. Consequently, assessment of their health status is essential to their survival. Determination of gestational age can be made by utilizing the standardized assessment tool developed by Lubchenco and others (Figs. 22-9A and B). This tool has been known to be a very effective instrument for recording the infant's physical and neurological status. It has been accepted as an excellent means of identifying the immature infant. Early identification permits early intervention based on priorities.

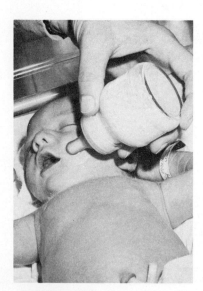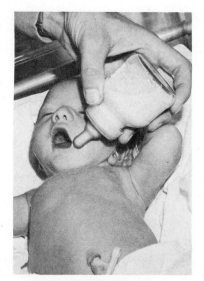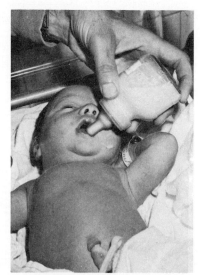

FIGURE 22-6. The rooting reflex. Left, Touch cheek. Middle, infant opens mouth and turns head toward source of stimulation. Right, sucking response is elicited. (Reprinted with permission from Clark, A. L., and Affonso, D. D.: *Childbearing: A Nursing Perspective,* 2nd ed. Philadelphia, F. A. Davis, Co., 1979, p. 593.)

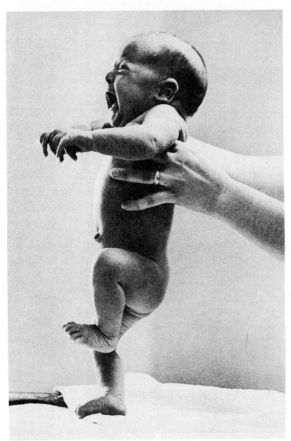

FIGURE 22-7. The stepping response (also called placing). (Reprinted with permission from Clark, A. L., and Affonso, D. D.; *Childbearing: A Nursing Perspective,* 2nd ed. Philadelphia, F. A. Davis Co., 1979, p. 595.)

INFANT

Health History

Interviewing to obtain data on the health and developmental status of infants (birth to 1 year) most logically involves the parents or the child's caretaker. It is most desirable to have both parents present during the initial interview and if possible at future interviews. The interview process itself provides the nurse with an excellent milieu for observing parental skills which require a constant changing of behaviors to accommodate the rapidly changing development of the infant. The nurse should keep in mind that one observation is not sufficient. Excellent parental skills at one developmental stage might be totally inadequate for a subsequent stage. It is essential for information of this nature to be recorded to provide a baseline for assessing the appropriateness of future parental ability. Also this knowledge facilitates the development and implementation of a health teaching plan.

Developmental milestones and behavior during infancy are essential for the adequate monitoring and counseling required for both the parent and the child. Finally, the patterns of sleep, feeding, nutrition, and play as well as immunizations should be noted in the health record.

Physical Examination

Parents are always eager to learn about their infants. Encouraging participation during the physical examination is an excellent way of educating parents. Knowing what the nurse is examining and looking for is also reassuring. Normal variations are more readily understood and accepted with this approach. It also increases the parents' ability to assess their own child's health and judge the quality of health care they are receiving. Infants are usually examined on the examining table with parents in close attendance. All of the child's clothing should be removed to allow for complete inspection. The order in which the examination is conducted is dependent on the behavior of the infant and the preference of the examiner. The key factor that must not be violated is that of consistency. Consistency in format assures that the examiner will not overlook a step in the process. Also needed when dealing with children is a repertoire of interpersonal skills which will foster the interest and cooperation of the infant and parent.

Development

During the first year of life the infant experiences a rapid increase in physical growth which should be plotted on anthropometric charts and standardized growth charts at each health visit (Figs. 22-2, 22-3, 22-4, and 22-5). Accurately plotted growth charts depict graphically the range and normalcy of the infant's physical status. Longitudinally plotted charts are more effective than putting a note on the record because the full scope and pattern of the child's progress can be seen at a glance. Developmentally the motor control of the infant proceeds in a cephalocaudal direction, from proximal to distal and from gross motor to fine motor. The sequence of these developmental processes is orderly

A

PHYSICAL FINDINGS — WEEKS GESTATION (20–48)

Physical Findings	Findings by gestational weeks (20–48)
VERNIX	APPEARS (~20–21) · COVERS BODY, THICK LAYER · ON BACK, SCALP, IN CREASES (~38) · SCANT, IN CREASES (~41) · NO VERNIX (~44–48)
BREAST TISSUE AND AREOLA	AREOLA & NIPPLE BARELY VISIBLE, NO PALPABLE BREAST TISSUE · AREOLA RAISED (~35) · 1-2 MM NODULE (~36–37) · 3-5 MM (~38–39) · 5-6 MM (~39) · 7-10 MM (~41–42) · ?12 MM (~45–48)
EAR — FORM	FLAT, SHAPELESS · BEGINNING INCURVING SUPERIOR (~34) · INCURVING UPPER 2/3 PINNAE (~36) · WELL-DEFINED INCURVING TO LOBE (~42–48)
EAR — CARTILAGE	PINNA SOFT, STAYS FOLDED · CARTILAGE SCANT RETURNS SLOWLY FROM FOLDING (~33–35) · THIN CARTILAGE SPRINGS BACK FROM FOLDING (~36–37) · PINNA FIRM, REMAINS ERECT FROM HEAD (~42–48)
SOLE CREASES	SMOOTH SOLES ? CREASES · 1-2 ANTERIOR CREASES (~32) · 2-3 ANTERIOR CREASES (~34–35) · CREASES ANTERIOR 2/3 SOLE (~36–37) · CREASES INVOLVING HEEL (~38–40) · DEEPER CREASES OVER ENTIRE SOLE (~42–48)
SKIN — THICKNESS & APPEARANCE	THIN, TRANSLUCENT SKIN, PLETHORIC, VENULES OVER ABDOMEN, EDEMA · SMOOTH THICKER NO EDEMA (~33–34) · PINK (~36–38) · FEW VESSELS (~39) · SOME DESQUAMATION PALE PINK (~40) · THICK, PALE, DESQUAMATION OVER ENTIRE BODY (~42–48)
SKIN — NAIL PLATES	AP-PEAR (~21) · NAILS TO FINGER TIPS (~32–34) · NAILS EXTEND WELL BEYOND FINGER TIPS (~42–48)
HAIR	APPEARS ON HEAD (~21–23) · EYE BROWS & LASHES (~25–26) · FINE, WOOLLY, BUNCHES OUT FROM HEAD (~29–33) · SILKY, SINGLE STRANDS LAYS FLAT (~37–38) · ?RECEDING HAIRLINE OR LOSS OF BABY HAIR, SHORT, FINE UNDERNEATH (~45–48)
LANUGO	AP-PEARS (~21) · COVERS ENTIRE BODY (~24–28) · VANISHES FROM FACE (~34–36) · PRESENT ON SHOULDERS (~38–40) · NO LANUGO (~45)
GENITALIA — TESTES	TESTES PALPABLE IN INGUINAL CANAL (~30–33) · IN UPPER SCROTUM (~37–38) · IN LOWER SCROTUM (~43–44)
GENITALIA — SCROTUM	FEW RUGAE (~31–34) · RUGAE ANTERIOR PORTION (~36–37) · RUGAE COVER (~40–41) · PENDULOUS (~45)
GENITALIA — LABIA & CLITORIS	PROMINENT CLITORIS, LABIA MAJORA SMALL, WIDELY SEPARATED (~30–34) · LABIA MAJORA LARGER NEARLY COVERED CLITORIS (~36–38) · LABIA MINORA & CLITORIS COVERED (~43–44)
SKULL FIRMNESS	BONES ARE SOFT (~23–25) · SOFT TO 1" FROM ANTERIOR FONTANELLE (~30–32) · SPONGY AT EDGES OF FONTANELLE, CENTER FIRM (~35–37) · BONES HARD, SUTURES EASILY DISPLACED (~39–40) · BONES HARD, CANNOT BE DISPLACED (~44–48)
POSTURE — RESTING	HYPOTONIC, LATERAL DECUBITUS (~22–24) · HYPOTONIC (~27–28) · BEGINNING FLEXION THIGH (~30–31) · STRONGER HIP FLEXION (~32–33) · FROG-LIKE (~34) · FLEXION ALL LIMBS (~36–37) · HYPERTONIC (~39) · VERY HYPERTONIC (~44)
RECOIL — LEG	NO RECOIL (~24–26) · PARTIAL RECOIL (~34–35) · PROMPT RECOIL (~42)
ARM	NO RECOIL (~27–29) · BEGIN FLEXION NO RECOIL (~34–35) · PROMPT RECOIL MAY BE INHIBITED (~36–37) · PROMPT RECOIL AFTER 30° INHIBITION (~43–48)

Weeks gestation scale (top and bottom): 20 21 22 23 24 25 26 27 28 29 30 31 32 33 34 35 36 37 38 39 40 41 42 43 44 45 46 47 48

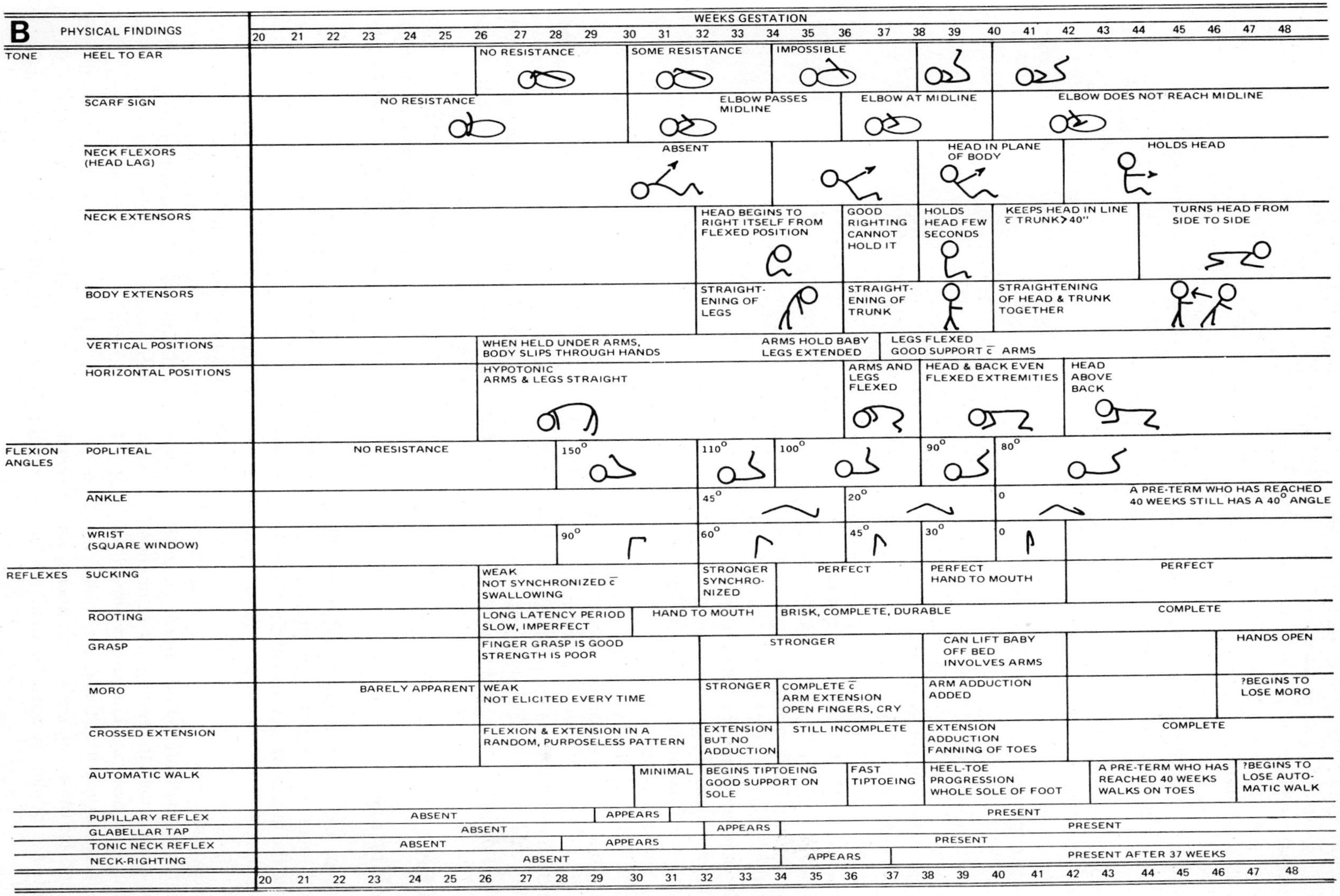

B

WEEKS GESTATION

TONE

| PHYSICAL FINDINGS | 20 | 21 | 22 | 23 | 24 | 25 | 26 | 27 | 28 | 29 | 30 | 31 | 32 | 33 | 34 | 35 | 36 | 37 | 38 | 39 | 40 | 41 | 42 | 43 | 44 | 45 | 46 | 47 | 48 |

FIGURE 22-9. Clinical estimation of gestational age—an approximation based on published data. A, Examination to be done in the first hours after birth. B, Confirmatory neurologic examination to be done after 24 hours. (Reprinted with permission from Kempe, C. H., Silver, H. K., and O'Brien, D. O. (eds.): *Current Pediatric Diagnosis and Treatment*, 5th ed. Los Altos, Calif., Lange, 1974.

379

and predictable. Predictable milestones must be recorded for baseline data. The Denver Developmental Screening Test (Fig. 22-1) is a useful overview of the key developmental milestones. Normally all developmental skills proceed on a continuum. For example, in the *gross motor* area the infant first holds up his head, then head and chest followed by rolling over, sitting with support, sitting without support, crawling, standing with support, cruising, standing alone, and finally walking. In the area of *fine motor* coordination, the infant first follows an object with his eyes, can bring hands to meet, reaches for offered objects, reaches for objects purposely, uses both hands equally, and transfers objects; hand dominance becomes evident particularly when he exhibits pincer grasp.

Language development commences with the birth cry. Almost immediately small throaty sounds are emitted followed by cooing, laughter, squealing and repetitious sounds. By the end of the first year some sounds are distinguishable. Cognitive development is highly related to the acquisition of language. Both cognitive and language development are highly dependent on the infant's interaction with the environment. Parents must be counseled on the need to initiate and sustain stimulation and interaction with significant others.

Recent studies suggest that bonding of the infant is the first stage in the personal and social development of the child. From attachment to the mother and father, the infant then proceeds to meet the outside world, smiling responsibly (social smile), followed by stranger anxiety, and separation anxiety.

TODDLER

Health History

The assertive, exploratory behavior of the toddler (ages 1 to 3) requires a special understanding and sensitivity to the uniqueness of the child in this stage of development. Assessment of the toddler is most effectively accomplished over a period of time. Widening the time frame permits the establishment of an accepting climate and allows time for the child to become familiar with the setting, the equipment, and the nurse. It also provides an increased opportunity for assessment of the parent-child relationships and for observing the growth and development of the toddler. If baseline data are not

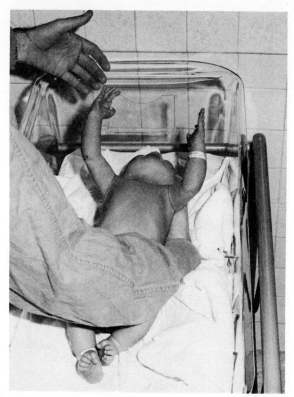

FIGURE 22-8. The Moro reflex. (Reprinted with permission from Mead Johnson Laboratories, Evansville, Indiana.)

available, a complete history should be obtained, including prenatal and neonatal data, approximate dates developmental milestones were achieved, whether immunizations are up to date, and a history of communicable diseases. The child's nutritional state and feeding patterns should be obtained. Finally, interactions of parents and the child should be closely observed to detect clues of possible child abuse or neglect.

Physical Examination

Education during the physical examination should be directed toward both the parent and the child. The child can understand simple terms and names of body parts. The examination may be conducted with the child sitting on the parent's lap or on the examining table whichever helps to diminish anxiety. Palpation of the abdomen should always be done with the child in supine position. Growth and development can also be assessed during the physical examination. This affords the nurse an excellent opportunity to counsel and teach the parents how to stimulate their child's physical, social, language, and cognitive development, as well as, the principles of accident prevention. Dates should also be recorded in regard to sleep pattern, methods of discipline, toilet training, temper tantrums, and coping behaviors exhibited when under stress.

Development

The achievement of early developmental milestones is essential for the child to reach optimal development in the exciting, expansive, exploring toddler years. The sense of trust acquired in infancy provides the security for the toddler to begin to acquire a sense of self (autonomy). This is accomplished by venturing into the environment, finding out about the world, learning to separate, achieving bladder and bowel control, and expanding communication skills. Among other accomplishments of this age, the toddler acquires increased motor skills allowing the child to attend to personal needs such as self-feeding, dressing, and mobility.

PRESCHOOLER

History Taking

The interviewer should assess the preschooler's (3 and 4-years-old) physical, motor, mental, language, play, and emotional characteristics through interviews with parents or guardians. It is important to note the needs of the child such as rest, nutrition, and immunizations. Elicit from the parents information concerning different relationships the preschooler develops with siblings, parents, and strangers. Ask the preschooler simple questions such as name and address and counting. Assess toilet habits. Nutritional status and concomitant teaching should be carried out.

Physical Examination

The preschooler grows proportionately in height and weight. The pulse rate is normally 80 to 110, with respiration rate of 30 per minute. The blood pressure is usually around 90/60. The vision in the preschooler tends to be around 20/50 or 20/40. The preschooler begins to master musculoskeletal control, such as walking backwards and heel-to-toe walking.

Development

The preschooler experiences great pleasure and eagerness for socialization. Development of a sense of initiative is the task of this age. Mastery of special skills of muscle coordination and movement are obvious. The child can walk downstairs as well as upstairs, stand on one foot, and skip. Routine is the preschooler's world. He requires routine eating habits, exercise, and rest. Communication patterns and behaviors become more mature. This is the age of why? Three and 4-year-old children tend to conform to the expectations of others. This age group gains increasing ability to handle potentially harmful situations. Cognitive development is still preoperational.

SCHOOLCHILDREN

History Taking

The interviewer should explore the family relationships of the schoolchild (5 to 12-years-old) and the influence they have on him as well as the influence of the peers on the schoolchild. It is important to also obtain a history of the family developmental tasks, such as working together to achieve common goals and providing for parental privacy and space for children's play. The history should include an assessment and comparison from earlier stages of physical changes and needs, nutrition, rest, safety and health protection. Schoolchildren can be interviewed alone and together with their parents about their self-concept, communications, and their emotional and intellectual development. It is important to note the child's adaptation to entry in school or interactions with schoolmates. It is also important to explore the schoolchild's relationship with his friends and siblings.

Physical Examination

The schoolchild exhibits considerable physical changes at a slower rate. Weight and height vary considerably among these children. By age 12, the brain has reached the size of an adult brain. The once childish face also begins to mature into that of an adult. The jaw bones grow longer and more prominent.

The temperature, pulse, and respiration approach adult norms. At the same time the blood pressure averages around 108/68, and the heart becomes larger. For instance, the apex of the heart can now be palpated at the fifth interspace, again closer to the adult norm, whereas earlier the apex could be palpated at the fourth intercostal space. Neuromuscular and musculoskeletal changes develop closer to that of the adult. For this reason the schoolchild is better coordinated and begins to become more involved in sports. The visual acuity of schoolchildren approaches 20/20; they are able to read small print, and they begin to develop skills in the written language. Because lymphoid tissues reach their height of development in the schoolchild exceeding the adult, there is an increased prevalence of sore throats, upper respiratory infections, and ear infections. This is due to the increased vulnerability of the mucous membrane to congestion and inflammation. The sebaceous glands of the skin mature and the incidence of acne increases. Along with this prepuberty phenomenon comes the secondary sex characteristics. Fat distribution increases along with height.

This is the time for the female growth spurt. The female develops breast tissue, broadening of the hips, and appearance of pubic hair. During the later phase of prepuberty, menses may begin. The male develops pubic hair, his voice changes, and the size of the genitalia increases.

Development

Decreasing dependency and a sense of industry characterizes the schoolchild. It is important to consider the age when dealing with a schoolchild. There is a marked difference between a 6-year-old and a 12-year-old. During these years, the child is learning basic adult concepts and is learning to handle strong feelings and impulses in a constructive manner. Another task of this period is adjusting to the changing body image and self-concept in terms of the masculine and feminine social roles. Physical growth is slow, but fine motor skills continue to increase slowly.

SUMMARY

Health assessment and health supervision of children are important areas of nursing practice that have become more comprehensive in scope. The literature documents the increased kinds and quality of health care provided by nurses. Nurses providing child health care should have a strong theoretical base and experience in child health settings. This chapter has provided a relatively short synopsis of the extensive literature available to nurses who function as providers of child health care. It is important for those nurses who will provide primary health care services to children to utilize textbooks and guides that are more specific to the child health specialty.

REFERENCE

1. Schmidt, J.: *Attorney's Dictionary of Medicine and Work Finder.* New York, Matthew Bender Co., Inc., 1962. Cumulative supplement and revision, May, 1975, p. 27.

BIBLIOGRAPHY

Apgar, V.: The role of the anesthesiologist in reducing neonatal mortality. *N. Y. State J. Med.* 55:2365, 1955.

Barnard, K., and Douglas, H. B.: *Child Health Assessment.* Bethesda, Md., U.S. Dept. Health, Education, and Welfare, December 1974.

Campbell, C.: *Nursing Diagnosis and Intervention in Nursing Practice.* New York, John Wiley and Sons, 1978.

Chinn, P., and Leitch, C.: *Child Health Maintenance.* St. Louis, C. V. Mosby Co., 1974.

Fraiberg, S.: *The Magic Years.* New York, Charles Scribner's Sons, 1959.

Frankenburg, W. K., and Dodds, J. B.: Denver developmental screening test. *Pediatrics* 71(2):181–191, 1967.

Kempe, C. H., Silver, H. K., and O'Brien, D. O.: *Current Pediatric Diagnosis and Treatment,* 3rd ed. Los Altos, Calif., Lange Medical Publishers, 1974.

McCain, F.: Nursing by assessment not institution *Am. J. Nurs.* 65:82–84, 1965.

Murray R., and Zeitner, J.: *Nursing Assessment and Health Promotion through the Life Span.* Englewood Cliffs, N. J., Prentice-Hall Inc., 1978.

Mussen, P. (ed.): *Carmichael's Manual of Child Psychology,* 3rd ed. New York, John Wiley and Sons, Inc., 1974.

Scipien, G., et al. (ed.): *Comprehensive Pediatric Nursing.* New York, McGraw-Hill, 1975.

Zuidema, G., and Judge, R.: *Physical Diagnosis—A Physiological Approach to the Clinical Examination,* 3rd ed. Boston, Little-Brown, 1974.

CHAPTER 23

Chapters 18—22 have presented the first phase of assessment, the collection of data. This chapter discusses the logical result of assessment, data analysis and problem identification. (The term "nursing diagnosis" will be used to describe "problem identification" in this chapter.) Making a nursing diagnosis is somewhat like solving a jigsaw puzzle with data collection as the springboard for action and the nursing diagnosis as the blueprint for action.

The purpose of this chapter is to present the concept of nursing diagnosis, its purpose, focus, and value in the nursing process. The time at which a nursing diagnosis is formulated and the knowledge and skills necessary for its development will be discussed. Also, the forces that influence, and help to define, and clarify nursing diagnosis will be addressed.

TOWARD A NURSING DIAGNOSIS

The term and process of nursing diagnosis is now very much emphasized. It has been incorporated

NURSING DIAGNOSIS OF HEALTH CARE PROBLEMS

M. Patricia Fasce, M.S., R.N.

into the American Nurses' Association "Standard for Nursing Practice" and appears in the revised Nurse Practice Acts of most states. At a recent National Conference on Nursing Diagnosis, a small group was established to define and classify nursing diagnosis. What are the reasons for this recent emphasis and what are the compelling forces that have influenced the establishment of nursing diagnoses? For one, as the roles of nurses have expanded, they have also become more independent. Consequently, the nurse must assume responsibility for identifying health problems that will be responsive to nursing intervention and independently search for better methods to identify needs and consequent problem areas.

Nursing must be visible and accountable in its unique contributions to health care in wellness and illness. Dodge addressed other compelling forces and suggested how nursing diagnosis could be the answer to them:

1. Justification as a profession by having a scientific body of knowledge uniquely its own.

Nursing diagnosis can be the means of discovery.
2. Delineation of the specific contribution that nurses make in health maintenance and identifying health states. Nursing diagnosis would determine goals in wellness and in illness.
3. Quality assurance in practice. Nursing diagnosis would be a valuable vehicle for evaluating nursing practice.
4. Definition of unique services that justify the existence for and retaining control in professional nursing. Nursing diagnosis will clearly identify specific activities and nursing roles.
5. Desire for a systematic and logical method of reasoning in practice to assure quality of care. Nursing diagnosis as a process would offer this as well as personal fulfillment.
6. Government pressure to determine services for which it is paying, and with the advent of national health insurance and third-party payments, nursing diagnosis will delineate those services and justify their need for existence.
7. Better informed health consumer who wants

accountability for care received and to know what professional nursing has to offer that is not offered by any other group. Nursing diagnosis would be the area of expertise with its special knowledge and skills and utilized process.[1]

Gebbe and Lavin[2] suggested that a defined and classified nursing diagnosis is one way to improve the assessment of health care needs and consequent problem areas. For example, with a specific nursing diagnosis in mind, data collection would be easier and more specific.

Nature of Any Diagnosis

Diagnosis, regardless of who makes it, is a conclusion about an undesirable state. *Webster's New International Dictionary* defines *diagnosis* as "the act of identifying a disease from its signs and symptoms; an investigation or analysis of the cause or character of a condition, situation or problem; and a statement of conclusion concerning the nature or cause of some phenomena."[3] A *phenomenon* is an observable fact, known through the senses rather than thought or intuition, or an exceptional, unusual, or abnormal person, thing or occurrence.

What distinguishes the nursing diagnosis from that of the physician and other health team members? (These differences will be examined in detail later in this chapter.) The similarities include the method of gathering information, making connections with the information, recognizing a pattern, and coming to a conclusion. The differences are in the focus of concern, subject matter, area of expertise, and the particular knowledge and skills needed for diagnosis.

Nursing—a Foundation for Diagnosing

The philosophy and working definition of nursing influence the way in which the nurse views the roles, behaviors, and focus in assessing and diagnosing. Bloch presents a clear definition of nursing practice that is appropriate to the nursing process and relevant to nursing diagnosis. The practice of registered nursing means:

The collection of data about the health status of individuals, families, or communities; the defini-

tion of nursing problems (where nursing problem refers to health problem which is expected to be responsive to intervention by registered nurses); and the planning, implementation and evaluation of intervention designed to solve the identified nursing problems. The purpose of such data collection, problem definition and intervention is to maintain health to prevent disease and to promote recovery from illness and disability.[4]

Nursing assumes many roles in practice, such as teacher, counselor, nurturer, comforter, protector, communicator, technician, and diagnostician. The problems that confront nurses require different roles according to the needs that must be met.

Concepts and Theories

Individuals have many needs—physiological, interpersonal, sociocultural, and spiritual. They are also exposed to many stressors—intrapersonal, interpersonal, or extrapersonal—that threaten these needs from being adequately met. If they are inadequately handled, then problems arise, and some type of outside assistance is required.

The nurse must determine which needs are problem areas that nursing intervention can resolve. To do this, the nurse must have in mind a framework of relevant theories and concepts, such as Maslow's[5] "hierarchy of needs," Erikson's[6] "eight ages of man," and Selye's[7] "theory of stress and adaptation." Relevant concepts are homeostasis,* crisis, and need gratification.

Little and Carnevali[8] suggested that in assessment, functional coping deficits in the areas of strength, endurance, sensory input, knowledge, desire, courage, skill, dexterity, and support systems should be considered. Saxton and Hyland[9] and Bower[10] suggested that stress-adaptation as a theoretical model for nursing assessment and diagnosis should be used.

It is suggested here that the student who has just been introduced to the concepts of assessment and diagnosis review the areas mentioned above as well as other models relating to the common needs of man and choose a conceptual model that will give the needed guidance and structure.

---

*See Chapter 6. Opinions vary as to whether the term homeodynamics or homeostasis should be used.

COMPONENTS OF A NURSING DIAGNOSIS

Definition of Terms

There is lack of consistency and clarity in the use of terms to describe the components of nursing diagnosis, and this can be particularly confusing to the beginning student. In the discussion of nursing diagnosis, many terms which are crucial to the process must be defined, such as health problems, health needs, client problems, nursing problems, nursing needs, and assessment. For example, the terms "needs" and "problems" are often used interchangeably, when in fact they mean different things. There is also confusion about the definition of assessment. Some authors have formulated working definitions which are applicable to this subject.

Bloch addressed the issue of clarity and overlap with the terms "needs," "problems," and "assessment" and pointed out important distinctions in the following definitions:

> Nursing problem is a patient health problem that is expected to respond to nursing intervention.
>
> Health problem is a deficit or potential deficit in the health status of the individual, family, or community, that is believed to be in need of correction or anything of concern to the patient or the care provider.
>
> Health need refers to the action necessary to solve the problem; a problem is solved by meeting a need. The distinction is made between a need and a problem. Not all needs are problems, only those needs that cannot be met. (If you state the client's health problems as needs, you are not clearly indicating the specific problem that made you feel there was a need; instead you are stating an objective rather than a problem.)
>
> Assessment in nursing is considered to be two separate processes: (1) data collection without the interpretation; and (2) problem definition (or the making of diagnosis) where judgment is made from the data by critical analysis and interpretation.[4]

Clark offered some definitions which are relevant and applicable to the discussion and view of nursing diagnosis held in this chapter.

> High level wellness is maintaining homeostasis as well as pursuing goals beyond basic needs.
>
> Illness is an imbalance that results when a person adapts unsuccessfully to complex interactions of physical, emotional, sociocultural and spiritual stressors.
>
> Homeostasis is a healthy stable state where no undue imbalance is present between a person's internal and external environment.
>
> Needs are physiological, safety, interpersonal, and self-actualization factors that motivate people to seek balance between the internal state of their body and external environment.[11]

Saxton and Hyland[9] defined stress and adaptation as applicable to diagnosing.

> Stress is any factor that requires a response and produces some change.
>
> Adaptation is the anatomical, physiological, or psychological responses which occur as a reaction to and a defense against stress. These defenses are efficient or inefficient and create new stresses to which further responses are necessary.

The Focus

The specific concern of a nursing diagnosis is with the unhealthful responses (problems) that result from unmet needs and with those factors that contribute to the unhealthful response. It is a problem, for example, with adaptation to stress. These responses can be actual or potential. Actual problems are those currently existing. Potential problems are those which are anticipated if preventive measures are not taken.

Lewis[12] identified problem areas that should concern the nurse in her assessment of problem areas: clients' responses to health and illness-related experiences, problems of discomfort and dysfunction, physiological and psychological imbalances, problem reactions to illness, inability to cope successfully with life experiences, inability to accept change in life style as a result of disease or treatment, unrealistic expectations about disease prognoses or treatments, inconsistency between potential and actual solutions, unhealthful practices, inappropriate solutions, or undiagnosed problems.

Nursing diagnosis is the key to successful nursing care because it concentrates specifically on what needs to be changed and what is preventing that change.

What It Is Not

There are some areas that are mistakingly considered to be a nursing diagnosis but which are not. Little and Carnevali[8] identified these and gave examples of how they could be turned into a nursing diagnosis. According to these authors nursing diagnosis is:

1. *not* the reiteration of a medical diagnosis but the responses to change in life style as a result of the disease. For example, diabetes is the *medical diagnosis,* but potential insulin shock related to not eating the complete breakfast after insulin is the *nursing diagnosis.*
2. *not* the diagnostic test but the client's concern or stress related to the test. For example, the *medical diagnosis* is a barium enema x-ray, but worry related to possible inability of retaining enema during the x-ray is the *nursing diagnosis.*
3. *not* the medical treatment but the unhealthful responses from the adjustments necessary as a result of the treatment. For example, the *medical diagnosis* is a low sodium diet; however, disregard to salt restriction related to dislike of or lack of knowledge of the diet selection is the *nursing diagnosis.*
4. *not* the equipment but again the unhealthful response as a result of it. For example, the *medical diagnosis* is skeletal traction, but redness of sacrum related to patient weakness and inability to raise self off back with trapeze is the *nursing diagnosis.*
5. *not* the broad concept label but the specific response(s) indicating the concern. For example, the *medical diagnosis* is immobilization, hypokalemia; however, too many questions have to be asked to determine specific concerns or problems that need changing. In the latter, is the hypokalemia from lack of intake, replacement, excessive loss and what is going on that *nursing* can resolve without a medical order.
6. *not* the *nurse's* problem with the client. For example, the client is demanding of the nurse's time and seeks constant attention of the nurse on duty. One must identify the meaning behind this behavior in order to resolve it.

Medical versus Nursing Diagnosis

The true difference between a medical and nursing diagnosis lies in the cause and focus of the problem. Medical diagnosis is concerned with the disease pathology and its underlying mechanisms and problems that will only be resolved through medical intervention. Nursing diagnosis, as stated previously, is concerned with the difficulties and unhealthful responses as a result of the disease which can be handled independently by nursing interventions.

To illustrate the difference between medical (m.d.) and nursing (n.d.) diagnoses, some examples are listed below.

1. m.d.—fractured femur.
   n.d.—anxiety related to fear of falling in learning crutch walking.
2. m.d.—emphysema.
   n.d.—client resistant to halting smoking related to lack of understanding of hazards of smoking.
3. m.d.—myocardial infarction.
   n.d.—client annoyed at bedrest restrictions related to denial of disease process and its resulting limitations.
4. m.d.—leukemia.
   n.d.—client nauseated related to effects of the chemotherapy.

These examples illustrate how the nurse can take a medical diagnosis, apply her own academic information, and arrive at a nursing diagnosis.

INTERDEPENDENCY OF MEDICAL AND NURSING DIAGNOSES

What concerns the nurse will be of concern to the physician and vice versa. Nursing and medical diagnoses exist concurrently and should work together. Medical diagnosis can become a nursing diagnosis, and a nursing diagnosis can become a medical diagnosis. For example, insulin shock once medically stabilized presents areas of concern for the nurse, such as fear of potential insulin shock related to inability to determine insulin dosage, skipping meals, or not eating the complete meal as indicated, and ignorance of the signs, symptoms, or the cause of insulin shock. In this example the medical diagnosis is a stressor and a generator of the nursing diagnosis. An example of a nursing diagnosis becoming a medical diagnosis would be: the observation of a client's inability to cough and deep breathe compounded by severe weakness which eventually resulted in hypostatic pneumonia.

Little and Carnevali[8] pointed out how the nurse's knowledge of the pathophysiology and psychopathology of the medical diagnosis will alert her to the actual and anticipated discomforts, functional disabilities, and prognoses, so that realistic expectations can be made. For example, knowledge of the mechanisms or pathophysiology related to poor circulation would lead to the anticipated problem of poor tissue healing; an understanding of the pathophysiology of deficient sensory nerve functioning would help the nurse with a diagnosis related to inability to feel painful stimuli; or if the client had hyperthyroidism, the nurse may arrive at a nursing diagnosis of insomnia due to increased metabolism from the disease.

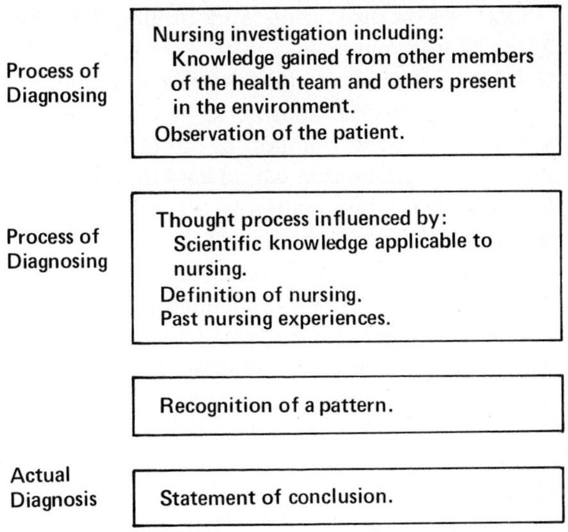

DEVELOPMENT OF A NURSING DIAGNOSIS

Making a nursing diagnosis is a deliberate conscious act of scientific inquiry and problem identification that involves combining data collection, knowledge, and skills. It is not based on intuition, although intuition can be a valuable asset. The nursing diagnosis will be as accurate as the data, the practitioner's knowledge base, and essential skills, and past experience will allow.

Durand and Prince[13] see nursing diagnosis as two steps as outlined in Figure 23-1. First, the process of diagnosing, and second, the decision or actual diagnosis. The diagnosis is formulated after the following criteria are met:

1. The pattern is recognized in responses.
2. The responses are unhealthful.
3. The unhealthful response can be changed to a more healthful one.
4. Nursing intervention can make the change.

Knowledge Base

Facts do not exist in isolation; they develop in relationship to each other and must be analyzed against some theoretical framework. Previous men-

FIGURE 23-1. The steps of a nursing diagnosis.

tion has been made of relevant theory and concepts. Also mental screening must occur against different bodies of knowledge, the social and physical sciences, their scientific principles and principles of nursing and, comparisons of normal and abnormal responses. This implies certain cognitive processes and other supporting skills.

COGNITIVE PROCESSES

Using the wealth of information implied from the data collected involves a movement between observations and stored knowledge. Four cognitive processes—analysis, synthesis, inductive and deductive reasoning—occur.

Inductive reasoning is making generalizations from specific evidence. For example, a client with a recent amputation demonstrates certain behaviors such as sadness, withdrawal, depression, or anger. These would lead to a general conclusion of grief from loss and altered body image.

Deductive reasoning is making specific observations from generalizations. For example, a client with a new colostomy (generalized condition) might demonstrate specific problems such as repulsion to the looks of the colostomy, inability to change collection bag because of intolerance of odor, restrictions on social interactions related to fear of odor coming from the bag, and skin excoriation related to secretions around the stoma.

Synthesis is organizing and putting together pieces of information to make a sensible whole, allowing for pattern recognition. For example, excessive perspiration, exposure to heat for long periods of time, administration of diuretics, and the presence of hypotension would lead to the conclusion of possible hyponatremia, dehydration, and anticipated hypovolemic shock.

Analysis is pulling apart or separating a whole into its parts, that is, an examination of the components of a complex situation; for example, in depression, noticing the behaviors that led to this problem such as loss of appetite, apathy, withdrawal, or unkempt appearance.

Skills

Supporting the cognitive processes are other skills that enhance a more accurate, sophisticated nursing diagnosis. These include the skills of observation, communication, interviewing, and technical expertise; these in turn require imagination, creativity, curiosity, and objectivity.

Deterrents

Marriner[14] addressed some common problems besides those listed above, including lack of reflection on the client's verbalizations and behaviors, and stereotyping (which alters objectivity and can lead to value judgments and clichés). Instead of listing facts as they exist, the nurse lists what she thinks the facts are. Little and Carnevali[8] state that certain problems result when the facts are recorded incorrectly. This can result from (1) not differentiating cues from inferences; or (2) permitting preconceived ideas from a label erroneously given to a client which influences objectivity in planning care.

Statement of the Problem

The statement of conclusion is the communicator for the subsequent plan of action. Criteria for good problem statements include:

1. A precise and neutral view of the problem.
2. Only the client's problem should be described.
3. Problems should be identified as actual or potential so that they are dealt with as such.

4. Problems should be stated in such a way that objectives or goals can be determined.
5. Problems should be clear to all who read them.
6. Problems stated should reflect the specific area of concern of the client or the nurse.
7. Problems should be as brief as possible. Durand and Prince[13] identified different types of statements which can be seen in the examples given. They can be descriptive, etiological, physiological, psychological, symptomatic, anticipated (from a medical diagnosis), complications of a primary illness, a result of hospitalization, or the same as a medical diagnosis in an emergency situation. The authors give good examples of each.

There is no single way of stating a nursing diagnosis. Mundinger and Jauron[15] suggested that nursing diagnosis be a two part statement.

1. The actual or potential unhealthful response (which indicates what has to be changed) and the derived outcomes.
2. The contributing factors to the unhealthful response (which indicate what is preventing the change). The nursing actions are based on these factors.

Examples of nursing diagnosis statements using this format would be:

Constipation related to:
    inability to sit on the bedpain without pain;
    lack of privacy when using the bedpan;
    lack of mobility from forced bedrest;
    little roughage in the diet;
    low fluid intake.
Anxiety over passing final examinations related to:
    missing class content.
Inadequate sleep related to:
    noise in the environment;
    frequent nursing care activities;
    worry about family at home.
Cough related to:
    tickling in throat;
    increased secretions;
    increase in smoking;
    dryness in the environment.

Depression related to:
   loss of breast;
   husband's upset over the loss.
Frustration related to:
   inability to dress self without assistance.
Inadherence to diet restrictions related to:
   dislike of diet selections;
   inadequate knowledge;
   inconvenience caused when a guest in others'
      homes.
Loneliness related to:
   separation from family;
   lack of visitors.
Grief reaction related to:
   loss of job;
   termination of friendships;
   loss of goals;
   loss of self concept;
   loss of body image;
   forced change in life style.
Nausea related to:
   chemotherapy
Potential hypostatic pneumonia related to:
   reluctance to deep breathe and cough.
Reluctance to turn and cough related to:
   fear of incisional pain.
Potential decubiti on back related to:
   inability to turn off back by himself.

Mundinger and Jauron[15] pointed out mistakes to avoid in writing the nursing diagnosis:

1. Writing them in terms of needs instead of problems. For example, needs to increase fluid intake instead of stating the specific problem or response demonstrated which makes this a concern.
2. Using the words *due to* rather than *related to*, which could be legally hazardous.
3. Reversing the two part statement by putting the contributing factors first. For example, odors in the room causing inability to eat meals rather than inability to eat meals related to odors in room.
4. Writing a response that is not necessarily unhealthful. For example, a client has just lost his job and is expressing anger. This is an expected response and is not necessarily unhealthful and therefore may not be a problem for nursing diagnosis.

5. Writing an unhealthy response in such a way that it cannot be changed. For example: writing a nursing diagnosis related to inability to speak due to a complete laryngectomy.
6. Writing two parts of a statement which say the same thing. For example: inability to have bowel movement related to constipation.

Classification

A National Conference on the Classification of Nursing Diagnoses was first held in 1973 to begin the work of classifying those health problems most commonly identified by nurses and treated by means of nursing interventions. Gebbie and Lavin[16] have edited the proceedings of this group. Since that time, two additional national conferences have been held, and further nursing diagnoses and defining characteristics have been identified. A task force headed by Dr. Marjory Gordon of Boston College is continuing this work.

Table 23-1 alphabetically lists some of the nursing diagnoses on which the conference group agreed were client problems or concerns identified by nurses that can be resolved by some type of nursing intervention.[17] These diagnoses are now in the process of being categorized into classes and subclasses so that patterns and relationships can be seen. This group is attempting to establish a con-

TABLE 23-1. Tentative List of Nursing Diagnoses

Alterations in faith	Manipulation
Altered relationship with self and others	Mobility, impaired
Altered self-concept	Motor uncoordination
Anxiety	Noncompliance
Body fluids, depletion of	Pain
Bowel function, irregular	Regulatory function of the skin, impairment of
Cognitive functioning, alterations of	Respiration, impairment of
Comfort level, alterations in	Respiratory distress
Confusion (disorientation)	Self-care activities, ability to perform
Deprivation	Sensory disturbances
Digestion, impairment of	Skin integrity, impairment of
Family's adjustment to illness, impairment of	Sleep-rest pattern, ineffective
Family process, inadequate	Susceptibility to hazards
Fear	Thought process, impaired
Grieving	Urinary elimination, impairment of
Lack of understanding	Verbal communication, impairment of
Level of consciousness, alterations in	
Malnutrition	

sistent nomenclature for these diagnoses and eventually substitute either a number or abbreviation so that they can be computerized.

The work by this group has been started but in order to develop a comprehensive and valid classification, nurses must become familiar with these diagnoses and test them in the actual practice setting. It cannot be left just to those in research. Nurse educators will orient their nursing content around the nursing diagnoses.

PURPOSE AND VALUE

The hope is to develop a diagnostic classification and a comprehensive list of nursing diagnoses or labels that are similar to the standard nomenclature used for medical diagnoses. This would facilitate and provide a language commonly accepted by all nurses and would eliminate the need for the summary statements now present. For example, in medicine the medical diagnosis, diabetes mellitus is concise, self-explanatory, and has the same significance to all physicians. They all agree that it has a certain pathology, etiology, signs, symptoms, and a specific time at which to validate the course of treatment and prognosis. Thus, categorizing established labels for nursing diagnosis could accomplish the same type of thing. Therefore, this diagnostic system would be a frame of reference for nurses, indicating what data to collect or what parameters must be present to arrive at this diagnosis. It would also indicate nursing approaches.

In utilizing this system, the nurse will have to learn what manifestations would place the diagnosis in a certain category. For example, to use the label "anxiety" would require that the nurse know what parameters indicate anxiety and what data must be collected. If categorized under moderate versus high level anxiety, the nurse must know the specific criteria which would delineate two levels.

For educators, skills of diagnosis and critical thinking will have to be taught and content will be the nursing diagnoses and their manifestations. For the future practitioners of nursing, this system would be conducive to computerization by substituting numbers or abbreviations for labels. Gebbie and Lavin[16] present in detail the proceedings of the first conference and the mechanics of classifying present nursing diagnoses.

SUMMARY

Nursing diagnosis is a client-centered approach, and the client often can be the most valuable resource in pinpointing the problem and appropriate care.

Nursing diagnosis, a scientific process, can offer much satisfaction and challenge in practice. It requires knowledge of basic human needs, an understanding of human behavior, and a good solid foundation of supporting sciences and principles of nursing. As a cognitive process it helps develop observational, interviewing, and diagnostic skills and encourages logical thinking, problem solving, and conceptualization.

Nursing diagnosis assures individualized care for the client. For the practice of nursing, it spells out the domain of nursing activity, accountability, and its justification as a profession. It also provides a good vehicle for future research in nursing practice and education.

REFERENCES

1. Dodge, G. H.: Forces influence move toward nursing diagnosis. *A.O.R.N.J.* 22(8):4, 1975.
2. Gebbie, K., and Lavin, M. A.: Classification of nursing diagnosis. *Nurs. Outlook* 23:96, 1976.
3. *Webster's New International Dictionary of English Language,* 2nd ed. Springfield, Mass., G. C. Merriam Company, 1961.
4. Bloch, D.: Some crucial terms in nursing—what do they really mean? *Nurs. Outlook* 22:689, 1974.
5. Maslow, A.: *Toward a Psychology of Being.* New York, D. Van Nostrand Company, 1962.
6. Erickson, E.: *Childhood and Society,* New York, W. W. Norton and Company, 1963.
7. Selye, H.: *The Stress of Life.* New York, McGraw-Hill Book Company, 1956.
8. Little, D. E., and Carnevali, D. L.: *Nursing Care Planning,* 2nd ed. Philadelphia, J. B. Lippincott Company, 1976.
9. Saxton, D. F. and Hyland, P. A.: *Planning and Implementing Nursing Intervention.* St. Louis, C. V. Mosby Company, 1975.
10. Bower, F. L.: *The Process of Planning Nursing Care—A Theoretical Model.* St. Louis, C. V. Mosby Company, 1972.
11. Clark, C. C.: *Nursing Concepts and Processes.* Albany, N.Y., Delmar Publishers, 1977.
12. Lewis, L.: *Planning Patient Care,* 2nd ed. Dubuque, Wm. C. Brown Company, 1976.
13. Durand, M., and Prince, R.: Nursing diagnosis: process and decision. *Nurs. Forum* 5:4, 1966.

14. Marriner, A.: *The Nursing Process*. St. Louis, C. V. Mosby Company, 1975.
15. Mundinger, M., and Jauron, G.: Developing a Nursing Diagnosis *Nurs. Outlook*, 23:96, 1975.
16. Gebbie, K. M., and Lavin, M. A.: *Classification of Nursing Diagnosis*, St. Louis, C. V. Mosby Company, 1975.
17. Gebbie, K., and Lavin, M.: Classifying nursing diagnoses. Am. J. Nurs. 74:250, 1974.

BIBLIOGRAPHY

Aspinall, M. J.: Nursing diagnosis—the weak link. *Nurs. Outlook* 24:32, 1976.
Bircher, A. U.: On the development and classification of diagnosis. *Nurs. Forum* 14:1, 1975.
Dodge, G. H.: What determines nursing versus medical diagnosis? *A.O.R.N.J.* 22(7):1, 1975.
Dodge, G. H.: Current works to define, classify nursing diagnosis, *A.O.R.N.J.,* 22(9):4, 1975.
Gordon, M.: Strategies in problem concept attainment: a study of nursing diagnosis. Ph.D. dissertation, Boston, Mass., 1972.
Komorita, N.: Nursing diagnosis: *Am. J. Nurs.* 63:83, 1963.
Kraegal, J. M.: A system of patient care based on patient needs. *Nurs. Outlook* 20:2, 1972.
Mayers, M. G.: *A Systematic Approach to the Nursing Care Plan*. New York, Appleton-Century-Crofts Publishers, 1972.
Nichols, M. E., and Wessells, V. G.: *Nursing Standards and Nursing Process*. Mass., Contemporary Publishers, 1977.
Roy, Sr. C.: A diagnostic classification system for nursing. *Nurs. Outlook* 23:2, 1975.
Rothberg, J. S.: Why nursing diagnosis? *Am. J. Nurs.* 67:1040, 1967.
Walter, J. B., Pardee, G. P., and Molbo, D. M.: *Dynamics of Problem-Oriented Approaches: Patient Care and Documentation*. Philadelphia, J. B. Lippincott Company, 1976.
Wrobel-Vaughan, B. C., and Henderson, B.: *The Problem Oriented System in Nursing—A Workbook*. St. Louis, C. V. Mosby Company, 1976.
Yura, H., and Walsh, M. B.: *The Nursing Process,* 2nd ed. New York, Appleton-Century-Crofts, 1973.

CHAPTER 24

The plan of care is the third phase of the nursing process. It is based on a thorough assessment of the client and family and an accurate diagnosis or statement of the problems to be solved. The first two phases provide the data; the plan provides the continuity of care. Without a plan, each person caring for the client or family must read the data and make separate diagnoses and plans for the shift, day, week, or anticipated length of contact; or the client must repeat the data to each person who comes to care for him, making him wonder about hospital communication. Each contact in this instance is a new experience for both the client and the nurse. When there is no written plan, it is not possible to know if all the needs of the client are being met. Needs and concerns could be missed unless a particular worker happened to ask the right question at the right time or the client volunteered the information. A written plan built on a complete, systematically obtained data base helps eliminate these problems. A plan also provides direction for auxiliary workers who might not have the knowledge to make their own plans.

PLAN OF CARE

Carol V. Hayes, M.Ed., R.N.

The following factors contribute to the success of a nursing care plan:

1. Completeness of the data base.
2. Completeness of the problem list or accuracy of the nursing diagnosis.
3. Knowledge base of the writer, including anatomy, physiology, pathophysiology, nutrition, and nursing techniques.
4. Specificity of the nursing approaches to solve the problems.
5. Creativity and imagination of the writer.
6. Involvement and commitment of writer and staff to carrying out the plan as well as the involvement of the client and family in constructing the plan.
7. Anticipated length of contact with the client.
8. Communication system of the health care agency.

Each of these factors will be discussed in detail (items 1−7 in this chapter and item 8 in the next chapter).

NURSING CARE PLAN

Data Base

As stated earlier in this text, the data base is obtained through several techniques—observation, interview, and physical examination (inspection, auscultation, palpation, percussion). To plan the care of the client, the data base must be complete. If it is not completed in one contact with the client then the first problem to be solved is "incomplete data base." "Other problems which can be identified from the available data are listed and dated accordingly. When the defined data base has been recorded, problem 1 is resolved, and the date entered on the list."[1] As long as the data base is incomplete, according to whatever criteria are established by the agency, the plan of care will be incomplete.

The data base should be completed as soon after admission as possible. The nursing history begins with an introduction to the client that typically takes the following form: "My name is Miss Hayes and

I am going to be your nurse while you are here. I'd like to ask you some questions, the answers to which will help us plan your care." If the history is taken after the client has already been in the hospital for a few days, he may wonder what the basis of his nursing care had been during that time.

Problem List

The next factor that influences the effectiveness of the plan of care is the completeness of the problem list or the accuracy of the nursing diagnosis. The process of arriving at either diagnosis or problem statements will not be discussed here in detail; however, the more knowledge the nurse brings to her job, the more easily problems can be conceptualized. (See Chapter 23 for discussion of nursing diagnosis.) This writer prefers the use of problem statements because they make it possible to use the scientific method or problem-solving approach in combination with the problem-oriented recording system.

Stage 1 of the scientific method or problem-solving approach is data collection. Usually this means taking a nursing history, but the process can be less extensive or formal than that.

Stage 2 is statement of the problem or a "nursing diagnosis." "The term problem is used to mean a question proposed for solution or consideration; anything required to be done. A problem is any condition or situation in which a patient requires help to maintain or regain a state of health or to achieve a peaceful death . . . the problem must be based on data obtained from the patient, the family and/or other members of the health team."[3] It does not always refer to an undesirable state, but does always refer to something with which the client needs assistance.

Stage 3 is an analysis of the problem which involves surveying existing knowledge relevant to it. It calls upon the knowledge base of the nurse and may require use of the library for research to be sure all identifiable factors or phenomena contributing to the problem are studied.

Stage 4 is selection of the phenomena to be studied. Factors found in the literature thought to apply to the current situation are separated from irrelevant factors.

In *stage 5*, induction, data collected from the client are categorized according to the factors se-lected. Observation, description, and classification are the processes used in this phase.

Stage 6 is statement of hypotheses. From all the previous study and thought, using the data classified according to the phenomena selected, the nurse should list the reasons thought to account for the client's problem. These hypotheses are only possible explanations for the existence of the problem: all ideas should be considered.

Stage 7, deduction, consists of two parts: (1) a statement of postulates (assumptions or consequences) which begin with the word *if*; and (2) testing each postulate by observation, study, and experiment.

Stage 8 is a "clarification of the relationship of the verified hypotheses to the initial problem." Here the results of postulate testing are analyzed and a conclusion made that either confirms or refutes hypotheses stated in stage 6. This is an evaluation of both the nurse's thoughts and the progress of the client. If hypotheses are not validated, attempts must be made to discover the reason. Some reasons for lack of validation are: (1) the statement of the problem was incorrect; (2) the problem was not studied appropriately (e.g., the wrong phenomena were selected for study); (3) the hypotheses were inadequate or incorrect; (4) the postulates were inadequate or incorrect leading to collection of inappropriate data and thus incorrect results. If the hypotheses are found to be incorrect, others must be chosen and the process of testing is repeated.

Stage 9 is generalization to other situations. This entails the application of findings to unknown but similar situations, being careful to avoid generalization from too few instances.[3]

Each of the nine stages of the problem-solving approach follows logically from the previous one, hence the parts of the method are dependent on each other, rather than independent. Table 24-1 illustrates the kind of information which goes into each stage; it is not meant to be a thorough treatment of the problem but merely illustrative of the method.

The nursing diagnoses listed in *Classification of Nursing Diagnoses*[4] can also be thought of as problem statements and are thus also amenable to solution by the problem-solving approach. Becknell and Smith state, "diagnosis is defined as: investigation or analysis of the cause or nature of a con-

TABLE 24-1. Problem-Solving Approach

Stage	Process
1. Data collection	Nursing history of Mr. Brown. Not repeated here. Data from it are listed in the various categories below.

2. Statement of the problem	1. Efficient physiological functioning requires that waste substances be eliminated from the body.
	2. Patterns of elimination vary among individuals due to:
	  a. early childhood training
	  b. eating patterns: kinds of food, fluid intake
	  c. activity
	  d. presence of disease conditions
	  e. stress
	  f. environment-privacy, time of usual defecation; use of bedpan; toilet
	  g. medications; laxatives
	  h. medical and surgical treatment and some diagnostic procedures.

3. Analysis of the problem	Survey existing knowledge; research.
4. Selection of the phenomena to be studied	1. Usual pattern of elimination. 2. Type and amount of food usually ingested and changes in this pattern during hospitalization. 3. Fluid intake. 4. Activity. 5. Use of mechanical aids and laxatives. 6. Stress; environmental factors. 7. Medications, medical treatment and diagnostic procedures. 8. Age. 9. Medical diagnosis.
5. Induction (observation, description and classification)	1. Usually soft formed stool daily *after breakfast.* 2. At home, a typical day's meals include, breakfast (6 am): 6 oz prune juice, coffee, toast and jelly; lunch (11:30 am): sandwich, cookies, ice tea; dinner (5:30 pm): chicken, greens, rice or potatoes, cake or pie and coffee. Six oz of prune juice at 9:30 pm. Drinks approximately 2 qt fluids daily (counting drinks with meals). 3. Mr. Brown has been in the hospital for 3 days. During this time he has been NPO for diagnostic procedures and has not had breakfast for 3 days. He has returned to the unit too late to receive a late tray. Between the time he returned to the unit and the time lunch was delivered, he has munched on chocolate candy. When lunch was delivered he stated that after waiting so long he was no longer hungry. However he did eat half of his meat and drank the beverage. For dinner, he has eaten approximately ⅔ of the meat and vegetables, has left his salad as there has been no dressing on it. (He did not ask for dressing because he didn't want to bother anyone.) When his prune juice was brought to him at 10:00 pm he was asleep. The nurse left the prune juice at his bedside and then removed it at 12:00 pm because he was then NPO. 4. Mr. Brown is on bedrest. His activity at home consists of sitting in a chair or sitting up in bed. He does walk to the bathroom.
6. Statement of relevant hypotheses	1. Mr. Brown has not had a bowel movement because of lack of the bulk, roughage, and fluids to which he is accustomed. 2. Mr. Brown has not had a bowel movement because he will not ask for the bedpan and thus delays urge to defecate.

TABLE 24-1. Continued

Stage	Process

7. Deduction	1. Formulation of postulates.
	    a. If Mr. Brown follows the regime listed below he will have a bowel movement daily.
	        (1) Eats one green salad and two leafy vegetables daily.
	        (2) Drinks 3000 ml daily.
	        (3) Uses the bedpan when it is offered at 6:30 am.
	        (4) Drinks 6 oz of prune juice at 6:00 am and 9:30 pm daily.
	    b. Mr. Brown has completed his diagnostic tests and can resume his usual food and fluid intake.
	2. Test each postulate.
	    (1) *Day 1*: Mr. Brown was given his prune juice at 6:00 am and 9:30 pm. He has eaten one green salad and two green leafy vegetables and his fluid intake was 3030 ml.
	    (2) *Day 2*: Mr. Brown drank his prune juice and coffee at 6:00 am. He was given the bedpan at 6:30 am and promptly produced a soft, formed brown stool. During the day, Mr. Brown ingested one green salad and two green leafy vegetables and 2990 ml fluid. He drank his prune juice at 9:30 pm.
	    (3) *Day 3*: Mr. Brown drank his prune juice and coffee at 6:00 am. He was given the bedpan at 6:30 am and promptly produced a soft, formed brown stool.

8. Clarification of the relationship of the verified hypotheses to the initial problem	The above observations and testing verify hypothesis 1. (Hypothesis 2 not tested.)
9. Generalization to other situations	Maintaining an individual's usual patterns (prehospitalization) may help prevent any disturbance or alteration in the pattern.

dition, situation, or problem; a statement or conclusion about the nature or cause of a phenomenon."[5] Mitchell[6] reserves the term diagnosis for those problems to which a cause can be attributed and uses the term problem when causation is not known. With the work being done by the National Group for Classification of Nursing Diagnoses perhaps the nursing profession will be able to accept one group of statements and terms, thus avoiding confusion and semantic arguments. For the purpose of this chapter, *problem* is the term most likely to be used and is seen as synonymous with the term *diagnosis*.

ESTABLISHMENT OF GOALS

The identification or establishment of goals (short or long-term) or a statement of nursing care objectives is the next element in a plan of care. Once the problem is identified then the nurse thinks of what

she specifically hopes the client will do that will indicate that the problem is being solved; this is stage 7 of the problem-solving method. It is too easy to identify problems and write nursing orders, approaches, or actions and not think of what behavior to expect from the client that will show the problem has been solved. *Webster's 20th Century Unabridged Dictionary* defines goal as "the end or final purpose . . .," and objective as "something aimed at or striven for." The two words, goal and objective, will be used interchangeably in this chapter. A great deal of nursing care is focused on meeting immediate needs, so most objectives will be short-term. Additional objectives can always be set when the immediate ones have been achieved, so that the long-term concerns can usually be met in short steps. Whether the goal is long or short-term, it is important that the behavior expected from the client is stated in specific, achievable terms. "The primary purpose for stating nursing care objectives in patient behavioral terms is to provide a means of evaluating patient progress and the effect of nursing care on the patient. Nursing care is evaluated in terms of whether or not it achieved what it set out to do—that is, whether we 'get to where we are going' in managing or solving the patient's nursing problems or whether we do not."[7] Becknell and Smith state very clearly the criteria for correctly written objectives, including "a statement of the *behavior* expected to be demonstrated, the *conditions* under which the behavior is expected to occur and the *criterion* for determining acceptable performance. The subject expected to demonstrate the behavior must also be stated. Usually this is the patient but it may be a family member or other significant person. If the nurse expects some physiologic behavior then the subject is the skin, the weight, and so forth."[8]

Knowledge Base

One of the main influences on the quality of the plan of care is the knowledge base of the writer. Obviously all the knowledge needed for a plan cannot be included in this chapter, but the more the nurse knows the better the plan will be. A nurse cannot be limited to one fundamentals text or one medical-surgical nursing text for the knowledge she may need for a particular problem. Many books, articles, and individuals may have to be consulted before a plan can be developed.

Most knowledge comes from the various sciences, including anatomy, physiology, pathophysiology, microbiology, chemistry, psychology, sociology, pharmacology, and nutrition. For example, to plan preoperative teaching a nurse should have knowledge of the structures being operated on, complications likely to occur after manipulation of these structures (immediate and long-term), as well as the effects of medications and anesthesia.

Knowledge of the medical and nursing procedures required by clients is also important. The medical procedures are those performed by doctors as well as those delegated to nurses; the nursing techniques are those nurses perform independently. The plan of care is limited in its completeness if the nurse has not mastered a variety of techniques to apply to the solution of the client's problems. Although the nurse will not be performing many medical procedures, she needs to know what

medical treatments are planned and be familiar enough with them to write instructional plans for her clients. She should also know how to explain procedures that nurses or aides will carry out so she can write specific directions in her plan (see specificity of approaches below).

Knowledge of the role of the nurse, the philosophy of nursing practice, and the policies of the agency can influence the plan of care. The nurse should know when she must request an order for a procedure from the physician or when she can order the procedure herself. The list of permitted procedures is similar in most institutions, but it is likely to vary in important details so the nurse should become familiar with the policies of the agency in which she is studying or practicing. If, for example, an agency has a policy that all heat or cold applications must be ordered by the physician—that is, the nurse can not independently order warm compresses to the area of phlebitis from an intravenous infusion—then the plan is dependent on the availability of the physician and his approval. On the other hand, if she can do this independently, she can begin to promote the comfort of the client as soon as she identifies the need or when the client reports pain. Most invasive procedures, such as enemas or catheterizations, and all medications, even when needed for solving nursing problems, must be ordered by the physician. Every situation cannot be covered in this chapter, but each nurse should know this information when she is writing her plan of care.

Knowledge of the humanities and social sciences is also important. These fields teach us about how values and beliefs are acquired and the influence they have on behavior. For example, it may help the nurse whose client has suffered a loss of self-esteem to devise ways to help him regain it. Also, it must be emphasized that the nurse develops *herself* as a person during the study of philosophy, religion, art, and music, which consequently enriches her interactions with clients. She should be fully aware of her own values and beliefs so that she can keep them separate from those of the client. Knowledge of this nature may not directly produce specific nursing approaches as much as it indirectly shapes the nurse's general being and manner of approach.

The plan is often affected by agency policies which will definitely vary from agency to agency.

In some agencies, one nurse is alone responsible for formulating, modifying, and updating the plan; other workers contribute their ideas but no one changes the plan without the nurse's permission. In other agencies, all who care for the client are equally responsible, each adding ideas or modifying approaches no longer in effect. Unfortunately, under the latter system it is easy to assume that someone else has taken the responsibility for updating the plan often with the result that no one has updated it. Also, assigning accountability and evaluating both the nurse and the plan are more difficult. However, regardless of the form of organization, it is important that data obtained from the client are known to all the workers, organized into problems or diagnoses, and used to develop a plan which is communicated, evaluated, and revised as necessary.

Nursing Approaches to Problem Solving

A nursing care plan consists of a client problem or diagnosis, the subjective and objective data which document the problem, an assessment or conclusion concerning that problem, and the specific approaches which the writer of the plan anticipates will solve the problem. All of these categories must be as complete as possible.

The subjective, objective, and assessment categories, which are discussed more fully in the next chapter, consist of the following. Subjective data are those thoughts, feelings, and activities which the client himself reports. Objective data are those things which can be measured or are obtained by the nurse's own observation; they can be validated by others. Also included are descriptions of specific actions taken by the nurse, or medical orders. The assessment category contains a summary of the nurse's thoughts. It can include the "analysis of the nature of the problem or a probable explanation for the existence of the problem (stage three of the scientific method), an explanation of why the plan will deviate from the usual management of the problem due to conflicts with other interacting problems, the thoughts relative to whether or not nursing intervention should be instituted, and a prediction of the probable result of initiating nursing intervention."[9] The assessment category is where the conclusion, drawn from the data presented in the subjective and objective categories, is stated

(stage 8 of the scientific method); it is a bridge between data and action, containing thoughts, rationale, and hypotheses as well as conclusions or diagnosis. For example, if the data lead to the conclusion of anxiety, then the plan must show evidence of dealing with anxiety; if the assessment is an hypothesis about the meaning of a particular form of behavior, then the plan should contain the further data to be collected to confirm or refute the hypothesis. All the parts of the plan must interlock.

SPECIFICITY OF THE PLAN

We turn now to the actual writing of the directions for care, the approaches the nurse should take with the client, the specific nursing orders. Think of the plan as a series of directions or prescriptions which will cut down the time and effort of deciding daily how and what to do for each client. This is especially important if the client has a particular way he wishes something done and becomes upset if the procedure varies.

Specificity of the plan is important for another reason. It gives everyone the same frame of reference or goal. For example, the phrase "force fluids" is open to as many interpretations as there are readers. To one, it may be a directive to be harsh and literally forceful with the client, while to another it may mean gentle persuasion. One may interpret the amount required as 1000 ml, whereas another may think it should be 3000 ml. Thus, the same client could get quite different nursing care from each nurse, and the ideal continuity would certainly be lost. When the physician's orders read only "force fluids," the nurse can either request a specific amount from him—1500, 2000, or 2500 ml or select an amount based on her own knowledge; however, she must convert the physician's general order into a specific nursing order. The nursing order actually would be, "carry out the fluid plan at the bedside," which would have the specific amounts and kinds of fluids to be given at specific times. All nurses then will know at any hour of the day how to manage the client's fluid intake. Even if the specific amount of fluid is stated in the original medical order, a fluid plan is necessary to provide continuity of care.

For each problem, specific orders or directions are written which the nurse expects to be useful in solving the problem. Routine hygienic care need not be detailed in the plan nor should medical orders be merely repeated as nursing orders.[10] If further orders are needed to clarify or indicate exactly how the medical orders will be carried out, then nursing orders are written. Sleeplessness is an example of a problem that could require both medical and nursing orders: the physician writes the order for a sleeping medication, while the nurse writes her own orders for back rub, pre-sleep activity and either leaves the sleeping pill order to the medication nurse or writes one of the following orders specifying the degree of freedom the patient has regarding his own medication. "Give the sleeping pill at 10 pm," or "Ask the patient at 10 pm if he wants the sleeping pill." The nurse's knowledge of the necessity for promoting independence of clients in general, as well as the meaning to the individual client of choosing care or having care given without asking, will influence the exact statement of the nursing order.

Nursing orders are written in the form of imperative sentences. The verbs are specific ones that tell the reader exactly what to do. Many nursing articles and texts use the word "encourage" as a guide to action. Unfortunately, this word does not tell the reader specifically what to do, and, is therefore, not useful to the writer of nursing orders. It takes considerable thought to state what the nurse should do to "encourage a patient to eat, drink, or ambulate," but that effort must be made if the plan of care is to be useful to the nurse or the client. Thus, an order might read: "Ask the patient to drink 120 ml of water or juice every hour between 6 am and 10 pm," or "Ask the patient if he wants his pain medication before or after he ambulates." Other words that are *not* specific enough to be the action verbs for nursing orders are "allow," "let," "have," "permit," "teach," "maintain," "prevent," and "provide." Even a word that sounds specific, like "assist" does not tell the nurse what has to be done to help the client; she is therefore left to either interpret it herself or ask the client to tell her how she can assist him, two things the plan was designed to avoid. "Reassure" is the other nonspecific word used so often in the literature which, like "encourage," is made up of many actions rather than defining a specific action.

"Listen," "reflect," "find out (specific information for the client)," "bring pain medication to patient as close to the exact time as humanly possible" are all ways that can "reassure" clients. The author of the plan uses her knowledge of interpersonal relations, communications skills, and the client to answer the question, "What do I think would 'encourage' him to do what I want him to do?" She then specifies those verbs that apply. If the writer of the plan cannot state orders specifically enough for another reader to carry out, then she says so in the order or states that she alone will administer the nursing care for this problem. Very often the specific actions can be identified in the process of administering the care and then orders can be written for others to follow. For example, one of the author's clients was struggling with the problem of grief and anxiety. The plan of care for this problem was as follows:

Problem 7: Grief and Anxiety

3-20-78   2:00 PM

Subjective: "My mother died in December 1975, and my neighbor who did everything for us just died. I feel sad a lot; I feel scared inside most of the time. Doctors, hospitals, and thoughts of an operation make me nervous. I've been called uncooperative, and guess I was."

Objective: Talked in quiet, soft voice most of the time; lay quietly in bed, looking at and playing with fingers. No tears evident.

Assessment: Pt has suffered two significant losses recently and also has altered body image so grief is inevitable. Do not think she has been able to express any anger; she seems too controlled for that. Fear could be from anger or just from necessity of unfamiliar and painful treatments. If she has too much fear, suspect she will "run away" from us.

Plan: 1. Ask pt. qd how she is feeling; listen and focus on feeling rather than on why she might feel a certain way. 2. Explain procedures before doing anything and tell her where she is going if she has to leave ward. 3. Tell her what kinds of sensations she might experience if she's never had the experience before. 4. Try to get her to raise her voice in anger or to cry if she looks like she could. (I can't be any more specific on how to do this, sorry.) C. Hayes, R.N.

The parenthetical sentence shows how this author explained the lack of specificity in the order to the reader. Two subsequent progress notes state, in the objective data category, how the author "tried to get her to raise her voice in anger or to cry if she looks like she could.''

Problem 7: Grief and Anxiety

3-27-78   11:00 AM

Subjective: "I'm not as scared as I was, as nothing drastic is going to happen right away. I'm more scared than I would be at home though." When asked, talked about father moving to Florida, to farm, when she was 2; she and mother moved to country (seven acres) when he died; stayed pretty much by themselves. She doesn't drive—never learned how; minister comes to call once in a while; she doesn't go to church; doesn't garden; would like to grow some roses. Had horses—last one died 2 years ago. Worked since high school at home making shell jewelry until she stopped about 6 years ago. She and mother mostly read, watched TV all day "although mother did a lot of things around the house." Talked about change in helpfulness of some neighbors after Mr. Cross died.

Objective: Attempted to have pt talk more about herself; had to ask fairly direct questions, but she answered with more than one sentence. Speaks in a monotone; not able to detect any change in character of voice with particular subjects.

Assessment: Sounds like quite a lonely, certainly isolated life, focused around mother who is no longer present. It will take quite a lot of effort on her part, I suspect, to develop a life of her own.

Plan: Continue to try to have pt. talk more about herself and hopefully her feelings. C. Hayes, R.N.

Problem 7: Grief and Anxiety

3-28-78   1:00 PM

Subjective: "I'm just not going to stay here and go through all of this; I have four different doctors and four different stories, they're not going to do the IV yet, I don't know why. It's not going to do any good to be treated. It won't work out anyway. Nothing has for me for the past 10 years, I don't know why it would now. I might as well go home. I'm going to die anyway. I'm eating more than I ever have and am still losing weight, so I'm not even making progress there. Why

can't the fistula just be cut out? They can see where it is.''

Objective: Tears in eyes when talking about nothing working out for the past 10 years. Stopped when I reflected she'd lost everyone.

Assessment: Feelings are strong, close to surface and come out with very little provocation; has little tolerance for discomfort (perhaps has so much all the time, any more is too much); Sees and comments on lack of consideration we sometimes have; needs a fairly structured, consistent environment to keep feelings under control.

Plan: Will have to think about how to achieve consistency, if even possible. Will wait for change in physicians (4-1-78) before trying anything. Otherwise will continue to listen to feelings and try not to get angry with her. C. Hayes, R.N.

The knowledge the writer has of the nursing techniques available and the independence with which she can apply the techniques will influence the quality of the plan. If the problem is "impairment of skin integrity: potential," but the nurse lacks knowledge of the nursing techniques which prevent skin breakdown, the plan will be inadequate. If she writes, "turn patient every four hours" but leaves off "gently massage all bony prominences with lotion after turning patient," she will not solve her problem. The necessity of knowing policy regarding independent nursing functions has already been discussed.

Creativity and Imagination of the Writer

Creativity and imagination are two abilities that also influence the quality of the nursing care plan, but unfortunately rules can not be written for their use. Not everything that can help solve a problem is already known and written in a book. Nurses must look at some problems from a fresh perspective to see solutions. Maybe hospital or agency rules and policies need to be bent every once in a while; for example, the nurse may occasionally cook a special food herself to tempt a client's appetite instead of depending on the hospital kitchen to do so, since a surprise brought to a long-term client can relieve the monotony of his diet. The more open we can be to all possibilities, the more variety we will have in our plans, the more interesting our work will be, and the more likely we are to meet clients' needs. If we confine ourselves to textbooks, we will miss a lot, although it goes without saying that all approaches in the plan must be consistent with safe practice.

Involvement and Commitment to the Plan

Involvement and commitment are two other personal characteristics that influence the plan. Involvement means the capacity to become close to the client and his family without losing the ability to act in their best interests. A nurse is too involved when she is unable to act because her feelings rather than her professional judgment and knowledge are guiding her. Being drawn so deeply into the feelings of a client and his family as to feel overwhelmed by all that is happening is part of learning to become a nurse. Each nurse must learn to recognize the clues that tell her when she is reaching her limits. If a nurse protects herself from closeness before she even feels it, she is less likely to think of nursing orders that will promote closeness. Thus, the approaches selected will depend on how free the nurse is, how willing she is to take chances for her clients, and how fully committed she is to their progress.

Any successful plan must involve the client's family and significant others. If the family is not available to help set goals and priorities, then they should at least be informed of them. Ideally the family is part of the planning from the beginning, but that is not always possible—that is, the plan may have to be written without the family's input. If the plan is one which will be carried out at home, then the family must naturally be involved in it for it to work. It does no good, for instance, to order range of motion exercises to be done by the daughter twice a day without considering her work schedule. It is beyond the scope of this chapter to mention all the specifics which must be taken into consideration for writing a plan which is to be carried out at home or which involves more than one client, but it should be realized that a complete data base must be collected, including the determination of the capabilities of any health provider for the tasks required.

Duration of Contact with Client

The plan also depends on the anticipated length of contact with the client. A 3 day hospitalization does not allow time for major behavior modification. At the least, the immediate needs and concerns of the client should be considered. When caring for such a client, the data base may consist only of the client's understanding of the reason for admission, his expectations, what he does to ensure sleep and elimination, any problems he may have with these daily activities, and how he feels about asking for help. The interview may then close with the question, "Is there anything you want us to know about you in order for us to take better care of you while you are here?" If the client has very particular ways of managing his sleep and elimination, a more complete data base should be obtained because it is likely that he has particular ways to manage his other activities.

SUMMARY

The selection of nursing orders depends on the personnel and equipment available to carry out the plan. If there is no physical or occupational therapist to consult, then orders cannot be written to do so. An order to use a "portolift" to assist a client from bed to stretcher cannot be written if such a device does not exist in the institution or home, regardless of how appropriate such an order might be. In other words, a nursing care plan should include everything that is feasible and legal with nothing hypothetical, theoretical, or illegal. Too often the plan is written for an ideal situation inviting discouragement when it cannot be carried out. If there is no relationship between the nursing care plan and the actual care given the client, then a mere formality has been carried out.

The plan of care is only the third phase of the nursing process. Implementation is the fourth phase. The plan is carried out as written. The orders will either be successful or unsuccessful in meeting the objective or solving the problem. If the orders are successful, the problem will be solved or show evidence of improving; if the problem is not changing, the orders will probably have to be changed. New data that arise need to be evaluated to detect new problems, which then require a plan of care with implementation of the plan and evaluation of its success. Evaluation is the fifth stage of the nursing process which can lead to additional data collection and repetition of the whole process.

Documentation of the nursing process occurs in the client's written record. The next chapter will cover the subject of writing progress notes as well as other aspects of the client's record and the communication system.

APPENDIX

The data base used in this appendix is the one discussed by Becknell and Smith.[1] The client, Mr. A. B. Cero, was reluctant to participate in the taking of a nursing history with a student. The author engaged the client in conversation one morning and was able to obtain the data shown. These data, however, are incomplete; because a thoracotomy was under consideration, involving an extended period of incapacity in the hospital during recovery, a complete data base was necessary. The illustration shows how the problem—incomplete data base—is covered in the plan of care.

Mr. Cero was discharged before the complete data base was obtained so his plan of care remained incomplete. It will never be known what problems went unsolved due to the incomplete data base. It is hoped that none of the omissions were serious.

Nursing History

10-29-74   8:30 AM

Vital statistics: First STH* admission for Mr. Albert B. Cero, 65-year-old, white male, married, from south, Florida.

Understanding of illness: "Two or three months ago I had walking pneumonia and that's when my trouble started. I don't feel bad, but I don't have the zip or energy to do what I'm used to doing—like trimming my 600–700 ft hedge; I'm still working and doing all my own care, but something's not right. My doctor wanted to operate on me, but I wanted another opinion, that's why I'm here. I don't have any shortness of breath or anything. I don't know what 'it' could be."

Expectations: Expects a bronchoscopy (my word)

---

*Abbreviation for name of hospital.

today. "I hope I'm knocked out for it. I don't remember anything about the other one I had. I don't see any reason to suffer anxiety if I don't have to. I hope I don't need an operation, and if I do I guess I could go home to have it. I want to get my strength back and feel like my old self again. If I can't, I'll be all washed up—finished—I'll need a gun." Wants shot for pain when he asks for it; wants to know what is expected of him, and what sensations he will have.

Brief social-cultural history: Is an auto mechanic, owns his own shop; is still working. Education not elicited. Lives with his wife. Has at least one son. Other immediate family members not determined, nor were concerns about his family. Wife is here in a motel. Most significant person not elicited.

Significant data in terms of:

1. *Sleeping pattern*: not determined. Stated he had no problem sleeping, did nothing routinely to help him sleep.
2. *Elimination pattern*: Has BM qd p̄ cup of coffee. States he tends to get "constipated" (meaning not determined) when he "lies around" like he is now. Thinks he might need some milk of magnesia tonight. Voiding not asked about.
3. *Breathing*: "I have no shortness of breath, unless I walk a long distance (length not determined) or exert myself (meaning not elicited). I think that is only normal, don't you?" Rhythm even, rate and muscles used not determined. No accessory muscles used, no audible sounds. Auscultation not done. Cough forceful, expiratory wheeze, tightness heard. Pt has mucous but I did not see it.
4. *Eating and drinking*: No data elicited at all at this time.
5. *Skin integrity*: Arms and face tan, legs white; dry on arms and legs, rough on arms and hands, smooth on legs, firm turgor. Healed scars on arms. "I get banged up a lot in my work." States he has no open wounds. Back, chest, and bony prominences not observed. States no special care for skin—just soap and water. Type and time of bath, shaving schedule, and care of teeth not elicited at this time. Pt has upper and lower dentures. He needs no assistance at this time.

6. *Activity*: Walking not observed, nor range of motion. States he has no limitations.
7. *Recreation*: Fishing mentioned; other activities not elicited at this time.
8. *Interpersonal and communicative patterns*: Did not ask how he feels in new situations. He sat in chair, feet crossed at ankles, arms resting on arms of chair, rubbing hands together, looking at them, picking at fingernails, looking out window when answering questions, looking at me when I asked questions. Answered questions with elaboration, volunteered information; seemed to evade mentioning "lung" or being too specific about his illness. Did not ask questions, or change subject, spoke distinctly.
9. *Temperament*: "I really try to keep from getting mad as I don't get over it easy at all. Being taken advantage of makes me mad. I walk away from situations to avoid getting mad." Did not ask him if others would know if he was mad. Said he did not get or feel nervous.
10. *Dependency-independency patterns*: (1) For self—"everything I can." (2) For others—not elicited. (3) Others for him—not elicited. Did not elicit directly how he lets others know what he wants. He did say "when I ask for a shot for pain, I really want it because I really need it. I can take a lot of pain, so I don't ask for a lot of medication, but when I need it, I need it." Did not obtain how pt feels when he asks for or accepts help.
11. *Senses*: States he uses glasses for reading; otherwise no vision or hearing problems. Handedness not obtained. Only prosthesis is false teeth.
12. *Statement of that which makes pt feel safe, protected, care for*: not elicited at this time. C. Hayes, R.N.

PROBLEM LIST

Problem	Date First Noted	Resolved
1. Incomplete data base.	10/29/74	
2. Speaks of illness as "it" or "trouble."		
3. Possibility of surgery.		

4. "Constipated" if lies around.   10/30/74
5. Dry skin.

Progress Notes

10-29-74   1:00 PM

Returned from bronch. Appeared to be shaky all over with no control of lower extremities, but pt stated he was all right and would be fine when wife came. VS stable. Tol. liq. well, stated he would wait for dinner tonight. 3:00 PM no more shaking. J.T., R.N.

INITIAL PLAN OF CARE

10-29-74   1:20 pm

Problem 1: Incomplete Data Base

Subjective: No data.

Objective: Interviewed pt "surreptitiously," meaning I did not explain that I was taking a nursing history; this made it difficult to obtain some information. Do not have the following data:

1. Members of immediate family, any concerns about family; ascertain education level.
2. Most significant person.
3. Times to go to sleep and arise.
4. Meaning of "constipated."
5. Length he can walk s SOB and what exertion is to him.
6. Description of breathing.
7. Eating and drinking patterns, and all related data.
8. Shaving pattern, type of bath he prefers.
9. Care of teeth and whether he sleeps with them in or not.
10. Ability to walk and range of motion.
11. Recreational activities.
12. How he feels in new situations.
13. If others would know he was angry.
14. Things he does for others and wants, permits and likes others to do for him.
15. How he lets others know what he wants.
16. How he feels about asking for or receiving help.
17. What his dominant hand is.
18. What makes him feel safe, comfortable, cared for.

Pt, according to a student report to me, had requested nursing history be done at times other than when student had wanted to do it. Talked freely to me this AM.

Assessment: There are two or three possibilities as to patient's hesitancy (apparently) with the student: didn't want to be taken care of by a student; the times she chose were inconvenient; she gave him a choice and he took it as a way to exercise control over his situation. I didn't want a formal interview situation for fear of pushing him away, so am not sure I will be able to obtain the above data.

Plan: Each time I am with pt, at least once a day, will attempt to elicit the missing data by questioning him and will record obtained data under this problem.

Problem 2: Illness Is "It" or "Trouble"

Subjective: "I don't know what "it" could be; my trouble started 2−3 months ago."

Objective: No data at this time.

Assessment: Pt is avoiding or putting off facing the full implications of his disease; if a phenomenon stays unmentioned, the phenomenon is less real and therefore less threatening. Change in descriptive phrases may indicate changes in meaning of disease to pt.

Plan: Listen to and record phrases pt uses to describe illness.

Problem 3: Possibility of Surgery

Subjective: "I wasn't ready to have an operation. I may go home to have it, if it's recommended. I want to know what sensations to expect and what I need to do."

Objective: Surgery not scheduled yet.

Assessment: A pt can cooperate better if he knows what he's supposed to do and will be less frightened by strange sensations if he knows what to expect.

Plan: Will write out the preop teaching I will do when surgery is scheduled. Will ask pt if he has any questions about what I tell him or what the doctors have told him. Will ask pt to cough so I can examine sputum: will listen to breath sounds in AM to see how clear lungs are.

Problem 4: "Constipated" if Lies Around

Subjective: "I don't have any problems unless I lie around like I'm doing now."

Objective: Has a MOM order, activity ad lib, regular diet.

Assessment: Want to prevent constipation or impaction while pt undergoes diagnosis and treatment.

Plan: Ask pt tomorrow after breakfast if he had a BM and chart on bedside graphic sheet. Ask about eating and drinking patterns to see if diet will assist with prevention.

Problem 5: Dry Skin

Subjective: No comments made about his skin.

Objective: Skin on arms and legs felt dry to me.

Assessment: Dry skin is more susceptible to breakdown than moist skin.

Plan: Ask if patient has lotion at bedside and ask him to use it on arms and legs qd after bath. Feel pt's skin qd to see if softness has increased. C. Hayes, R.N.

10-30-74   1:30 PM

Problem 1: Incomplete Data Base

Subjective:
1. "I have 2 sons—one in Winter Haven and one in Key West. I have no concerns about my family or about my business. I only want to get well."
2. "I didn't finish college—quit after 2 years."
3. Breathes with abdominal muscles.
4. Takes shower and shaves night before bed. Is shaving and bathing in am here in hospital; says skin is too sensitive to shave in am and then go outside.
5. Brushes teeth with paste 3−4 times a day. Sleeps with teeth in. Takes them out only when told to.
6. Walk (gait) is steady, no limitations in ROM.
7. Figures he'll usually get what he needs, or he works for what he wants, "I've missed out on some things because I wouldn't ask for help."

Objective: Conversed with pt and obtained above info.

Assessment: No comment at this time.
Plan: Continue to collect data per initial plan.

Problem 2: Illness Is "It" or "Trouble"

Subjective: "I feel much better than when I came in here. I was really depressed. Maybe this will turn out to be only a fungus instead of something more serious meaning losing a lung or part of a lung. The thing is, I don't feel sick. I was really dreading test yesterday, but it wasn't so bad."
Objective: Looked at me when talking, rubbed hands together. Coughed and cleared throat 2−3 times. Moved around more when talking about "fungus" and losing lung.
Assessment: He is talking more specifically about disease, but is hoping it will not be too bad. Maybe hoping it won't be cancer?
Plan: Continue initial plan of care. Chart feelings in this problem unless they belong specifically to another problem.

Problem 3: Possibility of Surgery

Subjective: "I still have to decide, if surgery is recommended, whether to have it here or in South. I don't know what I'll do."
Objective: Awaiting results of bronchoscopy. Auscultation—faint breath sounds at apices R=L. Louder sounds toward bases; seem diminished on right. Maybe some rales right axillary line—not sure. Did not see sputum.
Assessment: No comment today.
Plan: Await decision to operate; chart comments from pt about surgery in this problem.

Problem 4: "Constipated" if Lies Around

Subjective: "I'm all taken care of. Moved my bowels about an hour ago—took some prune juice this morning." Eating and drinking patterns: coffee and cereal (6:30−7:00 AM); an egg, grits, and toast after getting to work (9:00−10:00 AM); lunch between 2:00−3:00 PM: meat, 1−2 vegetables; dinner 7:30 PM: meat, vegetables; eats preserved figs and biscuits at least once a day. Drinks 1−2 qt water, 5−6 cups coffee qd.
Objective: No data except to tell pt he had a laxative order.

Assessment: Pre-hospital diet adequate to prevent constipation, seems to be managing this one himself.
Plan D/C problem. Ask about BM and record on graphic. Reactivate if pt needs help.

Plan 5: Dry Skin

Subjective: No, I haven't been using lotion.
Objective: Has lotion at bedside. Skin smooth and soft on arms; legs not observed.
Assessment: Think skin is not as dry as I thought it was yesterday.
Plan: Look at skin tomorrow; if still smooth and soft, d/c problem. C. Hayes, R.N.

10-31-74   1:35 pm

Problem 1: Incomplete Data Base

Subjective: "I'm right handed."
Objective: Asked question.
Assessment: As long as pt is doing things for himself, I will probably not obtain rest of data. If he is scheduled for surgery, I will try to complete data base.
Plan: Record any data obtained during interaction with pt.

Problem 2: Illness Is "It" or "Trouble"

Subjective: "I just wish I knew what to do. I keep thinking maybe it's a fungus left over from my pneumonia. I know that can happen. I keep hoping it won't come to having surgery, but I'm afraid it will. I don't know why I'm so scared of an operation. I'm not usually afraid of things. Afraid of what they'll find, of kicking the bucket, of not being able to be fixed up. I've got things to straighten out, like stocks and bonds my wife doesn't know about; we've never talked about them. If I go home (like for the weekend) I'd never come back. No, I'm not ready to talk about it yet."
Objective: Used reflection technique.
Assessment: Am almost sure pt is thinking he has cancer but doesn't want to think about it and therefore is not ready to talk about it yet.
Plan: Continue to listen and record.

Problem 3: Possibility of Surgery

Subjective: See problem 2. "Can you tell me when those x-rays are scheduled?"
Objective: Going to have quantitative lung scan tomorrow.
Assessment: Work-up continues; comments regarding surgery seemed more appropriate under problem 2 today.
(Problem 5 not evaluated today. Will do tomorrow.) C. Hayes, R.N.

11-1-74   1:00 PM

Problem 1: Incomplete Data Base

No data obtained today.

Problem 2: Illness Is "It" or "Trouble"

Subjective: "I had that scan today. I think it's a fungus. I've been told everything's negative so far. I'm afraid it will come to surgery if nothing definite is found. That's the way it was at the other hospital."
Objective: Smiled, looked away, shifted position, and shook head yes when I said, to his comment about fungus "and trying not to think about the other things it can be, right?"
Assessment: Still unable to consider possible diagnoses other than fungus.
Plan: Continue

Problem 3: Possibility of Surgery

No additional data today.

Problem 5: Dry Skin

Subjective: "I guess it is kind of dry; yes, I could use the lotion each day. I haven't been using it."
Objective: Skin is mildly dry, some white flaking on legs. Asked pt to use lotion qd p̄ bathing.
Assessment: No comment. Can't evaluate effectiveness of lotion until pt uses it.
Plan: Evaluate on 11-4-74

11-4-74   11:20 AM

Problem 1: Incomplete Data Base

No additional data collected today.

Problem 2: Illness Is "It" or "Trouble"

Subjective: "I was disappointed I couldn't go home. There is something there; they've got a couple more tests planned. The pain I have is like a sore throat. That's what I think it is. It's just next to my windpipe here and goes toward my R ear and over the top of my head. I've been to a chiropractor and three EENT specialists to find out the trouble. I think that's what's making the mucous. The ear doctor here is going to look at it, I think. They gave me skin tests. They don't show anything, I don't think. My x-rays from Friday were misplaced, so Dr. Green couldn't talk to me Sat. like he said he would. I'd like to get better and get out of here."
Objective: Pointed to throat area that is sore, showed areas of skin testing, rubbed hands together and looked at them q 2−3 minutes, coughed 2−3 times, wheezey sound, forceful. Used word fungus and mentioned lung, I think, in regard to x-rays; pt has yet to mention lung to me specifically.
Assessment: Continues to avoid speaking of his disease specifically. I have a feeling he is thinking about it a lot, but can't talk about it, at least not with me. Don't know if he is discussing more specific possibilities with his wife or not.
Plan: Continue initial plan.

Problem 3: Possibility of Surgery

Subjective: No comment.
Objective: When pt talked about further tests, I did not ask about surgery. Dr. Smith says doctors are thinking of an expl. thoracotomy on 11-6-74 or 11-7-74 if diagnostic work-up can be completed.
Assessment: Think pt will be upset to have surgery but will do what he has to do to get better.
Plan: Do preop teaching 11-5-74 (if surgery is scheduled). C. Hayes, R.N.

NURSING DISCHARGE SUMMARY

11-5-74   10:30 AM

This was the first STH admission for Albert B. Cero. He was here for diagnosis of a suspicious area in his lung. Pt was able to do all his own physical care when he was admitted and when he was discharged. A nursing history was never completed. The unobtainable data are listed in the chart and could be obtained on a subsequent admission. The most outstanding features, to me, with Mr. Cero were his appearance, at least, of independence and his lack of putting any name other than "fungus" to his illness. He never told me his problem was related to his lung. I knew it was and never specifically asked, but I found it interesting that he never spontaneously mentioned it. I had a feeling never fully validated, that he thought a lot about having cancer but could not talk about it, at least not with me. This was the main problem we worked on. I did not see him the day of discharge, so I do not know his reaction (feelings and thoughts) to the diagnosis. No further nursing care is needed at this time. C. Hayes, R.N.

(Discharge summary not written according to SOAP format as recommended in next chapter)

REFERENCES

1. Becknell, E., and Smith, D. M.: *System of Nursing Practice.* Philadelphia, F. A. Davis Co., 1975 p. 74.
2. *Ibid.,* p. 16.
3. *Ibid.,* p. 165.
4. Gebbie, K. M. and Lavin, M. A., (ed.): *Classification of Nursing Diagnoses.* Proceedings of the First National Conference, St. Louis, C. V. Mosby Co., 1975.
5. Becknell and Smith, p. 68.
6. Mitchell, P. H.: *Concepts Basic to Nursing,* 2nd ed. New York, McGraw-Hill Book Co., 1977, p. 82.
7. Becknell and Smith, p. 95.
8. *Ibid.,* p. 92.
9. *Ibid.,* p. 88.
10. *Ibid.,* p. 69.

CHAPTER 25

The communication system in a health care agency is the last link in the nursing care plan. If the plan is not communicated verbally and in writing, it will not be possible to completely and accurately inform all concerned.

When information is obtained from a client by a professional person, moral and legal obligations exist to keep that information confidential—to be shared only with others who also are involved in his care. It should not become gossip shared over a cup of coffee, discussed in an elevator, or in one's dormitory with nonmedical personnel. This can sometimes be a burden, but if the nurse feels a need, she can confide in her supervisor or teachers. The material in a client's chart should be factual or if speculative, clearly identified as such. Conclusions are based on data, and there should be opportunities for others to add additional data and make their own conclusions.

A record can be subpoenaed as evidence in a court of law; therefore, the information it contains can be the basis for questioning and decision-making. Consequently, the record should be exact. Un-

COMMUNICATION

Carol V. Hayes, M.Ed., R.N.

fortunately, there are innumerable ways in which the chart can be unclear. For example, as many as three or four ages for the client may be recorded; descriptions of wounds and their locations may vary; variable methods of recording dates may be used, or dates and times may be omitted altogether. Writing is often illegible, with misspelled words and confusing time sequences. Phrases like "ate well," "activity tolerated well," "poor day," "vital signs stable," are used without description or specificity.

CHARTING

Nursing Notes

Kerr, in her excellent article on the legal implications of nurses' notes, stated the reasons why these notes are so important.

1. When orders are written, the nurses' notes hold the only clue as to whether the orders were carried out and what the results were.

2. Nurses' notes are the only notes written with both time and date and strictly in chronological order. Since several people chart on each chart, each must get his charting done promptly in order to have the record chronological.
3. They also offer the most detailed information regarding the patient.[1]

Kerr also discussed the importance of charting on each line rather than squeezing information between lines. "Most important of all, your records must tell the truth. Nothing will make a hot seat of the witness chair any faster than to have written something that someone else can prove was not true. Make your notes as factual as possible."[2] She gave a brief guide for the observations to record. "Write what you see, . . . write what you hear, . . . write what you smell, . . . write what you feel"[2] (by palpation not emotion). She also cautioned against the use of "basket terms," such as "good night," "feeling better than yesterday," "patient is restless," because of the variety of meanings these terms can have. "When you write a conclusion, your charting has changed from a record of factual observations to a record of your opinions. Personal opinions have no place on a medical record. You are in real jeopardy if you put yourself in the position of having made a medical opinion. Even so-called nursing opinions can cause trouble. If you make it a habit to write facts instead of conclusions, you will allow those who review your notes to come to the same conclusions you have, but you will never have to explain to any attorney how you came to that conclusion without any documentation to substantiate your opinion."[2] For example, it is better to chart subcutaneous crepitus—an observation, that is, something one can feel or hear—rather than subcutaneous emphysema, which is a diagnosis.[2]

A well-written note is a pleasure to read; a poorly written note is frightening. It takes time, concentration, knowledge, skill, and proofreading to write an *accurate* record, but this is a responsibility all nurses have. If you "have always been a poor speller," then carry a pocket dictionary; if you have always had poor handwriting, then practice writing legibly, allowing enough time to write slowly so it can be read.

Symbols and Abbreviations

The chart is not the place to exercise creativity in the use of symbols and abbreviations. Each agency usually has a list of acceptable abbreviations similar to those in Table 25-1. While this list is not exhaustive, it is quite representative. These abbrevi-

TABLE 25-1. Abbreviations

Abbreviation	Meaning	Abbreviation	Meaning
a	before	MOM	milk of magnesia
aa	of each	N/G	nasogastric
ac	before meals	NPO	nothing by mouth
ad lib	as desired	OOB	out of bed
AM	morning	OD	right eye
bid	twice each day	OS	left eye
BM	bowel movement	OT	occupational therapy
BP	blood pressure	OU	both eyes
BR	bathroom	oz	ounce(s)
BRP	bathroom privileges	p̄	after
c̄	with	pc	after meals
C	centigrade	po	by mouth
cc	cubic centimeter	PM	afternoon
cm	centimeter	PRN	whenever necessary
ECG	(also EKG) electrocardiogram	pt	pint
EEG	electroencephalogram	PT	physical therapy
fl	fluid	q	every
gal	gallon	qd	every day
Gm	gram	qh	every hour
gr	grain	qid	four times daily
gtt	drop	qod	every other day
H or hr	hour	qt	quart
hs	hour of sleep	ROM	range of motion
ht	height	RT	radiotherapy or radiation therapy
ICU	intensive care unit	Rx	treatment or therapy
IM	intramuscularly	s̄	without
I and O	intake and output	sc	subcutaneous
IPPB	intermittent positive pressure breathing	SOB	shortness of breath
IV	intravenously; also used to refer to the intravenous infusion set-up	s̄s̄	one half
		stat	at once
Kg	kilogram	Tbsp	tablespoon
L	liter	tid	three times daily
lb	pound	TPR	temperature, pulse, and respiration
mg	milligram	VS	vital signs
ml	milliliter	wt	weight
mm	millimeter		

Adapted from Becknell, E., and Smith, D.: *System of Nursing Practice.* Philadelphia, F. A. Davis Co., 1975, pp. 167–168.

ations are understood by others in the medical field so they have communication value. Abbreviations that are idiosyncratic to the writer destroy the communication attempt and thus the point is lost for which they were intended.

Most charts are written in what is known as telegraphic style. Short phrases or incomplete sentences are used to cut down on space and redundancy. Generally, the subject of the sentence is understood to be the client so the word "client" rarely needs to be used. However, if other family members or health workers have been referred to, then the word "client" will have to be repeated to make the sense clear to the reader; for example: "Has living father, one sister and one brother. Client lives alone." If "client" was not used in this case, it would be unclear as to who lived alone, the client or his brother.

Because the chart is a legal record, erasures and other obliterations are prohibited. If an error is made, a single line is drawn through it, and the word "error" is written above immediately followed by the writer's initials; the note is then continued with the correct material. Erasures or obscuring a word with ink could be questioned if the chart is used as evidence in a law suit.[3] Some beginning students write out a rough draft of their charting to correct the errors that are bound to occur initially. However, because there is not always enough time, it is better not to depend on a rough draft. It is most efficient to think through a note and write it correctly the first time. Instructors vary in their requirements, so students will have to find out which method is expected of them.

Necessary Information

The client's hospital record contains material which the nurse should not only understand but also know how to find and use. The sequence will vary among institutions or agencies as will the forms used, but the substance is essentially the same. The data which can be found in most client records are listed in Table 25-2. It is suggested that the student compare this information with that found in her client's record, looking for differences and similarities in how the data are recorded and the forms that are used.

Agencies have different policies regarding the color of ink and how often a nursing note has to

TABLE 25-2. Data Found in Most Client Records

Medical history and physical examination
Nursing history and plan of care
Physicians' orders
Laboratory and x-ray results
Reports of operations
Medical and nursing progress notes
Consultation reports including dietary, occupational, and physical therapies as well as other physicians
Medication, vital signs, and intake and output records
Flow sheets and checklists
Emergency room records
Identifying information from the patient, such as name, address, insurance policy numbers, next of kin
Permission sheets for various procedures

occur on a chart. There are times when a note must occur: for example, on admission; when the client has returned from a diagnostic procedure or the operating room; when he declines any ordered treatment or medication; when an abnormality occurs; and when measures do not produce the expected result (e.g., pain medication offers no relief or a sleeping medication does not result in sleep). If the client is involved in any accident, that should be described. In the Problem-Oriented System of Charting, many of these notes would be related to problems. Sometimes a specific problem has not been identified; in these instances either a problem is identified or the note is entitled "Additional Data," and the SOAP format (Subjective, Objective, Assessment, and Plan categories) is applied. All notes must have a complete date, the time the note was written, and a signature which consists of first initial, last name, and status of the writer. The signature should be placed just below the body of the note so that no one can enter in additional material. If the note and signature do not take the entire space, a line should be drawn from the signature to the edge of the page.

Note Format

Notes can take several forms, and each agency has a system to follow. Notes can be described by the title of the person who writes them, such as nurses' or physicians' progress notes, or by the style, such as narrative notes or SOAP notes. Nurses and physicians can write separate narrative or SOAP notes or they can write joint progress notes, either in a narrative or SOAP format. A narrative note is written in paragraph form with no specific form to it—

that is, there is no attempt to separate portions of the note. It often includes several topics, and if not carefully written, can be difficult to follow, or so general as to be meaningless.

Many agencies are now using the Problem-Oriented System as developed by Weed.[6] This is a logical system with specific rules which, when followed, gives a complete picture of the client. It is based on a complete data base (or an acknowledgment of an incomplete data base). From the data base, however it is defined by the agency or group of practitioners, client problems are identified.

There can be one or more problem lists and set of progress notes; that is, one for nursing and one for medicine. A combined list is the ideal situation for giving a comprehensive, nonrepetitious picture of the client. In agencies where there is only one list and one set of progress notes, the physician is usually responsible for the final, permanent problem list; however, all health team members contribute to the "working problem list" and chart in the progress notes. The Appendix illustrates a nursing problem list and progress notes.

After the data base is obtained, it should be reviewed for the problems the client has that will require attention from nursing and other health care workers as discussed in Chapter 23 and 24. Problem statements are not easy to write, but it is important to learn to record these well as the rest of the system follows from the problem statement. On the other hand, the client's care can not be held up while the perfect statement is composed. State the problem in the best way possible; when further data are obtained, the statement may be rewritten and the title changed.

PROBLEM-ORIENTED SYSTEM OF CHARTING

SOAP Format

The plan of care is written in the SOAP format, pulling together all the data from various parts of the history that relate to one problem and set the rationale for the problem. If there are no data to support a problem, then maybe one does not exist and the statement of the problem is hypothetical or from a textbook rather than from the client. *S* stands for the subjective category which contains all the things the client says, such as his feelings,

ideas, pain, and his report of events. The purpose of this category is to capture the client's point of view. *O* stands for the objective category, including those things that can be measured, validated, observed, and described. Actions taken by the nurse, reports of consultations with other health care workers, physician's orders and progress notes, and comments from the client's relatives or other visitors are also recorded here. *A* stands for the assessment category which contains the conclusions drawn from the subjective and objective data. Because this is the intellectual component of the note, it does not include data but statements from texts or research literature which are the rationale for the conclusions drawn or the plan to be followed. It also includes the diagnosis, the reason why something is going to be done, and hypotheses about the meaning of the data. *P* stands for the plan of care section and includes objectives, goals, specific nursing directions for the client's care, his education, or directions to collect further data.[5]

Initial Plan

In the initial plan of care, the subjective data are those things the client said in the nursing history. The objective data are the observations made during the history, the physical examination findings obtained by the nurse or doctor, the medical orders that exist at the time which will help or hinder the solution of the problem, and the laboratory data. (If the nurse has seen the client before the physician, there may be no medical orders; in this case, the plan would contain nursing orders to obtain medical orders rather than orders to administer them.) The assessment category contains the nurse's thoughts about the meaning of the data and the conclusions she can draw from these data. If there has been comment from the client about "fluttery, uneasy feelings inside, feels scared most of the time," with objective data along the lines of "swinging legs, smoked six cigarettes in 1 hour, scratching arms and legs every 2—3 minutes; no visible rash or lesions on skin" the assessment can then be "feeling anxious." It is not a correct assessment *to repeat* merely what the client said. In the above example, conceivably the client could have said, "I feel so anxious all the time." Objective data could be the same; assessment now has to be something other than "feeling anxious," as the client has said that already. In this instance the assessment might be a hypothesis as to the cause of anxiety or a statement about the effect of his anxiety on other parts of his care. It is also possible, that data are too scarce initially to draw any conclusions in which case, a comment to that effect is made.

Specific Plan

Once the assessment is complete with all possible meanings likely for the data available, the specific plan for the problem is written. Its success depends on those things covered in Chapter 24. If time is limited, it may only include the immediate actions to be taken, with additional actions to be added at a later date. However, if possible, it should include all those things thought to be appropriate to solve the problem. If the writer lacks knowledge about a particular problem and techniques to solve it, the plan should say "Go to library and read about prevention of joint deformities in paralysis." Also it should state that the nurse is going to consult a dietician, social worker, or minister, as well as the criteria by which the problem will be evaluated and the frequency of charting that will be done on a particular problem.

The plan guides the activities of the nurse in her subsequent visits with the client. If she has done her work thoroughly in writing the initial plan and the client's condition is relatively stable, her work flows rather easily, and it is not too time consuming to write progress notes which are the next part of the Problem-Oriented System.

Progress Notes

Progress notes contain the documentation of the care administered. If it is not recorded that the plan of care has been carried out, it is as if it was not, and the effect of nursing on the progress of the client has been lost. The data in progress notes validate the suitability of the plan or offer clues as to how the plan must be changed. Progress notes are also written in the SOAP format. The subjective data category now contains the client's comments about the problem since the nurse last saw him. If he does not spontaneously offer the data desired, the nurse should ask questions to elicit it. She decides when she writes the plan of care what data she is going to need to evaluate the problem. He can tell her about his pain, his feelings, his worries, his understanding of his illness, his schedule, various tests, operation and sequence of events, how he slept, how much he ate, and his appetite. The objective data can be most simply stated as "carried out initial plan," if indeed that is what the nurse has done. If she had plans for teaching the client a new skill or informing him about his operation and surrounding events in which she had stated the exact content she was going to cover (and she covered it as she had written it), then she does not repeat it. If there have been any exceptions (additions or deletions), those should be charted. If there are none, she merely charts, "Carried out initial plan." Objective data are any medical orders that are different from the ones available when the initial plan was written; any observations of the client's behavior that corroborates or contradicts his statements in the subjective category, medications taken that relate to the problem or validate the client's statements, as well as direct observations made of the portion of the body with which the problem is concerned such as wounds, decubiti, phlebitis, edema, or pulses. If the client has had a test, operation, or other procedure, and the nurse wants to record that, it goes in this category. Again, the assessment category contains the conclusion which can be drawn from the two data categories. Comments about improving, doing better, normality, abnormality as well as more standard diagnostic type phrases such as anxiety, depression, or healing go in this category. No data should appear in this category; nothing can be mentioned that has not been alluded to previously in the data categories. Incorrect and correct assessments are illustrated in some of the examples of SOAP charting which follow. The plan section either contains "continue plan" or the changes that are necessary based on the data and assessment. The plan is what is going to be done, not what has been done. (That is now objective data.) The nursing directions in the plan fall into one of three categories, of which the nurse should be aware when she is writing her directions:

1. Plans for collection of additional data to better define a problem or facilitate its management.
2. Plans for dissemination of information pertinent to the management of a problem.
3. Plans for the nursing "treatment" of a problem.[6]

When the nurse is going to collect data, she needs to state exactly what data are to be gathered, how, when and from what source.[6] Dissemination of information includes teaching clients and families. When this is the plan, "precisely what information is to be imparted to whom, how, when, and by whom must be written. When appropriate, the plan should include what is expected of the individual as a result of receiving the information."[7] Plans for the nursing "treatment" of a problem include all the material about nursing objectives and orders discussed in the previous chapter; in fact all the things related to the plan of care cited in the former chapter apply to this part of the Problem-Oriented System.

Charting Examples

I. Subjective data in objective category
  A. *Objective*: Experienced pain when abdomen palpated; moved leg freely without pain.

   Comment: Pain is always a subjective experience or a conclusion. In the above example, objective data might be the patient's facial expression or bodily movements when the abdomen was palpated or the leg was moved.

II. Assessments without data to support them
  A. *Problem 1*: Pain in lower left abdomen
   Subjective: Says he's had pain in L lower abdomen since last evening. It is a constant, dull burning sensation.
   Objective: Demerol 50 MgIM q4h prn available for pain. Charted as having been taken three times in past 24 hours. Points to area lateral to umbilicus, takes deep breath, and closes eyes tightly when abdomen touched.
   Assessment: Is being treated for diverticulitis but has normal hematocrit and white blood count so observation is very important.
   Plan: Ask patient to report any change in location or character of pain. (Not intended to be a complete plan for this problem).

   Comment: "Normal" is a conclusion. In order to conclude that the hematocrit and white blood count are normal, the most recent laboratory figures have to

be mentioned in the objective data category and in this instance they are not.
  B. *Problem 2*: Expects surgery
   Subjective: No data.
   Objective: Patient went to surgery at 12:00 noon for simple unilateral mastectomy. Nursing history was obtained this AM. Patient had preop teaching consisting of turning, coughing, deep breathing, and their purposes, possible tubes she may have, such as IV, Foley catheter or Hemovac. She was informed of decreased arm mobility and the importance that exercises will have.
   Assessment: Patient seems prepared psychologically and emotionally for her surgery.
   Plan: Ask patient postoperatively if her preop instruction helped decrease her anxiety. (Not intended to be a complete plan.)

   Comment: Without subjective data to indicate the patient's feelings or state of emotional health, no conclusion about her psychological preparation can be drawn in the assessment category.

III. Nursing orders (plans of care) that are not specific. (These do not all relate to the same problem.)
  A. *Plan*: (1) Teach patient about exercises and range of motion. (2) Watch for abscess formation. (3) Watch for fistula formation to bladder or other adjacent organs. (4) Observe carefully for signs of infection. (5) Encourage patient to exercise his leg four times a day. (6) Discuss diet.

   Comment: *Teach* is a broad term encompassing objectives, content, methods, and evaluation. Each of these need to be stated exactly so the reader knows what was attempted and how achievement would be known. *Watch for* and *observe* are usable words if their objects are specific. In the above examples, fistula and abscess formation are conclusions or diagnoses, not observations. One would "watch for" or "observe for" redness, heat, swelling, listen for patient's comments about increased pain. The data to be collected should be stated exactly so that each reader knows what to look for. In that way complete data can be obtained.

IV. Conclusion in objective data category

A. *Problem 3*: Anxiety

Subjective: "I really feel good especially since the Reach for Recovery lady was in."

Objective: Pt (patient) shows no signs of anxiety or depression; was laughing and joking with doctors on rounds this morning. Reach for Recovery volunteer was in today and instructed pt on exercises and bra comfort.

Assessment: Pt appears in good spirits and eager to get well.

Plan: Continue to monitor pt for signs of anxiety.

Comment: "Pt shows no signs of anxiety or depression" is a conclusion, not a description. To avoid this kind of error, the nurse needs to ask herself, "What did I observe to lead me to this conclusion?" In this example, the nurse has also written the behavior and she could have saved herself time by not putting the conclusion in the incorrect category. She now has a repetition between the objective and assessment categories and when this occurs, one of the categories is incorrect—in this instance, the objective category. The comment in the assessment category is correct, although whether there are data to support the "eager to get well" conclusion could be debated.

A better example of conclusions in the objective category rather than description is the next one.

B. *Problem 4*: Right arm edema

Subjective: No data.

Objective: No further increase in edema; edema is decreased. No symptoms of infection.

Assessment: Arm is doing well.

Plan: Continue to monitor patient for an increase in edema.

Comment: "Increase," "decrease," and "no symptoms of infection" are all conclusions. What is the circumference of the arm? What does the arm look like in terms of redness, or drainage, or feel like in terms of temperature? Those are the data the nurse needs in the objective category, then the conclusions she has can be placed in the assessment category. This note is also an illustration of an inadequate plan. How will the nurse monitor for an increase in edema? Will she use the patient's verbal statement that the arm is more or less swollen on a particular day? Will she use her own eyes, and say it looks more or less swollen? Will she measure the arm at particular places on specific days? The latter plan, of course, is the most specific one.

V. Correctly written progress note.

A. *Problem 2*: Tentative surgery

Subjective: "I think I understand about the operation now, and a nurse from the intensive care unit came down to my room to explain what goes on in the unit."

Objective: Carried out initial plan (which is a specific detailed plan of what is expected of the patient, sequence of events, sensations he will experience).

Assessment: Pt seems adequately prepared for surgery.

Plan: Following surgery debrief the pt by asking him if the preop teaching was beneficial in preparing him, if anything happened which wasn't expected and how he feels the surgery went.

Comment: This note has the data in the correct categories, the assessment is based on data and the plan is specific (see Appendix for other examples of progress notes).

Discharge Summary

The last part of the Problem-Oriented System is the discharge summary. It is a summary of the client's care and recommendations for further care. It can serve as a source of written instructions for the family or personnel in another hospital or extended care facility if the client is transferred; it also can be the nursing referral for the public health nurse. The nurse must review the entire record when writing the discharge note and thus "she may see relationships and gain insights that were not evident to her at an earlier time."[8] The content of the note will depend to some degree on the client and his condition. If the note is serving as a referral to community or institutional personnel, more information will be needed about ways that have been helpful in working with the client, his family or significant others as well as the interactions between the client and his family than if the client is being discharged home without need for further assistance at this time.[8] Institutions may have a form to fill out, or one can be written according to the format used in the illustration at the end of this chapter.

If the Problem-Oriented System is being used, the discharge summary is written according to the problems identified from the data presented by the client. Resolved problems are merely listed by title and number, the date first noted and the date resolved. Problems that are still active are summarized in SOAP format; recommendations for further care are placed in the Plan Section.[9] An "other recommendations" section[10] can be used not only for suggestions and assessment of continuing care that do not fit under specific problems such as who will be assuming primary responsibility,[10] but also for a statement of the client's present status of self-care that also does not fit into a particular problem. For example, the statement might be "Client and his wife will be assuming responsibility for care upon discharge. No specific care is needed so no problems are anticipated. Client can do all his own physical care and has regained pre-hospitalization eating, sleeping, and eliminating patterns."

Discharge planning starts upon admission of the client to the agency or institution by gathering data pertinent to the home situation. As the client's care progresses, it becomes clearer what his limitations and needs might be for care after discharge. As soon as the needs are known, investigation has to occur into the details of the home and community resources if these data are not complete. For example, who is at home to assist the client with ambulation, food preparation, or toileting if he is unable to do any of these alone? Are there funds for a continuing supply of bandages or medications? Does a local social agency have to be contacted for assistance? Can the client even go home? Maybe a nursing home would be best and so forth. Unless the hospital nurse follows a client to home, she will have to make a referral to a public health or visiting nurse. The following criteria warrant a public health referral:

1. Open wound requiring dressing change.
2. Change in function:
   a. colostomy, ileostomy, ileoconduit.
   b. amputation.
   c. diabetes.
   d. motherhood.
   e. stroke.
   f. terminal illness.
3. Client hospitalized for a long time who lives alone.
4. Client confined to bed for one reason or another.

The above list is not meant to represent all the circumstances for which a referral might be made. There could be any number of other reasons for a referral. The hospital care of the client is not complete until it is clear that he is going to have the care he needs at home. It takes skill on the part of the nurse to plan her care in such a way as to have the client ready for discharge by the time the doctor decides it is time for him to go home. Too often, without collaboration with the nurse, the doctor discharges the client because he is surgically healed, or medically well and the nurse is left to complete her discharge planning and implement her plan as quickly as possible. In the ideal situation, the nurse and physician plan together and with other health team members for the discharge of the client, each aware of the others' objectives of care, and the degree of attainment achieved. In this way the client receives complete care and the nurse, physician and health team have met their professional responsibilities. For a more detailed look at discharge planning and process see Chapter 45.

OTHER METHODS OF HOSPITAL COMMUNICATION

Flow Sheet

One other form of chart material exists in the Problem-Oriented System and that is called a flow sheet (Fig. 25-1). This is a sheet that can be used to record rapidly changing data or when one wants to see the relationship between numerous data. Intensive Care Units almost always use flow sheets on which to record frequent vital signs, IV intake, urinary output, blood gas results, and levels of consciousness. It would be entirely too time consuming to record these data in narrative or problem-oriented notes each time they are collected. Also, the relationships between the various data would not be so obvious. At the end of an 8 hour or longer period of time, the data can be summarized in regular problem-oriented fashion. Weights, measurements of a decubitus, or an edematous limb are other kinds of data that lend themselves to a flow sheet and periodic summary.

Bedside Checklist

Related to flow sheets are bedside checklists on which standard expected nursing techniques are listed and against which the nurse or auxiliary personnel can place a mark when the technique is carried out (Fig. 25-2). Many techniques lend themselves to this method of charting from bed baths to ambulations, to Foley catheter care and even preoperative teaching. These things are done regardless of what is wrong with the client or whether he wants to know or not. Certain items, such as Foley catheters, nasogastric or chest tubes, and even intravenous feedings require care from the nurse to insure proper functioning. The care required is fairly standard, varying only slightly from institution to institution; however, it is the same in all situations within an institution or agency.

When care depends on an item instead of the individuality of the client, the particulars of care can be written in a procedure book, rather than repeated on each client's chart, and the item can be checked off on the bedside checklist with the understanding that the care was given as established by the nursing service department of the agency. The particulars of care can be called criteria, and it is understood that if the item is checked off, the criteria have been met. For example, the criteria for appropriate Foley catheter care are as follows: the drainage bag hangs below the bladder; the tubing is free of kinks; the catheter is taped to the thigh; the meatus is cleansed each day with an appropriate antiseptic, such as betadine, the client's fluid intake is between 2500–3000 ml (assuming no medical orders for fluid restriction, including NPO).

Each time the catheter is checked off on the bedside checklist, it is assumed the above criteria have been met. Nasogastric tubes, chest tubes, IV's, and wounds all lend themselves to having specific criteria developed and then charting of their care is a check mark next to the item rather than writing the specific care given each day. Routine hygienic care, activity, diet orders also lend themselves to a checklist format as the example of a checklist illustrates. The written portion of the chart then becomes pertinent data about the client not a list of activities carried out.

Often specific directions for care are written out from the chart and left at the bedside so each worker knows how to do the particular care and does not have to ask the client how it should be done. Fluid plans, dressing changes, how to achieve particular positions in bed, various rituals the client may have are some of the care items that lend themselves to this technique.

Kardex

The Kardex is yet another form of communication. This particular format varies from agency to agency, but its purpose is to provide an up-to-date copy of the physician's orders on each client so the nurse does not have to consult each chart each day. The physician's orders are transcribed from the order sheet to the Kardex by a ward clerk with discontinued orders being erased. Many times the Kardex also contains the nursing care plan, the objectives, and nursing orders (Fig. 25-3).

Verbal Communication

The above discussion concerns the written forms of communication most often used in health care agencies. There are also verbal forms of communication used. These are shift reports and team conferences. A shift report is given by nurses going off duty to the nurses coming on duty to provide continuity of care. The nurse going off duty describes the current condition of each client, their orders, and any events that might be anticipated on the next shift. Special concerns of the client are often discussed, and specific care needs may be pointed out. The format and content can vary from place to place.

A team conference is usually for the purpose of

THOMAS JEFFERSON UNIVERSITY HOSPITAL
CRITICAL CARE FLOW SHEET

Part 1

Date _____   Weight _____

ADDRESSOGRAPH

TIME	TEMP.	Heart Rate / Rhythm	RESP.	PRESSURES									MEDICATIONS
				B.P. Cuff									

FIGURE 25-1. Critical Care Flow Sheet, Part 1. (Reprinted with permission of Thomas Jefferson University Hospital, Philadelphia.)

THOMAS JEFFERSON UNIVERSITY HOSPITAL   Part 2
CRITICAL CARE FLOW SHEET

IV SOLUTION and MEDS	Time up	7 - 3	3 - 11	11 - 7

ADDRESSOGRAPH

VENTILATION DATA				ABG'S						INTAKE							OUTPUT				
TYPE	% O₂	Tidal Vol.	PEEP / IMV	pH	pO₂	PCO₂	HCO₃	O₂ Sat.		PO	IV	IV	IV		Blood Plasma		CHEST TUBES / Hr / Total	URINE / Hr / SP. GR			

24 Hour Intake

24 Hour Output

FIGURE 25-1. Critical Care Flow Sheet, Part 2.

SHANDS TEACHING HOSPITAL AND CLINICS
GAINESVILLE, FLORIDA
NURSING CHECK LIST

	DATE															
	TIME	N	D	E	N	D	E	N	D	E	N	D	E	N	D	E
Bath	Self Bed Bath															
	Partial Bed Bath															
	Bed Bath By Nurse															
	Tub - Shower															
Activity	Bedrest															
	Chair How Long?															
	Ambulant															
	Ambulant With Help															
	Dangled How Long?															
	Weight															
	Evening Care															
Specimens Tests Therapies																
Treatments																
	Initials - Signature															
Food Taken	Type															
	Total															
	Partial															
	None															
	Signature - Days															
	Signature - Evenings															
	Signature - Nights															

15-0373-0

FIGURE 25-2. Bedside checklist. (Reprinted with permission of Shands Teaching Hospital and Clinics, Gainesville, Florida.)

discussing the nursing care of a specific client by the persons responsible for his care. The client may be presenting a nursing care challenge to the staff or have an unusual disease, new treatment, or none of these things. It may be the policy of that staff to discuss each client briefly at each conference to make sure all necessary care is being administered. Suggestions for care may be entered in the Kardex so that they are available to those unable to attend. Ideally such a conference occurs every day, but the work load often makes this impossible and fewer are held. Some meetings are held every week on each unit where one client, his concerns, and care are discussed. Often hospital-wide patient conferences are held once a month, the responsibility for which rotates from unit to unit. These conferences are a way to improve the care of clients and contribute to the continuing professional growth of the nurse.

Communication among health care professionals is very important. It should be done accurately, concisely yet completely, and utilizing whatever forms or methods are necessary to promote continuity of the client's care. An example of a nursing history, problem list, initial plan of care, progress notes with the addition of new problems and a discharge summary is presented in the Appendix.

APPENDIX

Nursing History

ADDRESSOGRAPH

2-21-78   9:10 AM

Vital statistics: This is the first STH* admission for 67-year-old white woman from north Florida.

Understanding of illness: "Doctor says I have a blockage in my artery right here (rubs right side of neck). I was having trouble with my legs and that's why I went to the doctor; in examining me, he found blockage. I think I have some vascular problems—numbness in fingers and legs don't work right—I attributed it to age. Since I've been here I've developed a lot more aches and pains. Maybe I haven't sat still at home so much. I keep

---

*Abbreviation for name of Hospital.

active. I don't go to the doctor right away. I can't stand to stay in bed. I'm like a yo-yo—up and down all the time." Trouble with leg—means like a cramp from hip on down; pain was short duration; had pain last week. Holds on so she won't fall and never has fallen from this. Has continued with own housework: cooking, light housework, working with potted plants. Has a constant pain from heart surgeries on lower L. rib cage. Starts around 10:00 AM: "my nerves start up by then; I'm a very nervous person. I have to keep busy. Nothing else to do about it." Has taken pills, but they put her in a "stupor," so she gets along the best she can. Takes Tylenol if she has a "touch of arthritis" (hands). (Did not go into heart surgery c̄ pt.)

Expectations: Going to have artery checked and maybe heart valve studied. "I didn't know valve could become abnormal." Otherwise don't know what will be done. "I'm a worrier, and I don't like being in hospital. I hope nothing has to be done to the valve." Hopes to be put in good shape again—as good as they can. "Don't want surgery if I can avoid it, but I don't want a stroke either. Hate to put my family through the ordeal of heart surgery again." Expectations of nurse: would like a softer mattress and to be in a room by herself—worries about roommate. Couldn't think of anything else.

Brief social-cultural history: Has worked outside home only once on Welcome Wagon. Otherwise has been a homemaker. Completed 2 years of college—didn't like it. Been married 45 yrs. Has two grown daughters. Lives with husband. No concerns about family. Family most significant. Wouldn't want to have to choose between husband and children.

Significant data in terms of:

1. *Sleeping pattern*: Retires 11:30 PM; arises 2:30–3:00 AM; reads for 2–3 hours then goes back to sleep until 9:00 AM. If sleeps all night, arises around 7:00 AM. No trouble going to sleep, but trouble staying asleep. "Don't know why—I'm just wide awake after a couple of hours. If I read until 2:00 AM, I'll sleep all night. I'll nap during the day in my chair so this pattern of sleep doesn't bother me." Drinks Sanka at 2:00 AM; no other pre-

Form 0007-00 (Each) (Rev. 8/28/70)

DIET	I & O	MISCELLANEOUS	A

WT.

BEDREST _____

BRP _____

OOB _____

SIDERAILS _____

FRACTIONALS

DRAINAGE DEVICES

COMPLETE CARE _____

PARTIAL _____

SELF _____

DATE OF
LAST RITES

ADDRESSOGRAPH

V.S.　　　TRANSPORT BY　　　CONDITION

DATE	PATIENT PROBLEMS	NURSING ORDERS	B

FIGURE 25-3A–D. Sample of a Kardex.

DATE	TREATMENTS	DATE	TREATMENTS	**C**

DATE
SURGERY   SERVICE

NAME   DR.   DX.   ROOM

NURSING SERVICE CARDEX SUPPLEMENT CARD   **D**

DATE	LABORATORY TESTS	DATE	STUDIES	DATE	DIAGNOSTIC PROCEDURES

NAME   FORM 0007-01(EA.)3/31/70 sleep rituals; also no meds. Feels she gets enough sleep. Uses two pillows (has own pillow c̄ her).

2. *Eliminating pattern:* Usually has one BM q̄ AM p̄ coffee. May also have a BM late in afternoon. Has virtually no difficulty c̄ constipation. Eats spinach, but has cut out beans and lettuce. Had a BM today. Even if she travels for a couple of days and does not have a BM, she will go spontaneously when she gets home. Did have trouble when in hospital once. No trouble voiding.

3. *Breathing:* No trouble with breathing. Breathes through her mouth and feels she breathes shallowly from upper chest. Coughs only if she has a bad cough. Cough is shallow, nonproductive, only moderately forceful. Noiseless rhythmic breathing, no signs of distress; rate not determined. Feels short of breath if bends over head first. Smokes half pack/day for 40 years or so.

4. *Eating and drinking:* 12:00 noon–12:30 PM first meal—meat, vegetables, salad, dessert, beverage; 6:30–7:00 PM—sandwich, bowl of cereal c̄ banana, cottage cheese, soup. May have something to drink during morning but no set schedule. Drinks Sanka, hot or iced tea, water, maybe small glass milk. Doesn't drink juice much; orange juice gives her indigestion. Drinks approx. 1 qt/day. Likes spicy foods, desserts; sauerkraut is only dislike. No problems eating or drinking; no assistance needed.

5. *Skin integrity:* Bruises easily. Is on Coumadin. Skin is smooth, soft, firm, and very slightly dry. Uses lotion on skin every day. Has healed sternotomy and thoracotomy scars from heart surgery. No open areas that she knows of. Takes tub bath but only if someone is in house. May take a sponge bath during cold weather. Had two friends die from head injuries slipping in tub. No assistance needed. Can use only Palmolive dish soap and Tussey deodorant; Noxema on face, Caress soap, Lifebuoy at home. Has full dentures. Scrubs dentures c̄ Comet, uses Clorox, tooth paste, 2–3 times a day. Keeps them in all the time except to brush.

6. *Activity:* States she has full ROM; no restric-

tions noted in shoulders, hip, knees. No difficulty walking. No assistance needed.

7. *Recreation:* Has grandchildren over to spend night and plays with them. Goes to river place, fishes, reads a lot (books and magazines), watches TV.

8. *Interpersonal and communicative patterns:* "I have no unfamiliar situations; I've been places like this hospital before. I accept new situations. If I can't cope with something I leave it alone or if I don't like someone I stay away from them." Answers questions, volunteers information, elaborates at great length. Asked no questions; speaks clearly. In bed during interview, twice turned on side toward interviewer, once got up to take a sip of juice; rubbed stomach, epigastric area most of the time; talked with eyes closed sometimes; frequency not determined. Much gurgling in intestinal juices during interview.

9. *Temperament:* Gets disgusted with "give aways" in country. Says she doesn't get violently angry. When I first asked her what makes her mad she said, "You don't want to go into that." Doesn't do anything when angry—talks to commentators perhaps. Husband provokes her—doesn't make her mad. "We never fight, we have a difference of opinion, that's all." She tells him if provoked. Thinks she would say something if she didn't get what she needed and felt disgruntled. Has hollered for help when she couldn't reach bell cord. Is highly nervous inside, tied-up in knots; attributes this just to herself, that is, meaning born nervous; "Have no reason to grow into it. Had a fine family. Maybe due to my heart condition." Keeps busy to keep from thinking about herself.

10. *Dependency and independency patterns:* *For self:* I hate to go to the beauty parlor, but I do that every week; like to go grocery shopping; make the decisions that affect only me. *For others:* Take food to them, see, visit others. *Others do for her:* Be nice, thoughtful, come see her, speak to her, call her up. Doesn't usually tell anyone what she wants; goes to town to get what she wants;

doesn't share problems. If can't do something, asks for help. Is not hesitant.

11. *Senses*: No problems hearing; wears glasses mostly for reading. R handed. Menopausal.

Statement of that which makes pt feel safe, protected, cared for: "Her own bed in her own house." Come talk to her; children, husband and neighbors are good to her (unable to be more specific).

Additional data: "Ever since I was 4-years-old, until after I had the heart operation in 1960 I've been sickly. Had growing pains; had pneumonia 4× by the time I was 4-years-old. Even after the heart operation, I had such terrible pain I could hardly stand it. When the second operation was done, seems like the pain all congealed in this one place (lower left rib cage)."

Patient went to have an echocardiogram after completion of nursing history. C. Hayes, R.N.

PROBLEM LIST

Problem	First Noted	Resolved
1. Expects tests.	2-21-78	3-02-78
2. Feelings of nervousness.	2-21-78	3-02-78
3. Lack of understanding of drug administration.	2-22-78	
a. Coumadin		2-24-78
b. digoxin		3-02-78
4. Red area on hip.	2-25-78	2-28-78
		C. Hayes, R.N.

INITIAL PLAN OF CARE

2-22-78   8:20 AM

Problem 1: Expects Tests

Subjective: "I'm going to have my artery (neck) checked and my heart. Didn't know something could go wrong with the valve. I thought it was good forever. I don't think I could put my family through another operation. Otherwise I don't know what tests will be done."

Objective: Echocardiogram done 2-21-78. Carotid arteriogram scheduled for 2-23-78.

Assessment: Perhaps an explanation of procedures will help keep her nerves under control (see problem 2).

Plan:
1. On 2-22-78 review procedure for carotid arteriogram.
   a. She will receive a medication before going to x-ray that will help her feel drowsy.
   b. She will lie on an x-ray table which will probably be hard.
   c. The area on her neck will be washed and towels will surround the area, perhaps covering her face.
   d. She will receive a local anesthetic which will probably sting. She will feel pushing as needle and catheter are inserted. There might be pain, just how much I don't know. There will be a hot feeling when the dye is injected. The radiologist will tell her when that will happen and will also tell her what he wants her to do during the procedure.
   e. There are virtually no side effects from the procedure when it is over. Note: There are complications so I think I will not say this about side effects.
2. Answer any questions she has. Accompany her to the procedure if possible. Ask her how it went when it is over.
3. Keep informed about any other tests scheduled and write a plan of instruction for them.

Problem 2. Feelings of Nervousness

Subjective: "I'm a very nervous person. I have to keep busy. I can't stand to stay in bed. I'm like a yo-yo. Since I've been in the hospital, I've developed a lot more aches and pains. I must have been born nervous as I have no reason to grow into it. Had a fine family. Maybe it's due to my heart condition." Keeps busy to keep from thinking about herself. Says she'll holler for help, that she's not hesitant to ask for things she can't do herself. Sleep is interrupted by a wakeful period if goes to sleep before midnight but not if she stays awake until 2:00 AM.

Objective: Moved from back to side 2–3 times during interview; got up to drink juice; elaborates her answers to questions.

Assessment: I don't think we will be able to make her less nervous. I think our job is to help her keep it under control. Would like to know the thoughts she has about herself; would like to know what she feels like inside. Wonder if sleep will be a problem while here even though she does not consider it so at home. The inactivity of the hospital could cause considerable discomfort.

Plan: Ask her each day how her nerves are. Ask how she slept. Keep her informed as to what plans there are for her. Ask if she has enough reading material or other things to stay busy with; listen to whatever other concerns she might have. C. Hayes, R.N.

PROGRESS NOTES

2-22-78   12:50 PM

Problem 1: Expects Tests

Subjective: "Will the test hurt? Are there any long term effects from the test? I got this thing (Holter monitor) yesterday after the echocardiogram. I hope they come by soon to take it off."

Objective: Found out from clerk in x-ray that she is scheduled for an arch study rather than carotid arteriography, so did not carry out plan exactly as written. Said I did not know how much pain there would be, probably some, but a numbing medicine would be used. The test would be done from the groin and she might have some of the hair shaved off there. She would have a hot feeling; the radiologist would tell her the hot feeling was coming, that there were some complications which the doctor would tell her about (did not feel I could give a yes or no answer to her question so got into complication but not fully). Could not tell her when the test will be tomorrow.

Assessment: Am not sure that she has expressed her feelings about the test. Maybe she will have more to say after it's over.

Plan: Accompany pt if possible tomorrow.

Problem 2: Feelings of Nervousness

Subjective: "My nerves are fine today. I took a sleeping pill last night and slept all night. I didn't get any sleep the night before. I got my third roommate. It's so noisy. No, don't try to get me another room. I'm settled here and don't want to be disrupted."

Objective: Asked how her nerves are. Did not carry out rest of plan today.

Assessment: Think emotions are under control at the moment.

Plan: Continue initial plan.

Problem 3: Lacks Understanding of Drug Administration

A. Coumadin

Subjective: "I thought when the figure on my blood was high it meant I could clot more easily. I never understood where I could bleed from. It is not easy to keep track of my blood through the lab. I have to get down there, then walk a long way to the lab then call back in the afternoon or call my doctor if the lab won't give me the results and the nurse won't tell me, only she can't get the doctor to call me. I just gave up having it checked, and just took the same amount. I didn't know it could vary so.

Objective: PT today 13.0/10.8. Dr. Jones told pt she would be regulated while she's here.

Assessment: Not in therapeutic range and needs help in finding a way to get prothrombin time checked and dosage adjusted accordingly.

Plan: On 02-23-78 or 02-24-78 explore with pt all the alternatives we can think of for getting pro-time checked on a regular basis. One I think of is having the nurse call the pt if dosage needs to be regulated. Probably better however for pt to take the initiative. Am not sure what all the alternatives might be.

B. Digoxin

Subjective: "I haven't had my Lanoxin since I've been here. I was told to take my pulse before taking the pill, but I'd get confused between what I'd feel in my chest and what I'd count at the wrist so I gave up. I've just gone on taking the pills twice a day."

Objective: Pulse 56 radially, slightly irregular (just the faintest hesitation between some beats).

Assessment: Wonder if pt can be taught to take her pulse or perhaps husband can learn so pt does not overdose herself.

Plan: On 02-24-78 ask pt to try to count pulse radially and see how accurate she is and what feelings and concerns she has about the task. Do this with husband present and see if he can count pulse accurately. Suggest a public health referral to them, for follow up instruction after discharge.
C. Hayes, R.N.

02-23-76   1:45 PM

Problem 1: Expects tests

Subjective: "I was a little nervous about the test, worrying if it would work out all right, if I could hemorrhage—all those things he told me about. My headache's gone, I've passed my water, my leg doesn't hurt, lunch tastes good. Feel sleepy now." Never actually answered if she felt prepared.

Objective: Arch aortography performed this AM. Puncture site sealed, no swelling, discoloration or bleeding. During procedure pulse 62, Resp. 14; lay quietly on table with eyes closed. Did wince and cry out with pain during cannulization. Vital signs now P60 B/P 90/72. Ate all lunch. Asked if she felt prepared.

Assessment: Did not appear outwardly nervous during test; seems relaxed now. Don't think anymore tests are scheduled; only protimes.

Plan: Find out each day if any tests are scheduled and explain as needed.

Problem 2: Feelings of Nervousness

Subjective: "My nerves were pretty tense yesterday but aren't too bad today. When my nerves are acting up, I feel tight, tense inside all the time. I took a sleeping pill last night and slept well. I have a good book over there to read. Hope I remember to keep my leg straight during sleep." Mentioned neighbors.

Objective: Eating lunch; talking about home things, the news.

Assessment: I concur with her comment that she's not very nervous today.

Plan: Continue.

Problem 3: Lacks Understanding of Drug Administration

Objective: Did nothing with this problem today so pt can get over aortography. Will carry out plans tomorrow. C. Hayes, R.N.

02-24-78   10:45 AM

Problem 1: Expects Tests

Subjective: "I'm just a little sore there. Otherwise, I'm ok."

Objective: Groin area dry, no bruising, no hematoma.

Assessment: No apparent residual effects from aortogram.

Plan: Chart only if new tests are scheduled.

Problem 2: Feelings of Nervousness

Subjective: "My nerves are all right today. My roommate had a lot of company last night which tired me out a lot. I took a sleeping pill and slept all night so they didn't keep me awake. It was just noisy with them all here. No problems I haven't had for 3−4 years."

Objective: Lying in bed; smoked one cigarette; no excessive motions, moving legs or arms.

Assessment: Can't get a real feeling of a lot of nervousness from pt. She either controls the expression of it very well or is not feeling as much as she indicated she felt in nursing hx.

Plan: Continue.

Problem 3: Lacks Understanding of Drug Administration

A. Coumadin

Subjective: "I'll just have to make time to go to the hospital to have the blood drawn. It's just a matter of making a schedule and doing it. I get to the beauty parlor each week, I can get to the hospital. No, we don't need a public health nurse to check on us."

Objective: Still being regulated; yesterday 11.0/14.1. Up to 10 mg Coumadin qd.

Assessment: No comment. Think she will participate in the weekly lab studies.

Plan: D/C this aspect

B. Digoxin

Subjective: "I always have so much trouble counting my pulse. I don't think I catch them all. I can feel it over my heart best. Yes I feel each beat as you count it."

Objective: First time she counted pulse she got 55, 2nd was 64. I got 73 each time. I counted out loud while she palpated radial and temporal artery. She closed her eyes during this and moved more in bed. Told her to practice today.

Assessment: I think she's nervous about doing this and suspect she will not practice and will have a hard time doing it tomorrow.

Plan: Ask her to take pulse tomorrow and see how she does. C. Hayes, R.N.

02-25-78   11:05 AM

Problem 2: Feelings of Nervousness

Subjective: "My nerves are fine. I slept well."
Objective: Dalmane taken last night.
Assessment: Seems calm.
Plan: Continue.

Problem 3: Lacks Understanding of Drug Administration

B. Digoxin

Subjective: "I got 55. I probably missed a lot; this time I got 63. I'll work on it."

Objective: I got pulse of 73 first time. Husband counted and said he got 66. I retook pulse and got 68. More irregular first time than second time I took it.

Assessment: I think husband can count pulse and pt was probably correct her second time. Need to find out anticipated dosage and be sure she

should not take drug if pulse below 60, as we would do here.

Plan: Talk with Dr. Jones as soon as I can about anticipated discharge dosage so my instructions to pt are correct.

Problem 4: Red Area on Hip

Subjective: "I have this sore place where she gave me a shot before x-ray the other day. It is really sore. I have these hard places on my buttocks and she should have given it to me lower. It'll go away. I don't want a hot pack on it. I can't lie on my side too well."

Objective: Red, warm, raised, circumscribed area on left upper outer quadrant of left buttock. Nurse who gave injection said she used a 22 × 1½ needle. Location of area is outer aspect of upper outer quadrant. Suggested pt sit in tub.

Assessment: Area certainly looks sore. Believe technique and location were correct. I have a hypothesis that use of a 1 inch needle is likely to cause this type of situation, but these data do not confirm that. Think warmth would help area feel better.

Plan: Look at area on 02-28-78 to see if there is any change.

Additonal Data

Subjective: "I told you I had no trouble with my bowels usually or if I did it's because I'm going but not like I usually do. I don't like prune juice. Do you have MOM tablets? Maybe I will need to take something."

Objective: MOM 30 ml prn ordered. Suggested pt take it; told her she needed to ask for it so she would not get constipated.

Assessment: Hope she does not avoid the laxative and get into trouble.

Plan: Check with her on 02-28-78 and see if she has had a satisfactory BM. If not, make constipation problem 5.

Problem 3: Lacks Understanding of Drug Administration

B. Digoxin

Objective: Talked with Dr. Jones who said pt would go home on 0.25 mg digoxin qd and she should not take it if pulse is below 60.

Plan: Will incorporate the above in my instruction on 02-28-78. C. Hayes, R.N.

02-28-78   9:35 AM

Problem 2: Feelings of Nervousness

Subjective: "I'm tired today. I didn't sleep well. I had the heebee jeebies. I went out to lunch yesterday. I was with people who make me nervous, and driving in traffic makes me nervous; also a lady told me about her grandson who was admitted here and not expected to live and my own grandson has been sick. I know that got me upset. I feel ok today. I read. I didn't take a pill last night."
Objective: No Dalmane recorded as given.
Assessment: Sounds like a normal reaction and not out of hand.
Plan: Continue.

Problem 3: Lacks Understanding of Drug Administration

B. Digoxin
Subjective: "I've been practicing taking my pulse from all angles. I can practice better when I don't have all these distractions. I won't take the pill if my pulse is below 60."
Objective: Did not have pt count pulse with me today. It was 58–59 and quite irregular when I took it. Told pt she would only be on one pill a day and that if her pulse was below 60 at the time she should take her pill she shouldn't take it, not worry about it for that day and try it again the next day.
Assessment: I think she understands. Will check her out tomorrow to be sure.
Plan: Ask pt on 03-01-78 to count pulse and report it to me. (I will take it too.)

Problem 4: Red Area on Hip

Subjective: "My hip is not really sore, just a very little bit. I consider it cured."
Objective: Area is just barely a bit more pink than surrounding skin; not raised or warm.

Assessment: Resolved.
Plan: D/C
Additonal Data
Subjective: "I've gotten all cleaned out. I took milk of magnesia and a glass of prune juice that night (02-25-78) and I really went. No problems now."
Objective: MOM charted as given 02-25-78.
Assessment: Seems to be resolved.
Plan: None.
Also, pt wants to ask Dr. Jones if she can continue to take her Donnatal if she has stomach distress. A note is left for him at her bedside. I'll try to ask him about it myself. C. Hayes, R.N.

03-01-78   10:40 AM

Problem 2: Feelings of Nervousness

Subjective: "I slept well last night. I took a pill after having had the heebie-jeebies all day. I don't feel that way today. I'm looking forward to getting home."
Objective: Dalmane charted as given last evening. Sitting in chair, smoked two cigarettes during visit.
Assessment: Nerves still seem under control.
Plan: Continue.

Problem 3: Lacks Understanding of Drug Administration

B. Digoxin
Subjective: "My pulse was 65 today. I'll take my pulse everyday and if below 60 I won't take the pill. No, I won't worry about it all day. I'll be more careful about taking care of myself."
Objective: I got 68 when I took pulse.
Assessment: Think pt knows what to do and will do it.
Plan: Ask tomorrow if she has any questions about home care.
Additional Data:
Subjective: "Yes, I asked Dr. Jones about the Donnatal. He said I could take it, although it did interfere with the action of Coumadin. I don't take too much of it—only if I feel churned up inside."

Objective: No data.
Assessment: Pt took care of situation herself.
Plan: None. C. Hayes, R.N.

03-02-78 10:30 AM

Problem 1: Expects tests

Subjective: No comment.
Objective: Pt being discharged today. No tests scheduled.
Assessment: No need for problem.
Plan: Discontinue.

Problem 2: Feelings of Nervousness

Subjective: "I feel good today. No, I don't have the heebie-jeebies today nor did I yesterday. I slept well; I'm ready to go."
Objective: Things packed, pt dressed.
Assessment: No evidence of nerves being a problem—either today or really during hospitalization—at least that I saw or heard about.
Plan: Discontinue.

Problem 3: Lacks Understanding of Drug Administration

B. Digoxin
Subjective: "I think I understand what I'm supposed to do. I'm glad to have the list so I don't have to remember what you said. You've been very helpful. I had one of those 'fading away' spells yesterday."
Objective: Saw pt with Dr. Jones this morning to review all medications. She's not to take potassium, just at least one glass of juice to cover diuretic effects of digoxin; take one digoxin pill a day if pulse over 60; no diuretic unless ankles swell and she thinks she would feel better; no evidence of heart being in failure; can eat what foods she desires; take 12.5 mg of Coumadin qd; get blood tested every couple of days; Coumadin will be regulated by Dr. Green. All these things were written in list form for her to take with her. Dr. Jones said if spells were a problem, she could come back anytime.
Assessment: Think pt has a better idea of health management and is better regulated. Think she will carry out plans. Hope spell was not serious omen.
Plan: Discontinue. C. Hayes, R.N.

NURSING DISCHARGE SUMMARY

03-03-78 8:45 AM

This was the first STH admission for a 67-year-old married woman. She was admitted on 02-20-78 for investigation of a blockage in her right carotid artery and discharged home on 03-02-78.

1. Expects tests: noted 02-21-78; resolved 03-02-78.
2. Feels nervous all the time: noted 02-21-78; resolved 03-02-78.
3. Lack of understanding of: Coumadin—noted 02-22-78; resolved 02-24-78. digoxin—noted 02-22-78; resolved 03-02-78.
4. Red area on hip: noted 02-25-78; resolved 02-28-78.

Additonal data (other recommendations): The patient and her husband are assuming primary care for her health on discharge. She has a list of instructions to follow. During hospitalization, the patient did her own care, stayed out of bed most of the time, had one episode of feeling constipated, treated with MOM and prune juice with good results. I feel the patient and her husband are able to be responsible for the care and anticipate no problems. C. Hayes, R.N.

REFERENCES

1. Kerr, A. H.: Nurses' notes: that's where the goodies are! *Nurs. '75* vol. 5:34, 1975.
2. *Ibid.*, p. 35–36.
3. Wood, L. A.: *Nursing Skills for Allied Health Services*. Philadelphia, W. B. Saunders Company, vol. 1, p. 101.
4. Weed, L.: *Medical Education and Patient Care*. Cleveland, Case Western Reserve University, 1970.
5. Becknell, E. P., and Smith, D. M.: *System of Nursing Practice*. Philadelphia, F. A. Davis Company, 1975, pp. 87–88.
6. *Ibid.*, p. 89.
7. *Ibid.*, p. 91.
8. *Ibid.*, pp. 117–118.
9. *Ibid.*, pp. 118–119.
10. *Ibid.*, p. 119.

CHAPTER 26

Evaluation of nursing care is an essential component of professional practice. The goal of evaluation is to determine whether the client has met the objectives which were established during the development of his nursing care plan. Evaluation also serves as a basis for revising the plan of care.

EVALUATION PROCESS

The evaluation process has three components:

1. Determining the criteria which will be used in measuring achievement of objectives.
2. Gathering data relevant to the identified criteria.
3. Making judgments about the achievement of objectives on the basis of the data obtained.

Determination of Criteria

The evaluation process is initiated when the nurse develops her plan of care by identifying her long

EVALUATION OF NURSING CARE

Barbara A. Beeker, Ed.D., R.N.

and short-term objectives. Criteria which will be used to determine the degree to which the client has achieved these objectives must be defined at this time. You will remember from Chapter 24 that criteria for determining acceptable performance are essential components of correctly written objectives.

Criteria serve two purposes: (1) they provide a guide for the kind of data that should be collected; and (2) they provide the standard by which to judge this data.[1] Esssential characteristics of a criterion are measurability and specificity. Consider the following objective for an infant admitted to the hospital with vomiting and diarrhea: "Adequate hydration will be maintained." This would not tell the nurse what data to collect while caring for this patient. However, if the objective was restated as, "Adequate hydration will be maintained as evidenced by: (1) normal skin turgor; (2) full fontanel; and (3) urinary output of × ml/24 hours," any nurse caring for this infant would know exactly what data to collect. It is critical to have well-de-

fined, clearly stated criteria to guide the next step of the evaluation process, the collection of data.

Data Collection

Data are collected so that judgments can be made about the achievement of objectives. The type of data to be collected will depend on the criteria previously established. Both objective and subjective data may be necessary. You will remember from Chapter 25 that subjective data are those which the client and his family report, while objective data are factual information compiled from the nurse's observation.

Whenever possible data should be quantitatively measurable; for example, "Pulse increased from 68 to 92 after climbing 10 stairs." Obviously the more quantifiable and objective the data, the better for purposes of evaluation. The ideal data need no interpretation by the observer; for example, laboratory reports, pulse, and blood pressure. Subjective data from the client or data depending on observed interpretation, such as degree of restlessness, are less preferable. However, such types of data must be used frequently in nursing. When this is the case, Taylor suggests that "it is advisable to use more than one source, such as patient interview and a staff conference, to provide some opportunity to verify information."[2]

Recalling the infant with vomiting and diarrhea, it is evident that the criteria specified for adequate hydration call for the collection of objective rather than subjective data. It is also evident that the criterion related to urinary output is much more quantitative than that related to skin turgor.

In some cases, it is necessary to collect both objective and subjective data. For example, if the objective was "client will indicate relief from pain," subjective data are obviously needed. A statement by the client that "it hurts more now than it did before breakfast" is an example of appropriate subjective data. Appropriate objective data would include such observations as decreased restlessness, decreased pulse and respirations, and changes in facial expression which are indicators of pain relief. Again, note that some criteria, namely pulse and respiration, are more quantitative than the criterion facial expression.

Data must be clearly and concisely recorded if they are to be useful for evaluation. The Problem-Oriented System of charting described in the preceding chapter provides an effective structure for recording. The type of data to be recorded will determine if it is more appropriate to use progress notes in the SOAP format or a flow sheet. In any event, it is essential that everyone caring for the client provide adequate documentation of the care provided and the client's response to that care. Without such data, the evaluation process cannot proceed to its final step, making judgments about the achievement of objectives.

Evaluating Achievement of Objectives

Providing that the criteria for determining if an objective has been met were clearly defined when the nursing care plan was developed and the appropriate data have been collected and recorded, it is relatively easy to determine whether or not an objective has been achieved. Again, we can look at the example of the infant with diarrhea and vom-

iting. If the flow sheet on his urinary output indicated an output of over $\times$ ml per 24 hours and the SOAP notes consistently indicated a full fontanel and good skin turgor, the nurse could easily make the judgment that the objective "maintenance of adequate hydration" was achieved.

Both the nurse and the client should have an active role in determining whether objectives have been achieved. The Standards of Nursing Practice of the American Nurses' Association provide a means for determining the quality of nursing care by specifying that "the client's/patient's progress or lack of progress toward goal achievement is determined by the client/patient and the nurse."[3] Since the client has been an active participant in planning his care, it seems logical that he should be involved in evaluating the effectiveness of such care. Evaluation results in one of the following conclusions:

1. The client has achieved the objective or is moving satisfactorily toward achievement of the objective.
2. The client has made little or no progress toward achieving the objective.

Subsequent nursing actions are dependent on these conclusions.

MODIFICATION OF THE PLAN OF CARE

If the evidence leads to the conclusion that an objective has been achieved, the nursing actions related to that objective may be discontinued if the underlying problem no longer exists. For example, when the objective, "The patient will test his urine for sugar and acetone four times a day," has been achieved, the nurse could discontinue the nursing actions related to that objective. However, continuing with the nursing orders even though they have been successful in meeting an objective is sometimes indicated. For example, if the nurse were caring for a client with dehydration due to an elevated temperature and excessive perspiration, an objective might be "The patient will maintain a fluid intake of 2500 ml per day." Even if the nurse determines that the objective has been achieved, the nursing actions related to this objective would be continued as long as the dehydration continued.

If the client has not reached an objective but

seems to be moving satisfactorily toward its achievement, the nursing actions should definitely be continued. Re-evaluation of the objective's achievement would take place at a later point in time.

If the client has made little or no progress toward meeting an objective, the nurse must try to determine what happened and take appropriate action. The Standards of Nursing Practice specify that "The client's progress or lack of progress toward goal achievement directs reassessment, reordering of priorities, new goal setting, and revision of the plan of care."[3]

An initial step would be for the nurse to determine if the nursing care prescribed was actually carried out. Since the client may have been cared for by many nurses, it is important to look at the totality of his care. There are two major reasons why the nursing care prescribed may not have been carried out: (1) the nursing orders may not have been clear enough to guide the other staff members in providing care, and (2) external constraints, such as a shortage of staff, may have interfered with the implementation of nursing orders.

Unless nursing orders are clear each staff member may have a different interpretation of the order, inhibiting the delivery of consistent care. For example, if a nursing order reads "force fluids," inconsistencies might result in such areas as:

1. The amount of fluid the client receives: one nurse might decide he needed 1800 ml, while another might decide he needed 2500 ml.
2. The manner in which fluid intake is distributed over the 24 hour period: one nurse might decide the intake should be evenly distributed over the three shifts, and another might decide the client should receive more during the day and the evening than at night.
3. The approach to the client: one nurse might be reminding the client every hour of the need to drink something, while another nurse might encourage the client to accept the responsibility for increasing his fluid intake.

It is easy to see why the objective may not be met. A nursing order which reads: (1) "Maintain intake at 2500 ml/24 hours;" (2) "Divide intake—1200 ml days, 900 ml evenings, and 400 ml nights;" or (3) "Monitor client's adherence to agreed upon plan for fluid intake which is at his bedside;" provides much more definitive guidelines. If it appears that the nursing orders were not clear, restatement in more definitive terms is indicated.

It is not uncommon for external constraints to hamper the implementation of nursing orders, especially when these constraints were not taken into account when planning care. For example, a plan for forcing fluids which includes providing the client with 100 ml of fluid every hour and varying the type of fluid offered each time may be appropriate for a nursing student caring for one client during hours when the dietary department is open. However, such a plan would be inappropriate if there is very limited staffing and a limited variety of fluids available during evening and night shifts. If the identified constraints cannot be overcome, and often realistically they cannot be, it is necessary to develop a plan which is more realistic and achievable in light of the identified constraints. What if the plan of care has been carried out as designed but an objective still has not been met? The nurse must re-evaluate each step of her plan of care to determine where revision is needed.

In relation to her assessment and the resultant nursing diagnosis the nurse would ask such questions as: (1) Was the data base adequate enough to justify the nursing diagnosis I made? (2) Do I now have additional data that changes my diagnosis? (3) If the nursing diagnosis changes, it is obvious that new objectives and new nursing actions must be developed. In relation to the objectives developed the nurse could raise such questions as: (1) Were my objectives appropriate? (2) Were they realistically achievable within the constraints imposed by the agency, the client, and the family? If the answer to such questions is no, the objectives need revision. Similarly in reviewing the nursing actions prescribed, the nurse could ask: (1) Were the actions prescribed directly related to the objectives? (2) Were alternative nursing actions identified and adequately considered in deciding which actions to prescribe? Depending on her answer to these questions the nurse could develop new nursing actions or decide to try one of the alternative actions she previously rejected.

Obviously once the needed revisions are made and the new plan implemented, evaluation will be necessary again to determine if the objectives have been met. Thus it becomes evident that planning, giving, and evaluating nursing care is an ongoing dynamic process with constant interaction between the parts. Evaluation is a critical component of this process because it enables us to determine whether the care has been effective, and it serves as a basis for revising care.

REFERENCES

1. Little, D. E., and Carnevali, D. L.: *Nursing Care Planning*. Philadelphia, J. B. Lippincott Co., 1976, p. 231.
2. Taylor, J.: Measuring outcomes of nursing care. *Nurs. Clin. North Am.* 9:344, 1974.
3. American Nurses' Association: Standards of nursing practice. *Am. Nurse* 6:11–12, 1974.

BIBLIOGRAPHY

Becknell, E. P., and Smith, D. M.: *Systems of Nursing Practice*. Philadelphia, F. A. Davis Company, 1975.
Block, D.: Evaluation of nursing care in terms of process and outcome: issues in research and quality assurance. *Nurs. Res.* 24:256–263, 1975.
Bower, F.: *The Process of Planning Nursing Care*. St. Louis, C. V. Mosby Co., 1972.
Ethridge, P., and Packard, R.: An innovative approach to measurement of quality through utilization of nursing care plans: *J. Nurs. Admin.* 76:25–31, 1976.
Mayers, M. G.: The patient's response as a test of good planning, in *A Systematic Approach to the Nursing Care Plan*, edited by Mayer M. G., New York, Appleton-Century-Crofts, 1972.
Mitchell, P. H.: *Concepts Basic to Nursing*, 2nd ed. New York: McGraw Hill Book Co., 1977.
Nicholls, M., and Virginia W.: *Nursing Standards and Nursing Process*. Wakefeld, Mass., Contemporary Publishing, Inc., 1977.
Pardee, G., et al.: Patient care evaluation is every nurses job. *Am. J. Nurs.* 71:1958–1960, 1971.
Walter, J., Pardee, G., and Molbo, D. (eds.): *Dynamics of Problem-Oriented Approaches: Patient Care and Documentation*. Philadelphia, J. B. Lippincott Co., 1976.
Yura, H., and Walsh, M. B.: *The Nursing Process*. New York, Meredith Corporation, 1973.

PART 5:
PROVIDING BASIC
HEALTH CARE

To administer safe nursing care effectively, there are certain procedures with which nurses must be acquainted. Part 5 introduces the student to the most common of these. While many of these interventions are seen primarily in the hospital setting, a large proportion of them are implemented in community settings.

All nursing care is based on principles from the behavioral, social, and natural sciences. While a review of some of the major principles from these areas is incorporated in the following chapters, it is assumed that the student has been introduced to all of these subjects. While studying the following chapters, the student must remain cognizant of the fact that client teaching and promotion of independent functioning are always major components of care. Furthermore, legal aspects and the rights of clients must always be a consideration in the delivery of this care.

These chapters alone certainly will not provide the student with manipulative skill and clinical expertise. This will take varying amounts of experience as well as the guidance of other skilled personnel, particularly instructors. It is hoped, however, that the student nurse will be able to apply her knowledge to develop some of the functional aspects of nursing care.

CHAPTER 27

Think about yourself and the one other person that you know best. Observe the effects on you (or on the other person) of the interaction with the psychosocial milieu. This psychosocial milieu consists of space, objects, people, and events that are part of the immediate world of the individual human being. The results of the interaction between person and milieu at any given period of time can range from (a) nearly nothing to (b) a total change in that person's existence.

There is a reason that I suggested considering yourself as well as one other person placed interchangeably in the same position. In a way, your observations are those of a social psychologist who studies human interactions.[1] You should be able to see, understand, predict, and hopefully even control events. By imagining yourself in the position of a person being studied, tested, or treated, you might gain a clearer understanding of that person's feelings. Basing your observations on more than one person will help you to realize that there is a uniqueness in each person's reaction to the world,

THE PSYCHOSOCIAL MILIEU

Carl J. Cooper, Ph.D.

but at the same time, that there are laws of behavior common to all human beings. Behavioral scientists, such as social psychologists, have been working to discover these laws. The implications of understanding them are most important in nursing care.

Begin your observations with the extreme—*no environment*—a situation in which the interaction between person and world is minimized. How would you and your friend react to nothing? As a volunteer in an experiment on sensory deprivation, as much of the data to your senses as possible is eliminated without physically damaging your eyes, ears, and skin receptors. You lie on a cot in a quiet room, wearing gloves and cardboard cuffs in such a way that it is nearly impossible to recognize objects by touching them; in fact, you may not even be sure you are touching anything. You wear earphones which allow only the steady, unchanging, low-pitched humming sound called *white noise*. A plastic visor is over your eyes, admitting light but no visual perceptions. Enough time is allowed for the needed physiological events. What do you

think would happen to you over the period of an hour, a day, or a week? Heron[2] found that all kinds of psychological distortions occurred, such as anxieties and hallucinations. In fact, if you were offered $50.00/day for all the consecutive days in a sensory-deprived state such as the one described, you would probably find that after the first day or two spent catching up on all the sleep you have missed as a nursing student, you would almost certainly find the experience so traumatic that you would not be likely to last longer than 3 or 4 days! Sensory input is *essential* to daily existence.

HOSPITALISM

Sensory Deprivation

What has all this talk about sensory deprivation to do with nursing care? Consider the very young among your clientele, that is, the infant. The psychosocial milieu of a hospitalized infant can easily become second cousin to a sensory deprivation experiment of a most prolonged and disastrous type. The high-walled cribs or bassinets; the lack of visual, auditory, and tactile stimulation; the relative lack of communication with and touching by a caring adult can lead to a situation of pure hell for the child. Spitz[3] calls the resultant syndrome *hospitalism*. What is seen in their behavior is listlessness, lethargy, and apparent depression. What happens over the long run is likely to be serious developmental retardation. Harlow and Harlow[4] with their fascinating research on rhesus monkeys provide further evidence to suggest that the long range effect of prolonged social deprivation (let alone total sensory deprivation) can be serious defects in personality development. As a result of the observations of people like Spitz,[2] Harlow,[4] Ribble,[5] and others, most hospitals that work extensively with pediatric clients have evolved some plan where the parents can spend a considerable amount of time with their sick children. The ideal situation is one in which the parents can arrange to live-in during hospitalization.

The information on sensory deprivation may have implications for nursing care with adults, even though the extremes of situation-caused hallucinations, anxiety, and depression are not likely to appear in most normal hospitalizations. If, however, you or the friend that you observed in the first part of this section were to be hospitalized, think of the possible effects. Being ill enough to require such care is in itself anxiety-producing. At their worst, the surroundings could actually work against appropriate nursing care. You would be essentially isolated from much of the stimulation that you ordinarily receive. It is possible that after a time, effects similar to those noted by Heron[2] or Spitz[3] might be felt by you. The differences between individuals (you or the friend you have chosen to observe) would cause some differences in how the milieu affected you, but it is quite likely that a long stay in the hospital would have negative emotional results. These results could easily be a mild psychological depression, which in itself may have an effect on treatment.

Sensory Overload

In a modern hospital, it is just as likely that instead of being placed in a situation of sensory deprivation, the opposite could occur. A bombardment of sights, sounds, smells, discomfort, pain, questions, and instructions might easily overload the client in his attempts to understand what is happening. A person who is already anxious about being hospitalized may find this type of situation overwhelming.

To illustrate the effects of sensory overload, perform the following simple experiment. The next time you are in a situation where two or more conversations are going on simultaneously within earshot, such as at a restaurant or a party, try to focus on everything that is being said by people in two different conversations. You will be able to hear sounds from both people but will be able to concentrate on only one of the persons speaking at any given moment; more likely, you will find yourself switching back and forth between the two. It will be just about impossible to attend to both conversations at the same time. Try to concentrate on three or four words said by two different people at the same time and try to be aware of the meanings of these words in context of the two separate conversations. You cannot! If you try to keep it up you will probably be totally confused by *both* conversations.

Now think of the hospital. The client is trying to interpret tremendous amounts of data simultaneously, including his own physical feelings, new sights and sounds, diagnostic and other technical jargon that everyone else seems to understand, as well as conversations in the background that cannot quite be heard clearly. The confusion that you felt in trying to perceive two conversations at once is mild compared to that of the hospitalized person in a sensory overload situation. Remember also, you were only playing; the client's situation is real. Symptoms of the confusion caused by sensory overload may not be particularly easy to notice. Think of the bewilderment that you might feel if you were trying to interpret all kinds of strange sights, sounds, and feelings when you were in a new and stressful situation. Someone who knows you well could probably detect that you were confused from the way you were acting. He or she would see that you appeared anxious—possibly more so than the situation seemed to call for—and that you had some difficulty in selecting the most important information from all that you were trying to perceive.

In nursing care the problems of anxieties due to

sensory overload might be reduced by seeing to it that the client is not overwhelmed by too much that is new all at once. Explanations should be clear and simple. By carefully observing the nonverbal responses made by the client to the situation (see Chapter 18 on the observation of nonverbal behavior) the competent nurse is often able to detect when he is confused by the total surroundings. She can then attempt to slow things down a bit and help to clarify the information already received.

INVASION OF PRIVACY

You might answer the question, "How old are you?" without giving it a second thought or you might feel that it was really none of anyone's business—that is, that your privacy was being invaded. Most people do not like to have strangers, or even friends, intrude on certain emotional and physical areas that they consider personal and private. There are bitter complaints when the government or the newspapers go too far in their investigation into the private lives of people. Recent feminist literature[6] discusses how important it is that the person not be considered an object free for manipulation, but that any close relationship between people depends on a genuine respect for and an understanding of the privacy rights of the person.

Physical Space

People are made very uncomfortable when their private physical space is invaded.[7] Observe that when two people are talking to each other while standing still, there is usually some distance between their faces. You will notice that in a party situation when several groups of couples are talking, each of the pairs has about the same distance separating them. (In some cultures, as in some South American and some Arabic countries, this distance is smaller, while in others, such as northern Europe, it tends to be greater.) To continue the experiment, while you are talking with another person try moving back an inch or two, without being too obvious about it; then move a bit closer. What does the other person do? The social psychologist Brown[7] reported a situation in which he was manipulated into moving across an entire room simply by having his physical privacy invaded an inch or two at a time when his partner deliberately slid his

chair (a little at a time) closer to Brown's chair. Notice also in your experiment whether or not *you* feel uncomfortable when your face is too close to someone else's face in a casual conversation.

The implications for nursing care seem obvious. Many times certain aspects of a person's privacy must be invaded as part of the total care plan. The health team must have information about the client that is ordinarily personal and private. Touching and moving the person almost as an object is often necessitated by the treatment. The nurse must perform her duties, but she should be aware of individual needs. To make things even more complicated is the fact of individual differences in privacy needs. On one extreme is the client who needs almost total attention and is willing, almost insisting, to delve into and discuss his entire physiological and personal history. At the other extreme is the client who wants to be left entirely alone to sleep, read, and perhaps to participate in essential tests and take necesssary medication.

SUMMARY

As mentioned earlier in this chapter, the psychosocial milieu consists of relationships with everything in the immediate world of the individual. It is important that the *nurse-client relationship* be viewed separately from the *nursing care plan*. Many psychologists argue that the quality of this relationship can have a major effect on the results of treatment. The difficulty lies in pinpointing exactly what it is that the nurse should observe and what she should do in order to help create an optimal psychosocial milieu. However, it is not possible in a short chapter in an introductory text to provide more than the briefest overview of some of the issues involved in manipulating the client's psychosocial world.

The hospitalized client is likely to respond to everything in his environment with increased anxiety. It is quite possible that the interaction between client and health care personnel adds stress to an already stressful situation and increases the anxiety felt by the client. Ideally, it will not. Nurses can benefit greatly from supplemental course work and experience in psychological counseling as a complement to their professional nursing education. The ability to watch and listen is an invaluable tool that aids the nurse in her determination of whether or not the psychosocial milieu is helping with the treatment plan of a specific client. Experience in observation and interpretation is really the only way (with good supervision) that this can be developed. The client will give you clues when something is wrong by his reaction to you and the situation. As you progress in your education and career, you will learn how to interpret these communications and to respond to them in more meaningful and appropriate ways.

The entire psychosocial milieu is quite significant to the total nursing care situation. The particular relationship between nurse and client should be influenced by the needs for appropriate stimulation without overloading sensory systems and the client's ability to process the information received. This must all be balanced by an awareness of the needs for privacy. The actual physical setting within the hospital room must also be considered. Comfortable furniture, correct temperature, appropriate noise, silence when necessary, and even the colors (not bland and probably not too vivid) conceivably have some bearing on the emotional as well as physical aspects of the nursing care plan.

Our psychosocial milieu is flowing and dynamic. Needs and responses vary from person to person and even for the same person at different times. An awareness of these needs and changes can easily add to the effectiveness of any nursing care plan, because being *aware* means that you know you must *adapt*.

REFERENCES

1. Raven, B. H., and Rubin, J. Z. *Social Psychology: People in Groups.* New York, John Wiley and Sons, 1977.
2. Heron, W.: The pathology of boredom. *Sci. Am.* 196:52, 1957.
3. Spitz, R. A.: Hospitalism: an inquiry into the genesis of psychiatric conditions in early childhood, in *The Psychoanalytic Study of the Child,* vol. 1, edited by Freud, A., Hartman, H., and Kris, E., New York, International Universities Press, 1945.
4. Harlow, H., and Harlow, M. K.: Social deprivation in monkeys. *Sci. Am.* 207:207, 1962.
5. Ribble, M. A.: Infantile experience in relation to personality development, in *Personality and Behavior Disorders,* vol. 2, edited by Hunt, J. M., New York, Ronald Press, 1944.
6. Boston Women's Health Book Collective: *Our Bodies Our Selves.* New York, Simon and Schuster, 1973.
7. Brown, R.: *Social Psychology.* New York, Free Press, 1965.

BIBLIOGRAPHY

Spitz, R. A., and Wolf, K. M.: Anaclytic depression: an enquiry into the genesis of psychiatric conditions in early childhood, II, in *The Psychoanalytic Study of the Child,* vol. 2, edited by Freud, A., Hartman, H., and Kris, E., New York, International Universities Press, 1946.
Suedfeld, P.: The benefits of boredom: sensory deprivation reconsidered. *Am. Sci.* 63:60, 1975.
Bloch, D.: Privacy, in *Behavioral Concepts and Nursing Intervention,* edited by Carlson, C. E., Philadelphia, J. B. Lippincott Company, 1970.

CHAPTER 28

The initial relationship between the nurse and the client begins with his arrival on a nursing unit and serves as a foundation for future therapeutic interactions. Comprehension of the entire admission process, as well as appreciation for the special needs of the client at this time, are prerequisites to carrying out, in a holistic fashion, the nursing responsibilities required by the agency. Although health care agencies vary in their established admission procedures, the hospital admission will be used as a model here.

ADMISSION PROCESS

The physician initiates the preadmission process after advising the client of his need for hospitalization. The physician or his designee calls the hospital to arrange for an admission date. Information must be provided to the hospital regarding the urgency of the client's need and the estimated length of his

ADMISSION OF THE CLIENT

Nancy S. Sypert, M.S., R.N.

stay. Admission personnel then assess the availability of beds and assign an admission date.

Today, space in most hospitals is at a premium, and the assigned admission date is often inconvenient for the client. The necessity of hospitalization is usually disconcerting, forcing the client into rapidly modifying his self-image; rather than being a relatively healthy individual, he is now so ill that he requires the kind of specialized care provided by a hospital. (This process and the factors that impinge upon it have been discussed in detail in Chapter 4, "The Client as a Person.") The rapidity with which a client must enter the hospital may not allow him sufficient time to make the necessary employment, financial, family, and home arrangements. This adds to his sense of personal "crisis." If the client's admission is elective, rather than urgent, he may have adequate time to adapt to his new self-image and to plan for the interruption in his routine. However, in these instances he may also be uncomfortable about his inability to expedite resolution of

his health problem once he feels "ready," and this lack of control enhances his anxiety.

Once the admission reservation is made, the physician provides the hospital with as much information as he has with regard to the client's background. If there is adequate time, some hospitals will mail a pre-admission form to the client requesting additional information to facilitate the admission process. This information might include, for example, his preference for a private or semi-private room or his smoking habits. Some hospitals send information to the client prior to admission, explaining the policies of the institution and often including a sample floor plan of a nursing unit. In some instances, a nurse from the unit to which the client has been assigned calls him on the day before admission to introduce herself and answer any questions he might have.

The client may be transported to the hospital on the day of admission by ambulance, bus, or automobile. His journey to the hospital may be very short, in the case of a community based facility, or very long, which is frequently true of clients entering a large medical center. He generally is accompanied by one, or perhaps several, relatives and friends, as well as various personal possessions.

The client generally gives his name to an admitting receptionist who greets him and asks him to take a seat in a designated reception area. At this time, a hospital record number is assigned, and an Addressograph plate, which identifies all further records, is made. The client is then interviewed by specially trained personnel who confirm all pre-admission data. Information is obtained with regard to the client's insurance coverage, and the client may be required to sign a promissory note and to pay a deposit against the cost of his hospitalization. The client is requested at this time to deposit any valuable items, such as jewelry or large amounts of cash with the admitting office. He is also required to sign a form consenting to treatment. This admission consent provides for medical treatment (with the exception of surgical or experimental procedures and some diagnostic procedures), nursing care, and release of information to third-party payers.

When these procedures are completed, an identification band, on which the client's name, admission date, and hospital record number are printed, is fastened on his wrist. The client is then either escorted, usually by hospital volu teers, or directed to the hospital laboratory where blood is drawn to obtain baseline data pertaining to hematocrit or hemoglobin, blood count differential, and a serological test for syphilis. If necessary, the client is escorted to the radiology department for a baseline chest x-ray or to the cardiology department for an electrocardiogram.

All of the admission procedures mentioned thus far take place before the client ever reaches the nursing unit. There is often a great deal of delay in carrying out these procedures (Fig. 28-1); in fact, they can take several hours or even an entire day. As Chapter 4 pointed out, such delays ignore the client's sense of urgency, caused by his physical, emotional, and social crises and enhances his anxiety. Some hospitals, recognizing the needs of the client, encourage the physician to perform laboratory tests in his office prior to admission. The client can then bring the data with him to the hospital. Some institutions also provide the option of sched-

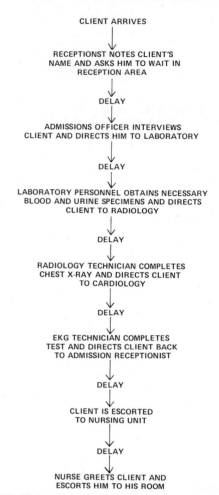

ADMISSION TO THE HEALTH CARE AGENCY

CLIENT ARRIVES

RECEPTIONST NOTES CLIENT'S NAME AND ASKS HIM TO WAIT IN RECEPTION AREA

DELAY

ADMISSIONS OFFICER INTERVIEWS CLIENT AND DIRECTS HIM TO LABORATORY

DELAY

LABORATORY PERSONNEL OBTAINS NECESSARY BLOOD AND URINE SPECIMENS AND DIRECTS CLIENT TO RADIOLOGY

DELAY

RADIOLOGY TECHNICIAN COMPLETES CHEST X-RAY AND DIRECTS CLIENT TO CARDIOLOGY

DELAY

EKG TECHNICIAN COMPLETES TEST AND DIRECTS CLIENT BACK TO ADMISSION RECEPTIONIST

DELAY

CLIENT IS ESCORTED TO NURSING UNIT

DELAY

NURSE GREETS CLIENT AND ESCORTS HIM TO HIS ROOM

FIGURE 28-1. The admission process.

uling the admission interview on the day before admission. When these choices are provided for the client, he can exercise some control of the activities surrounding his hospitalization, and his sense of personal crisis may be decreased.

ASSIGNMENT TO THE NURSING UNIT

After the initial admission procedures have been completed, the client is either directed or escorted to the nursing unit to which he has been assigned. Very often the sight which greets him is one of bustling activity, with nurses and other hospital personnel rushing past him, barely glancing in his direction. He very quickly forms the impression, perhaps the correct one, that his presence is viewed as an unwelcome intrusion. As Smith has pointed out:

> The desk clerk at any first class hotel, besides offering a greeting, expresses some sort of awareness that the guest has, for some reasons, chosen this hotel for his stay. It is perfectly ordinary procedure for him to say: "We hope your stay will be a pleasant one."[1]

As institutions that serve the public, certainly hospitals should be cognizant of the fact that their "guests" pay very dearly for their "hotel rooms" and have a right to demand courteous and prompt attention to their needs.

With this in mind, the nurse should recognize that admission to the hospital is a time of perhaps overwhelming anxiety. The client may be fatigued from a long journey to the hospital and may have been even further exhausted by those admission procedures which took place prior to his arrival on the nursing unit. Those procedures, at the very least, invaded his privacy and took from him many of the accoutrements of his identity. He has come to the hospital supposedly to have his health needs cared for; yet, his needs may have been thus far relegated to low priority status. The nurse who first greets the client and admits him to the nursing unit can begin to meet many of his needs and plan his care in a holistic fashion which restores his sense of identity and self-esteem.

A *need* is defined as "a lack of something requisite, desirable, or useful; a condition requiring supply or relief."[2] A client's needs may be classified as affective, cognitive, and biological.

Affective Needs

The client's first impressions of the nursing personnel often provide the framework within which he chooses to interact with all health professionals during his hospitalization. As Schwartz and others have stated, "As long as the . . . staff can demonstrate their ability to care for him, the patient feels relatively safe."[3] A nurse who admits the client can help him to feel safe and begin to establish the necessary trusting relationship. Chalmers[4] pointed out many little things which are often neglected and

which are so important in the formation of impressions about the quality of care. She recommends that expected new admissions should be assigned to individual nurses at the start of the shift. When this is done, the client "benefits by a nurse who has been expecting him and made preparation for his arrival."[4] Preparations should include some thought as to the client's prospective roommates (e.g., if he is to be placed in a room with someone who smokes several cigars each day). The client's bed and room can be made to appear inviting when the bed is turned down, clean towels are available, and a water pitcher and glass are on the nightstand. The temperature of the room should be comfortable, and window curtains could be opened to make the room appear sunny and cheerful.

The appearance of the nurse is just as important as that of the hospital room. A nurse whose uniform is wrinkled or dirty, whose shoes are scuffed, and whose hair is awry gives the client the impression that she is barely capable of caring for herself, much less him. The nurse who is assigned to admit a new client should leave instructions with the ward clerk to be promptly notified of his arrival. She should greet him by name in a relaxed and friendly manner, introduce herself, and escort him to his room. If there are other clients in the room, it is appropriate to make introductions. The client should then be given an opportunity to unpack whatever belongings he has brought with him, because he will probably feel more comfortable in the new surroundings if, for example, his shaving kit is nearby and a picture of his family is in sight. Unless a client will soon require extensive physical care or diagnostic tests, it is not necessary for him to undress and put on a hospital gown or pajamas at this time. He may feel more comfortable in his own pajamas or he may wish to remain dressed until bedtime. These options should be provided. The admitting nurse should recognize that the client may desire assistance in unpacking and changing clothes, especially if he is quite fatigued. On the other hand, he may wish to be alone for a short time to rest and grow accustomed to his new environment. These options should also be offered to him.

Cognitive Needs

While the nursing measures which have been discussed thus far can relieve a great deal of the client's initial anxiety, interventions designed to meet his need for knowledge, his cognitive needs, will further alleviate anxiety and facilitate his becoming more comfortable in the hospital setting. A client cannot adapt to that which he does not understand. Schwartz and others have stated that, "the mental health of human beings consists very largely of the conviction that they are able to predict the future correctly."[3] Since the hospital is an unfamiliar environment, the client requires some concrete information upon which he can base predictions of his future during hospitalization.

Porter and others[5] have identified a hierarchy of clients' needs for information. Their study indicated that information about hospital routines and rules were of primary importance to a newly admitted client. This included such things as when meals are served, visiting hours, visiting limitations (i.e., in terms of the age and the number of visitors allowed), the time of physician rounds, and when he can expect to be awakened in the morning.

Second in importance was information about physical surroundings. This might include the location of the nurse call light and instruction of how it works; the location of the bathroom, nursing station, and day room or lounge; how the electric bed controls work; and the operation of television or radio controls.

Information about the social environment was third in priority. The client should know, for example, who will be taking care of him, who wears what color uniform, who is the appropriate person to ask for pain medication, and who should he complain to if his meals are not satisfactory.

Least important to the client was information about the patient role. Perhaps this is because clients hear a great deal prior to hospitalization from friends and relatives about how to act and who to talk to. Clients also may feel they have no *right* to know what is expected of them—that is, that they are entirely at the mercy of the medical and nursing personnel. Concrete information must be given to the client by the admitting nurse regarding his right to refuse a medication or treatment, his right to knowledge of his illness, the rationale for treatment, and his right to actively participate in his care. He also needs to know any expectations the particular hospital or its staff have of him, such as informing his nurse if he leaves the nursing unit for any reason.

As it was previously stated, the client's cognitive needs must be met upon admission to the nursing unit. A hierarchy of needs was presented and serves as a convenient means of classification. However, as Taylor has stated, "information needs are unique to each patient's background, status, hospital sophistication, and to his disease and the way in which he interprets his disease."[6] Therefore, a nurse admitting a new client must be observant of clues indicating what *his* priority of needs is.

Biological Needs

It is the responsibility of the admitting nurse to gather some baseline data about the client's physical status. Generally, after the client has been allowed some time to settle in his room and the nurse has assessed and met his needs for information, she verifies that laboratory specimens have been obtained and that other routine admission tests, such as a chest x-ray, have been performed. She then measures the client's height and weight. It is important that these are determined by exact measurement rather than relying on the client's statement of his usual height and weight, since dosage of medication, intravenous fluid therapy, and other treatments are calculated on the basis of these measurements. It is equally important that these initial data are obtained on the same scale which the client will use throughout his hospitalization, since there can be a major variance among scales.

Next, the nurse must take the client's vital signs. These include blood pressure, pulse, respiratory rate, and temperature. Again, it must be remembered that these are baseline data, and their accuracy is imperative. Equipment should be in excellent working order, and no shortcuts should be taken. The timing of taking vital signs is also important. O'Dell reported a study conducted at the Walter Reed Medical Center in Washington, D.C. which indicated that "anxiety during admission does affect these readings, some of them significantly."[7] In the study, blood pressure and pulse measurements taken on admission were significantly higher than measurements obtained 6 hours after admission, while temperature and respiratory rate remained relatively the same. It seems wise, therefore, for the nurse admitting a new client to assist him in coping with his anxiety prior to attempting to establish baseline data regarding vital signs.

In addition to obtaining the data discussed

above, the admitting nurse has the responsibility of beginning the client's chart. Vital signs should be recorded on the graphic sheet. Specimens or requests sent to the laboratory should be documented, as well as any medications or treatments which have been given. The nurse should also record any subjective or objective data which she may have obtained during her interactions with the client so far.

At this point, the admitting nurse must begin to plan for the ongoing holistic care of the client. Of absolute necessity to the accomplishment of this goal is taking a nursing history. Little and Carnevali define a nursing history as "a written record of specific information about the patient, providing data upon which to assess the existing or potential nursing care needs or patient problems, as a basis for planning and giving nursing care."[8] The nursing process and use of the nursing history are discussed elsewhere in this text, and therefore will not be dealt with here. However, the timing of the nursing history is essential to obtaining accurate and complete data. The nurse who admits a new client should keep in mind that a tired or anxious client will not be likely to cooperate in giving the necessary data.

SUMMARY

When a nurse has admitted the new client to the nursing unit, she must notify the client's physician of his arrival. At this time, she should be prepared to provide the physician with baseline data in terms of the client's affective, cognitive, and biological needs and to request whatever information from him that she needs to begin to administer care.

As hospitals grow larger and larger, the reams of paper which are shuffled from place to place in an attempt to meet the agency's needs sometimes bury the client. He is stamped, numbered, filed, and assigned to a slot. Wu quoted a patient who said, "outside of the hospital you're somebody; in here you're nobody."[9] Certainly, it must fall to nurses, as caring professionals encountering the client when he is admitted, to intervene in a manner which aids him in retaining his self-esteem and which assures him that he is, indeed, a very important "somebody."

REFERENCES

1. Smith, R. K.: Depersonalization inexcusable. *Nurs. Outlook* 18:15, 1970.
2. *Webster's Seventh New Collegiate Dictionary.* Springfield, Mass., G. and C. Merriam Co., 1965, p. 565.
3. Schwartz, L. H., and Schwartz, J. L.: *The Psychodynamics of Patient Care.* Englewood Cliffs, N.J., Prentice-Hall, Inc., 1972, p. 228.
4. Chalmers, H.: Return to basics: first impressions stick. *Nurs. Mirror* (Suppl.), 1977.
5. Porter, A., et al.: Patient needs on admission. *Am. J. Nurs.* 77:112, 1977.
6. Taylor, C. D.: The hospital patient's social dilemma. *Am. J. Nurs.* 65:96-97, 1965.
7. O'Dell, M. L.: Are routine admission signs really reliable? *R.N.* vol. 38 OR/ED: p. 23, 1975.
8. Little, D. E., and Carnevali, D. L.: *Nursing Care Planning.* Philadelphia, J. B. Lippincott Company, 1969, p. 66.
9. Wu, R.: *Behavior and Illness.* Englewood Cliffs, N.J., Prentice-Hall, Inc., 1973, p. 70.

CHAPTER 29

One of the most frequent tools utilized by the nurse to assess a client's condition is the observation of specific objective signs that indicate the status of body functioning. Because the temperature, pulse, respirations, and blood pressure are controlled by the vital organs and are essential to life, they are referred to as the *vital* or *cardinal signs.* These signs are usually fairly stable, but will change, often significantly, when deviations occur in the body's functioning. The changes in the vital signs serve as clues or indicators that a disturbance has taken place. Variations point to the possibility of an alteration of or interference with: fluid and electrolyte balance (e.g., decreased circulating blood volume, circulatory overload, acidosis, alkalosis), oxygenation of body tissues (as in cardiovascular and respiratory conditions), stress and emotional status (depression, elation, fear, and anxiety), and immunity and susceptibility (barriers) to infection (e.g., childhood illnesses, bacteriogenic diseases, injury, and tissue trauma).

The vital signs are measured and recorded at the time of initial contact with the client or upon his

THE ASSESSMENT OF VITAL SIGNS

Arlyne B. Saperstein, M.N., R.N., and
Margaret A. Frazier, M.S., R.N.

admission to an agency. This serves as a *baseline reading* or data base. Vital signs taken during the remainder of the period when the client is undergoing care or treatment can then be compared to the original findings for evaluation. Careful periodic monitoring of the vital signs ensures that nurses remain in tune with any significant alterations that take place. The timing of the intervals between the measurements of the vital signs varies according to the specific agency's policies and the condition of the client. Naturally, the more serious the client's condition, the more frequently they should be obtained. Critical situations require constant monitoring of vital signs.

The healthy individual's vital signs fall within a set range designated as "normal." Even within this range, there are variations from one person to another. For instance, a temperature that is normal for one individual may be subnormal for a different person or slightly elevated for yet another. Many factors influence the vital signs. These include age, sex, weight, metabolic rate, health status, illness, time of day or month, increase or decrease in phys-

ical activity, environmental changes such as room temperature, humidity, and weather, stressful or anxiety-provoking incidents, ingestion of drugs (especially stimulants and depressants), and pain.

BODY TEMPERATURE

Regulation

HEAT PRODUCTION

The temperature of the body in warm blooded (homeothermic) animals, including man, results from a balance between heat production and dissipation. Heat production, a *chemical* process, is the outcome of *metabolic activity;* the more the metabolism is stimulated, the more heat will be produced. Oxidation of nutrients (proteins, fats, and carbohydrates) liberates energy, therefore heat. It is for this reason that in colder climates a person will need heartier meals to "provide enough fuel for the furnace" when facing low temperatures and the need for more heat production and warmth.

Heat and cold sensitive nerve receptors are found in the skin. When they register that we are feeling cold, a message is sent to the brain and appropriate actions to conserve and produce more heat are initiated. The thermoregulatory center in the brain, the *hypothalamus,* coordinates all of the processes that must occur for temperature control. Its action is much like that of a thermostat; neurons sensitive to heat are located in the hypothalamus and when cooled will increase heat production. When signals from the skin receptors are sent, the "setting" of the thermostat will be altered as necessary for regulation of the temperature to take place. To increase heat production, sympathetic nerves in the posterior hypothalamus are stimulated, causing a decrease in the activity of sweat glands, vasoconstriction of the blood vessels in the skin (cutaneous vessels), and cutis anserina or pilo-erection (gooseflesh) to occur. Peripheral vasoconstriction decreases heat loss by allowing less blood to flow near the skin surface where it can be cooled and keeping it in the deeper, more insulated areas of the body. As the sympathetic nervous system is stimulated, there will also be an increase in the metabolic rate as epinephrine and norepinephrine are produced. In addition, the skeletal muscles receive signals from the posterior hypothalamus to contract (involuntarily), and the resulting shivering will increase the production of heat. Voluntary muscle contraction or tensing also generates large amounts of heat as fat and glucose are burned. The more strenuous the exercise, the more heat will be yielded. Temperature will rise temporarily since the heat cannot be eliminated as fast as it is produced. In all physiological states, except arduous exercise, the liver is the prime source of heat due to the diversity and magnitude of basal metabolic processes required for life which it carries out. It follows that the temperature of the liver is the highest in the body.

HEAT LOSS

While heat production is essentially chemical in nature, heat loss occurs via the following *physical* processes:

1. Radiation, or the interchange of energy from one object, through the air, to another object.
2. Conduction, the transfer of heat from one object to another through direct contact.

3. Evaporation, the vaporization of a liquid in the presence of heat.
4. Convection, the transference of heat through liquids or circulating air.

The hypothalamus again is called into action when it receives the message that cooling mechanisms are necessary. The parasympathetic nervous system is stimulated resulting in heightened activity of sweat glands. Perspiration increases; the skin is cooled as evaporation of sweat (moisture) takes place. Peripheral vasodilation increasing radiation, conduction, and convection occurs. Approximately 85 percent of body heat is lost via the skin (radiating surface area) while the lungs and urinary and digestive excretions account for the remaining 15 percent.[1] Metabolic activity is slowed and muscle relaxation (decreased tonus) takes place. Perhaps this is why the activity and pace of life appears to be slower and more relaxed in areas where warm weather is prevalent.

Factors Affecting Temperature

"Normal" temperature must refer to a range rather than a single point on a scale, since for every individual that particular point is different. Although 98.6° Fahrenheit (37° Celsius or Centigrade) refers to the statistical average of oral temperatures, it may be within normal limits if the temperature is 1 degree above or 2 degrees below that value.[2] Not only does temperature differ from person to person, it is different in the same person when various factors are introduced.

ENVIRONMENTAL CONDITIONS. The temperature of the body tends to be lower in cold weather and higher in hot weather. When the temperature and humidity of ambient air is elevated or the person is submerged in water hotter than that of the body, then radiation cannot take place and the temperature rises. Vaporization of perspiration and convection are dependent upon air currents (circulation) and on the amount of surface area (skin) exposed to the air.

AGE. An infant's temperature is labile since his hypothalamus is immature. Wide rapid swings in temperature in relation to environmental conditions and amount of clothing or coverage are common.

Children's temperatures will often be ½ to 1 degree Fahrenheit higher than that of adults since their physical (muscular) activity and metabolic rates are higher. In old age vascular changes which decrease blood flow—sedentary activity, lessened muscle tonus, diminished appetite, and loss of body insulation (subcutaneous tissue)—account for less heat production and a lower temperature.

PHYSICAL ACTIVITIES. Any activity that stimulates the endocrine glands and increases basal metabolic rate significantly will vary the temperature during and immediately following it. Examples are exercise, sexual intercourse, and eating.

EMOTIONAL ACTIVITY. Any strong emotional state can cause a rise in the temperature of the body since glandular secretions, and thus, metabolic rate, increase.

CIRCADIAN (DIURNAL) RHYTHM. In the early hours of the morning, when the body is at rest, the temperature is at its lowest point. As activity increases, so does the temperature, reaching its peak in late afternoon or early evening. People who work at night and rest during the day demonstrate the reverse in their temperatures; the highest point occurs in the morning and the lowest in the evening. This is known as an *inverse* temperature.

MENSTRUATION, OVULATION, AND PREGNANCY. The body temperature rises from ½ to 1 degree Fahrenheit at the time of ovulation and remains elevated until it drops just prior to the next menstrual cycle. For women whose cycles are *extremely* regular, temperature readings can assist them in calculating when they ovulate. By taking their temperature at the same time every morning (upon arising) and keeping a graph or chart of these temperature readings, a pattern emerges and ovulation may be pinpointed with some accuracy. This record is known as a *basal temperature chart.* During pregnancy, since metabolic activity is high, the body temperature may remain elevated approximately 1 degree.

ROUTE OF MEASUREMENT. A temperature measured rectally usually registers from ½ to 1 degree Fahrenheit (0.28 to 0.50 degree Celsius) higher than by mouth. Temperatures taken via the axillary (armpit) method read approximately ½ degree Fahrenheit lower than the oral temperature.[3]

Divergence from Normal

Just as an exact "normal" point cannot be designated for body temperature, the specific point at which an elevated temperature becomes a *fever* (*pyrexia* or *hyperthermia*) and a lowered temperature becomes *subnormal* (*hypothermia*) is difficult to establish. For the sake of practicality, anything below 97°F (36°C) orally, is considered subnormal and above 100°F (37.8°C) orally, is considered *febrile* (having a temperature elevation). Again remember that this varies from individual to individual; the person whose temperature is usually found in the low-normal range will be hyperthermic at a lower temperature than the one who runs a higher normal reading.

Pyrexia occurs when there is a disproportionate amount of heat production in relation to heat loss; that is, heat is produced at a faster rate than it is eliminated. The symptoms which may accompany the febrile state are increased pulse and respiratory rates, general malaise (discomfort or achiness), pale, dry skin (later flushed) which is hot to the touch, chills, loss of appetite (anorexia), nausea, constipation, and occasionally diarrhea, thirst, headache, restlessness, coated tongue, decreased urinary output, concentration of the urine, insomnia, irritability, weakness, and in *hyperpyrexia* (temperature above 105°F) delirium, coma, and convulsions. The latter is seen more often in children (up to age 5) and is not necessarily related to the severity of the illness.

In hyperpyrexic states, damage can occur to the central nervous system causing irreparable harm and loss of function, if not death. Equally as traumatic, severe hypothermia can prevent functioning or destroy tissues by depressing metabolism. Symptoms of hypothermia are reduced pulse and respiratory rates, paleness, cyanosis, coldness of skin to the touch, loss of feeling, and unconsciousness.

There are three specific periods or stages in the *course of a fever:*

1. *The invasion or onset* is that time when the temperature is rising until the maximum point has been reached. This stage can be either

gradual or sudden, depending on the cause of the fever. Each disease has a characteristic pattern that the course of the fever follows, which is sometimes so distinctive that the physician automatically thinks of that particular disease when the pattern is described.

2. *The fastigium or stadium* is the highest point of the fever. The period includes the time when the fever remains fairly constant, but it varies in some fevers.

3. *Defervescence* is the decline of the fever until the normal range is reached. This stage, too, can be gradual (*lysis*) or sudden (*crisis*) and is also very characteristic of the causative condition.

In describing fevers, they are categorized by certain behaviors:

1. A *sustained, continuous,* or *constant fever* is a raised temperature that remains almost without variation at an elevated point.

2. An *intermittent fever* consists of alternating periods of elevated temperature and returns to normal or subnormal, within the same day.

3. A *hectic fever* is a form of intermittent fever in which the swings between the highest and lowest points are very wide.

4. *Remittent fever* is a fever with wide fluctuations, but one which does not return to normal until the fever has subsided.

5. *Relapsing fever* is a recurrent fever in which the temperature will alternate between elevation and periods of normalcy that last for a day or more.

Measurement

Body temperature is measured using either a thermometer or one of a variety of devices that determine oral or skin temperature. The *clinical thermometer* is a glass tube containing mercury within a bulb at one end. When the bulb comes in contact with body heat, the mercury, a liquid metal, expands and rises up the stem of the instrument. A narrowing in the base of the stem keeps the mercury from flowing back into the bulb. The mercury must be forced back into the bulb by forceful snapping movements. A temperature scale, calibrated in tenths of a degree is etched along the stem of the thermometer. The curvature of the instrument magnifies the mercury column and scale for ease of reading. The shape of the bulb determines the site of placement and the rapidity of registration. The greater the surface area of glass surrounding the mercury (as with the long slender bulb), the more rapidly the mercury will heat and expand. See Figure 29-1 for both calibrations and bulb shapes. Rounded or blunt bulbed thermometers are used for rectal temperatures, since there is less likelihood of injury (puncture) to the rectal mucosa than with the long bulb which is used for oral or axillary temperatures. See Table 29-1A (at the end of the chapter) for the steps involved in measurement of body temperature with a clinical thermometer.

In addition to the clinical thermometer, there are alternative devices for temperature measurement. These include an *electronic thermometer* which gives an accurate reading in just seconds. Plastic disposable sheaths cover the probe, virtually elim-

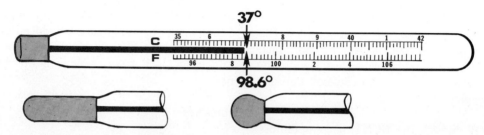

FIGURE 29-1. The thermometer with both Fahrenheit and Celsius (centigrade) temperature scales. The blunt bulb can be used for both oral and rectal insertion. The elongated bulb (bottom, left) is found on an oral thermometer. The round bulb (bottom, right) is found on a rectal thermometer.

inating the possibility of injury, infection, or cross-contamination among clients. Some of the electronic thermometers must be prewarmed prior to use. Readouts are either flashed digitally or read from a needle on a stationary scale. Other devices are *heat sensitive discs or tapes* that are used primarily for infants. The tape, which is applied directly to the abdomen, changes color with change in temperature. If pyrexia or hypothermia is indicated, then temperature must be taken with a thermometer to gauge the accurate amount. Additionally, a variety of disposable devices for temperature measurement are now on the market.

ORAL. Choice of route depends on specific considerations. Oral temperatures are the easiest to obtain but cannot be used if the client is not able to hold the thermometer safely and readily in his mouth. This would be the case in the weak or debilitated person, the unreliable individual, as in infants, children, or adults who are uncooperative, confused, irrational, or unconscious. Oral temperatures also are contraindicated in cases of inability to breathe through the nose, as in nasal congestion, acute colds, the presence of nasogastric tubes, and diseases or surgery of the nose or mouth.

RECTAL. A rectal temperature is usually ordered when accuracy is vital, especially with clients who have an elevated temperature that must be watched closely. They are contraindicated for clients who have fecal impactions, diarrhea, or diseases, conditions, or surgery of the rectal or perineal area.

AXILLARY. When both oral and rectal temperatures are not possible, as in severely burned clients, infants in hospitals where rectal temperatures are not permitted, or for any other reasons, then *axillary temperatures* will be taken.

Treatment of Deviations

Fever is believed by some authorities to be beneficial or constructive in that it not only warns us of a physical disturbance, but it also serves to protect the body by causing the environment to be too hot for the pathogenic (invading) organism to survive. It can be quite destructive, too, as in the case of sunstroke. Hypothermia, with its resultant depression of metabolic activity, can be used constructively, as in certain surgical procedures where the body is purposefully cooled considerably, lessening the body's need for oxygen consumption. Hypothermia, as in cases of extended periods of exposure to extreme cold, can also be harmful.

In any case, when extremes are reached in hypothermia and hyperthermia, treatment must be instituted before irreversible damage or death occurs. Treatment should be specific, of course, to the nature of the causative illness or condition, but the fever or hypothermia also will usually be treated symptomatically.

In the case of hypothermia, the vital signs should be measured, recorded, and reported at frequent intervals; the more severe the condition, the more frequently they should be obtained. Provisions for warmth and insulation should be made with blankets and hot water bottles. The latter will require a physician's order. In addition, he may order hot drinks and an increase in physical activity if this is feasible.

Similarly, in the case of pyrexia, the physician determines the course of treatment. Vital signs are taken in a similar fashion as stated above; if the temperature is high or if chills occur, the frequency of measurement should increase. (If chills are present, then warmth should be provided during that period.) The client needs rest, and the environment should be conducive to relaxation with limitations of exercise and activity. Since the client may be quite weak, he must be carefully observed and protected against falls and injury. The use of side rails is advisable. Antipyretic drugs, such as aspirin (acetylsalicylic acid) or Tylenol (acetaminophen) are usually prescribed. Cooling the body may be done by lowering the temperature of the environment or by the application of cool compresses. Sponging the body with cool water increases evaporation and therefore, heat loss. The addition of alcohol to the water increases the rate of evaporation. If giving an alcohol and water (or plain water) sponge, keep the parts not being sponged covered to avoid severe chilling, and provide for privacy. The temperature should be closely monitored to avoid a crisis-like defervescence. Fluids are usually encouraged; intake and output are measured, and urinary elimination is observed for amount and concentration. The physician should be informed of the client's status throughout the duration of treatment.

RESPIRATIONS

The student is referred to Chapter 36, "Maintenance of Respiratory Status and Pulmonary Functioning," for a detailed review of basic respiratory function. Included in that chapter are: anatomy and physiology; neurological and chemical regulation and control of the pulmonary system; influences affecting the quality of respirations; and causes and effects of respiratory dysfunction, including conditions and mechanisms of respiratory impairment. Nursing care measures most frequently employed to assist in prevention of dysfunction and restoration of optimal levels of functioning are also explored. It is recommended that the student review the process of respiration before progressing further in this chapter.

General Considerations

When assessing a client's respirations there are many aspects that must be considered. Under normal conditions, respirations are quiet, easy (without effort), relaxed, and uniform. Many factors can change that normal pattern. Any time that the *metabolic rate* of an individual is increased (for any reason), the respiratory rate will increase accordingly. Conversely, when the metabolic rate drops, the respirations decrease. When the body's *demand for oxygen* increases or the availability of oxygen decreases, it must be supplied with more, and thus, stimulation of respiration occurs. Placement in an atmosphere that has a high oxygen concentration may decrease respiratory rate. *Drugs* or *medications* and *illnesses* are capable of changing (including raising or lowering) respiratory patterns. (Illness usually increases the rate because of the demands on metabolism; however, there are certain conditions that can depress respiration.)

In addition to rate, depth, character (quality), and patterns of respiration, the nurse should observe body parts that specifically relate to the respiratory process. Skin *color* is an important clue to physiological status. *Cyanosis* is a dusky or bluish tinge; it may be seen over the entire body surface when it is marked, but it usually appears in areas with a rich superficial blood supply. While the lips, earlobes, and nailbeds are excellent sites to observe and are commonly checked for cyanosis, the gums, buccal mucosa and the area beneath the tongue give the most definitive picture. This is especially true with regard to people with deep pigmentation of the skin.

The *configuration and symmetry of the chest* can indicate the presence of chronic respiratory problems. Along with this, a *position of comfort* taken to ease difficult breathing should be noted. Increased *involvement of musculature* other than the diaphragm in adults for respiratory effort is noteworthy. In infants, symptoms of respiratory difficulty or distress include *intercostal* and *sternal retractions, seesaw respirations, chin lag, nasal flaring,* and an audible expiratory *grunt* (Figure 29-2 demonstrates rating of respiratory distress in infants.)

Rate and Depth

While the newborn breathes approximately 30 to 40 times per minute, the *rate* slows down through the years until adulthood, at which time it is approximately 16 to 20 times per minute. (Some state that 12 is the low normal limit, while others believe that 22 is the normal high limit.) Pulse rate and respiratory rate usually correspond to one another; the ratio is about one respiration to four or five heartbeats.

Depth refers to the amount (volume) of air exchanged with every respiration. The normal adult's *tidal volume* averages approximately 500 ml of air. Depth should remain fairly even from breath to breath. *Shallow* and *deep* are the most common terms used when referring to depth.

The following terms relate to rate and depth of respirations:

bradypnea. Very slow breathing.
hyperpnea. An increase in the rate of respirations that are deeper than usually found during normal periods of activity.
hyperventilation. Increased rate and depth of respirations causing increased air inspiration and expiration. Carbon dioxide depletion occurs and must be reversed to combat decrease in blood pressure and dizziness which results.
hypopnea. A decrease in both rate and depth of respirations that is abnormal.
hypoventilation. Decrease in the rate and depth of respiration.
oligopnea. An extremely slow respiratory rate with either shallow or abnormally deep breathing.

Upper Chest	Lower Chest (Intercostal Retraction)	Xiphoid Retraction	Dilation Of Nares	Expiratory Grunt

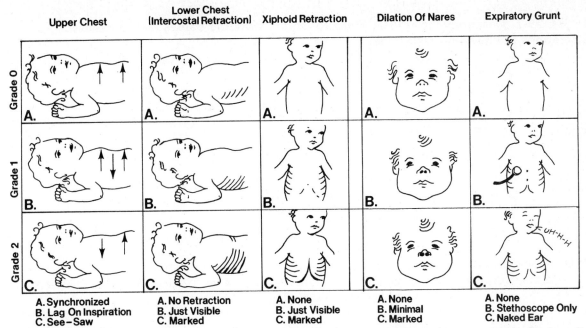

A. Synchronized B. Lag On Inspiration C. See-Saw	A. No Retraction B. Just Visible C. Marked
A. None B. Just Visible C. Marked	A. None B. Minimal C. Marked
A. None B. Stethoscope Only C. Naked Ear	

FIGURE 29-2. Evaluation of the respiratory status of the infant is determined by assigning a grade of 0, 1, or 2 to each of the five criteria shown. Totaling the grades will give a a score of 0 to 10. 0 indicates—no respiratory distress, 10—indicates extreme distress. (Courtesy of Ross Laboratories.)

polypnea. Very rapid (panting) breathing.
tachypnea. Very rapid breathing.

Character or Quality

In describing respirations, the ease or difficulty of breathing is observed. In conjunction with this are the sounds that relate to breathing. The following terms are descriptive:

apnea. The absence of respirations.
dyspnea. Difficult or labored breathing. Respirations are rapid, and individual appears frightened; may gasp for breath.
eupnea. Normal breathing.
orthopnea. Difficulty breathing in positions other than standing or sitting erect.
sighing. A breath characterized by a slow, audible expiration which follows a deep inspiration.
stertor. Breathing that is labored and accompanied by snoring sound.
stridor. Harsh, high-pitched, crowing sound on inspiration.
wheezing. Difficult breathing accompanied by wheezing sounds.

Patterns

Associated with certain conditions there are distinct patterns of respiratory behavior that can be identified. The more common ones are:

apneustic breathing. A short and ineffectual attempt at expiration follows a prolonged inspiration.
Cheyne-Stokes respiration. Alternation of cycles of increasingly rapid and deep respirations with periods of apnea that vary in length (often seen just prior to death but can occur for other reasons).
Kussmaul's respirations. Labored, gasping respirations of increased rate and depth, associated with diabetic coma.
paradoxical respirations. Lung deflation occurs upon inspiration, with inflation upon expiration.

It is important that the nurse describe respirations that vary from normal carefully. Recording of respiratory rate alone is insufficient information for client assessment. For a description of the method for measuring respirations see Table 29-1.

The Assessment of Vital Signs 459

TABLE 29-1. Measurement of Vital Signs to Obtain Baseline Values and to Assess Alterations in Physiological Status

Anticipated Accomplishment	Scientific Principles/ Rationale	Specific Considerations

A. Measurement of Body Temperature by Oral, Rectal, and Axillary Routes

Anticipated Accomplishment	Scientific Principles/ Rationale	Specific Considerations
1. Minimization of the spread of microorganisms: cleansing of nurses' hands.	Resident bacteria and other microorganisms on hands can be transmitted by direct contact or with objects that come in contact with client.	
2. Decrease client's anxiety by explaining procedure.	Fear of unknown and lack of information are major factors in heightened anxiety states.	Ascertain: 1. clients level of understanding; 2. age; 3. previous experience with procedure. Most adults are not anxious about procedures if they *know* they are painless. May be concerned about frequency with which vital signs are taken or results. Use of rectal route may concern adults. Small children may be more alarmed at sight of thermometer than procedure, especially if it is first experience.
3. Select route of measurement and appropriate thermometer.	Accuracy of measurement and safety of client are prime concerns. Rectal thermometers have short, round bulbs, minimizing chance of perforating rectum. Oral and axillary thermometers have long slender bulbs; surface of bulb containing mercury is larger; therefore, less time is needed to heat (and thus expand) mercury.	Considerations for use of rectal or oral route: 1. Can client breathe through nose without difficulty or discomfort? 2. Is there infection, disease, lesions, injury, or trauma (such as surgery) to nose, mouth, rectum or perineum? Is there diarrhea? 3. Can client assume responsibility for holding glass thermometer in mouth safely for prescribed time? 4. Does client have elevated temperature?

Implementation	Recommendations	Observations
Wash hands using aseptic technique.		
Explain to client in understandable terms, reasons for and steps of procedure.		Does client appear anxious or ask questions as to why temperature is being taken (i.e., "Do you think I have a fever?"). Does client appear relieved or more confident after explanation?
Check with physician if there is a question about route ordered. Check agency policy.	Oral route is never used in infants, small children, irrational, unreliable, confused, combative, weak, or comatose adults.	

TABLE 29-1. Continued

Anticipated Accomplishment	Scientific Principles/ Rationale	Specific Considerations
4. Minimization of spread of microorganisms: cleansing of thermometer (removal of antiseptic storage solution).	Antiseptic (chemical solutions) usually have disagreeable taste; may also be irritating to mucous membrane of mouth, rectum, and skin. Some solutions may temporarily alter skin temperature. Hot water causes expansion of mercury. Possibility of spread of microorganisms is reduced by moving from "clean" to "dirty" area. (Bulb of thermometer is cleaner than fingers prior to taking client's temperature.)	How is thermometer stored? If sterilized and enclosed in wrapper, no cleansing or wiping is necessary. If stored in antiseptic solution, remove solution before insertion.
5. Return mercury to point in column lower than anticipated body temperature. (Proceed to step 8 for use of oral route. Steps 6 and 7 relate to rectal temperatures.)	Mercury column must be forcibly lowered manually. If body temperature is lower than point on scale, mercury will not lower itself automatically to new reading.	Use well lighted area to assure correct reading.
6. Lubrication of thermometer.	Smooth insertion of thermometer into rectum is facilitated with lubricant to decrease friction and discomfort. Also decreases the possibility of irritation of mucous membrane which can cause stimulation of rectum and expulsion of thermometer.	
7. Correct positioning of client for measuring rectal temperature.	Unobstructed visualization of anus facilitates insertion of thermometer and avoidance of discomfort if hemorrhoids are present.	Meet client's need for privacy.

Implementation	Recommendations	Observations
Rinse thermometer with water.	Use *cold* water. Hot water may break thermometer.	
Dry thermometer by wiping from bulb end toward fingers.	Use clean facial tissue for drying thermometer.	
Read point at which mercury level matches temperature scale.	Hold thermometer at eye level and rotate until mercury column can be clearly visualized.	
If necessary shake thermometer until mercury level is below 96°F. (35.5°C.)	Grasp thermometer *securely* with thumb and forefinger and shake downward sharply using wrist action. (Avoid standing near furniture to eliminate possibility of hitting glass against objects and breaking thermometer.)	
Lubricate thermometer with K-Y jelly or suitable alternative.	With applicator or tongue blade, place lubricant on facial tissue to spread lubricant on tip and up 1 inch of thermometer stem (shaft). If lubricant comes in single use disposable packets, open end and dip thermometer into packet.	
Place client in Sim's (side-lying) position after providing for privacy.		Note presence of hemorrhoids.

TABLE 29-1. Continued

Anticipated Accomplishment	Scientific Principles/ Rationale	Specific Considerations
8. Insertion of thermometer.	Internal body heat is greater than at periphery since cooling takes place via skin. Blood transports heat to body tissues. Rectum gives most accurate reading of internal temperature because of rich blood supply and no exposure to air. Small sublingual pockets also give accurate reading (if the mouth is kept closed) since this too has rich blood supply. Injury could result if client rolls over on thermometer and it breaks.	Place thermometer in area with good blood supply and least possible exposure to air. Has client ingested hot or cold food or fluids, chewed gum, or smoked in last 20 to 30 min? (If so, wait for 20–30 min.)
	Chance of exposure to air is greater with oral and rectal routes since these are not actually enclosed cavities. Moisture conducts heat. Bath water and friction may alter temperature.	Axillary temperatures are used when oral and rectal routes are contraindicated or when agency policy dictates. This is least hazardous of routes, but least accurate. Thermometer must remain in place longer. Is axilla moist or dry?
9. Minimization of the spread of microorganisms: cleansing of thermometer after removal.	Reduction of spread of microorganisms from client to nurse move from "clean" to "dirty" area. (Bulb of thermometer is more contaminated than fingers after taking the client's temperature.) Cleansing thermometer of material facilitates accuracy of reading.	

Implementation	Recommendations	Observations
Oral: Place thermometer in client's mouth, under tongue in small sublingual pocket. Thermometer is held in place by client's lips.	Instruct client to keep mouth closed and not bite down on thermometer. Leave in place 7 to 8 min. (Some say 5 to 7, others 7 to 10. There is great controversy in literature on time for accurate registration.)	While thermometer is in place, assess other vital signs (unless taking rectal temperature in Sim's position) and observe client for color, condition, etc.
Rectal: Insert thermometer gently 1½ to 2 inches into anus.	Ask client to breathe deeply to relax sphincter and ease insertion. Leave in place 3 min. (Some say 2, others 5.) Do not leave infant or child alone with thermometer in place. With infants, small children, and unreliable adults, hold thermometer in place.	
If perspiration present, wash and dry area and wait 10 min. Insert thermometer in apex of axilla between inner aspect of arm and chest.	Pat dry rather than rub; friction raises temperature. Have client hold arm across chest to keep thermometer in place. Leave for 10 min.	
Remove thermometer. With tissue clean from fingertips down to bulb once. Discard wipe.		

TABLE 29-1. Continued

Anticipated Accomplishment	Scientific Principles/ Rationale	Specific Considerations
10. Ascertain body temperature reading		
11. Record temperature reading and report as necessary.	Vital signs, especially variations, are indicators of client's status when looked at as part of a whole clinical picture.	Contrast reading with baseline, previous reading, and standard "normal" values.
12. Store thermometer.		Store according to accepted agency procedure. Some thermometers are used once and returned to central supply for sterilization. Others use one thermometer/client throughout stay. Storage containers also differ.
B. Measurement of Respirations		
1. Ascertain that client is at rest.	Respiration increases with increases in metabolic rate.	Has client experienced stress, exertion, or heightened emotion recently?

Implementation	Recommendations	Observations
Read thermometer as in step 5.	Do not shake thermometer down until after temperature reading is recorded, allowing for double check (i.e., if distracted momentarily).	
Record in manner appropriate to agency.	Record on work sheet if no bedside chart exists. Do not cast to memory.	
Report significant findings or variations to appropriate personnel.	Transcribe on graphic sheet in client's record.	
Temperature reading is oral unless designated otherwise. Ⓡ next to temperature indicates rectal; Ⓐ axillary. (In some institutions, ink color designates route.)	If writing temperature in narrative, include °F or °C after numeral for absolute accuracy. To convert from Fahrenheit to centigrade: $$°C = \frac{(°F - 32)}{9} \times 5.$$ To convert from centigrade to Fahrenheit: $$°F = \frac{9}{5}°C + 32.$$	
Replace thermometer in designated receptacle if to be used again. Cleanse and disinfect as per designated procedure.	Usually thermometer is cleansed by washing with soap and rinsing with cold water, dried, and returned to disinfecting solution.	
Be sure client is in comfortable position (at rest).	Respirations are best counted immediately after pulse while client is seated or recumbent.	Does client appear at rest?

TABLE 29-1. Continued

Anticipated Accomplishment	Scientific Principles/ Rationale	Specific Considerations
2. Count respirations.	There is both voluntary and involuntary control of breathing. When one knows that their respirations are being counted, they become aware of their breathing and tend to control it to a degree.	
3. Record and report respirations	Respirations are valuable indicator of physiological status when viewed in relation to whole picture of client.	Compare with baseline reading for significant changes and with standard "normal" values.
C. Measurement of Heartbeat		
1. Provide for client's comfort.	Physical and emotional stresses alter (usually increase) rate which is reflected in heart rate.	Has client had recent exercise, exertion, or period of heightened emotion? If taking a radial pulse, be sure arm is supported. If taking apical pulse, area at tip (apex) of heart should be accessible.
2. A. Count pulse by palpation.	Superficial pulses usually lie over bony prominence. Normal pulse is obliterated if compression is too forceful. Not enough compression makes measurement difficult.	Choice of site depends on its accessibility and condition of client.

Implementation	Recommendations	Observations
Count number of complete cycles of respiration/min (inspiration and expiration). (One cycle equals one respiration.)	While holding client's wrist (or while stethoscope is in place against chest), begin counting respirations. If client is unaware that respirations are being counted and believes that pulse is being taken, count will be more accurate.	Assess quality and character of respirations.
Record and report significant findings or alterations to appropriate personnel.	Record on worksheet if no bedside chart. Transcribe on graphic sheet in client's record.	

Implementation	Recommendations	Observations
Explain procedures. Place client in comfortable position (at rest).	Dorsal recumbent or a sitting position (semi-Fowler's or Fowler's) are usually positions of comfort or rest appropriate for taking radial pulse. Do not extend client's arm with no support. Place client's arm across chest to facilitate counting respirations after taking pulse. It also gives arm a base of support.	Does client appear at rest?
	Supine position is best for accessibility to client's chest. (Provide for privacy as needed).	If client has orthopnea, do not use supine position. Use position of comfort that affords ease in respiration. (Difficulty breathing will cause anxiety, increasing heart rate.)
Place two or three fingertips over pulse site and apply moderate pressure.	Do not place thumb over pulse because thumb has own pulse.	
Count regular pulse beat for 30 seconds and double amount for the rate/min. Count irregular pulses for full min.	Use watch with sweep second hand. Time must be exact for counting heart rate.	Assess rate, rhythm, volume, and if applicable, pattern of pulse. Observe color and other characteristics but attend to time.

TABLE 29-1. Continued

Anticipated Accomplishment	Scientific Principles/ Rationale	Specific Considerations
B. Count pulse by auscultation.		A stethoscope is needed for this procedure.
	Heartbeat is best heard over apex of heart (over ventricles). Apex is to left of sternum, usually just below nipple line.	If diaphragm is cold to touch, warm by holding in hand. There are two heart sounds for each beat. Do *not* count as two beats!
3. Record and report heartbeat.	Heartbeat is valuable indicator of physiological status when viewed in relation to whole picture of client.	Compare with baseline reading for significant changes and with standard "normal" values.

D. Measurement of Blood Pressure

Anticipated Accomplishment	Scientific Principles/ Rationale	Specific Considerations
1. Minimization of the spread of microorganisms: cleansing of nurse's hands.	Resident bacteria and other microorganisms on hands can be transmitted by direct contact or with objects that come in contact with client.	
2. Decrease client's anxiety by explaining procedure.	Fear of unknown or lack of information are major factors in heightened anxiety states.	Ascertain: 1. client's level of understanding; 2. age; 3. previous experience with procedure.
3. Recognize factors which alter blood pressure.	Stress, emotional reactions, food, smoking, change in climate, bladder distention, fecal impaction, physical exertion, pain, and sex may influence blood pressure.	Ascertain client's: 1. emotional status; 2. physical status (e.g., exercise, meals, or cigarettes in last 20–30 min).
4. Select site of measurement.	Forearm is usually the recommended site, as it is readily available and the supply of appropriate blood vessels is plentiful.	If the client is supine, repositioning of arm may be needed since arm is already at heart level.

Implementation	Recommendations	Observations
Cleanse both ear tips and diaphragm (disc) with antiseptic before use. Place diaphragm or bell end of stethoscope (either type will be suitable) directly over apex of heart. Count for full min.	Cleanse ear pieces with appropriate antiseptic (e.g., alcohol) to decrease possibility of transmission of ear infection. Ear pieces usually feel more comfortable and afford better sound quality if placed so tips are facing forward in external (outer) ear.	Assess the quality and character of apical pulse.
Record in manner appropriate to agency. Report significant findings or alterations to appropriate personnel. Pulse is assumed radial unless identified as from another site.	Record on worksheet if no bedside chart. Transcribe on graphic sheet in client's record.	
Wash hands using aseptic technique.		
Explain to client in understandable terms reasons for and steps of procedure.		Does client appear anxious?
Control or avoid stimuli as much as possible.	Adults and children should be in quiet surroundings. Clothing should not constrain area where pressure is taken. Client should not alter position for 5 min preceding reading.	Any factors noted that influence blood pressure should be recorded with findings.
With client in dorsal recumbent position, support arm and place horizontally at heart level.	It is preferable to take pressure readings on left arm. If not possible, use right arm.	There may be physical reasons why one or both arms cannot be used (e.g., casts, burns, traction, or intravenous infusion).

TABLE 29-1. Continued

Anticipated Accomplishment	Scientific Principles/ Rationale	Specific Considerations
		If forearm is inaccessible, blood pressure can be taken on thigh.
		In clients experiencing cardiovascular difficulties, take pressure readings in both arms and in one or both legs.
5. Select method and appropriate equipment.	Most prevalent method of indirect arterial blood pressure is auscultatory technique using sphygmomanometer and stethoscope.	Two types of sphygmomanometers are: mercury gravity and aneroid manometer. Each includes an inflatable rubber bladder in a cloth cuff, inflating bulb, pump, manometer, and pressure valve. Bladder is used to occlude an artery. Cuff must be correct width for diameter of extremity. If cuff is too narrow, pressure reading will be high; too wide a cuff lowers pressure reading. Cuff should be 20% −25% wider than diameter of limb.
		Examples of cuff widths: 2.5 cm, 5 cm, 8 cm; birth—12 yrs of age; 12 cm to 14 cm; average adult; 18 cm to 20 cm; obese person or thighs. Cuff should be long enough to encircle extremity and fit securely.
		Mercury gravity mamometer: Manometer is glass tube calibrated in mm connected to a receptacle of mercury. When the cuff is inflated (pressure is placed on the bulb), mercury rises in tube. Upper surface of mercury has convex curve termed meniscus. Pressure is indicated by position of meniscus.

Implementation	Recommendations	Observations
	Record site of each reading so that all readings are taken at same site.	Blood pressure readings on thigh may show a recording of 20 mm Hg higher than when taken on arm.
After determining method, select appropriate size cuff.	Cuff size is determined by diameter of limb. In extremely obese clients, apply cuff around forearm and ascultate over radial artery. Cuff should be made of material that exerts even pressure throughout surface of cuff.	Inflatable rubber bladder and pressure bulbs should be carefully examined for leaks.
	Column of mercury must be in vertical position for accurate reading.	Watch carefully for loss of mercury. Edge of mercury meniscus should be exactly at zero.
Reading is taken at eye level within 3 feet.		Distortion in reading, (i.e., it appears higher or lower than it actually is) occurs if meniscus is

TABLE 29-1. Continued

Anticipated Accomplishment	Scientific Principles/ Rationale	Specific Considerations
		Aneroid manometer: Manometer utilizes metal bellows connected to calibrated dial with needle showing pressure. When pressure is applied to bulb, bellows expand and contract. In this way, gears are rotated causing needle to move. Aneroid manometer is calibrated against mercury gravity manometer.
		Stethoscope: Stethoscope is described in Chapter 21.
		Stethoscope is necessary to hear sound caused by blood flowing through vessels as pressure in blood pressure cuff is released.
	Indirect arterial blood pressure may be taken by palpation technique.	This method is recommended when ascultation technique is impossible (e.g., health worker has hearing impediment or noisy environmental conditions exist).

Implementation	Recommendations	Observations

read from below or above eye level. Be sure cuff, tubes, valves, and air vents are free of dirt to prevent inaccurate readings.

Maintain accurate calibration by yearly check.

Bell of stethoscope should be placed directly over selected artery.

Do not depress stethoscope with unnecessary pressure (occlude artery) or too lightly (unable to hear).

Cleanse ear tips, diaphragm disc, and bell with antiseptic before and after each use.

Alcohol is recommended for cleansing ear pieces, diaphragm disc, and bell of stethoscope. Cleansing helps to prevent possibility of contraction and transmission of infection.

Ear tips of stethoscope are placed in external ear canals. Ear tips are available in different sizes.

Obtain pressure by placing index and middle fingers on selected artery while sphygmomanometer cup is inflated to 30 mm Hg above point where pulse is obliterated. Release valve on pressure bulb so air pressure is slowly released. Reading at point pulse reappears upon deflation of cuff— gives systolic pressure; record reading as such.

TABLE 29-1. Continued

Anticipated Accomplishment	Scientific Principles/ Rationale	Specific Considerations
	The Flush method is utilized to determine arterial blood pressure in infants.	
6. Techniques to determine blood pressure.	To take blood pressure accurately and quickly, health worker requires theoretical knowledge and psychomotor skills.	It is suggested that client be in appropriate position.
		In taking blood pressure on thigh, palpate popliteal artery and place stethoscope on artery.
		Deflating a cuff at a faster or slower rate may cause erroneous readings.

Implementation	Recommendations	Observations
Client should be in a comfortable position. Appropriate blood pressure cuff is applied to limb (wrist or ankle). Elevate part and apply bandage on exposed part. Blood is occluded from visible part of inflated cuff. Inflate cuff above client's average blood pressure.	If infant is crying, systolic pressure may be increased.	
Remove bandage, one health worker slowly deflates blood pressure cuff while another assesses pale extremity for first flushing of limb. Average (mean) between systolic and diastolic pressures is recorded at point where flushing occurs. Record readings as such.	Have two health workers perform this technique. If only one is available, it is imperative that the manometer and limb be situated so that both can be observed simultaneously.	
Having assessed the site (e.g., brachial artery), method, and appropriate equipment for measurement, gather necessary equipment.	Check client's record or ask client what his "normal" blood pressure usually is.	
If blood pressure is to be taken on thigh, client lies in either supine or prone position.		When taking blood pressure, note in client's record specific positions in which reading was taken.
To prevent uneven pressure, place deflated cuff evenly and snugly around extremity; lower margin of cuff should be 2−3 cm above antecubital space.	Health worker should be situated so dial of aneroid manometer or mercury column is clearly visible.	Position monitors so client cannot observe fluctuations in monitor readings and have false perceptions of his blood pressure reading.
After palpating selected artery (e.g., brachial artery) with fingertips, place stethoscope on artery where palpable pulse was noted.	Note previous statements related to stethoscopes.	Readings may be affected if stethoscope is touching either cuff or clothing. Systolic pressure is slightly higher in popliteal artery than brachial artery.
Inflate cuff to 20−30 mm Hg above client's "normal" pressure. Deflate cuff slowly and evenly (2−3 mm Hg per sec)	Once blood pressure cuff valve is released, continue deflating cuff until monitor reads 0 mm Hg. If necessary to repeat pro-	Due to blood not flowing through vessels during inflation period, client may state extremity feels numb.

The Assessment of Vital Signs 477

TABLE 29-1. Continued

Anticipated Accomplishment	Scientific Principles/ Rationale	Specific Considerations
	Korotkoff Sounds:*	
	Phase 1: sound begins with faint, clear, rhythmic tapping or thumping which gradually increases in intensity—systolic pressure.	
	Phase 2: sound is murmur or swishing quality.	
	Phase 3: sound is crisper and more intense.	
	Phase 4: sound is distinct, abrupt muffling (soft, blowing quality)—i.e., diastolic pressure.	
	Phase 5: sound is no longer heard—second diastolic pressure.	
7. Record and report blood pressure.	Blood pressure is valuable indicator of physiological status when viewed in relation to whole picture of client.	Compare with baseline readings for significant changes and with standard "normal" values.

*Kirkendall, W. M. et al.: *Recommendations for Human Blood Pressure Determination by Sphygmomanometers*. The American Heart Association, New York, 1967, p. 13.

Implementation	Recommendations	Observations
until first sound appears—i.e., systolic pressure. This is phase 1 of the Korotkoff sounds.	cedure, allow minimum of 1–2 min between inflations so venous circulation returns to extremity.	When repeating procedure, carefully check that cuff position has not changed.
Continue to deflate blood pressure cuff until sound becomes muffled—i.e., diastolic pressure.	Phase 4 is recommended by the American Heart Association as best index for diastolic pressure.	
Continue to deflate blood pressure cuff until all air is released, remove cuff, cleanse properly and return to proper storage facility.		
Record in manner appropriate to agency; report significant findings or alterations to appropriate personnel.	When pressure readings in phases 4 and 5 are same, agencies will record systolic and diastolic pressures in one of following ways: 120/80/80 or 120/80. It is not unusual to have a difference between phases 4 and 5. If this does occur, record both first and second diastolic readings (e.g., 120/80/76). This method of recording is approved by World Health Organization and American Heart Association. Record on work sheet if no bedside chart. Transcribe on graphic sheet in client's record.	
Blood pressure readings are assumed to have been taken on brachial artery unless designated differently.		
Extremity and position of client during pressure reading should be specified in the recording (e.g., L.A. 120/80/78 standing).		

PULSE AND BLOOD PRESSURE

Since both of these measurements deal with the circulatory system they will be looked at together for ease of presentation. The circulatory (cardiovascular) system is a closed one containing approximately 5 or 6 L of blood (in the adult). The left (side of the) heart pumps oxygenated blood that it has received from the lungs (via the pulmonary veins) into systemic circulation via the aorta. The right heart pumps deoxygenated blood that it has received from systemic circulation (via the venae cavae) to the lungs via the pulmonary arteries.

The conduction system of the heart, including the sinoatrial node, generates electrical impulses and transmits them, causing the heart to contract and controlling its rate and rhythm. One complete cycle of the heart's action consists of a contraction (*systole*) and a period of relaxation (*diastole*); this cycle is referred to as a *beat*. During intrauterine life, the heart rate of the fetus will average 120 to 160 beats a minute. At birth, the rate will be about 130 to 140. As the individual ages, the heart rate slows until adulthood is reached. A rate between 50 and 100 beats per minute is considered to be within the "normal" range by the American Heart Association. The average adult's heart rate is approximately 60 to 80; the female's rate being approximately five to ten beats faster per minute than the male. In extreme old age, the rate once again becomes somewhat faster. As with temperature and respirations, the heart rate increases as the metabolic rate increases. Therefore, all factors that affect metabolic rate influence the rate of heartbeat. As the rate increases in relation to metabolic activity, so does the *cardiac output*—that is, the amount of blood pumped into the aorta each minute. Normally when the person is at rest, about 5 L will be pumped every 60 seconds. Increases are dependent upon the needs of the tissues for oxygenated blood.

Whereas veins have walls that are thin, arteries have thicker walls that are elastic in nature. As a person ages, this elasticity is lost. When the left ventricle contracts, blood is ejected into the aorta with a great deal of force. To allow for the increased intra-arterial pressure, the aorta distends, sending a shock wave through the arteries. Each time a wave (pulsation) travels along the arteries that are fairly close to the periphery of the body it can be palpated, especially if the artery is located directly over a bony prominence. The most easily palpated arteries are illustrated in Figure 29-3.

Blood exerts pressure on the walls of all of the blood vessels. Peak pressure is found in the left ventricle during systole. This pressure decreases as it goes from arteries to capillaries to veins (where the pressure is the lowest). The *central venous pressure* (pressure of blood in the right atrium) can be measured via the intravenous introduction of a sterile catheter, by way of the subclavian vein (or the jugular), into the superior vena cava. This diagnostic tool is certainly far less common than the indirect measurement of the arterial blood pressure. The amount of blood (*stroke volume*) of the contraction, the diameter and elasticity of the arteries (which gives resistance to the cardiac output) and the viscosity of the blood (which is determined by the amount or percentage of erythrocytes [*hematocrit*] in the blood) are factors influencing the blood pressure. When referring to the blood pressure, the terms *systolic* pressure and *diastolic* pressure are used to indicate the pressure during contraction (systole) of the ventricles and the pressure during relaxation (diastole) of the ventricles. *Pulse pressure* is the difference between the two amounts. All of these pressures are measured in millimeters of mercury (mm Hg). When measured in the brachial artery (the preferred site), the normal range for an adult is 90 to 145 mm Hg with an average reading of 120 mm Hg for the systolic pressure, and 60 to 90 mm Hg with an average of 80 mm Hg for the diastolic pressure. Therefore, the average reading is written 120/80. Average pulse pressure is 30 to 40 mm Hg, although some believe the range to go as high as 50 mm Hg. If the blood pressure reading were 120/80, the pulse pressure would be 120 minus 80 or 40 mm Hg. The average systolic pressure in childhood is approximately 90 to 110 mm Hg. Diastolic pressure after age 5 is approximately 60 to 80 mm Hg.

Consistent with the other vital signs, the blood pressure varies with age, weight, activity, exercise, stress, emotional status, circadian rhythm, and positional changes, as when the individual stands up after being in a reclining position.

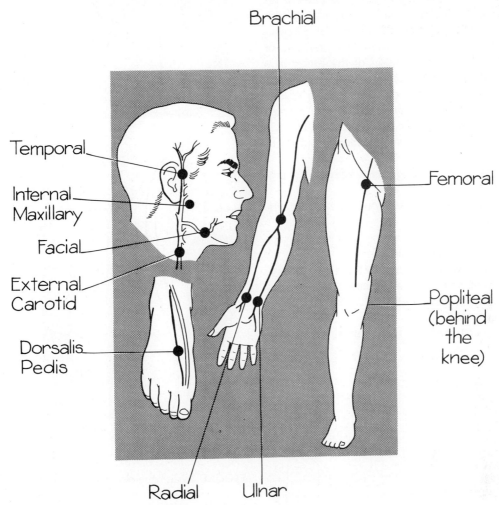

FIGURE 29-3. Common sites for palpation of pulse.

Measurement

No instruments are needed in the measurement of the pulse unless an *apical pulse* or a fetal heart tone is being obtained. Fetal heart tones are obtained by placing a specialized stethoscope (fetoscope) on the pregnant abdomen. The heart rate of the fetus is usually discernible after 5 months gestation. The apical pulse is measured with a stethoscope that is placed over the apex of the heart. Rather than feeling, or in this case hearing, one pulsation as when taking a palpated pulse, the nurse will hear two heart sounds which make up a single beat. Occasionally, the physician will order an apical-radial pulse, especially if the radial pulse is irregular. In this case, two individuals are needed—one to take the radial pulse and one to take the apical pulse. One timepiece is used, and counting for a full minute begins at a predesignated time to insure that both are counting for exactly the same period of time. A difference between the two counts is called *pulse deficit.* Table 29-1C illustrates the methods for taking palpated and apical (auscultated) pulses.

When assessing the pulse, it is looked at in terms of *rate, rhythm, and volume (amplitude).* Heart rate has already been discussed above. Rhythm is normally constant or regular; the intervals between beats and the force of the beat are equal. Volume refers to the ease with which the pulse can be obliterated by pressure of the fingers over the pulse.

If obliteration occurs very readily, the pulse is referred to as *low-tension, small, weak, feeble, soft,* or *thready* (filiform). One that is difficult to compress or obliterate is known as *full, high-tension,* or *bounding.* Similarly, palpation of the artery in a healthy young individual reveals a smooth, round, soft, elastic vessel. The elderly client with vessels that have become sclerotic demonstrates a *hard, tortuous, wiry,* or *cordlike* feeling artery. The following terms are descriptive in relation to pulsation:

bigeminal pulse. A long pause follows two regular beats.

trigeminal pulse. Three regular beats are followed by a pause.

collapsing pulse. Rapid and complete disappearance of a feeble pulse.

Corrigan's (water-hammer) pulse. Jerky, strong beat with a sudden collapse.

dicrotic pulse. Two arterial pulsations are felt for one heartbeat.

intermittent pulse. Occasional beats are skipped.

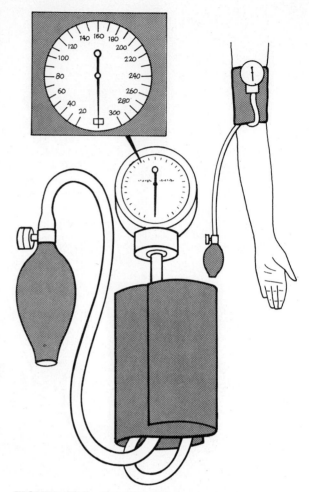

FIGURE 29-5. Aneroid sphygmomanometer.

irregular pulse. Varies in force and rate (when rhythm is irregular, *arrhythmia*).

bradycardia. A heart rate below 50 beats a minute.

tachycardia. A heart rate above 100 beats per minute.

The two most frequent terms associated with blood pressure are *hypertension* and *hypotension.* Hypertension is referred to as persistent blood pressure elevation over 140/90, according to the World Health Organization. The systolic pressure or the diastolic pressure, or both, can be elevated in this condition. Both males, females, adults, and children can be hypertensive. Early diagnosis and treatment are vital as this disease can result in stroke (cardiovascular accident; CVA) congestive heart failure, and renal disease. Therefore, the

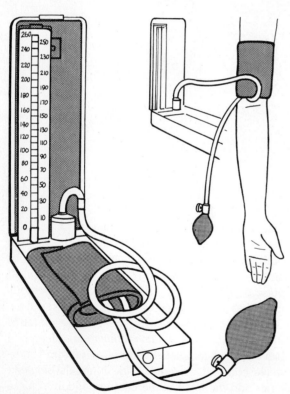

FIGURE 29-4. Sphygmomanometer—mercury manometer type.

value of screening programs and education of the public is apparent.

Hypotension is accepted as being persistent blood pressure readings of lower than 95/60. If the individual is healthy and displays no other symptoms than the reading alone, then there is usually no cause for alarm. The condition causing the hypotension determines if initiation of treatment is necessary or urgent. Table 29-1D and Figures 29-4 and 29-5 describe the equipment needed and the methodology used in measuring indirect arterial blood pressure.

REPORTING AND RECORDING

Reporting of vital signs to the proper personnel is of great importance. Once a baseline has been established with which to compare all readings, the nurse should have no difficulty in noting significant changes. Any change in a measurement which appears to be abnormal or suspicious should be reported at once to the appropriate person, usually the physician. Failure to attend to the clues that the client's body is exhibiting can be harmful and possibly fatal to him. Certainly the omission of a report or recording of meaningful data would constitute negligence on the part of the nurse.

To report or record vital signs, the nurse should be familiar with terminology as it is used in the agency with which she is associated. Certain terms are similar and often misused by personnel. It is safer and perhaps wiser to report in a descriptive manner, indicating the signs and symptoms, complaints, and behaviors as observed, rather than labeling. Recording varies from agency to agency, but each institution has its own style and forms for recording. Figure 29-6 shows a sample of a graphic

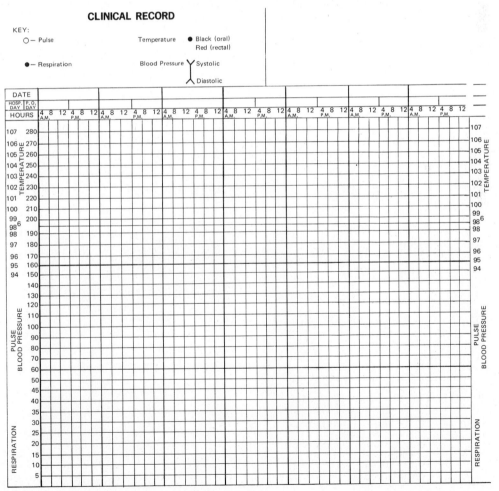

FIGURE 29-6. Graphic sheet for the recording of vital signs.

sheet for the recording of vital signs. It cannot be overemphasized how important it is to record the cardinal signs and accompanying related observations with extreme accuracy. To do so often assists in the physician's process of diagnosis, thereby hastening the initiation and implementation of a course of treatment.

REFERENCES

1. *Taber's Cyclopedic Medical Dictionary,* 13th ed. Philadelphia, F. A. Davis Co., 1977, p. T-14.
2. *Ibid.,* p. F-17.
3. *Ibid.,* p. T-13.

BIBLIOGRAPHY

Beaumont, E.: Blood pressure equipment. *Nurs. '75* 5(1):56, 1975.

Blainey, C. G.: Site selection in taking body temperature. *Am. J. Nurs.* 74:1859, 1974.

Fowler, N. O.: *Inspection and Palpation of Venous and Arterial Pulses.* New York, American Heart Association, 1970.

Gruskin, A.: Clerical evaluation of hypertension in children. *Primary Care* 1:233, 1974.

Guyton, A. C.: *Textbook of Medical Physiology,* 5th ed. Philadelphia, W. B. Saunders Co., 1976.

Jarvis, C. M.: Vital signs. *Nurs. '76* 6(4):31, 1976.

Kirkendall, W. M. et al.: *Recommendations for Human Blood Pressure Determination by Sphygmomanometers.* New York, American Heart Association, 1967.

Leifer, G.: *Principles and Techniques in Pediatric Nursing,* 3rd ed. Philadelphia, W. B. Saunders Co., 1977.

Nordmark, M. T.: *Scientific Foundations of Nursing,* 3rd ed. Philadelphia, J. B. Lippincott Co., 1975.

Roberts, S. L.: Skin assessment for color and temperature. *Am. J. Nurs.* 75:610, 1975.

Sparks, C.: Peripheral pulses. *Am. J. Nurs.* 75:1132, 1975.

Tate, G. V., et al.: Correct use of electric thermometers. *Am. J. Nurs.* 70:1898, 1970.

CHAPTER 30

GLOSSARY

abduction. The lateral movement of the limbs away from the median plane of the body, or the lateral bending of the head or trunk. The lateral movement of digits away from the axial line.

active exercise. A form of bodily movement which the client performs without supervision or an assistant.

adduction. Moving a limb toward the midline of the body.

assistive exercise. A form of bodily movement which the client performs assisted by another individual or some mechanical device such as a pulley or a weight.

atony. Debility or lack of normal tone.

atrophy. The wasting of tissues or organs. Atrophy of muscle tissue may result from interruption in nerve supply or from a disorder invading motor centers of the brain, motor pathways of the spinal cord, motor neurons of the cord, or their endings in muscle; disuse may occur following immobilization of joints; or pathological conditions involving muscles directly. Some conditions are hereditary and of unknown etiology.

BODY MECHANICS

Jacqueline F. Freitas, M.S., R.N.

balance. A state of equilibrium.

body mechanics. Mechanical correlation of the various systems of the body. Efficient use of the body as a machine and as a means for locomotion.

contracture. A condition of fixed high resistance to the passive stretch of a muscle; may result from fibrosis of tissues surrounding a joint.

dorsiflexion. The act of bending or flexion toward the dorsum or back (opposite of plantar flexion); may also be applied to straightening or extending the toes.

extension. A movement which brings the members of a limb into or toward a straight condition. The opposite of flexion.

eversion. Turning outward.

exercise. Functional activity of the muscles, voluntary or otherwise.

external rotation. Turning or moving away from the center.

flexion. The act of bending or condition of being bent, in contrast to extending.

gravity. Property of possessing weight.

hyperextension. Extreme or abnormal extension (past the normal range of motion or position of the joint).

hypertrophy. Any increase in size as a result of functional activity.

internal rotation. Turning or moving inward toward the center.

isotonic (muscle-setting). Having the same tension or tone.

inversion. Turning inward.

lever. Rigid bar used to modify direction, force, and motion.

mechanical. Pertaining to the action of forces which produce motion.

motion. A change of place or position; movement.

passive exercise. Form of bodily movement which is carried through by the operator without the assistance or resistance of the client. Same as relaxed movement.

plantar flexion. The act of bending or turning the toes or foot upward; opposite of dorsiflexion.

position. Manner in which a body is arranged.

posture. Attitude or position of the body.

pronation. 1. The act of turning the hand so that the palm faces downward or backward. 2. The act of lying face downward.

rehabilitation. Process of restoring or undergoing restoration, to health or maximal efficiency.

resistive exercise. Form of supervised bodily movement which offers resistance to muscle action.

rotation. Process of turning on an axis.

supination. 1. The act of turning the palm or foot upward. 2. Act of lying flat on the back.

therapeutic exercise. Form of supervised bodily movement for the purpose of restoring function to diseased or injured tissue.

tonus. The normal state of partial contraction of muscle which determines firmness.

weight. Measurement of heaviness or mass.

The capacity to be independent and care for one's self is generally considered to be a desirable goal in life and is something that most individuals take for granted. Anyone who has been confined to bed for any period of time or has had an extremity immobilized in a cast or traction soon appreciates the ability to move body parts freely and at will.

The significance of the relationship of body parts to moving about and carrying out the usual routines of life such as sleeping, eating, standing, walking, sitting, and lifting is seldom associated by most individuals with the term *body mechanics*; however, body mechanics is closely related to these daily activities. It is through the coordinated use of muscles and joints that the motion necessary for our mobility and for our independence is produced and achieved.

In this chapter, basic concepts and scientific principles of body mechanics are presented and discussed as they relate to the postures and movements of nurses and their clients. Because assistive equipment is frequently necessary to maintain good posture and body mechanics, therapeutic devices and mechanical aids for client care are also described.

PRINCIPLES OF BODY MECHANICS

Posture

Posture is the position of body parts, and body mechanics is the coordinated use of body parts to produce motion and maintain balance. Body me-

chanics involves the application of physical laws to the human body both at rest and during activities. Utilization of good body mechanics enables the nurse to conserve energy, prevent injuries to herself or others, and to add to the client's comfort and well-being.

Body mechanics is closely related to posture in that correct posture aids normal physiological functioning and requires minimal energy output. Correct body mechanics and posture are achieved by application of knowledge of mechanical and physical laws to activities which require movement of body parts.

Principles

The principles of body mechanics consist of the laws of gravity, balance, motion, leverage, force and friction. These mechanical laws are basic to all body movements.

GRAVITY. Gravity, the mutual attraction the earth has for a body and a body has for the earth, affects all body movement. Exerted in a vertical direction downward toward the center of the earth, it pulls on the weight center of all body parts. For this reason, the *center of gravity* is the center of the body's weight. In other words, the center of gravity is the point within the body around which the mass of the body's weight is equally distributed. Man's center of gravity, in a standing position with both hands at his sides, is found at approximately 55 percent of the body's total height. The *line of gravity* passes through the center of gravity downward in a vertical direction. The body's muscular effort works against the pull of gravity and increases in proportion to the distance the line of gravity shifts away from the center of the *base of support*. Body weight is centered at the line of gravity which passes through the base of support, and balance is easily maintained (Fig. 30-1).

BALANCE. A body is in balance when its center of gravity is over the base. *The larger the base, the more stable the body. The nearer the line of gravity is to the center of the base, the more stable the body. The greater the weight, the more balance.* The center of gravity shifts with changes in body position. When one part of the body moves away from the line of gravity in one direction, the center of gravity shifts in that direction. Therefore, *the*

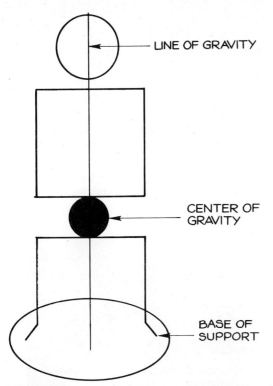

FIGURE 30-1. Schematic drawing showing the line of gravity, center of gravity, and the base of support.

base should be enlarged in the direction of the moving force to allow for the shift of the center of gravity without the line of gravity falling outside the base. Widening the base of support gives greater stability and should be done without interference to or strain on joint movement or muscles. Another consideration is the direction of the force exerted by the individual against the ground. *If the shift of the center of gravity puts it beyond the base, another body part must move in the opposite direction to bring the center of gravity back over the base or balance will be lost. The lower the center of gravity, the more stable the body. Forward or backward rotating motion increases stability.* (Note, if external weights are added to the body, they become part of the total body weight and affect the location of the center of gravity by moving it in the direction of the added weight.)

MOTION. Motion is a change in position or place, direction, and speed. There are two types of motion: *linear* (motion in a straight line) and *angular* (motion around an axis). A body or object is put into motion when a force of sufficient strength is applied and overcomes its inertia or inactivity. In the early eighteenth century, the mathematician, Sir Isaac Newton (1642–1727), formulated what are now known as *Newton's laws of motion*. The first of these basic mechanical laws is the *law of inertia*: a body in motion or at rest tends to remain in motion or at rest unless acted upon by a force. Newton's second law is the *law of acceleration*: when a body is acted upon by a force, the resulting change in acceleration or speed is directly proportional to the force and the direction of the force. A small push on a large object will accelerate it slowly, and a large push on a small object will accelerate it rapidly. The third law is called the *law of reaction*: for every action force, there is an opposite and equal reaction.

LEVERAGE. The body moves by use of a leverage system. The *lever* is a rigid bar that turns around a fixed axis which is called a *fulcrum*. To operate, a lever must have a *fulcrum*, an *effort* (E) or *power force* (P), and a *resistance* (R) or *weight force* (W). Muscles are attached above and below joints and work as the effort or power force of a lever with the joints acting as the fulcrum and the bones the lever arm. Levers are classified according to the position of these components.

First Class Lever. The fulcrum is situated between the effort or power and the resistance or weight (e.g., triceps brachii muscle).

$$\text{E or P} \times \underline{\qquad\qquad} \times \underline{\qquad\qquad} \times \text{R or W}$$
$$\text{Fulcrum}$$

Second Class Lever. The resistance or weight is situated between the fulcrum and the effort or power. (There is no evidence of a second class lever in the human body.)

$$\times \text{R or W}$$
$$\text{E or P} \times \underline{\qquad\qquad\qquad} \times \text{Fulcrum}$$

Third Class Lever. The effort or power is between the resistance or the weight and the fulcrum (e.g., biceps brachii muscle).

$$\times \text{E or P}$$
$$\text{Fulcrum} \times \underline{\qquad\qquad\qquad} \times \text{R or W}$$

Body Mechanics   489

FORCE. Force is a pull or push applied to alter the state of motion of a body. To be produced, one body or object must always act on another. The types of force that cause a body to move are *internal* (the force is produced by the body itself) or *external* (the force is produced by another). Examples of external force are another person or machine and the downward pull of gravity. As noted, a body is put in motion when a force of sufficient strength overcomes the body's inactivity. Some additional *principles of force* are:

1. The greater the size of the object exerting the force and the faster it is moving, the greater the force exerted.
2. The longer the force is applied to an object, the greater the force exerted.
3. The greater the distance over which momentum may be gained, the greater momentum possible.
4. The more assistive muscles used, the more force gained.
5. The fewer nonassistive muscles used, the less energy wasted.
6. The stronger the muscles used for work needing a great deal of force, the more efficient the effort and the less the muscular strain.
7. The more continuous or orderly the movement, the more force gained.
8. The more fully a muscle is extended, the greater force it can exert.
9. The faster the muscle contraction, the greater the speed at the end of the moving lever and the greater force resulting; the slower the speed of muscle contraction, the less energy required.
10. If linear motion is wanted, the more closely through the center of gravity the force is exerted, the less force needed to move a given object.
11. The further from the center of gravity the force is exerted, the less force needed to rotate the object.
12. If one point of an object is fixed, it will rotate regardless of where the force is exerted.

FRICTION. A final factor that modifies motion and is usually required for movement to start is friction, the opposition of one object's movement across the surface of another. It may be caused by roughness of two surfaces, adhesion of one surface to another, or irregularities of two surfaces. Friction is reduced when the amount of surface contact between the two surfaces is reduced.

APPLICATION OF PRINCIPLES TO NURSING PRACTICE

The practice of nursing involves standing, lifting, and moving other persons and objects. The nurse must understand and apply principles of body me-

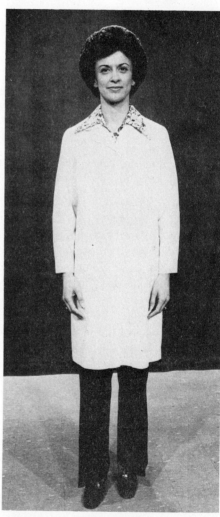

FIGURE 30-2. Good standing position. Body is straight; head is erect and in line with spine; chest is forward with arms by the side and elbows slightly flexed; feet are apart with knees flexed with one foot slightly forward.

chanics in order to administer safe and effective care. The following competencies reflect the nurse's understanding and ability to apply principles of body mechanics to practice.

Standing and Walking

Variations in body build may make ideal posture difficult to attain. In good standing position, the body is straight, not tense, and body parts rest one upon the other in a vertical column. The head is erect, on a straight line with the vertebral column, and the chest is forward and elbows slightly flexed. The feet are apart with one foot forward to broaden the base of support. The knees like the elbows are also slightly flexed (Fig. 30-2).

The process of walking involves two phases, swinging and weight-bearing. From a standing position, weight is shifted to the left leg, and the right leg is lifted and brought forward with the foot dorsiflexed; the right heel is placed on the floor followed by the ball of the right foot. Weight is then shifted to the right leg. The right leg is now weight-bearing, and the left leg swings forward to repeat the phases. In correct position, the advancing leg is not turned outward as it is placed forward, and the patella faces forward with the foot in the same direction. A heel to toe gait allows body weight to be smoothly shifted. With correct posture, the center of gravity of each body part is directly over its supporting base; muscular effort on one side of the body is equal to that on the opposite side. Posture may be improved with practice. Emphasis on correct posture is important since poor posture leads to strain and fatigue.

Moving, Lifting, and Carrying Objects

A heavy object is better moved by pushing or rolling than lifting. To move an object, keep it in motion and avoid frequent stops and starts. If possible, plan the activity ahead of time, try to reduce friction, face the direction of movement, and take advantage of the body's lever action.

To *push* an object, get close to it, bend knees according to its height, and place one foot forward and one back. Place hands on the object at chest height, and push by leaning your shoulder against it and then straighten. To *pull*, stay close to the object, holding it near the center, and crouch with one foot in front of the other. The back should remain straight, and in the process of pulling, reverse leg positions.

When it is necessary to *lift* an object, prepare by "setting the pelvis" (retract the abdominal muscles and contract the gluteals). Stand or stoop as close to the object as possible with feet apart, forming a solid base of support; the closer the object is to the body's line of gravity, the less energy is needed to do the lifting. Bend at the hips and knees and lift by extending the lower extremities. Lift in a straight line while keeping the back straight, and carry the load close to the body (Fig. 30-3A and B).

To *bend*, keep the trunk straight and feet spread apart for a broad base of support to maintain balance. To *reach* for an object, establish a base of support by placing feet wide apart. Keep the body centered over this base and avoid twisting or turning the trunk. To *carry an object*, relax the elbows and keep the object close to the body. Stand straight with feet about 18 inches apart for good balance and support; avoid bending over.

Moving, Lifting, or Transferring Clients

As noted, a basic principle always applied to lifting is "the closer the lifted weight is to the line of gravity of the body, the less energy force is required to do the work." When it is not possible to bring the weight close to the line of gravity, the principles of leverage should be used.

To move or lift a client, get assistance; it will take at least two people to reposition a client who is completely helpless or not allowed to move. To facilitate the client's cooperation and to decrease her anxiety, be certain that the client always understands how and when she will be lifted or moved. Avoid uneven pulling movements; use smooth, even, continuous motions that will make the move more comfortable for the client and reduce the possibility of injury to the nurse or the client. A turning sheet, which is discussed in the section on assistive equipment, facilitates this type of move.

UPWARD OR DOWNWARD. The nurse and her assistant should stand on opposite sides of the bed at the level of the client's chest. Each places

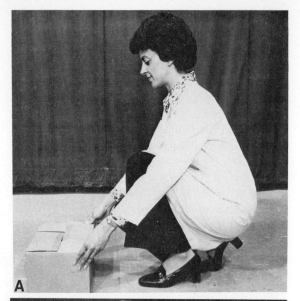

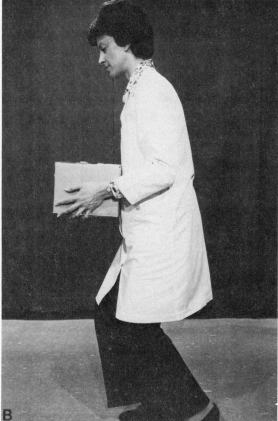

FIGURE 30-3. Correct positions for lifting. A, Correct "stooping" position to lift a box, bending at the hips and knees with back straight. B, Rising from the "stooped" position to standing. Back is straight, and knees are in the process of straightening but still slightly flexed. The box is held close to the body.

one arm under the client's shoulder, and the other under the thigh. While standing erect with knees slightly bent, turn toward the direction of movement with feet positioned in that direction (Fig. 30-4). Using a prearranged signal, let your assistant know you are ready to move the client; straighten the knees, keeping the back as straight as possible. Note that the moving or lifting is done by the straightening of the legs not with the arm or back muscles. This basic maneuver is used to lift or move a client toward the head or foot of the bed.

FROM SIDE TO SIDE. This maneuver can usually be done by one person. Explain to the client what is going to be done and position her arms *over her chest*. Stand at the left side of the bed if the client is to be moved to the left and the reverse if moving the client to the right. Facing the client's head and shoulders, brace one leg or thigh against the bed, and flex the hips and knees. Stabilize the pelvis by contracting the abdominal and gluteal muscles (known as "setting the muscles" or "the internal girdle" referred to in the section on lifting). Flexion of the hips, knees, and ankles allows the stronger leg muscles to do the work of pulling the client toward the side of the bed. If the spine were bent, most of the work would be placed on the back which does not have the mechanical advantage of the leg muscles. Place one hand under the client's head and reach under the far shoulder. Place the other hand and arm farther down under the shoulders. Move the upper part of the client's body toward you, then move the hips in the same manner by placing your hands and arms under the heaviest parts. Place one hand under the knee and the other under the ankle, and move each leg, one at a time. (These steps may have to be repeated to move a very heavy client.) If two people are moving the client, both stand on the same side of the bed and carry out the procedure as described with the same foot positioned forward and legs braced against the bed.

TO SIDE-LYING POSITION. After assessing the client's need for repositioning, begin by placing her in the center of the bed using the method described above. Stand at the left side of the bed if the client is to be turned to the left. Cross the right leg over the left with the right knee slightly flexed. The lower arm should be in abduction and external rotation with the elbow flexed and the upper arm

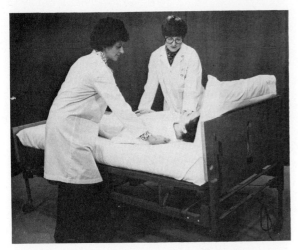

FIGURE 30-4. Basic position to move client. Two nurses are standing on opposite sides of the client's bed. Each having one arm under the client's shoulders and the other arm under her thighs. The nurses' backs are straight and bodies turned slightly towards the direction of movement (head of the bed). Their knees are slightly flexed, feet apart with one foot forward toward the head of the bed.

in adduction and internal rotation across the chest. (The reverse is true for turning to the right side.) The nurse reaches across the client and places one hand behind the far shoulder; the other hand is placed behind the far hip. The client is then gently rolled toward the nurse (Fig. 30-5). The nurse's weight is shifted from the forward leg (braced against the bed for stability and leverage) to the other leg as she rolls the client toward her. Readjust the client's position as necessary.

TO A SITTING POSITION. With the client lying on her back, stand on the right side. (Note, stand on whichever side is more convenient. Reverse leg and arm positions for moving the client from the opposite side.) While facing the client, the nurse places her left leg forward and right leg back. Braced against the bed, both knees are flexed. The right hand and arm are placed under the client's right shoulder or upper back. The nurse's hand is extended completely under the client's shoulder so that the thumb is on the neck, and the fingers are between the scapulae. Placing the left hand on the bed for support, the nurse lifts the client by pushing against the bed with her left arm. Body weight is shifted from the forward foot to the rear one as lifting takes place.

FROM BED TO STRETCHER. Align the stretcher with the bedside, and be certain that both the bed and the stretcher are in a locked position. If there are no locking devices, another person must hold the stretcher in place by leaning against it. After explaining the procedure, instruct the client to slowly slide her hips, shoulder, head, and then legs and feet onto the stretcher. Offer help as needed. (Note, the same procedure is followed for moving the client from one bed to another.)

Helpless Clients. A *three-man lift and carry* is useful for tranferring helpless or dependent clients to a stretcher or another bed. The nurse should review the transfer procedure with assistants before entering the client's room. There must be agreement as to how the signals will be given for such moves as lifting and lowering. A safe transfer is dependent upon a cooperative effort. Allowing room for maneuvering, place the stretcher at a right angle to the head or the foot of the bed. After adjusting the bed to its maximum height, the nurse and her assistants line up along the side of the bed facing the client. The person closest to the client's head places her hands and arms under the neck and back securing the far shoulder and arm. The sec-

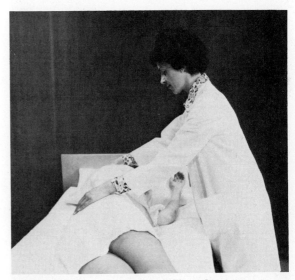

FIGURE 30-5. The nurse turns the client onto her left side. The client's right leg is crossed over the left, and the knee is slightly flexed. The right arm is adducted and internally rotated. The left arm is abducted and externally rotated. The nurse is reaching across the client with one hand behind the right shoulder and the other on the hip. The client is rolled toward the nurse.

ond person places her hands and arms under the hips and buttocks, giving support to the sacral area. The third person places her hands and arms under the client's thighs and ankles (Fig. 30-6A). The three-man team starts with the same foot forward flexing their hips and knees. On signal, they straighten their knees, lifting the client and turning him toward them for support (Fig. 30-6B). The team then carries the client to the stretcher (or the other bed).

FROM BED TO CHAIR. If a wheelchair is used, bring it to the client's bedside. It is important to be familiar with the wheelchair's design and how it is adjusted and locked. Help the client to a sitting position with the legs dangling over the side of the bed. If the client is unable to push herself up, assist her by supporting the trunk with your arms. Maintain a position as described previously on pulling and lifting. To assist the client from a sitting to a standing position, the nurse places her arms around the client's upper trunk while the client places her arms on the nurse's shoulders. To maintain balance, the nurse's feet should be apart; the knees are flexed and placed against the client's for additional support. As the client stands, the nurse's knees go from a flexed to an extended position. Turning the client with her back to the wheelchair, the nurse flexes her knees and hips, keeps her back straight, and lowers the client into the chair.

Accident Prevention

Work related back injuries and other accidents caused by lifting and moving are preventable. The following considerations and actions will be of utmost importance in accident prevention.

1. Consider the weight, size, shape, and mobility of all persons or objects before any move.
2. Plan ahead and know the distance and obstacles involved.
3. Use common sense and ask for assistance if the weight of the object is too heavy.
4. Make use of available aids such as carts, dollies, and lifts.
5. Good balance and a broad base of support are obtained by placing the feet far apart straightening the legs while lifting.
6. Always get close to what you are going to lift and avoid reaching.
7. Avoid strain by keeping the back straight, bending at the knees and hips, shifting the position of the feet rather than twisting the body, and by continuous, smooth movements.

It is most important to apply the principles of body mechanics to all positioning and moves. Instructing the client in what is going to be done and how it will be done will decrease her anxiety and

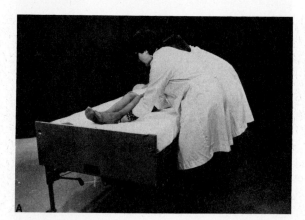 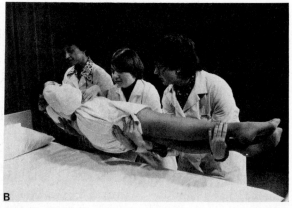

FIGURE 30-6. Three-man carry. A, A nurse and two assistants are lined up by the same side of the client's bed. The nurse has her hands and arms under the client's neck and back, securing the far shoulder. One assistant has her hand under the client's hips and buttocks, and the other assistant is holding the client's thighs and ankles. All are standing with their backs straight, knees slightly flexed, and feet apart with the same foot forward. B, The nurse and her assistants standing, holding the client in a position so that she is turned slightly toward them.

enlist her assistance and cooperation. The instruction of others in these principles will decrease the possibility of accidents and injury to the client and coworkers.

APPLICATION OF PRINCIPLES TO CLIENTS

The client's position in or out of bed affects body posture and capacity for movement. Poor positioning decreases her ability to freely move muscles and joints. Clinical conditions may also cause restriction of motion and interfere with positioning. The nurse involved in planning, providing, and directing rehabilitative care uses her knowledge of body mechanics to assist the client toward a goal of independence. The client's rehabilitation potential is determined by the quality of the nursing care received. Plans of care based upon and including principles of body mechanics help the client gain, maintain, or regain the maximum level of motor functioning.

Joint Motion Exercises

Prolonged immobility or inactivity causes *changes* to occur in muscles and joint structures. Therefore, unless contraindicated, joints and major muscle groups are taken through active, active assistive, or passive exercises daily. These exercises maintain and promote muscle strength and joint function and are as essential to client care as correct body positioning. The nurse uses her understanding of the therapeutic value of exercise (and specifically range of joint motion) to recognize the effects of immobility or disuse phenomena. She then implements measures to prevent further restrictions and complications. Some important considerations in joint motion exercises are:

1. Extremities are supported and held at the joints.
2. All movements are done slowly and smoothly and without discomfort to the client.
3. A joint should not be moved beyond its free range of motion; movement should be stopped if there is pain.
4. When holding an extremity, avoid grasping of the muscle "belly" unless absolutely necessary as in some arthritic conditions.

The five different types of exercise—active, active assistive, passive, resistive, and isotonic (muscle-setting)—are defined in the glossary at the beginning of this chapter. However, they are restated here because the importance of these exercises, particularly with bedridden clients, cannot be overemphasized.

Active exercises, which are performed by the client without assistance, involve the contraction of muscles and the movement of joints. The goal of these exercises is to promote and maintain muscle strength in addition to maintaining joint motion. *Active assistive* exercises are performed by the client against resistance to motion produced by another person or a mechanical device. *Passive* exercises, which are performed for the client by another person, do not promote or maintain muscle strength but assist in preventing contractures. *Resistive* exercises are performed by the client against resistance to motion produced by another person or a mechanical device. *Muscle-setting* exercises are performed by the client with no movement of body parts. For example, in the quadriceps setting exercise, the knee is extended and maximum tensing of the quadriceps muscles is produced without the movement of the knee joint. The client may be instructed to press the back of the knee against the bed to facilitate this "tensing." Quadriceps setting is a specific exercise for the client in traction or in a cast. Abdominal and gluteal setting are also important isotonic exercises for the immobilized client.

Range of Joint Motion

Range of motion refers to the extent of movement present for any given joint. The following words—all of which have been defined in the glossary at the beginning of this chapter—describe range of motion: *adduction, abduction, flexion, dorsiflexion, plantar flexion, extension, hyperextension, pronation, supination, rotation (internal* and *external), inversion,* and *eversion.*

Passive joint motions—that is, those that are performed for the client by another person—do not maintain muscle tone but assist only in preventing contractures. These motions are illustrated in Figures 30-7 through 30-18 and are described in detail in the accompanying legends. In all of these ex-

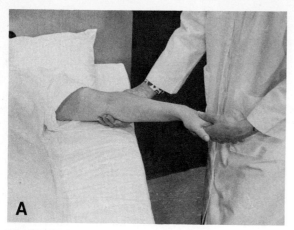 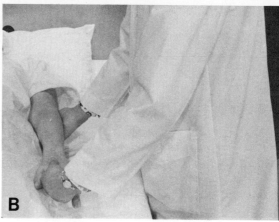

FIGURE 30-7. A, Abduction of shoulder: the nurse places one hand on the client's elbow and holds her other hand. Keeping the arm straight, the nurse moves it away from the side of the body above the head. B, The nurse returns the client's arm to her side.

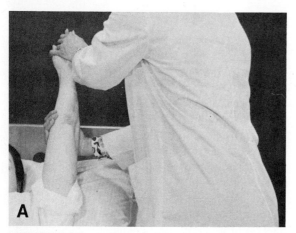 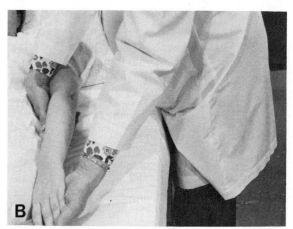

FIGURE 30-8. A, Flexion of shoulder: holding the client's arm above the elbow with one hand and her hand with the other, (as in Fig. 30-7A), the nurse lifts the arm upward from the side of the body until it is alongside the head. B, Extension of shoulder: the client's arm is returned to a position by her side.

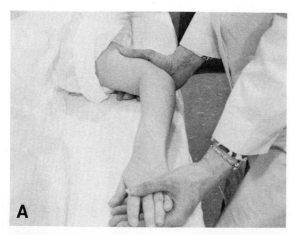 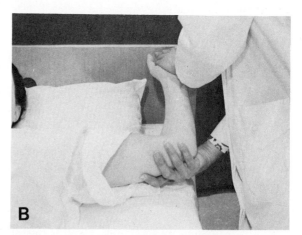

FIGURE 30-9. A, Internal rotation of the shoulder: the client's arm is in a position of abduction (at shoulder height) with the elbow bent at a 90 degree angle with palm of the hand towards the feet. Holding the client's hand and placing the upper arm against the mattress, the nurse brings the forearm down on the mattress. B, External rotation of the shoulder: the nurse brings the client's arm back up from the position of internal rotation so that the palm and lower arm now face backwards.

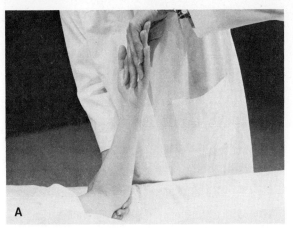 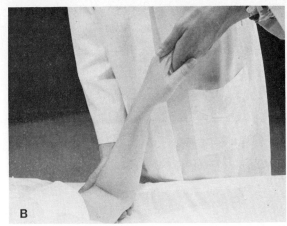

FIGURE 30-10. A, Supination of forearm: the nurse positions the client's elbow at the waist, with the arm flexed at a 90 degree angle. The hand is supported as in a "hand-shake" and the other hand supports the client's flexed elbow. The palm of the hand is then turned upward toward the face. B, Pronation of forearm: the client's palm is now turned downward (back toward the feet).

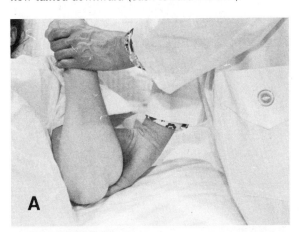 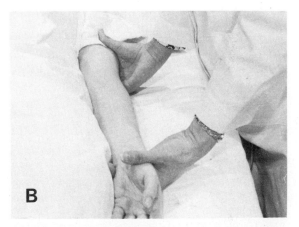

FIGURE 30-11. A, Flexion of the elbow: the client is positioned with the arms at her side, palm up. The nurse places one hand under the client's wrist and the other above her elbow; the elbow is then bent, bringing her forearm and hand toward her shoulder. B, Extension of the elbow: the client's elbow is straightened by returning the arm to a resting position in bed.

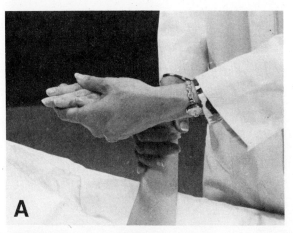 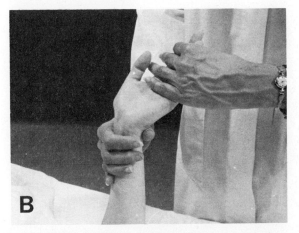

FIGURE 30-12. A, Flexion of the wrist: the nurse holds the client's wrist with one hand and her hand with the other hand. The client's upper arm rests on the bed with the elbow flexed. The client's hand is first bent forward by moving the palm of the hand toward her forearm. B, Extension of the wrist: the client's hand is now bent backwards so that the palm is facing upward.

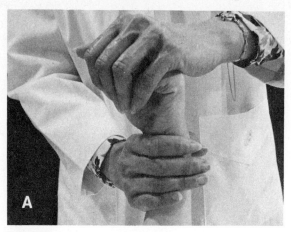 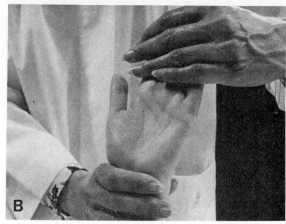

FIGURE 30-13. A, Flexion of the fingers: the client's position is the same as for flexion of the wrist with the extended wrist supported by the nurse's hand. The nurse places her other hand over the back of the client's hand and fingers and bends the fingers to make a fist. B, Extension of the fingers: the client's fingers are straightened from the "fist" position.

FIGURE 30-14 Flexion of knee and hip: the nurse places one hand under the client's knee and with the other hand supports the heel of her foot. The knee and hip are flexed as the nurse lifts the leg off the bed and moves it back toward the head as far as it will go. (The knee is then straightened by lifting the foot upward and lowering it to the beginning position.)

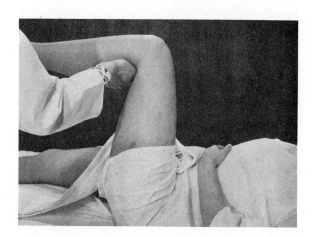

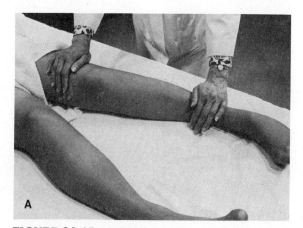 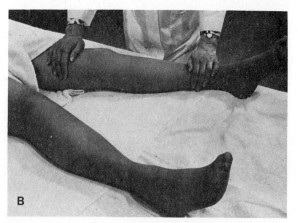

FIGURE 30-15. A, Internal rotation of the hip: the nurse places one hand above the client's ankle and the other hand above her knee. The thigh and lower leg are rolled inward to the center or midline of the body. B, External rotation of the hip: the leg is returned to a neutral position and then rolled outward.

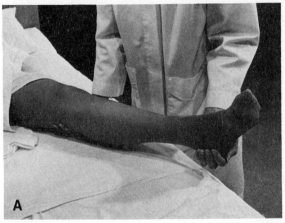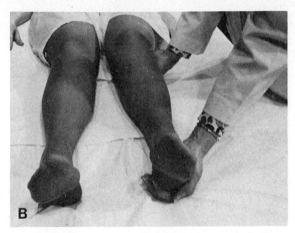

FIGURE 30-16. A, Abduction of the hip: the nurse places one hand under the client's heel and the other under the knee. While holding the leg straight, it is lifted a few inches from the mattress, then moved toward the edge of the bed. B, Adduction of the hip: the leg is moved from the abducted position at the edge of the bed toward the client's body to the beginning position.

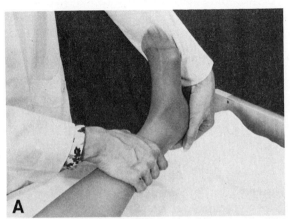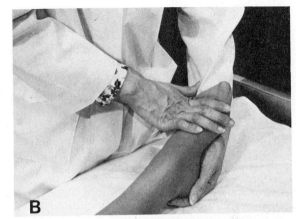

FIGURE 30-17. A, Dorsi-flexion of the foot: the nurse rests the client's foot on her forearm and holds the heel with one hand and places her other hand above the ankle. Using her forearm, she pushes against the bottom of the foot, moving it toward the client's leg. B, Plantar flexion of the foot: the nurse brings the foot back to the beginning position and places her hand on top of the client's foot under the toes and pushes the foot down.

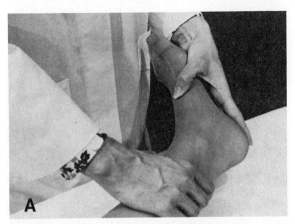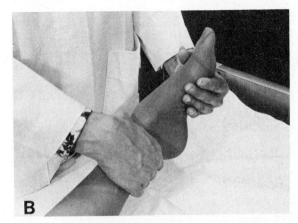

FIGURE 30-18. A, Eversion of the foot: with one hand, the nurse holds and places her fingers on the bottom of the client's foot and places her other hand on the ankle. She turns the whole foot away from the center of the body so that the sole is facing outward. B, Inversion of the foot: the foot is then turned so that the sole is turning inward toward the center of the body.

amples, the client is lying in a supine position with her head on a pillow.

Posture of Bedridden Clients

Clients dependent upon others for physical care require protection from injury to their neuromusculoskeletal system. Clients who are unconscious, weak, debilitated, or immobilized for a specific therapeutic reason may have impaired motor or sensory functioning. To maintain good body posture and prevent joint stiffening and muscle wasting in these clients, position changes are required. A client's position is changed every 2 hours, day and night, or more frequently if indicated, to prevent fatigue, contractures, and continuous pressure on any one body part. The position should be a comfortable one with the client's hips and knees slightly flexed whether she is on her side, back, or abdomen. Position changes from flexed to extended hips and knees are important to prevent contractures. To move the client smoothly and maintain normal body alignment, support is provided for the head, extremities, and joints; body parts are held gently but firmly. A firm mattress and springs prevent the body from sagging and promote correct alignment. The ideal mattress allows the client's hips and shoulders to maintain the spine in a straight position and evenly distributes support for the whole body (Fig. 30-19). A bedboard is required for the mattress that is less than ideal.

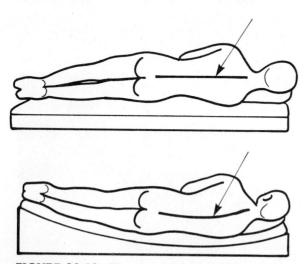

FIGURE 30-19. The ideal mattress allows the client's hips and shoulders to maintain spine in a straight position and evenly distributes support for the whole body.

A footboard is used to position the client's feet when she is lying on her abdomen or back. The footboard should be several inches higher than the toes, supporting the foot at a right angle to the lower leg and keeping the toes in extension. Footboards and cradles prevent bed linen from being drawn tightly over the feet; tight bed linen causes discomfort, restriction of movement, and foot deformities; for example, plantar flexion, tightening of the heel cord, or a shortened Achilles tendon.

ANATOMICAL ALIGNMENT

Gravity tends to pull downward on any body part that is not supported. The resulting stress forces joints into hyperextension, shortens or stretches tendons, and strains the muscles attached to any unsupported parts. *Normal anatomical alignment between body parts is referred to as correct posture.* Alignment, regardless of the position the client is in, should be balanced with minimal muscle tension; all parts must be supported without pressure, strain, or sagging. "Supine," "prone," and "side-lying" are the three basic, anatomically correct positions for the client who is lying in bed.

Supine Position (Dorsal or Back-lying)

The client lies on her back; her head is in a straight line with the spine, and face and toes point upward. The arms may be flexed at the elbows with hands at her side, or one arm may be positioned over the head to relax the back and shoulder muscles. A pillow placed under the head will provide support; a small pillow under the legs will aid in muscle relaxation (Fig. 30-20).

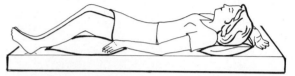

FIGURE 30-20. Client lying on her back (supine position), in good body alignment with a small pillow under her head for support; head is in straight line with spine. One arm is positioned at her side, relaxed, elbow slightly flexed. Other arm is flexed over head. A small pillow is placed under her legs.

As noted, gravity tends to pull the knee joints into a state of hyperextension. If the client lies on her back with knees extended for any length of time, pressure is felt, and leg weight pulls on the pelvic girdle tilting it forward. This pull transfers to the lower back and will result in a backache. A small pillow placed under the knees will release this pull and will position the lower back flat against the mattress. If this is ineffective, another very small pillow or support individually sized to fill the space between the client's back and the bed may be used.

Other aids used in positioning clients are: (1) a footboard and cradle, which hold the bed linens off of the client's toes and maintains the feet in a functional position; (2) a folded bath blanket placed under the calves of the legs, which lessens pressure on the client's heels and may be used to slightly flex the knee joints without undue pressure on the popliteal spaces; (3) small towel rolls or "trochanter rolls," which support and maintain the legs in a neutral position and prevent external rotation of the client's hips or thighs. The client's position is checked by standing at the foot of the bed and ascertaining that all body segments are in a straight line. An imaginary straight line from the middle of the client's forehead through the center of the body and between the ankles should be noted. The client's head should be in line with the spine, and the shoulders and hips should be at right angles to this imaginary line. Flexion of the hips should be minimal. The heels must be positioned so that there is no pressure under them, and the toes should point straight up.

Prone Position (Face-lying)

The prone position is opposite that of supine. The client lies on her abdomen with toes suspended over the end of the mattress. Usually no pillow is placed under the head since an elevated head in this position causes strain on the spine. A small pillow placed under the client's legs will prevent pressure on the toes and hyperextension of the feet. In addition, it will relax the muscles of the legs and support the areas between the knees and ankles. In female clients, a small pillow placed under the lower chest prevents pressure on the breasts. Position is checked for the imaginary straight line using the same method as in the supine position (see above).

The client's head should be positioned laterally in good alignment with the rest of the body. The arms should be abducted and externally rotated with elbows flexed; the legs should be in a neutral position with the toes over the mattress as described above (Fig. 30-21). In this position, the areas that must be checked for pressure points are the ear, tips of the shoulder blades, breasts with females, genitalia with males, anterior iliac crests, knees, and toes.

Side-lying Position (Lateral)

In this position, the client is on her side; the head is in line with the spine and the body is straight. A pillow should support the head; another pillow may be placed near the head to support the arm. A pillow folded in half and tucked against the client's back will support or maintain this position, keeping her from rolling over onto the back. Placed lengthwise between the client's legs, another pillow serves to keep the upper leg from exerting too much pressure on the lower leg preventing strain and maintaining normal anatomical alignment of the body (Figs. 22A and B).

This position is checked by looking at the client's back while standing alongside the bed. The client's head should be in line with the spine; the spine should be straight; and the hips and shoulders should be at right angles to the spine. Pressure

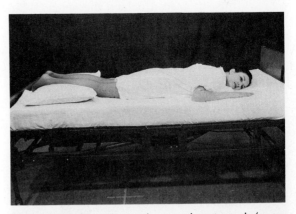

FIGURE 30-21. Client is lying on her stomach (prone position) with no pillow under the head, which is positioned to the side. A small pillow should be placed under the chest for female clients. A small pillow is under the lower legs to keep the toes off the bed and relax the leg muscles.

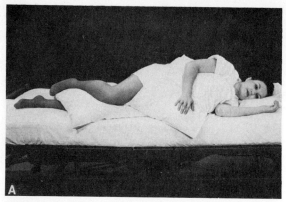 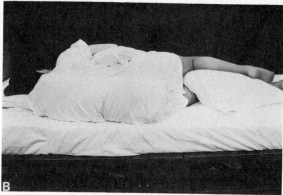

FIGURE 30-22. The front (A) and back (B) views of the side-lying position with the head on a small pillow. The body is in a straight line, a pillow is between the legs with the lower leg slightly flexed and the upper one in more flexion. The lower arm is alongside of the head, and the upper one is flexed and positioned on a pillow. Note, pillow behind client (B) is to prevent her from rolling over.

points that must be observed are the ear, trochanter (hip), and lateral malleolus (ankle).

Sitting in Bed or Chair

While sitting in bed, the client may be positioned at various angles. For example, specific orders may be written to elevate the head of the bed 45 to 60 degrees (Fowler's position); 30 degrees (semi-Fowler's position); 90 degrees (high Fowler's position). Raising the head of the bed flexes the client's hips while supporting the back (Fig. 30-23). If it is necessary to increase support and maintain alignment, a pillow may be placed behind the small of the

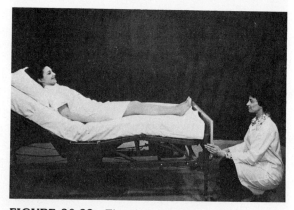

FIGURE 30-23. The client is sitting in bed with the bedrest raised to a comfortable position. Pillows are behind the head and back, the knee rest is raised slightly to provide support for the client's legs.

back. A pillow under the client's head keeps it in line with the rest of the spine. The client's legs may be extended in front with the lower section of the bed raised to slightly flex the knees and hips, eliminating pressure on the knee joint which results from the hyperextension caused by gravity. In some agencies, a physician's order is needed to flex the lower section of the bed. The client's arms are supported by placing the lower arms on pillows with elbows flexed. A footboard supports the feet as described above for other positions. When checking this position (while standing at the side of the bed), the client's spine should be in normal alignment with all body parts well supported. Then, standing at the foot of the bed, note the imaginary straight line position with the client's shoulders and hips at right angles to the spine.

Maintaining good posture while sitting in a chair allows the client's feet to rest flat on the floor with hips and knees flexed at right angles. Body weight is placed on the client's ischial tuberosities, and body alignment should be like that maintained with good standing posture. The arms of the chair support the client's forearms without causing any elevation of the shoulders (Fig. 30-24).

Standing

A correct standing position with the body in anatomical alignment lowers the center of gravity, promotes and maintains balance, and conserves muscular energy. In standing, as in all positions,

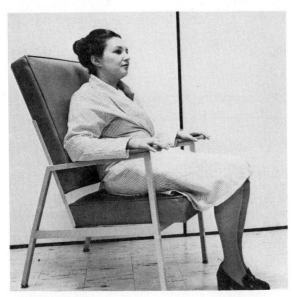

FIGURE 30-24. The client in correct sitting position in a chair with feet flat on the floor, knees and hips at right angles, and back supported by the chair. Body weight is resting on the client's ischial tuberosities and proximal portion of thighs. A "captain's" type chair is good for positioning.

physiological systems function most effectively when the body is in correct alignment.

A description of the correct standing position has been presented previously (see Fig. 30-2).

Other Positions

In addition to the usual positions (prone, supine, and side-lying) described above, the client is often placed in other *positions for reasons of comfort, therapeutic effect, or because they are necessary for the implementation of certain examinations or diagnostic procedures.*

DORSAL POSITION. In the dorsal position, the client lies on her back without any elevation of the head. This position is frequently used postoperatively, and in this instance, the client's head may be turned to one side in case of vomiting.

DORSAL RECUMBENT POSITION. In the dorsal recumbent position, the client lies on her back with the head and shoulders elevated on a pillow. The knees are bent, and the feet are flat on the bed.

LITHOTOMY POSITION. This position is the same as the dorsal recumbent position except that the legs are apart, and the client's feet are elevated and held in position manually or placed in stirrups. This position is used during catheterization and gynecological examinations and procedures (Fig. 30-25).

SIM'S POSITION. This is a semiprone position in which the client lies on her left side with the upper arm held forward and the lower arm extended behind the back. The lower leg is slightly flexed, and the upper one flexed higher at the hip and knee. A small pillow is placed under the head, and a second pillow may be used under the upper leg at the flexed knee. This position is used during the administration of an enema as well as for other purposes (Fig. 30-26).

FOWLER'S POSITION. In Fowler's position, the head of the bed is elevated 45 to 70 degrees, depending upon individual needs. The client's knees may or may not be flexed. Unless contraindicated, for example, if the client had circulatory or vascular problems, the bed may be raised in the center to provide for knee flexion (Fig. 30-27).

KNEE-CHEST POSITION. In the knee-chest position, the client is placed in a kneeling position with the head and shoulders down on the bed or examination table. The head is held toward one side and a small pillow provided for comfort. This position is used for gynecological and rectal ex-

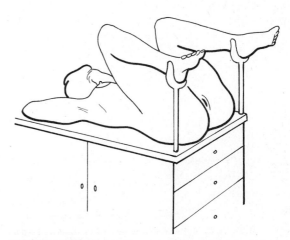

FIGURE 30-25. Lithotomy position.

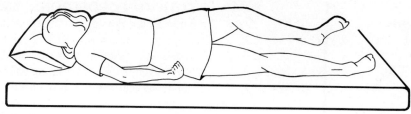

FIGURE 30-26. Sim's position.

aminations and procedures. Other positions may be more desirable to use since it is difficult to maintain this position for any length of time; clients frequently express embarrassment when placed in this position (Fig. 30-28).

TRENDELENBURG POSITION. In the Trendelenburg position, the client lies on her back with the foot of the bed elevated. The head and shoulders remain lower than the hips and legs (Fig. 30-29). According to some authorities, clients suffering from *hypovolemic shock* (decreased circulating blood volume) respond more favorably to a modified Trendelenburg. This position is accomplished by elevating the client's legs to a 45 degree angle with knees straight and the pelvis somewhat higher than the thorax. A pillow can be placed under the head.

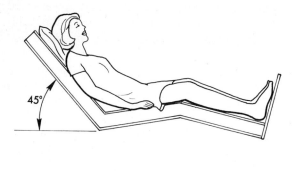

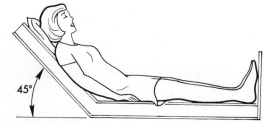

FIGURE 30-27. Fowler's position.

Educating Clients in Body Mechanics

A teaching program is part of every client's plan of care. As a health educator, the nurse must instruct clients in ways to maintain their health and sense of well-being. The teaching plan is developed following an assessment of the client's life style and learning needs.

Health teaching in body mechanics involves an explanation of the principles of body mechanics and how they apply to the client's daily activities. Posture, sitting, standing, walking, and lifting are integral parts of how a person works, plays, sleeps, and carries out the activities of daily living. The teaching plan is concerned with the basic principles of body mechanics and their interrelatedness to these daily activities. Consideration should be given to the following:

1. How to correct and improve body posture.
2. The application of body mechanics to all daily activities.

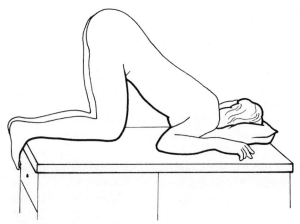

FIGURE 30-28. Knee-chest position.

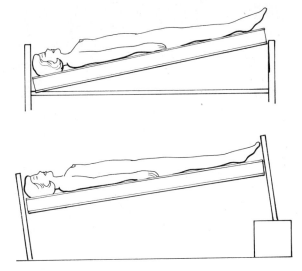

FIGURE 30-29. Trendelenburg position.

3. The effects of clothing and the type and fit of shoes on posture and body movement.
4. An explanation of the need for regular health examinations as a preventive measure to maintain physical ability to carry out daily activities.
5. The correct use of exercise and the avoidance of overexercise.
6. The use of body mechanics to prevent accidents at work and in the home.

As a role model, the nurse is in a strategic position to encourage good health habits (including body mechanics) and to teach those preventive health measures that will promote the client's highest level of functioning, enabling him to reach his maximum rehabilitative potential.

MECHANICAL AIDS

In caring for clients, the nurse frequently uses therapeutic devices and mechanical aids to promote good body positioning and to facilitate the safe and therapeutic movement and ambulation of clients.

Positioning

TURNING SHEET

The turning sheet is used to position clients unable to move themselves. A turning sheet is made by folding one large sheet lengthwise and then in half. The closed end of the sheet is placed under the client's shoulders extending it from above the shoulders to below the buttocks. The sheet is then rolled tightly toward the client by two people standing at opposite sides of the bed. Both people then grasp the rolled sheet at the hip and shoulder areas, and the client is lifted in any direction or positioned on either side. The turning sheet is left under the client and changed only as necessary when soiled.

TROCHANTER ROLL

A trochanter roll is used to prevent the client's hips from externally rotating. Made with a bath blanket or towels, depending upon the size of the client, it is placed under the greater trochanter of the femur in the hip-joint area (Fig. 30-30A). If a bath blanket is used (one or two if required), it is folded lengthwise in thirds; the outer edge of each side is then rolled under the client's hip and thigh. Sandbags may also be used to prevent external rotation of the hip.

A trochanter roll may also be used to maintain proper position of the hand and to avoid contractures (Fig. 30-30B).

FOOTBOARD, CRADLE, AND PILLOWS

As previously described, a footboard and cradle are used to keep bed linens off of the toes and to maintain correct positioning of the client's feet at right angles to the legs when in a supine or prone position (Fig. 30-31).

Pillows of varying sizes and shapes are useful to support and maintain correct body alignment. For example, a small pillow may be placed under the lower part of the client's back in the lumbar area when in the supine position, or under the head when in the prone position. If different size pillows are not available, foam rubber pads, towels, bath blankets, synthetic materials, or any other type of supportive padded material may be used and shaped as desired by placing it in a pillowcase and folding to size.

TRAPEZE

A trapeze helps the disabled, weak, or immobilized client to move in bed and change position, facili-

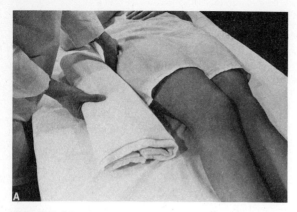
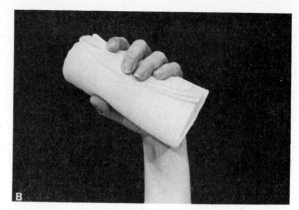

FIGURE 30-30. Trochanter Rolls. A, a bath blanket may be used as a trochanter roll by folding it lengthwise in thirds and rolling the outer edge of each side under the client's hip and thigh. B, a hand towel or washcloths folded lengthwise in thirds may be used as a roll to maintain proper position of the hand.

tating self-care. The trapeze may not be indicated for all clients because of specific medical conditions or rehabilitative goals. In some cases, clients have become extremely dependent upon its use and have not exercised important arm and shoulder muscles needed for ambulation with crutches or walkers.

Moving and Ambulating

TRANSFER BOARD

A transfer or sliding board is used to move a client from bed to chair (or chair to bed or to toilet) and

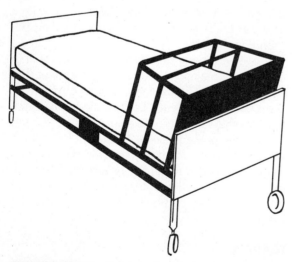

FIGURE 30-31. Footboard and cradle. A footboard and cradle placed on the bed is used to elevate bed linens and to maintain position of the client's lower extremities.

is useful for clients whose muscles are not strong enough to lift themselves. Any type of smooth, lightweight polished board may be used. One side of the board is placed under client's buttocks and the other on the surface of the chair, bed, or wherever the transfer is being made. The client then is able to lift herself with her hands to move the buttocks and slide across the board.

HYDRAULIC LIFT

The hydraulic lift makes it possible for one person to safely lift and move a dependent person (Fig. 30-32). It is essential that the nurse be completely familiar with this device before using it to move a client. Anyone who is to use the lift should be transported in it first to become familiar with the sensation of being lifted and carried in this manner, as it may be a frightening feeling for many people. Always demonstrate and explain the use of the lift to the client before the transfer. The lift may have a one piece sling seat that supports the client from head to knees. Other lifts have a two-piece sling set, with one sling under the buttocks and thighs, and the other behind the back or shoulders. The slings may have web straps or chains that hook to a wide-angle swivel bar. The positioning of the slings is very important since some sliding may occur as the client is lifted. (Note, since the swivel bar is apt to be close to the client's face, eyeglasses should be removed if worn by the client.) It is most often necessary for two practitioners to be in attendance while this device is used.

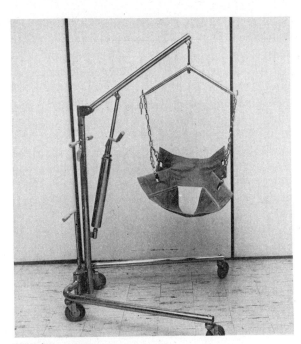

FIGURE 30-32. Hydraulic lift.

TURNING FRAMES

Lateral turning frames such as the "Stryker" or "Foster" frame are used to facilitate the care of a client whose condition requires immobilization of the spine. These are frequently used in the treatment of clients with spinal cord injuries or other back conditions and provide a means to turn and change the position of the client frequently. These devices have an anterior and posterior frame fitted on a standard with a pivoting device. Generally, one person may turn the frame. However, for security and support, it is recommended that two people are present during this procedure. The frame is turned in a smoothly maneuvered manner after the client has been instructed accordingly.

Although lateral turning frames have traction accessories available, a vertical turning frame, the "Circ-O-Lectric" bed used when it is necessary to apply cervical traction. As the vertical turning frame is rotated, the weights hang free, providing continuous traction. The "Circ-O-Lectric" bed is electrically controlled. Therefore, the nurse should practice turning an empty bed slowly and smoothly before attempting the procedure with a client. Positioning for clients on turning frames is essentially the same as that of the client in a regular bed, with consideration given to correct body alignment in the supine and prone positions.

CRUTCHES

Crutches are supports used to assist clients requiring aid in walking because of injury or disease in the lower extremities. The client who uses crutches will need special instructions on how to use them correctly. Usually this instruction is given by the physical therapist; however, the nurse must also have some knowledge of the use of crutches.

Exercises to prepare the client for crutch walking include quadriceps and gluteal setting, and push-ups. The client may also be taught the use of weights and other muscle strengthening exercises for the upper extremities.

Types

There are two types of crutches. *Axillary* crutches fit under the upper arm, and *Canadian* or *Lofstrand* crutches fit around the forearm by means of a metal cuff (Fig. 30-33).

Axillary crutches provide more adequate support than the Canadian type. The Canadian crutch has some rehabilitative advantage in that the client has to depend more on her own muscles than on the crutches. In addition, the Canadian crutch, which has no axillary bar, provides less chance of crutch paralysis (axillary muscle damage).

To measure the client for axillary crutches, place the client in a standing position. Measure the length from the axilla to a point 6 inches (15 cm) out from the side of the foot (heel). (If the client is lying down, measure the length from the axilla to the foot and add 2 inches [5 cm]. It is desirable to have a two-finger width between the axillary fold and the armpiece. An alternative method is to subtract 15 inches (40 cm) from the client's total height.

For Canadian crutches, adjustment is made to allow the elbows to bend at approximately a 30 degree angle with the crutch tip 6 to 8 inches (15–20 cm) to the side and in front of the foot.

With the axillary crutches, the handpiece on the crutches should allow a 30 degree elbow flexion as noted for adjusting the Canadian type crutch. The client's wrist is extended and the hand, dorsiflexed. Other considerations to be made include: the use

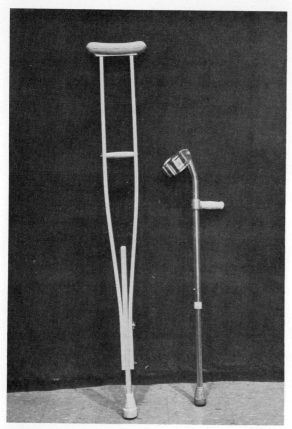

FIGURE 30-33. Two types of crutches: Left, axillary; Right, Canadian or Lofstrand.

of rubber tips on the crutches to prevent slipping (these tips should be checked and replaced if worn down and no longer safe); pads may be used over the axillary bars to prevent undue pressure on the ribs and arm; clients should be advised to wear well-fitting shoes that provide support and have firm soles; clients should also be advised to remove loose rugs or other obstacles from their environment and to avoid waxed or wet floors to prevent slipping or falling. A client should not be allowed to use crutches alone until she has demonstrated the ability to use them safely and correctly. *Correct posture is essential for effective and safe crutch walking.*

Common Postural Defects

Postural defects frequently seen in the client using crutches include rounded shoulders, slumping, stooped back, flexion at the hips and knees, exter-

nal rotation of the hips, and eversion of the feet. Although factors such as fatigue and muscle weakness contribute to these defects, the nurse must teach and encourage correct crutch walking posture. A correct posture is one in which the client stands as straight as possible; the head is held straight and high, and the pelvis is in line with the feet. The crutches are placed approximately 4 inches (10 cm) in front and 4 inches (10 cm) to the sides of the feet. This posture provides a stable base of support, for the body weight is borne largely by the client's hands (never by the axilla). The axillary bar is held close to the client's body against the rib cage and grasped there by the adductor muscles of the chest. This is the pivot point for crutch motion.

Crutch Gaits

The selection of a crutch gait is determined by the type and severity of disability and the client's physical condition, muscle strength, and body balance. The *four-point gait* is a simple, slow, safe, and stable gait that allows the client's weight to be constantly shifted. It is used for clients who can move each leg separately and can bear partial weight on both lower extremities. The sequence is *right crutch, left foot, left crutch, right foot* (Fig. 30-34). There are three points of support on the floor at all times.

The *two-point gait* requires more balance since there are only two points of support for the body at any one time. It may also be used by clients who can move each leg separately and are allowed to bear weight on the lower extremities. The two-point sequence is *right crutch* and *left foot* (together at the same time) then *left crutch and right foot* (together at the same time) (Fig. 30-35). If a person cannot bear weight on a lower extremity or may only bear minimal weight, the *three-point gait* is advised. In this gait, *both crutches and the weaker leg move forward together*, then the *stronger leg is brought forward* (Fig. 30-36). To use this gait, the client's arms must be strong enough to support the body weight, and she must have good balance. Other types of gaits, such as the *swing-through* and *tripod*, which are taught to clients with severe lower extremity involvement, are not commonly used.

In addition to learning a specific gait, the client must also be instructed in how to go up and down stairs and how to sit and rise from a chair with the

FOUR—POINT CRUTCH GAIT

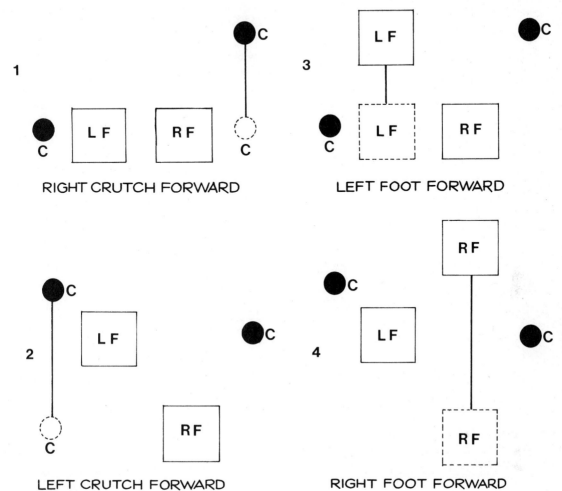

FIGURE 30-34. The four-point crutch gait is a simple, slow, safe and steady crutch gait that provides three points of support at all times.

aid of crutches. *To go downstairs*, crutches are lowered one step. The involved (or disabled) leg is advanced to the step first followed by the uninvolved leg. This insures that the uninvolved leg shares the body weight being borne by the arms. *In going upstairs*, the uninvolved leg goes up to the next step first, then the crutches and the involved leg follow. *To sit in a chair*, the crutches are held at the hand pieces for control, and the client bends forward slightly while assuming the sitting position. *To stand up*, both feet are placed in a wide base of support as close to the chair as possible. The crutches are grasped at the hand pieces, and the

client pushes down on the hand pieces as she raises herself from the chair.

CANES

To fit the client for a cane, the client's elbow is flexed 25 to 30 degrees, and the cane is adjusted until the handle is level with the greater trochanter of the femur (hip). When at the proper length, the cane will allow for the same degree of elbow flexion noted above. As weight is put on the client's hand, the elbow is extended.

When a cane is used, it is held in the hand op-

TWO-POINT CRUTCH GAIT

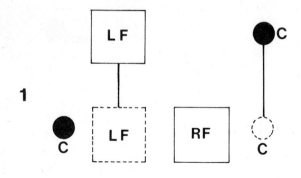

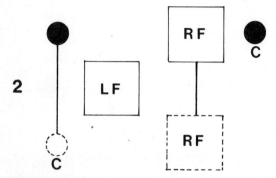

FIGURE 30-35. The two-point crutch gait is used by clients with balance who are allowed to bear weight on the lower extremities.

posite the involved extremity and is advanced at the same time as the involved extremity. Therefore, the body weight is taken partially on the cane and the involved extremity as the uninvolved leg moves forward. *Going upstairs*, the client steps up with the uninvolved leg, then places the cane and involved leg on the step. When going downstairs, the procedure is reversed; the cane is held close to the body to prevent leaning.

The standard cane is available in adjustable or sized aluminum and solid wooden canes. The *three-legged* or *four-legged cane* has a handgrip like that on a shovel and a tripod base. These are usually made of aluminum and are most helpful for the elderly client who may walk slowly and have poor balance (Fig. 30-37). As with crutches, all canes should be checked for safety, replacing worn rubber tips whenever necessary.

WALKERS

A walker will provide more support than a cane and is useful for supplying additional security and support to ambulating clients. Walkers may become a disadvantage if clients become too dependent on them and are unable to ambulate without their use. Another limitation is that walkers cannot be used on stairs.

There are two basic types of walkers available. The *standard walker* (Fig. 30-38) is a rigid four-legged frame. The *reciprocal walker* is similar to the standard, but has an additional hinge mechanism

THREE-POINT CRUTCH GAIT

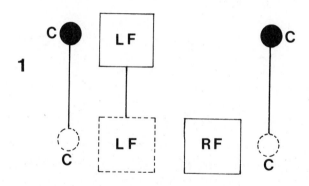

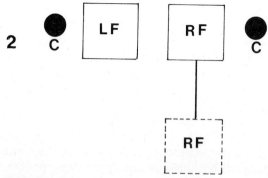

FIGURE 30-36. The three-point crutch gait is used by clients who cannot bear any weight or who may only bear minimal weight on a lower extremity.

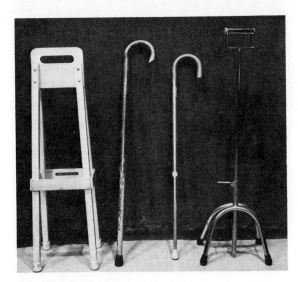

FIGURE 30-37. Variety of canes.

that allows for each side of the walker to be moved independently. This feature allows for more maneuverability. In selecting a walker, individual needs of the client should be considered. Some walkers have wheels; however, this type is considered inadvisable since wheels reduce stability and make the walker a potential hazard. The safety considerations that apply to crutches and canes can be applied to walkers.

WHEELCHAIRS

Many factors must be considered when a wheelchair is selected for an individual client. Frequently, the ordering of wheelchairs is done by someone highly trained and skilled in assessing the client's problems and his requirements in a chair.

Available in adult, extra-wide, junior, and child sizes, there are several types of wheelchairs. The *universal* chair has larger wheels in the back and may be used both indoors and outdoors (Fig. 30-39). This type facilitates easier transfers and can be tilted to go up and down stairs. For *amputees*, there is a chair with rear wheels that are set farther back. This type of chair maintains safe balance by compensating for the loss of client weight in front due to the amputated limbs. The *power-driven* chair should only be used for clients without the ability to self-propel.

Many types of accessories for wheelchairs are

available. When selecting these, the needs of the client for accomplishing daily activities are evaluated as well as the requirements for maintaining correct posture, body alignment, and comfort. Selection of accessories is best accomplished by a trained person. However, the nurse should be familiar with basic information on the use of those features which are used for positioning, comfort, and safety. Every wheelchair has *brakes* for safety. *Adjustable backrests* may be obtained for the client who cannot sit upright at all times; a removable *headrest* extension will give additional back and head support. *Adjustable legrests* are also available for elevating legs if necessary. *Footrests* with heel-loops or supports will prevent the client's feet from slipping off the footrest. Foam rubber *seat cushions* in 2 or 4 inch heights promote comfort and correct positioning (Fig. 30-39).

STRETCHERS

In addition to transporting clients, stretchers are useful for those clients unable to sit up in a conventional chair or wheelchair because of large casts, appliances, or physical limitations. Clients are po-

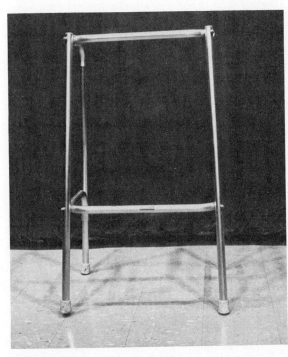

FIGURE 30-38. Standard walker.

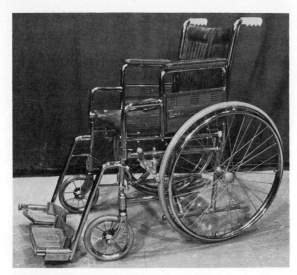

FIGURE 30-39. Universal wheelchair.

sitioned on stretchers as they are in bed. Therefore, many stretchers have features similar to those of a bed—for example, a means of raising the head and foot, side rails, and gatches. A major consideration in the use of stretchers is safety. Safety straps must be fastened even if side rails are in the up position. When moving a stretcher, always stand at the client's head; push the stretcher with the client moving feet first. As with a wheelchair, the stretcher's brakes should always be locked in place when it is standing still.

Clients confined to wheelchairs or stretchers for long periods of time, especially the debilitated and disabled, require frequent position changes to maintain motion, muscle strength and tone, and to stimulate circulation. It is the nurse's responsibility to plan care that includes activities that will prevent deformity and deterioration of muscle tone and strength and will encourage the client to do as much for herself as possible in the way of self-care. As previously discussed and described, proper body alignment is basic for all positioning postures. The principles of body mechanics and the maintenance of body alignment apply to the client who is confined to a wheelchair or stretcher and are essential in enhancing their potential for correct body posture.

BIBLIOGRAPHY

American Rehabilitation Foundation: *A Handbook of Rehabilitation Nursing Techniques in Hemiplegia*. Minneapolis, American Rehabilitation Foundation, 1964.

Bilger, A., and Greene, E. H.: *Winters' Protective Body Mechanics: A Manual for Nurses*. New York, Springer Publishing Company, Inc., 1973.

Broer, M.: *Efficiency of Human Movement*, 3rd ed. Philadelphia, W. B. Saunders Company, 1973.

Browse, N. L.: *Physiology and Pathology of Bed Rest*. Springfield, Ill., Charles C Thomas, 1965.

Brunner, L. S., and Suddarth, D. S.: *Textbook of Medical Surgical Nursing*, 3rd ed. Philadelphia, J. B. Lippincott Company, 1975.

Brunnstrom, S.: *Clinical Kinesiology*, 2nd ed. Philadelphia, F. A. Davis Company, 1966.

Larson, C. B., and Gould, M.: *Orthopedic Nursing*. 8th ed. St. Louis, C. V. Mosby Company, 1974.

LeVeau, P.: *Williams and Lissner: Biomechanics of Human Motion*, 2nd ed. Philadelphia, W. B. Saunders Company, 1977.

National League for Nursing: *Rehabilitative Aspects of Nursing. A Programed Instruction Series. Part 1: Physical Therapeutic Measures. Unit 1: Concepts and Goals*. New York, National League for Nursing Research and Studies Service, 1966.

National League for Nursing: *Rehabilitative Aspects of Nursing. A Programed Instruction Series. Part 1: Physical Therapeutic Nursing Measures. Unit 2: Range of Joint Motion*. New York, National League for Nursing Research and Studies Service, 1967.

Nordmark, M. T., and Rohweder, A. W.: *Scientific Foundations of Nursing*, 3rd ed. Philadelphia, J. B. Lippincott Company, 1975.

Public Health Nursing Section, Colorado State Department of Public Health: *Elementary Rehabilitation Nursing Care*. Washington, D.C., U.S. Department of Health, Education and Welfare, 1966.

Taber's Cyclopedic Medical Dictionary, 13th ed. Philadelphia, F. A. Davis Company, 1977.

Yates, J. A.: *Moving and Lifting Patients: Principles and Techniques*. (Rehabilitation Publication No. 720) Minneapolis, Kenny Rehabilitation Institute, 1970.

CHAPTER 31

GLOSSARY

abscess. Self-contained pocket of purulent material.

active immunity. State of immunity produced when the body produces its own antibodies.

agent. Any factor which can cause disease.

antibody. A plasma protein formed after contact with an antigen.

antigen. A substance that stimulates the formation of antibodies.

antisepsis. Prevention of sepsis by inhibiting the growth and multiplication of pathogenic microorganisms.

antiseptic. Mild disinfectant.

asepsis. Absence of pathogenic microorganisms.

attenuated. Having reduced virulence of pathogenic microorganisms.

bactericidal. Chemical which kills bacteria.

bacteriostatic. Chemical which prevents the growth and multiplication of bacteria.

Betadine. Iodide disinfectant solution.

clean. Free of pathogenic microorganisms.

communicable disease. Disease capable of being transmitted from person to person.

ASEPSIS

Ramona Mae Leslie, M.S., R.N., and
Christine S. Pakatar, M.S., R.N.

contamination. State of uncleanliness.

cross-contamination. Transfer of infectious material from one location to another.

debridement. Removal of dead or damaged tissue.

disinfectant. Chemical which destroys microorganisms but not necessarily their spores.

disinfection. Chemical process which destroys microorganisms but not necessarily their spores.

enteric. Pertaining to the gastrointestinal tract.

environment. Set of conditions which allows an agent to flourish in a host.

epidemic. Disease incidence in excess of expectations.

epidemiology. Study of disease in populations.

fomites. Inanimate objects capable of harboring microorganisms.

fungus. A parasitic or saprophytic plant.

germicide. Chemical which destroys microorganisms.

host. A person who receives an agent.

immune system. Body defense mechanism against specific diseases.

immunization. Artificial method of enhancing the body's internal defense system.

incidence. Measurement of disease occurrence.

incision. Surgically induced wound.

infection. Body response to invasion by pathogens.

inflammation. Tissue response to injury or infection.

isolation. System of barriers designed to inhibit cross-contamination.

keloid. Overproduction of scar tissue.

medical asepsis. Techniques used to inhibit the growth and multiplication and to prevent the transfer of pathogenic microorganisms.

microorganism. Organism that can only be seen by using a microscope.

mold. A type of fungus.

morbidity rate. Disease rate.

mortality rate. Death rate.

neonate. A newborn infant between birth and four weeks of age.

nosocomial infection. Hospital-induced.

pandemic. Epidemic of worldwide proportions.

parasite. Any organism living in or on another organism.

passive immunity. State produced when antibodies are introduced artificially, and the body does not produce its own antibodies.

pathogen. Disease-producing organism.

prodromal. Preclinical.

purulent. Containing pus.

pus. Product of inflammation containing leukocytes, necrotic tissue, and pathogens.

resident bacteria. Skin bacteria that cannot be removed by chemical or mechanical means.

resistance. Decreased probability that agent invasion will be successful in the host.

sanguineous. Pertaining to blood.

scar. A mark left by healing of tissue.

sequelae. Aftereffects of disease or injury.

serosanguineous. Pertaining to serum and blood.

serous. Pertaining to serum.

sterile. Free of all microorganisms and their spores.

sterile field. Small area rendered free of all microorganisms and their spores.

sterilization. Physical or chemical process which destroys all microorganisms and their spores.

surgical asepsis. Techniques used to kill microorganisms and their spores.

susceptibility. Increased probability that agent invasion will be successful in the host.

symbiosis. Relationship of two organisms which is beneficial to each.

transient bacteria. Skin bacteria that can be removed by chemical or mechanical means.

virulence. Measurement of disease severity.

virus. Submicroscopic organism capable of growing only in living cells.

wound. Disruption in the integrity of the skin or mucous membrane.

HISTORICAL PERSPECTIVES

The recognition and prevention of disease has interested man for centuries. Even when diseases were believed to be caused by demons, miasmic vapors, or as punishment for sins, preventive measures were instituted which effectively curbed the spread of some diseases. The Romans devised public water and sewage systems, early examples of public sanitation; the Jewish culture has a sanitary code of health and dietary laws dating at least from the writing of the Book of Leviticus. The Bible records the isolation of persons with leprosy (Hansen's disease), a technique which persists to this day for control of some communicable diseases.

Throughout the Middle Ages, cholera, syphilis, and plague periodically ravaged the world population. During the London Plague in 1665, more than 68,000 Londoners died. Fear was rampant, and many possibilities for control were tried; however, the flea-infested rats, which transmitted the disease, remained unidentified as the main problem.

General lack of progress marked the years until the invention of the microscope, and it was nearly two centuries later before the great discoveries about infectious disease began. Early proposals and theories were not well received. In 1854, John Snow proposed that cholera was transmitted by contaminated water and contact with cholera victims, based on his famous study of London's two water supply systems. Semmelweiss, in Vienna, was ridiculed for suggesting that puerperal fever and maternal deaths were the result of doctors not washing their hands before performing deliveries, particularly after they examined cadavers.

At the same time, Florence Nightingale was attending British casualities of the Crimean War in Scutari. Although she never subscribed to the "germ theory," she did believe in scrupulous cleanliness and humane treatment. Fatalities among the soldiers decreased dramatically, mostly because her methods effectively reduced the incidence of infection. In the United States during the Civil War, a staggering two-thirds of the deaths among the military were due to disease not wounds. Although this was recognized, sanitary conditions in military hospitals and detention camps were horrendous, and no organized effort emerged to correct the situation.

As the nineteenth century progressed, Pasteur finally disproved the "theory of spontaneous regeneration," and Lister's research on microorganisms led to theories about wound infection. Koch proposed his "postulates of disease causation," lending more credence to the scientific search for cause and effect of communicable diseases.

By 1900, the "germ theory" was widely accepted as valid. Immunization was demonstrated as a valuable adjunct in the control of infectious disease. Social consciousness was being raised, sanitary conditions were improving, and the prevailing feeling was one of optimism. Man, indeed, was the master of his destiny.

The effect of the 1918–1919 influenza pandemic was devastating. It ran unchecked, killing 5,000,000 people worldwide, and 500,000 in the United States. There were more casualities from the influenza pandemic than there had been military casualities during World War I. A similar event was predicted, though it never materialized, in 1976, leading to the largest immunization program ever attempted in the United States. During the 1940s, the "miracle" antibiotic drugs held promise for the final control of all infectious disease. However, indiscriminate use of these drugs has created new problems.

Man's search for the cause, control, and prevention of infection continues, but the battle has not been won. Smallpox has been conquered worldwide. Diphtheria, pertussis, tetanus, and poliomyelitis are no longer major health problems in the United States, but *Staphylococcus, Streptococcus,* and *Rubella,* to name only a few concerns, still pose important threats. The control of infection remains as important as ever.

EPIDEMIOLOGY OF INFECTION

Infection is the body's response to invasion by pathogenic microorganisms. These pathogens can be identified and classified according to type: bacterium, mold, protozoa, rickettsia, and virus. All pathogens are parasites in the sense that they obtain their nourishment from the host they have invaded.

Epidemiology is the study of disease causation, and the epidemiologic approach looks at the who, what, where, when, why, and how of infectious disease.

An agent is any factor which can cause disease. In the case of an infectious disease, the agent is one of the pathogens already mentioned. The host is the person who receives the agent. The environmental component refers to the set of conditions and circumstances which allow the agent to flourish in the particular host at any given time (Fig. 31-1). If all of the parts are present and operative, an infectious disease will occur. If, on the other hand, anyone or more of the parts is altered or removed, an infectious disease will not occur.

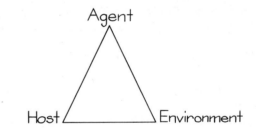

FIGURE 31-1. Components of the disease process.

The sequence of an infectious disease can also be thought of as a chain starting with the agent (Fig. 31-2). The following list comprises the links of this chain.

1. The *agent* is a pathogenic microorganism. It must be present in sufficient quantity and virulence to cause disease.
2. The *reservoir* is the location where the agent can grow and multiply. This can be a human or other animal who is prodromal or clinically ill with the disease or who harbors the agent, in which case he is called a carrier. The reservoir can also be an inanimate object, such as soil.
3. The *portal of exit* is the way in which the agent escapes from the reservoir. Most commonly, in humans, the escape is through the

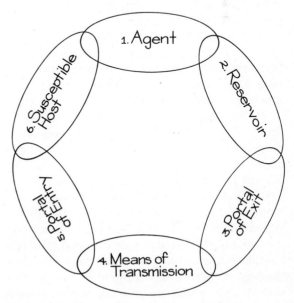

FIGURE 31.2. Sequence of infectious disease.

gastrointestinal, genitourinary, or respiratory tracts; the conjunctivae; and open skin lesions.

4. The *means of transmission* refer to the method by which the agent is passed from the portal of exit to the portal of entry. The methods can be direct or indirect. Examples of direct transmission are direct contact by touching, venereal means, or by inhaling droplets from an infected person. Indirect transmission can occur when contact is made with any object that harbors the agent. If the object is alive (e.g., fly or mosquito), it is called a vector. If it is an inanimate object, it is called a fomite.

5. The *portal of entry* is the way in which the agent enters a new host. Most commonly in humans, the entry is through the respiratory or urinary tracts, the mouth, conjunctivae, breaks in the skin, or bites.

6. The *susceptible host* is one whose resistance is lowered to point that the agent will be able to gain a foothold. Resistance is related to general health status, heredity, nutritional status, state of immunity, age, and sex.

Because it is true that a chain is only as strong as its weakest link, it follows that the chain should be broken wherever it is weakest. It is this principle that governs the choice of control methods. If more than one link can be interrupted or altered, the probability for control is enhanced even further.

The characteristics of an infectious disease can vary widely. It is arguable as to whether the variations are mostly agent, host, or environmentally related. Agent-related properties arise from the nature of the agent and its virulence in the host. Many of the infectious diseases are relatively mild, short-lived, and self-limited. They leave no permanent sequelae in the majority of the population, and one course of the illness confers permanent immunity. Mumps is an example of such a disease. On the other hand, an infectious disease can be a severe, long-term affair, with all kinds of sequelae. Bulbar poliomyelitis, for example, frequently causes permanent neurological damage, including paralysis.

While it is common to consider many infectious diseases as nonserious, it is important to remember that even uncomplicated ones can cause untoward and unwanted consequences. For example,

mumps can cause sterility in the adolescent or adult male; measles can damage the eighth cranial nerve; rubella can cause congenital anomalies in the fetus when contracted during the first trimester of pregnancy; and untreated gonorrhea can lead to pelvic inflammatory disease. Thus, none of the infectious diseases should be viewed casually, and efforts to prevent or control all of them are worth pursuing.

Host-related properties in response to a pathogenic agent include an infinite number of factors. The host's susceptibility to the invading agent is the primary factor. Susceptibility is directly related to the host's resistance. Susceptibility is the combination of factors that increases the probability that agent invasion will be successful. On the other hand, resistance is the combination of factors that decreases the probability. In epidemiological terms, the factors are called risk factors, and one aim of disease control is to decrease the host's probability of risk. Immunization is one common method of reducing risk. The general health status of an individual is a strong influencing factor. Everyday observation shows repeatedly that some individuals are less prone to the development of infectious disease than others. Intact skin reduces the chance for pathogenic invasion, as does the proper functioning, with appropriate defense mechanisms, of the body systems. Heredity may play a part in this mechanism, although it has been difficult to prove, and the research is incomplete. The incidence of nosocomial infections is well established. Although ease of transmission is definitely a contributing factor, the debilitated state of the hospitalized client is an additive factor.

The well-nourished individual, who is neither overweight, nor underweight, has greater resistance than the malnourished person. This is probably due to interference with antibody production during protein synthesis in the poorly nourished person. Age, also, mediates resistance. The very young and the elderly have less resistance to infectious disease than do the rest of the population, as indicated statistically by the Center for Disease Control of the U.S. Public Health Service. It is interesting, however, that the 25−34 age group had a higher than expected incidence of morbidity and mortality during the 1918−1919 influenza pandemic.

Sex has been implicated in susceptibility and resistance, although it is unresolved as to why some infectious diseases are more prevalent in one sex than the other, and also why morbidity is higher in females and mortality is higher in males. A current theory revolves around sex-linked heredity, although opportunity for exposure may be equally important.

Environment-related factors include anything which enables an agent to complete its activity within the host. Proper sanitation accounts for the control of many infectious diseases simply because the agent can not be transmitted from improperly treated food, water, or excreta. Climate and geography influence the spread of disease. The diseases of malaria and yellow fever are endemic in the tropics and unknown elsewhere unless introduced by a visitor or traveler.

The foregoing paragraphs only highlight some factors and their interrelationships. The work of meshing these factors and relationships for a better understanding of infectious disease properly belongs to the study of epidemiology. However, it is important for the nurse to be as aware of these factors as possible. The symbiotic relationship of agent, host, and environment must be operative for infectious disease to occur and flourish. Therefore, the practitioner must understand the factors and relationships to make realistic plans for the control and prevention of infectious disease.

INFECTIOUS DISEASE CONTROL

Prevention and control of infectious disease are planned to render the agent ineffective, to increase the resistance of the host, or to change the environment.

Control of Agent

It is clearly impossible to eradicate all of the possible agents from the face of the earth. However, public measures for disease control, especially sanitation and environmental controls are instituted to reduce the number of agents, as well as to interrupt their normal environment. Well-implemented programs have had notable success, especially in the developed nations of the world, although much remains to be accomplished in underdeveloped nations.

Resistance of Host

Outside of maintaining the host's optimum state of health and limiting his exposure to infectious dis-

ease, the main avenue for increasing his resistance is by increasing his immunity. Immunity is a state of protection against disease. Disease does not develop because the plasma cells have been stimulated to form antigens which in turn produce antibodies. Antibodies have specificity—that is, a set of antibodies must be developed for each disease. The antibodies must be adequately developed and be present in sufficient quantity to afford protection.

Each individual possesses some natural immunity which is acquired in several ways. The major part of natural immunity is due to the body's inherent defense system. Aiding this system are the natural barriers of the skin, mucous membranes, and cilia in the respiratory tract. Also, gastric acidity, the inflammatory response, lysozyme in the tears, white blood cells, macrophages of the reticuloendothelial system, and the lymphatic system enhance this mechanism. Clients who have lost these defenses for one reason or another are more susceptible to infection. For example, a client with a decubitus ulcer is much more prone to develop a *Staphylococcus aureus* or *Pseudomonas* infection than a client whose skin is intact. When the polymorphonuclear leukocytes are suppressed or rendered immature by immunosuppressive drugs or leukemia, the resistance is lowered. In addition to natural immunity from body mechanisms, there is species immunity. Humans do not contract distemper, and lower animals seem to be immune from most human diseases.

Finally, the newborn has natural immunity which is acquired from the mother, because of placental transfer during fetal life, which continues if the infant is breast-fed. Although this immune protection is adequate for the neonate and young infant, it is important to realize that the immunity is temporary, lasting a few weeks or months, at best, and the immunity only includes those diseases for which the mother has acquired active immunity. Therefore, it is necessary to institute an adequate immunization program early in life to insure continuous protection.

Immunity may also be acquired either by contracting a disease or by immunization. Immunity so acquired is classified as being either active or passive. Active immunity occurs when the body is stimulated to produce its own antibodies. Having a disease, such as mumps or chickenpox, will produce this result. It should be noted that not all agents stimulate this body response. *Gonococcus neisseria,* for example, does not, and one course of gonorrhea does not confer immunity. Reinfection is not only possible, but probable unless treatment of the client and all sexual partners is adequate.

The same result can be induced by immunization with a vaccine or a toxoid. These preparations are killed, attenuated, or inactivated antigenic materials. Examples are: typhoid and pertussis vaccines (killed); oral-Sabin-poliomyelitis and measles vaccines (attenuated); and tetanus and diphtheria toxoids (inactivated).

Generally, active immunity is long-term. When active immunity comes from having had the disease, immunity lasts a lifetime. It is rare to hear that someone had mumps more than once. Immunization with a vaccine or toxoid lasts for several years and requires boosters at periodic intervals to stimulate the body to reproduce antibodies.

Passive immunity is acquired from antibodies produced from an outside source. The usual preparations are antitoxins and antisera derived from immunized humans or animals. This protection is immediate and complete and is used for people who are susceptible or have been exposed to infectious disease. They may also be used in the treatment of those who have contracted the disease. Examples are diphtheria and tetanus antitoxins. This protection is valuable in certain instances, but the effect is temporary, and the body is not stimulated to produce its own antibodies. Some of these preparations are made with a horse serum base. Allergy for horse serum must be established before administration, lest an anaphylactic reaction be precipitated.

Schedules for immunization are suggested by the various State Health Departments and may vary slightly. They include diphtheria, pertussis, tetanus (DPT), and poliomyelitis vaccines during the first year of life, with boosters at 1 year, and measles and rubella shortly thereafter. Boosters should be readministered at the time of school entry. Tetanus boosters should be given at least every 10 years, although it is routine to offer a booster at the time of injury if the last tetanus was administered 5 years or more ago, or if the individual is not certain when the last administration occurred. Vaccination for smallpox is no longer required in the United States because the disease is declared officially quiescent.

Immunization is an important part of pediatric practice. However, it is not exclusively a childhood procedure. When the World Health Organization predicted the swine flu pandemic in 1976, the Surgeon General of the United States convened a meeting of the health officers of all the states and territories. The need for a program was assessed, a plan drawn up, and the project was implemented. The evaluation phase will provide material for graduate students for years. Part of the planning stage included identification of high-risk groups, the elderly and the chronically ill, especially those with respiratory problems. The high-risk groups were immunized during the first phase because of priority needs. It was a good example of the epidemiological approach to an identified health problem.

Immunization is effective. Logically, a method for disease control that is widely accepted as effective should be universally implemented. Unhappily, this is not the case. Public ignorance and apathy abound, and nearly every community health nurse knows that the struggle to have every child fully immunized is never ending. Part of the problem stems from the very success of immunization. The effects of poliomyelitis, for example, have not been seen or experienced by young parents or their peers. They see little reason to subject their children to a procedure for protection against an elusive agent that they never expect to materialize. Also, the necessity for return visits to a physician or clinic to complete a series is seen as bothersome. Neither argument is valid, and nurses continue to share responsibility for promoting immunization as one effective tool in infectious disease control. Federal and state health agencies are becoming concerned about this problem. The U.S. Public Health Service plans to step up its public education and information programs, and many State Health Departments are requiring full immunization as a prerequisite to public school entry.

Control of Environment

Public measures to control the environment are unquestionably an important part of this arm of control. However, this section is concerned with those concepts and techniques which are specifically geared toward client situations. It has already been stated that the ill individual is at greater risk for the development of infectious disease than is the healthy individual. When ill people are housed together in one site, the probability of the development of infectious disease increases proportionately, and the need for specific, scientifically-based control measures can be clearly demonstrated. These measures include surveillance of personnel and the environment, the integrity of practitioners, and the practice of asepsis.

Most health care facilities have an organized program for infectious disease control. There is usually an infection control committee which is charged with the responsibility for implementing the program. Their activities range from case-finding to monitoring personnel and clients, and the committee usually includes an epidemiologist, who may be a nurse. They are responsible for data collection about identified and potential outbreaks of infectious disease, planning, and implementation of specific measures for disease control, and evaluation of the overall program. They monitor clients and conduct surveillance of personnel, looking especially for breaks in technique.

The integrity of individual practitioners is crucial to an effective program. It is necessary for every nurse to develop an "aseptic conscience," and to expect no less from her colleagues. When one realizes that nosocomial infections develop in 3 percent of institutionalized clients and that one of every 100 hospital admissions develops bacteremia, for which the mortality rate is 30 to 50 percent, the scope of the problem becomes obvious. Widespread and often indiscriminate use of antibiotics has unleashed new strains of bacteria which are resistant to known chemotherapeutics. *Staphylococcus, Streptococcus, Pseudomonas,* and *Proteus* are present, active, and increasing in incidence and virulence. When the antibiotics were introduced in the 1940s, it was thought that the problem of infectious disease would be largely overcome. Aseptic techniques were relaxed, and the concept of an "aseptic conscience" was seen as less important than previously. However, the problem is not going away, and it seems unlikely that it will disappear in the future.

Part of personal integrity also includes the nurse's care of herself. If she is ill with an infectious disease and works in a client-centered setting, she increases the risk of spreading the disease to her clients. Since the client is already at risk, it is unwarranted and unsafe for her to needlessly expose him to further risk.

A further nursing responsibility is education and counseling about good health practices. These activities are primarily aimed, but not limited, to clients. Clients do not come to the health setting with the same background and knowledge as the health professional. They should, however, leave the health setting with complete information. Because the nurse has more extensive contact with clients than any other member of the health team, she must assume this responsibility. A "once-over-lightly" review is insufficient. Development of client teaching plans is discussed elsewhere, but it is worth reiterating that clients who understand the disease process and the rationale for treatment are more likely to comply with a prescribed regimen. Time, interest, and knowledge on the part of the nurse is likely to increase the client's efforts toward better health practices.

Finally, the concept of asepsis needs to be explored. The remainder of the chapter will focus on the creation and maintenance of asepsis, including appropriate techniques.

ASEPSIS

Asepsis is the absence of pathogens. The concept is divided into medical asepsis and surgical asepsis. The broad goal of medical asepsis is to reduce the number of pathogens and inhibit their transmission. Medical asepsis encompasses all of those procedures which constitute the "clean" technique. The broad goal of surgical asepsis is to eliminate all microorganisms and their spores. As such, the techniques are "sterile." Before proceeding, it is necessary to fully understand the basic difference between medical and surgical asepsis. Usually the details are specifically spelled out for individual client situations. However, this is not always true, and the nurse must be able to rationalize and plan a correct course of action based on what needs to be accomplished. This point cannot be overemphasized. Many of the nursing skills suggested for the maintenance of asepsis tend to become ritualistic. The various steps of the procedures as written in this chapter constitute a safe way to carry out asepsis. However, modifications and adaptations can be made in individual situations, so long as the basic principles of asepsis are not violated.

Medical

Many studies have confirmed that handwashing is the single most effective aseptic practice for the pre-

TABLE 31-1. Medical Aseptic Handwashing to Maintain Medical Asepsis

Anticipated Accomplishment	Scientific Principles/ Rationale	Specific Considerations
1. Remove all jewelry from hands and wrists, except a plain ring.	Microorganisms harbor on inanimate objects.	
2. Stand away from sink.	The sink is a fomite.	
3. Turn on water and adjust to desired temperature.		Temperature of the water is not a key element.
4. Wet hands and wrists.	Gravitational pull moves organisms.	
5. Apply emulsifying agent.	Emulsifying agent removes skin oils, and reacts with protein of microorganisms to enhance destruction.	Institutional policy governs choice of cleansing agent.
6. Scrub hands and wrists.	Friction action is most effective part of handwashing technique. Transient microorganisms are removed by friction.	
7. Rinse thoroughly.	Running water acts as the vehicle to carry away microbial products.	
8. Dry hands and wrists with paper towels.		Hand lotion may be used to prevent excessive drying of skin.
9. Use dry paper towels to turn off faucets.	Faucet is considered contaminated.	This step is not necessary if sink has knee operated controls.

vention of cross-infection. Other medical aseptic procedures to be considered are: disinfection methods and isolation techniques.

HANDWASHING

The skin harbors transient and resident microorganisms which have the potential to become pathogenic if the right circumstances exist. Transient bacteria, which are acquired by daily contact with animate and inanimate objects, can be readily removed by correct handwashing using soap and water. Resident bacteria adapt to the skin environment and penetrate in and around sebaceous glands. Resident bacteria cannot be removed by any method of mechanical scrub or by the use of antiseptics. Therefore, it is impossible to sterilize the skin. Any method or solution capable of sterilizing the skin would destroy the dermal layers. Nevertheless, properly executed handwashing procedures can reduce the number of microorganisms and inhibit their transfer. Handwashing as an aseptic technique interrupts the epidemiological triangle at all points: agent, host, and environment.

Implementation	Recommendations	Observations

Keep hands downward.

Use a generous portion.

Scrub each hand with other hand front and back interlacing fingers to cleanse between them. Clean fingernails.	This step should take 2 min at minimum.	

Work from area of wrist to fingertips. Discard towels.		Observe hands for cuts, scratches, or scrapes.

It is recommended that hands be washed: (1) at the beginning of the workday; (2) between client contacts; (3) during the performance of nursing activities such as handling dressings, catheters, urinals, bedpans, specimen collection, even when gloves are used; (4) after working in an isolation area; (5) after coughing or sneezing; (6) before and after eating; (7) after using the toilet; and (8) at the end of the workday.

The key elements for adequate handwashing are running water, an emulsifying agent, and friction, with friction the most important factor. Friction mechanically removes microorganisms from the skin. The emulsifying agent removes the oily residue of the skin with its collection of microorganisms and also interacts with the protein portion of the microorganism. Running water carries the products away.

Since the skin is the body's first line of defense against invading microorganisms, care should be exercised to prevent any injury or cracking of the skin from handwashing measures. The use of brushes to scrub the hands is not recommended because of the increased probability of trauma to the skin and nail beds. To keep the skin soft and pliable, an emollient hand cream or lotion applied to the hands following handwashing is highly recommended. To avoid contamination of clean hands, it is preferable to have a sink and soap dispenser with knee operated control.

The procedure for handwashing may need to be adapted in some community-based settings. For example, if running water is not available, water should be poured over the nurse's hands during the rinse phase by a second person. Soap and paper towels should always be carried in the bag of the community health nurse. Even, if adaptation is necessary, the rationale for handwashing remains constant (Table 31-1).

MICROBIAL CONTROL

Disinfection and sterilization are methods utilized for microbial control. Disinfection implies that a chemical process is used to destroy pathogenic microorganisms but not necessarily their spores. Germicides are substances used to accomplish disinfection. The term disinfectant describes a chemical germicide that is used on inanimate objects (fomites). They can destroy pathogenic microoranisms. Antiseptics are weaker chemicals than disinfectants. Antiseptics are safe to use on the skin and mucous membranes. Antiseptics are used to inhibit the growth and activity of pathogens. It is not possible to truly disinfect the skin. Bacteriostatic agents inhibit the growth of bacteria, whereas bactericidal agents destroy bacteria. These terms are not synonymous with disinfectant or antiseptic.

Sterilization is a physical or chemical process used to kill all microorganisms and their spores. The most common methods used to achieve sterilization are: (1) steam under pressure (autoclave), (2) dry heat, (3) boiling, and (4) ethylene oxide gas. Other methods used are flaming, ultraviolet rays, and sonic disruption (use of sound waves). Steam under pressure is the best known and most widely used method (Tables 31-2 and 31-3).

Sterilization of materials in home-based settings is possible. Some materials, such as linens can be baked in an oven, using the guidelines suggested for "dry heat." The oven should be thoroughly clean, and the door must fit tightly. Far more common is the method of moist heat, or boiling, which can be used to sterilize instruments, tubes, or catheters.

It must be ascertained that the materials will not

TABLE 31-2. Disinfection

Compound	Type	Effective Against	Selected Uses
Alcohol	Disinfectant and antiseptic	Vegetative organisms and tubercle bacillus	Skin antisepsis, cleaning thermometers, instruments and needles
Phenolic compounds (hexachlorophene)	Disinfectant	Vegetative bacteria, tubercle bacillus	Hospital housekeeping, when added to a detergent
Quaternary ammonium (aqueous zephiran chloride)	Disinfectant and antiseptic	Gram positive organisms	Limited except in hospital kitchens for disinfection; inactivated by contact with soap
Glutaraldehyde* (cidex)	Disinfectant	Spores, tubercle bacillus	Instruments with lenses, heat-sensitive equipment, anesthesia equipment
Iodine + iodophors (Betadine)	Disinfectant and antiseptic	Spores, fungi, viruses, bacteria, tubercle bacillus	Skin antisepsis (as tincture of iodine), mucous membrane antisepsis (as Iodophor)
Chlorines	Disinfectant	Spores, only in neutral or acid solutions	Cleaning compounds, disinfection of water
Formaldehyde Bard-Parker (formalin)	Disinfectant	Spore forms of bacteria	Instrument disinfection, especially transfer forceps

*Often called "cold sterilization."

TABLE 31-3. Sterilization

Method	Temperature	Time	Selected Uses
Steam under pressure (autoclave)	121°C 126°C 134°C	15 min/15 lbs/sq in 10 min/10 lbs/sq in 3 min/29.4 lbs/sq in	All equipment: supplies except plastics, delicate-lensed instruments, and substances impregnated with petroleum and powders
Boiling*	100°C	10–20 min	Instruments, equipment: main use in home-based setting
Dry heat	170°C 150°C 120°C	60 min 150 min 8 hr	Glassware, linen, petroleum-impregnated gauze, and powders
Ethylene oxide gas	Below 60°C	See manufacturer's recommendation	Materials damaged by water: plastics and rubber

*Spores are not destroyed.

be destroyed by boiling; this information should be written on the original packages. Whatever is to be boiled should be washed with soap and water and rinsed thoroughly. The pan chosen for boiling must be clean and large enough to accommodate the instruments so that they are entirely immersed in water. A second pan is used to boil the tip and most of the handle of a hemostat, which will be used to remove the instruments from the boiling water. Both of these pans should be stainless steel or aluminum. Enameled pans may be used, providing they are not chipped or dented. The boiling time is counted from the time that the water starts to boil vigorously and must be timed for at least 10 minutes. When this time has elapsed, the unsterile handles of the hemostat are grasped with a hot-pad, and it is removed from the water, taking care to keep the hemostat tips pointed downward. The hemostat is then used to lift the other boiled items, one at a time, from the other pan. They are placed on an already prepared sterile field, after allowing them to air dry for a few seconds, so that the sterile field will not become wet and thereby contaminated. (See the discussion of concurrent and terminal disinfection in the following section.

ISOLATION

Isolation is a protective practice. Either the environment needs to be protected from the pathogens of the client or the client needs to be protected from the environmental pathogens. All isolation procedures derive from this basic concept.

The Center for Disease Control in Atlanta divides isolation into five categories. These are based on epidemiological studies of the most common infections and diseases encountered among the American population (Table 31-4).

The Laminar Air-Flow or Life-Island Units are extreme forms of protective (reverse) isolation. These systems are used when a client's immune system is severely compromised or lacking and are designed to maintain an environment that is as sterile as possible. The Laminar Air-Flow room has an air filtering system which filters all known microorganisms. All persons (staff and visitors) wear sterile garb, and all supplies are sterile. In the Life-Island Unit, the air entering the plastic canopied bed is sterilized. The nurse works through portholes which are encased with sterile sleeves. Everything that comes in direct contact with the client must be sterile.

Although the nurse does not always make the decision of whether or not to institute isolation, it is her responsibility as a case-finder, to institute this practice if her assessment deems it necessary. She uses the nursing process to assess the agent, host, and environment; identify the problem; and develop and implement appropriate plans. Assessment of host factors includes evaluation of the client's general condition and changes due to the onset of infectious process. Observable changes include: (1) appearance of skin lesions, (2) inflamed and purulent drainage from a wound, (3) coughing greenish yellow sputum, (4) elevated temperature and respiratory rate, and (5) sudden onset of fre-

TABLE 31-4. Isolation

Type of Isolation	Indications for Use	Recommendations*
Respiratory	Pathogens transmitted by airborne route; examples: pulmonary tuberculosis; rubella; rubeola; mumps; meningococcal meningitis; chicken pox	1. Private room 2. Masks for personnel and visitors 3. Mask on client when transported (i.e., x-ray) 4. Special handling of sputum and paper tissues
Enteric	Pathogen transmitted through direct or indirect contact with infected fecal material; examples: salmonellosis; shigellosis; infectious and serum hepatitis; E. coli gastroenteritis	1. Private room with private bath preferable 2. Gown and glove precautions for personnel and visitors when touching client or objects in room 3. Double-bag linen, objects used by client, and objects used in care of client 4. In cases for infectious or serum hepatitis, special precautions are used for contaminated needles and syringes
Wound and skin	Pathogen is transmitted by direct contact with lesion; examples: impetigo; staphylococcal skin and wound infections	1. Gowns and gloves for personnel and visitors coming in direct contact with client 2. Double-bag articles that have been in direct contact with client
Strict isolation	Pathogens are highly communicable and transmitted by contact and airborne routes; examples: staphylococcal pneumonia; extensive staphylococcal and streptococcal infected burns; rabies and plague	1. Private room with closed door 2. Gowns, gloves and masks for personnel and visitors 3. Special handling of all articles coming out of room
Protective (reverse)	Pathogens from environment pose threat to client with lowered resistance; examples: leukemia, agranulocytosis; extensive burns; clients on immunosuppressive therapy	1. Private room with closed door 2. Laminar Air-Flow or Life-Island Units 3. Sterile supplies and linen 4. Sterile gowns, gloves, and mask for personnel and visitors

*When possible use disposable equipment and utensils for all types of isolation.

quent yellow-green watery stools. Assessment of agent factors includes: (1) probable causative microorganism, (2) mode of transmission, (3) portals of exit and entry, and (4) pathogenicity and communicability of microorganisms. For example, if a nurse working in a newborn nursery observed that an infant passed a thin watery yellow-green stool, accompanied by an increase in body temperature and poor skin turgor, she should suspect that the infant harbored a diarrhea producing pathogen in his gastrointestinal tract. She makes this nursing diagnosis even before the causative organism is identified. Her decision to institute isolation precautions is based on her knowledge of the agent and host factors already enumerated. Assessment of the environment is an ongoing process. The nurse must be vigilant in identifying lapses in aseptic practices that result in cross-contamination. In the above situation, it is imperative that the other infants in the nursery be provided with a safe environment.

Once the decision about isolation is made, appropriate preliminary activities are instituted. To minimize the traffic in and out of the area, equipment and supplies should be readily available in a portable cabinet outside the unit. Although the use of specific articles is determined by the type of isolation ordered, isolation tags, plastic bags, and linen bags should always be on hand. Agencies generally follow or adapt the guidelines and cards with directions and description of the various types of isolation measures from the Center for Disease Control. These cards are posted at the entry point of the isolation unit. The cards should be clearly visible so that all persons entering the unit are aware of the procedure (Table 31-5).

There will be times when clients on isolation need to be transported to other areas of the institution for specific tests or treatments. To contain the client's microorganisms to himself, the following plan for transportation should be adopted.

1. Cover the transporting vehicle with a clean sheet before entering the isolation unit.
2. Assist client onto vehicle.
3. Cover client with another clean sheet to cover the entire body except for the face. If the client is on respiratory, strict, or protective isolation masks should be worn by the client and the transporter.
4. Ideally the corridor is cleared of all traffic.
5. Call the department receiving the client to notify them that the client is on isolation precautions.
6. After the client returns to the unit, the transport sheets are removed and discarded in the linen receptable in the client's unit.

Concurrent and Terminal Disinfection

Concurrent disinfection includes all of the ongoing procedures used in the maintenance of medical asepsis. The specific practices will depend upon the nature of the agent, mode of transfer, pathogenicity, and communicability, as well as the susceptibility of the host. Terminal disinfection includes the procedures used when isolation is discontinued for an individual client. Disposable items are discarded using the appropriate methods (e.g., double-bagging). Furniture items are cleaned with a germicidal solution, according to institutional policy. All items in the room which can not be adequately disinfected must be discarded. Clients or their families need to be informed that items, such as stuffed, nonwashable toys; cosmetics; and reading material can not be disinfected and therefore will have to be destroyed.

Teaching the Client

The probability of successful isolation practices increases in proportion to the number of people carrying out correct isolation procedures. The nurse has the responsibility for sharing her knowledge about isolation to the client and others who are likely to come in contact with him. This includes family, visitors, and other health team members.

Too often the nurse and other personnel rely upon the card posted outside the isolation unit to take the place of the responsibility to teach precautionary procedures. The information on the card is explicit and useful particularly to those familiar with isolation techniques because it aids in the recall of a large body of knowledge. It is a mistake to presume that the client, family, and visitors possess this same knowledge. It is important for the nurse to assess the need for a teaching plan accordingly. The rationale for each precautionary measure related to the infectious process should be reviewed with the client, family, and visitors. It is important for the nurse to assess the need for a teaching plan and plan accordingly. There is more likely to be compliance with the restrictions when the reasons for specific procedures are understood. Observations of correct practices by all concerned will validate the effectiveness of the teaching plan. The same principles of teaching control of infection apply to nurses in community-based settings.

Social Isolation

Others have referred to the psychological effect of remaining in isolation as the phenomenon of sensory deprivation. This effect is more accurately described as social isolation, which is a form of perceptual monotony. The basis for this rationale is that the client still has his sensory capabilities, but he is placed in an environment which is totally foreign and rigidly controlled. Also, this environment precludes most social interactions and is likely to be visually boring.

Reactions to social isolation vary widely, from apathy to anger, and may include such responses as listlessness, irritability, restlessness, depression, regression, hostility, crying, withdrawal, and rebellion. Any reaction can occur at any age, but certain responses occur more frequently during developmental stages. A good knowledge base of growth and development helps the nurse to identify responses and plan appropriate interventions. For example, an expected response to social isolation in the adolescent would be rebellion. He may also exhibit hostility and anger. Developmentally, the adolescent is striving for independence and ego identity. Peer relationships have priority. The nurse can appeal to these feelings by encouraging visitation by peers, allowing ventilation of fears, and explaining the necessary restrictions. It would also be worthwhile to encourage his sense of self-importance by allowing him to participate in the plan of care, insofar as it is safe and practical. Staff members should make a planned team effort to interact

TABLE 31-5. Isolation Technique to Maintain Medical Asepsis

Anticipated Accomplishment	Scientific Principles/ Rationale	Specific Considerations
Preparation for entering the unit. 1. *Gowning:* Wash and dry hands.	Skin harbors microorganisms. Hand washing removes transient microorganisms.	
Open the gown.	Gown is barrier which inhibits cross-transference of microorganisms.	Sleeve and body length of gown should cover arms and uniform.
Don the gown.	Moisture facilitates movement of microorganisms.	If gown becomes wet, it is considered contaminated.
2. *Masking:* Wash and dry hands.		Not necessary to repeat if it has already been done before donning a gown.
Place mask securely over nose and mouth.	Mask is barrier which inhibits cross-transference of microorganisms. Moisture favors growth of microorganisms.	Both disposable and fabric masks become damp from normal respiratory secretions.
3. *Gloving:* Open glove package on flat surface.		
Don gloves.	Clean gloves protect nurse from contamination in environment. Sterile gloves are worn to reduce transfer of microorganisms and cross-contamination when sterile or surgically clean environment is desirable.	Gloves should not be powdered. Donning procedure is same for sterile or nonsterile gloves.

Implementation	Recommendations	Observations
Use medical aseptic hand washing technique.	Remove jewelry.	
Grasp inside of back of neck opening.	Inside gown is considered contaminated.	
Slide arms into sleeves. Tie neck strings at back of neck. Overlap waist and tie strings in front, if possible.		
Remove nursing cap. Tie securely at back of head, high enough for comfort and to hold mask in position. Change mask when it becomes damp.	Use each mask only once. Mask should not be allowed to hang around neck. If nurse is ill with respiratory disease, mask is not effective protective barrier.	
Grasp one glove at folded edge. Locate thumb and put one glove on. Pick up other glove by placing fingers under folded cuff. Insert fingers and pull on securely.	If glove is torn, either change gloves, or place another glove over torn one.	

TABLE 31-5. Continued

Anticipated Accomplishment	Scientific Principles/ Rationale	Specific Considerations
Activities within the unit. 4. *Vital Signs:* Prepare equipment.	Paper towel acts as a barrier and avoids necessity for touching watch.	Thermometer, sphygmomanometer and stethoscope should remain in isolation unit for duration of client's stay. Thermometer is discarded at end of isolation period. Stethoscope and sphygmomanometer may be double-bagged and returned to designated area for sterilization.
Take vital signs.		

5. *Disposition of contaminated materials.*
  Double bagging:
  Tie knot at top of bags containing linen, trash, disposable equipment, used utensils, or instruments.
	Knotted-bag makes a closed-system barrier for contaminated materials	A second person and a second bag should be available outside unit.

Place contaminated bag inside a second bag, knot-side down.	Protection is increased for persons outside isolation unit.	
Label bag.	Protection against mixing contaminated materials with non-contaminants.	Tag or sticker attached clearly stating type of isolation.
6. *Collection of Specimens.* Prepare equipment.		
Collect specimen.		
Remove equipment.		

Implementation	Recommendations	Observations
Watch used for counting pulse and respirations is carried into unit on clean paper towel and placed where it can be seen. After vital signs have been taken, wash hands and pick up watch from clean side of paper towel. Discard paper towel, taking care to touch only clean side.	Clean equipment after each use.	
Record, when outside unit.		
	As a minimum, bags should be discarded every 8 hrs.	
A second person stands outside unit and holds second bag. Cuff of "clean" bag is unrolled over enclosed "contaminated" bag and sealed by second person.	Second bag is folded into a deep cuff that can be held from inside of fold.	
Second person does labeling.	Label should be large and bright enough to be easily visible.	
Label specimen container and laboratory slip with type of isolation before entering unit. Place container in clear, plastic bag.		
Follow double-bagging procedure (above).	Specimen container must be maintained in upright position to avoid spillage.	

TABLE 31.5. Continued

Anticipated Accomplishment	Scientific Principles/ Rationale	Specific Considerations
7. *Preparation for Exiting from the Unit.*		
Remove gloves.	All removal procedures follow principle that surfaces touching nurse are considered clean. All surfaces exposed to client are considered contaminated. When client is on protective (reverse) isolation, above principles are reversed.	Removal procedure is same for sterile or nonsterile gloves.
Wash hands.		Follow medical aseptic hand washing technique.
Remove mask.		
Exit room.		
Wash hands.		

socially as well as professionally with the client. Contacts should be brief but frequent.

Generally, isolation is a self-limited short-term therapy, but this does not mean that the nurse can overlook her responsibility to meet the client's needs for social interaction. When the client is on reverse isolation, the time span is usually considerably longer. The client's needs will be greater, and the nurse can anticipate that the reactions will be intensified.

Surgical

There are many situations when the nurse will use surgical aseptic techniques to control the source and transmission of pathogenic microorganisms. Some of the more commonly used procedures are urinary catheterization, dressing changes, wound care, and parenteral procedures. It is important to distinguish between what is and what is not sterile and what can never be sterile. For example, the floor is considered to be the most contaminated area of the environment. Also, the entire area sur-

rounding the client is not sterile, with the possible exception of the environment in a Life-Island Unit. Even then there is the potential for contaminating the environment because the client harbors endogenous microorganisms. A further distinction needs to be made between what is sterile and what is surgically clean. Whereas sterility is the absence of all microorganisms and spores, surgically clean implies that there is a marked reduction in the number of microorganisms present (Fig. 31-3). Examples of moving from the contaminated state toward surgical cleanliness are surgical handwashing and donning a sterile gown.

Surgical handwashing is used when the arms and hands have become grossly contaminated, before entering a protective (reverse) isolation unit and in obstetrical and operating suites. A preliminary handwashing, using medical aseptic techniques, is completed with two adaptations: (1) include the area from elbow to fingertips, instead of wrist to fingertips; and (2) do not dry hands and arms. Using either the sterile scrub brush with a cleansing agent or a sterile Betadine-impregnated sponge,

Implementation	Recommendations	Observations
Grasp wrist edges and pull gloves off, inside out, in one motion. Discard in appropriate receptacle.	Avoid touching skin of hands.	
Untie strings. Discard in appropriate receptacle.	Touch ties only.	
Use clean paper towel when touching inside door knob of unit. Discard in appropriate receptacle placed just inside unit.		

start the cleansing action at the fingertips and work toward the elbows. Scrub each area for 2 minutes. Under running water, rinse hands and arms, keeping hands elevated so that rinse water will continue to flow from hands and elbows (i.e., from the cleaner area toward the more contaminated area). Hands and arms are dried with a sterile towel, being careful that the towel edges do not touch any object or surface. During and after the procedure, the hands and arms should be maintained in a position above the waist and below the neck. Drop the used towel into an appropriate receptacle.

Gowning for sterile procedures follows the same pattern as gowning in medical asepsis. In adapting the activity for surgical asepsis, it is recommended that the following be noted. The gown is held by its upper half and away from the body as it unfolds. A second person ties the neck and waist strings.

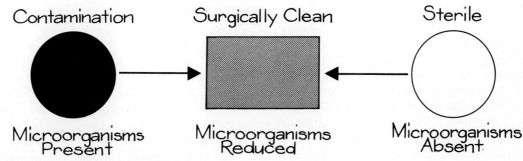

FIGURE 31-3. Relative states of cleanliness.

TABLE 31-6. Handling Sterile Equipment

Anticipated Accomplishment	Scientific Principles/ Rationale	Specific Considerations
Opening sterile package:		
1. Validation of sterility.	Outdated goods are not considered safe.	With prepackaged goods, effective date for sterility is checked. Package is examined for tearing.
2. Place package on flat surface.	Sterile supplies are wrapped so potential for contamination is minimized during unwrapping phase.	
3. Open package.		Inside surface of wrapper provides a sterile field.
4. Add supplies as needed.		Supplies are added as close to center of sterile field as possible.

Both sets of strings should remain at the back of the body because the back is considered a contaminated region.

The use of transfer forceps, placed in a disinfectant solution has been discontinued in many agencies. The solution and container are potential reservoirs for contaminants, especially when technique is poor. When used, the following guidelines apply. If forceps touch unsterile surfaces, including the top edges of the container, which is not covered by solution, the forceps should be resterilized before return to the container. The tips of the forceps are always held in a downward position so that the solution does not flow upward to the unsterile handles. Clean and sterilize the forceps and container and replace the disinfectant at least once *every 24 hours.* See Table 31-6 for the method used in the handling of sterile equipment.

WOUND CARE

A wound is any interruption in the integrity of tissue or mucous membranes. If there is a disruption in the continuity of the skin or mucous membrane, the wound is considered "open." The wound is classified as "closed" when the skin or mucous membrane is intact. Whether a wound is classified as "contaminated" or "clean" depends upon the presence or potential for infection. All wounds are at risk for the development of infection. Contami-

Implementation	Recommendations	Observations
Check date on package and code established by agency.		
Folds must be facing upward so that top flap will fold away from nurse.		Be sure surface upon which equipment is placed is dry.
First, unfold top flap, then side flaps, and finally, flap nearest nurse.	1 inch from edge of wrapper, and all edges falling over edges of flat surface are considered contaminated.	Ascertain that equipment is properly wrapped.
Unwrap similarly wrapped packages in same manner. All four corners are dropped downward, and gathered around wrist. Approaching from side of sterile field, drop item onto field. Large items may be transferred with sterile forceps. Commercially wrapped dressings are pulled open at the indicated edge, turned upside down, and allowed to drop onto field.	Do not allow corners to touch sterile field or any outer package surfaces.	

nated wounds are more likely to become infected because they are generally unexpected or accidental. Clean wounds usually are intentional and result from a surgical incision in a controlled environment. Table 31-7 lists the major types of wounds and their characteristics.

A wound automatically stimulates the inflammatory response. Histamine is released into the surrounding tissue causing the body to mobilize its internal defenses against infection. Local symptoms of this response which are observable are heat, redness, pain, swelling, and limitation of movement. When the body's defensive reactions are unsuccessful, a wound infection develops. If purulent exudate (pus) is present as a result of an infection and is successfully walled off, an abscess forms. When the pus spreads to the surrounding tissue and the area of inflammation is ill-defined, a state known as cellulitis exists. Infrequently, in the presence of infection, a tract between two organs or from an organ to the surface of the body is formed. This formation is called a fistula.

Healing

The mechanism of wound healing is an intricate process. If, however, the blood supply is adequate and there is no necrosis or foreign substances to deter progress, healing will proceed at a maximum rate. Wound healing can occur on three levels: (1)

Table 31-7. Major Types of Wounds

Type	Example	Open	Closed	Clean	Contaminated	Remarks
Intentional:						
Surgical incision	Any incision necessary for surgery	X		X		
Stab	For drainage of boil or carbuncle For drainage (bile)	X		X	X	
Accidental:						
Abrasion	Scrape on knee	X			X	
Contusion	Bump on head		X		X	
Laceration	Cut on hand from broken glass	X			X	
Puncture	Stepping on nail	X	X		X	May close rapidly after puncture; high risk for tetanus
Penetrating	Bullet wound	X	X		X	May close rapidly after penetration; high risk for internal damage and infection
Fracture	Leg injury	X	X	X	X	Open considered "contaminated;" closed considered clean

primary, (2) secondary, or (3) tertiary intention. The simplest form of wound healing is primary intention (primary union). This is generally seen following surgical incisions. The damage to tissue is minimal because the wound edges are smooth and can be brought together (approximated) to form an even line. During this phase the hemorrhage clot which forms following tissue injury, releases fibrinogen molecules. These molecules form a network of fibers that knit together. New epithelial cells and blood vessels fill in the spaces. The resulting scar on the surface of the skin can be observed and described as thin and linear.

Secondary intention which is sometimes referred to as the granulation phase is a type of healing which occurs when the wound is infected and healing is delayed. There is pus present and more granulation tissue is required to fill in the defect. It is impossible to approximate the skin edges. The gap between the edges slowly fills in with granulation tissue which is interlaced with a new capillary supply. Tissue grows up from the bottom and in from the sides. Epithelium may cover the granulation tissue on the surface. The results are an insensitive scar which is uneven and wide.

Healing by third intention or secondary closure occurs when a wound is kept open for drainage or to rid the body of necrotic tissue by debridement. This may also be the condition resulting from the spontaneous disruption of a previously closed wound and may require a secondary closure. With tertiary closure, there is a long delay in final tissue repair and healing. Consequently, the scar is wide and deep. Occasionally, there is extensive scar formation irrespective of the type of healing. This aberration is called a keloid.

Some of the factors which influence the rate of healing are nutrition, age, the amount of tissue damage, the vascularity of the region, foreign bodies, the immune response of the client, the state of wellness that exists with the client, and mechanical interferences. Although the tissue of the young client heals more rapidly, the nutritional requirements remain the same for all age groups. Protein is the only nutrient that promotes growth and regeneration of tissue. A high protein diet is indicated during the healing process. Also, vitamin C and adequate caloric intake favor healing. This is especially important for clients whose resistance is lowered as a result of chronic illness or debilitation.

Mechanical Interruptions

Mechanical interruptions refer to those things which are not ordinarily part of the healing process, including any foreign bodies, such as a sponge, inadvertantly left in the operative site or a drain purposely inserted to promote drainage of purulent material and speed healing. Drains may be tubes or catheters coming either from the operative site itself or a nearby stab wound. The most commonly used type is the Penrose drain which is usually sutured to the skin and further secured with a safety pin. Occasionally, a cigarette drain is used (gauze which is placed inside the Penrose drain) to facilitate drainage. These drains form open systems, and as such, the dressings require more frequent changes or reinforcements. The danger of sepsis is increased because of capillary action which increases the possibility of microorganisms transported into the wound as well as to the outside environment. A closed system of wound drainage that is commonly used is the Hemovac. This is used when there is a large amount of fluid (usually lymph) that would interfere with tissue granulation.

Another mechanical feature that affects wound healing is the suture material used. During surgical procedures, sutures are used to bring tissue edges together or to control bleeding. Ligatures (ties) are sutures without a needle that are used to tie off blood vessels. Sutures are absorbable or nonabsorbable. Absorbable sutures used are plain or chromic catgut. Chromic is specially treated to last longer. Nonabsorbable sutures such as silk, cotton, nylon, wire, mersilene, and Dacron are permanent types which are used on the skin and are intended for removal. A heavy suture usually made of nylon, metal clips, or wire used to support the approximated wound edges for 2 or 3 weeks is called a retention suture. The wound is weakest between 3 to 6 days postoperatively; therefore, it is common practice to leave skin sutures in place for 7 to 10 days.

Nursing Care

Nursing care of wounds usually includes the application of sterile dressings which are protective barriers. Sometimes the physician prefers not to place a dressing over a wound because the dressing may act as a mechanical interference. Studies have

TABLE 31-8. Changing Dressings to Protect Wounds and Promote Healing

Anticipated Accomplishment	Scientific Principles/ Rationale	Specific Considerations
1. Check physician's order.		Physician may want to change initial or subsequent dressings.
2. Prepare client.	Anxiety is reduced and cooperation is enhanced if client is fully aware of procedure.	Dressing changes should be coordinated with other activities to conserve client's energy. Large or disfiguring wounds may be disruptive to client's body image.
3. Collect sterile supplies and equipment.	Use of sterile equipment and supplies inhibits introduction and transfer of microorganisms.	Selection of supplies depends upon size, nature, location and drainage of wound. Some institutions may use disposable equipment. In others, nurse or CSR (Central Supply Room) will prepare dressing tray or cart.
4. Wash hands.	Skin harbors microorganisms and handwashing removes transient microorganisms.	Use medical aseptic handwashing technique.
5. Prepare environment.	Client could become chilled if there is a draft. Microorganisms are everywhere and can be transmitted by air currents.	Some institutions provide a treatment room where all dressings are done.
6. Place equipment on overbed table and unwrap.	Respiratory tract harbors microorganisms, and they are transported by air currents.	All equipment and supplies should be placed in center of sterile field.
7. Open antiseptic solution and pour adequate amount into sterile container.	Microorgamisms move through wet materials by capillary action.	
8. Loosen tape.		Ascertain if client is allergic to tape.

Implementation	Recommendations	Observations
Validate that procedure is being carried out for correct client.	Nurse may reinforce dressing with or without specific orders to change dressing.	
Explain procedure to client.	Medicate 30 min before procedure, if it is likely to be painful.	Assessment of client's physical and psychological states is ongoing throughout procedure.
Include: Instruments: scissors, 2 hemostats, forceps. Gauze, dressing material. Antiseptic solution and container. Plastic bag. Tape.	Second hemostat is used during dressing removal. Include binder to support wound if client is obese. Consider Montgomery straps for draining wounds and frequent dressing changes.	Check sterile supplies for current dating and intact packaging.
	Remove jewelry on hands and wrists prior to handwashing.	
Close windows. Close door or curtains around unit. Assure privacy. Keep traffic to minimum. Clear area to be used as the work space.	Wait at least 15 min after floor has been swept or washed.	
	Supplies to be used last are placed at bottom of pile. Do not cough or sneeze over the wound or sterile field. Limit talking.	
Pour from side of sterile field instead of across field. Avoid spilling.		
Pull tape gently, especially if area is hairy.		Check skin under tape for irritation.

TABLE 31-8. Continued

Anticipated Accomplishment	Scientific Principles/ Rationale	Specific Considerations
9. Remove soiled dressing and discard in plastic bag.	Sealing dressing in plastic bag inhibits spread of microorganisms.	Wear gloves if dressing is grossly contaminated.
10. Don sterile gloves.	Mechanical barriers impede cross-contamination.	
11. Cleanse wound area.	Gravity causes fluids to flow downward. A warm, dark, moist environment enhances growth of microorganisms. Skin can be injured by chemical and mechanical actions.	If irrigation is indicated, position client so flow of fluid will be downward.
12. Apply new dressing.	Sterile field rapidly moves from sterile, toward surgically clean upon exposure to atmosphere.	Exercise care that drain is not inadvertently removed. Cover suture line adequately in all directions, at least 2 inches around the edges. Place heaviest part of dressing at lower end of wound.
13. Secure dressing.	Microorganisms cannot move themselves but can be moved by physical or mechanical means.	If dressing moves significantly, it should be considered contaminated and should be replaced.
14. Remove gloves.		
15. Assure that client is comfortable.		

Implementation	Recommendations	Observations
Use one of hemostats if there is copious drainage. Dressing may be picked up in center if it is dry, with a hemostat or a gloved hand.	Irrigate with normal saline if dressing sticks to suture line. Yellow or green drainage is cultured.	Look for evidence of inflammatory infection, skin excoriation, hemorrhage. Note color, odor, amount, character of drainage. Serous drainage is clear. Serosanguineous drainage is pink or red tinged. Yellow or green drainage indicates infection.
Do not touch skin with gloved hands.	If contamination is suspected or unknown, maxim is, "If in doubt, throw it out."	
Use sterile hemostat, 2 × 2 gauze and antiseptic solution. Gently wipe each side of wound, from incision outward, with separate sponges. Discard after use. Allow to air dry.	Use of cotton balls for this step is *not* recommended.	
Only plain gauze touches skin. Dressing should be secure, but not so tight that circulation is impeded. Cotton filled dressings should be used when there is copious drainage. Avoid touching the wound with anything not sterile.		
Apply tape. Ends should extend several inches beyond dressing.		
Discard in plastic bag.		
Straighten covers of bed. Reposition client so he is comfortable.		

TABLE 31-8. Continued

Anticipated Accomplishment	Scientific Principles/ Rationale	Specific Considerations
16. Care of equipment.		
17. Record and report findings.		

demonstrated that clean surgical incisions heal just as well without a dressing nor is the incidence of infection increased. Other physicians prefer dressings on all wounds. When there is drainage from a wound the dressing is necessary. Whether or not the wound is dressed, strict surgical asepsis is the goal in caring for the wound (Table 31-8).

The dressing is used to absorb drainage, provide a seal against microbial invasion or escape, and to apply pressure and protect the wound against further injury. Pressure is used for the control of hemorrhage and to promote drainage from dependent parts. Wounds, such as skin grafts or plastic surgical repairs are fragile, and injury to the wound edges should be avoided.

WET DRESSINGS. Wet dressings are often ordered for wounds which are infected. The moisture of the dressing collects the exudate by capillary action, and this acts to mechanically clean an area. Granulation proceeds more favorably.

WOUND IRRIGATION. When wounds are grossly infected, irrigation is a common procedure. The solutions used are mild antiseptics, sterile normal saline, or sterile water. A syringe is used, and the solution is either squirted directly onto the wound or a catheter is threaded into the wound to introduce the solution. In either case, the solution should be directed in such a way that the flow will be favored by gravity. The plan is to work from a clean area toward a contaminated area. Irrigations are usually continued until return flow is clear. Occasionally, following irrigation the wound may be packed, with a sterile absorbent material that may or may not be medicated.

BANDAGES. Bandages are coverings which are used to hold dressings in place and to provide even pressure to support body parts. Gauze rolls may be used to supplement or replace tape, especially in small, awkward areas such as the fingers. Kling bandages are made of stretchy gauze, which can be molded to fit around a part. An advantage is that it adheres to itself and will stay in place. Ace bandages are elasticized and are commonly used to provide even pressure on the limbs. An Elastoplast is similar, but has one adhesive side. A binder is a form of bandage, usually used to cover and support larger areas. The fabric is a heavy muslin, flannel, or cotton twill. Common types are the T-binder, the scultetus binder, breast binder, and the triangular binder (sling).

SUMMARY

In summary the major emphasis of this chapter is the control of infection in health care facilities and community-based settings. Various concepts and principles for the maintenance of asepsis have been discussed. Implementation of the concepts and principles by specific procedures is also discussed.

Implementation	Recommendations	Observations

Wash used instruments and place in area to be returned for resterilization. Discard plastic bag in appropriate receptacle.

Record time of procedure. Provide observations of wound healing, drainage, client reactions, and any unexpected findings. Report any unusual findings immediately.

Adaptation of procedures is possible, but the principles remain constant.

The professional nurse monitors many factors, including her own practice. Her main goal is to achieve a homeostatic equilibrium among the agent, host, and environment so that an infectious disease cannot occur.

BIBLIOGRAPHY

Allan, K. G.: *Surgery, Principles and Practices,* Philadelphia, J. B. Lippincott Company, 1961.

Auld, M., et al.: Wound healing. *Nurs. '72* 10:36, 1972.

Beland, I., and Passos, J.: *Clinical Nursing: Pathophysiological and Psychosocial Approaches,* 3rd ed. New York, Macmillan Publishing Company, Inc., 1975.

Benenson, A. (ed.): *The Control of Communicable Disease in Man.* 12th ed. American Public Health Association, 1975.

Castle, M.: Isolation: precise procedures in better protection. *Nurs. '75* 5:50, 1975.

Chavigny, K. H.: Nurse epidemiologist in the hospital. *Am. J. Nurs.* 4:638, 1975.

Domsicz, H. J.: OR nurse's role in control of prevention of infection. *AORN J.* 25:233, 1977.

Fox, M., et al.: How good are handwashing practices? *Am. J. Nurs.* 74:1676, 1974.

Greene, V. W.: Microbial contamination control in hospitals. *Hospitals* 43:78, 1969.

Goldman, J. M., et al.: The use of plastic isolators to prevent infection in neutropenic patients. *Postgrad. Med. J.* 52:558, 1976.

Henderson, V., and Nite, G.: *Principles and Practices of Nursing.* 6th ed. New York, Macmillan Publishing Company, Inc., 1978.

Department of Health Education and Welfare: *Isolation Techniques for Use in Hospitals.* 2nd ed. Washington, D.C., Public Health Service for Disease Control, 1976.

LeMaitre G., and Finnegan, J.: *The Patient in Surgery: A Guide for Nurses.* Philadelphia, W.B. Saunders Company, 1970.

Lentz, J.: The nurse's role in extending infection control to the community. *Nurs. Clin. North Am.* 5:165, 1970.

Myers, M. B.: Sutures and wound healing. *Am. J. Nurs.* 71:1725, 1971.

Wenzel, K.: The role of the infection control nurse. *Nurs. Clin. North Am.* 5:89, 1970.

Wilson, M., and Minzer, H.: *Microbiology in Patient Care,* 2nd ed. New York, Macmillan Publishing Company, Inc., 1974.

CHAPTER 32

The provision of nursing care requires that the nurse be familiar with societal expectations and norms. This knowledge assists her in understanding the needs and demands of the client, his family, and his peers. While the norms of our society are fairly well accepted, there are clients whose individual philosophy and life style deviate from that of the majority; in fact, their "beliefs" may conflict with others, including those of the nurse.

People have always been concerned with their personal appearance. In this country, for instance, the emphasis is on youth, beauty, and cleanliness. The media continuously remind the public of the need to be clean, smell sweet, to look masculine or feminine, or to be generally inoffensive. While many people subscribe to this, there are also many who disagree. Examples of people who vary from the "norm" might be (1) the child who must be coerced into bathing, (2) the woman who prefers not to shave her legs or underarms, or (3) the individual who frequently has stains or odors emanating from his attire.

PERSONAL HYGIENE, COMFORT, AND SAFETY MEASURES

Arlyne B. Saperstein, M.N., R.N.,
Margaret A. Frazier, M.S., R.N., and
Mary Ellen Sullivan, M.S., R.N.

While good personal hygiene may give most people a feeling of well-being, there are others who believe that cleanliness and bathing are not only unnecessary but detrimental to their health. In general, however, it is fairly well accepted that poor personal hygienic practices may lead to illness; the frequent use of soap and water is an important factor in the prevention of the spread of disease. This is true both for the client and the health care worker, particularly those in a hospital setting who are especially vulnerable to infection. The awareness of the relationship between cleanliness and infection (disease) control should be a primary consideration of nursing care.

The manner in which a client responds both to his illness and to his treatment regimen (including hospitalization) is influenced by his personal standards of cleanliness and personal appearance. Individuals who are fastidious about their personal hygiene are often traumatized when their usual routine is temporarily or permanently interrupted. Clients often exhibit signs of discomfort or anxiety when this occurs. These clients experience the same symptoms when their surroundings are unkempt or in disarray. While nurses today are not responsible for the same housekeeping tasks of their predecessors, they are still responsible for maintaining an environment which is as comfortable (physically as well as psychologically) as possible for the client. This may entail teaching auxiliary members of the staff how to clean and disinfect the client's unit, utilizing her knowledge of scientific principles, to help them understand why this function is valuable.

In summary, the client's social and cultural background, his family experiences, peer pressures, and life style, as well as the immediate situation and its requirements for adaptation or change, influence the emphasis which he places on hygienic practices and his reaction to the treatment plan and provision of care. The nurse and the other members of the health team must be sensitive to the client's feelings and assist him to cope with his anxieties by encouraging the resumption of normal daily activities to the extent that his condition or health status permits. Whether in the hospital or in the home, the main objective of care for both the client and the nurse is the attainment and maintenance of the maximum level of *independence* and self-care. Encouragement, support, education, and supervision all fall within the realm of nursing care in assisting the client with this objective and in the performance of the activities of daily living necessary for his comfort and integrity. Accurate assessment of the client's capabilities, confidence, and functioning enables the nurse to implement a plan of self-care.

HYGIENIC PRACTICES

Mouth

Care of the mouth is important to both physical and psychological well-being, particularly when an individual is ill. Dirty teeth containing crusts, tartar, or food particles are unsavory and uncomfortable. Not only does halitosis (bad breath) occur when mouth care has been neglected, but the gums and teeth deteriorate as well, making chewing difficult and inadequate; detrimental effects on the digestion of nutrients may result. In addition to frequent dental checkups and follow-up care, conscientious oral hygiene decreases the incidence of periodontal disease and tooth decay.

Brushing the teeth removes the major causes of tooth decay: plaque (a film on the teeth), bacteria, food particles, sugar, and acids. In combination, these have a deleterious effect on the tooth enamel. Therefore, brushing (and flossing which will be discussed below) at least twice a day, preferably after each meal, reduces the possibility of dental problems.

The minimum equipment needed is a *toothbrush* and *dentifrice*. While dental creams are the most popular, tooth powder, salt, or bicarbonate of soda can also be used for tooth brushing. Polishing agents, which contain abrasives that supposedly are not injurious to the teeth, battery powered toothbrushes and pulsating water jet gum massagers are examples of the devices on the market for dental care. Most hospitals provide a toothbrush and toothpaste as part of the admission pack.

The nurse may, depending upon the need of the individual client, either provide the client with all of the necessary equipment to brush his own teeth (i.e., brush, toothpaste, floss, emesis basin, towel,

and water) or do it for him. It may require some practice before the student feels comfortable providing oral care. When brushing the client's teeth, a soft brush with rounded bristles is recommended; a small brush should be used with pediatric clients. All surfaces of the teeth should be brushed with the brush held at a 45° angle to the gums. Small strokes are used so that no surfaces, especially those in the back of the mouth, are missed, and only a few teeth at a time are brushed. In addition, the tongue is brushed lightly, particularly when it is coated.

Dental floss is advocated for the removal of food particles between the teeth. The use of waxed or unwaxed floss is a personal preference. Approximately one foot of floss is removed from the container and wrapped around the middle or index fingers, anchoring it and giving control to the person who is doing the flossing; a short piece of floss is left with which to work. The floss is pulled from side to side after moving it downward to the gums at the base of each tooth. The floss should never be forced into the gum tissue; roughness can cause bleeding. The mouth should be rinsed thoroughly after flossing.

The value of *mouthwash* is debatable. In most cases, there is no way that a germicidal or antiseptic effect can be insured; mouthwash simply provides a pleasing way to rinse the mouth. If a mouthwash has been provided by a hospital pharmacy and the strength of the preparation is not stated on the label, the nurse should check with the pharmacist and dilute it accordingly.

Dentures should be removed at least once a day for cleaning. The timing of this, whenever possible, should be determined by the client's preference. Most clients require privacy as they are *sensitive* about anyone, especially family and friends, seeing them without their dentures. The dentures should be placed in a cup made specifically for cleaning purposes and covered with water or a commercial preparation specific for denture cleansing. Whenever they are taken out of the mouth, they must be kept in a safe place. When cleaning dentures, hold them securely to avoid breakage. In fact, the nurse should place a face cloth in the bottom of the sink and fill it with water to prevent breakage when brushing. Most products made for brushing dentures contain a mild abrasive or a foaming agent, which is rinsed off with cool water. (Note, preparations which are manufactured specifically for dentures are not to be used orally.) While the dentures are being cleaned, the client, if able, should rinse his mouth as needed. If the client needs assistance in replacing the dentures, the insertion is facilitated if the dentures are wet. Naturally, if the client is able, it is easier for him to replace them himself.

In caring for clients who are restricted in the ingestion of foods and fluids, mouth care takes on an even greater significance. Not only does it refresh the mouth, it also lubricates it, preventing dryness and cracking of oral mucous membranes. In addition to care of the teeth, tongue, and gums, the lips must also be moistened. Use of glycerin and lemon swabs is effective for this purpose.

Nares

Clients who have respiratory problems, are receiving oxygen therapy, or who have a nasogastric tube in place may need special attention to the nares. The main objective is keeping the airway clear and unobstructed. If there is crusting of the anterior nares, it can be softened and removed gently with a cotton ball saturated with water; oily substances should *not* be inserted in the nose. Excoriation or irritation of the skin around the nose may be soothed or relieved by the application of petrolatum jelly or cold cream. If the mucous membranes are very dry, then vigorous or harsh nose blowing should be discouraged. Facial tissues should be readily available to the client.

Eyes

If the client's eyes are open for an extended period of time (e.g., in comatose clients), special care is needed to counteract the problems which may result, including irritation, crusting, ulcer formation, and drying of the conjunctiva and cornea. Often the physician writes an order for either irrigation (with sterile normal saline) or lubrication (with a sterile ophthalmic preparation). Crusts are softened and removed in the same manner as discussed under care of the nares; however, sterile water, rather than tap water is used.

Many clients wear corrective lenses. While eyeglasses are still the most prevalent, contact lenses have become extremely popular. Both can be lost or damaged (usually due to scratches). Since they are rather costly, care should be taken to keep them in a safe place when they are not worn. Cleanliness is a major consideration. The nurse must make certain that the client does not sleep with contacts in place or wear them for long periods of time.

Hair

An aspect of personal hygiene that occasionally presents problems is the care of the hair. This is particularly true in cases of extended hospitalization, limited activity, or weakened states. The removal of dirt, excess oil, and dead cells can be partially accomplished by hair brushing. In addition, circulation and nourishment of the scalp are improved by increased stimulation of the tissue. When an individual is ill, his hair is treated in much the same manner as when healthy. However, it is not unusual for the hair to seem limp or lifeless when illness is present. Also, when bedridden, the hair may become matted or tangled. For most people, shampooing every few days is sufficient. Shampooing on a daily basis is not necessary except in cases of extreme oiliness or due to personal preference or habit. Shampoos can be given to the bedridden client; in many institutions a physician's order will be necessary for this procedure. A number of commercial products (troughs) are available for washing the hair of a client who is in a reclining or sitting position. These can be used at the sink or while the client is in bed. The trough is positioned in such a way that the water flows into a suitable receptacle. When no trough is on hand, pillows that are encased in waterproof material can be used to simulate the device. Care must be taken not to allow water or shampoo into the client's face or eyes; a wash cloth over the eyes often eliminates this problem. If water in the ears also is irritating, then cotton balls can be placed in the external canal for protection. The water temperature should be warm; the client whose judgment is trustworthy can test the water temperature himself. All soap must be removed when rinsing the hair and scalp. Towel drying should be followed by an electric hair dryer whenever possible to prevent chilling. After shampooing, the client is kept warm until the hair has dried. Dry shampoo can also be used; while it does not replace regular shampooing, it can decrease some of the discomfort. Long, matted, tangled, or curly hair can present problems since they take a great deal of time to shampoo, comb, brush, and dry. Cream rinses should be used when the hair is snarled. When all attempts at removing knots or tangles have failed, cutting the hair (with a doctor's order) may be necessary. The client's hair should be arranged in a suitable manner. Curly hair is most easily combed with a wide tooth comb. Do not use ribbons or childish hair styles unless specifically requested by the client. When combing a client's hair, any deviations from normal (e.g., pediculosis capitis [head lice] or dandruff) should be noted and reported.

Nails

An aspect of hygienic care that is often overlooked is the care of the fingernails and toenails. An orange stick can be gently and carefully used to keep the nails clean, and an emery board, to keep them a suitable length and shape. Fingernails are usually shaped in an oval; toenails are cut straight across, decreasing the chance of infected hangnails or ingrowth. If cutting or clipping with a nail clipper is necessary, the nails should be soaked in a warm, soapy solution for softening prior to cutting. A physician's order is necessary for this procedure. Acetone can be utilized to remove nail polish. A diabetic's nails must be handled carefully because of circulatory problems and the risk of complications such as gangrene (a physician's order is always required with diabetics).

Shaving

Whenever possible a client should do his or her own shaving. Barber or beauty shop services are quite convenient, if available, particularly in the hospital setting. Often the client prefers to have a family member assist him with this task. When shaving the male client, it is helpful to determine the direction in which the beard grows, by running the fingers over his face and neck; if resistance is felt then the fingers are going against the grain, and if none is felt, the fingers are moving with the grain. A closer shave is obtained by shaving against the grain; if with the grain, the shave will be more comfortable. Following this, the face should be washed with soap and hot water. This removes both dirt and oil from the beard and softens the beard, making shaving easier and decreasing the likelihood of nicking. Shaving cream or soap lather is applied to the beard. Holding the skin taut, the razor (which must be sharp) is drawn across the beard in quick, short strokes while being held at a slight angle to the face. Any excess soap should be removed with

a damp towel at the end of the shave. It is quite comforting to have a warm damp towel placed over the beard for a few minutes after shaving. An astringent lotion applied gently after this will close the pores and feel soothing. Obviously the use of an electric razor if available is both faster and safer.

The same principles hold true for shaving the female's legs and underarms. Care must be taken so as not to nick delicate skin. It is helpful to ask the client how she prefers this procedure to be performed.

Skin

Because the skin is our outer line of defense, protecting us from injury and infection and playing a major role in body temperature (heat) regulation, it is important that continuous efforts are made to maintain its integrity. The effect of limited activity associated with bedrest or immobility, is a decrease in circulation, especially to the portions of the skin and underlying tissues that are in direct contact with the surface of the bed. A decrease in the circulatory functioning reduces the oxygenation and nutrition of the cells, as well as the elimination of waste materials. As a result, the tissue breaks down. The first sign of this is redness and mottling. If the process continues, a pressure sore (decubitus ulcer) forms. The areas most often affected are bony prominences pressing against a hard surface (the mattress); the trochanters of the femur, the scapulae, the elbows, ankles, knees, heels, and the sacrum and coccyx. Anything which increases the pressure against the skin (mechanical irritants), such as wrinkled sheets, crumbs in the bed, rubber rings that are supposed to keep the part off of the mattress, and casts, as well as any chemical irritant, such as urine, feces, perspiration, and wound drainage, are predisposing factors in the formation of decubiti. Once a pressure sore is established the possibility of infection is likely. Reversal of the ulcer is extraordinarily difficult to accomplish and in some cases so extensive that surgical debridement and grafting are required. It is therefore obvious that the prevention of this condition is of utmost importance. Preventive measures utilized by health care workers include: (1) adequate nutrition: the client who is likely to form an ulcer needs a high vitamin and protein diet; (2) turning the client: position changes alleviate pressure areas; (various types of appliances and devices successfully decrease pressure (e.g., alternating air mattresses, Circ-O-Lectric beds, Stryker frames, water beds, sheepskin protectors, and lambswool) (Figs. 32-1A and B); (3) gentle massage or back rubs: (Fig. 32-2) increase circulation; (4) meticulous skin care keeps the skin free of irritants; and (5) range of motion exercises increase circulatory and muscular functioning. (Range of motion exercises, turning, positioning, and provision of proper body alignment for maintenance of the integrity of the skin as well as prevention of contractures and deformities are discussed in Chapter 30, ''Body Mechanics.'')

There are probably almost as many remedies for treatment of decubiti as there are workers. The treatment depends upon the extensiveness of the ulceration, the degree of involvement of subcutaneous tissues, and the condition of the client. Most treatment modalities require a physician's order; their popularity varies from institution to institution. While some physicians and nurses advocate some of these treatments, others are distinctly opposed to their use. The following is a list of some measures that have been used in the treatment of skin that has broken down and the area surrounding the ulcer:

1. Irrigations or compresses utilizing a prescribed solution such as sterile normal saline or Dakin's solution.
2. Applications of ointments such as boric acid, zinc oxide, vitamins A and D, and various antibiotic preparations.

3. Applications of liquid preparations such as Maalox, Gelusil, 1 percent mercurochrome.
4. Applications of powders such as karaya and sulfonamides.
5. Applications of heat via heat lamps.
6. Exposure to air.
7. Application of a sterile dressing.
8. Positioning to keep pressure away from the affected area.

Bathing

Bathing serves more purposes than simply cleansing the skin. It is extremely useful in assisting the individual to feel better about himself; it is refreshing, relaxing, soothing, and even sedating; it improves circulation, therefore is healing and nutritive; and it may relieve a variety of symptoms associated with skin disorders, such as dryness, scaling, peeling, itching, and oiliness. The various types of baths are described below.

1. The *cleansing bath* or *complete bedbath* is administered to the client who cannot for a variety of reasons, bathe himself. The nurse gives the entire bath with little or no assistance from the client (Table 32-1).
2. The *partial bath* is provided for the client who can do a portion of the bathing himself. The nurse is usually called upon to bathe the client's back, buttocks, and possibly his legs.

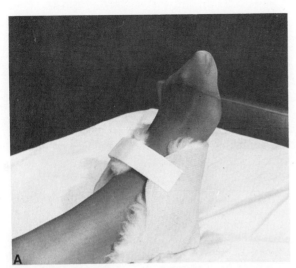
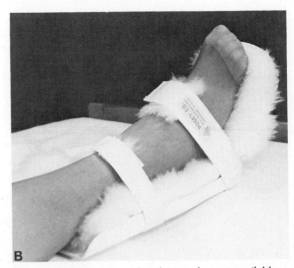

FIGURE 32-1. Sheepskin heel protectors; two of the many types of protective sheepskin devices that are available.

Personal Hygiene, Comfort, and Safety Measures   **549**

TABLE 32-1. Bed Bath and Back Rub for Adults and Adolescents to Cleanse Skin, Refresh and Relax Client, Improve Circulation, and Increase Muscle Tone

Anticipated Accomplishment	Scientific Principles/ Rationale	Specific Considerations
1. Organization and preparation for procedure.	Time and energy are saved making procedure less traumatic and exhausting for client and nurse if several trips to gather equipment are eliminated and nurse does not have to bend over to carry out procedure. An explanation prior to implementation reduces anxiety and fosters cooperation and independence of client.	Is this first time client has been bathed by another individual? Is client reliable to test water temperature?
2. Provision of privacy and prevention of chilling.	Drafts, low ambient air (room) temperature and evaporation of water from exposed skin will cause chilling. While individuals vary, most clients have a need for privacy.	What is temperature of room? Procedure should be done at time when client is not scheduled for tests or other procedures so no interruptions occur and client does not feel rushed.
3. Remove dirty linens.	Floors are contaminated with microorganisms. Spread of microorganisms from client to client (cross-contamination) can occur via the health worker's clothing.	Do not place linens on floor. Do not allow dirty linen to come in contact with uniform or apparel.
4. Position client for ease of administering bath.	Reaching across bed to bathe far side of client is inconvenient and makes use of proper body mechanics difficult	Can client assist in moving himself?
5. Cleanse client's head and neck.	Contamination is avoided when cleansing proceeds from the "clean" to the "dirty" areas. (See Chapter 31 on medical and surgical asepsis.)	Client should be encouraged to wash his own face if able and there are no medical contraindications. Client's preference (as well as assessment of dryness or oiliness of client's skin) determines if soap is used on face.

Implementation	Recommendations	Observations
Assemble needed equipment at client's bedside: basin of water, soap, wash cloth, two towels, comb, brush, lotion, powder, deodorant, and clean bed linens, including client gown.	Ask client if he needs to void or defecate prior to beginning procedure. Client's bed should be raised to comfortable working level for nurse. Bath thermometer must be used to avoid burning client. Temperature of water should range from 110–115°F (43.3–46.1°C). If client is reliable, then allow him to test water for comfort and preference.	
Explain procedure to client while preparing equipment. Raise bed to most convenient level.		
Provide for privacy and warmth by: closing door, pulling curtains around bed, or placement of screens. Replace top sheet and spread with bath blanket for both privacy and warmth.	Ask client to hold top edge of bath blanket securely. Reach under, pull top sheet and spread toward foot of bed, and remove.	
Remove client's gown and place in laundry bag or hamper. Remove pillow (and pillow case) unless client feels discomfort without it or it is medically contraindicated.	Keep laundry bag outside client's room and do not place dirty linens on other bed or bedside tables.	Observe client's skin integrity (i.e., redness, mottling, breaks, abrasions, bruises, color, and lesions) as client undresses or is assisted to undress.
Move client or assist him to side of bed closest to you.	Leave side rail up on far side of bed to prevent falls.	
Wash eyes first, proceeding from the inner aspect (canthus) to outer. Cotton balls or different areas of wash cloth should be used for each eye. After cleansing eyes, continue with rest of face, ears, and neck.	Hold wash cloth securely or in such a manner that edges do not dangle or drip on client's face. Fold wash cloth around hand and tuck it in to form a mitt to avoid this problem.	Assessment of characteristics of each area being bathed can be done readily during bath.
	Soap is not used for eyes. If client has dry skin, oil may be ordered by physician to be added to bath water.	Observe texture and dryness (or oiliness) of skin, especially of face.

TABLE 32-1. Continued

Anticipated Accomplishment	Scientific Principles/ Rationale	Specific Considerations
6. Cleanse upper extremities.	Wet bedding can be uncomfortable and chilling.	Range of motion exercises of arms may be done at this time if necessary. (See Chapter 30 on body mechanics.) Does client have an IV line in place? Care must be taken not to dislodge needle, catheter, or tubing.
7. Cleanse chest and breasts.	A good medium for bacterial proliferation is a dark, warm, moist area. Breakdown and infection of skin are more likely to occur under these conditions and in presence of debilitation.	Provide for privacy; many women feel embarrassment when their breasts are exposed. Place a towel over areas of chest that are not being washed.
8. Cleanse abdomen and anterior thighs.	Chilling occurs when a large surface of skin is wet and exposed to air (evaporation).	Prevent exposure of large surface area while washing abdomen and upper thighs.
9. Cleanse legs and feet.	Soaking feet softens toenails, facilitating toenail care.	Range of motion exercises on legs may be done at this time if necessary. (See Chapter 30 on body mechanics.)
10. Provide clean water of proper temperature.	Water that has cooled can chill client and feel quite uncomfortable.	Is client reliable to test water temperature?
11. Cleanse posterior aspects of client's body.	Circulation is improved with application of friction, assisting in prevention of decubiti.	Can client turn himself? Do usual pressure points show signs of decreased circulation?

Implementation	Recommendations	Observations
With towel placed under arm on far side, wash entire arm, including underarm (axilla). Rinse off soap, and dry arm well using second towel. Arm nearest nurse is then washed and dried in same manner.	Wash basin or small bowl may be placed in a secure position on bed for soaking client's hands. Dry well after soaking. Nail care can be done after soaking as needed.	
Wash and rinse chest well. Dry thoroughly, especially under pendulous breasts.	Breast self-examination can be taught to client at this time. Small amount of powder or cornstarch applied under pendulous breasts decreases friction and minimizes breakdown.	Observe breasts and nipples for unusual discharge, lumps, and dimpling of tissue.
With a towel over chest, fold bath blanket down to pubic area. Wash, rinse, and dry abdomen, including umbilicus. With towel covering chest and abdomen, fold bath blanket over to each side; wash, rinse, and dry each anterior thigh individually.		Observe umbilicus for any drainage or crusting.
Begin with distal leg. With towel under leg, protecting linens, wash, rinse, and dry each leg individually. Client's foot can be placed in basin while washing leg. Keep other leg covered with bath blanket while washing leg. Dry well between toes.	It is sometimes easier for both client and nurse if feet are soaked in basin while client is seated in chair (provided there are no contraindications to this activity).	Assess for reddened areas (pressure points) on heels and ankles.
Clean wash basin; refill. Check temperature of water with bath thermometer.	Client should be allowed (if reliable) to check water temperature for comfort.	
With client close to you, turn him or assist him to turn on his side or abdomen (condition permitting). Wash, rinse, and dry thoroughly neck, back,		Observe for reddened, mottled, or broken-down areas, especially around coccyx, sacrum, and scapulae.

TABLE 32-1. Continued

Anticipated Accomplishment	Scientific Principles/ Rationale	Specific Considerations
12. Back care.	Massaging tissue causes vasodilation, improving circulation, and increasing muscle tone. Lotion or powder reduces friction, allowing hands to glide along skin more readily.	Back rubs can either relax or stimulate client; what purpose does this backrub have and what would be most beneficial to client? Usually in morning, stimulating rubs are used; at bedtime or if client is in pain, relaxing rub may reduce need for sedation or pain medication. Particular attention must be given to pressure points and areas subject to breakdown.
13. Cleanse anogenital area.	Urine, feces, and discharge contain irritating substances which can contribute to tissue breakdown. Cleansing the female from front to back avoids contamination of urethra with fecal material.	Is client able to cleanse himself properly? Is retention catheter in place, which would require further observation and care? Cornstarch may be ordered and applied to reddened areas or those places where skin rubs together and may become irritated. Cornstarch is soothing to skin.
14. Provide for comfort and warmth.	Therapeutic effect of bath is relaxation and comfort. Chilling after bathing is likely and should be prevented.	Is there an IV line in place in hand or arm? If so, assistance will be needed by client in threading solution and tubing through arm of gown or pajamas. If client can help (and has no IV line), he should be encouraged to put on his own gown.
15. Decrease possibility of cross-infection.	Microorganisms are communicated from one client to another by health worker's hands. Handwashing reduces number of microorganisms on skin.	

Implementation	Recommendations	Observations
shoulders, buttocks, and posterior thighs. (Have bed protected with towel.) Turn client to other side to wash remainder of back.		
Prone position is preferable if comfortable for client and not contraindicated, otherwise place client on side. Circular motions are used while rubbing client's neck. For restful backrub, begin at coccyx with long strokes; move slowly upward toward scapulae: then move downward using wide strokes in a circular manner. For stimulating rub, use shorter strokes gently squeezing tissue with fingers. (See Fig. 32-2)	Pouring cold lotion directly onto back has a chilling effect; this is alleviated by rubbing lotion between palms of hands before applying. Powder may be used in place of lotion to facilitate back rub. Always keep hands in contact with client's skin.	Observe to see if back rub is relieving tension and producing a relaxing effect or if stimulation is occurring.
Wash, rinse, and dry genitals thoroughly, proceeding from front to back in female client. Utilize a different area of wash cloth for each stroke. Do not reuse parts of wash cloth that have already been contaminated. On male clients gently retract foreskin while cleansing the penis.	If client can cleanse himself, allow him to do so in private. Provide him with water, soap, and a washcloth. This may be appropriate time to teach female client principles of perineal care. Side rails are raised while client is unattended.	Observe for reddened or irritated areas.
Place a clean gown on client and tie or snap closed.	Client's hair can be groomed at this time if he is not too exhausted at end of procedure.	Is client warm, comfortable, chilled, or exhausted?
Remove dirty equipment and soiled laundry; discard. Wash and dry hands thoroughly. If client can tolerate procedure, make bed at this time.	Lotion may be used on hands to reduce dryness, cracking and irritation (which can become infected) that may result from frequent handwashing.	

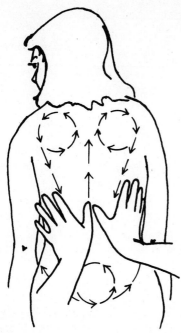

FIGURE 32-2. Direction of massage in backrub procedure. (See Table 32-1, step 12, for description of backrub.)

3. The *self-administered bath* is performed by the client himself. The nurse's responsibility is to provide the client with the necessary articles for bathing, to assure privacy, and to wash his back if necessary.

4. The *infant bath* is usually a sponge bath (at least until the cord has fallen off). After the cord is no longer attached (it is never removed forcefully), the infant can be bathed in a small tub or basin provided support is given to the head, neck, and body. No attempt is made to remove the cheeselike substance (vernix caseosa) found on the skin at birth since this has a protective function. Usually the vernix disappears in 24 hours; if allowed to remain longer than 48 hours, irritation of the skin may occur. Blood and mucus found on the skin at birth, however, are removed in the initial bath which is usually given after the infant's temperature has stabilized. Care of the cord is often done at bath time. This consists of applying an antiseptic (such as 70 percent isopropyl alcohol) to dry the cord; usually it will dry out and detach within 5 days after birth. Air

drying is also advocated. Cord care procedures vary from agency to agency, however, any foul odor, oozing, or bleeding should be reported to the physician and noted. The use of powder, oil, lotions, and heavily perfumed soaps make the baby smell the way we expect him to but is actually more harmful than helpful; powder can be aspirated into the infant's lungs, and the oils and locations may clog the pores (Table 32-2).

5. *Shower baths* may be taken by clients who are ambulatory provided there are no contraindications and the physician is in agreement. Because the client is alone for a period of time while in the shower, the nurse must be judicious in determining that he is capable of taking it. Her responsibility includes pointing out the emergency call light and explaining its use, adjusting the temperature of the water, making sure that a bath mat is provided outside the shower, and that all necessary equipment is assembled.

6. *Tub baths* can be taken only by persons who have the agility to get in and out of the bathtub or by those who can be safely assisted in and out of the tub and can be supervised closely. If a nonskid bottom is not available, a towel can be placed in the bottom of the tub to decrease the possibility of slipping. Once again, just as in the shower bath, the emergency call light must be demonstrated to the client and his safety insured.

7. *Sitz baths* provide wet heat for clients with a variety of perineal or rectal conditions. The treatment increases circulation to the affected area and promotes healing and comfort. The client is seated in a small tub designed to contain the buttocks and hips only; portable models are available that can be used in the client's room or on the toilet for usually 15−20 minutes. The water temperature ranges from 100−115°F (37.8−46.1°C), depending on the treatment. The client should be observed for any untoward symptoms such as dizziness.

8. *Medicated baths* are used for a number of reasons, each with its own action and purpose.

9. *Soothing baths*, also known as *cooling, an-*

tipruritic, or *emollient baths*, include sodium bicarbonate, cornstarch, bran or oatmeal, and Alpha-Keri. The temperature of the water as well as the amount of medication varies according to the purpose of the bath, the consistency desired, and the preference of the prescriber. Instructions are found in the doctor's orders, the procedures manual of the agency, or on the container in which the medication is packaged.

10. *Stimulating baths* include saline (sea salt) and mustard baths.
11. *Antipyretic baths* include alcohol and tepid water.
12. *Therapeutic baths* are utilized for relaxation of the client, for alleviation of muscle aches and strains, and to reduce the temperature of the body. These include whirlpool baths, sitz baths, sponge baths, hot water baths, and certain soaks. Once again the temperature range varies according to the nature of the treatment.

The Client's Bed

A discussion of the client's bed is included here since during a prolonged illness, it often becomes the focus of his whole world and all of his activities. While the bed must provide comfort and safety (i.e., side rails) for the client, it must also be convenient for the health care worker. Hospital beds must have firm mattresses for support; most are sealed within a plastic waterproof covering, making both cleansing and disinfection simpler, and decreasing the possibility of allergic reactions in clients who have this predisposition. In addition, waterproofing is necessary with the incontinent (bedsoiling) client. Hospital beds can be electrically or manually operated; their height can be controlled, as well as the position of the head and foot of the bed.

Pillows can be made of a variety of materials, each of which has positive and negative attributes. For the most part, whichever material is chosen for use will also be covered with plastic waterproofing for the same reasons that the mattress is covered. While most hospitals use standard-sized pillows, pillows of many sizes and shapes are seen. These are primarily used for support, positioning, and comfort.

When making up hospital beds, nearly all will require a top and bottom sheet, pillow case, and spread. Depending on the client's individual needs, however, other forms of linen are also used. Plastic (or rubberized) drawsheets which cover the area from the client's shoulders to his knees are covered with a cotton draw sheet; these are utilized with incontinent clients, making the necessity of changing of the bottom sheet less frequent. A cotton draw sheet (or pull sheet) can be utilized with or without the plastic sheet for the purpose of turning or moving the weak or helpless client. Lightweight blankets (thermal blankets have become quite popular) are utilized as needed for warmth. Contour (fitted) sheets are most often used as the bottom sheet since they give a tight, more comfortable fit. Colorful linens, which are less reminiscent of hospitals than the traditional whites, are more pleasing to the eye. Children in particular respond well to colored or printed bed linens and hospital gowns.

Cribs and *bassinets* should be designed for safety and comfort. The side rails are meant to contain the infant in such a manner that he cannot become wedged between the bars and so that falls cannot occur when he is left unattended. An additional safety feature that can be added to cribs is the crib net (Fig. 32-3) which prevents active children from climbing out over the bars or side rails. Crib mattresses are covered in plastic waterproofing for the same reasons discussed above; pillows, when used for toddlers (infants do not sleep with pillows) are also protected in this manner. While contour sheets are preferred since they are not undone as readily, bassinets often utilize a pillow case as the sheet.

(See Tables 32-3, 32-4, 32-5, and 32-6 for bedmaking procedures.)

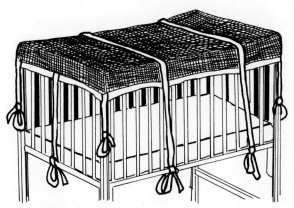

FIGURE 32-3. Crib-net.

TABLE 32-2. Infant Bath to Cleanse Skin, Observe, Assess, Touch, and Stroke the Infant

Anticipated Accomplishment	Scientific Principles/ Rationale	Specific Considerations
1. Decrease possibility of cross-infection.	Handwashing (use of friction, soap, and running water) helps to prevent spread of disease and infection by reducing number of microorganisms present on skin.	
2. Organization and preparation of materials for procedure.	Having all equipment gathered facilitates rapidity with which infant bath can be done—avoiding leaving infant unattended for any length of time.	Room temperature should be warm—approximately 75–80°F (23.9–26.7°C). Avoid drafts.
3. Preparation of infant for procedure.	Infants' (especially newborn) mechanisms for temperature regulation are immature, thus they can become chilled quite rapidly once undressed or uncovered. While on their backs, newborns cannot raise their heads. If anything falls back in throat, airway becomes obstructed in this position. Infants receive gratification from putting things in their mouths; they will automatically put objects they can grasp into their mouths.	Infants must never be left unattended if on a surface from which they may roll. Newborns should not be left in back-lying position when not being directly supervised. While infant is undressed, weigh him if necessary, making undressing more than once unnecessary.
4. Cleanse infant's head and neck.	Proceed from "clean" to "dirty" areas to minimize possibility of cross-infection and disease. Infant's skin is irritated easily; infants are quite susceptible to infection. Soap is drying to infant's skin.	Infant usually has many fatty folds and creases; these must be washed and dried quite carefully to avoid irritation and tissue breakdown in addition to bacterial growth. Anything placed over infant's face causes him to become quite anxious, making him feel as though he is smothering; do not drag wash cloth across infant's face.

Implementation	Recommendations	Observations
Wash and dry hands thoroughly, using procedure for correct handwashing described in Chapter 31 on medical and surgical asepsis.		
Assemble all necessary equipment: shirt, diaper (and pins if necessary), sterile water, sterile cotton balls, basin, mild soap, receptacle for dirty laundry, wash cloth, and towel.	Water for bath should be approximately 100–105°F (37.8–40.6°C). A bath thermometer should be used to avoid burning infant's tender skin.	
Gently remove shirt and diaper. Cover infant with blanket. Discard soiled shirt and diaper.	Infants do not like anything over their faces; therefore, remove shirt carefully so as not to give infant a feeling of smothering. Place closed safety pins (if used) outside of bassinets so infants cannot place them in their mouths.	Observe for reflexes, skin condition, characteristics and amount of stool or urine in diaper. Observe for drainage from eyes, redness, crusts, or irritation. Note blemishes or markings.
Using a sterile cotton ball saturated with sterile water (and wrung out) for each eye, wipe from inner aspect (canthus) of eye in outward direction. Discard each cotton ball after one wipe. Wash infant's face without soap using soft wash cloth. Wash, rinse, and dry thoroughly ears and neck.	Do not use soap on face because of its drying effect. Soap should be removed carefully.	Observe for rooting and sucking reflexes.

TABLE 32-2. Continued

Anticipated Accomplishment	Scientific Principles/ Rationale	Specific Considerations
4A. Cleanse infant's scalp.	Gentle massage of scalp increases circulation.	Infants usually enjoy having their hair washed. Depending upon age of infant amount of support of head and neck needed will vary.
5. Cleanse upper and lower extremities, trunk, back, and buttocks.	Bacteria proliferate in dark, warm, moist areas; irritation, cracking, and bacterial invasion cause breakdown and infection of infant's tender skin.	Consider age of infant. Is cord still attached? What reflexes should (or should not) be present?
6. Cleanse genitalia and anus.	"Dirtiest" or most contaminated areas are cleansed last to avoid contamination of "clean" areas.	Is male infant circumcised? Vaseline gauze is used as a dressing on fresh circumcisions.
7. Provide for comfort and warmth.	After bathing, infants' temperatures may drop quickly due to immaturity of their heat regulatory centers and process of evaporation of water from surface of skin.	If in hospital what is their procedure for wrapping infants?

Implementation	Recommendations	Observations
Wash, rinse and thoroughly towel dry hair and scalp using a small amount of gentle nonperfumed soap. Hair can be gently combed or brushed.	Hold infant in "football hold" with arm along infant's back and hand cradling head and neck. Infant is held securely against nurse's hip leaving her other hand free.	Observe for cradle cap, crusting, marks on scalp, condition (status) of fontanels (soft areas at junction of bony suture lines of the infant's skull); there is one on anterior (top of skull) and one on posterior surface.
Wash and rinse arms, hands, legs, feet, trunk, back and buttocks. Dry thoroughly, especially in creases and folds of skin. If cord is still attached, follow agency procedure for cord care. In home 70% isopropyl alcohol can be swabbed on base of cord.	Hands can be used rather than a wash cloth to apply soap to body. This allows for both pleasurable contact between infant and nurse, and allows lumps or lesions to be felt more readily with fingertips than through wash cloth.	Observe other reflexes (e.g., grasp or Moro), at this time. Note any markings, lesions, or bruises. If cord is still attached, observe for oozing, bleeding, or foul odor.
Wash, rinse and dry genitalia. For females, use single cotton balls (moist) from front to rear (or use each corner of wash cloth). Gently retract foreskin of penis to cleanse male. Cleanse anus last.	Keep infant's genitalia covered with towel or clean diaper while undressed; urination occurs fairly frequently and may soak surroundings, including nurse.	Observe for oozing, bleeding, and normal voiding if circumcision is present. Note vaginal discharge in female infant.
Dress infant in clean shirt and diaper. Wrap in blanket and tuck in. Discard dirty laundry in appropriate manner.	Sheet of bassinet should be changed at end of bath. If convenient, a second person can change this while infant is being held, or nurse can change it herself by placing infant on one side of bassinet, changing other side, and then moving infant to clean side and finishing other side.	

TABLE 32-3. Making an Unoccupied (Open) Bed to Provide Cleanliness and Physical and Psychological Comfort for Client

Anticipated Accomplishment	Scientific Principles/ Rationale	Specific Considerations
1. Decrease possibility of cross-contamination and spread of infection and disease.	Handwashing (the use of soap, friction, and running water) helps in prevention of spread of disease and infection by reducing number of microorganisms on hands.	
2. Organization of materials and preparation for procedure.	Time and energy expended are reduced by having all necessary materials together prior to beginning procedure. Muscle strain and fatigue are not as likely when proper body mechanics are used.	What are client's individualized needs (e.g., incontinent client might require rubber drawsheet, cotton drawsheet to cover rubber sheet, and disposable linen saver pad)?
3. Remove dirty linens, pillow and pillow case in a manner that will not encourage cross-contamination.	Fluffing of linens will scatter microorganisms through the room via air currents.	
4. Reposition mattress correctly if necessary.		Is top edge of mattress up as far as head of bed as it should be?
5. Make up bottom of bed on one side.	Mitering (squaring corners of sheet) reduces slipping of sheet and maintains a tight and secure fit for longer time than one that has only been tucked in.	Straight sheets used as bottom sheets should have the corners mitered (Fig. 32-4).

Implementation	Recommendations	Observations
Follow procedure for correct handwashing (See Chapter 31 on medical and surgical asepsis.)		
Gather materials: two sheets (one for bottom which may be either contour sheet or straight sheet and one for top sheet), drawsheet, pillowcase for each pillow, spread, and blanket, if necessary. Raise bed to convenient working level for nurse (usually highest level).	Use good body mechanics. (See Chapter 30 on body mechanics.)	
Dirty linen is removed carefully without fluffing or holding against uniform or wearing apparel. Place soiled linen in laundry bag or linen hamper outside client's room.	Client's pillow can be left on a chair while bed is being made. Do not put it on floor or on overbed table.	As they are removed, check dirty linens to be certain that client's personal items such as dentures, jewelry, money have not fallen into folds or been placed under pillow.
Holding side of mattress firmly at center and end at foot, slide the mattress up to head of bed.	Some mattresses are equipped with handles on sides, making this procedure easier. It is faster and simpler to have assistance of second person when moving mattress.	
Bottom sheet is centered on bed and then unfolded lengthwise so smooth side is facing upward (away from hem). Bottom edge of sheet reaches as far as edge of mattress at foot of the bed but will not extend any further; top edge is tucked under head of mattress and top corner is then mitered. Drawsheets (rubber and cotton), if used, are then placed so top	Smooth side of sheets, that will touch client's skin, should face client for his comfort.	

TABLE 32-3. Continued

Anticipated Accomplishment	Scientific Principles/ Rationale	Specific Considerations
6. Make up top linens of bed on same side (as step 5.)	Nurse's energy and time spent are reduced by eliminating need to go from one side of bed to other repeatedly.	When centering top linens, some excess should be allowed for lengthwise pleat that will be made when completing bed.
7A. Complete making other side of bed (bottom linens).		If bottom sheet is pulled tightly when tucking it in, bed will look and feel smoother and neater against client's skin.
7B. Complete making other side of bed (top linens).	When top linens pull feet downward, they are forced into an unnatural position and "foot drop" (a permanent deformity) will occur.	Clients who are ambulatory or who can get in and out of bed at frequent intervals often will not need a toe pleat. Clients who are confined to bed for long periods of time will undoubtedly benefit from inclusion of toe pleat in top covers.
7C. Completing top linens.		Folded sheet keeps rough edges of blanket and spread away from client's skin, reducing possibility of irritation.

Implementation	Recommendations	Observations

edge is approximately where client's shoulder or upper chest is located and bottom edge approximated at level of knees. Sheets are all tucked in at same time from head of bed to foot on that side.

Top sheet is centered in same fashion as bottom sheet with smooth side down. Blanket (if used) and spread are also placed on bed in this manner. Top edges will match edge of head of mattress, and bottom edges will all be tucked under foot of mattress together and then mitered. Sides of top linens are not tucked in but allowed to hang freely at side of bed.

Bottom sheet and drawsheet(s) are tucked and mitered as on previous side.

Top linens should be folded away from current side of bed to allow nurse to complete making the bottom sheet(s).

A lengthwise pleat approximately 3 inches is created in center of top linens (Fig. 32-5). They are then tucked in and mitered as they were on other side.

At head of bed, top sheet is folded back over top edges of blanket and spread.

TABLE 32-2. Continued

Anticipated Accomplishment	Scientific Principles/ Rationale	Specific Considerations
8. Replace clean pillow(s) on bed.	Since pillow(s) has been contaminated by contact with client, it should not come in contact with nurse's uniform or wearing apparel as this would foster cross-contamination.	Open end of pillow case should face away from doorway for a neater looking bed.
9. Facilitate client's safe reentry into his bed.	Falls are common accidents. When bed is at convenient level for client to reenter, possibility of a fall is diminished.	Shorter clients may have difficulty getting into bed that is at high level.
10. Prevention of cross-infection and spread of disease.	Handwashing will reduce number of microorganisms now on nurse's hands from contact with client's contaminated linens.	

TYPES OF BEDS AND RELATED EQUIPMENT

For the client who must spend all of his time in bed, special attention must be given to the condition of his skin and his musculature. As discussed earlier, the skin is prone to breakdown and necrosis when subjected to inactivity; muscle tone also diminishes during periods of confinement. To reduce the detrimental effects of bedrest, numerous kinds of equipment and apparatus, used in conjunction with preventive measures, are employed. Some of these are discussed below.

Air beds and *alternating pressure mattresses*, while maintaining support of the client's entire body, provide continuous pressure change. This is accomplished by a process of alternating inflation and deflation of air or water-filled channels. In this manner, no area or points of the body are subjected to constant pressure, thus, decreasing the possibility of tissue breakdown due to mechanically induced circulatory insufficiency.

In addition to their comfort, *water beds* assure that all body parts are supported equally since the client is "floating in water." The main drawback of the water bed is that the support is so evenly maintained by the surface of the water matching the body's curvature that no air can circulate between the mattress and the skin.

A number of beds and frames can be used to vary the client's position either electronically or manually. These devices make turning and positioning more convenient and less traumatic than it might be in the standard hospital bed. Some of the more common apparatus include the *Circ-O-Lectric* (circle) *bed* (Fig. 32-6), the *high-low tilt bed*, the *cardiac* (chair) *bed*, *Stryker frames* (Fig. 32-7), and *Foster frames*. Each of these has its own characteristics and functions; the choice of one is made by taking into consideration the special needs and problems of the individual client and matching them as well as possible to the plan of care that is constructed to satisfy these needs.

SAFETY

When the client places himself in the hands of the health care worker (and thus, the agency to which

Implementation	Recommendations	Observations
Place clean pillow case(s) on pillow(s) and position at head of bed.	Pillow can be placed on bed and case slid onto it. Pillow should not be held under chin as this brings it into contact with nurse's uniform or apparel.	
Top linens are fanfolded (like fan or accordion), leaving top edges nearer to foot of bed (lower half of bed). Place bed at its lowest height so client's return to bed is not difficult.	Do not forget to reattach client's signal light cord in a convenient position within his grasp. Also provide him with ability to reach electronic bed position control if appropriate.	
Wash hands thoroughly after disposing of dirty linens in appropriate place.	Unit should look neat when bed has been made. Provisions for tidying unit should be facilitated.	

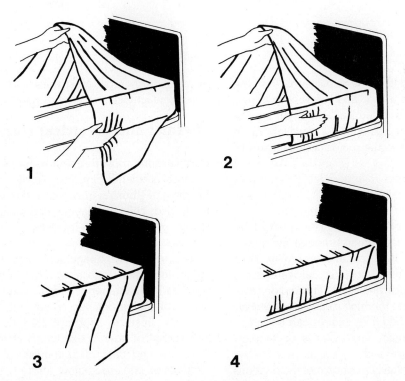

FIGURE 32-4. Four steps in making a mitered (square) corner.

TABLE 32-4. Making a Closed (Empty) Bed to Prepare a Clean Bed and Protect Bottom Linens and Top Sheet from Dust until Ready for Use

Anticipated Accomplishment	Scientific Principles/ Rationale	Specific Considerations
1. Prepare bed as described in steps 1 through 7B in Table 32-3, Making an Unoccupied (Open) Bed.		
2. Protect bottom linens and top sheet.		
3. Placement of pillow on bed.		
4. Facilitation of client's entering bed upon admission.		If client enters on stretcher, bed can be raised to highest position for convenience of health care workers assisting with client's transfer.

this worker is associated), he expects that his care will be delivered in a safe and effective manner. The responsibility, both ethical and legal, for the client's safety and well-being most often falls upon the nurse, since she is the major control agent of his environment.

While anyone is open to injury, debilitated clients and those unable to take responsibility for their own well-being and safety are the most accident prone. The prevention of accidents is accomplished by careful maintenance of environmental factors as well as education of the client and his family. Most accidents are preventable in that their causes are due to carelessness or oversight. The major categories of accidents are *thermal, electrical, chemical*, and *mechanical*. In addition, injuries can be *radiologic* and *bacteriologic*. The latter is covered in Chapter 31 on medical and surgical asepsis. Radiologic accidents are usually a concern of the divisions of an agency dealing with nuclear medicine, x-rays,

or radiation therapy. Most nurses have little or no direct contact with this type of hazard.

Thermal and Electrical Hazards

Burns are the most frequent result of thermal and electrical accidents. *Fires* are usually due to careless handling of smoking materials and matches (smoking in bed, children playing with matches or flammable toys); explosions involving gases, faulty wiring, including frayed cords; overloaded electrical outlets; improper management of combustible materials; improper disposal of rubbish; defective appliances or machinery; and accidents associated with cooking and kitchen equipment. Fire prevention can best be accomplished by education. Knowledge of how to extinguish various types of fires, use and care of extinguishers, routes and methods of safe evacuation, ability to call for help, and care in the handling and management of

Implementation	Recommendations	Observations
		Only difference in open and closed beds is way in which top linens are completed.
Top edges of bedspread and top sheet are not folded back and fanfolded as in open bed, but are left in closed position— even with edge of head of mattress.		
Clean pillow is placed on bed as in step 8 of Table 32-3.		
Lower bed to its lowest height.		

equipment or flammable substances, as well as installation of early detection equipment systems help to avert many injuries.

Other causes of burns are *improper applications of heat,* (e.g., heating pads, hydrocollator packs, hot water bottles, hot compresses, hot baths, and

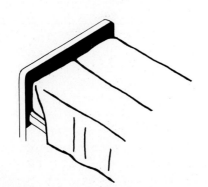

FIGURE 32-5. Toe-pleat in top linens.

heat lamps) and burns caused by live *steam* (predominantly in the kitchen and engineering departments but also associated with steam inhalators).

In addition to burns, severe *shock* or *electrocution* can result from accidents involving electrical equipment. These accidents most often are caused by defects in the equipment (or its wiring) or by careless usage (i.e., touching an electrical device with wet hands). Obviously, awareness of the hazards and strict adherence to safe technique are vital in the prevention of accidents of this type.

Chemical Injury

The most prevalent cause of injury in this category is *drug error, overdosage,* and *toxicity.* This problem, unfortunately, is seen all too frequently, both in clinical facilities and in the home. Along the same line, *poisoning* due to household cleansers, disinfectants, pesticides, lead paint and other chemical

TABLE 32-5. Making Recovery or Postoperative Bed to Permit a Rapid Transfer of Client from Stretcher and Provide Comfort

Anticipated Accomplishment	Scientific Principles/ Rationale	Specific Considerations
1. Prepare bottom sheets only on both sides of bed as described in Table 32-3.	Client who has undergone anesthesia may feel chilled in immediate postoperative period.	Is room cool? Consideration of procedure that client has undergone and anticipated reactions that may occur will help to determine what needs are for equipment, warmth and safety.
2. Place top linens on bed as in Table 32-3; however, do not miter corners or tuck under mattress.		
3. Provide a surface across which client can be slid without getting tangled in top covers or pillow.	When stretcher is alongside bed, fanfolded linens will be on side opposite stretcher.	Have pillow available but do not place on bed until after client is in bed and his need for it is ascertained.
4. Protect linens from any possible soilage.	Frequent reactions to anesthesia are nausea and vomiting.	
5. Facilitate ease of client's transfer from stretcher to bed.	There is less strain on workers who transfer client into bed if proper body mechanics are used.	Move any furniture in unit that will interfere with transfer away from line of travel of stretcher.

Implementation	Recommendations	Observations
	If room is cool, a bath blanket can be placed over bottom sheets and tucked in with them.	
	A bath blanket can be placed on bed along with placement of top sheet for additional layer that provides warmth. (Put bath blanket on first so it will come in contact with the client rather than top sheet.)	
Fold all layers of top linens at foot of bed together up toward center of bed, rather than tucking them in. Fold all layers of top linens at head of bed together down toward center of bed. Fanfold all top linens lengthwise to side of bed.	Do not put up side rail on far side of bed until client is returned to bed as this will interfere with his transfer into bed.	
Place a disposable linen saver pad at head of bed.	Place an emesis basin nearby.	
Leave bed in high position.	Signal cord needs to be attached to bed; however, if it interferes with transfer of client, it can be done immediately after client is returned to bed.	

TABLE 32-6. Making an Occupied Bed to Change Linen When Client is Unable to Get Out of Bed and Maintain the Integrity of Client's Body

Anticipated Accomplishment	Scientific Principles/ Rationale	Specific Considerations
1. Decrease possibility of cross-contamination and spread of infection and disease.	Handwashing (use of soap, friction, and running water) helps in prevention of disease and infection by reducing number of microorganisms on nurse's hands.	
2. Reduce anxiety of client.	Client who is less anxious will be more likely to cooperate and participate in self-care.	Occupied bed is usually made up immediately following bed-bath or whenever necessary.
3. Organization of time and materials and preparation of client for procedure.	Nurse's time and energy are conserved by eliminating extra trips to gather needed materials.	
	Possibility of back strain and fatigue are minimized by use of proper body mechanics. (See Chapter 30 on body mechanics.) Client is prone to chilling when uncovered (especially following a bath).	If there are no contraindications, bed should be flat with no elevation of head.
4. Return mattress to top of bed if necessary.	Proper use of body mechanics when moving heavy mattress and client will decrease possibility of injury or strain.	
5. Position client to allow one side of bed to be made.	Client must remain at far side of bed so proximal side of bed can be made.	Side rail on distant side of bed must be in place so that client cannot fall out of bed. A pillow can be placed under client's head if he is uncomfortable.

Implementation	Recommendations	Observations

Follow procedure for correct handwashing. (See Chapter 31, on medical and surgical asepsis.)

Explain procedure to client. Provide privacy by closing door of room, closing bedside curtains or providing screens around bed.

Gather equipment: two sheets, drawsheets, pillow cases, spread, client gown (if this needs changing or was not changed at end of bath).

Position linens conveniently in order they will be used. If this procedure is immediately following bed bath, this step should be accomplished along with gathering of materials for bath. Have laundry bag or receptacle for dirty linens located conveniently.

Raise bed to convenient height if this has not yet been done. Replace top linens with a bath blanket if this has not already been done. (See step 2 of Table 32-1, The Complete Bed Bath.)

Have two people use handles at sides of mattress or grasp mattress edges in center and at foot of bed; move mattress up towards head of bed.

Place or assist client into side-lying position at far side of bed. (See Chapter 30 on body mechanics for positioning of client.)

Client can steady himself by grasping side rail.

TABLE 32-6. Continued

Anticipated Accomplishment	Scientific Principles/ Rationale	Specific Considerations
6. Make bottom of bed on one side.	Side of linen which has come in contact with client should not touch clean linens when procedure is done properly, maintaining cleanliness of linens.	
7. Roll client over onto clean side of bed to facilitate making second side.		Prior to turning client, explain to him that he will roll over a thick hump of linens. Use care so that dirty linen does not contaminate uniform or wearing apparel.
8. Complete making other side of bottom sheets.	Wrinkled sheets add additional (uneven) pressure to tissues and predispose it to breakdown and formation of decubiti.	
9. Place top linens on bed as in steps 6 and 7A, B, and C of Table 32-3, Making an Unoccupied Bed.		Care must be taken not to fluff linens over client's face.
10. Provide for the client's comfort and safety.		Consider client's unique need for positioning (e.g., skin condition and pressure areas).
	Side rails are a major deterrent in preventing clients from falling out of bed.	
11. Decrease possibility of cross-contamination and spread of infection and disease.	Handwashing will reduce amount of microorganisms on nurse's hands which can be transmitted to other clients.	

Implementation	Recommendations	Observations

Undo bottom sheets and tightly roll them up to client's back. Apply clean bottom sheets, miter top corners and tuck in as with unoccupied bed. (See step 5 of Table 33-3, Making an Unoccupied Bed.) Roll excess material of clean bottom sheets (meant for other side of bed) and tuck beneath rolled dirty linen.

Place side rail in up position on completed side before moving client to that side. Assist client to opposite side of bed if he is unable to do so by himself. Change pillow case, and re-place pillow under client's head.

Remove dirty bottom sheets and place in laundry bag. Pulling clean bottom sheets as tightly as possible, miter and tuck in as with unoccupied bed.

Position client in a comforta-ble position. Attach the client's signal light cord to bed for easy access.
Place side rails in up position.
Place bed at lowest height.

If signal cord has no clamp, secure it using a safety pin. (Do not pierce cord with pin.)

Wash hands after disposing of contaminated linens in ap-propriate manner.

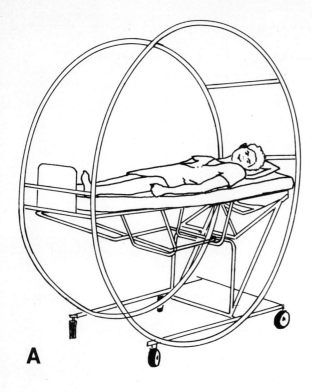

A

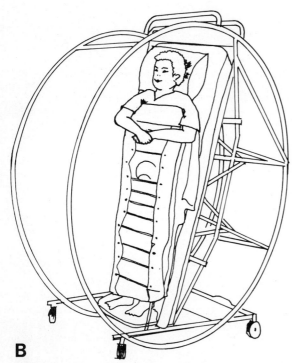

B

FIGURE 32-6. The Circ-O-Lectric bed. A, Client supine; B, client standing.

agents cause numerous injuries (especially to children) annually.

Asphyxiation by gas inhalation, damage to the skin, mucous membranes and the lungs by *contact with* or the *inhalation of* chemical and carcinogenic substances (e.g., asbestos, coal dust, and smoke) are other causes of chemical injury. Prevention of chemical injury revolves around the use of care in the employment and utilization of *all* chemical agents.

Mechanical Accidents

Falls are by far the major cause of mechanical injury; negligence in providing for safety precautions accounts for most of these accidents. Falling associated with beds, cribs, chairs, wheelchairs, stretchers, examining tables, bathtubs, and showers are the most frequent offenders. Judicious use of restraints, side rails and guard rails, as well as explanations and appropriate supervision, are the most effective precautions against these accidents. Slipping on wet or highly waxed floors and stairs are not unusual occurrences. Even when these factors are not involved, falls associated with ambulation occur; proper assistance and guidance can be an effective preventive measure.

Ineffective instruction in and usage of canes, crutches, and walkers also account for a number of falls each year. These too, require careful monitoring.

Improper handling of mechanical devices or use of defective apparatus can be another source of injury. Care in reading instructions, becoming acquainted with equipment that is unfamiliar, and periodic assessment of mechanical functioning are means of decreasing this type of hazard.

In the home, toys with sharp edges, with small pieces that can be swallowed, or with small openings in which tiny fingers can get caught account for many accidents each year. *Suffocation* due to the mechanical obliteration of air intake occurs primarily with children; frequent causes are playing with abandoned refrigerators and with plastic bags. Obviously education of the public is the best preventive measure in this type of accident.

The importance of knowledge of safety factors and principles of accident prevention cannot be overstated. The possibility for the occurrence of

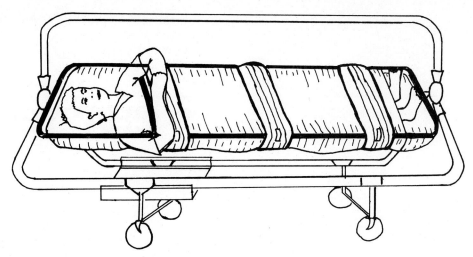

FIGURE 32-7. Stryker frame.

accidents exists not only in hospitals, but in homes, industry, schools, and all other aspects of the community. As health care workers the awareness of potential causative factors and their methods of control as well as the ability to provide safe care and implement programs of prevention are among the most important aspects of the nurse's professional responsibility.

SUMMARY

The provision of care that is physically and emotionally *comforting* as well as *safe* is of utmost concern to the nurse and the other members of the health care team. From the materials presented above it can be seen that *prophylaxis*, or *prevention*, is a key factor in the planning and implementation of sound client care. Many problems such as decubiti and accidents are preventable if only forethought and constant attention and awareness of the possibilities are manifested by the prudent practitioner.

Fostering of the maximum amount of independence possible for each client is another important aspect of care which may require patience and creativity. While allowing the client to be dependent when this is timely is certainly appropriate, the ability to discern, with the cooperation of the client, when independent activity must be encouraged and fostered will be one of the prime indicators of successful client care.

BIBLIOGRAPHY

Bower, F. L., and Bevis, E. O.: *Fundamentals of Nursing Practice—Concepts, Roles and Functions.* St. Louis, C. V. Mosby Co., 1979.

Dison, N.: *Clinical Nursing Techniques,* 3rd ed. St. Louis, C. V. Mosby Co., 1975.

Elhart, D., et al.: *Scientific Principles in Nursing,* 8th ed. St. Louis, C. V. Mosby Co., 1978.

Fuerst, E., Wolff, L., and Weitzel, M.: *Fundamentals of Nursing,* 5th ed. Philadelphia, J. B. Lippincott Co., 1974.

Gordon, J. E.: Circ-O-Lectric beds: Circumventing the trauma of positioning. *Nurs. '77* 7(2):42, 1977.

Gruis, M., and Innes, B.: Assessment: essential to prevent pressure sores. *Am. J. Nurs.* 76(11):1762, 1976.

Henderson, V., and Nite, G.: *Principles and Practice of Nursing,* 6th ed. New York, Macmillan Publishing Co., Inc., 1978.

Karchak-Keyes, M. S.: Four proven steps for preventing decubitus ulcers. *Nurs. '77* 7(9):58, 1977.

King, E., Wieck, L., and Dyer, M.: *Illustrated Manual of Nursing Techniques.* Philadelphia, J. B. Lippincott Co., 1977.

Kukuk, H.: Safety precautions: protecting your patients and yourself. *Nurs. '76* 6(7):45, 1976.

Leifer, G.: *Principles and Techniques in Pediatric Nursing,* 3rd ed. Philadelphia, W. B. Saunders Co., 1977.

Murray, M.: *Fundamentals of Nursing.* Englewood Cliffs, N.J., Prentice-Hall, Inc., 1976.

Sutton, A. L.: *Bedside Nursing Techniques in Medicine and Surgery,* 2nd ed. Philadelphia, W. B. Saunders Co., 1969.

Wallace, G., and Hayter, J.: Karaya for chronic skin ulcers. *Am. J. Nurs.* 74:6, 1974.

Wood, L. A., and Rambo, B. J.: *Nursing Skills for Allied Health Services.* Philadelphia, W. B. Saunders Co., 1977.

CHAPTER 33

Applications of heat and cold as therapeutic remedies are found in both professional health settings and the home. In the home, they are most frequently used for comfort and first aid for minor injuries. In the hospital, however, they have many functions. While most of the procedures that nurses perform using heat and cold are fairly simple, hazards are involved. (Complex and technical treatments, such as paraffin baths and ultraviolet treatments, are handled by specially trained personnel in the physical therapy department of the agency.) In fact, one of the most common accidents involving clients in the hospital setting is burns, often the result of the negligence of the health care worker, either in the implementation or the explanation of the procedure.

Heat and *cold* actually refer to the *energy* (*kinetic*) that is produced when molecules are in motion. When the molecules in a substance move rapidly, the substance is hot. The faster the movement, the warmer it becomes; the slower the molecular movement, the cooler the substance. Chemical re-

ADMINISTRATION OF THERMAL AGENTS

Arlyne B. Saperstein, M.N., R.N., and
Margaret A. Frazier, M.S., R.N.

actions usually occur more rapidly when heat is applied; thus, metabolic processes which are the result of chemical reactions also occur more rapidly with the application of heat. Conversely, metabolism is slowed by cold.

Heat transfer occurs through the processes of *convection, radiation,* and *conduction.* (These processes are also discussed in Chapter 29, "The Assessment of Vital Signs.") *Convection* refers to the transfer of heat through motion or circulation of liquids or gases, for example, whirlpool baths in which warm water circulates through the tub; the movement of the water transfers the heat. *Radiation,* or the transfer of heat (in waves) through space, is exemplified by the use of heat lamps. The closer one moves to the heat source (the light bulb), the more warmth one feels; thus, the heat is radiated from the bulb to the skin. *Conduction* occurs when one substance comes in direct contact with another—that is, the heat is transferred from one object to the other. Thus, when heat is applied to the body surface, the surface gets warmer; when

cold is applied to the surface of the body, the heat from the body is lost to the cold object, cooling the body. A *conductor* is an object or material in which there is a rapid transfer of heat; a poor conductor is known as an *insulator* (slow transfer of heat). Conduction and insulation are relative as all materials conduct heat, but the rapidity with which this occurs varies significantly. Metals and water, for example, are excellent conductors of heat, while air and fabrics are poor conductors.

Although heat and cold are applied locally to both small and large areas of skin, other parts of the body far from the site of application may be affected similarly due to the anatomy and physiology of the skin and the underlying structures. These effects occur when the temperature receptors in the skin (for both heat and cold) are stimulated, sending impulses by way of somatic afferent fibers to both the hypothalamus and the cerebral cortex. The result of this is an awareness in the individual that the temperature has changed; the reflex action that occurs—vasodilation or vasoconstriction—is the body's attempt to maintain normal body temperature. Irritation (excitation) of the cutaneous sensory nerve fibers occurs when applications 20°F below and 15°F above the usual surface temperature of the skin (93°F [33.9°C]) are made. The skin receptors adapt quite readily (and rapidly) to temperature changes, especially if the changes are not extreme. However, with slight temperature changes, the individual may be unaware of the sensation of temperature. Under these circumstances, clients may be injured quite easily since they are no longer aware of the application.

The skin's sensitivity to and tolerance for variations in temperature vary from one individual to another and from one body part to another. (Normally, areas of exposed skin are more tolerant of temperature changes than those usually protected by clothing.) Tolerance is influenced by the *duration* (length) and *amount* (size) of skin exposure to heat or cold, *age* (very young and very old individuals do not tolerate temperature extremes well), and physical *condition* (persons with poor circulation or diminished sensation, as in debilitated, comatose, or neurologically damaged clients, are less tolerant or unaware of extremes). The ability to withstand tissue damage or injury due to temperature extremes, which is perceived as pain, also varies from one individual to another. Temperatures below 40°F (4.4°C) and above 110°F (43.3°C) are considered beyond the general range of safety in direct thermal applications and may cause tissue damage in some individuals. For this reason, when applying heat and cold to a client where no specific temperature has been specified, these extremes should be used as maximum cutoff points.

In this chapter, applications of heat and cold are examined. The descriptive terms and the ranges for the various temperature applications are as follows: very hot, 105–115°F (40.6–46.1°C); hot, 98–104°F (36.7–40°C); warm, 96–98°F (35.6–36.7°C); neutral, 93–96°F (33.9–35.6°C); tepid, 80–92°F (26.7–33.3°C); cool, 65–80°F (18.3–26.7°C); cold, 55–65°F (12.8–18.3°C); and very cold (any temperature below 55°F [12.8°C]). The order for the application usually includes the general method to be used, the area of the body to be treated, the length of each treatment, and the frequency of the treatments. Again, temperature may or may not be indicated by the prescriber, leaving that decision to the nurse.

APPLICATIONS OF HEAT

Heat is applied therapeutically to relieve pain (analgesia), to relax muscles (antispasmodic), to hasten lymphatic flow and absorption of waste products, increasing healing and reducing edema (decongestion), to relieve tension and fatigue (sedation), and to increase the body temperature. When *moderate* heat is applied to the skin, the warmth causes dilation of the peripheral blood vessels, decreasing the viscosity of the blood. This increases the amount and speed with which blood is brought into an area, thus supplying more oxygen to the tissues (improving cellular nutrition) and increasing the removal of waste products. This encourages tissue repair, healing, and resolution of the inflammatory response by promoting phagocytosis (increased leukocyte production), suppuration (pus formation), and removal of debris from the area. Local application of heat for 20 to 30 minutes effectively achieves these actions; if prolonged, however, the skin cells can be weakened, making them more prone to damage or injury. After an hour, vasoconstriction occurs, rather than vasodilation—that is, the effects of prolonged heat application resemble the effects of the application of cold. (However, when an application of heat is removed and then replaced after an interval of time, vasodilation recurs.) *Very hot* applications, when used for *short times,* also resemble cold applications; blood supply decreases with resultant muscle tension or contraction.

Heat may be applied in moist or dry forms. *Moist heat* applications include compresses, packs, soaks, and baths. *Dry heat* can be applied via hot water bottles and heating and hyperthermia pads (Aquamatic K-pads). Somewhat higher temperatures are used with dry applications of heat, since water is an excellent conductor, making burns more of a likelihood. Clients should feel comfortable warmth during a heat application (unless sensory perceptions are impaired); the skin is usually pink and moist. If he complains that the treatment is too hot or if mottling of the skin occurs, adjustments must be made.

Heat is not applied when vasodilation would result in pain. For example, a hot compress would not be applied with headaches since the dilation of the blood vessels increases pressure against the cranial vault exaggerating the pain. Heat applications are not used in cases of malignancy since the increase in cellular metabolism is an undesirable effect. In addition, heat is contraindicated in the initial (acute) stage of trauma. Vasoconstriction is desired rather than vasodilation to retard edema. After the first 24 hours, heat is applied to increase the removal of the waste products and facilitate provision of nutrients and thus healing in the area. Along the same lines, heat would not be used in acute inflammatory responses, such as appendicitis, because of the possibility of rupture due to increase in suppuration.

Moist Heat

PACKS AND COMPRESSES

Hot moist packs and compresses are similar in nature; the pack is an application of a moistened cloth to an area of the body, and the compress is the application of a moist dressing (gauze) to a less extensive body area. Both are applied at the hottest temperature that the client can comfortably tolerate. (Again, individuals who have peripheral circulatory problems or who are unable to communicate the degree of heat or discomfort should be carefully watched; an application of approximately 105°F [40.6°C] should be used rather than that which the nurse "feels" would be comfortable.) Often these applications are ordered continuously, in which case they are changed as frequently as necessary to keep the application hot, depending on the nature of the dressing; this may vary from every 30 minutes to every 2 hours.

There are a number of ways to prepare the compress or pack. Since each agency may have a preferred method, only one will be described here. The designated solution which has been heated to the proper temperature is poured into a container holding the appropriate material (i.e., gauze and cotton). The compress is then removed and wrung out (using aseptic techniques) prior to the application. If the application must be sterile, then sterile forceps are used to handle the material.

There are various methods for maintaining heat in these applications; for example, after they are wrapped in waterproof material and reinforced with additional material, a hot water bottle or hyperthermia pad could be placed over the compress or pack to keep the warmth continuous. However, the danger of this method would be excessive exposure to heat because the moisture in the dressing acts

as a good conductor. A protective coating of mineral oil or petrolatum can be applied to the skin (except in cases where this heat application is for the purpose of vein distension prior to initiation of the venipuncture procedure) at the site of the application of the pack, or gauze may also be layered under the pack for additional protection. In addition to water or saline, a mild antiseptic or astringent solution (e.g., witch hazel or Epsom salts) may be prescribed for a compress. The temperature of the solution should be taken with a thermometer to avoid accidental burning. If the compress must be sterile, such as those used on eyes, wounds, or suture lines, the temperature of the solution (which must also be sterile) can be taken with a sterile thermometer, or a small amount of solution can be poured into a nonsterile container and measured for temperature with an unsterile thermometer. In applying sterile compresses, it must be remembered that *all* materials used, including insulation, must be sterile.

Hydrocollators

A special type of pack, called a Hydrocollator, is sometimes seen in the hospital setting. This pack contains silica gel, and is covered in canvas. It is stored and heated in a container that brings its temperature to 140°F (60°C) or higher. The pack, which can be rolled up or hinged to adapt its shape to bodily contours, retains its heat for at least 20 or 30 minutes without additional means. Care must be taken to wrap the pack well in insulating materials since the high degree of heat in the pack could severely burn the individual.

When applying hot moist packs or compresses, it is important to keep the client warm and out of drafts since he may experience a chilled feeling. The body must be kept in proper alignment to avoid complications and provide for comfort.

SOAKS AND BATHS

Soaks call for immersing a body part or area into water or solutions containing medication. In addition to medicating the afflicted area, soaks are used in the same instances as the local application of heat, particularly, local infections or sloughing wounds. A soak may or may not be sterile; if not, clean technique is used. Soaks are usually maintained for 20 minutes, during which the temperature of the water is kept constant by adding additional solution. The soaking body part should be kept in good alignment, just as with packs, for both comfort and avoidance of fatigue. Solutions used for soaks usually range from 105 to 110°F (40.6°C to 43.3°C), but physicians' orders vary.

The various types of *baths,* including *medicated baths* and *sitz baths,* are discussed in detail in Chapter 32, "Personal Hygiene, Comfort, and Safety Measures." The purposes of the different types of baths vary greatly from relaxation to promotion of healing after surgery or childbirth to treatment of a number of skin, rectal, and perineal conditions.

Dry Heat

HOT WATER BOTTLES

Hot water bottles or bags, which are used in both hospitals and homes, consist of a rubber bag and a stopper to retain water without leakage. Their action is based on conduction of heat. Although made of rubber, which is not an excellent conductor of heat, a good insulator, such as flannel, is used between the filled bag and the client's skin to insure that burns do not occur. The bag is filled approximately two-thirds full with water that ranges in temperature from 115 to 130°F (46.1 to 54.4°C). (With infants, 115°F [46.1°C] would be the maximum water temperature.) In a laboratory setting, a hot water bottle was filled with water measuring 115°F

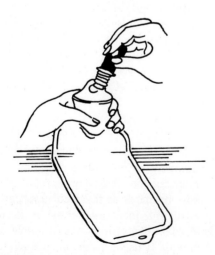

FIGURE 33-1. Expression of air from hot water bottle.

(46.1°C). The external temperature of the bag registered 104°F (40°C); however, when a bath towel was wrapped around the bag, the external temperature registered 102°F (38.9°C), falling within safe limits for heat applications.

Residual air in the bag is removed by resting the filled bag on a flat surface in such a way that the water in the bag is at the level of the mouth of the bottle (Fig. 33-1). The stopper is applied with the bag in this position. After sealing the bag, it is held upside down to be certain that there are no leaks. It is then covered with the insulating material before application to the specific affected area. The main disadvantage of this form of heat application is that water is heavy, making it uncomfortable for the client in certain situations.

HEATING PADS

Electric heating pads have become one of the more popular forms of dry heat application in both hospitals and homes. Their light weight makes them more comfortable than hot water bottles. Unfortunately, many people burn themselves with these pads because their sensitivity or awareness of the heat diminishes after they have been in place for a short time, and clients often increase the heat setting as this phenomenon occurs. Since a heating pad is an electrical appliance, there is always the danger of electrocution; perspiration occurring from the heat can short-circuit the pad if the wires become wet. Therefore, the heating pad should always be well insulated and covered by a waterproof cover. Care should be taken not to puncture the pad (especially with pins) or crush the pad, causing it to malfunction or overheat. In the hospital, heating pads with removable, washable covers are usually used to provide for asepsis between clients' usage. These pads may be preset to avoid the client's tampering with the temperature selection control, a very important safety feature.

AQUAMATIC K-PADS

Aquamatic K-pads or K-modules are devices which circulate distilled water through tubing contained in a pad. A control unit is used to vary the prescribed temperature which is usually 105°F (40.6°C) or less. (The use of a key which locks in the temperature prevents the client from changing the setting.) This device delivers dry heat if it is placed in a pillow case before applying it to the prescribed area. It can also be utilized to maintain moist heat applications by placing the pad over the moist compress. The pad is secured by ties made from gauze or special tape (twill). It is never pinned in place as the accidental puncturing of the tubing in the pad would render it useless. A careful reading of the directions before use reduces the possibility of errors. For correct and efficient functioning, the excess tubing should not be kinked or hung below the level of the control unit.

HEAT LAMPS

Local heat application can be made through the use of light bulbs or varying types of heat lamps. As stated earlier, radiation is the means of heat transfer in this method. Two main factors affect this type of application and its effectiveness: the size (wattage) of the bulb and the distance from the affected area of the body. Usually a 25 watt bulb can be placed approximately 1 foot away from the skin, a 40−60 watt bulb about 18−24 inches, and larger bulbs 24−30 inches away. These distances vary according to need and area of the body to be treated. In this method of heat application, the client who cannot discern temperature variations should be watched as the possibility of burns is great. Heat treatments are comforting and comfortable in that there is no weight involved and no direct contact with the skin. The client should be positioned in proper alignment and draped accordingly. Heat treatments of this type are approximately 15−30 minutes in length. This type of application is often seen postpartum (after childbirth) for the promotion of comfort and healing of the perineal area. If a wound is involved, extreme caution should be used in making sure that a bulb of fairly small wattage is used and that the client is cautioned to call the nurse if the area begins to feel too warm.

Although nurses do not give *diathermy* treatments, they should be aware of their use as they may see the treatment given on the hospital unit or down in the physical therapy department. Heat is produced in deep tissues by the use of ultrasound, short wave, and microwave diathermy. The treatments, which can also cause burns, are given by qualified therapists.

APPLICATIONS OF COLD

The local application of cold causes vasoconstriction to occur, tissue metabolism to decrease (with less need for oxygen and less accumulation of waste), and numbness or anesthesia of the skin. Applications of cold slow the flow rate and increase the viscosity of the blood; this, in conjunction with vasoconstriction, makes its use with hemorrhages apparent. Applying ice packs to stop nose bleeds has long been a home remedy. Cold is used to inhibit suppuration and inflammation during the first 24 hours of the inflammatory response. In some cases, it can be used to control (inhibit) microbial activity thereby retarding the infectious process. It is utilized as a comfort measure in the relief of pain associated with headache, muscle sprains, and bruises.

The application of cold causes the skin to appear pale and cool. If mottling, redness, discoloration, or blisters, which are indicative of tissue damage, occur, discontinue the treatment immediately, and report to the appropriate personnel and the physician.

Cold applied for an extended period of time causes vasodilation—that is, the effects of short-term local applications of heat. Excessive cold can cause tissue damage or death. As with the application of heat, a local cold treatment of 20−30 minutes is usually long enough to obtain a therapeutic effect.

COMPRESSES

Moist cold compresses are a means of applying cold to small areas of the body. The area to which the compress is applied determines the size and material used. Gauze or wash cloths are commonly seen as cold compresses. After being soaked in ice water, the compress is wrung out and applied to the affected area. They tend to need frequent changing since they are warmed by the body. Often the intervals between changes are about 2 minutes. A period of time is allowed to transpire between treatments (usually about 2 hours). The treatment itself should last about 15−20 minutes.

ICE BAGS

Ice bags and ice collars are another means of cold application to specific areas. The ice bag is filled with small bits of ice, making it easy to shape or mold to the contour of the affected area of the body. After filling the bag two-thirds full and removing the air, a cover is placed on the bag to absorb condensation on the outside. Application for approximately 30–60 minutes is usually effective. The bag is removed for about 1 hour and reapplied after being refilled with fresh ice. An ice bag can be made by using a plastic bag and tape; a commercially manufactured product is not necessary. In some agencies, a rubber (examining) glove is filled with ice chips, sealed with tape and applied to the affected area. This is used, for example, during the first 24 hours after childbirth on the mother's perineum to reduce edema as the filled glove fits more comfortably than an ice bag in this area.

ALCOHOL SPONGE BATHS

Alcohol (sponge) baths are discussed in Chapter 29, "Vital Signs." A systemic rather than a local effect is the goal of the alcohol bath which is used to lower elevated body temperature. A bath usually lasts approximately 30 minutes, using tepid water and alcohol mixtures. Cold wet wash cloths or ice bags are placed over areas with large superficial blood vessels (the axilla and groin), to aid in temperature reduction. Sometimes an ice cap on the forehead is comforting as is a warm hot water bottle on the feet. Care is taken not to chill the client while the bath is taking place. This is done by draping with a bath blanket all areas not involved in the process at the time.

HYPOTHERMIA BLANKETS

Another systemic application of cold is done with hypothermia blankets. Extended (prolonged) cooling is used in the treatment of certain conditions; deep (profound) cooling is seen as an adjunct to certain surgical procedures. With this method a mechanical device circulates a refrigerant through a network of coils in a large pad. The hypothermia blanket (Fig. 33-2) works under a similar principle to that of the Aquamatic K-pad. The client may be placed directly on the blanket, or a sheet, which protects the skin, may be placed between the pad and the client. In some cases (usually where profound cooling is taking place), the skin will be further protected from damage (i.e., frostbite) by applying a coat of oil. The client is then covered with another sheet. Occasionally the client is enclosed between two hypothermia blankets. In that case, the two blankets can usually be secured by ties or fasteners. Pins cannot be used because of the danger of puncturing the coils. A rectal probe monitors body temperature. After insertion to approximately 2 inches, it is taped in place. With some units the probe is associated with a thermostat which will keep the body temperature at a specific level. The physician orders the desired temperature of the body, the area to be cooled, the length of time of the procedure, and the amount of time for cooling to take place. Observation of the client is an absolute necessity; shivering often takes place, especially in the initial stages of the treatment. This may be treated with medication. The vital signs are watched closely; after the treatment has been discontinued, the temperature may continue to drop—usually 2°F. Support for both the client and his family is needed to allay fears and anxiety about the procedure and the condition of the client.

CONTRAST BATHS AND PACKS

Occasionally the alternating use of both hot and cold applications is seen. A local hot bath followed by a local cold bath is called contrast baths. Their purpose is to stimulate the circulation. This can also be achieved by alternation of hot water bottles and ice bags to a specific part.

Disposable hot and cold packs, which are used in emergency or first aid situations, are available today. The pack works by utilizing a chemical re-

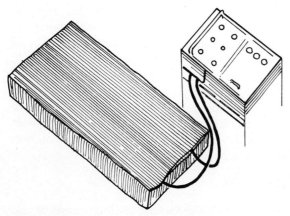

FIGURE 33-2. Hypothermia blanket and unit.

action. The bag, which is usually blue for cold or red for heat, is struck sharply against a hard surface or the edge of a table or countertop; it is then kneaded until the chemicals within combine. On mixing, their reaction causes the production of either heat or cold depending upon the nature of the chemicals involved.

SUMMARY

When applying thermal agents, it is important to remember that great care must be taken to safeguard the client from harm. Extremes in temperature or prolonged use of the agents are always potential sources of injury, in that the body's tolerance for temperature variations narrows as the duration increases. In addition, the greater the area of thermal application, the less tolerant the skin will be to the treatment. Caution must be used in following the procedures carefully; if there is any doubt as to any portion of the physician's instructions, this must be questioned and clarified before implementing the procedure. All observations, including the measurement of vital signs, the condition of the skin, and the responses of the client should be recorded and reported in the appropriate manner for the situation in which the procedure takes place.

BIBLIOGRAPHY

Dison, N.: *Clinical Nursing Techniques,* 3rd ed. St. Louis, C. V. Mosby Co., 1975.

Elhart, D., et al.: *Scientific Principles in Nursing,* 8th ed. St. Louis, C. V. Mosby Co., 1978.

Everall, M.: Cold therapy. *Nurs. Times* 72:144, 1976.

Fuerst, E., Wolff, L., and Weitzel, M.: *Fundamentals of Nursing,* 5th ed. Philadelphia, J. B. Lipppincott Co., 1974.

Leifer, G.: *Principles and Techniques in Pediatric Nursing.* Philadelphia, W. B. Saunders, Co., 1977.

Moore, J., et al.: The case of the warm, moist compress. *Can. Nurse* 71(3):19, 1975.

Nordmark, M. T., and Rohweder, A. W.: *Scientific Foundations of Nursing,* 3rd ed. Philadelphia, J. B. Lippincott Co., 1975.

Petrello, J. M.: Temperature maintenance of hot moist compresses. *Am. J. Nurs.* 73:1050, 1973.

Taber's Cyclopedic Medical Dictionary, 13th ed. Philadelphia, F. A. Davis Co., 1977.

CHAPTER 34

How often have you heard someone say, "I don't feel well. I think I'll go to the doctor and get a shot," or "I have a headache; I'm going to take an aspirin." We live in a society that is medication oriented. It is nearly impossible to open a magazine or watch television today without being bombarded by commercials offering relief from pain, headache, diarrhea, "irregularity," burping, bloating, and psoriasis. In any drugstore, there are aisles upon aisles of drug preparations that can be bought without a prescription or the advice of a knowledgeable health professional. Self-medication is certainly the rule rather than the exception. How many people do you know who do not have a single drug—that is, neither headache remedies, ointments, nose drops, nor birth control devices—in their home? The public has a very casual attitude toward the use of medicine. It is paradoxical that of all the areas of nursing practice, the administration of medications carries the greatest risk of error and calamity. This is an area that can hardly be treated casually.

ADMINISTRATION OF MEDICATIONS

Arlyne B. Saperstein, M.N., R.N., and
Margaret A. Frazier, M.S., R.N.

LEGISLATION

Until 1906 the sale and distribution of drugs was entirely unrestricted in this country. While some of the available preparations were fairly harmless, others were useless and often dangerous. The *Pure Food and Drug Act* of 1906 was the first federal legislation that attempted to prevent "the manufacture of adulterated or misbranded or poisonous . . . foods, drugs, medicines, and liquors" and to regulate traffic therein. This act gave the government the right to enforce official standards, that is, the United States Pharmacopoeia or USP, which was originally printed in 1820, and the National Formulary (NF). This law was clearly insufficient to protect the public.

In 1937, over 100 people died as a result of an anti-infective agent. The drug, sulfanilamide, was prepared with an untested solvent that proved to be toxic. It was because of this tragedy that the *Federal Food, Drug, and Cosmetic Act* of 1938 was passed. This law made it compulsory for all new

drugs to be tested before being marketed to insure safety. It further recognized the Homeopathic Pharmacopoeia of the United States as an official standard, taking its place with the USP and the NF. These three sources are still recognized today as legal standards.

In 1952, an amendment to the 1938 Federal Food, Drug, and Cosmetic Act was enacted. The *Durham-Humphrey Amendment* differentiated between prescription (those needing a physician's order) and over-the-counter drugs. It further stated that those drugs which could not be used without medical supervision must be labeled with a legend reading, "Caution, federal law prohibits dispensing without prescription." Refilling prescriptions could be done only when the physician authorized its renewal.

Once again, the same law was amended as a result of misfortune. In 1962, the *Kefauver-Harris Drug Amendment* was passed in response to the birth of deformed infants born to European women who had taken a sleeping medication, thalidomide, during early pregnancy. The amendment mandated that the compulsory testing must provide substantial evidence that the drug in question had the effect that it claimed to have. Thus, the government could now control efficacy of a drug as well as its safety.

The legislation of narcotics is a corollary to the discussion of drug control laws. In 1914, the Congress passed the *Harrison Narcotic Act* to control the manufacture, sale, transport, distribution, and importation of opium, coca (cocaine), and their derivatives. Revisions of this law extended coverage to all opium and cocaine products, as well as a variety of synthetic drugs that are similar to the original two narcotics. The *Drug Abuse Control Act* of 1965 further regulated the control and distribution of amphetamines, barbiturates, and habituating drugs, as well as others that cause depression, stimulation, or hallucinogenic effects on the central nervous system. A law entitled the *Controlled Substances Act* was passed in 1970 (although portions of it became effective in 1972), replacing the Harrison Act and all of its amendments. This law established five schedules or general categories of controlled substances (drugs). These include drugs for which there are no acceptable medical uses and those with varying (high to low) abuse potential. This act regulates the transportation, storage, prescription, and administration of these drugs. The ramifications of this act are great, particularly for nurses; guidelines to nursing practice and action in relation to the administration of controlled substances are clearly outlined.

Record keeping (including the client's name, the licensed prescriber's name, the drug, dosage, route, date, time of administration, and the nurse's signature) when administering these drugs from a stock supply, responsibility for the key to the storage cabinet, and accountability for the entire stock of controlled drugs belongs to the nurse. Any nurse convicted of a violation of any part of this act may be fined, imprisoned, and have her license revoked.

GOVERNMENT AGENCIES

The *Food and Drug Administration* is an arm of the Department of Health, Education, and Welfare (HEW). The primary function of this agency is to enforce the Federal Food, Drug, and Cosmetics Act. Its responsibilities include the insurance that foodstuffs sold in the U.S. are safe and pure; that drugs, apparatuses, and instruments used for therapeutic purposes are safe and effective; that materials used for cosmetic purposes cause no harm; and that all of the above are packaged with accurate labeling. An accurate reporting system is required of all firms manufacturing drugs. Also, information received by the FDA from other sources documents adverse reactions not formerly disclosed by research.

Another branch of HEW is the *Public Health Service* (PHS). The PHS regulates biologic products by the inspection and licensure of the manufacturers and the products. This department is known as the Division of Biological Standards of the National Institutes of Health.

The *Federal Trade Commission* (FTC) is an agency whose responsibility to the public with relation to drugs is to oversee and repress false and misleading advertising of nonprescription drugs.

Until July 1973, the Bureau of Narcotics and Dangerous Drugs enforced narcotic control. This was replaced at that time by the *Drug Enforcement Administration* (DEA) in the Department of Justice.

DRUGS

Classification

Drugs can be classified either by the system of the body that they affect, such as "drugs affecting the gastrointestinal tract," or by their *therapeutic action* which means (1) their effect on the body as a whole causes a specific, desirable result (i.e., vasodilation), (2) their effect on the causative organism itself (i.e., an anti-infective effect), or (3) their effect on the signs and symptoms of the illness (i.e., relief of pain). When speaking of the action of a drug, it should be noted that it may stimulate (increase) or depress (decrease) the activity of the cells. If the drug acts only at the site where it is applied, it is said to have a *local action;* if it is absorbed and distributed by the blood to all body parts, it is said to have *systemic action.* A drug can have both a systemic and local action, for instance, certain drugs are absorbed after being applied locally to the skin or mucous membranes. In addition, there are drugs that, although swallowed, have a local effect only, since absorption from the gastrointestinal mucosa does not occur. Table 34-1 lists many of the major classifications of drugs by therapeutic action. Remember that although a therapeutic or beneficial action is listed, most drugs have the potential of causing undesirable results as well as those that are expected. Knowledge of the action of drugs assists the nurse to recognize when an unanticipated effect has occurred.

Sources

It is helpful to be aware of the sources of drugs to understand the final product, as the original source influences the preparation and dosage of the drug.

Some drugs are obtained from *animal sources.* The body fluids, tissues, and organs are extracted from various animals (including man), and the products made from these are usually used as substitutes or replacements for deficiences in glandular secretions. Examples are insulin, thyroid, hormone, adrenocorticotropic hormone (ACTH), antitoxin serums, and gamma globulin.

Plants are probably the most widely used source from which relief of disease has been sought throughout history. Various parts of a plant are utilized: the bank, leaves, roots, oils, resins, gums, and tannins. Examples of these are digitalis (a glycoside which contains sugar), morphine (an alkaloid which is a nitrogenous substance), tinctures of opium and belladonna, cocaine, and senna (used for its laxative effect).

Mineral substances, such as metals, salts, clays, and radioactive isotopes are also used as drug sources. Examples are iodine, aluminum hydroxide, zinc oxide, magnesium citrate, and magnesium sulfate (better known as Epsom salts).

In modern medicine, many of the drugs that formerly could only be obtained from natural sources are now made artificially in the chemical laboratory. *Synthetic drugs* are usually more economical to manufacture and are free of the impurities that may occur in the natural drug form. Examples of laboratory-made drugs are sulfonamides, epinephrine, and oxytocin (the latter two also occur naturally). Certain antibiotics and vaccines are produced in the laboratory from *microorganisms*—bacteria, viruses, and *fungi*—such as penicillin, streptomycin, tetracycline, bacitracin, tetanus toxoid, polio (Sabin) vaccine, BCG vaccine (used for tuberculosis), influenza vaccine, and rubella (German measles) vaccine.

Drug Administration

The manner in which a drug is to be administered depends upon several considerations. (1) *What are the goals or objectives of the therapeutic plan?* Does the physician or dentist desire a local or a systemic effect from the drug (or both)? How quickly is the desired effect of the drug needed, and should the effect(s) last for a lengthy period of time or be of a short duration? (2) *What limitations or parameters are set by the client's physical and emotional state of being?* What is the client's level of consciousness and capacity for taking responsibility? Can he safely ingest oral feedings (liquids) and retain them? Can he swallow tablets? Does he have any conditions or disorders that prevent administration or affect absorption of drugs in the gastrointestinal tract, the mucous membranes, the genitourinary tract, the eyes, ears, nose, throat, skin, muscles, or lungs? (3) *What are the characteristics of the drug and its form(s) of preparation that also set certain guidelines or restrictions on its usage?* Can the specific drugs and the dosage ordered be administered safely and effectively via the desired route? Is the drug manufactured in the form preferred for this treatment program? Last, is the administration of this drug relatively uncomplicated and convenient for both the nurse and the client (and possibly his family)? Relative to this, for long-term drug therapy, is the client economically able to, intellectually capable of, and psychologically motivated to handle this particular mode of medication administration?

Drugs are prepared in a variety of ways. The drug form will be determined by the nature and properties of the drug, its intended purpose, and the route of administration. Many drugs come from the manufacturer in a number of forms to permit choices and alterations when needed in the plan of care.

In the manufacturing process, drugs may be combined with materials that are inert or therapeutically inactive. These substances, called *vehicles,* are the agents that carry the drug and give it its form or consistency.

TABLE 34-1. Classification of Drugs

Description	Effects/Actions
Adrenergic Agents (Sympathomimetics and Sympathetic Amines)	
Drugs that act similarly to sympathetic nervous system stimulants or parasympathetic nervous system depressants. They may behave similarly to antihistamines while others stimulate the central nervous system.	Affect musculature of heart (increasing rate and strength of contractions), blood vessels (vasoconstriction), eyes (dilation of pupils), urinary and gastrointestinal tracts (relaxation and decrease in muscle tone), and bronchi (dilation). Most glandular secretions are decreased.
Adrenergic Blocking Agents (Sympathoplegics, Sympatholytes, and Adrenolytics)	
Drugs that block secretion of norepinephrine and epinephrine, or nullify (antagonize) actions of sympathomimetic agents. Response usually seen with sympathetic nervous system stimulation is prevented by these drugs, thus their other name, *sympathetic depressants*.	Cause vasodilation, and increased peripheral circulation, decreased cardiac output, decreased blood pressure, and affect musculature of gastrointestinal tract and other smooth muscle tissue (increased tone).
Amebicides (Amebacide) and Trichomonacides	
Eradicates amebae.	Kills parasitic agent.
Analeptics	
Used for stimulation of central nervous system.	Respiratory stimulation, increased blood pressure, and vasoconstriction.
Analgesics	
One of the classifications of central nervous system depressants (along with sedative/hypnotics, anesthetics, and anticonvulsants). These drugs affect the brain (cerebral cortex and thalamus) by interference with nerve impulse conduction or alteration of pain perception.	Opium (and derivatives) narcotic analgesics may cause drowsiness (or in large dosages deep sleep), euphoria, clouding of mental and sensory functioning, constriction of pupils (miosis), depression of rate and depth of respirations and of the cough reflex, peripheral vasodilation, lowered blood pressure, smooth muscle relaxation, decreased peristalsis and therefore, constipation, nausea, and vomiting. These effects vary from drug to drug. Synthetic analgesics (like meperidine [Demerol]) have basically the same effects as opiates with less respiratory depression and addictive qualities.

Selected Uses	Selected Examples
For rapid increase of blood pressure (as in shock), as a mydriatic (dilates the pupils of the eyes), and for treatment of bronchitis, asthma, allergic conditions, and nasal congestion.	Epinephrine (Adrenalin), aminophylline, Wyamine, Isuprel, Sudafed, Afrin, Neo-Synephrine, and Visine.
For treatment of peripheral vascular diseases, hypertension, migraine and vascular headaches, and to decrease postpartum hemorrhage.	Ergotrate, Methergine, Sansert, Aldomet, and Regitine.
For treatment of acute and chronic amebiasis, disease caused by *Entamoeba histolytica* (a protozoan), and trichomoniasis, caused by a parasitic flagellate protozoan.	Carbarsone, emetine hydrochloride, Ipecac, and Flagyl.
To reverse respiratory depression that occurs when central nervous system depressants (such as barbiturates) have had toxic effect.	Metrazol, Coramine, Dopram, and Benzedrine.
Used to treat various intensities of pain (from mild to severe), reduce coughing, relieve diarrhea, and provide sleep when pain prevents it.	Morphine sulfate, Dilaudid, Demerol, Talwin, codeine phosphate, Hycodan, Darvon, aspirin, Tylenol, and paregoric.

TABLE 34-1. Continued

Description	Effects/Actions
Anesthetics	
General anesthetics produce unconsciousness and loss of sensation by depressing the central nervous system. Local anesthetics are not central nervous system depressants but act by blocking conduction of impulses to the brain from nerves to which they are injected or applied, producing loss of sensitivity to pain with no accompanying loss in consciousness.	General anesthetics cause: loss of pain sensation; loss of consciousness; changes in pupil size (dilation), corneal and light reflexes, and eyeball movement; changes (depression) in respirations, pulse, and blood pressure; and muscular relaxation. Local anesthetics cause: insensitivity to both pain and changes in temperature, (nerve endings are deadened) and vasodilation.
Antacids	
Mineral drugs that reduce or neutralize hydrochloric acid in stomach.	Direct neutralization of or buffering of gastric acid. Astringent action (when some drugs combine with acid) adds protection for ulceration; delaying of emptying time of gastric contents occurs.
Anthelmintics (Helminthics)	
Drugs used to rid body of parasitic worms.	Each drug has its own action or effects, including direct killing of parasite, paralysis of its muscles, inhibition of its metabolism or its growth, or sterilization of adult female parasite.
Antiarrhythmic Agents	
Drugs used to treat cardiac arrhythmias (alterations in rate and rhythm of heart).	Drugs vary in their actions, including stimulation of vagus nerve, reduction of heart rate, and cardiac output, increase in strength of contractions, depression of myocardial excitability (irritability), prolonging of refractory (muscle relaxation) period of heart, and facilitation of atrioventricular node conduction.
Antibiotics (Bacteriocidals and Bacteriostatics)	
A synthetic or natural drug which kills microorganisms or inhibits or prevents their growth. Broad spectrum drugs are effective against a number of microorganisms, while narrow spectrum drugs have activity specific to only a few microorganisms.	These drugs block cell wall formation or synthesis of protein or enzyme formation in microorganism, therefore obstructing or interfering with its metabolism.

Selected Uses	Selected Examples

For induction and maintenance of loss of sensation and consciousness. Used during surgery when muscle relaxation is mandatory. For loss of pain sensation topically (at skin surface) or in specific area or region of body.

Cyclopropane, nitrous oxide, Trilene, ether, Penthrane, halothane, Pentothal, Brevital, Surfacaine, Nupercainal ointment, Novocain, Xylocaine, Butyn, and Pontocaine.

For treatment of hyperacidity (heartburn), and peptic ulcers; to decrease pain caused by hyperacidity and to promote healing of an ulcer. (Certain drugs can be used for their laxative effect.)

Aluminum hydroxide, magnesium hydroxide, calcium carbonate, and sodium bicarbonate.

To treat cases of infestations of nematodes (roundworms), including ascariasis, trichonosis, pinworms, hookworms, and threadworms, *Platyhelminthes* (flatworms or tapeworms) and trematodes (flukes), the most notable schistosomiasis or bilharziasis.

Piperazine citrate (Antepar), Vermox, gentian violet, Povan, Mintezol, Antiminth, and Caprokol.

Treatment of various cardiac arrhythmias, including atrial and ventricular tachycardia and fibrillation, atrial flutter, premature systoles, and extrasystoles, sinus bradycardia and arrest, sinus tachycardia, conduction defects, and heart block.

Digoxin, quinidine, Dilatin, lidocaine, Isuprel, Inderal, and atropine.

For treatment of diseases or infections caused by bacteria, gram-positive or gram-negative organisms, spirochetes, and rickettsial diseases. They may also be used prophylactically in the presence of viral infections to prevent bacterially caused secondary infections or in debilitated persons to prevent infection.

Penicillin, streptomycin, tetracycline, Kantrex, Keflin, Erythrocin, Chloromycetin, Lincocin, bacitracin, and neomycin.

TABLE 34-1. Continued

Description	Effects/Actions

Anticholenergic Drugs (Parasympatholytics and Cholinergic Blocking Agents)

Drugs that antagonize acetylcholine, affect and cause depression of parasympathetic nervous system, and have an effect similar to sympathetic nervous system stimulants.

These agents counteract vagal stimulation, increasing heart (and thus, respiratory) rate, relax smooth muscles, reduce peristalsis, decrease glandular secretions (such as saliva, gastric juices, and bronchial secretions), and dilate pupils (mydriasis).

Anticoagulants: Thrombolytics

Anticoagulants are agents that inhibit coagulation of blood. In case of blood clots, thrombolytic drugs cause them to dissolve more rapidly.

Interfere with the process of coagulation. Prevents prothrombin synthesis, reducing amount found in the blood.

Anticonvulsants

Agents which prevent or are used in treatment of seizures or convulsions, usually caused by neurological disorder—epilepsy.

These drugs depress (selectively) the brain's motor center or raise the seizure (stimulation) threshold in the neurons of the central nervous system.

Antidepressant (Psychic Energizers and Psychoanaleptics)

Drugs used as mood elevators in clients with depression. These drugs are divided into two main classes, tricyclics and monoamine oxidase (MAO) inhibitors.

Although actions are somewhat uncertain, it appears that these drugs increase levels of norepinephrine (when insufficient in amount it is thought that depression occurs), and serotonin (thought to be related to sensory perception and sleep) in the brain.

Antidiarrheics

Drugs which inhibit diarrhea and hypermotility of the gastrointestinal tract.

Slows motility of intestine; peristaltic activity is inhibited by effect on intestinal musculature.

Antiemetics

Drugs that are used to prevent or treat nausea and vomiting.

Control vertigo by action on vestibular apparatus of the ear, or vomiting by depression of the medulla (chemoreceptor trigger zone).

Antiflatulents (Carminatives)

Agents used for relief of gastric or intestinal distention caused by gas.

Many of these drugs change the surface tension of gas and cause bubbles of air to coalesce. They prevent air pockets from forming in the gastrointestinal tract.

Selected Uses	Selected Examples
To dilate pupils; to reduce smooth muscle spasm (antispasmodic), such as spasms of the bladder, stomach, and gallbladder, to decrease secretions; to treat bronchial asthma, peptic ulcers, hypermotility of the gastrointestinal tract, and parkinsonism.	Atropine sulfate (belladonna), hysocyamine, scopolamine, Valpin, Bentyl, Banthine, Pro-Banthine, Cogentin, Artane, and Mydriacyl.
Treatment of thrombophlebitis and pulmonary embolism to prolong clotting time. Prophylactically to prevent stroke.	Dicumarol, Coumadin, and heparin sodium.
To control seizures and prevent occurrence of convulsions in grand mal, petit mal, and psychomotor forms of epilepsy.	Dilantin, Milontin, Tridione, Valium, and phenobarbital.
To treat psychotic and neurotic types of depression and anxiety.	Elavil, Parnate, Tofranil, Sinequan, and Ritalin.
Treatment of diarrhea, flatulence, and gastrointestinal hypermotility.	Kaopectate, Pargel, kaolin, Lomotil, and bentonite magma.
To treat and prevent nausea, vomiting, vertigo (dizziness or loss of equilibrium), and motion sickness.	Compazine, Dramamine, Antivert, Atarax, Torecan, Tigan, and Vistaril.
To treat abdominal distention (flatulence). (Usually used with antacids.)	Simethicone, Ilopan, activated charcoal, bentonite magma, oil of peppermint, aluminum hydroxide gel, and bismuth subgallate.

TABLE 34-1. Continued

Description	Effects/Actions
Antifungals, Fungicides, and Fungistatics	
Drugs used to kill or check growth of fungi or yeasts.	Interference with cell membrane functioning or with cell division.
Antihistamines	
An abnormal amount of histamine is released into body tissues in cases of hypersensitivity and acute allergic reactions. These drugs antagonize (counteract) effects of histamine in structures, while having no effect on histamine release or synthesis.	Prevention of vasodilation, formation of edema, and itching. Increased permeability of capillaries, central nervous system depression, causing drowsiness and in some cases, sedation and muscle relaxation.
Antihypertensives (Vasodilators and Ganglionic Blocking Agents)	
Agents which reduce blood pressure by causing vasodilation to occur.	These drugs work by lessening resistance to blood flow through relaxation (dilation) of vasoconstricted peripheral vessels. They decrease effects of the sympathetic nervous system on the musculature of arterioles (blocking impulses of the sympathetic nervous system) causing vasodilation, or they have direct action on arteriolar smooth muscle.
Antihypotensives—See Adrenergic Agents	
Anti-inflammatory Agents	
A drug that counteracts or diminishes inflammatory reactions (or their effects). Many also have analgesic or antipyretic effects as well. Corticosteroids are known for their anti-inflammatory effects.	Little is known about anti-inflammatory action of drugs. Lowering of the prostaglandin (fatty acid derivatives) levels may have to do with the drugs' effects.
Antimalarials (Plasmodicides)	
Anti-infective agents which prevent or cure the disease, malaria.	Causes destruction of asexual forms of malarial parasites. Prophylactically makes blood noninfective to the mosquito (*Anopheles*).
Antiparasitics	
Agents used to rid the skin of infestation with mites.	Kills eggs (nits) and adult forms of pediculi.

Selected Uses	Selected Examples
Used to treat infections caused by *Candida* organism; and mycotic infections such as histoplasmosis, coccidioidomycosis, and cryptococcosis.	Nystatin, Mycostatin, Fungizone, and griseofulvin.
To treat symptoms of allergies caused by release of histamine, inflammation and congestion of nasal mucosa due to coryza (common cold) and allergic reactions, asthma, itching (pruritus), conjunctivitis, motion sickness, nausea, and parkinsonism.	Dimetane, Benadryl, Chlor-Trimeton, Phenergan, and Pyribenzamine.
To treat hypertension (mild to severe), peripheral vascular disorders, migraine headaches, arteriosclerosis, and angina pectoris.	Reserpine, Cyclospasmol, Paveron, Apresoline hydrochloride, amyl nitrite, Isordil, papaverine, Unitensen, Ismelin sulfate, and Aldomet.
For treatment of rheumatic diseases such as rheumatoid arthritis and rheumatic fever, lupus erythematosus, gout, and post-traumatic inflammatory conditions.	Aspirin, Indocin, Butazolidin, Nalfon, Naprosyn, cortisone, hydrocortisone ointment, Depo-Medrol, Solu-Cortef, and prednisone.
For prophylaxis or treatment of malaria and treatment of lupus erythematosus, rheumatoid arthritis, and amebiasis.	Primaquine phosphate, quinine sulfate, and Atabrine.
To treat pediculosis (lice) and scabies.	Sulfur, gamma benzene hexachloride (Kwell), Benylate, creosote ointment, and xylene ointment.

TABLE 34-1. Continued

Description	Effects/Actions
Antipruritics	
Drugs that relieve itching. Relief is usually temporary.	Ointments or lotions are applied topically for local relief of itching. Corticosteroids can be injected locally or antihistamines administered orally for their antagonistic effect against histamine.
Antipyretics	
Drugs which reduce elevated body temperatures.	These drugs lower body temperature in febrile states only. They do not lower normal temperatures. They act on the hypothalamus, and it is thought that they affect (lower) the thermostatic setting. Peripheral dilation increases heat loss, and the temperature, therefore, drops. A mild analgesic action also accompanies the antipyretic effect. Some of these drugs also have anti-inflammatory properties.
Antiseptics and Disinfectants (Germicides and Bactericides)	
Chemical agents which prevent growth of microorganisms and can be applied to living tissue. Disinfectants destroy microorganisms (although spores may survive). Used in varying strengths, some may be applied to living tissue. Usually they are used on inanimate objects.	Actions vary and are not always known, but most agents affect by chemical reactions with the enzyme systems, protein or protoplasm of the microbe.
Antitoxins, Toxoids, and Vaccines	
Antitoxins are agents (serums) containing specific antibodies which provide short-term passive immunity to a disease, either preventing its occurrence or diminishing its severity. (Passive immunity means that antibodies come from a source other than the individual himself.) Serum is obtained from blood of animals in which infection with a disease has been initiated causing antibody formation to take place, or from blood of persons who have recovered from the disease. (These are known as immune serums.) Toxoids and vaccines are agents containing antigens that are live (but diminished in virulence), dead, or partially detoxified. These cause active immunity (production of antibodies within the individual's bloodstream) to occur.	The body's defense against disease, or its immune response, occurs when antibodies interact with antigens (foreign substances [protein], toxins, and bacteria) to which they are specific or sensitive. The result, depending on the type of antibody, can be neutralization of the antigen's toxins, clumping (agglutination) of bacteria, rupturing (lysis), or dissolving of the bacterial cell, or a coating of bacteria that facilitates the process of phagocytosis.

Selected Uses	Selected Examples
Treatment of skin disorders or allergic reactions that cause itching and pruritus vulvae.	Temaril, Tacaryl, Forhistal, hydrocortisone ointment, and calamine lotion.
Treatment of pyrexia and mild pain or discomfort.	Aspirin, Tylenol, Tempra, Arthropan, and phenacetin.
Various agents each have their own use, including disinfecting utensils and environmental objects, as well as destroying microorganisms that have contaminated food or water supplies. For cleaning skin, mucous membranes, and wounds, for treatment of burns, and to prevent gonococcal infection in the newborn's eyes.	Ethyl alcohol, isopropyl alcohol, Dakin's solution, iodine (Betadine), ammoniated mercury ointment, Merthiolate, silver nitrate solution, hydrogen peroxide, potassium permanganate, cresol, phenol, pHisoHex, benzalkonium chloride, Cēpacol, genetian violet, Burow's solution, boric acid, formalin, and Furacin.
Toxoids and vaccines are prophylactically used to prevent a person from contracting a disease by causing his body to produce antibodies specific to that disease. Antitoxins are usually used to prevent, or make less severe, an illness in an individual who has already been exposed to it.	BCG vaccine (tuberculosis), diphtheria toxoid or antitoxin, DPT (diphtheria and tetanus toxoids and pertussis vaccine), immune serum globulin, measles virus vaccine, mumps virus vaccine, rubella virus vaccine, Sabine vaccine (attenuated polio virus), rabies vaccine, influenza virus vaccine, typhoid vaccine, smallpox vaccine (for use out of the country), and typhus vaccine.

TABLE 34-1. Continued

Description	Effects/Actions

Antitussives (Demulcents and Emollients)

Agents that inhibit or prevent coughing.

These drugs work by protecting (coating) mucous membranes from mechanical irritation caused by coughing or by depression of the medulla (cough center) preventing the cough reflex.

Astringents

Agents which when applied to skin or mucous membrane cause shrinkage (contraction) of tissue and therefore, a decrease in secretions or discharge.

These drugs influence both osmosis, by changing surface tension of cells, and precipitation (coagulation) of protein. They reduce oiliness of skin, excessive perspiration, itching and chafing of skin, swelling, and stop bleeding from minor cuts.

Cardiotonics (Cardiac Glycosides)

Drugs which increase the strength of myocardial contraction and thus increase efficiency of the heart.

The vagus nerve is stimulated, causing more forceful pumping action, increasing cardiac output and improving circulation. Pulse strengthens and slows. Edema, cyanosis, and respiratory difficulties subside with greater cardiac efficiency.

Carminatives:—See Antiflatulents

Cathartics (Laxatives and Purgatives)

Drugs which encourage or cause bowel evacuation. A laxative is a mild cathartic; a strong cathartic is called a purgative.

Saline cathartics: the solution has high osmotic pressure; water is retained in the intestine, increasing bulk and fluidity of stool, and thus, promotion of peristalsis. Edema is reduced by loss of fluid from blood and tissues.

Bulk cathartics: volume of feces is increased by nonabsorbable substances.

Stimulant or irritant cathartics: chemical substances that directly stimulate the smooth musculature of the bowel, thereby increasing its contractility.

Emollient or lubricant cathartic: a fecal softener; stool passes more readily through the intestine due to decrease in friction when feces are emulsified or reabsorption of water is prevented by addition of the agent.

Selected Uses	Selected Examples
To reduce pain and irritation by supressing coughing (especially nonproductive) associated with acute or chronic upper respiratory infections or allergic diseases.	Codeine, Hycodan, Tuss-Ornade, Romilar, glycerin, Tessalon, and Sucrets.
To treat symptoms of various skin conditions and forms of dermatitis. Also, in certain cases, to treat mucous membranes of the throat and eye to relieve inflammatory symptoms. To stop bleeding from minor cuts (as in shaving).	Zinc oxide, calamine, witch hazel, alum, aluminum acetate solution, aluminum hydroxide gel, tannic acid, boric acid, sodium borate, and styptic pencils.
Treatment of failing (decompensating) heart (congestive heart failure) and heart with atrial flutter or fibrillation. Used in cases where ventricles are not emptying properly (due to insufficient contraction of the myocardium) therefore causing decreased cardiac output.	Digoxin (Lanoxin), Cedilanid, digitoxin, gitalin, and ouabain.
Treatment of occasional (as opposed to chronic) constipation; as preparation for surgery or diagnostic procedures; to treat specific gastrointestinal disorders.	Fleet enema, milk of magnesia, Epsom salts, magnesium citrate, methylcellulose, Metamucil, bran, cascara sagrada, Modane, Senokot, castor oil, Dulcolax, glycerin suppositories, Ex-Lax, Surfak, Colace, and mineral oil.

TABLE 34-1. Continued

Description	Effects/Actions

Cholinergic Agents (Parasympathomimetics and Parasympathetic Stimulants)

Drugs which behave like or simulate the actions of acetylcholine (which is needed for transmission of nerve impulses), thus causing parasympathetic nervous system stimulation	Decreases rate and conductivity of the heart, causes vasodilation, increases smooth muscle tone (contraction), increases most glandular secretions, relaxes the bladder, constricts the pupils, and reduces intraocular pressure

Counterirritants

Agents which relieve irritation in a deeper structure by causing a local irritation or inflammatory reaction.	By topically irritating the skin (superficial irritation), circulation is increased; this in turn relieves irritation or inflammation of structures located adjacent to or beneath the skin.

Cycloplegics, Mydriatics, and Miotics

Cycloplegics are drugs which render adjustment of the eye to vision at different distances (accommodation) impossible. Mydriatics dilate the pupils. Miotics constrict the pupils.	Cycloplegics paralyze the ciliary muscle, thus paralyzing accommodation. Mydriatics cause pupil dilation and increased intraocular pressure. Miotics cause stimulation of the ciliary muscle, resulting in spasm of accommodation, constriction of the pupil, and decrease in intraocular pressure.

Cytotoxic Agents (Antineoplastic Drugs)

A drug that is poisonous to both normal and cancerous (neoplastic) cells. The latter, because of greater activity and faster proliferation, are affected more by these drugs.	Alkylating agents: interfere with cell reproduction (mitosis) by linking with the cell's nucleic acid and damaging the cell's DNA.
	Antimetabolites: cell metabolites' functions are mimicked or replaced by the drug causing cell metabolism to stop functioning. Natural products, including antibiotics, enzymes, hormones, and plant alkaloids interfere with cell division by stopping it at a certain phase, or by catabolyzing certain substances needed for metabolism, or by making environmental conditions unfavorable for cellular growth. Certain forms of cancer are destroyed by radioactive isotopes.

Selected Uses	Selected Examples
Treatment of urinary retention occurring after surgery or childbirth, glaucoma, myasthenia gravis, specific types of constipation or abdominal distention, as the antidote for the effects of belladonna (atropine) or scopolamine.	Urecholine, prostigmin bromide, Ilopan, Tensilon, pilocarpine hydrochloride, and Phospholine Iodide.
To relieve inflammation or irritation of structures beneath the skin, as muscles or joints, as in rheumatic conditions, arthritis, and sciatica.	Methylsalicylate (oil of wintergreen), and chloroform liniment.
To permit ophthalmoscopic examination for errors of refraction and scrutinization of the eye's inner structures (including retina and optic disc). To treat specific conditions or diseases of eyes. (For example, miotics are useful in treating glaucoma, and mydriatics relieve ciliary spasm.)	Atropine sulfate, homatropine, scopolamine hydrobromide (hyoscine), cyclopentolate hydrochloride (Cyclogyl), pilocarpine hydrochloride, Floropryl, Humorsol, acetylcholine chloride.
Chemotherapy is used alone or in conjunction with other therapy (as radiation) in treatment of cancer.	Cytoxan, nitrogen mustard, 6-mercaptopurine, methotrexate, vinblastine, L-asparaginase, and radioactive iodine.

TABLE 34-1. Continued

Description	Effects/Actions
Demulcents, Emollients, and Protectives	
Drugs which coat, protect, and soothe skin and mucous membranes.	Demulcents are colloidal substances that coat and protect mucous membranes and tissue.
	Emollients are fatty (oily) substances which soften, coat, protect, and soothe skin; and reduce pain and itching locally.
	Protectives are used to form a film on the skin to prevent irritations or cover raw or abraded skin surfaces.
Diuretics	
Drugs that increase the production of urine and decrease extracellular fluid.	Promotes sodium excretion (as well as chloride and potassium) by decreasing rate of (or preventing) water and electrolyte absorption in the renal tubules.
Emetics	
Agents that cause vomiting.	Directly irritate (stimulate) mucous membranes of the gastrointestinal tract, or stimulate the chemoreceptor trigger zone in the medulla of the brain (vomiting center).
Emollients—See Demulcents, Emollients, and Protectives	
Expectorants	
Drugs which assist with removal of mucus, secretions and exudate from the respiratory tract.	Loosen or liquefy tenacious mucus and increase its removal from the lungs. Some may reduce inflammation and assist with healing of mucous membranes. Bronchial secretions may be reduced.
Germicides—See Antiseptics and Germicides	
Hematinics (Hematopoietics)	
Drugs that increase the amount of hemoglobin in the blood, and stimulate production of blood cells.	Replacement of deficient iron will correct anemias caused by loss of or erythrocyte destruction. Replacement of inadequate vitamins or minerals needed for manufacture of blood cells in bone marrow will correct deficient production.

Selected Uses	Selected Examples
To treat the throat and reduce coughing; to soothe inflamed or abraded skin; to form a protective barrier from drainage in clients with stomas (as in colostomies); treatment of skin ulcerations.	Cold cream, acacia, glycerin, tincture of benzoin, and karaya.
To control edema (especially that which accompanies cardiac disease); in treatment of specific types of hypertension, hepatic disorders, certain renal disorders, and premenstrual retention of fluid.	Diuril, Hygroton, Diamox, Thiomerin, Lasix, Aldactone, and mannitol.
For induction of vomiting (emesis) when a toxic substance has been swallowed.	Ipecac, mustard, copper sulfate, and apomorphine hydrochloride.
To treat respiratory conditions, such as bronchitis, which are associated with viscous pulmonary secretions, and irritation of mucous membranes.	Robitussin, potassium iodide solution, terpin hydrate elixir, eucalyptus oil, Mucomyst, and ammonium chloride.
To correct anemias (iron deficiency or blood cell production deficit types). (Copper, manganese, cobalt, nickel, and zinc may be added to iron preparations to aid in their utilization.)	Fer-In-Sol, ferrous sulfate, Imferon, Jectofer, and liver injection.

TABLE 34-1. Continued

Description	Effects/Actions

Hemostatics (Coagulants)

Agents that control or stop oozing, bleeding or hemorrhage.

Topical agents (gelatin) absorb blood and then are slowly absorbed systemically. Systemic agents inhibit plasminogen activators or aid thrombin formation from prothrombin.

Hormones (The specific hormones are too numerous to list, therefore, they will be treated generally.)

These substances are produced by tissues, organs and mainly, by endocrine glands. Carried via the blood, they either stimulate or depress functional activities and processes. Hormones used for replacement therapy come from animal sources or are synthesized in the laboratory.

Specific hormones, when lacking or out of balance will cause mild to severe symptoms, depending on the hormone itself and how drastic the imbalance. Replacement will usually decrease or prevent symptoms.

Hypnotics (Somnifacients and Soporifics), Sedatives, and Tranquilizers (Ataractics, Ataraxics, Antianxiety Agents, and Antipsychotic Agents)

Hypnotics are drugs that cause sleep to occur (also known as somnifacients or soporifics). High dosages of barbiturates have a hypnotic effect. Sedatives are calming and quieting in effect and may produce drowsiness. Low dosages of barbiturates have a sedating effect. Determination of hypnotic as opposed to sedative effect is mainly based on dosage.

Hypnotics and sedatives depress the central nervous system, and interfere with nerve impulse transmission to the cerebral cortex. In addition to motor center depression, there may be (in large dosages) depression of vital organs, affecting heart rate and respirations. Therefore, depending on the drug and dosage, effects may include drowsiness, sleep, loss of muscular coordination, changes in reflexes, decreased awareness of and response to stimuli, and changes in vital signs with possible respiratory depression.

Tranquilizers are psychotropic drugs (affecting the mind) that calm or quiet the individual with less likelihood of drowsiness (as with sedatives). They can be classified as antianxiety agents or antipsychotic agents.

Tranquilizers have a muscle relaxant effect, certain anticonvulsant properties, reduce mental activities and response to stress, and may have antiemetic qualities as well as decreasing hyperactivity and aggressive behavior. They usually do not depress the central nervous system.

Immune Serums—See Antitoxins, Toxoids, and Vaccines

Laxatives—See Cathartics

Miotics—See Cycloplegics, Mydriatics, and Miotics

Mydriatics—See Cycloplegics, Mydriatics, and Miotics

Oxytocics—See Hormones

Selected Uses	Selected Examples
To control bleeding in individuals with defective clotting (as in hemophilia) or to control capillary oozing or bleeding (as during surgical procedures).	Gelfoam, thrombin, Hemofil, Proplex, and fibrinogen.
Use of these substances is for correction of deficits or imbalances that cause disorders or disease. (For example, insulin is used in the disease diabetes.) In addition, they are used in antineoplastic therapy, and in labor, delivery and postpartum (after delivery) care to promote uterine contractions (assisting the labor process and controlling postpartum hemorrhage).	Ovarian hormones, estrogen, progesterone, insulin, pituitary hormone (posterior pituitary hormones—oxytocics), adrenal hormone, and thyroid hormone.
Hypnotics and sedatives: to control disorders in which convulsions may occur, to cause anesthesia, for preoperative and postoperative rest and reduction of anxiety, for certain cases of insomnia, and as an adjunct in treating specific conditions, such as certain cardiac disorders, and gastrointestinal disturbances.	Amytal sodium, Brevital, Butisol sodium, Nembutal, Seconal, Luminal sodium (phenobarbital), pentothal sodium, paraldehyde, Noctec, Placidyl, Delmane, Doriden, Quaālude, and calcium bromide.
Tranquilizers: to treat tension, anxiety (mild to moderate with antianxiety agents, severe agitation with antipsychotic agents), to treat symptoms of neuroses and psychoses, delirium tremens (in alcohol withdrawal), muscle spasms, arthritis, certain convulsive conditions, asthma, and vomiting.	Librium, Valium, Equanil (meprobamate), Mellaril, Thorazine, Prolixin, Trilafon, Sparine, Compazine, Stelazine, Haldol, lithium carbonate.

TABLE 34-1. Continued

Description	Effects/Actions
Protectives—See Demulcents, Emollients, and Protectives	
Purgatives—See Cathartics	
Sedatives—See Hypnotics, Sedatives, and Tranquilizers	
Somnifacients—See Hypnotics, Sedatives, and Tranquilizers	
Soporifics—See Hypnotics, Sedatives, and Tranquilizers	
Stimulants (Central Nervous System)	
Drugs which increase activities of organs or systems.	By stimulating the central nervous system (vasomotor and respiratory centers of the medulla) and cerebral cortex, they increase heart and respiratory rates, motor activities, and alertness. They also elevate the mood, sometimes to the point of mild euphoria. Fatigue and appetite are suppressed. Dilation of the pupils and bronchi and contraction of sphincter of the bladder are effects of amphetamine stimulants.
Sulfonamides	
Bacteriostatic agents used to fight gram-negative and gram-positive microorganisms.	Interference with growth (multiplication) of specific bacteria. They do not destroy mature microorganisms.
Toxoids—See Antitoxins, Toxoids, and Vaccines	
Tranquilizers—See Hypnotics, Sedatives, and Tranquilizers	
Vaccines—See Antitoxins, Toxoids, and Vaccines	
Vasoconstrictors—See Adrenergic Agents	
Vasodilators—Also See Antihypertensives	
Agents which dilate the peripheral blood vessels or those in the heart, various organs, and skeletal muscles.	Relaxation of the muscles surrounding peripheral capillaries and arteries, increasing the peripheral circulation and blood flow to the extremities. Nitrates and nitrites (coronary vasodilators) decrease the blood pressure and stroke volume of the heart and decrease heart muscle hypoxia.

Note: Placebos, although not a drug classification, are mentioned here to alert the student to the use of inert substances (usually sterile water, sterile normal saline for injection, or sugar pills). The purpose of the administration is for psychological effects only; the client thinking he has been given a particular medication

Selected Uses	Selected Examples
To treat obesity (by controlling appetite), some cases of chronic exhaustion or fatigue, specific abnormal patterns of behavior, urinary problems (such as incontinence), fainting (to stimulate respirations), narcolepsy, certain metabolic deficiencies, shock and collapse (to stimulate cardiac and respiratory functioning), and to overcome effects of depressant overdosage.	Spirits of ammonia, Benzedrine, caffeine, Dexedrine, Desoxyn, Ritalin hydrochloride, Metrazol, Tenuate, Preludin hydrochloride, and Dopram.
Treatment of certain infectious disorders such as urinary tract and respiratory infections, burns (with wound infection), bacillary dysentery, ophthalmic infections, chancroid, vaginal infections, toxoplasmosis, and meningococcal meningitis.	Sulamyd sodium, Thiosulfil, Gantrisin, sulfa, sulfadiazine, Sultrin, and Silvadene.
According to type of vasodilator administered, for treatment of peripheral vascular disease, dysmenorrhea, diabetic vascular disease, angina pectoris, hypertension, asthma, coronary insufficiency, and to relieve intestinal, bronchial and urethral colic.	Cyclospasmol, Vasodilan, Pavabid, Roniacol, amyl nitrite, Isordil, nitroglycerin, Maxitate, and Unitensin acetate.

will occasionally "feel better." The use of placebos must be ordered by a physician. Their use is quite controversial.

ORAL ROUTE

Provided there are no contraindications to the oral route, such as with unconscious clients or those who have been designated as having "NPO" (nothing by mouth) status, this is certainly the simplest and most frequently used method of administering medications. It is probably the most inexpensive route since no special equipment, such as syringes, needles, and alcohol swabs are needed for administration. This route is also considered to be the least traumatic. Further, depending upon the rate of absorption the safety factor is greater with the oral route under certain circumstances since vomiting or gastric lavage (cleansing out the stomach) could prevent the absorption of any drug remaining in the stomach. In the following paragraphs, dosage forms used in the administration of oral medications are discussed.

Tablets

A drug in powdered or granular form is compressed or molded into the shape of a flattened disk (or other configuration that the manufacturer believes make it attractive or distinctive, such as a triangle). *Uncoated* tablets will readily disintegrate after being swallowed, while *coated* tablets may be more palatable (the coating is often flavored and the drug within it, bitter) and have a longer shelf-life as the coating protects the drug from environmental influences. Drugs that irritate the stomach and cause nausea or those that would be destroyed if they came in contact with the acidic secretions in the stomach are also coated. This *enteric coating* will not dissolve in the stomach but is soluble in the alkaline contents of the small intestine where the drug is ultimately absorbed. This same principle is used in the manufacture of certain *long (prolonged) action* or *controlled (sustained) release* oral medications. An enteric coated tablet may have an outer layer of the same drug compressed around it; the outside layer dissolves first, and at a later time, the inner tablet dissolves, repeating the dosage. In another of these long-acting drug forms, the medication is carried in an insoluble, inert plastic vehicle that is quite porous; the drug is very slowly released as the tablet moves along the gastrointestinal tract. This dosage form has the advantage of being administered less frequently than single dose forms of the same medication, thereby saving time and effort for both the client and the nurse.

For clients (adults and children) who experience difficulty swallowing tablets, certain drugs are placed in a chewable form. Calcium, vitamin, and iron preparations can be found in this form. Many antacids are also produced as chewable tablets, making them easy to carry and take without water and also hastening the disintegration process giving more rapid action of the drug. In addition, aspirin can be obtained in the form of chewing gum.

Pills are drugs in the form of a powder or pellet that has been molded into a spherical shape. This form is rarely seen today; when tablets are referred to as pills, it is actually incorrect.

Capsules

Medications (one or more) that are placed within a container made of gelatin to keep the bitter or unpleasant flavors of the drug from being tasted are called capsules. Hard capsules are made up of two halves and contain the drug(s) in powdered form. Soft capsules usually contain a liquid medication and are therefore sealed closed. Capsules can also be prepared as long-acting drug forms. Tiny beads of a drug are encased in different thicknesses of a coating. These are mixed with uncoated beads and placed in a gelatin capsule. The uncoated pellets are the first to dissolve and be absorbed, and the remainder dissolve at varying intervals of time. Any one of these time-release drugs (including the tablets referred to previously) should never be modified, (i.e., crushed or halved) to make swallowing easier for the client, as the risk of overdosage is increased. If they cannot be swallowed, the physician should be notified so that another form of drug can be prescribed. (Some prolonged action drugs also come in liquid form.)

Troches (Lozenges)

Troches are drug preparations that are usually mixed with mucilage and sugar and formed into disks or similar shapes. These are meant to be held in the mouth, much like a sucking candy, and dissolved.

Sublingual tablets are small tablets which are placed and kept under the tongue and allowed to dissolve. The drug has a systemic effect after being absorbed through the rich network of capillaries found in this area.

Like sublingual tablets, *buccal tablets* are not swallowed. They are held between the cheek and the gums (or teeth). Absorption through the mucous membrane in the buccal cavity is meant to be slow. Clients should be instructed not to disturb sublingual or buccal tablets, not to chew them, and not to swallow food or fluids while the tablet is in place.

Powders

Drugs are ground finely into powders or prepared as granules. In some cases the drugs are dispensed as premeasured single dosage forms in little paper packets. (This is rarely seen today.) The drug may also be obtained in bulk form with instructions as to an amount that is to be measured out and stirred in water until dissolved. Some of these powders are effervescent. The drug is combined with an acid (citric acid) and an alkali (sodium bicarbonate) which when dissolved in water react together and yield carbon dioxide bubbles or effervescence. Certain of these effervescent powdered drugs are now formed into tablets which when dropped into water have the same result.

Solutions

Solutions are a homogeneous mixture of a drug (the solute) and water (the solvent). Concentrated (saturated) solutions are made by adding large quantities of very soluble drugs to the solvent. An *aromatic water* is a solution that has had a volatile material, such as cinnamon oil, added to disguise the unpleasant taste of the solute. A *liquor* contains a nonvolatile material dissolved in water. *Syrups* are sugar solutions to which a flavoring such as orange or chocolate is added to hide unpleasant tasting drugs. Pediatric medications are often mixed with syrups to make them palatable to children. However, the danger in this practice is that they often taste so good that the child, if he manages to obtain a large enough quantity of the medication, often swallows it all, suffering an overdose. Extreme care must be taken to keep medications out of the reach of children and to explain to them (even the very young) that this is medicine, not a delicious drink.

SUSPENSIONS. Insoluble drugs are contained in a liquid. When the suspension is of two liquids that cannot be mixed (immiscible), such as an oil (fat) and water, the preparation is an *emulsion*. Because of the nature of their manufacture, the droplets of oil remain suspended. When a solid inorganic or mineral substance is suspended in water the result is a *magma* or a *gel*. These substances are very viscous. After standing, the particles will settle, and the suspension must be shaken well to disperse them again.

ALCOHOL. The drug (solute) is mixed with alcohol (solvent). *Elixirs* are solutions that contain a drug (and sometimes more than one), sugar, alcohol, water, and flavoring. *Spirits* are alcoholic (or *hydroalcoholic*) solutions containing volatile materials as the solute. A *fluidextract* is a concentrated preparation of a vegetable drug manufactured so that its strength is 100 percent. In other words, 1 ml of a fluidextract will always contain one gram (1000 mg) of the drug. (An *extract* is a very concentrated preparation made by evaporating the alcoholic solvent until a thick syruplike fluid or powder is remaining.) *Tinctures* are vegetable drugs that are dissolved in alcohol and are usually made in 10 percent or 20 percent strengths. If the solution contains a strong (potent) drug, the tincture is prepared as a 10 percent solution. One ml of the tincture will contain 0.1 Gm (100 mg) of the drug. Twenty percent solutions are made from the drugs which have a lower potency. One ml of the tincture will contain 0.2 Gm (200 mg) of the drug.

PARENTERAL ROUTE

Parenteral drug administration refers to the injection of a medication, even though the term literally means by any route other than enteral (intestinal). When rapid action of a drug is necessary, when a client is not capable of taking a medication orally, or when the drug of choice may be destroyed by the secretions in the gastrointestinal tract, the parenteral route is used. Although a very necessary mode of drug administration, it carries with it a greater risk than the other routes. Once a medication has been injected, it obviously cannot be retrieved. Because the rate of absorption is rather rapid, counteracting the effects of the drug is very difficult. Also, the skin is a natural defense against invasion by bacteria. Penetration by a foreign body (the needle) increases the possibility of introducing microorganisms, another factor that escalates the hazards involved. Incorrect placement of the needle and properties of the solution injected can cause temporary or irreversible damage to the structures beneath the skin (Fig. 34-1).

Intravenous Injections

The most rapid action occurs with *intravenous injections* (in a vein). When a drug is administered by this route, absorption is *immediate*, as it is placed directly into the circulating blood, making it, by far, the most dangerous method of medication administration.

Intravenous injections are used in emergency situations when there is no time to waste waiting for absorption to take place. In nonemergency situations, this route is utilized when an individual has circulatory problems which would make absorption of a drug from other tissues (such as subcutaneous tissue or muscle) sluggish, or when a medication that is harmful to other tissues, causing sterile abscesses and tissue necrosis, is being used. Nurses'

responsibilities in regard to intravenous medication administration varies from state to state and from institution to institution. Intravenous infusions and administration of medications are discussed in detail in Chapter 35, "Fluid and Electrolyte Balance—Administration of Parenteral Fluids."

Intramuscular Injections

Intramuscular injections have the fastest rate of absorption after the intravenous route. The medication is placed into large muscle bodies, making it less painful than subcutaneous injections (see below) since there are not as many nerve endings in this site. The amount of solution that can be injected varies with the size of the muscle body involved. Up to 5 ml may be given into deep, heavy adult muscles, but it is preferable to divide the dosage into two portions and inject in two sites. The greater the volume injected, the longer absorption will take. Drugs that would be irritating to subcutaneous tissues are injected into muscles. Many of these drugs are oily suspensions and cannot be deposited safely into the circulatory system since the solute is insoluble.

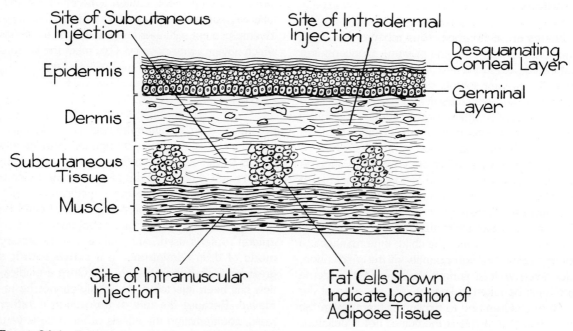

Figure 34-1. Cross section of skin and underlying structures.

Hypodermic and Intradermal Injections

Hypodermic injections (subcutaneous) are those in which the medication is injected into the tissue beneath the skin. Absorption time is longer than that of the intramuscular injection. A maximum amount of 2 ml can be given to an adult in an area with a good supply of subcutaneous tissue and normal peripheral circulation. Irritating drugs cannot be given because they are both painful (due to large numbers of sensory nerve endings) and can cause necrosis and sloughing off of the affected tissue.

Intradermal (intracutaneous) injections are administered by depositing very small amounts of the drug (usually 0.1 ml) into the upper layers of the skin and forming a wheal. The site of choice is usually the inner surface of the forearm. Effects are local rather than systemic as in the other parenteral categories listed above. As absorption is quite slow, this route is usually utilized for the testing of skin for drug sensitivity and allergen desensitization, as well as for tuberculin testing (Fig. 34-2).

Intraspinal Injections

The remainder of the parenteral drug routes are performed by qualified physicians with the assistance of the nurse. Intrathecal (intraspinal) injections are instillations of a drug (usually a local anesthetic or an anti-infective agent) into the subarachnoid space (between the innermost of the three meninges, the pia mater, and the middle membrane, the arachnoid). The technique that is used is the one that is seen when a lumber puncture is done with entrance into the spinal canal through a vertebral interspace. *Epidural injections* are similar to intrathecal in that they are usually done for local anesthetic purposes and entrance is through a vertebral interspace. In this type of injection, the drug is placed into the epidural space between the outer membrane covering the spinal cord, the dura mater, and the periosteum which lines the inner surfaces of the vertebral canal.

Intracardiac, Intraarterial, Intrasynovial, Intraperitoneal Injections

Intracardiac injections are made directly into the heart muscle. This procedure is seen in certain cases of cardiac arrest where a small amount of

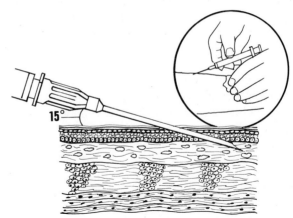

Figure 34-2. Intradermal route of medication administration. Note 15 degree angle of needle to skin and bevel of needle facing upward. Wheal will be produced when solution is injected. The skin is not wiped or massaged with alcohol when injection is completed. However, a sterile wipe may be used to gently blot area.

epinephrine (a cardiac stimulant) is instilled using a 4 inch needle.

Intraarterial injections are done during specific procedures where a dye or radiopaque substance must be injected into an artery for radiological examination or in certain cases where cytotoxic drugs are injected directly into a tumor's blood supply.

Intrasynovial (intraarticular) injections are instillations of corticosteroid hormones into a joint for anti-inflammatory purposes. In cases of acute bursitis cortisone or local anesthetic agents may be injected into the bursae; similarly, injections into tendons are also done for local drug action.

Intraperitoneal injections are used to remove toxic substances from the peritoneal cavity in cases of renal failure or in specific types of poisoning; it may also be used to decrease ascites (accumulation of serous fluid) in the peritoneum due to certain conditions, as in some cases of cancer. The procedure involves the passing of chemical solutions through the peritoneal cavity.

INHALATION

A local or a systemic effect may be obtained when volatile drugs are inhaled as gases or vapors. Absorption is quite rapid; drugs are passed into circulation via the mucous membrane lining, the lungs, and the alveoli. Medications administered by inhalation are for specific respiratory diseases and infections, including mucolytic detergent agents which liquefy secretions that are tenacious and may be obstructing respirations, antibiotics for local pulmonary contact, bronchodilators which ease labored respirations in asthmatic or emphysematous conditions, and oxygen which is administered for various respiratory or cardiac conditions. Drugs which relieve syncope (fainting) and angina pectoris (pain associated with the heart) are inhaled, as are many of the general anesthetics. Aqueous preparations are utilized for inhalation. An oily substance would be unsatisfactory since damage to the pulmonary tissues occurs when oils are inhaled. Administration of these drugs is done through the following devices. (1) *Nebulizers,* which can be used alone (they work much like a hand held atomizer) or in conjunction with a compressed air or oxygen supply, cause very fine droplets of the drug to be inhaled as a mist. (2) *Jet humidifiers* (which can be used in conjunction with *croupettes* for infants and children) produce a very fine mist in the surrounding atmosphere (particularly confined areas as the croup tent or a room). (4) *Vaporizers* produce warm or cold, moist, and medicated vapors. (5) *Inhalers* contain a medication that is inhaled as a vapor when one end is inserted into the nostril. (6) *Spray bottles* deliver droplets of medication when held upright and squeezed. (7) *Aerosols* propel a liquefied form of drug through a valve. (8) *Ampules,* when crushed and held under the nostrils, release the drug in vapor form to be inhaled.

TOPICAL ROUTE

Almost all drugs administered topically (externally) have a local rather than a systemic effect. Tissues directly under the area of application may be affected by certain drugs, but absorption into circulation rarely occurs because of the natural protective qualities of the skin. Most drugs are applied to the skin to treat various dermatologic conditions, to cleanse the skin, for antisepsis, vasoconstriction, counterirritation, and for comfort and soothing effects. Dosage forms commonly used for topical medication administration include: *soaks, compresses* (or *wet dressings*), and *baths* utilizing solutions (i.e., aqueous preparations containing a nonvolatile drug). Soaks and compresses are dis-

cussed in more detail in Chapter 31, "Asepsis" and in Chapter 33, "The Administration of Thermal Agents." Medicated baths are discussed in more detail in Chapter 32, "Personal Hygiene."

LOTIONS. Lotions are watery suspensions which are used to stop itching (antipruritic effect), to soothe, protect, cool, dry, or lubricate skin. They are usually not to be used near mucous membranes, especially the eyes, or on areas that have serum exuding (weeping) since they can clog the tissue. In most cases lotions are applied in a thin layer with a gauze pad; care is taken to apply the lotion gently but firmly, by patting or stroking on. Lotions are not rubbed on as this is quite irritating.

CREAMS. Creams are very soft preparations (between liquids and solids in consistency) that are considered semisolid. While most creams protect the skin (emollient action), others soften or lubricate it. These substances are applied to the affected area in smooth and long strokes with the flat portion of the fingers. In both applying and removing creams, follow the direction in which the hair grows to avoid inflammation of the hair follicles due to irritation.

OINTMENTS. Ointments are fairly similar to creams but may be thicker in consistency. They are usually manufactured with an oily or lanolin base, although other vehicles are used depending on the action and stability of the drug incorporated into it. Ointments are used to treat certain dermatologic conditions, especially those requiring a prolonged local effect of the agent. Since the vehicle is fatty, it softens or liquefies when it is in contact with warmth and keeps the drug in contact with the skin for an extended time. Ointments protect and lubricate skin. Because they hinder the evaporation process that normally occurs via the skin, they should not be applied to wounds that are draining. Applying and removing ointments from the skin is the same as with creams. If lesions are present, the nurse should not apply the medication with bare hands. A soft gauze pad can be used. With both creams and ointments, a tongue blade is used to remove the desired amount from the container rather than dipping in the fingers; this eliminates the possibility of contaminating the rest of the product in the jar.

POULTICES. Poultices (pastes), while infrequently seen, are still in use in certain cases, particularly as a home remedy. These, like ointments are spread on a piece of material and then applied to the skin. Often the vehicle is flour or starch. The effects can be drying or protective, and in some cases, provide relief for inflammation.

PLASTERS. Plasters are solid preparations that mix a drug with a vehicle such as resin or a rubber mixture. When in contact with the skin, the body heat softens them and they adhere to the skin. Plasters serve as either counterirritants or as simple adhesives.

POWDERS. Powders are usually inert substances (although they may be vehicles for therapeutic agents such as antifungal drugs) that are finely pulverized and have an adhesive action which helps them to cling to the skin. They are protective and serve to decrease friction when applied to skin areas that tend to rub against an opposing surface.

VAGINAL AND URETHRAL ROUTES

The action of vaginal and urethral medications is primarily local; however, some systemic effects do occur when the drug is absorbed through the mucous membranes. Drugs applied to the vagina are instilled directly in the form of *tablets,* globular shaped *suppositories, creams, jellies,* or *foams.* These are usually anti-infective agents, antipruritics, or hormone preparations. *Solutions* are used for balancing the pH of the vaginal secretions (which are normally acidic) or for cleansing, antisepsis, preparation for surgery or the local application of heat; *douches,* or vaginal irrigations (discussed below), are the mode of administration for solutions.

Clean technique (see Chapter 31, "Asepsis") is usually used for vaginal applications and irrigations, since the vagina is not a sterile area. A glove is worn on the hand that separates the labia if an applicator is used for administration of the drug form. If the fingers are being used to insert the drug, both hands are then gloved. The client should void prior to this procedure. The lithotomy position (see Chapter 30, "Body Mechanics") is used for vaginal applications; careful draping is essential to provide privacy. Directions are provided with the medication as to the filling and use of accompanying applicators. The filled device is inserted into the vagina to an approximate depth of 2 inches; when the plunger is depressed, the medication within the applicator is propelled into the vaginal canal. The appliance is then removed, and the client instructed to maintain a supine or dorsal recumbent position. Insertion without an applicator is done in the same manner, using the forefinger to push the tablet or suppository into the correct position. Since these drugs soften and melt after insertion, drainage occurs; a perineal pad will absorb some of this discharge.

The *vaginal douche* utilizes a can or bag which holds up to 2 L of solution, tubing, and a special nozzle designed to fit the curvature of the vagina. (These often come in disposable sets.) Antiseptic or astringent solutions are used, but normal saline and tap water is also ordered; the temperature ranges from 100 to 110°F (37.8 to 43.3°C). Holding the apparatus over the sink, solution is run through the tube to remove the air and lubricate the nozzle. After explaining the procedure, providing for privacy, and draping the client who has been placed on a bedpan in lithotomy position, the nurse *gently* inserts the nozzle into the vagina. The can is held (or hung) just above the client's hips to provide a fairly slow flow of solution. Forceful flows can be traumatizing to the vaginal tissue. The nozzle should be turned or rotated slowly while the irrigant is flowing to assure that all surfaces are reached. Many authorities believe that douching should be done only when absolutely necessary (i.e., for medical purposes such as in preoperative preparation or treatment of infection) as this procedure washes away the body's normal defenses found in the vaginal secretions.

URETHAL DRUGS

Urethral drugs come in the form of long, slender suppositories with pointed ends. Their purpose is for local anesthesia or soothing of traumatized tissue. Sterile techniques (see Chapter 31, "Asepsis") must be used as the bladder is a sterile cavity, and prevention of the introduction of microorganisms into this orifice is essential. Again, the client voids before being placed in lithotomy position and draped. Cleansing of the meatus is done as with catheterization. (See Chapter 42, "Maintenance of

Urinary and Intestinal Elimination.'') The suppository, after lubrication with a water soluble lubricant or sterile water, is inserted with gloved (sterile) hands. Painful spasms usually occur with expulsion of the suppository as a result. Therefore, a sterile sponge should be held over the meatus until these subside. Since voiding will also expel the drug, the client should not urinate for approximately half an hour if possible.

Bladder instillations are done via irrigations through a catheter. (See Chapter 42, "Maintenance of Urinary and Intestinal Elimination.'')

RECTAL ROUTE

Medications are administered rectally in the form of *suppositories* and *liquid instillations.* The latter, which usually take the form of small (150 ml or less) *retention enemas,* are retained in the rectum for approximately 30 minutes. (For enema procedure, see Chapter 42, "Maintenance of Urinary and Intestinal Elimination.'') There is less likelihood that irritation or inflammation of the rectal mucosa will occur with instillation of solutions since their absorption is faster than that of the solid medications. The problem is that many clients have more difficulty retaining the fluid bulk than they do the smaller suppository.

Suppositories are bullet or conically shaped with a rounded end that facilitates easy insertion. Bases of cocoa butter, lanolin, wax, polyethylene glycols, glycerin, or gelatin are used as vehicles for the medication. Since they melt in warm temperatures, they are usually stored in the refrigerator until used. After explaining the procedure, providing privacy, and draping the client, he is placed in Sim's (sidelying) position. (See Chapter 30, "Body Mechanics''.) The anus is exposed by drawing back the upper buttock; the lubricated suppository is then inserted by the nurse with her gloved hand. Finger cots rather than the glove can be worn on the thumb and forefinger. The suppository is pushed along with the forefinger until it has passed the anal sphincter (insertion to a depth of approximately 2 inches). The client should retain the suppository for at least 20 to 30 minutes, to allow it to melt completely and for absorption to take place. When the rectal agents are expelled too soon, there is little or no drug action. Administration of rectal medications is most successful after a bowel movement or be-

tween meals, as eating will increase peristalsis and the likelihood of expulsion.

Rectal drugs are usually used when an antiemetic effect is needed, for local analgesia, as a preoperative medication causing relaxation or sleep in children before administering a general anesthetic, and for induction of bowel movement. Years ago enemas were given for nutritive purposes. Sugar solutions and predigested proteins were instilled for absorption through the rectal mucosa. Whiskey enemas were also used for sedation. Occasionally, solid medications, such as tablets, can also be administered by this route, but for maximal results, these are best dissolved and given in the form of the retention enema.

OPHTHALMIC MEDICATIONS

Medications instilled in the eyes are local in action. Usually they are intended for dilation or contraction of the pupils, treatment of infections, and for soothing of irritation or itching. These drugs are found in the form of *solutions, suspensions,* and *ointments.* Solutions for ophthalmic use are manufactured to be *isotonic* with the tears—that is, they have a concentration of electrolytes which will exert an equal osmotic pressure as the solution to which they are compared (the tears). They are packaged in *bottles with a dropper,* in *squeeze vials* with a built in dispenser, or in *tubes* with special tips for the administration of ointments. If they have been refrigerated, rolling the tube between the hands will warm the drug. Even though the eyes have more than one defense against invasion of microorganisms (the lashes keep foreign bodies out and conjunctival secretions have certain protective qualities), they remain subject to infection. Therefore, ophthalmic drugs are *sterile,* and the object in their administration should be avoidance of contamination and protection of the eye against injury or irritation. Along the same line, the nurse's hands must be washed, and the dropper is never inverted once solution is drawn up to avoid the possibility of small rubber particles mixing with the drug.

Because the cornea is quite sensitive and easily traumatized, care must be taken not to apply medication directly onto it; thus, the ophthalmic agents are deposited into the *conjunctival sac* of the lower lid while the client is in supine position or is seated. The client looks upward while the nurse pulls the lower lid down and away from the eye with her thumb only. The number of drops ordered are instilled into the center of the pocket that is formed; the tip of the dropper never touches the eye or the lip (Fig. 34-3A). Any unused drug in the dropper is discarded. With ointments, the process is the same. A small amount of ointment is squeezed onto a sterile gauze pad to insure that no crusts have formed in the tip of the tube. A very thin band of ointment is then deposited across the conjunctival sac from the inner canthus (at the lacrimal duct) toward the outer corner (outer canthus) of the eye (Fig. 34-3B). Ophthalmic medication (both drops and ointments) are distributed evenly when the lower lid is released and the eye blinks. No attempt should be made to rub the eye after the application of the drug, although a clean tissue can be used to gently blot excess medication beginning at the inner canthus of the closed eye and moving outward. When medication has been instilled in both eyes, a separate tissue must be used for each eye to avoid cross-contamination.

Irrigations of the eye (*conjunctival irrigations*) are used for removal of excess secretions in the treatment of eye infections. Sterile saline or an ophthalmic antiseptic solution is used; the amount needed varies with the condition being treated. If a large amount of the solution is necessary, a soft bulb syringe is used; in cases where small amounts will suffice, an eye dropper is utilized. The most effective position for the client is side-lying with the affected eye toward the mattress, allowing the solution to flow from the inner canthus downward toward the outer canthus. An emesis basin placed under the cheek acts as a receptacle for the solution. The client directs his eyes upward; the lower conjunctival sac is everted as described above and the solution is dropped or allowed to flow from no farther than a height of 4 inches across the sac. Again, the irrigating tip must never touch the eye. If both eyes are to be irrigated, the client must turn toward the opposite side to treat the second eye. The solution is *always* directed from inner canthus toward the outer canthus.

OTIC MEDICATIONS

Otic medications have a local action and are used as anti-infectives, local anesthetics, and cleansing agents. Unless the tympanic membrane has been

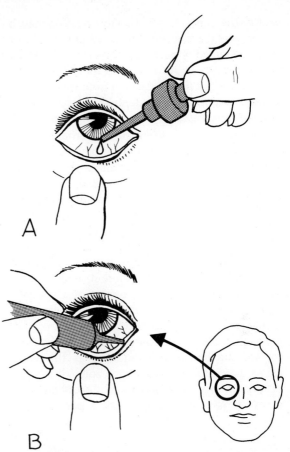

Figure 34-3. A, Administration of ophthalmic solutions to conjunctival sac. B, Administration of ophthalmic ointment to conjunctival sac from inner canthus to outer canthus.

ruptured or penetrated (accidentally or surgically), the ear is not considered a sterile area. In the case of a break in the membrane, special care must be taken in instillation so as not to introduce microorganisms or foreign material from the external ear to the inner ear. A dropper is used to instill drug solutions into the external auditory canal.

After washing her hands, the nurse positions the client in the side-lying position with the affected ear facing upward. The pinna (auricle) is pulled in an upward and posterior direction to straighten the external auditory canal and facilitate the instillation of the drops. In infants and small children, the pinna is directed downward and posteriorly. The drops, which should be at body temperature to avoid the discomfort or dizziness caused by extreme temperatures, are directed toward the inner wall of the canal. A small cotton pledget may be placed gently and *loosely* in the vestibule but must never be forced or pushed into the canal. The client should remain on his side for a short time to prevent the loss of the medication from the ear.

Irrigations of the ear (external auditory canal) are done in most cases for both cleansing and for local application of heat. Warm (approximately 105°F [40.6°C]) antiseptic solutions or physiologic saline are utilized for the procedure. It is preferred that the client be seated if at all possible, although he could lie down if necessary. He is draped to protect him from getting wet and is asked to hold an emesis basin under the ear to collect the irrigant as it flows out. His head is tilted slightly toward the affected ear, and the external auditory canal is straightened as described above. The solution, which is contained in either a soft bulb syringe or a special irrigating set designed for the ear, must flow very gently and is directed toward the side or roof of the canal (Fig. 34-4). It is never forced in or aimed toward the tympanic membrane as this would cause discomfort or dizziness or both. (If this does occur, the procedure should be discontinued and a report made to the appropriate personnel, in-

cluding the physician). After the prescribed amount of irrigant (which varies but may be 0.5 L) has flowed in and out of the ear, the client's ear is gently patted dry, and he is asked to lie on the side of the affected ear to allow any further drainage to occur.

NASAL MEDICATIONS

Nose drops and sprays are used for the purposes of decongestion (vasoconstriction with shrinkage of the mucosa allowing for sinus drainage), local anesthesia, and hemostasis (the arrest of bleeding). The position of choice is lying on the back with the head hyperextended, which is accomplished by placement of pillows under the client's shoulders, allowing the head to fall backwards. If allowed, a client could lie flat on his back with the head hanging over the edge of the bed. This position is not as comfortable as the other. If necessary, the client may remain seated with his head extended backwards. Correct positioning is important because drainage of the medication into the nasopharynx occurs when incorrect positioning is used. The prescribed number of drops are instilled in each of the nares. The dropper should not touch the nose as this may induce sneezing. With children, infants, or uncooperative clients, the dropper should have a rubber tip or tubing at the end to avoid injury (Fig. 34-5). Ideally, a new dropper is used for each nasal instillation. The client should remain in position for 3–5 minutes to avoid loss of the drug. With nasal sprays, the client is seated, and the tip of the bottle inserted into the nares. A gentle squeeze is given the bottle which directs the flow of atomized drug into the nasal passages. Drugs given via the nasal route should be expectorated rather than swallowed.

THROAT MEDICATIONS

In addition to troches, mentioned earlier, drugs are delivered to the mucous membranes of the throat in the form of *sprays, painted applications, gargles,* and *irrigations.* To allow for certain procedures (diagnostic and surgical) in which the gag reflex would interfere with instrumentation, a local anesthetic may be sprayed on the throat. In cases of pharyngeal pain and swelling, associated with irritation and infection, anesthetics and antiseptics may be applied by spraying or ''painting'' with a

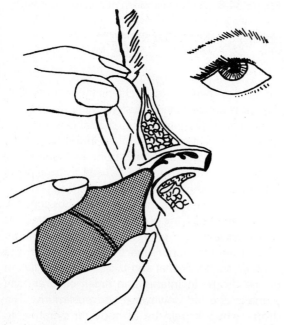

Figure 34-4. Otic irrigation (irrigation of external auditory canal).

long cotton-tipped applicator. The client should be asked to tilt his head back. A good light source is used to visualize the affected area, and a tongue depressor is used to keep the tongue down and out of the line of vision. Both the applicator and the tongue depressor should be discarded since many potentially dangerous microorganisms are harbored in the mouth and throat.

Gargles

Antiseptic or *saline gargles* are occasionally ordered to relieve irritation and to remove secretions in the throat. Actually, these may be appropriate for use in the oropharynx but for reaching most of the affected areas of the throat are not as satisfactory as *irrigations*. In fact, strong antiseptics are often overused, resulting in irritation and destruction of the natural defenses found in the oropharynx. Irrigations take a long period of time and can be tiring to a client who is already in a weakened condition. This procedure, in which the client must be seated in front of a sink or basin, is also done to remove thick secretions from the throat. Local application of heat is another purpose. Physiologic saline or antiseptic solutions which range from 100 to 120°F (37.8 to 48.9°C), according to the client's preference and tolerance, are allowed to flow *very gently* against the affected tissues. An irrigating can with a nozzle and a clamp on the tubing are used to direct the flow; the height of the can determines the force of the solution, so that it is usually placed only slightly higher than the client's mouth. A forceful stream could cause gagging or increase the irritation. The client, if able, controls the nozzle and the clamp, turning the flow on and off in a manner that is comfortable for him. He holds his breath while tilting his head forward over the basin and allows the irrigant to flow over the throat. Turning his head from side to side while the irrigant is flowing facilitates the procedure. The amount of solution needed varies from individual to individual, though amounts up to 2 L are sometimes used.

Actions and Dosages

When dealing with the administration of medications, it is important to keep in mind that people usually react in similar ways to the same drugs. However, on occasion an individual exhibits symp-

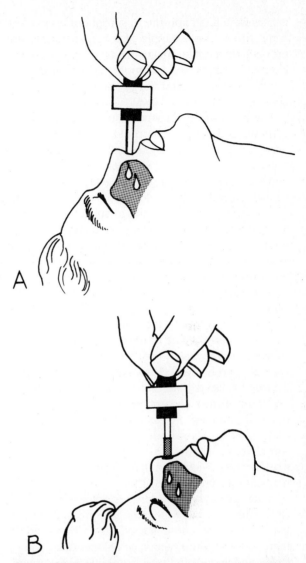

Figure 34-5. Instillation of nasal medications. A, When drops are administered to the adult, the head is in hyperextension. B, For the administration of nose drops to a small child, use a rubber protector on tip of glass dropper.

toms and behaviors that are not anticipated with a specific drug or at a certain dosage level. Many factors combine to influence the actions or effects of drugs and their dosage.

The *condition of the drug* itself is a factor. Drugs are altered and can decompensate when their shelf-life (period of potency) has expired. Not only age, but environmental conditions can change the characteristics of a drug. Lack of refrigeration when it is necessary and exposure to sunlight or air modify some drugs. For example, if a cap is not closed properly on a bottle, a solvent may evaporate, leaving the remaining solution more concentrated than normal and increasing the possibility of overdosage.

The *route of administration* influences drug absorption and action. The rapidity with which the drug can be diffused across cell membranes, the presence of food in the stomach, and the rate of peristaltic activity of the gastrointestinal tract are all considerations in the oral route. Site of injections (i.e., intravenous as opposed to subcutaneous) affects absorption time; the former being absorbed immediately and the latter taking a great deal longer. Condition of the various tissues into which the drug is injected and permeability of cell membranes are considerations in parenteral drug administration.

Dosage forms vary the effects and absorption time of drugs. The size of the drug particle and the substances with which they are mixed (i.e., bases, vehicles, and binders) determine the length of time it takes to disintegrate and the acceleration or retardation of their absorption. While most of these materials are inert or relatively harmless in nature, there may be some individuals with a particular sensitivity or allergy to the agent. Although there may be no problem with the drug itself, the vehicle may cause a problem.

When more than one drug is administered to a client within an interval of time, the presence of the two agents may cause the effects to be different than had each drug been given alone. *Additive effects* or *addition* is the total (sum) effect seen when the individual effects of each drug are added together and viewed as a whole. When two drugs with similar actions are administered together they may produce an effect which is greater than the total effects of each of the drugs had they been acting alone. This is known as *synergism*. *Potentiation* also gives a total effect that is greater than the two drugs above; however, these drugs are dissimilar in their individual action. When opposite effects occur—that is, one drug counteracts or decreases the effects of another—the effect is known as *antagonism*.

After several doses of a drug have been administered, it accumulates in the body because excretion is out of balance with absorption. When the drug's disposal is slower than its absorption, the outcome is known as a *cumulative effect.*

Drugs are given for a specific primary purpose or *therapeutic effect,* but many drugs have *side effects* (desirable or undesirable) as well. For instance, two side effects of drugs given for analgesia or pain relief are sedation and respiratory depression. The sedative effect may be positive in that rest is provided for the client. However, if there is a problem with oxygenation, then the respiratory depression may be a very dangerous side effect. The undesirable side effect is also known as an *untoward effect.*

Clients may exhibit an unusual or unexpected reaction to a drug. This *idiosyncrasy* is often an effect that is the reverse of the one that was anticipated (a *paradoxical* effect), for instance, stimulation rather than the expected relaxation. An *allergic reaction,* in which an individual responds to a drug he had taken previously (or its vehicle) with an unusual or abnormal reaction such as rash, itching, swelling, difficult breathing, or shock (*anaphylaxis*), is known as *hypersensitivity.*

Factors associated with the individual rather than the drug include *age* (infants, children, and the elderly are more susceptible to overdosage and unusual reactions), *sex* (women, being of lower body weight than men and having additional considerations such as menstruation, pregnancy, and lactation, may need less of a drug), *physical condition* (during health and during many disease states, including pain, cellular and systemic responses to drugs will differ, changing the dosage requirements), and *emotional status* (the "state of mind" of an individual will be reflected in drug and dosage requirements; for example, the severely anxious psychotic individual will need a great deal more of a tranquilizing agent than the person who needs the same drug for mild anxiety or control of nausea). When certain drugs are given to clients over a prolonged period of time, equal doses of the drug are found to have a diminishing effect, and dosages must be increased to get the same results. This phenomenon is known as *tolerance. Cross-tolerance* occurs when resistance is increased for drugs with very similar actions as well as to the original drug. If physiologic changes occur so that the cells are not only able to function when high levels of the drug are present but cannot function without the drug's presence, then *physical dependence* has occurred. When combined with an emotional need and desire for the drug as well as a tendency to increase the dosage, *addiction* results. *Habituation,* on the other hand, is the term used when an individual desires the drug and may feel a psychologic need for it but usually does not continue to increase the dosage.

RULES OF MEDICATION ADMINISTRATION

Although the *order* for a drug must come from a *physician,* it is the responsibility of the nurse to carry out the order in an *intelligent, responsible,* and *legal* fashion. The nurse's most valuable tools are her *knowledge* and her *judgment.* Mistakes may occur, but they can be minimized if the basic rules of medication administration are learned well, incorporated into daily practice, and followed conscientiously in every situation. This does not discount flexibility in certain emergency situations, but even in these, the margin of error is reduced when the safety factors have become ingrained.

The following general rules of medication administration apply in the preparation and distribution of drugs in any dosage form or by any route. (Since abbreviations are frequently used in medication administration, a list of commonly used abbreviations is given in Table 34-2).

TABLE 34-2. Common Abbreviations Used in Relation to Pharmacology

Abbreviation	Meaning	Abbreviation	Meaning
ā	before	os	mouth
aa	of each; equal parts	OU	both eyes
ac	before meals	oz	ounce
ad	up to; to	p̄	after
ad lib	freely as desired	pc	after meals
am	morning	per	by; through
amt	amount	po	by mouth
aq	water	PRN	as necessary; when required
bid	twice a day	pt	pint
c̄	with	pulv	powder
cap	capsule	q	every
cc	cubic centimeter	qam	every morning
cm	centimeter	qd	every day
comp	compound	qh	every hour
d	day	q2h	every two hours
dc (D/C)	discontinue	qid	four times a day
dr	dram	qn	every night
elix	elixir	qod	every other day
ext	extract	qs	as much as is required (quantity sufficient)
fl	fluid		
Gm	gram	R	rectal
gr	grain	℞	treatment or therapy
gtt	drop	s̄	without
h or hr	hour	sat	saturated
(H)	hypodermic (subcutaneous)	Sig or S	write on label
hs	hour of sleep (bedtime)	sol	solution
IM	intramuscular	sos	one dose if necessary
IV	intravenous	sp	spirits
L	liter	ss (s̄s̄)	one half
lb	pound	stat	immediately
m	minim	syr	syrup
mg	milligram	tab	tablet
MOM	milk of magnesia	tid	three times a day
NPO	nothing by mouth	tinct or tr	tincture
N/S	normal saline	TO	telephone order
OD	right eye	U	unit
OS	left eye	ung	ointment
		VO	verbal order

Physicians' Orders

All drugs must be specified by a written order from a licensed physician or dentist. The components of the physician's order are: the date when the order is written (and the time in the case of narcotics); the name of the drug which in most cases is the *official* or *generic name* (listed in the USP or NF) as opposed to the *trade name* (the name assigned to a drug by the manufacturer); the exact dosage and its route of administration; the frequency of administration; and the signature of the physician.

In certain cases a drug order will be written for a single (one time) administration only. If it is to be given immediately, it is known as a *"stat" order.* Drugs which can be given at the nurse's discretion when she feels the client needs them (within certain time intervals) are called prn (as necessary) orders. An example would be a drug for pain relief which the doctor orders every 4 hours prn. The nurse can give the medication to the client when in her best judgment she feels this is appropriate; she can give it at intervals of no less than 4 hours or may not give it at all if there appears to be no need for it.

Although it is ideal to have a written order, there are certain instances where a *verbal* or *telephone order* must temporarily suffice. For example, in an emergency, a physician may give a verbal order. There is no time during crises or life-threatening situations to find the chart or physician's order sheet for his signature. When the emergency is over, however, he should be asked to put these verbal orders into writing. Even when the nurse is quite familiar with the physician, telephone orders are extremely risky. However, in an emergency, the nurse may have to call the physician in which case she writes, with the physician's name, "telephone order" and then countersigns her name, the date, and time. This, too, will be signed by the physician when he arrives at the scene. Accepting a drug order by telephone in any other situation should be avoided since there have been numerous cases of fraud in which the clients, their relatives, or friends have decided that a medication was necessary and called it in to the nurses' station.

TRANSCRIPTION OF MEDICATION ORDERS

The ultimate responsibility for accurate transcribing of a doctor's written order onto the *Kardex,* which includes the plan of care for the client, and onto *medicine* (or *identification*) *cards,* belongs to the nurse. Even if the actual transcription is done by another worker, the nurse must check it for accuracy and then date and initial it indicating that this has been done. It is at this point that many errors are caught. The nurse must be familiar with drugs, their actions, side effects, and their average dosages, since a misplaced decimal point can mean a significant difference between too little drug for therapeutic action and toxicity due to overdosage. A nurse not catching an incorrectly written order is as responsible as the prescriber if a legal action is brought by a client. It, therefore, behooves the nurse to obtain information on each and every drug with which she is unfamiliar. A copy of the *Physicians' Desk Reference* (PDR) which annually lists drugs in current usage and information on their action, uses, composition, dosages, routes of administration, contraindications, and side effects is usually found on most units where drugs are given. An alternative source that may also be utilized is the *hospital formulary;* this resource is a book containing information on all of the drugs accepted for usage in the agency. If a reference cannot be found, a call to the hospital pharmacy is in order to obtain the desired information about a drug. Whenever there is a question about a drug order, it is the nurse's responsibility to contact the physician who ordered the medication and indicate that there is some clarification needed.

The medicine card may vary from institution to institution, but should contain the *full name* of the client, his *room* (and *bed number* if applicable), the *name of the drug,* the *dosage, frequency* (and *times*) and *route of administration,* the *date ordered* (and the *expiration date* if applicable), and the *initials of the transcribing nurse.* This card will be used for information in the preparation of a drug, to accompany the drug and assist in client identification during its administration, and in the recording of the drug's administration. A separate medicine card is used for each drug.

There are many systems used for filing of medicine cards. Frequently a board with 24 individual compartments, one for each hour of the day, is used; cards are placed in the compartment or slot when the medication will next be given. If preparing 10:00 am medications, for example, cards will be removed from the 10:00 am slot; after the medication has been administered and recorded, the card is returned to the slot where it will be used for the next dose.

Prescriptions

Along the same lines as the medication order, a *prescription* for a client must be signed by the physician or dentist. Nurses must be familiar with the components of the prescription in case she is requested to write one (to be signed by the physician before giving it to the client) or to read it and explain the directions for use to the client. The prescription is an order to a pharmacist as to how a drug should be prepared and supplied. It contains: (1) the *client's full name and address;* (2) the *date* written; (3) the *superscription* or symbol ℞ (Latin recipe); (4) the *inscription,* that is, the name and quantity of the desired drug; (5) the *subscription,* that is, the directions to the pharmacist for mixing or preparing (compounding) the drug (this may or may not appear on prescriptions, depending upon the drug and its form); (6) the *transcription or signature* indicated by the abbreviation *Sig* (from the Latin *signa* which means "write"), that is, directions to the client on the label; and (7) the *prescriber's name* (doctor's signature). The prescriber must also indicate on the prescription how many times it can be refilled. Doctor's order sheets and prescriptions are *legal documents* that can be entered in court as evidence in cases involving medication errors, negligence or malpractice.

Calculation of Dosage

In the United States two systems of weights and measures are used—the *metric* and the *apothecary.* Frequently a drug will be ordered using one system of measurement, and the labeling will appear in the terminology of the other system. The units used in these systems are different and not compatible; therefore, to calculate dosages, a *conversion* must take place. Very simply stated, conversions change the terminology used for equal quantities of a drug from one system to the other. Even though tables are available with these conversions listed, the ability to understand and convert measurements is a valuable and necessary skill for all nurses (Tables 34-3 and 34-4).

Liters (volume), grams (weight) and meters (length) are the basic units of measurement in the metric (decimal) system. All other units are derived

TABLE 34-3. Commonly Used Approximate Equivalents

Weight		Volume	
Metric	Apothecary	Metric	Apothecary
1 Gm	= 15 gr	1 ml	= 15–16 minims
0.06 Gm	= 1 gr	1cc	= 1 ml
4 Gm	= 1 dram	0.06 ml	= 1 minim
30 Gm	= 1 oz	0.5 ml	= 8 minims
1 kg	= 2.2 lbs	0.3 ml	= 5 minims
		4 ml	= 1 fluidram
		30 ml	= 1 fl oz
		500 ml	= 1 pt
		1000 ml (1 L)	= 1 qt

from these units by dividing or multiplying by powers of 10. When dividing or making subunits, which are smaller than the basic unit, the Latin prefixes *deci,* or 0.1 (1/10), *centi,* or 0.01 (1/100), and *milli,* or 0.001 (1/1000) are used to identify the subunit. When multiplying or increasing the number of basic units, the Greek prefixes are added; *deka* or 10 times the unit, *hecto* or 100 times the unit, and *kilo* or 1000 times the unit. Abbreviations commonly used are: Gm (gram), mg (milligrams), L (liter), and ml (milliliters).

In the apothecary system, the basic units of weight are the *grain* (gr), *dram* (ʒ), *ounce* (℥),

TABLE 34-4. Approximate Equivalent Weights

Apothecary			Metric
gr xv	= 1.0	Gm =	1000 mg
gr x	= 0.6	Gm =	600 mg
gr 7½	= 0.5	Gm =	500 mg
gr v	= 0.3	Gm =	300 mg
gr iii	= 0.2	Gm =	200 mg
gr 1½	= 0.1	Gm =	100 mg
gr 1	= 0.06	Gm =	60 mg
gr ¾	= 0.05	Gm =	50 mg
gr ½	= 0.03	Gm =	30 mg
gr ¼	= 0.015	Gm =	15 mg
gr ⅙	= 0.010	Gm =	10 mg
gr ⅛	= 0.008	Gm =	8 mg
gr 1/12	= 0.005	Gm =	5 mg
gr 1/15	= 0.004	Gm =	4 mg
gr 1/20	= 0.0032	Gm =	3 mg
gr 1/30	= 0.0022	Gm =	2 mg
gr 1/40	= 0.0015	Gm =	1.5 mg
gr 1/50	= 0.0012	Gm =	1.2 mg
gr 1/60	= 0.001	Gm =	1.0 mg
gr 1/100	= 0.0006	Gm =	0.6 mg
gr 1/120	= 0.0005	Gm =	0.5 mg
gr 1/150	= 0.0004	Gm =	0.4 mg
gr 1/200	= 0.0003	Gm =	0.3 mg
gr 1/300	= 0.0002	Gm =	0.2 mg
gr 1/600	= 0.0001	Gm =	0.1 mg

and *pound* (lb). Measurement of fluids is done in the units *minims* (℧), *fluidrams* (ℨ), *fluidounces* (℥), *pints* (pt), *quarts* (qt), and *gallons* (C). When indicating units of measure in the form of symbols, Roman numerals are used to state quantity. For instance ℨ ii reads 2 drams and grv reads 5 grains. Roman numerals are not used for subunits, and fractions are written. For example gr ⅛ reads one-eighth of a grain.

Household measurements are not used in the medical unit; however, when instructing clients to measure medications at home, these measurements are the most practical, being familiar and easy to implement. Although the order for a drug may read 1 dram (ℨ i) or 4 ml, the client is instructed to measure one teaspoonful (tsp) or 5 ml since this is the closest household measurement available. Similarly, drops (gtt) and minims (℧) are said to be equivalent for home use, although they do differ.

Before dosage can be calculated, both the required amount of the drug and the amount or dosage that is on hand must be expressed in the same system of measurement (metric or apothecary). It is suggested that a programmed textbook be used to review the process of conversion from one system to the other without the use of a table.

When both the desired dosage, or amount ordered (D), and the amount you have, or dosage on hand (H), are expressed equivalently, then the calculation of the necessary amount can be figured. A formula using ratio and proportion is set up: D (amount ordered):X (amount to be administered) = ratio of strength (dosage in units: amount of solution or tablets).

EXAMPLE. The doctor's order reads: give 30 mg of codeine sulfate po (by mouth) q3h (every 3 hours). The label (dosage on hand) reads codeine sulfate, gr ¼. (There is one-quarter of a grain in each tablet.)

1. Convert grains to mg (or if preferred mg to gr). The objective is to state the formula in equivalents of the same measurement system:

    ¼ gr × 60 (there are 60 mg in 1 gr)

    $$\frac{1}{4} \times 60 = \frac{60}{4} = 15 \text{ mg}$$

    1 tab = 15 mg

2. State formula using information about dosage desired and that on hand:

    $$\frac{30 \text{ mg (D)}}{X \text{ (amount needed)}} = \frac{15 \text{ mg \ (H)}}{1 \text{ tab}}$$

    $$30 = 15X$$
    $$2 = X$$

3. Answer: give two tablets.

EXAMPLE. The doctor's order reads: give 75 mg of meperidine hydrochloride IM (intramuscular injection) q4h (every 4 hours). The label (dosage on hand) reads Demerol (meperidine hydrochloride) 50 mg/ml.

1. This step is unnecessary since both factors are stated in metric measurements.
2. State formula using information about dosage desired and that on hand:

    $$\frac{75 \text{ mg (D)}}{X \text{ (amount needed)}} = \frac{50 \text{ mg (H)}}{1 \text{ ml}}$$

    $$75 = 50 \text{ x}$$
    $$1.5 = \text{ x}$$

3. Answer: give 1.5 ml of solution.

For calculation of pediatric dosages the physician uses one of several formulas to arrive at the desired dosage. The nurse should be able to use these formulas to understand the process of determining small dosages, especially since drug errors tend to be far more disastrous in children than in adults. In the past, age was the determinant. This is rarely used today. *Clark's rule* is one that calculates pediatric dosages from the adult dose, based on weight. This is more accurate than the methods using age. The formula is:

$$\frac{\text{weight of child in pounds}}{150} \times \text{adult dose}$$
$$= \text{child's dose.}$$

An even more accurate system being used by many physicians today is based on body surface area (BSA). Using a graph that estimates the BSA from the height and weight of the individual, a pediatric dosage is determined.

Preparation of Medication

After washing her hands, the nurse is ready to prepare the medication for administration to the client. Using the medication card as a guide, the *label* on the dosage form is *checked against the order* (as stated on the card) *three times*. This rule must never be broken as it is one of the best safeguards against error. The label and medicine card are crosschecked before the container is removed from the shelf, before the drug is removed from the container, and before the container is replaced on the shelf. If a label cannot be clearly read (for any reason), the container and its contents should be returned to the pharmacy unused. The risk of making an error should never be taken, *even* if the nurse is fairly certain of the contents of the container. *Accuracy in measurement of the dosage is absolutely necessary.*

To pour *oral medications,* a suitable container for delivering the drug to the client is needed. Tablets, capsules, troches, and sublingual and buccal tablets are placed in tiny paper or plastic cups. Powders and granules are measured into a cup but are not mixed with water until at the client's bedside. Liquids are poured into plastic or wax coated paper cups with calibrations on their sides for easy measurement. Each medication is placed in an individual container. The medication card is always kept with the drug; they should not be separated. Solid dosage forms are poured from the bottle into the cap. The correct number of tablets is then transferred to the medicine cup; the drug should not be touched by the nurse. Liquids are poured at eye level until the bottom of the concave meniscus that forms on the surface is exactly level with the appropriate marking on the calibrated cup. When pouring liquids, pour on the side away from the label, so as not to stain it and make it illegible. For very small doses a minim cup is used, or a syringe can be used since its calibrations measure very small amounts accurately. Drugs are sometimes measured by a dropper which is calibrated by the manufacturer of the drug or the pharmacist. Droppers cannot be interchanged with those that accompany another drug since the size of a drop containing a specific dosage amount for one drug will vary from that of a different drug. After placing the appropriate number of drops in a medicine cup, any drug remaining in a dropper is discarded, not returned to the bottle.

Before drawing up solutions for *parenteral medication administration* suitable equipment must be collected. *Syringes* are chosen according to the amount of drug to be injected. Amounts from 1.0 ml and up use syringes that have a 2 ml or 3 ml capacity (unless the amount is greater than 3 ml and then a 5 ml syringe is chosen). The 2 and 3 ml syringes are calibrated in both minims and tenths of ml. For amounts that are less than 1.0 ml, a *tuberculin syringe,* which is calibrated in tenths and hundredths of a ml, is used. *Insulin syringes* are calibrated in scales of 40, 80, and 100 U/ml, since the dosage of the drug, insulin, is ordered in U rather than in ml. *Needle sizes* are measured in terms of *length* and *gauge* (diameter of bore). Determination of the size to use is based on the depth to which the needle must go in order to reach its intended destination. The size of the client (how much subcutaneous fat is present) as well as the site of injection will be the factors that influence choice of length. For intramuscular injections (IM), how far does the needle have to be inserted to reach a muscle? For the average size adult, a 1½ inch needle will usually suffice in most deep muscle sites. An obese client might require a 2 inch needle while a very thin individual may need a 1 inch to 1¼ inch needle. An injection into the deltoid muscle might require only a ¾ to 1 inch needle in the average size adult. For children, a 1 inch needle usually suffices for IM injections. These are all based on averages, but each client must be considered individually since size of the client and amount of subcutaneous tissue varies. For subcutaneous injections (sc), a ⅝ inch to ¾ inch needle is generally used in adults. A ⅝ inch needle is the usual size for children.

Gauge is determined by the viscosity of the solution to be injected. The thicker the solution, the thicker the needle, and vice versa. Needle gauges for injection of medications run from 27 (the thinnest needle bore) to 17 (the thickest). Medications used for intramuscular injection tend to be more viscous and will usually require a 21 or 22 gauge needle in adults and a 21 to 23 gauge needle for children. Subcutaneous injections in adults usually need approximately a 23 to 25 gauge needle and a 25 gauge needle for children. Intradermal injections call for 25 to 27 gauge, ½ inch needles. The entire needle shaft (including the tip), the tip of the syringe, and the inside of the barrel (body) and shaft of the plunger must be kept sterile. If any of these parts are touched (contaminated), they are discarded.

Solutions are packaged in a variety of containers: single dose ampules, single dose vials, multiple dose vials, and single dose disposable cartridges (Fig. 34-6 and 34-7).

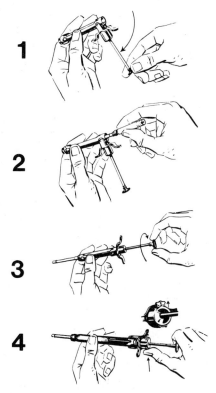

Figure 34-6. Loading a cartridge-needle unit syringe. 1. Grasp barrel of syringe in one hand. With other hand, pull back firmly on plunger and swing the entire handle-section downward so that it locks at right angle to the barrel. 2. Insert cartridge-needle unit, needle end first, into the barrel. Engage needle ferrule by rotating it clockwise in threads at front end of syringe. 3. Swing plunger back into place and attach end to the threaded shaft of piston. Hold metal syringe barrel—not glass cartridge— with one hand and rotate plunger until both ends of cartridge-needle unit are fully, but lightly, engaged. To maintain sterility, leave rubber sheath in place until just before use. 4. The 2-cc syringe can be used for a 1-cc syringe. Engage both ends and push the slide through so the number "1" appears. After use, the syringe automatically resets itself for 2 cc. (Courtesy of Wyeth Laboratories, Philadelphia, Penna.)

To draw up medication from an *ampule,* the medication trapped in the tip (or upper portion of the ampule) is tapped down into the lower position by light flicking with the fingertips. Scored ampules are prepared by the manufacturer to open without needing filing. These have a line drawn around the neck of the ampule. (If the ampule is not scored, this must be done by the nurse with a small file.) The neck of the ampule is covered with a sterile sponge or alcohol swab and the top snapped off and discarded. It is not recommended that the top be removed using bare fingers. The alcohol swab also cleanses the neck of the ampule. The contents of the ampule should be inspected for minute particles of glass before drawing up the solution. The needle is carefully inserted well into the ampule. The plunger is pulled back until the desired solution has been drawn into the syringe. (The ampule can be tipped to a 45 degree angle if necessary to withdraw the contents.) After removing the needle from the ampule the dosage is checked for accuracy and the protector sheath replaced over the needle to maintain its sterility until given to the client.

To remove medication from a *vial* (single or multiple dose), the rubber diaphragm is cleansed with 70 percent alcohol. An amount of air equal to the amount of solution to be removed from the vial is injected into the vial, increasing the air pressure in the vial, and thus, making the fluid withdrawal easier. This is best accomplished by drawing up the necessary amount of air, and with the vial standing on the work surface, inserting the needle into the vial just above the surface of the fluid and injecting the air. In this manner, the air goes into the air in the vial and does not bubble through the solution which would make its subsequent removal more difficult. The vial and the syringe are then inverted and the required amount of solution drawn up in the syringe. The needle should not be withdrawn until the accurate dosage is in the syringe. After removing the needle it is then capped with the sheath to retain its sterility.

Directions for mixing sterile solutions from *powders* are enclosed with the packaging. They consist of drawing up a specific amount of a designated solvent and injecting this into a vial or ampule containing the drug in powder or crystalline form. The vial is agitated or twirled between the hands until completely dissolved and the designated amount of solution withdrawn as above.

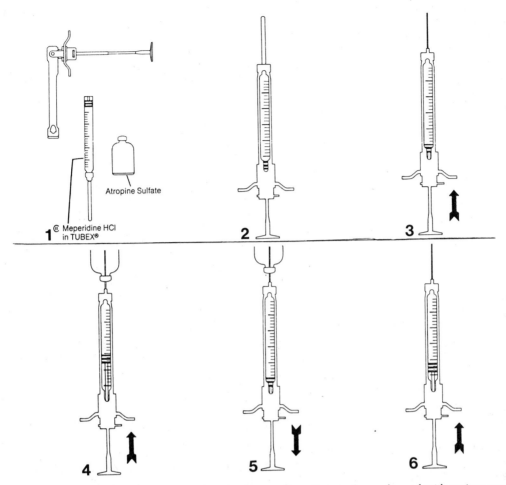

Figure 34-7. Mixing of fluids in Tubex sterile cartridge-needle units may be performed with various medications of no more than 2½ cc total liquid volume. The dosages of meperidine and atropine sulfate are selected arbitrarily to illustrate the mixing technique and not recommendations of a specific regimen. Nor can any specific recommendations be made for compatibility or duration of stability.

WARNING: Incompatible compounds should not be mixed in cartridge-needle units. Before initiating mixing procedures, please consult the appropriate source materials for specific incompatibilities and contraindications.

1. Assemble injection materials. Check labels and verify medications order. Convert the atropine order from grains (1/150) to cc which in this case will be 1 cc. Cleanse diaphragm of vial in usual manner. 2. Load syringe and hold it in a vertical position, needle end up. 3. Remove needle sheath. Rotate glass cartridge until calibrations are visible. Now adjust the rubber piston so that its surface that is in contact with fluid is opposite 2½ cc calibration. 4. Still holding syringe vertically, insert needle into the vial of atropine. Inject 1 cc of sterile air into vial. The 1 cc (1/150 gr) of atropine cannot be easily withdrawn until an equal amount of sterile air is injected into the vial. 5. Draw plunger back exactly 1 cc. When cartridge has filled with exactly the amount of atropine that you wish (in this case, 1 cc), remove needle from vial. You now have 1 cc of meperidine combined with 1 cc of atropine. Note, during mixing procedure, an air space between contents of vial and cartridge have been maintained to help prevent accidental infusion of contents from one receptacle to the other. 6. Expel excess air, leaving a bubble (about 1/10 cc) if this is to be an IM injection. Replace needle sheath until time of injection. (Courtesy of Wyeth Laboratories, Philadelphia, Penna.)

Administration of Medication

After readying the medication and collecting any necessary items, such as additional alcohol swabs and straws, the drug and the matching medication card are carried (on a tray) to the client's room. *Correct identification of the client* is imperative. The client is asked to state his name. When a client's name is called out, many clients, especially when they are drowsy, will answer to the wrong name. Errors are avoided when he states his name to the nurse. The name on the medicine card is then compared to the name on the client's identification band. This is a double check that further eliminates the possibility of error. Once identification of the client has been established, the medication can be administered. Fresh water should be provided with capsules and tablets. (Sublingual and buccal med-

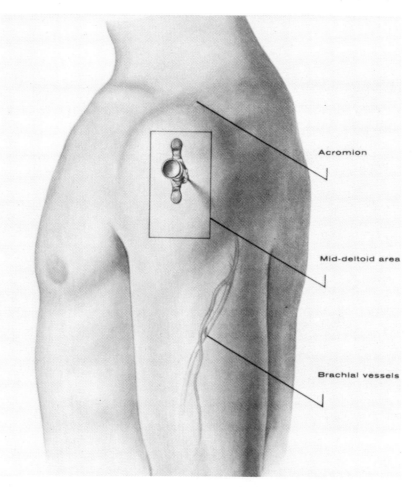

Acromion

Mid-deltoid area

Brachial vessels

Figure 34-8. The mid-deltoid area intramuscular injection site. A site often chosen for its ease of access is the deltoid area which can be employed when the patient is either standing, sitting, or prone. While the deltoid muscle forms a fairly large triangle on the shoulder prominence, the actual area available to a shoulder injection is limited, since there are major bones, blood vessels and nerves to be avoided. The recommended boundaries of the injection area form a rectangle bounded by the lower edge of the acromion on the top to a point on the lateral side of the arm opposite the axilla or armpit on the bottom. The two side boundaries are lines parallel to the arm one-third and two-thirds of the way around the outer lateral aspect of the arm. Care should be taken to avoid not only the acromion, clavicle and humerus, but also the brachial veins and arteries and the radial nerve. It is recommended that the number and size of injections made at this site be limited. The area is small and cannot tolerate repeated injections and large quantities of medication. (Courtesy of Wyeth Laboratories, Philadelphia, Penna.)

ications and troches are given without water; instructions for their placement should be given to the client.) Water is not used to dilute cough syrups; the client should not drink fluids for approximately 15 minutes after taking them.

Remain with the client until he has swallowed all capsules or tablets. If the client does not want to take the medication immediately, it should not be left in the room but brought back at a later time. A nurse should record as administered only those drugs which she has actually seen taken by the client. Although fairly infrequent, there have been some unfortunate incidents where clients have saved up their oral medications and committed suicide by overdosage. This possibility is decreased when drugs are not left unattended in a client's room. (The exception to this rule is when the physician orders that drugs be left at the bedside for the client's self-medication).

Parenteral administration requires selection of an appropriate site. Intramuscular injections in an adult are given in the mid-deltoid area (Fig. 34-8), the

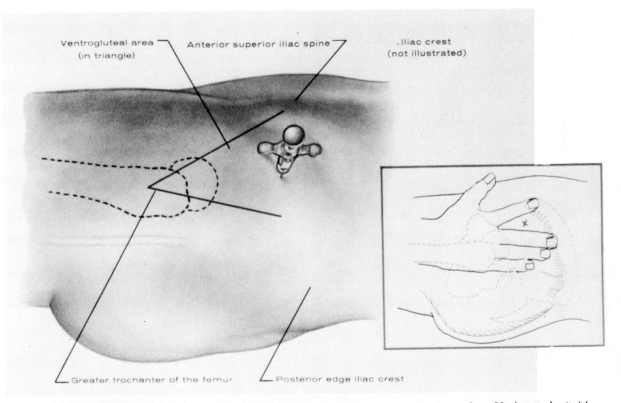

Figure 34-9. The ventrogluteal area intramuscular injection site. The ventrogluteal area (von Hochstetter's site) has been accorded growing recognition as a site removed from major nerves and vascular structures. The subcutaneous fatty layer is relatively shallow and there is good gluteal muscle density. Because anatomic landmarks are easily identifiable around the ventral area of the gluteal muscles, this site is also recommended for injections in children. Although especially suitable for a patient lying on his back, this site is also accessible with the patient lying prone, on his side, or standing.

The patient should always be sufficiently exposed to enable adequate identification of anatomic landmarks. Palpate to find the greater trochanter, the anterior superior iliac spine and the iliac crest. When injecting into the left side of the patient, place the palm of the right hand on the greater trochanter and the index finger on the anterior superior iliac spine. (Use the left hand to delineate the site when injecting into the patient's right side.) Spread the middle finger posteriorly away from the index finger as far as possible along the iliac crest, as shown in the straight-line drawing above. A "V" space or triangle between the index and middle finger is formed. The injection is made in the center of the triangle with the needle directed slightly upward toward the crest of the ilium. (Courtesy of Wyeth Laboratories, Philadelphia, Penna.)

ventrogluteal area (Fig. 34-9), the mid-portion of the vastus lateralis (Fig. 34-10), and the gluteus medius (Fig. 34-11) (although this site is not approved of in many institutions). IM injections in children are given in the anterior, mid-lateral thigh (Figs. 34-12 and 34-13) and occasionally in the deltoid. Injections into the gluteus should not be given prior to the age of 4 and then only when acceptable according to institutional policy. The main concern in IM injections is avoidance of damage to nerve bodies and also the avoidance of giving the drug intravenously rather than into a muscle.

Subcutaneous injections can be given in numerous sites on the upper arms, thighs, back, gluteus, and abdomen. When a client receives daily injections (such as insulin), it is helpful to absorption and maintenance of tissue integrity to rotate the site of injection. Figures 34-14, 34-15, and 34-16 illustrate the steps for an IM injection and Figures 34-17 and 34-18 for subcutaneous injections. The main differences in the two injections are the needle length and angle of insertion.

Upon completion of all medication administrations, date, time, drug, dosage, route, and site (if applicable) must be recorded. If a medication is missed or refused, this is also noted. The reason for missing the dose (for instance, while the client is at the x-ray department) is stated. If refused, it is helpful to discuss the reasons for the refusal with the client. Sometimes it is simply confusion or lack of understanding that is the underlying cause of refusal. A simple explanation will often allay fear or alleviate concerns. Observations of any unusual reactions or complaints should also be noted in the client's record.

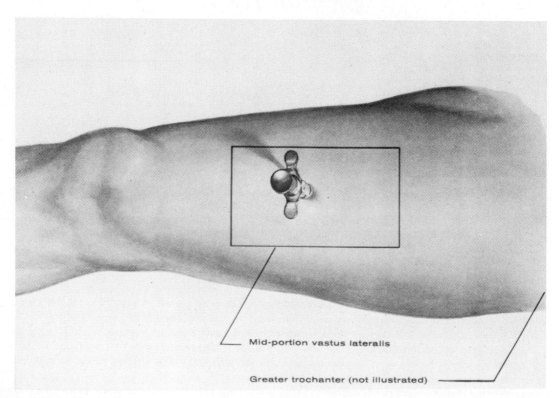

Mid-portion vastus lateralis

Greater trochanter (not illustrated)

Figure 34-10. The vastus lateralis intramuscular injection site. Another site recommended for its relative safety and freedom from major nerves and blood vessels is the vastus lateralis. This injection area is bounded by the mid-anterior thigh on the front of the leg, the mid-lateral thigh on the side and is a hand's breadth below the greater trochanter at the proximal end and another hand's breadth above the knee at the distal end. Although it is easier to give an injection in the vastus lateralis when the patient is lying on his back, it is acceptable to use this site when he is in a sitting position. The entire area should be exposed to permit identification of anatomic landmarks pertinent to this site. This site may also be used for pediatric patients. (Courtesy of Wyeth Laboratories, Philadelphia, Penna.)

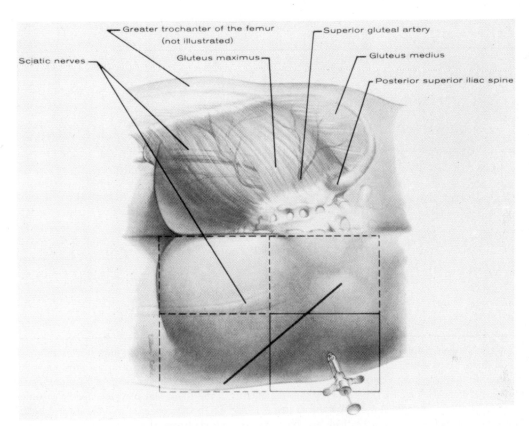

Greater trochanter of the femur
(not illustrated)

Sciatic nerves

Gluteus maximus

Superior gluteal artery

Gluteus medius

Posterior superior iliac spine

Figure 34-11. The gluteus medius intramuscular injection site. The posterior gluteal area is possibly the most commonly considered site for injections. In defining this site for injection purposes care should be given to restrict injections to that portion of the gluteus medius which is above and outside of a diagonal line drawn from the greater trochanter of the femur to the posterior superior iliac spine. Extreme caution should be observed to ensure that the boundary line is maintained, avoiding the hazard of possibly injecting into either the sciatic nerve or the superior gluteal artery. The patient should be lying face down. A "toe-in" position relaxes the muscles. The injection site should be clearly exposed. Under no circumstances should there be any compromise with correct technic. Do not hurry, do not let modesty tempt you to give this injection to a person who is bending over a table or with his clothing only partially removed from the injection site. The needle is inserted perpendicular to the flat surface on which the patient is lying—needle penetration should be on a direct back-to-front course. (Courtesy of Wyeth Laboratories, Philadelphia, Penna.)

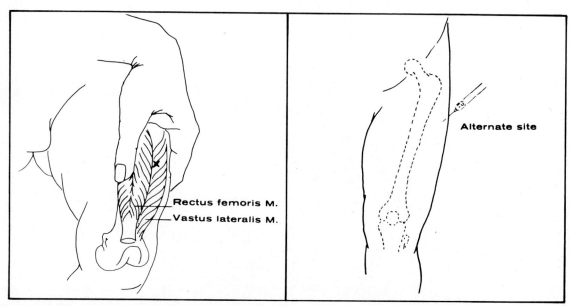

Figure 34-12. Pediatric intramuscular injection sites. The quadriceps femoris is the largest muscle group in the anterolateral thigh. The vastus lateralis is the major muscle of this group and is located on the most lateral aspect of the thigh away from major nerves and vessels. The anterior surface of the mid-lateral thigh is therefore a suitable site for intramuscular injections in this area. Survey the overall size of the thigh and plan the needle insertion depth accordingly. In very small infants, needle insertion to just a 1 inch depth will penetrate into the muscle belly.

The infant lies on his back. Grasp the thigh and compress the muscle tissue as shown. This helps to stabilize the extremity and concentrates the muscle mass. Using the position shown, the left arm helps to restrain the struggling patient. The needle penetrates the gathered muscle mass on the lateral portion of the anterior thigh and is directed on a front-to-back course. This is removed from the medial portion of the thigh where major nerves and vessels are located among the deeper layers of the muscle tissue (see Fig. 34-13). An alternate injection site in this area is the anterolateral surface of the upper thigh. When this location is used, the needle is directed distally and inserted obliquely at an approximate 45 degree angle to the horizontal and long axes of the leg. The needle should not penetrate deeper than 1 inch. Compressing the muscle tissues between the fingers amasses the musculature at the site of injection. (Courtesy of Wyeth Laboratories, Philadelphia, Penna.)

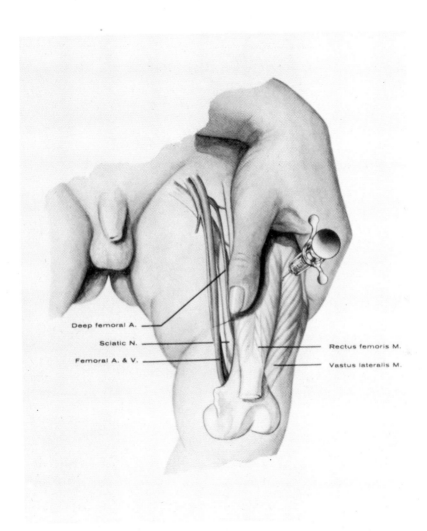

Deep femoral A.

Sciatic N.

Femoral A. & V.

Rectus femoris M.

Vastus lateralis M.

Figure 34-13. Anatomy of site of pediatric injections. (Courtesy of Wyeth Laboratories, Philadelphia, Penna.)

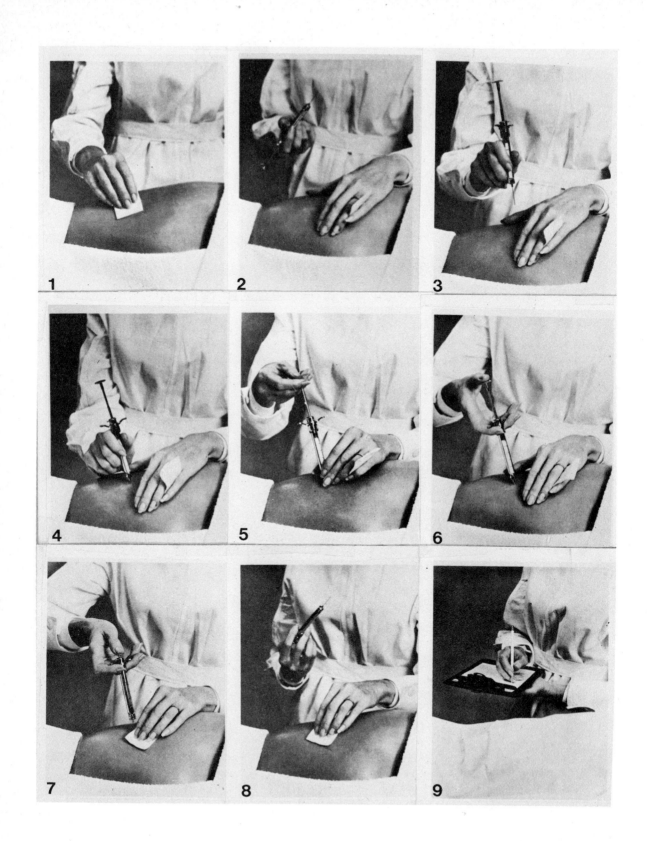

1 2 3
4 5 6
7 8 9

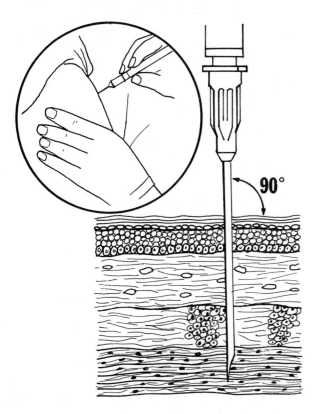

Figure 34-15. Intramuscular route of medication administration. (*See* insert for IM administration in deltoid muscle.) Note 90 degree angle of needle to skin. Needle tip is in muscle tissue.

Figure 34-14. Giving the intramuscular injection. 1. Using an alcohol sponge or swab, cleanse an area approximately 2 inches square around the proposed injection site. 2. With the index finger and thumb of the left hand spread or tense the skin in the injection area. 3. Holding the barrel of the syringe in the right hand in a dart or pencil grip, introduce the needle into the skin with a quick thrust. 4. Once the surface of skin has been punctured by the needle, the remainder of the penetration of the needle through the skin and into the muscle should be with a firm and steady pressure. In the case of average or heavy clients it is preferable to retain the pressure on the skin around the injection site with the thumb and index fingers of the left hand for the entire time the needle is being inserted. In thin clients, on the other hand, it is often preferable to release the pressure of the left hand once the puncture has been made, and change to a slight pinching grip in order to firm the injection site and avoid the possibility of going too deep and striking a bone, nerve or blood vessel. 5. Once the desired depth of insertion has been reached, steady the syringe tip with the left hand and with the right hand pull back or out on the plunger approximately ¼ inch for a few seconds, to see if any blood can be aspirated back into the syringe. Should blood appear in the syringe, the needle should be withdrawn and the entire syringe, needle and solution discarded. Preparation of the injection would be begun again. 6. If no blood appears, the position of the fingers on the right hand can be shifted so that the thumb covers the head of the plunger and the index and middle fingers are hooked under the side grips on the syringe barrel. With a firm pressure on the thumb, move the plunger slowly downward into the syringe as far as it will go. (The small air bubble that is last to disappear is an important part of the injection, since it helps to spread medication, clear the medicine from needle, seal injection site, and prevent tracking of medication as the needle is withdrawn.) 7. After the medication has been injected, apply pressure against the injection site with the alcohol sponge in the left hand as the needle is withdrawn by the right hand; this reduces the risk of medication leaking into the subcutaneous tissues and possibly forming abscesses. 8. Then proceed to cleanse the injection site, by massaging the area with the sponge to remove any blood or medication that might be present. If rapid absorption is desired, massaging should be continued for about 2 minutes. 9. After the injection has been given, it is important that all the information be recorded on the client's chart. This should include: the hour of injection, name of the medication, amount and strength, method of administration, specific site including which side of the body, any unusual reaction and your signature. No injection is complete until this has been done. (Courtesy of Wyeth Laboratories, Philadelphia, Penna.)

Administration of Medications **635**

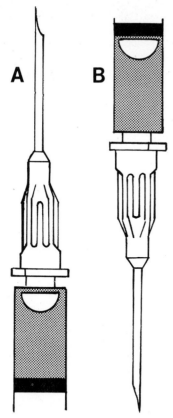

Figure 34-16. A, 0.2 ml of air is added to the syringe when preparing intramuscular injection after accurate dosage has been drawn into syringe. B, Note that the syringe is inverted as it will be during injection. Air bubble will now be administered after all solution has been injected, clearing medication from needle, preventing leakage of fluid back through subcutaneous tissue upon removal from site; thus insuring that solution remains in muscle where absorption is intended.

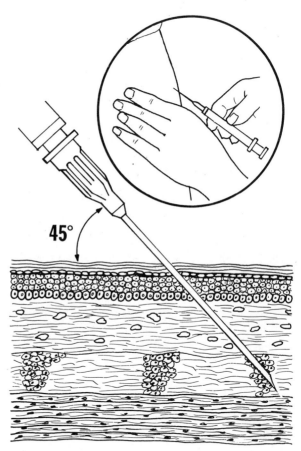

45°

Figure 34-17. Subcutaneous route of medication administration. After cleansing skin with alcohol, subcutaneous tissue is "pinched up." The needle is rapidly inserted to desired depth at a 45 degree angle to skin. By pulling back on the plunger (aspiration), it can be seen if the needle is located in blood vessel. Should blood appear, needle is withdrawn and injection preparation is begun again. Inject solution by slowly depressing plunger. Apply pressure against the injection site with alcohol sponge and rapidly withdraw needle. Massaging area with sponge will help to increase rate of absorption. Injection information is then recorded on client's record.

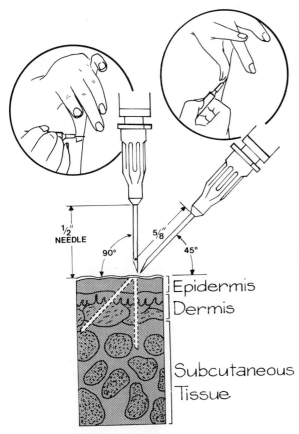

Figure 34-18. Subcutaneous and deep subcutaneous injections. The ⅝ inch needle is injected at a 45 degree angle to the skin. The ½ inch needle is inserted at a 90 degree angle to the skin. Because of the shortness of the needle length, it remains within the subcutaneous tissue, not the muscle. (Note inserts depicting angles of needle to subcutaneous tissue of upper arm.)

In the figure, labels read: ½" NEEDLE, 90°, ⅝", 45°, Epidermis, Dermis, Subcutaneous Tissue.

SUMMARY

The area of medication administration is one in which errors are unfortunately made with great frequency. The way to decrease these errors is through learning correct techniques for preparing and administering drugs and by a continuous, deliberate effort to maintain high standards of practice in this area. Because of the continuous barrage of new drugs on the market, it is very difficult if not impossible, to keep up with all current medications.

However, knowing the sources where information can be obtained and then utilizing them is a step in decreasing error potential. The "five rights"—(1) the right drug; (2) the right dose; (3) the right route (or method); (4) the right time; and (5) the right client—if kept in mind will increase accuracy. The nurse should be aware of the laws that protect her and those that protect the client and his rights. When one understands one's role and how the law works in relation to its implementation, then care is taken to achieve the highest level of safety possible. The nurse does not have to fear administering medications; it can be a challenging and interesting aspect of nursing care. She should, however, have a healthy respect for the hazards involved in this procedure and the need for both keen observation and good judgment.

BIBLIOGRAPHY

Asperheim, M. K., and Eisenhauer, L.: *The Pharmacologic Basis of Patient Care,* 3rd ed. Philadelphia, W. B. Saunders Company, 1977.

Bergersen, B. S.: *Pharmacology in Nursing,* 13th ed. St. Louis, C. V. Mosby Co., 1976.

Dison, N.: *Clinical Nursing Techniques.* St. Louis, C. V. Mosby Co., 1975.

Elhart, D., et al.: *Scientific Principles in Nursing,* 8th ed. St. Louis, C. V. Mosby Co., 1978.

Falconer, M., et al.: *The Drug, the Nurse, the Patient,* 6th ed. Philadelphia, W. B. Saunders Company, 1978.

Fuerst, E., and Wolff, L.: *Fundamentals of Nursing.* Philadelphia, J. B. Lippincott, 1974.

Henderson, V., and Nite, G.: *Principles and Practice of Nursing,* 6th ed. New York, Macmillan Publishing Co., Inc., 1978.

Loebl, S., Spratto, G., and Wit, A.: *The Nurses Drug Handbook.* New York, John Wiley and Sons, 1977.

Miller, B., and Keane, C.: *Encyclopedia and Dictionary of Medicine, Nursing, and Allied Health,* 2nd ed. Philadelphia, W. B. Saunders Co., 1978.

Plein, J., and Plein, E.: *Fundamentals of Medications,* 2nd ed. Hamilton, Ill., Drug Intelligence Publication, Inc., 1974.

Rodman, M., and Smith, D.: *Pharmacology in Drug Therapy in Nursing.* Philadelphia, J. B. Lippincott Co., 1968.

Taber's Cyclopedic Medical Dictionary, 13th ed. Philadelphia, F. A. Davis Company, 1977.

CHAPTER 35

NATURE OF HOMEODYNAMICS

Homeodynamics, the critical balance maintained by the human organism, is affected by a varied combination of physiologic and psychologic factors. Indeed, entire books have been devoted to the examination of the interrelated stressors that may disrupt the essential wholeness of body functions. Such disturbances of psychic and bodily function may either emanate from or cause disease states. Some 40 years ago, Hans Selye, the father of stress theory, formulated the models that occur in conjunction with stress. As a consequence of his research, specific physiologic events that occur as a result of varied environmental and internal stressors have been described. Thus, an examination of the physiologic and psychic components of stressor anxiety added useful information to psychiatric theory concerning neurotic and psychotic states. Moreover, a number of disease states are now recognized as having the potential to disrupt bodily processes and, hence, homeodynamics.

FLUID AND ELECTROLYTE BALANCE: ADMINISTRATION OF PARENTERAL FLUIDS

Genevieve Fitzpatrick, M.S., R.N.

Diabetes is one such disease state which may interrupt complex bodily endocrine functions with resultant acidotic states. The triad of diabetes symptoms illustrates the fluid and electrolyte disturbances this stressful disease causes: *polyuria* (excessive urination), *polydipsia* (excessive thirst), and *polyphagia* (excessive hunger). These three symptoms may cause an infinite variety of electrolyte disruptions. The prediabetic individual may also encounter such stress as overwhelming infection, which may play a significant role in disease causation. From the above discussion, the reader may conclude that a logical, even necessary, point of departure for any discussion of fluid and electrolyte problems and nursing procedures must be stress models and their impact on homeodynamics.

Selye's original model, which related the physiologic consequences of stress, has withstood the test of time. It has been refined by many investigators and is now used as the basis for many modern postoperative routines. Selye discerned that under stress organ systems are involved in a complex interplay which he called "General Adaptation Syndrome" (GAS)—that is, the body's attempt to cope with stress. He also theorized that the inadequate ability to cope would result in specific disease states, such as arthritis and asthma. Figures 35-1 and 35-2 are graphic representations of this stress model.

Two crisis theorists, Aguilera and Messick,[1] have developed an assessment tool, the crisis paradigm. If this behavioral model is superimposed on the physiologic model of Selye, the nurse might examine the totality of the impact of stress on the client. For example, the client whose anxiety is multiplied and unrelieved due to maladaptive coping skills and a distorted perception of the upcoming surgery may be in crisis. This person may as a consequence suffer fluid and electrolyte shifts of enormous proportions during complex surgery. Thus, the body's usual response to stress is magnified by this additional unrelieved anxiety. The balancing factors of a psychic nature as described by Aguilera and Messick (perception of the event,

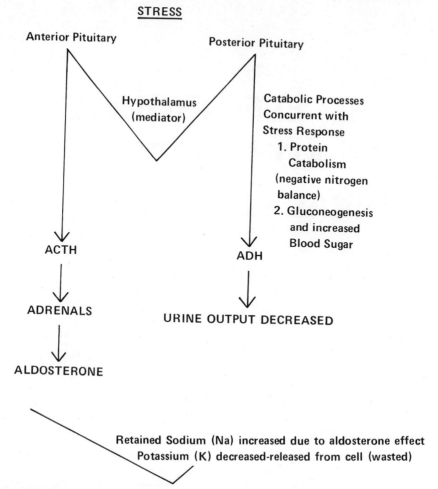

STRESS

Anterior Pituitary   Posterior Pituitary

Hypothalamus
(mediator)

Catabolic Processes
Concurrent with
Stress Response
1. Protein
    Catabolism
(negative nitrogen
balance)
2. Gluconeogenesis
   and increased
   Blood Sugar

ACTH   ADH

ADRENALS   URINE OUTPUT DECREASED

ALDOSTERONE

Retained Sodium (Na) increased due to aldosterone effect
Potassium (K) decreased-released from cell (wasted)

FIGURE 35-1. Graphic representation of stress model.

coping skills, and situational supports) should then be considered with those physiologic balancing factors that maintain dynamic equilibrium. The hospitalized client must be carefully assessed within this frame of homeodynamics from the moment of admission. Those factors that increase anxiety, such as language barriers, sensory deprivation (the blind or deaf client), and clouded perceptions, regarding the plans of care as elaborated by the physician and nurse, must be identified and relieved. Those factors that disturb physiologic balance, such as long-term drug therapy and uncontrolled or chronic disease states (e.g., diabetes, kidney disease), must be identified and considered in respect to the po-

tential for further complicating the body's adaptive responses. Failure to assess these disturbances will affect the entire rehabilitative process of the client. Thus, the implications for nursing care in every setting become apparent.

In summary, homeodynamics must be evaluated in terms of total body response to psychological and physiological stressors. Intelligent evaluation is based on an understanding of the organism in equilibrium. The aim of the following discussion is to select and detail only one aspect of the total fabric of the human organism's balanced state: fluid and electrolyte considerations. It is hoped the reader will look elsewhere in this text for the myriad

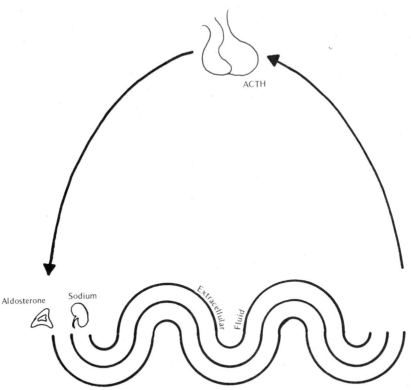

FIGURE 35-2. Negative feedback mechanism. Decreased sodium in the ECF results in the release of ACTH from the anterior pituitary which causes an increase in aldosterone. Aldosterone in turn causes the retention of sodium. (Reprinted with permission from Stroot, V. R., et al.: *Fluids and Electrolytes: A Practical Approach,* 2nd ed. Philadelphia, F. A. Davis Co., 1977, p. 64.)

psychic and physiologic factors that comprise a holistic understanding of the homeodynamic response. (See Chapter 6, "Homeodynamics and Stress".)

BODY FLUIDS AND ELECTROLYTES

Before the reader considers the nursing procedures related to fluid and electrolyte concepts, he must review the basic vocabulary and physiology of this aspect of homeodynamics.

The major component of the body weight in both adults and children is water, comprising 40−75 percent of adult weight and 70−85 percent of the child's weight. This water is distributed within (intracellular—¾ of total) and without (extracellular—¼ of total) the cells (Fig. 35−3). Extracellular water

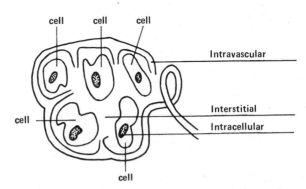

FIGURE 35-3. Intracellular water distribution. (Reprinted with permission from Dickens, M. L.: *Fluid and Electrolyte Balance: A Programmed Text.* Philadelphia, F. A. Davis Co., 1974, p. 39.)

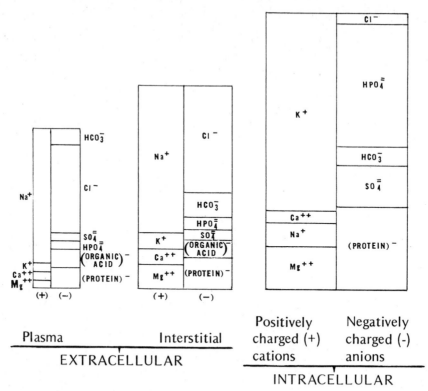

Positively   Negatively
charged (+)   charged (-)
cations   anions

Plasma   Interstitial

EXTRACELLULAR

INTRACELLULAR

FIGURE 35-4. Relationship between the amounts of fluid within the body fluid compartments. Cation and anion relationships. (Reprinted with permission from Dickens, M. L.: *Fluid and Electrolyte Balance: A Programmed Text.* Philadelphia, F. A. Davis Co., 1974, p. 41.)

TABLE 35-1. Electrolytes, Chemical Symbols, and Functions

Electrolyte	Chemical Symbol	Function
Cations:		
Sodium	Na^+	Major extracellular cation; fluid balance; osmotic pressure
Potassium	K^+	Major intracellular cation; neuromuscular excitability; acid-base balance
Calcium	Ca^{++}	Neuromuscular irritability; bones; blood clotting
Magnesium	Mg^{++}	Enzyme systems
Anions:		
Chloride	Cl^-	Major extracellular anion; fluid balance; osmotic pressure
Bicarbonate	HCO_3^-	Acid-base balance
Proteinates		Osmotic pressure; acid-base balance
Organic acids		Intermediary cellular metabolism
Phosphates	HPO_4^{--}	Major intracellular anion
Sulfate	SO_4^{--}	Protein metabolism

Adapted (with permission) from Stroot, V. R., et al.: *Fluids and Electrolytes: A Practical Approach.* Philadelphia, F. A. Davis Co., 1975, p. 7.

is located in plasma, interstitial spaces (spaces between cells), and lymph (specialized interstitial fluid) (Fig. 35–4). Dissolved in solution within the body fluid are a number of positively (cations) and negatively (anions) charged particles called electrolytes (Table 35-1). The major anions of extracellular fluid are: chloride (Cl) and bicarbonate (HCO_3), and the majority of plasma proteinate. Intracellular anions include sulfates (SO_4) and phosphates (HPO_4).

The major extracellular cation is Na^+ (sodium), and the major intracellular cation is K^+ (potassium). Because positively and negatively charged particles balance when electrolytes are placed in solution (water), these charges are measured in equivalents. One-thousandth of an equivalent, or a milliequivalent, is the convenient laboratory measure of the dissolved molecules. Laboratory data about concentration of electrolytes generated in milliequivalents per liter serve as a basis for determining fluid and electrolyte replacement needs of the hospitalized client (Table 35-2).

Extracellular fluid and its electrolyte components

TABLE 35-2. Chart of Normal Laboratory Values

Tests	Values	Tests	Values
Hematology:		**Blood Chemistry:**	
Blood count (red)	F 3.8−5.8 million/cu mm M 4.4−6.4 million/cu mm	Blood urea nitrogen (BUN)	10−20 mg/100 ml
		Calcium	8.5−10.5 mg/100 ml
Blood count (white)	5,000−10,000/cu mm	Chloride	95−105 mEq/L
Hct	F 37−47% M 40-54%	CO_2	24−32 mEq/L (adults)
Hgb	F 11−15 gms% M 12−17 gms%		18−27 mEq/L (children)
		Creatinine	0.5−1.5 mg/100 ml
		Creatinine clearance	100−130 cc/min
Urine Chemistry:		Electrolytes: sodium (Na)	135−145 mEq/L
		potassium (K)	3.5−5.0 mEq/L
Addis count, RBCs	Less than one half million	chloride (Cl)	95−105 mEq/L
WBCs	Less than one million	CO_2	24−32 mEq/L
Casts	Less than 5,000 (hyaline)	Glucose (fasting)	65−110 mg/100 ml
Calcium	50−300 mg/24 hours	Lactic dehydrogenase (LDH)	100−225 Technicon units
Catecholamines	Up to 100 mEq/24 hours	Osmolality	275−330 mOsm/kg
Chlorides	170−250 mEq/24 hours	Phosphorous	2.5−4.5 mg
Creatinine clearance	100−130 cc/min	Potassium	3.5−5.0 mEq/L
LDH (lactic dehydrogenase)	0−8,000 units	Protein	6.8 gm/dl
17-OH corticosteroids	5.5−12 mg/24 hours (adult)	Sodium	135−145 mEq/L
	3 mg/24 hours (up to 10 years)	Urea clearance	Standard 40−68 cc/min Maximal 64−99 cc/min
17-ketosteroids	5−15 mg/24 hours (female)	Uric acid	2.5−8.0 mg/100 ml
	7−20 mg/24 hours (male)	Total protein	Under 0.15 gms/24 hours
	21 mg/24 hours (children under 6)	**Blood Gases:**	
	3 mg/24 hours (6−10 years)		(Mean) (Range)
Potassium	27-123 mEq/24 hours	pH	V:7.37 (7.32−7.42)
Sodium	43−217 mEq/24 hours		A:7.40 (7.35−7.45)
Sugar (quan.)	negative	pCO_2	V:46 (42−55) mm Hg
			A:40 (34−46) mm Hg
Urea clearance	Standard 40−68 cc/min	H_2CO_3	V:1.38 (1.26−1.65) mm/L
Urea nitrogen	2.7−9.9 gms/24 hours		A:1.20 (1.02−1.38) mm/L
Uric acid	600 mg/L	HCO_3	V:26 (24−28) mEq/L
Urine osmolality	270−900 mOsm/kg; mean 550 mOsm/kg		A:24 (22−26) mEq/L
		pO_2	V:40 (Varies with pH) mm Hg
			A:90
		O_2 Sat	V:62 (55−71)%
			A:98 (over 90)%

Adapted (with permission) from Stroot, V. R., et al.: *Fluids and Electrolytes: A Practical Approach.* Philadelphia, F. A. Davis Co., 1975, pp. 215-216.

provide a proper nutrient environment for body cells, contribute to essential cellular activities and relieve the cells of their waste products. Bodily secretions and excretions derive fluids and electrolytes primarily from the extracellular fluid (ECF).

Transport and Osmolarity

The concepts of passive transport and osmolarity must be reviewed to understand the complexities of the fluid and electrolyte transportation system within the body. Passive transportation is accomplished by diffusion, osmosis, and filtration. *Diffusion* is movement of ions from areas of higher solute concentration to lower solute concentration. *Osmosis* is the primary mechanism by which intracellular exchanges take place as solutes, and solvents diffuse through a semipermeable membrane. *Filtration* occurs as a consequence of hydrostatic pressure which moves solutions from greater to lesser pressure areas.

Osmotic pressure is determined by solute concentration or osmolarity, and *oncotic pressure* refers to the unique moving force of the proteinate

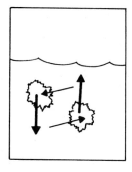 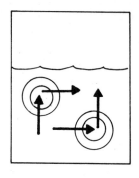 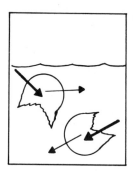

A. Hypertonic   B. Isotonic   C. Hypotonic

FIGURE 35-5. Comparison of solution (large arrows indicate greater movement). A, Osmotic pressure or pull of the solution surrounding cell causes more water to move out of the cell than into the cell. B, Solution and cells have equal movement of fluid. C, Osmotic pressure or pull of the solution within the cell causes more water to move into the cell than out of the cell. (Reprinted with permission from Stroot, V. R., et al.: *Fluids and Electrolytes: A Practical Approach,* 2nd ed. Philadelphia, F. A. Davis Co., 1977 p. 6.)

molecules within the plasma (Fig. 35-5). Disorders of the extracellular fluid composition and movement account for a number of the fluid and electrolyte imbalances that the nurse will observe in clinical practice. The remainder of these imbalances may be classified as acid-base disorders which reflect deviations from the normal alkalinity or acidity of body fluids as expressed by the pH (or hydrogen ion concentration) within the body. These minute concentrations of hydrogen ions are responsible for maintaining the normal ratio of bicarbonate to carbonic acid within the body (20:1) (Fig. 35-6). The normal pH of ECF is 7.35−7.45. Acidotic states

are reflected in a pH below 7.35, while alkalotic states occur at a level above 7.45. Apparently minor mathematical deviations, however, in the pH level may cause death if they persist. For example, fatalities occur at pH levels above 7.8 or below 7.0. pH is primarily regulated by the kidneys and lungs by resorption of bicarbonate and excretion of ammonium chloride (NH_3Cl) and conservation or wasting of carbon dioxide (CO_2), respectively. Fluids and electrolytes in normal health states remain distributed as previously described. Intracellular and extracellular electrolyte composition is equally distributed under normal circumstances. Fluids and electrolytes are maintained in balance by a number of bodily systems. The organs of homeodynamics include: the lungs, kidneys, adrenals, and other endocrine glands, the central nervous system, skin, gastrointestinal tract, and blood. The means by which these organs maintain homeodynamics are summarized briefly. The lungs adjust the level of PCO_2 to temporarily compensate for carbonic acid bicarbonate ratio disturbances. The kidneys excrete or retain bicarbonate sodium and chloride to compensate for acid/base disturbances.

The central nervous system elaborates antidiuretic hormone, stimulating aldosterone production by the adrenals. Mineral corticoid and glucocorticoid production may affect essential fluid and electrolyte changes when the organism is under stress (such as that generated by surgery). The skin via its evaporating power and insensible perspiration

20 bicarbonates : 1 carbonic acid

FIGURE 35-6. Acid-base balance. Blood pH is 7.4. (Reprinted with permission from Stroot, V. R., et al.: *Fluids and Electrolytes: A Practical Approach,* 2nd ed. Philadelphia, F. A. Davis Co., 1977 p. 85.)

may either conserve or excrete fluid. The gastrointestinal tract in the normal course of events absorbs and utilizes water and nutrients from food stuffs. Blood contains a hemoglobin buffer system within the red blood cells and plasma. The weak acids and alkali salts which act as buffers are protein by-products (Fig. 35-7). The endocrine glands by elaboration of a number of hormones exert profound effects on homeodynamics and fluid and electrolyte balance. In addition, thirst and hunger may be symptoms generated by the body in an attempt to restore fluids. Thus, the athlete drinks fluid to compensate for abnormal fluid losses generated by stressful activities.

Finally, a clear understanding of usual fluid and electrolyte gains and losses is essential to the nurse's conceptualization of disease states that abnormally deplete or overload the body with fluid and electrolytes.

Imbalances

Water is *gained* by food and fluid intake and by oxidation of nutrients within the body. Fluid and electrolytes are normally *lost* via the lungs (evaporation-breath), and the body fluids such as tears, urine, and insensible perspiration, as well as the intestinal fluid present in the stool.

Imbalances, which are a result of deviations from these gains and losses, may be minor or life threatening. For example, severe dehydration can result in death, whereas fluid depletion may be restored by the impetus of thirst and have no perceptible effects. Severe diarrhea with consequent loss of sodium and potassium may cause a life threatening metabolic acidosis, whereas one or two bouts of loose stools may be readily compensated. It has been estimated that up to a liter of fluid with electrolytes may be lost by perspiration alone in the febrile client. Inasmuch as the nurse's educative mission demands a great deal of health teaching, the importance of nutrition in maintaining fluid and electrolyte equilibrium and preventing imbalances deserves mention. Failure to observe and report such losses may result in irrevocable damage to the body's homeodynamics. Malnutrition may exist even in the individual who considers himself well-fed. The importance of the Basic Four and its basis for a health diet rests, to a great extent, on the fact

that these food groupings provide a large number of essential electrolytes in addition to meeting the body's fluid needs.

SIXTEEN BASIC IMBALANCES

Sixteen basic imbalances have been elaborated by Methany and Snively.[2] The imbalances, which derive from the prior discussions of location and distribution of fluid and electrolytes, are listed below with examples of the nursing actions that should be triggered by these imbalances.

1. *Plasma to interstitial fluid shift of extracellular fluid.*
    a. *Example:* The client, who was admitted to the hospital following massive crushing injury in a car accident, presents with the following symptoms: cold extremities, low blood pressure, pallor, tachycardia, weak pulse, increased hemoglobin, and increased red blood cell count. This imbalance may be corrected by parenteral administration of dextrose, plasma, or a plasmalike electrolyte solution.
    b. *Immediate nursing actions:* Observations on plasma administration as discussed under parenteral therapy procedures should be made. Complications may include allergic responses and post-transfusion reactions ranging from chills and fever to contaminant responses such as septic shock. Record and monitor intake and output.
2. *Extracellular fluid volume deficit.*
    a. *Example:* The client is admitted with a question of intestinal obstruction. Within the past 2 weeks, she has lost 20 pounds. Her body temperature is 97. Her urine output has been scanty for the past 24 hours. Her hemoglobin is 15 as opposed to a 12.2 baseline value.
    b. *Immediate nursing actions:* Make the nursing diagnosis of a possible fluid imbalance, and report all of these symptoms which relate to the basic deficit. Note the condition of the client's skin since dry skin is related to this deficit. The

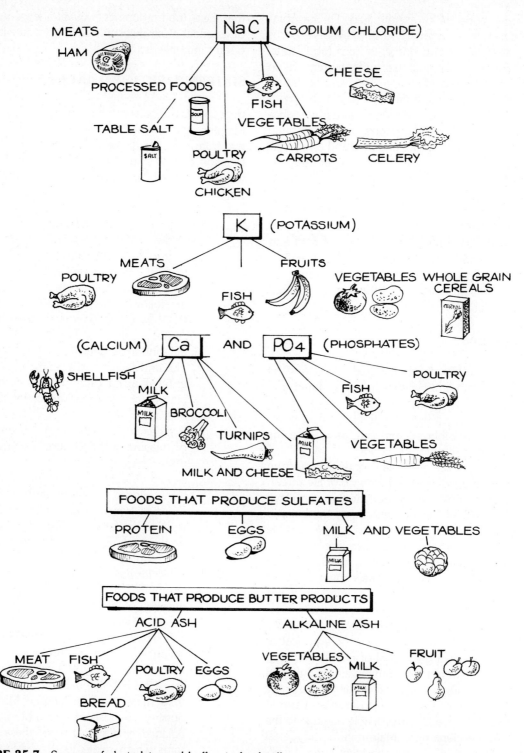

FIGURE 35-7. Sources of electrolytes and buffers in foodstuffs.

client should be placed on NPO (nothing by mouth) as the physician will order appropriate parenteral fluid administration. Record and monitor intake and output.

3. *Extracellular fluid volume excess.*
   a. *Example*: The client presents with congestive heart failure and renal disease. He has recently gained 20 lbs. On auscultation, you detect with a stethoscope moist rales in his lungs. His hemoglobin is 9.2 compared to a baseline of 13.2 for this client.
   b. *Immediate nursing actions*: Restrict fluid intake, position client for proper aeration, assess all vital signs, and report findings immediately. Record and monitor intake and output.

4. *Sodium deficit of extracellular fluid.*
   a. *Example*: The client has just had gastrointestinal surgery. He has been permitted nonelectrolyte ice chips and has been taking them almost constantly since surgery to alleviate oral discomfort due to a nasogastric tube. He appears apprehensive. In addition, you note oliguria, complaints of abdominal cramps and a urine specific gravity of 1.008.
   b. *Immediate nursing actions*: Stop ice chips, and report all of the above symptoms and your vital sign assessment to physician. Record and monitor intake and output.

5 & 6. *Sodium excess of extracellular fluid and potassium deficit of extracellular fluid.*
   a. *Example*: The client has been admitted with a diagnosis of "diarrhea of questionable etiology." Signs and symptoms include anorexia and diarrhea of 2 weeks duration. Skin is flushed. Laboratory values include a plasma chloride of 115 mEq/L, specific gravity of urine of 1.040 and an ECG (electrocardiogram) with a flattened T wave. (T waves represent repolarization of the ventricles—altered with potassium loss).
   b. *Immediate nursing actions*: Make a nursing diagnosis of a possible imbalance based on other likely symptoms, such as soft, flabby muscles and decreased urine output. Assess other vital signs and re-

port immediately. Record and monitor intake and output.

7. *Potassium excess of extracellular fluid.*
   a. *Example*: The client has been on an intravenous infusion with 20 mEq of potassium. You discover when you come into his room that his IV has been infusing at a rate of 60 drops/minute rather than 16 drops/minute (a maxidrip is on the IV). You note that your client is nauseated, very irritable, and has diarrhea. (Remember that such hyperkalemia may also occur with blood administration due to breakdown of stored red blood cells. Therefore, hyperkalemia symptoms should be noted if plasma or blood products are administered as in case 1). The ECG at this time displays a widened QRS (because depolarization of the ventricles takes longer). The ST segment is elevated.
   b. *Immediate nursing actions*: Put the client on a "Keep vein open" (KVO) intravenous infusion rate, and notify physician. Record and monitor intake and output.

8. *Calcium deficit of extracellular fluid.*
   a. *Example*: The client is admitted with a diagnosis of acute pancreatitis. He complains of abdominal cramps, muscle cramps, and tingling at the ends of fingers. Carpopedal (hand and foot) spasm is noted (Trousseau's sign).
   b. *Immediate nursing actions*: Report symptoms immediately, based on nursing diagnosis of a possible electrolyte problem consequent to a pancreatic disorder with the above symptoms. An additional laboratory test, the Sulkowitch test, on urine may be ordered by the physician or nurse. No precipitation indicates calcium deficit.

9. *Calcium excess of extracellular fluid.*
   a. *Example*: The client is admitted with a diagnosis of multiple myeloma and pathologic bone fractures. She has deep bony pain, severe flank pain and muscle hypotonicity. Sulkowitch test shows heavy precipitation.
   b. *Immediate nursing actions*: Client should receive no calcium by any route, includ-

ing IV fluids. After mental and vital sign status examination, report findings. Record and monitor intake and output.

10. *Primary base bicarbonate deficit of extracellular fluid (metabolic acidosis).*
    a. *Example*: The client is a diabetic admitted with a systemic infection and high fever. He exhibits Kussmaul's breathing (deep sighing respirations), stupor, weakness, plasma pH of 7.1, urine pH of 4. He is exhibiting signs of metabolic acidosis (diabetic coma acidosis).
    b. *Immediate nursing actions*: Prophylactic measures as for any client who is stuporous or potentially convulsive should be carried out. Follow physician "stat" (immediate, at once) order for insulin administration. Insulin effectively blocks ketoacidosis by minimizing fatty acid release from fat cells. Assess and report vital signs. Record and monitor intake and output.

11. *Primary base bicarbonate excess of extracellular fluid (metabolic alkalosis).*
    a. *Example*: The client complained of "heartburn" of several weeks duration with concomitant ingestion of large quantities of antacids. He is admitted to the hospital with nausea, vomiting, and diarrhea as his primary signs and symptoms. In addition, he is confused and twitching. His ECG (electrocardiogram) shows a sinus tachycardia (rapid heart beat).
    b. *Immediate nursing actions*: Use precautionary measures as for any client with convulsion potential. Assess and report vital signs immediately. Assess client for concomitant hypokalemia. Monitor and record intake and output for deficient replacement and imbalance correction.

12. *Primary carbonic acid deficit of extracellular fluid (respiratory alkalosis).*
    a. *Example*: The client is admitted to the emergency room with a psychiatric diagnosis of "acute anxiety state". Shortly after admission your client lapses into unconsciousness. His plasma pH is 7.6, and he is twitching.

    b. *Immediate nursing actions*: Administer sedatives as ordered; as client regains consciousness use crisis intervention principles such as reinforcement of adaptive coping mechanisms and positive feedback; allow ample opportunity for verbalization of current stresses to reassure client and reduce hyperventilation. Observe and record respiratory patterns at rest and awake.

13. *Primary carbonic acid excess of extracellular fluid (respiratory acidosis).*
    a. *Example*: The client is admitted with a diagnosis of chronic obstructive pulmonary disease (COPD). He is admitted with a history of emphysema (15 year duration). He is dyspneic, cyanotic, weak, and disoriented. His plasma bicarbonate is 34 mEq/L.
    b. *Immediate nursing actions*: Since low arterial oxygen (PO_2) is providing the drive for this man's respiration, oxygen administration must be kept at a low liter flow (2L/min) to prevent respiratory arrest. Assess and report all other vital signs. Place him in a position that promotes comfortable respiration. Prepare for bicarbonate buffer administration to combat acidosis.

14. *Protein deficit of extracellular fluid.*
    a. *Example*: The client is admitted with a diagnosis of a bleeding peptic ulcer. She is pale, fatigued, and has poor muscle tone. Her plasma albumin is 2.5 gm/100 ml.
    b. *Immediate nursing actions*: Prepare for blood transfusion administration, emergency measures for shock as Trendelenburg position, and for gastric ice lavage. Assess mental status. Assess and report vital signs immediately.

15. *Magnesium deficit of extracellular fluid.*
    a. *Example*: The client presents with a history of chronic alcoholism and is admitted with symptoms of disorientation and Chvostek's sign (facial nerve response to stimulation with resultant facial grimace).
    b. *Immediate nursing action*: Prepare for corrective parenteral fluid and electrolyte

administration. This client may be a candidate for total parenteral nutrition as well. Institute safety precautions as for any client with convulsion potential. Assess and report vital signs. Monitor and record intake and output.

16. *Interstitial fluid to plasma shift of extracellular fluid.*
    a. *Example*: Your client is admitted following an industrial accident in which multiple fractures and blood loss have been sustained. Your client exhibits air hunger, peripheral vein engorgement, moist lung rales, weakness, and pallor. His hemoglobin is 9.0.
    b. *Immediate nursing actions*: Assess and report vital signs and other significant laboratory values. Prepare for anticipated blood transfusion administration. Avoid positions that will increase symptoms such as rales. Assess and report mental status. Institute safety measures as with any client with depleted sensorium.

The preceding examples present only some basic representations of the common fluid and electrolyte imbalances. The reader is cautioned to remember that most fluid and electrolyte problems are mixed and complex as in the following example:

A 60-year-old woman has a ureterosigmoidostomy. Following surgery, she exhibits weakness, disorientation, and alteration of respirations (deep, rapid breathing). Her K is 3.5; her HCO_3 is 14; pH is 6.8; plasma chloride is elevated at 121 mEq/L. This client represents a combination fluid/electrolyte problem. Her problem is hyperchloremic hypokalemic, metabolic acidosis (base HCO_3 deficit). Urine with its acid pH and high chloride content is reabsorbed from the intestine. The buffer bicarbonate is depleted causing the pH of the blood to drop. Essential potassium is either excreted with chloride by the kidneys in large amounts or washed away with urine from the intestinal ureteral implant site. Thus, the mixed imbalance results. Concomitant problems must always be assessed if there is a clear cut picture of a major imbalance.

Intravenous Therapy and Venipuncture

The intravenous route of administration of parenteral fluid and medication serves a number of purposes related to correction of the major fluid and electrolyte imbalances described. Total parenteral nutrition or hyperalimentation restores nutrients for the nutritionally depleted client. The central venous pressure line serves as an effective monitoring technique of the cardiac effects of intravenous fluid. Both of these latter techniques are performed by physicians. Therefore, nursing responsibilities for assisting and maintaining these intravenous mechanisms will be discussed. The nursing procedure of venipuncture is utilized in the placement of heparin locks, intravenous needles for administration of standard IV solutions such as D/5W (dextrose in water—a 5 percent solution), intravenous medications and blood products, and drawing blood for laboratory tests.

Hypodermoclysis is *rarely* used in the infant or adult with poorly accessible veins. (It is included here since it is still sometimes used.) Extracellular fluid products are injected into the subcutaneous tissues of the client. Solutions administered by this route are ordered by the physician. Some of the solutions which may be safely administered include: specific strengths of saline solutions (such as isotonic saline 0.9 percent) with 2.5 percent dextrose and varying strengths of Ringer's and Ringer's lactate solutions with 2.5 percent dextrose. Electrolyte-free sugar solutions and solutions that may promote fluid shifts or pH alterations (due to variance from usual body pH) are contraindicated. Hyaluronidase is a useful substance injected into the site of hypodermoclysis to increase the fluid absorption rate and decrease discomfort at the clysis site. Tables 35-3 and 35-4 accompanying this chapter will detail nursing responsibilities for parenteral procedures commonly performed by nurses.

Total Parenteral Nutrition

Total parenteral nutrition is a hypertonic nutritive solution administered via a large blood vessel. Many hospitalized clients are in a catabolic (breaking down needed nutrients) nutritive state by reason of surgery or disease state. The usual intrave-

Table 35-3. Intravenous Infusions to Restore Fluid and Electrolyte Balance, and Provide Nutrients for Tissue Repair and Protein and Glucose in Depleted Clients

Anticipated Accomplishment	Scientific Principles/ Rationale	Specific Considerations
1. Check original physician order to prevent administration error and obtain solution ordered. Check amount, fluid type, sequence of solution (if other IVs to be given before).	Improper solution administration may cause fatal fluid/electrolyte complications.	Note any medication to be added to solution. Check compatibility of solution if medication is to be mixed in another reservoir and piggyback to main line. If solution is blood, check to be sure typing and cross-matching done.*
2. Place client at ease by explanation of procedure.	Stress contributes to fluid/electrolyte imbalance.	Emphasize the fact that IV therapy or blood transfusion is almost "routine." Reassure client that he is not failing to progress.
3. Wash hands carefully before assembling equipment and before beginning procedure.	Soap emulsifies bacteria. Careful handwashing decreases contamination and possibility of cross-infection.	Follow a specific procedure that includes all surfaces of hands and wrists.
4. Completely assemble equipment and inspect integrity of system as well as keeping procedure time at a minimum.	Anxiety is heightened by several trips to collect equipment; if bag is leaking or bottle is cracked, solution is contaminated.	For short-term IVs, metal needles are usually used, and "butterfly" plastic tipped needles with short bevels. The gauge of the needle is always smaller than vein. Long-term IVs, catheters, or plastic needles are used (variously called angiocaths).
5. Bring assembled equipment to bedside; arrange bedclothing to expose site and arrange for proper lighting; position yourself close to injection site.	Adequate lighting and exposure facilitates accurate venipuncture.	Stand comfortably close to site of injection to promote proper angle of needle insertion.

*In some institutions only specially prepared RNs may initiate IVs and hypodermoclysis. In addition, some state nurse practice acts have specific conditions under which RNs must operate for giving IV solutions.

Implementation	Recommendations	Observations
Add ordered medication to ordered solution, calculate flow rate on basis of doctor's order. For microdrip set, use 60/60 × amount of solution; for maxidrip, use 10/60 × amount of solution.	Obtain ordered solution. Add medication if ordered. Check integrity of bag/bottle. Check appearance of solution and check labels against physician's order. Number sequenced solutions serially rather than daily.	If blood, check label against client's blood type and Rh factor as well as client's name on name band.
Explain purpose stressing positive aspects of replacement and nutrition to hasten recovery or prepare client for surgery.	Validate client's understanding. Avoid frowning, expressions of concern, or body language that indicates client is "failing."	Note client's responses to explanations, messages of anxiety, or discomfort.
Handwashing with aseptic solution.	Repeat handwashing before beginning procedure.	Note breaks in skin or any superficial lesions which necessitate wearing gloves.
Use arm board for all IVs. For blood, a wide gauge needle, such as #19 or #18, is used; an administration set is selected, with micro- or maxidrip chamber; skin prep solution is assembled, Betadine or other antiseptic ointment for site of needle insertion and bp-cuff or tourniquet to distend veins and solution to be administered.	Size of vein is basis for needle selection. Special blood administration sets with filters must be used for blood and blood products.	
Use bedside lamp and overhead lighting. Identify proper vein site from Figures 35-8 to 11.	Room should be comfortable temperature.	

Table 35-3. Continued

Anticipated Accomplishment	Scientific Principles/ Rationale	Specific Considerations

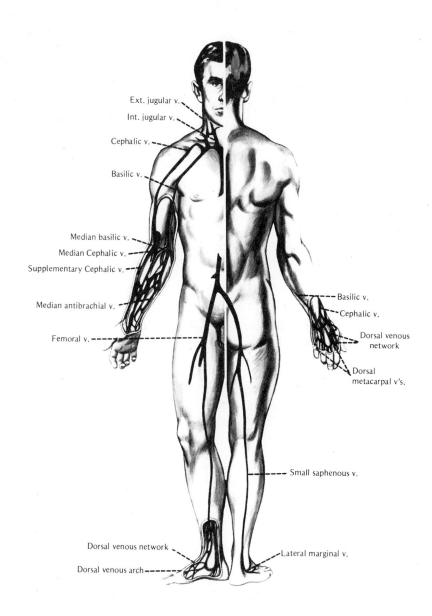

FIGURE 35-8. Anterior and posterior superficial veins used for rapid injection of drugs and intravenous infusion of blood or fluids. (Reprinted with permission from Venipuncture and Venous Cannulation, Abbott Laboratories, 1971.)

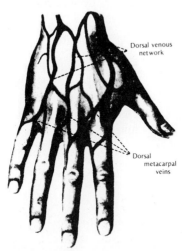

FIGURE 35-9. Several suitable sites for venipuncture on the back of the hand. (Reprinted with permission from Venipuncture and Venous Cannulation, Abbott Laboratories, 1971.)

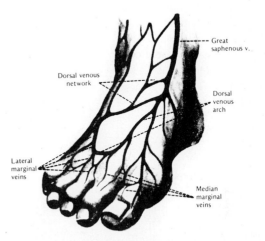

FIGURE 35-10. Accessible venipuncture sites in the area of the foot. (Reprinted with permission from Venipuncture and Venous Cannulation, Abbott Laboratories, 1971.)

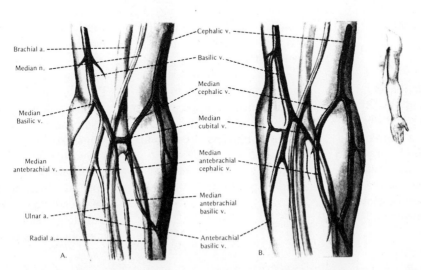

FIGURE 35-11. The relationship of superficial arteries and nerves illustrated by two common vein arrangements of the antecubital fossa of the left arm. (Reprinted with permission from Venipuncture and Venous Cannulation, Abbott Laboratories, 1971.)

Fluid and Electrolyte Balance 653

Table 35-3. Continued

Anticipated Accomplishment	Scientific Principles/ Rationale	Specific Considerations
6. Identify client by name band; double check solution against original order and chart name.	Misidentification of client and solution accounts for large numbers of IV administration order errors.	Ask client to state his full name; always double check *original* order.
7. Hang IV bag/bottle on IV pole; attach infusion set (Fig. 35-12); expel air from tubing; check solution.	Before inserting needle, infusion should be adequately prepared to easily attach needle to set with minimum possibility of introducing contaminants.	Recheck solution for cloudiness or particles, leakage, or cracks in bottle/bag. Squeeze drip chamber to fill it about ½–¾ full.

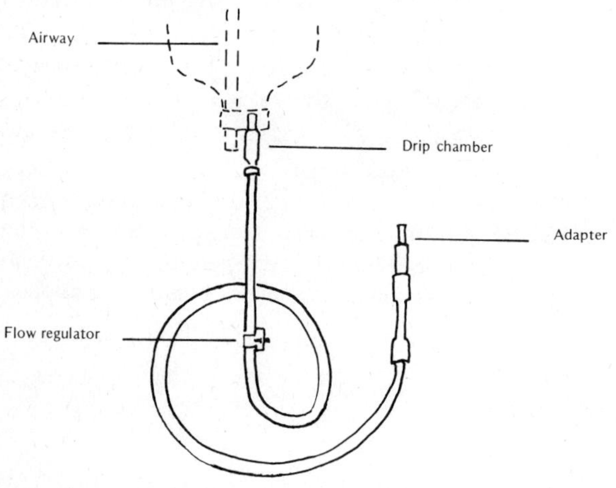

Airway

Drip chamber

Adapter

Flow regulator

FIGURE 35-12. Basic administration set. (Reprinted with permission from Stroot, V. R., et al.: *Fluids and Electrolytes: A Practical Approach,* 2nd ed. Philadelphia, F. A. Davis Co., 1977 p. 222.)

8. Prepare skin site.	Rotary motion, mechanical friction with antiseptic solutions is bacteriostatic.	Apply solutions vigorously to cleanse skin area.
9. Insert needle (bevel up at 45° angle, Fig. 35-13) after dilating veins and skin prep; remove tourniquet if applied.* See Figures 35-8 to 35-11 for usual sites of venipuncture; leg sites are avoided when possible because of danger of thrombi or phlebitis.	Dilated veins are easy to identify and enter. Skin preparation minimizes infection due to skin puncture. Holding bevel up at angle is an aid to following course of distended vein and avoiding puncture.	Dilate veins by lowering extremity below heart, or have client make a fist to distend veins. Apply a tourniquet 6 inches above desired site (immediately before insertion), or apply warm applications (a few minutes before insertion). With catheters, follow hospital or manufacturer's practice for in-

*In drawing blood much the same procedure for intravenous therapy is followed except a syringe or "vacutainer" apparatus is attached to the needle and tourniquet removed; blood is drawn, needle and reservoir (syringe) are removed, and pressure is applied to puncture site. Small "Band-Aid" is applied.

Implementation	Recommendations	Observations
Complete identification by stating to client that you will be starting IV. State solution to be used.		
Fill drip chamber; clear tubing of air. Cover adapter end of tubing with plastic set cover. If no air bubbles, discard bottle. For bag, remove plastic cover from outlet. Attach infusion set. For bottle remove rubber diaphragm. Insert infusion set if air bubbles are heard.		
Apply antiseptic solution according to institution's policy.	Cover entire venipuncture site with margin of safety.	
Apply pressure around selected vein manually to help it dilate. Place needle at an angle in subcutaneous tissue next to vein; insert needle in vein from the side at an angle. Remove tourniquet. Apply IV tubing.	Radial pulse should be palpated when tourniquet is applied. Blood backflow in tubing after tourniquet removal indicates you have placed needle intravenously. Butterfly needles should be taped down before IV tubing is connected.	If blood is to be infused, normal saline solution is usually started then blood administered via blood administration set which contains a special filter (to filter out clots and impurities). Albumin administration should likewise be through a filter set.

Table 35-3. Continued

Anticipated Accomplishment	Scientific Principles/ Rationale	Specific Considerations

INTRAVENOUS INFUSION TECHNIQUE

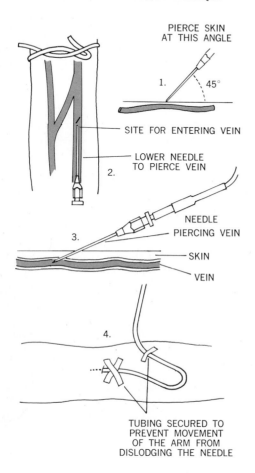

sertion. Apply antiseptic ointment around needle/catheter insertion site; tape needle to skin to securely fasten it in vein.

TUBING SECURED TO PREVENT MOVEMENT OF THE ARM FROM DISLODGING THE NEEDLE

FIGURE 35-13. Technique for initiation of venipuncture and intravenous therapy. (Reprinted with permission from *Taber's Cyclopedic Medical Dictionary*, 13th ed. Philadelphia, F. A. Davis Co., 1977, p. I–43.

10. Apply IV tubing and reservoir to inserted needle, apply arm board, monitor flow.	Arm board properly applied stabilizes needle in vein, prevents puncture of vein wall or dislodging of needle. Place tubing in a "V" and tape both sides of the "V" down to further anchor IV in vein; also by taping IV tubing beyond needle or catheter site, you prevent pulling on catheter/needle and dislodging it.	If *blood or albumin* is in reservoir, a special filter set should be used with IV tubing. An isotonic solution of saline is usually used as a "flush" for such substances before and after administration. Vital signs are carefully monitored before, during, and after administration of blood or albumin. Depending on client diagnosis, flow rate may need adjustment to avoid

Implementation	Recommendations	Observations

Apply IV tubing using aseptic technique. Tubing should be free of air. Always carefully identify client before hanging solution to be infused, and double check blood type when hanging blood and blood products.

Arm board application: (1) Pad arm board for comfort (some are prepadded). (2) Use two

Some IV therapists suggest using two clamps. The metal cap from a bottle serving as a second clamp, should first clamp fail.

Time tapes: either provided by manufacturer or made by nurse are useful monitoring techniques. A quick reference for determining whether or not IV is "on time" or infusing at

Nurse should monitor flow frequently (three times an hour) to avoid circulatory over load or failure to detect complications. If complaints of burning or pain at site of needle insertion, check flow rate, check for phlebitis, red streak from needle insertion site, pain, redness, and swelling. Discontinue IV and report.

Fluid and Electrolyte Balance **657**

Table 35-3. Continued

Anticipated Accomplishment	Scientific Principles/ Rationale	Specific Considerations
		circulatory overload or other complications related to volume. Check site of insertion in vein.
		Check flow rate. Is it flowing at proper rate? Pinch tubing or rubber flash ball beyond needle insertion site to elicit blood return. Take tape off down to needle site insertion, if uncertain, to check site for needle in vein. If no blood back flow and swelling near needle insertion site, infiltration is a probability and IV must be discontinued and restarted. Compare skin of both arms to determine if swelling is present. Skin of infiltration area is swollen, taut, and cold.
		Blood transfusion sets: approximately 15 gtt/cc (or as stated on container with tubing). Blood setups: always include a filter set (recipient set), and an IV solution administration set with a Y site and long tubing. Prior to transfusions, clients generally have the following tests performed in addition to typing, usually an hour long procedure, cross-matching, Rh factor, Coombs' test (for antibody screening). Donor tests are similar but also include tests for syphilis and hepatitis.

Implementation	Recommendations	Observations

pieces of adhesive, one longer than the other; press together and use exposed adhesive ends to fasten arm board to arm. Nonadhesive portions only should be against client's skin; apply firmly *not tightly,* and leave small free space between arm and arm board.

Always consider local policies or procedures in nursing procedure manuals *before* following general suggestions stated here.

Check local policy for rate determination using local IV sets.* Very slow: 15–28 gtt/min; 80–160 cc/hr; slow: 28–42 gtt/min; 160–240 cc/hr; average: 42–56 gtt/min; 240–320 cc/hr; and fast: 56–70 gtt/min; 320–400 cc/hr.

Average rates for blood sets with 15 gtt/cc: very slow: 20–40 gtt/min; slow: 40–60 gtt/min; average: 60–80 gtt/min; and fast: 80–100 gtt/min. A special pump may be used for fast infusions.

proper rate. Blood and blood products are usually started by nurse, IV therapist, or physician.

Do not lower bag/bottle below bed—butterfly needles have small lumen so blood backs into tubing and clots, requiring a restarting of IV with all new equipment. Usually *any* IV reaction necessitates sending entire set, tubing, needle and remaining solution, to bacteriology lab for culture studies to determine contaminant cause of reaction. Use forms provided by local institution to report reaction.

Air in tubing: notify IV therapy nurse if available. If no such nurse available use aseptic technique, detach tubing from needle hub, and run solution and air into container; reattach immediately. If straight set up with Burrette (Buretrol) (containing medication for example), filter valve seals off

Observe client with any IV infusion (including IV medications) for symptoms of reaction, including nausea, flushed face, urticaria (rash) chills, and fever. If electrolyte infusion, check client's most recent lab values (if K is in infusion and serum levels of K are high, question physician). When client is ambulatory, have him hold arm and tubing at waist and use an IV pole with wheels with bag about 1 foot above head.

Blood transfusion reaction: save all tubing and blood in event of reaction for examination by laboratory. *Blood incompatibility reactions* occur within administration of 500 cc blood: kidney and chest pain, shock, dyspnea, elevated temperature, chills, and hemoglobinuria.

---

*Drops/cc oₓ macro/micro drip IV infusions sets: standard macro (maxi) drips = approximately 10 gtt/cc; pediatric micro (mini) drips = approximately 60 gtt/cc.

Table 35-3. Continued

Anticipated Accomplishment	Scientific Principles/ Rationale	Specific Considerations
		Needles used by nurses in parenteral therapy include: butterfly ¾ in, #21 (IV fluids), #19 (IV fluids), and blood and blood product administration.
		Blunt plastic over steel administration needle #18 (2 in). Angiocaths #20 and #18 (1¼ in).
		Heparin lock is often a #21 (¾ in) needle with small length, plastic tubing and rubber stopper in it. Used to administer heparin and for intermittent administration of antibiotics.
		IV Medication: IV medications are used to insure accurate quick therapeutic blood levels of medications and present no problems relative to absorption. All nurses must be aware of venipuncture techniques as described above, local policy regarding starting new IV medication, local state law about IV medications administration, and have in-depth understandings

Implementation	Recommendations	Observations
	reservoir and air when empty. If double set up with two IV reservoirs: empty bag may have air flushed into it after clamping off access to needle inserted in vein. Frequently transfused clients may have reactions. Always check hospital/institutional policy in respect to these rules of thumb; IV departments often have special procedures.	*Allergic reactions*: 200–600 cc blood administered: urticaria, hives, wheezing, edema of lips, mouth, throat, and face, flushed skin. *Febrile*: 100–300 cc blood: rapid elevation of temperature, chills, and headache.
In event of blood transfusion reaction: turn blood off at once. Turn on 0.9% sodium chloride or other KVO fluid used for flush. Notify doctor at once. Obtain urine specimen marked "blood reaction specimen." Notify IV team so blood may be drawn for examination according to local policy. Report according to local policy.	Blood is stored at approximately 40°F (4.4°C). Blood should be unrefrigerated no longer than 15 min before administration. Always keep blood container and IV set intact for 24 hours in case of delayed reaction. Blood transfusion is always charted by doctor or nurse stating it on client's parenteral therapy sheet with date, time (started and finished), type of blood or blood products, identifying number and type, amount received in units, person starting and removing, and any observations.	
IV Medication: If medication is premixed by pharmacy, usually a small gauge needle and IV tubing is attached to bag of medication and inserted into rubber cap of heparin lock. Prior to insertion of medication into heparin lock nurse must ascertain that heparin lock is in vein. Usually a small amount of heparin is inserted into lock after pulling back on plunger of	Do not combine drugs unless you have checked out compatibility. Always examine drug in solution for evidence of contaminants or precipitate. Blood is *always* given alone. No medications are added to it, and new tubing must be used to administer medications if blood has been administered prior to medication administration. *Check out* policies regarding	

Table 35-3. Continued

Anticipated Accomplishment	Scientific Principles/ Rationale	Specific Considerations
		of compatibility of drugs, proper solutions in which drug is to be diluted and administered, as well as all information about drug. Generally student nurses must be completely supervised in IV medication administration.
11. Remove IV as ordered by physician. Discontinue IV by removing needle from vein. Chart procedure on parenteral therapy forms. (Initiation, all monitoring, and discontinuation of IV infusions are *always* recorded on IV flow sheets and in nurses' notes.)	Infusion needle should be removed in a manner that avoids trauma to vein and prevents air from entering vein to minimize complications. Fluid, electrolyte and medication needs are calculated on basis of infusions already received by client and current laboratory studies.	In removing needle pull straight out of vein to avoid trauma to vein wall. Always chart procedure immediately *after* discontinuing IV. If IVs are numbered in sequence, chart number of IVs as well.

Implementation	Recommendations	Observations

syringe to elicit blood return as evidence of needle in vein. If drug not compatible with heparin, normal saline flush is used before and after medication administration.

IV medication should be labeled "for IV use." In IVs not utilizing a heparin lock, drugs may be added through alcohol prepared injection sites specifically meant for medication administration, with a short #19 needle while IV is dripping. All drugs prepared by nurse must be labeled with an appropriate medication label. Never give a *new* drug unless you have ascertained that in your setting the drug is approved for administration by nurses.

Clamp off IV tubing, remove all tape and arm board; remove needle. Place sterile dressing over puncture site. Do not place tape completely around arm as it will occlude circulation.

At beginning of procedure chart amount infusion started, time, type of solution, and observations.

At end of procedure, similarly chart amount received, time discontinued, type of solution and observations.

---

administering medications at your institution.

Drugs are diluted in IV fluid (usually 50 cc) before administration.

Observe site for any sign of phlebitis or swelling. Reactions to any IV therapy should be charted on parenteral therapy sheets as well as medication sheets for IV medications and appropriate nurses notes in addition to reporting such reactions to physician.

Table 35–4. Hypodermoclysis Used with Small Child, Infant, or Adult with Poorly Accessible Veins for Replacement of Extracellular Fluid Components to Maintain Fluid and Electrolyte Balance

Anticipated Accomplishment	Scientific Principles/ Rationale	Specific Considerations
1. Check original physician order to prevent administration error and obtain solution ordered.	Improper solution administration may cause fatal fluid/electrolyte complications.	Note contraindicated solutions such as hypertonic solutions or solutions that are contrary to body pH.
2. Place client at ease by explanation of procedure.	Psychologic stress may contribute fluid and electrolyte shifts reducing efficacy of procedure. Cooperation is enhanced by client understanding.	If client has depressed sensorium explanation should be brief, concise, focus on "feel" of procedure as prick with needle insertion.
3. Wash hands carefully to promote surgical aseptic techniques.	Soap emulsifies bacteria; careful handwashing decreases contamination and possibility of cross-infection.	Follow a specific procedure for handwashing that includes all surfaces.
4. Completely assemble equipment to prevent site exposure for longer than necessary.	Anxiety is increased by prolonging treatments. Possibility of superimposed infection is increased by exposure of site and equipment.	Equipment usually includes: solutions for skin preparation, such as Betadine and alcohol, and swabs for applying solution. Needles 19–22 gauge 1½ in long. IV tubing (with Y connecting tubes if more than one needle used).
		Luer syringe for small amount solution. Screw clamps to control flow of solution. Drip chamber to control rate as ordered. IV pole; container for waste solution; plastic or paper bag for discarded materials; dressing supplies; waterproof drapes to place under site; and hyaluronidase as ordered. Shaving equipment if site is hair covered.

Implementation	Recommendations	Observations
Obtain proper solution ordered.	Read order completely. Note amount and type solution before obtaining solution, before administering solution, and after administering solution to prevent error.	Note label of solution. Check against original order, observe solution for contaminants. (Hold solution up to light to check.) Check expiration date.
Explain purpose simply "to give needed substances to body to maintain or restore health." Indicate site for injection, type of equipment, length of procedure; validate client understanding by eliciting feedback; position client.	Stress meaning of procedure—that is, the procedure is common and does not mean client is seriously ill but needs fluids by another route. Avoid frowning, expressions of concern; stress that nurse will check frequently throughout procedure.	Note body language, nonverbal messages of anxiety, or discomfort.
Handwashing with aseptic solution.	Repeat handwashing before going to bedside.	Note breaks in skin or any superficial lesions which might necessitate wearing sterile gloves.
Bring assembled equipment to client's bedside.	Double check solution against original order before bringing to bedside. Small gauge needles slow down rate of flow. Hyaluronidase (if ordered) to be injected into tubing after initiation of infusion with small needle. Observe strict aseptic technique with handling and assembling equipment.	

Table 35–4. Continued

Anticipated Accomplishment	Scientific Principles/ Rationale	Specific Considerations
5. Selection of skin site that is easily accessible and may be maintained.	Clysis equipment if dislodged diminishes therapeutic effect. Causes reinsertion of needle. Poor positioning interferes with treatment efficacy.	Usual skin sites: places with good skin supply, easily manipulated including: thighs (front), upper abdomen, iliac crest, under breasts, and back (below scapula).
6. Preparation of skin to minimize bacteria.	Rotary motion mechanical friction with antiseptic solutions destroys pathogenic bacteria.	Use solutions and skin prep procedure per institutional policy.
7. Hang solution and tubing; expel air to permit easy attachment to needle after insertion.	Expelling air prevents air entering tissues; promotes better fluid flow. Preassembly of tubing and solution container prevents contamination in attaching tubing to needle.	
8. Insertion of needle and attachment of tubing.	Needle is inserted at an angle to prevent damage to adjacent or underlying structures.	Hang solution 36–40 in above bed.
9. Monitor flow rate throughout procedure.	Too rapid flow causes distention of skin site and subcutaneous tissue pressure. Sensations of discomfort and the position necessary to maintain the system may require frequent reassurance of anxious client.	
10. Remove needle to discontinue procedure; redress.	Puncture wound should be dressed to prevent infection.	
11. Record length of procedure and amount of fluid absorbed.	Fluid balance is computed from intake and output chart according to institutional policy.	

Implementation	Recommendations	Observations
Select site to avoid blood vessels and nerves. Prone position for injection at back (preferable for infant).	Positioning hints: dorsal recumbent best for thigh and breast location. Above crest of ileum, turn on opposite side with supporting pillows at back. Pull down covers to expose site, but drape client carefully around exposed site.	Note condition of skin; always shave hairy areas; select unbroken skin area.
Usual skin prep may include: pHisoHex, Betadine, alcohol scrubs, and Betadine ointment around injection site after needle insertion.	Follow skin prep policy exactly to minimize infection possibility.	
Tubing and reservoir assembled. Tubing kept sterile for attachment to needle after insertion.	Cover end of tubing with sterile protective cap.	
Needle inserted at angle into loose skin without fluid infusing during insertion.	Secure needle and dressing to skin with tape to prevent dislodging. Ask for client to report discomfort at site. Check for Novocain or hyaluronidase order to decrease discomfort at site.	Reposition client for comfort. Observe for discomfort that accompanies procedure, including burning, tingling sensations.
Flow may be monitored according to physician's order and last from ½ hour to 5 or 6 hours.	Rate of flow should prevent tissue disruption at needle site. Keep client as quiet as possible to prevent disruption of procedure.	Observe tissue around needle; abnormal distention at injection site should be reported immediately.
Apply pressure dressing after needle removal.		
		Note and record appearance of dressed site.

nous solutions administered may maintain fluid balance without appreciable nutritive value. A total of 2500 cc of isotonic 5 percent D/W provides a mere 500 calories per day. To raise nitrogen and caloric intake, promote anabolism and tissue repair and synthesis, amino acid, and electrolytes in dextrose solution (20–40 percent for adults and 10–30 percent for children), providing 2000–3000 calories per day, must be infused. Using strict asepsis the physician passes a radiopaque catheter into the external jugular vein or superior vena cava via the antecubital vein. The infused solution is also prepared under rigid aseptic conditions. The system used is a closed one which further prevents contamination. Nursing responsibilities include: changing infusion bottles, monitoring flow, changing catheter site dressings, charting completely all infusions, observing clients for complications such as catheter embolism, pneumothorax, hyperglycemia and metabolic acidosis (clients are usually on routine urine testing) air and blood emboli, fungal or bacterial sepsis, thrombophlebitis, nausea, vomiting, and diarrhea. The reader is referred to other specialty textbooks for in-depth information on this procedure.

CVP Monitoring

Central venous pressure monitoring is sometimes a nursing responsibility. The first level student will only perform this procedure in a supervised setting. (The reader is referred to references beyond this textbook for an in-depth treatment of this topic.)[3] A catheter is inserted into the superior vena cava or right atrium through the jugular, subclavian, or antecubital vein, as with the TPN (total parenteral nutrition) catheter. Monitoring equipment, including a water manometer set-up is attached to the catheter. Readings are taken using a special stopcock to fill the manometer with the IV fluid in a reservoir. The manometer is always aligned with the right atrium via the midaxillary line to obtain appropriate readings. Water pressure readings of 2–12 cm are an acceptable normal range. As with the TPN catheter, the nurse observes the client for complications especially related to large vessel phlebitis. In addition, intravenous infusions are monitored and recorded as with any client receiving parenteral fluids.

SUMMARY

Fluid and electrolyte considerations are pertinent to the entire topic of homeodynamics. The nurse, acting out of her expressive and instrumental role, must understand the role that fluid and electrolyte balance plays in maintaining the human organism in a healthy state. Specific procedures related to fluid balance and electrolyte maintenance have been discussed as relevant to nursing practice. The nurse's observational skills and ability to articulate and record the complexities of fluid and electrolyte procedures have been stressed as crucial to the restorative success of such therapies.

REFERENCES

1. Aguilera, J., and Messick, D.: *Crisis Intervention Theory and Methodology.* St. Louis, C. V. Mosby, 1978.
2. Methany, N. M., and Snively, W. D.: *Nurses Handbook of Fluid Balance,* 2nd ed. Philadelphia, J. B. Lippincott, 1974, p. 49.
3. Beyers, M., and Dudas, S.: *The Clinical Practice of Medical Surgical Nursing.* Boston, Little, Brown, 1977, pp. 331–333.

BIBLIOGRAPHY

Dickens, M. L.: *Fluid and Electrolyte Balance: A Programmed Text.* Philadelphia, F. A. Davis, 1974.

Fuerst, E. V., Wolff, L., and Weitzel, M. H.: *Fundamentals of Nursing.* Philadelphia, J. B. Lippincott, 1974.

Grant, J. S.: Patient care in parenteral hyperalimentation. *Nurs. Clin. North Am.* 8:165, 1973.

Kurdi, W. J.: Refining your IV therapy techniques. *Nurs. '75* 5(11):41–47, 1975.

McGraw Laboratories: *Parenteral Hyperalimentation.* Glendale, Calif., 1973. (FreAmine instructor /information booklet)

Seyle, H., The General adaptation syndrome and diseases of adaptation. *J. Clin. Endocr.* 6:117, 1946.

Sheppard, V., and Reed, G.: *Regulation of Fluid and Electrolyte Balance: A Programmed Instruction in Clinical Physiology.* Philadelphia, W.B. Saunders, 1977.

Stroot, V., Lee, C., Schaper, C. A.: *Fluids and Electrolytes: A Practical Approach.* Philadelphia, F. A. Davis, 1975.

Williams, S. R.: *Nutrition and Diet Therapy.* St. Louis, C. V. Mosby, 1977.

CHAPTER 36

GLOSSARY

adequate ventilation. Volume of air necessary to maintain carbon dioxide elimination.

aerosol. Suspension of droplets in a gas.

anoxia. Deprivation of oxygen.

apnea. Cessation of breathing.

asphyxia. Decrease in amount of oxygen and increase in amount of carbon dioxide in the body as a result of some interference with respiration.

asthma. Disease characterized by hypersensitivity of the airways.

bagging. Manual intermittent positive pressure breathing using an AMBU bag or other equivalent equipment.

Cheyne-Stokes. An irregular cyclic breathing pattern which is initially slow and shallow. The rate then increases until a certain point, then is decreased gradually until it stops for 30−60 seconds.

chronic bronchitis. A clinical disorder character-

MAINTENANCE OF RESPIRATORY STATUS AND PULMONARY FUNCTIONING

Sue A. Driscoll, M.S., R.N.

ized by excessive mucous secretion and a chronic productive cough.

chronic obstructive pulmonary disease (COPD). Diseases characterized by persistent resistance and obstruction of the airways to air flow.

compliance. Distensibility of the lung and chest wall.

constant positive pressure breathing (CPPB). A positive pressure above atmospheric maintained within the airways during inspiration and expiration in spontaneous breathing.

controlled ventilation. Manual or mechanical ventilation in which the frequency of breathing is determined by the machine.

cor pulmonale. Right ventricular hypertrophy secondary to lung disease.

dead space, anatomical. Volume of all gas conducting or nongas exchange passages in the lung.

dead space, physiological. Anatomical dead space plus volume of gas which does not undergo gas exchange due to nonperfused alveoli.

diffusion. Movement of a gas from an area of higher concentration to an area of lower concentration.

dyspnea. A subjective sensation of difficult or labored breathing.

endotracheal tube. Artificial airway passed into the trachea by nasal or oral route.

hyperpnea. An increase in rate and depth of respiration.

hyperventilation. Excessive ventilation of gas exchange units resulting in a fall in the arterial carbon dioxide value.

hypoventilation. Decrease in ventilation of gas exchange units resulting in a rise above normal in the arterial carbon dioxide value.

hypoxemia. Decreased arterial oxygen tension.

hypoxia. Decreased oxygenation at the tissue level.

intermittent mandatory ventilation (IMV). Periodic controlled ventilation with inspiratory positive pressure, with the client breathing spontaneously between controlled respiratory efforts.

intermittent positive pressure breathing (IPPB). Use of equipment that delivers inhaled air under positive pressure.

low flow oxygen. Use of low concentrations of oxygen.

lung perfusion. Volume of blood flow through the pulmonary capillary bed.

nebulizer. A piece of equipment designed to break up a liquid into a fine spray or mist.

orthopnea. Difficult breathing when lying flat, relieved when assuming erect position.

positive end-expiratory pressure (PEEP). A residual pressure above atmospheric, maintained at the airway opening at the end expiratory phase.

pulmonary physiotherapy. A group of maneuvers designed to prevent pulmonary complications and improve function, including breathing exercises, cough, postural drainage, percussion, and vibration.

respiratory insufficiency. Inability to maintain arterial oxygen level of 50 mm Hg or greater.

tachypnea. Rapid rate of respiration.

tidal volume (V_T). Volume of air exchanged with a normal breath.

total lung capacity (TLC). Volume of gas in the lung after full inspiration.

tracheobronchial hygiene. Measures to aid in removal of secretions from the airways (e.g., suctioning).

tracheostomy. Artificial external opening into the trachea.

ultrasonic nebulization. Use of high frequency sound waves to break up droplets of liquid into fine particles for inhalation.

ventilator (respirator). A mechanical device designed to assist or replace the client's spontaneous respirations.

ventilatory failure. Inability of the ventilatory effort to keep the arterial carbon dioxide value less than 50 mm Hg.

vital capacity (VC). The largest volume of gas measured on complete expiration after a maximal inspiratory effort.

The body cannot be sustained without provision for a continuous supply of oxygen from the atmosphere. The earth's atmosphere consists of approximately 20.95 volumes percent of oxygen, 78.09 volumes percent of nitrogen, and 0.031 volumes percent of carbon dioxide. Respiration is the process of exchange of oxygen for carbon dioxide; gas exchange is a major function of the lung. Ventilation refers to the movement of air in and out of the lung. The effectiveness of ventilation is measured in terms of the carbon dioxide value in arterial blood. Alveolar ventilation is that portion of the gas (air) molecules which actually undergo exchange with the pulmonary blood.

RESPIRATORY SYSTEM

Anatomically, the atmospheric air enters the upper airway (the nasal cavity, nasopharynx, and oropharynx) where it is warmed, filtered, and humidified. Air is then conducted into the lower airway (the larynx, trachea, and bronchi). The major bronchi continue to branch into smaller bronchi and bronchioles of less than 2 mm in diameter. Terminal bronchioles branch into respiratory bronchioles which have the gas exchange units clustered at their termination. These gas exchange units are called alveoli. The average adult lung has 300–400 million alveoli available for gas exchange.

The walls of bronchioles contain mucous secreting glands, supportive cartilage, and smooth muscle within their walls. There is a gradual transition from gas conducting units to gas exchange units.

Inspiration occurs due to a change in the relationship of alveolar pressure relative to atmospheric pressure. When the alveolar pressure decreases, inspiration is initiated. Air continues to flow into the lung until alveolar pressure is greater than atmospheric. The mechanics of breathing are accomplished by the active contraction of the muscles of inspiration (intercostals and diaphragm). The thorax is enlarged by the contraction of these muscles. Relaxation of the muscles occurs on expiration. The lungs consist of a right lung and left lung which are closely adhered to the thoracic walls by a thin layer of fluid between the parietal and visceral pleura. The relationship of the basic structures of the lungs is noted in Figure 36-1.

There are certain resistances to lung expansion. A familiar term in working with respiratory disorders

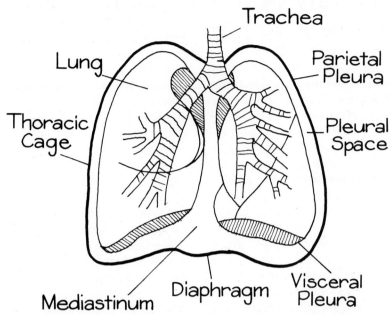

FIGURE 36-1. A schematic representation of the relationship between the lungs and the thoracic cage. The lungs within the thoracic cage are separated by the mediastinum. The heart and great vessels are located in this space. The parietal pleura is the lining inside the thoracic cage which covers the inside of the diaphragm and the inside lining of the thorax. The visceral pleura lines the surface of the lung. The space between these linings is known as the pleural space.

refers to the state of compliance of the lungs. Simply stated, compliance is the elastic resistance offered by expansion. The airways with their varying diameters, twists, and turns, cause frictional resistance to airflow. This resistance is negligible under normal circumstances. The tendency of the lungs to collapse or return to resting state after expansion is called *elastic recoil.*

Motor neurons send impulses from the respiratory centers initiating contractions of the muscles involved in the respiratory effort. The level of the alveolar ventilation is controlled by both neural and chemical influences. The neural respiratory center is located in the medulla oblongata of the brain stem. The intermittent bursts of activity in the respiratory center neurons initiate nerve impulses that travel via the phrenic nerve to cause contraction of the respiratory muscles. The coordination and depth of respiration are controlled by these neural influences. The increase in the alveolar ventilation is the result of an increase in the rate of amplitude of the impulses which results in an increase in tidal volume. Tidal volume is the amount of air exchanged in a normal breath.

The peripheral chemoreceptors, which are located at the bifurcation of the carotid arteries and along the aortic arch, are normally responsive to changes in oxygen tension values. Decreasing levels of oxygen tension in the arterial blood stimulates these receptors, and impulses are sent to the central respiratory center via the glossopharyngeal nerve and from the aortic body by way of the vagus nerve.

The integrity of the alveoli is maintained by a surface active material lining called surfactant. This phospholipid arises from cells within the alveoli and opposes the natural tendency of the alveoli to collapse. The formation of surfactant is dependent upon a normal perfusion of the blood to the alveoli and an intact metabolic process of the alveolar cells. The impairment of synthesis or excessive depletion of surfactant can result in alveolar instability. (This will be discussed in more detail later in this section.)

These are some of the basic influences which affect the quality of the inspiratory and expiratory phases of breathing. It is obvious from this brief overview that there are multiple and complex mechanisms regulating the respiratory effort.

CARDIOVASCULAR SYSTEM

Once the oxygen reaches the alveoli, it is transported to the tissues via the arterial blood. Deoxygenated blood returning from the tissue via the central venous system enters the right side of the heart. From that point, the blood is pumped into the right and left pulmonary arteries. The alveolar surfaces are surrounded by a dense network of capillaries. The deoxygenated blood passes through this capillary network, is oxygenated and passed back into the left side of the heart by way of the pulmonary veins. From the left side of the heart, the blood is pumped to the tissues via the arterial circulation.

The movement of oxygen from the gas phase into the liquid phase is accomplished by the process of diffusion. Diffusion is simply movement of molecules from one area of concentration to another. For oxygen to move across the gas liquid interface or alveolar-capillary membrane, a pressure gradient must exist. Thus the partial pressure of oxygen is greater in the alveoli than in the pulmonary-capillary blood. Conversely, the partial pressure of carbon dioxide is slightly greater in the pulmonary-capillary bed than in the alveoli. The rate at which the gas moves across the membrane is dependent upon: the degree of partial pressure difference; the surface area available for diffusion; the solubility of the gas through the barrier; and the thickness of the barrier to be crossed. A schematic representation of the alveoli and surrounding capillary structure is found in Figure 36-2.

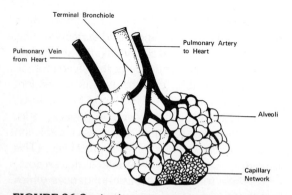

FIGURE 36-2. A schematic representation showing the relative relationship of the pulmonary circulatory bed to the alveoli. The alveoli are "bathed" in this capillary network.

Associated with the effectiveness of the pulmonary circulation is the state of the circulatory system. Perfusion represents the blood volume per minute which traverses the pulmonary capillaries. The average perfusion per minute is about 4–6 L. Normally less than 2 percent of the total pulmonary capillary blood flow bypasses the ventilated alveoli and does not undergo direct oxygenation. This includes blood supplying the heart muscle or myocardium and the lungs. This blood is mixed with the oxygenated blood. A portion of the venous return of the bronchial circulation is drained into oxygenated blood in the pulmonary veins. The thebesian veins drain from the heart muscle directly into the left side of the heart.

The cardiac output is capable of increasing more than four times its normal perfusion rate before there is a rise in pressure in the pulmonary arteries.[1] Such capacity is beneficial in reducing potential strain on the heart muscle or myocardium.

The final aspect of perfusion involves its relationship to the alveolar ventilation. This relationship is commonly referred to as the ventilation to perfusion ratio. The matching of alveolar ventilation to pulmonary blood flow determines the gas composition of blood leaving the lungs.

The adequacy of ventilation is determined by several factors which include: (1) the patency of the airways; (2) the compliancy of the lungs; (3) the number of alveoli undergoing aeration; and (4) the adequacy of thoracic musculature. The adequacy of perfusion is dependent upon: (1) an effective cardiac output; (2) low resistance to blood flow by the pulmonary arteries; (3) status of the microcirculation; (4) amount of blood available for perfusion; and (5) sufficient oxygen carrying capacity of essential components of the blood.

RESPIRATORY DYSFUNCTION: CAUSE AND EFFECT

It is evident that an intact cardiopulmonary system and intact neurological and musculoskeletal system are essential for proper pulmonary function. Thus, the maintenance of respiratory function necessitates a multisystem approach. Essentially dysfunction of the respiratory system relates to one or more of the following: (1) obstruction of the airway with or without hypoventilation; (2) alterations in the responsiveness of the muscles of respiration; (3) interference with the neurological control of respiration; (4) interference with the transport mechanism for oxygen, and (5) interference with adequate pumping capacity of the heart. Some of these conditions and the mechanism of respiratory impairment are discussed below. The nursing care measures most frequently employed to assist in prevention of dysfunction and restoration of optimal level of functioning is then discussed.

Pulmonary Disorders

UPPER AIRWAY OBSTRUCTION

Obstruction of the upper airway causes hypoventilation and limits the flow of air into the lungs. The response of the respiratory system is directly related to the degree of obstruction. Initially, the breathing pattern is slow and deep. If the obstructive mechanism becomes greater, then the respiratory rate increases and the respiratory depth decreases. Total obstruction results in cessation of respiration or apnea.

Trauma to the face and nose is one cause of upper airway obstruction. Fractures of the nose result in edema and obstruction of the nasal membranes. Edema is an increase in size or swelling. Mouth breathing is the alternative in simple fractures of the nose. If there is also trauma to the mouth and tongue, then obstruction of the oropharynx and nasopharynx is possible. One of the most common causes of airway obstruction results from the tongue occluding the airway. Emergency measures in care of obstructed airways are discussed in greater detail in Chapter 37, "Emergency Measures in Respiratory Obstruction and Arrest."

Severe facial injuries such as comminuted fractures of the mandible allowing displacement of the posterior tongue and glottis and comminuted fractures of the middle third of the face can cause dislodgement of the teeth and bone. Such fractures can also cause obstruction of the upper airway. Drainage of blood, saliva, and other debris into the larynx may also initiate spasms of the larynx.

External compression on the upper airway can be mediated by tumors; neoplasms of the thyroid gland; and tumors or polyps of the larynx, vocal cords, or trachea. Trauma to the larynx from a blow to the neck obstructs airflow by the potential for fractures of the larynx with subsequent swelling of airway structures. Obstruction to airflow may be partial or complete.

Coins and peanuts are often aspirated into the airway by children. Adult causes of *aspiration* are usually a bolus of food or a chicken bone, often as the result of the individual throwing his head back while laughing; food in the mouth then has a direct route to the airway. This situation is also referred to as the café coronary. The airway is occluded, apnea ensues, followed by cardiac arrest. Café coronary and cardiac arrest are also discussed in Chapter 37.

Instances of total acute upper airway obstruction may necessitate an incision into the trachea (tracheostomy). Such an opening bypasses the obstruction of the oropharyngeal or nasopharyngeal structures. Consideration of the precipitating factors involved and the degree of obstruction is contemplated for determining the need of an artificial airway. The more extensive the obstruction, the more labored the respiratory effort. Aspiration of foreign bodies produces choking, coughing, inspiratory sounds, restlessness, and apprehension. With severe laryngeal injury, a crowing sound or stridor accompanies respiratory efforts. Airway obstructions below the larynx are noted by a wheezing sound on inspiration and increased thoracic musculature effort.

A disease process most often encountered in children which causes various degrees of upper airway obstruction is called *croup*. Inflammation of the respiratory tract and edema (swelling) of the larynx are common. Formation of a false type of membranous tissue coats the lining of the upper respiratory tract. Acute laryngeal reaction with the potential for laryngospasm typically occurs at night. The child is awakened by an increased sensation of breathlessness, a barking type of cough, and stridor (noisy inspirations). Air hunger is noted visibly by increased thoracic musculature effort. High humidity is utilized to liquify secretions for removal.

Other types of respiratory infections of the upper airway can cause transient airway obstruction or irritation. The common cold with rhinorrhea (nasal drainage), watery eyes, and mild edema of the nasal passages is self-limiting. Respiratory dysfunction is not a major concern unless the process should move into the lower airways. Pneumonia is one example of an infectious process of the lower airways.

LOWER AIRWAY OBSTRUCTION

Lower airway obstruction relates to processes which affect the airways below the larynx and gas exchange units. Changes in airway dynamics, distribution of ventilation, adequacy of ventilation, and diffusing capacity are included in obstruction of the lower airway.

Bronchitis

Bronchitis is defined by excessive mucous secretions within the lower airways manifested by a recurrent productive cough on most days for a minimum of 3 months per year for greater than two successive years.[2] The constant presence of mucus in the airways increases overall resistance to airflow in airways of less than 2 mm in diameter. Continual irritation to the bronchi results in paralysis or destruction of portions of the tiny hair like projections of the lower airways called cilia. These cilia normally function to assist in propelling mucus toward the mouth for expectoration or swallowing. Secretions continue to be produced and may become thicker. A cough develops to assist the respiratory tract in removal of secretions. Such a cough is more common in the morning and is often called "smoker's cough." Cigarette smoking and certain environmental exposures on a long-term basis are precursors to the development of chronic bronchitis.

Recurrent bronchial infections increase the chance for interference with free movement of gas within the airways. The lungs become less distensible, expiratory and inspiratory resistance to airflow increases, and the volume of air that the lungs exchange decreases. Progressive airway involvement with increased obstruction of airways eventually leads to retention of carbon dioxide (hypercapnia) and to reduced arterial blood oxygen levels (hypoxemia). The hypoxemia is the result of a mismatching of available ventilation to the pulmonary capillary blood perfusing the alveoli. The air is partially wasted in these areas increasing the dead space (area not undergoing gas exchange). When this condition continues, alveolar hypoventilation with carbon dioxide retention results. The breathing pattern tends to be faster and more shallow, further contributing to the gas exchange problem. A later manifestation of long standing chronic bronchitis is right-sided congestive heart failure or *cor pulmonale*. This is discussed in greater detail later.

Emphysema

Emphysema is another form of lower airway obstruction characterized by a breakdown of the walls of the alveoli. There are fewer alveoli in number, but remaining air sacs are larger due to loss of structural integrity. These alveoli are very inefficient in gas exchange. Emphysema is a disorder of the alveoli while chronic bronchitis is a disease of smaller conducting airways or bronchioles. The individual with emphysema can move air into the lung but has increased difficulty with exhalation. This is known as air trapping and is a result of the loss of lung elasticity and collapse of small airways and alveoli on expiration.

The chest has an overdistended appearance often called barrel chest. Hyperinflation is a more correct term. Sputum production, unlike the individual with chronic bronchitis, is usually not a problem. The diffusion of oxygen and carbon dioxide is impaired by the loss of available surface area. Perceived shortness of breath is decreased when the breathing pattern is slower with emphasis on slow complete expiration. Rapid expulsion of air leads to increased airway collapse and obstruction to airflow. Development of emphysema relates to heredity factors, occupational exposure, cigarette smoking, or a combination of these.

Chronic Obstructive Lung Disease

Chronic obstructive lung disease (COLD) is the name given to a disorder which results in persistent obstruction of airways that cannot be ascribed to any specific disease entity. It is not uncommon for these individuals to have symptoms and structural changes commensurate with both emphysema and chronic bronchitis and a hypersensitivity of the airway characteristic in asthma. The first symptom is often the sensation of difficulty in breathing or dyspnea. Labored respirations, especially when accompanied by wheezes, are characteristic of airway obstructive disorders. Structural changes in the lung can be related to small airway alterations as well as loss of elasticity of the lung parenchyma and bronchioles, decrease in size of the capillary bed, and loss of alveolar structure with resultant air trapping.

Airway obstruction can also be mediated by increased mucous secretion as in chronic bronchitis.

Chronic airway disorders increase potential for development of infectious disorders of the lungs, further compromising lung function. Certain infectious, bacterial and fungal processes can produce airway obstruction and subsequently affect alveolar ventilation. *Pneumonitis* is one of the most common infectious processes of the airways. The causative organism varies from bacterial to viral in nature, but the respiratory alterations are similar. Examples of classifications of pneumonia are: gram-positive pneumococcal pneumonia; streptococcal pneumonia; staphylococcal pneumonia; gram-negative pneumonia; viral pneumonia; and interstitial pneumonia. Causative organisms enter the upper respiratory tract by inhalation and are deposited at various levels in the airways. Entrance of a foreign body increases the activity of the defense mechanisms of the lung. A series of events culminates with ingestion of bacteria by alveolar macrophages of the lung and mucociliary transport toward the mouth with subsequent increased sputum production. The coughing mechanism is part of the process of lung clearance. The lining of the walls of the airways becomes inflamed as a result of irritation of the invading organism. Physical symptoms vary in intensity depending on the causative organisms. However, the sputum is usually thick and viscous with a greenish, yellowish, or brownish cast. Hemoptysis (blood in the sputum) may be noted. Fever may or may not be present. Productive (or nonproductive) cough is usually present. Shaking and chills may accompany a fever. A pleuritic type of chest pain can develop as a result of constant coughing and irritation. Copious secretions interfere with the most effective distribution of air flow into the lung. Consequently, some alveoli may not reach their potential for efficient gas exchange. Arterial oxygen values can be decreased, and the individual senses a state of dyspnea.

The severity of lung involvement is related to the causative organism and the ability of the lungs to respond. For example, persons who smoke two packs of cigarettes a day can impair the lung's defense and clearance mechanisms. The mucociliary escalator responsible for propelling mucus toward the upper airway for expulsion is paralyzed for a period of time upon exposure to cigarette smoke.

A second type of bronchial obstruction which can become chronic and is often the result of recurrent respiratory infections is acquired *bronchiectasis*. On the other hand, congenital bronchiectasis may be related to an abnormal development of bronchial airways before birth. Severe pneumonia with acute infection can result in decreased ciliary movement and damage to the walls of the small airways. Resultant retained secretions contribute to weakening of the bronchial walls producing abnormal areas of dilation and accumulation of secretions. The normal flexibility of the bronchioles is lost when their elastic structure and muscular walls are destroyed. Scar tissue replaces this flexible tissue. If the walls of the bronchi are severely affected, then there may also be damage to the integrity of the bronchial circulation. These individuals have recurrent hemoptysis. Cough with copious sputum production is the most common presenting symptom of bronchiectasis.

Pulmonary tuberculosis is not infrequently associated with bronchiectasis. Tuberculosis is a bacterial type of infectious process. The route of entry is inhalation of the tubercle bacillus. Tuberculosis is spread by an infected person coughing or sneezing in the presence of another person. The inhaled bacteria deposits in the upper airways. The bacillus thrives in a high oxygen environment, and the respiratory system responds by setting up an inflammatory process. The infectious process is self-limiting and healed areas leave calcium deposits at the infection site. In severe cases, lung tissue cavitates, and there is loss of lung function. If not controlled by drugs, more and more areas of lung become involved, decreasing ventilation capabilities, reducing gas exchange, and compromising diffusion capabilities. Airway changes result from compression of bronchi by edema or compression due to edema of adjacent hilar lymph nodes. This decreases airflow to airways distal to the obstruction.

Fungus Infections

Fungus processes also affect airway dynamics and contribute to obstruction of the lower airways. Coccidioidomycosis and histoplasmosis are two examples. Coccidioidomycosis or valley fever is endemic to the American Southwest Sonoran desert region. It is spread by the spores of *Coccidioides immitis* located in the soil. These spores are inhaled with dust and are deposited in the airways. This sets up an influenzalike series of symptoms, including fever, cough, and malaise. Pulmonary changes are precipitated by resultant fluid or infiltrates in the alveoli and small airways. Cavitary lesions of the lung are not uncommon.

Histoplasmosis is another example of a fungus spread by inhalation of *Histoplasma capsulatum* found in the soil enriched by bat, chicken, or other bird excrement. The resulting inflammatory process culminates with nodules formed in the lung and edema of the lymph nodes. The formation of an interstitial pneumonia is not uncommon. Interstitial refers to that space which lies between the airways. The individual experiences shortness of breath, mild fever, sweating, and cough which may or may not be productive.

Allergic Reactions

Inflammatory process can also be mediated through allergic reactions. Allergic alveolitis which is also termed hypersensitivity pneumonitis occurs when organic dusts to which the individual is sensitive are inhaled. An allergic reaction is initiated within 4 to 6 hours after exposure. During the acute phase, there is a decrease in the ventilatory capacity of the lungs and a decrease in the diffusing ability between the gas liquid interface. Decreased diffusing capacity occurs in the response to inflammation and resultant increased thickness of the alveolar-capillary membrane. Body temperature is elevated, and a tendency toward rapid shallow breathing is not uncommon. Rapid and shallow breathing causes a blowing off of carbon dioxide and a tendency toward an alkalotic state in the body. Edema-like fluid may also be present in the alveoli, further compromising lung function. With repeated exposure to the allergen, a scarring or fibrosis of the lung tissue can result with an increasing stiffness of the lung itself and decreased lung volumes and capacities for ventilation. This condition is sometimes referred to in the general classification of pulmonary fibrosis. The gas liquid interface may also become fibrous decreasing the effectiveness of gas exchange. Farmer's lung (the result of exposure to moldy hay) and bird fancier's lung (the result of exposure to bird excreta or dropping) are two examples of allergic alveolitis.

A different form of allergic reaction which can result in respiratory dysfunction is *anaphylaxis* or anaphylactic shock. It is most closely associated with hypersensitivity to a drug with animal protein bases. Reaction is usually noted with injection of the second dose of the medication. An acute reaction ensues with edema and bronchoconstriction. Dyspnea, a feeling of tightness in the chest, and a cyanotic appearance are not unusual. A choking sensation and cough with asthmalike symptoms are present. Death is imminent without immediate treatment.

Asthma

Asthma is a chronic disease process mediated by hypersensitivity of an individual to specific antigen-antibody unions. Asthma may be classified as extrinsic (environmentally mediated) or intrinsic (internally mediated). The antigens cause edema and constriction of the airways. An increase in eosinophils and hypersecretion of mucus increases resistance to airflow. Conducting airways to terminal bronchioles are most directly affected. Hypersecretion of mucus with mucous plugging of airways decreases ventilation to alveoli distal to the plugs. Hypoxemia, with a slowly rising arterial carbon dioxide level, is not uncommon in prolonged severe attacks. The client breathes faster, and breathing is more labored.

Resistance to airflow increases with mucous plugging and airway edema. Wheezing or a whistling sound as air moves by the obstruction can be heard audibly during respiratory effort. Decreasing airway spasm and removal of accumulated secretions is necessary to improve ventilatory function. Asthma is a reversible airway disorder.

Cystic Fibrosis

Cystic fibrosis is an inherited disorder of metabolic derangement, involving the exocrine and mucous secreting glands. It is not reversible with treatment. The mucus is thick and sticky. Cystic fibrosis often is regarded as synonymous with the term mucoviscidosis. The most common changes within the lungs include: presence of copious amounts of mucopurulent sputum and lung congestion with dilation of the bronchi. Most individuals with cystic fibrosis die from respiratory failure due to overwhelming secretions and pulmonary congestion. Loss of functioning lung tissue and limitation of lung volumes result from compression of the lower airways and the lung tissue itself by congestion and edema.

Alterations in lung volumes with compression of airways due to edema, fluid, or hyperactivity of the airway musculature can result in certain processes referred to as complications. Atelectasis is simply described as a decrease in lung volume due to collapse of alveoli. Atelectasis occurs as a result of impingement on the airways proximal to a bronchial segment with deprivation of essential ventilation to alveoli distal to the blockage. The partial pressure of oxygen is greater in the alveoli than in the pulmonary capillary blood so diffusion continues to take place. Eventually alveoli collapse. The degree of atelectasis depends on the total area of lung involved. Dyspnea is a common finding as well as rapid shallow breathing in response to decreased lung volumes.

Consolidation and Compression of Lung Tissue

Inflammatory infiltrates within the lung can result in consolidation of the involved lung tissue. Pneumonia is one precipitating cause. The normal spongy lung is eventually transformed by the fluid filled alveoli into an apparent solid structure as opposed to an air filled structure. Dyspnea, increased rate of respiration, and chest discomfort with respiratory effort is not unusual. Greater area of lung involvement increases symptoms and further impairs adequate exchange of oxygen and carbon dioxide.

Fluid not only is able to accumulate in alveoli but also in the pleural space. The pleural space is that area between the surface of the lung (visceral pleura) and the internal lining of the thoracic cage (parietal pleura). Fluid in the intrapleural space behaves like a space occupying mass and decreases lung volume on the involved side. If sufficient fluid accumulates then the mediastinum, the space between the right and left lung, becomes displaced toward the unaffected side. Consequently, decreased lung volumes may also result on that side. This further restricts lung movement and decreases

effective ventilation and compromises pulmonary blood flow.

Compression of the lung tissue and the airways is not unusual in space occupying lesions and neoplasms. The degree of lung dysfunction is related to the extensiveness of the tumor and its location. Obstruction of the main bronchus results in severe pulmonary obstruction to the total lung area. Neoplasms in the periphery of the lung do not initially affect as much lung function. Bronchogenic carcinoma is classified by cell type. Lung dysfunction results from obstruction or compression of the airways. Fluid accumulated in the pleural space with compression of lung tissue is common. Frequent lung infections distal to the tumor are due in part to impaired lung clearance mechanisms. The changing lung picture includes diminished lung volumes, decreased diffusing capacity, chronic hyperventilation and decreased oxygen in arterial blood secondary to a mismatch of ventilation to perfusion.

Pneumothorax

Pneumothorax is the presence of air in the pleural cavity. Pneumothorax may be classified as spontaneous or traumatic. Spontaneous pneumothorax occurs as a result of a tear in a pulmonary air-containing structure which communicates to the pleura. Traumatic pneumothorax is often secondary to a blunt trauma to the chest wall or a penetration of the chest wall. The leakage of air causes the normally negative intrapleural pressure to become more positive. This situation allows pulmonary elastic recoil pressure, now unopposed, to collapse the lung.

Environmental Irritants

The inhalation of chemicals normally present in the environment as well as those found in occupational settings can result in alterations in ventilatory function. One group of disorders associated with exposure to toxic materials is known as pneumonoconiosis. Pneumonoconiosis is actually the result of deposition of dust in the lungs followed by a tissue reaction. The inhaled material varies. Exposure to coal dust, silica sand dust, asbestos, and aluminum dusts are examples. The length and time of exposure as well as the state of health of the individual affects the severity of the symptoms. The lung essentially reacts in two ways to this type of exposure: obstruction of the airways and restriction of the lung tissue.

The exposure to simple coal dust causes obstruction of the small airways and one form of anatomic emphysema. There is destruction of the walls of peripheral airways less than 2 mm in diameter caused by the years of dust deposition. Resistance of airflow is increased with a decrease in effective alveolar ventilation. Dyspnea results with the interference in gas exchange.

Constant exposure to silica sand dust, aluminum, metal dust, and asbestos can result in structural changes in the airways. Decreased diffusing capacity and decreased lung volumes with increased thickness of the alveolar-capillary membrane impair gas exchange.

Beryllium used in atomic energy is an irritant to the respiratory tract. A nonproductive cough, substernal pain, moderate degree of dyspnea, and chemical pneumonitis cause alterations in airway dynamics with obstruction and restriction of chest movement.

Certain chemicals in the gaseous state can also affect lung function. Three examples are: chlorine, fluorine, and inhalation of smoke. Chlorine gas is used as a bleaching agent in various industrial settings. Large concentrated doses can cause cramping in the musculature of the larynx, swelling of the mucous membranes, nausea, and vomiting. In severe instances, the individual can experience respiratory distress with: cough, hemoptysis, chest pain, dyspnea, and tracheobronchitis.

Excessive inhalation of fluorinelike chlorine may result in bronchospasm, laryngospasm, and fluid exudate in the lungs. Again, the severity of the symptoms is related to the concentration and the time of exposure.

Smoke inhalation as a result of fire causes a chemical bronchiolitis of the lower airways. The pulmonary damage is the result of incomplete combustion of burning materials. Toxic fumes from melting plastics, such as formica tops and plastic furniture, are not unusual. Incomplete combustion of wood also gives off toxic fumes.

Injury to respiratory mucosa is followed by sloughing or the separation of dead cells from the living tissue. Edema of the tracheobronchial tree with resultant pulmonary congestion and plugging of airways can cause development of atelectatic portions of the lungs. Carbon-tinged sputum is usually present with cough after smoke inhalation. Severe laryngeal edema and stridor may necessitate a tracheostomy. Pneumonia is not an infrequent complication of smoke inhalation.

Obstruction to the conducting airways and the alveoli can be mediated by various disease processes and various types of insults to the airway. The underlying mechanism for airway obstruction and the extent of obstruction in part determines the degree of associated pulmonary dysfunction. The return of function is dependent upon securing a patent airway and providing necessary respiratory support.

Neurological Disorders

The control of rate and depth of respiration is centered in the medulla oblongata of the brain stem. Interference with oxygenation to the brain tissue, trauma with resultant edema to the brain, and disorders affecting neurological functioning can affect respiration. For example, a traumatic blow to the skull in the area of the posterior occiput can cause trauma to the brain stem. If the pneumotoxic center in the pons is affected, then respiratory rate is slowed and respiratory depth is greater. If the vagus nerve is severed or severely traumatized, the uncontrolled apneustic centers in the pons result in prolonged inspiratory spasms termed apneustic breathing. Trauma or neoplastic processes to the spinal cord just below the medulla causes a very weak response to the stimulus for inspiration-expiration.

TRAUMA

Trauma to the skull can produce several resultant conditions: concussion, contusion, or fracture. A concussion is a state in which an individual has a brief period of unconsciousness. Consciousness returns within a few minutes with minimal residual alterations. The effect on respiration tends to be negligible. A contusion of the brain results in a bruise to cerebral tissue but without a break or laceration to this tissue. A skull fracture is a break in the continuity of the cranium. Such fractures may be closed or open. Open fractures result in potential for loose bone fragments and foreign bodies (bullets) to lacerate and penetrate brain tissue. Bleeding and edema with alterations in respiratory patterns sometimes accompany this type of injury.[3]

One of the most common complications following trauma to the brain is increased intracranial pressure (ICP). Edema of the brain tissue compresses the blood flow and decreases availability of necessary nutrients to delicate brain cells; loss of consciousness is common. Pressure in the cerebral spinal fluid is increased. Compression of brain tissue secondary to cerebral vascular accidents, trauma to the skull with subsequent damage to its contents, and space occupying lesions are potential causes for changes in patterns of respiration and production of ICP. Four commonly noted changes in respiratory patterns are found in Table 36-1. The effects of intracranial pressure changes on various areas of the brain can be in part determined by changes in the respiratory pattern.[3]

In Table 36-1, note that alterations in arterial carbon dioxide levels are sometimes seen. The chemical control of ventilation can be affected by changes in the arterial carbon dioxide, pH, and arterial oxygen values. Excess carbon dioxide will normally stimulate respiratory rate while low levels of carbon dioxide tend to decrease respiratory rate. In Cheyne-Stokes breathing, there is a cause and effect relationship. Carbon dioxide is rapidly inhaled followed by a pause in the respiratory effort until carbon dioxide builds up and respiration is stimulated. Metabolic derangements, such as diabetic acidosis, can result in alterations in the respiratory pattern. Respirations are rapid and deep in an effort to blow off carbon dioxide accumulated via the metabolic changes. This type of breathing is referred to as Kussmaul's respiration.

HEMORRHAGE, CEREBRAL INFARCTION, AND SHOCK

Hemorrhages and cerebral infarction (cerebral vascular accident; CVA) are associated with a narrowing of the cerebral vessels due to atherosclerotic processes. This process results in formation of a substance called plaque on the walls of the vessels with subsequent narrowing of their diameter. Respiratory dysfunction is dependent upon the location of the insult and the extent of the damage. The most important concern is a patent airway. CVA often has a sudden onset followed by an uncon-

scious or a confused state. It is possible for the tongue to fall back in the oropharynx and obstruct the airway or for aspiration of vomitus into the airway.

Certain cerebral dysfunctions can precipitate a state of neurogenic shock. There is a loss of neurogenic tone of the vessels, and vasodilation is produced. Brain damage or deep anesthesia, which depresses vasomotor centers in the medulla, can be an etiological cause.

Accidental electrocution is another form of shock. Electric current passes through the body resulting in a loss of consciousness, depression of the respiratory center, and cardiac standstill. Respiratory dysfunction by airway obstruction secondary to loss of consciousness is also possible.

SPINAL CORD INJURIES

In cervical spinal cord injuries, most often associated with diving and automobile accidents, there is an interruption of the nerve transmission from the brain to the muscle. Two nerve groups, the phrenic and vagus are integral in thoracic muscle response. Injury to the phrenic nerve causes paralysis of the diaphragm it innervates. Branches of the vagus nerve, which is the tenth cranial nerve, becomes part of the laryngeal nerve. Paralysis can cause hoarseness due to ineffective closures of the vocal cords. It is also known that branches of the vagus nerve are involved in regulation of airway diameter, cough reflex, and respiratory control. Direct injury or presence of compression mediated by a tumor can cause dysfunction of these processes. A compression of the spinal cord above cervical root four (C_4) may require artificial ventilation as autonomic respiratory control is interrupted.[4] Later, it is possible for the individual to be taught conscious control of ventilatory effort and manual methods for airway clearance.

DRUG AND CHEMICAL DEPRESSANTS

Depression of respiration can also be mediated by inhaled or ingested chemicals or drugs. There is a direct relationship between drug usage and respiratory function. Fluid in the lungs (pulmonary edema) can result from drugs with high sodium content, drugs that suppress cardiac output, as well

Table 36-1. Alterations in Respiratory Patterns Secondary to Neurological Deprivation

Type	Breathing Pattern	Lesion Location	Precipitating Causes	Arterial CO_2	Effects
Cheyne-Stokes	Increased rate followed by period of apnea then increased rate	Pons	Hypertensive cerebral vascular disease Infection Hemorrhage Laceration—contusion	Decreased (respiratory alkalosis)	Respiratory rhythm normal Respiratory response preserved
Apneustic	Prolonged inspiratory and expiratory pauses	Pons	Hemorrhage Trauma with contusion Cerebral vascular hypertension	Normal (35–45 mm Hg)	Disruption of respiratory rhythm
Ataxic (Biot's)	Random deep and shallow breathing Unpredictable pause	Medulla	Hemorrhagic infarction or embolus Contusion—laceration Cerebellar herniation into foramen magnum	Increased (hypoventilation)	Disturbance of rhythm between respiratory centers Decreased responsiveness to CO_2 stimulation Slowing respiratory rate
Central neurogenic hyperventilation	Hyperpnea Stertorous forced rate	Pons	Arterosclerosis Hypertensive cerebral vascular disease Infection Trauma	Decreased (respiratory alkalosis)	Uninhibited stimulation of inspiratory and expiratory centers of brain Rhythm preserved

as anaphylactic reactions. Oversedation with hypnotics, sedatives, narcotics, and barbiturates can lead to depression of the respiratory center.

Barbiturates and sedatives such as glutethimide (Doriden), secobarbital (Seconal), and pentobarbital (Nembutal) depress respiratory effort. Hypoventilation with retention of carbon dioxide becomes a problem as respiratory rate decreases with a more shallow breathing pattern.

The most common opiate overdose is diacetylmorphine (heroin). Excessive doses of heroin increase vascular permeability and increase the potential for pulmonary infiltrates into the alveoli.[5] Morphine sulphate in excessive dosages also depresses respiration and respiratory response.

Salicylate poisoning (aspirin) causes immediate alteration in respiratory functioning. First, stimulation of the respiratory center causes severe hyperventilation which causes respiratory alkalosis. Tachypnea and tachycardia with fever and hypoglycemia occur as the body moves into a state of metabolic acidosis.[3]

Inhaled chemicals can also be a source of respiratory depression. Gasoline inhaled in toxic doses behaves as a central nervous system depressant and in high doses, results in unconsciousness, coma, and finally failure of the respiratory system.

Carbon dioxide has a normal physiological function in the process of respiration. External inhalation of a 2−5 percent concentration for short durations increases respiratory rate and depth. Venous return to the heart is also enhanced due to decreased peripheral resistance. Excess carbon dioxide inhalation results in a state of acidosis and unresponsiveness of the respiratory center with increased carbon dioxide levels. Rate of breathing decreases and becomes more shallow with increasing concentrations.[6]

Neurological dysfunction can cause alterations in rate, depth, and rhythm of respiration. Such dysfunction can be mediated by tumors, infarctions, and disruption of cerebral vascular bed, infectious processes, and trauma among others. Essentially the edema or occlusion of a vessel decreases oxygen and the area it serves. Depression of the neural centers for regulations of respiration makes the brain less sensitive to rising levels of carbon dioxide. Unconsciousness, coma, and ultimately death can result without treatment.

Musculoskeletal Disorders

A condition which restricts the expansion of the chest wall increases the potential for impairing ventilation. Such disorders affect the mechanics of moving air into the lung and expelling air out of the lung. Lung volumes and capacities may be decreased. The elasticity or compliance of the lung is reduced so that the thoracic cage must have higher than normal inspiratory pressure to continue to maintain adequate alveolar ventilation.

Guillain-Barre syndrome is a relatively uncommon, reversible, paralytic disease. The cause is unclear. Motor disturbances with progressive weakness or paralysis of motor muscles begins in the lower extremities and gradually ascends toward the trunk muscles. There may or may not be trunk muscle involvement. If the vagus nerve becomes involved there is a loss of contractibility in bronchial smooth muscle, and thus there is interference with normal protective airway mechanisms. Pneumonia and atelectasis can be complicating factors. Paralysis of the muscles of inspiration decreases the ventilatory capability and may necessitate artificial life support. Symptoms gradually disappear. Residual muscle weakness is a concern.

Myasthenia gravis is another disorder resulting in muscle weakness and response. The cause may be a metabolic disorder. Essentially there is a defect causing inadequate transmission of impulses at the myoneural junction within the muscle fiber. The effects are marked weakness and easy fatigability of muscles. The disorder shows a definite affinity for muscles innervating the face and neck. Airway occlusion and aspiration are potential complications. Again, the individual may need artificial life support when there is involvement of the diaphragm and intercostal muscles.

Poliomyelitis, also known as infantile paralysis, is caused by a viral transmission. A virus seems to be the underlying mechanism for dysfunction. Bulbar poliomyelitis causes acute changes in respiratory function as the brain stem is involved. Swallowing and upper airway paralysis as well as generalized muscle weakness causes inadequate functioning of the muscles of the thorax.[7] Again, respiratory assistance may be necessary.

Muscular dystrophy is a chronic disorder which results in bilateral (both sides) symmetrical wasting of the skeletal (voluntary) muscles. There seems to be a strong hereditary tendency. The basic etiology is a metabolic defect in creatinine metabolism.[8] The progressive muscle wasting causes deterioration of muscle groups and eventually limits ambulation. Loss of muscle support also results in deformities of posture and trunk support. Respiratory dysfunction occurs due to a decrease in tidal volume and a reduction in lung capacities. Alveolar ventilation is decreased and increased potential for airway infection exists.

Respiratory muscle dysfunction can be artificially created with drugs. These drugs are known as curare type medications. One example of use is with clients on artificial ventilation who are asynchronous with the ventilator. Such a drug may also be employed during a difficult problem in intubation of a client with an artificial airway. Succinylcholine is one such drug. Its primary action is to interfere with the transfer of impulses from the motor nerve to the motor endplate. Muscle paralysis is the result. Apnea or cessation of breathing is the clinical outcome. Artificial ventilation is necessary to maintain respiration.

Trauma to the chest wall may also cause respiratory dysfunction. Nonpenetrating chest wall injury, such as a rib fracture, is one example. Pain limits inspiratory effort, and a shallow breathing pattern is assumed by the individual. With this pattern, there is potential for alveolar hypoventilation and infectious processes of the airways to develop as a result of inefficient airway clearance. Penetrating wounds of the chest wall can cause pneumothorax and thus decrease the lung size. The extent of lung involvement determines the degree of dysfunction. Alveolar hypoventilation with low arterial oxygen levels may be present. Clinically, the individual is short of breath and assumes a rapid shallow breathing pattern.

Surgical intervention into the chest wall, such as a thoracotomy, also results in a restriction of chest wall movement. Pain limits the desire of the client to take a deep breath, and the potential for alveolar hypoventilation exists. This can be further complicated by atelectasis and a pulmonary infection of the airways. Attention to effective lung clearance is important.

Deformities of the spine and thoracic cage can restrict lung volumes and capacities. Kyphoscoliosis is one such example. Kyphosis is an abnormal increase in convexity of the spine or a humped back appearance. Scoliosis is an abnormal lateral curvature of the spinal column. Restriction of chest wall movement increases potential for respiratory infections and alveolar hypoventilation. The volumes and capacities of air movement are decreased due to a structural abnormality.

Hypoxia and Hypoxemia

Hypoxia is a state of inadequate oxygen supply to the tissues. Hypoxemia is a decrease in arterial oxygen pressure. The causative factors in hypoxia are one or more of the following: (1) inadequate supply of oxygen in inspired air; (2) decreased circulatory capability; (3) reduction in oxygen carrying capacity of the circulation; (4) venous admixture by shunting of the circulation; and (5) histotoxic hypoxia.

Ineffective circulation is discussed in greater detail in the next section. Inadequate supply of oxygen in inspired air can be mediated by several causes. The air hunger experienced at high altitude is related to decreased partial pressure of oxygen as altitude is increased. The rapid and shallow breathing of hyperventilation, the most common response, is the body's attempts to increase minute ventilation and thus increase the supply of oxygen to the tissues.

Decreased availability of oxygen in inspired air can be caused by the presence of noxious gases or an enclosed airtight environment. Natural gas, whose major component is methane gas, causes displacement of the atmospheric air. Symptoms include shortness of breath followed by unconsciousness and death. Death is attributed to acute asphyxia, which is a lack of oxygen or an excess of carbon dioxide in the body. A closely related term is suffocation, which is an uncomfortable sense of air hunger due to a lack of oxygen. Natural gas and excess concentrations of nitrogen or helium are examples of simple asphyxiants which dilute the oxygen concentration of the atmosphere. Chemical asphyxiants also dilute the atmosphere and interfere with the body's ability to utilize oxygen. For example, carbon monoxide is able to diffuse across the gas liquid interface (alveolar-capillary membrane) about 200 times faster than oxygen by which means it decreases the ability of hemoglobin to carry oxygen. The result depends on how rich the environment is with this odorless and colorless gas. Small concentrations may cause headache and dizziness, but larger concentrations can produce unconsciousness and eventual death from tissue hypoxia.

Hydrogen cyanide behaves as a tissue asphyxiant. Cyanide inhibits the utilization of oxygen in tissue cells by interfering with the catalytic action of tissue enzymes that regulate the reactions of oxygen with substances in the cells.

Discarded refrigerators and mine cave-ins are examples of enclosed airtight environments. After the available oxygen is extracted from the air, the supply of oxygen is exhausted. Consequently, acute tissue hypoxia develops with death as the end result.

Drowning is death by acute asphyxia while submerged, regardless of whether or not liquid has entered the lungs.[9,10] Near drowning describes a condition of survival from submersion. Essentially, the pulmonary dysfunction is acute hypoxemia resulting from ineffective functioning of pulmonary surfactant thus allowing fluid to enter the alveoli. The fresh water drowning includes extensive hemodilution as a result of water passing from the lungs across the gas liquid interface and into the circulation. This can also cause strain on the myocardium. Salt water, on the other hand, causes persistent hypoxemia due to biochemical changes and damage to the lung parenchyma as a result of the presence of a hypertonic solution. Salt water causes transfer of plasma from circulating blood volume into the alveoli resulting in acute pulmonary edema.

Anemia is a condition which results in decreased hemoglobin concentration. The cause varies. Hemoglobin is the essential component for transporting oxygen in an easily dissociated chemical combination for release at the tissue level. Clinically, the individual experiences dyspnea with exercise as well as at rest. Complaints of low energy and malaise are common.

Oxygen carrying capabilities of the blood can also be disturbed by general anesthesia. During general anesthesia, pulmonary gas exchange is disrupted. Oxygen transfer from the alveoli to the blood is impaired and carbon dioxide retained unless there is a concomitant increase in the fraction of inspired oxygen as well as the minute ventilation. Anesthesia alters the alveolar distribution of gas in relation to the blood flow past these alveoli. A state of anesthesia with low tidal volumes potentiates mismatching of available oxygen with blood flow due to more uneven distribution of inspired gas at low tidal volumes. Thus, a transient hypoxemia postanesthesia is not uncommon with changes in the distribution of ventilation relative to the perfusion of pulmonary capillary blood.

Shunting

Alterations in the relationship of ventilation to blood flow is termed shunting or venous admixture. Shunts are classified into three categories: anatomical, anatomiclike, and physiological. Anatomic shunts are the result of abnormal vascular communications which allow blood to totally bypass the gas exchange units. Congenital heart disease, which is discussed later, is one example of anatomical shunting. The respiratory structure is essentially normal in relation to ventilation. The arterial carbon dioxide values can be maintained at nearly normal levels, but the oxygen values are decreased. Hypoxemia persists in spite of increased oxygen concentrations.

In an anatomiclike shunt there are areas of the lung which do not have adequate gas volumes for one of several reasons; therefore, pulmonary capillary blood bypassing these areas does not pick up additional oxygen. Atelectasis is one example. Anatomiclike shunts behave much like additional dead space.

Physiological shunting occurs when the pulmonary capillary blood flow passes by poorly ventilated alveoli and does not pick up the normal amount of oxygen; thus, there is a low ventilation to perfusion ratio. This is one of the most common causes of hypoxemia and is one of the underlying mechanisms for airway obstruction. Four different shunting situations can develop. (1) Alveoli are adequately perfused and adequately ventilated. (2) Alveoli are not perfused but adequately ventilated. (3) Alveoli are not perfused and not ventilated. (4) Alveoli are perfused but not ventilated. Any of the last three situations can cause alterations in the effectiveness of oxygenation and ventilation of the tissues.

HYPOVOLEMIC SHOCK

One example of impaired circulation resulting in an alteration in the relationship between ventilation and perfusion is hypovolemic shock, which is an acute loss of circulating blood volume through hemorrhage. Thus, there is a decrease in oxygen availability to tissues as well as the ability of the tissue to utilize the oxygen. The initial insult results in the body's effort to centralize the circulation to meet basic need of critical organs (heart, brain, kidneys, and lungs). The blood flow to peripheral tissues is decreased. Increased heart rate (tachycardia) and increased respiratory rate (tachypnea) by the body are attempts to increase the cardiac output. Success is limited unless blood loss is controlled and volume replaced. If the process continues, then eventually the cardiovascular system is unable to respond and blood pools in the tissues, resulting in cardiorespiratory failure. The system is unable to meet the tissue demands of the cells due to a lack of circulating blood volume.[11]

ADULT RESPIRATORY DISTRESS SYNDROME

Adult respiratory distress syndrome (ARDS) is an acute pulmonary dysfunction that is most often secondary to trauma to other organ systems. Terms like shock lung, postperfusion lung, and oxygen toxicity are synonyms for ARDS. Within 24 hours after the initial insult there is an alteration in the permeability of the alveolar-capillary membrane.[12] This is thought to be due to a dysfunction of the cells which manufacture surfactant. Surfactant assists in maintenance of alveolar integrity and prevents the transudation of fluid across the membrane. The alveoli become fluid filled and areas of atelectasis develop. Anatomiclike shunting causes hypoxemia. Presence of fluid in the alveoli affects pulmonary mechanics as well. The compliance of the lung is decreased, and the pressures required to open alveoli for given lung volumes increases. The work associated with breathing also increases. Without intervention, respiratory failure and death are inevitable. The most important precipitating clinical symptom is an increase in the respiratory rate in spite of the fact that the client seems to be doing well about 24 hours after the trauma to the system.

INFANT RESPIRATORY DISTRESS SYNDROME

The respiratory distress syndrome most often associated with premature infants previously was called hyaline membrane disease. Respiratory efforts are affected at birth. An audible expiratory grunt, accompanied by sternal retractions and labored breathing attempts, are common. Immaturity of the respiratory structure causes a decreased production of surfactant and instability of the alveoli with tendency toward alveolar collapse. Dead space ventilation is increased and proteinlike membranous strands are seen in the alveoli and airways in lung specimens obtained after death. There are many complicating factors which add to the total syndrome development and progression. These range from metabolic alterations to inability to maintain body temperature. More is being learned about the pathogenesis of this dread disorder of infants. Treatment can be successfully instituted in certain instances.

BODY TEMPERATURE CHANGES

Changes in body temperature are not confined to infants. Exposure to extremely cold temperature such as frostbite or immersion in very cold water can cause alterations in oxygen requirements. Hypothermia, a decrease in body temperature below accepted levels, is induced in hospital settings to reduce the oxygen demands by the body by decreasing the metabolic rate. Temperature is carefully monitored to stay within therapeutic levels. With frostbite, vascular changes can occur. The viscosity of the blood increases, capillary obstruction results followed by capillary shunting. The vasoconstriction with decreased flow and stasis progresses to sludging and increased potential for occlusion of vessels. Crystal type formations in the extracellular spaces of tissues can cause disruption of cellular metabolism and edema. Hypoxia results with impaired oxygen transport and oxygen utilization. Initially metabolism and oxygen requirements are increased in an attempt to maintain body temperature. Shivering is a mechanism that the body employs to maintain body temperature. Eventually, however, central nervous system function is depressed, and metabolic processes slow down.

Basal metabolic rate and oxygen consumption are increased with excess in body temperature or fever. With increased fever, oxygen is given up more readily to the tissue, thus blood leaving the tissue cells is more desaturated. Rapid breathing with tachycardia or increased heart rate are common symptoms of the body's attempt to meet the increased oxygen demand.

Often accompanying fever is a state of dehydration, which is a deficit of body water. Severe deficits can cause electrolyte imbalances which ultimately affect the acid base status of the body and respiratory functioning. Increased sodium levels decrease oxygen consumption. The oxygen consumption may either rise or fall with dehydration depending on the precipitating cause.[13] One effect of dehydration is drying of mucous membranes of the respiratory tract. This impedes pulmonary clearance mechanisms for removal of debris and mucus. As a result infection is possible as well as small airway obstruction. Dehydration can also cause metabolic alteration which results in the body trying to conserve or excrete carbon dioxide in response to an acidotic or alkalotic state.

THERMAL TRAUMA (BURNS)

Changes in basal metabolic needs and oxygen consumption is also demonstrated in thermal injury or burns to the surface tissue. Smoke inhalation which often accompanies the tissue burn is discussed earlier in this chapter. Tissue injury from burns is quickly accompanied by increased capillary permeability at the burn site and nonburned areas if enough surface area is involved. The extensive loss of intravascular volume subsequent to the capillary leak causes tissue edema within 48 hours postburn. The capillary permeability interferes with electrolyte balance and ultimately with oxygen consumption and carbon dioxide removal. Cardiac output is initially decreased with reduction in capillary flow and ultimately venous return. Oxygen pickup is then depressed, and oxygen utilization is depressed at the cellular level secondary to edema and cellular dysfunction. Basal metabolic rate is greatly increased to meet the body's response to the thermal insult. The edema of tissue can cause interference with mechanics of ventilation. Burns of the face and neck can cause laryngedema and need for an artificial airway to preserve an open airway. Burns of the trunk can cause restriction of movement and impair adequate levels of inhaled volumes of gas. Thus burns can cause mechanical as well as chemical dysfunction of respiration.[14]

Cardiovascular Disorders

The effectiveness of the respiratory system is dependent upon an intact pump (heart) and transport system (circulation). Congestion, occlusion, and congenital (birth) defects can alter the effectiveness of the heart and the circulation.

CONGESTION

Congestion of the circulation with fluid overload causes a strain on the heart and can lead to systemic and pulmonary dysfunction. Congestive heart failure (CHF) results when the heart muscle can no longer handle the circulatory load. There is a resultant increase in the diastolic pressure and volume in the left ventricle. This increased pressure is transmitted to the left atrium and into the normally low resistance pulmonary system. Dyspnea results due to the movement of fluid into the interstitium. This increased interstitial fluid decreases the compliance of the lungs and an increase in airway resistance with a resultant increase in the work of breathing. Alterations in the electrolyte sodium causes fluid retention further overloading the system. The resultant inefficiency of the heart leads to hypoxemia. Hypoxemia further stimulates the cardiac muscle which is already overloaded.

Pulmonary edema, a complication of this left-sided congestive heart failure, is the presence of fluid in the alveoli and the result of extreme vascular congestion. When this happens, not only is compliance decreased and airway resistance increased, but there is also alteration in normal gas exchange. The initial changes are hypoxemia with associated alveolar hyperventilation and reduced cardiac output. Thus, it is common for the arterial carbon dioxide to be normal or below normal. The individual experiences severe dyspnea with expectoration of pink-tinged, frothy sputum, and cough. Carbon dioxide retention is a later development if appropriate treatment is not instituted.

Cardiac failure can also occur as basically right-sided heart failure or cor pulmonale. Chronic obstructive lung disease is the most common precipitating factor in the development of cor pulmonale. In response to the hypoxemia of chronic obstructive lung disease, the number of red blood cells rises to increase the oxygen carrying capacity of the circulation. The increased number of red blood cells or polycythemia tends to cause the blood to become more viscous. This increased viscosity places a greater strain in the right side of the heart and increases pulmonary vascular resistance. Edema of the extremities and sudden weight gain are sometimes observed. Dyspnea is also noted. The underlying cause relates to lung dysfunction. The right-sided heart failure is a manifestation of that disorder.

OCCLUSION

A second complication of the increased viscosity of the blood with polycythemia is an occlusion of a blood vessel by a blood clot called a thrombus. If the thrombus detaches from the wall of the blood vessel and travels to another portion of the body, it is called an embolus. A pulmonary embolus is a blood clot that lodges in the lung. A portion of the pulmonary circulation is thus occluded, and a portion of ventilated alveoli do not have blood flowing past to pick up the necessary oxygen. The sudden onset of chest pain, increased respiratory rate (tachycardia), and possibly blood-tinged sputum (hemoptysis) are clinical signs of pulmonary embolus. Hypoxemia is common; however, overall ventilation to the lungs is increased thus arterial carbon dioxide values may be normal or decreased.

Another form of vessel occlusion occurs as a result of the narrowing of the internal diameter of a blood vessel. The decreased diameter is due to a deposit of lipids in the innermost tissue lining of the artery. This narrowing results in a disorder called arteriosclerotic or atherosclerotic heart disease (ASHD). This is an ischemic type of heart disease when the coronary vessels of the heart are involved. When a vessel becomes completely occluded or nearly occluded, the tissue which it serves becomes anoxic (lack of oxygen). If oxygen is not provided to that area quickly, then that tissue dies and becomes nonfunctional. Systemic atherosclerosis increases the workload on the heart and impairs cardiac output. Thus oxygen delivery capabilities can be decreased by an inefficient transport mechanism and potential for dysfunction of the pumping mechanism.

A myocardial infarction is an interruption of blood flow to the cardiac muscle. There is a resultant decrease in the total mass of contracting myocardium. An imbalance is created between the delivery capabilities for needed oxygen and the demand for oxygen. There is a mild hypoxemia which may be mediated by changes in the regional ventilation and perfusion, especially at the lung bases. Increased oxygen concentrations usually provide comfort to the client. Generally in an uncomplicated myocardial infarction, the pulmonary complications are minimal. Attention is paid to maintaining respiratory function and reducing strain on the heart by decreasing the body's oxygen needs. Complete bed rest during the initial period is necessary.

CONGENITAL ANOMALIES

In addition to congestion and occlusion of the vessels in the cardiovascular system, congenital anomalies of the heart can also contribute to respiratory dysfunction. During fetal life the lungs are bypassed as nutrients to the growing fetus are provided via the placenta. Special provisions are made for shunting the blood from the right to the left side of the heart. Between the right and left atria, there is an opening called the foramen ovale; after birth, this normally closes. In addition, between the pulmonary artery and the aorta, there is a tubular communication called the ductus arteriosus. A graphic illustration of these channels for blood flow is found in Figure 36-3. After birth, there is a flap which closes the foramen ovale, and the ductus arteriosus turns into a solid cord. The ductus venosus, also a fetal structure, receives a portion of the oxygenated blood from the placenta by way of the umbilical vein and dumps it into the inferior vena cava, thus mixing its blood with blood returning from the lower part of the body. Congenital dysfunction relative to a ductus venosus is very unusual.

Failure of the foramen ovale to close properly results in a right to left cardiac shunt. Due to this structural abnormality, a portion of the returning blood supply does not pass through the lungs for oxygenation. Rather, this deoxygenated blood passes directly into the left side of the heart where it mixes with oxygenated blood. In effect, this reduces the total oxygen tension in the arterial blood and causes severe hypoxemia with visible bluish cast to the skin (cyanosis).

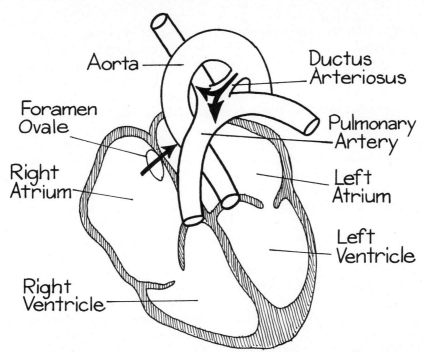

FIGURE 36-3. A schematic drawing of fetal heart structure prior to birth. After birth, the foramen ovale and the ductus arteriosus normally close off. If either does not close, blood is not properly oxygenated, and a shunt develops.

Tetralogy of Fallot is another example of congenital right to left shunt. It consists of an interventricular septal defect, a narrowing or stenosis of the pulmonary artery, a dextroposition of the aorta, and a right ventricular hypertrophy. Again there is a reduced blood flow through the lungs and decreased pulmonary pressure. Cyanosis and dyspnea are pronounced.

A patent ductus arteriosus creates a left to right shunt. Normally this closes off within 2–3 weeks after birth. If it does not, then the result is excessive pulmonary blood flow and subsequent pulmonary hypertension. Due to the left to right shunt, blood flow to the lungs increases with a resultant increase in the pulmonary arterial pressure and eventually to pulmonary vessel hypertension. Tachycardia, tachypnea, dyspnea, and fatigue are common symptoms.

NURSING RESPONSIBILITIES IN RESPIRATORY DYSFUNCTION

The care of the client with alterations in pulmonary function involves a multidisciplinary approach. It is common for client care to be coordinated among inhalation therapists, physical therapists, occupational therapists, nursing and social service personnel, and the physician. Integral to the development of a plan of care is the client and his family. Knowledge of adjunct measures to: promote pulmonary clearance, provide for improvement in ventilatory mechanics, and maintain adequate oxygenation by both the client and the staff are essential components in successful delivery of health care. The maneuvers designed to prevent pulmonary complications and improve function are known as pulmonary physiotherapy. These are discussed below.

Maintaining a Patent Airway

The client's ability to mobilize secretions is critical in the maintenance of a patent airway. Turning, coughing, and deep breathing maneuvers are utilized in the prevention and treatment of accumulated secretions. Compression of lung tissue is affected by gravity and weight. For example, a supine position tends to compress the lower posterior and anterior bases of the lung, resulting in greater potential for decreased distribution of ventilation to that area.[1] Therefore, position changes improve the overall distribution of ventilation and aeration of the lung units for gas exchange.

COUGHING

The *cough mechanism* is one means by which the lung facilitates removal of secretions. Coughing is generally a reflex stimulation of cough sensitive areas of the larynx and trachea triggered by an irritation. The sequence of events includes a deep inspiration followed by a quick tight closure of the glottis with a concomitant forceful contraction of the expiratory intercostal muscles and an upward thrust of the diaphragm. Pressure builds up against a closed glottis which subsequently opens, and air is expelled under force propelling liquid and solid matter from the lower respiratory tract toward the mouth. This autonomic cough reflex may be disturbed in certain disease states or conditions. Muscle paralysis, emphysema, fractures of the thoracic cage, head injuries with coma, and extensive surgical repair to the chest or abdomen are examples of such conditions. Surgery and its resultant pain decreases the client's desire to cough. Educating the surgical client in the promotion of an effective cough is an important part of the preoperative care plan.

It is helpful to teach the client how to splint the incisional area prior to coughing. Provision of adequate pain medication about 30 minutes prior to the treatment helps in promoting client cooperation. A pillow may be placed over the chest and abdominal area. The client wraps his arms around the pillow; when he coughs, the pillow provides support.

When muscle weakness is a factor, it is helpful to ask the client to take a deep breath, then exhale as far as possible. During exhalation, the nurse can place her hand or the client's hand on the area of the diaphragm and gently but firmly, push up and inward. This maneuver assists in building up pressure within the thorax for expulsion of air and secretions.

Individuals with long standing chronic obstructive lung disease tend to have less effective muscles of respiration. The diaphragm is flattened as a result of a hyperinflated chest. Lung compliance is increased, and airways are flabby due to loss of structure. Therefore, an assistive gentle cough after exhalation is more beneficial in mobilizing secretions

than is a forceful cough after a maximal inspiration. Forceful coughing at the end of inspiration tends to cause collapse of the airways with trapping of secretions behind the compressed airway.

Restrictive lung disorders result in a decreased compliance and "stiffer" lungs. Thus, deep inspiratory efforts are very difficult and short bursts of coughing are more effective and less fatiguing.

Coughing is more effective when the client is in a sitting position and sufficiently well hydrated to decrease the viscosity of secretions. Measures utilized to stimulate a voluntary manual cough are: (1) external stimulation over the trachea or "tickle" or (2) introduction of a suction catheter into the lower airway by a skilled practitioner. Care must be taken in this maneuver as laryngospasm can be induced.

While encouragement of coughing is generally the rule, there are instances where paroxysms (continuous attacks) of coughing are not beneficial. Frequent coughing, especially of a dry nature (such as irritation of upper respiratory tree), can cause fatigue and intercostal muscle discomfort. For this reason, cough suppressants or expectorants may be utilized to suppress cough. Careful evaluation of the client is essential as the cough is an important mechanism for removal of secretions. Cough suppressants act on the cough center and depress its activity, whereas expectorants are helpful in generating the flow of mucus and in promoting liquefaction of secretions, reducing muscular work associated with the cough.

In summary, the objective for coughing is to obtain the best results with the least amount of effort. If the client does not have the physical strength or is hampered by a restricting or obstructing defect, then special coughing techniques are of benefit in assisting the client toward an effective and energy efficient cough.

BREATHING PATTERNS AND EXERCISES

Breathing patterns tend to be individual, and most individuals are not conscious of their breathing pattern until dysfunction occurs. It is natural to periodically take a deep breath or sigh. This sigh mechanism is very important in promoting patency of the lung's gas exchange units. Periodic stretching of the alveolar ducts and alveoli promote the production of surfactant, a beneficial lipoprotein whose presence in the cellular structure of the alveoli (1) prevents collapse of the alveoli, (2) prevents capillary contents from entering the alveoli, and (3) contributes to the maintenance of alveolar integrity.

Instruction in deep breathing maneuvers is a beneficial component of preoperative teaching and prevention of postoperative pulmonary complications such as atelectatic pneumonias. Proper positioning facilitates the most effective breathing pattern. Sitting in an upright position allows for improved diaphragmatic function and increased expansion of the thoracic cage. Do not place pillows closely around the chest as this restricts chest excursion.

Emphasis is placed on deep inhalation, holding the breath for 1–2 seconds at the end of inspiration, followed by a slow prolonged expiratory phase. Provision of pain medication to postoperative clients helps promote the best effort. The client should be instructed to take 5–6 deep breaths every hour in conjunction with voluntary coughing measures.

Blow bottles are often used postoperatively to encourage the deep breathing maneuver. The objective is for the client to take a deep breath, put a tube connected to a bottle into his mouth and exhale forcefully, causing fluid to move from one bottle to the second bottle (Figure 36-4). The pressure generated forces fluid into the other bottle. This is a visual incentive with a reward—that is, seeing the fluid move from one bottle to the other bottle. The client is instructed to do this procedure five to seven times per hour. Instruction of the client in the proper use of the blow bottles is very important if they are to be used effectively or at all.

Segmental breathing exercises employ the idea of manual compression. Use of a gentle but firm manual compression to one specific area of the thorax on exhalation decreases the residual lung volume. The subsequent inspiratory effort tends to be deeper with greater lung volumes being exchanged with the respiratory cycle. Positioning of the hands is illustrated in Figures 36-5A and B. Care must be taken not to exert too much pressure. Careful selection of the client is necessary. Clients with rib fractures, post-thoracic surgery, or osteoporosis of the bone are not good candidates for this procedure.

Breathing exercises for clients with chronic lung dysfunction are primarily directed toward improv-

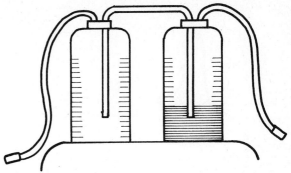

FIGURE 36-4. Blow bottles are used to assist client to deep breathe. The client blows into the tube connected to the bottle with the colored fluid inside. The pressure generated causes the fluid to move up the tubing within the bottle and move into the second bottle. The client then blows into the free tube of the second bottle and reverses the process.

ing muscle coordination and decreasing the muscular effort associated with breathing. The loss of elasticity of the lung and the resultant downward displacement of the diaphragm in chronic obstructive pulmonary disease decrease the efficiency of the breathing and often increase the muscular effort associated with moving volumes of air in and out of the lungs. Structural changes in the airways and the gas exchange units further interfere with complete exhalation. Thus, it is not uncommon for these clients to chronically use accessory muscles to accomplish respiration.

Breathing retraining is beneficial to these individuals. Inhalation is encouraged through the nose (if possible), while expiration is accomplished through a pursed lip breathing maneuver. By inhaling through the nose, the body's natural filtering and humidification mechanism is not bypassed. This is not always easy for a severely disabled client even though desirable. Pursed lip breathing, as shown in Figure 36-6, employs exhaling against a slight resistance, thus decreasing the potential for airway collapse. Expiratory effort should be approximately twice as long as inspiratory effort. Controlled breathing promotes an increase in coordination of breathing and an increase in confidence of the client that he can move air with greater effectiveness and less fatigue.

Several abdominal muscle building exercises are also utilized to increase breathing efficiency and muscle tone. In one such exercise, the client lies on

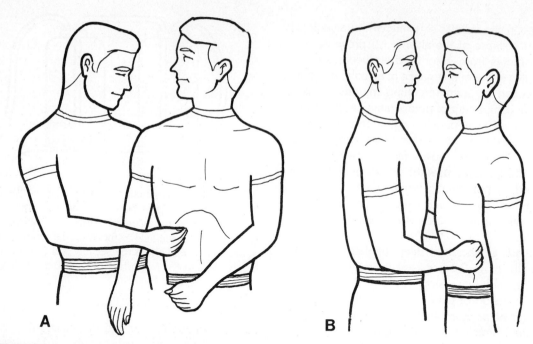

FIGURE 36-5. Segmental breathing. Placing the hands over the client's thorax at various positions as shown (A and B) and gently squeeze the thoracic cage as the client exhales. This maneuver assists more complete exhalation.

his back with the dominant hand on his abdomen just below the sternum, while the other hand is placed on the anterior chest. During inhalation the abdomen rises; on exhalation, the client expels air through pursed lips at which time the abdomen falls, pushing the diaphragm against the thorax.

In summary, the objective of breathing exercises in chronic obstructive respiratory disorders is to promote coordination of the breathing maneuver, muscle tone, and enhance full exhalation of inspired air. The effect of breathing exercises for the postoperative client is to decrease incidence of postanesthesia pneumonitis as well as the potential for secretion accumulation.

POSTURAL DRAINAGE, PERCUSSION, AND VIBRATION

Effective removal of secretions is increased by the use of postural drainage, percussion, and vibration. The use of positioning, gravity, and clapping techniques helps promote the flow of secretions and reduce energy expenditure. This maneuver is useful for clients with thick tenacious secretions which are difficult to mobilize, and is most often prescribed for clients with chronic lung dysfunction or

acute lung dysfunction resulting in decreased ability to remove excess secretions. Clients with the following conditions are unable to tolerate this procedure: (1) unstable cardiovascular function; (2) recent myocardial infarctions; (3) head injuries and resultant increased intracranial pressure; (4) unstable fractures of the spine; (5) pneumothorax; and (6) bullous emphysema. It may also be necessary to modify or limit the postural drainage treatment to accommodate a client's age or physical condition.

Effective drainage of secretions depends upon their location in the various lobes of the lung. Logically, it takes a longer period of time to facilitate removal of secretions from distal airways. The most acutely affected area should be drained first. Postural drainage, percussion, and vibration may be used for short-term sputum clearance such as in acute pneumonitis or acute bronchitis, or it may be a procedure taught to a client for home use. Clients with chronic lung dysfunction and copious sputum production such as bronchiectasis and chronic bronchitis with obstructive airway disease benefit by daily use of this procedure.

The viscosity of the sputum is a factor in effective removal. Fever and mouth breathing result in in-

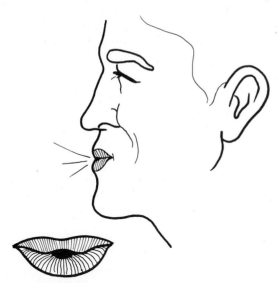

FIGURE 36-6. Pursed-lip breathing is a maneuver used by clients with obstructive lung disease. Exhaling through pursed-lips prolongs the expiratory phase and allows for a more complete exhalation. This results in a decreased amount of air trapped in the lungs on completion of exhalation.

sensible water loss and contribute to increased sputum viscosity. Mouth breathing bypasses the body's natural mechanism for humidification, increasing the drying effect on the respiratory tract. Supplemental oxygen further dries the secretions within the respiratory tract. Adequate hydration is necessary in liquefying secretions and promoting sputum clearance. In the absence of cardiovascular dysfunction or cerebral dysfunction, 2–3 L of oral or parenteral fluid per 24 hours is recommended.

Postural drainage is a physical means of enlisting the aid of gravity to assist in the transport of secretions from the smaller airways toward the main stem bronchus and the trachea for removal by coughing or suctioning. Various positions are employed for each segment of the lung as shown in Figures 36-7 to 36-15. Each position places a segmental bronchus in a vertical position so that gravity can assist in the drainage of that segment.

Percussion is the act of striking the chest wall rhythmically, with cupped hands (Figure 36-16) over the segment of the lung being drained. The oscillatory movements produced are transmitted to the airways where these sounds act to dislodge mucus in the airways and promote flow of secretions toward the trachea.

Vibration is the technique of applying manual compression and rapid tremor to the chest wall. The purpose is to further loosen and assist in the movement of secretions toward the trachea as well as aid in the process of exhalation.

In summary, postural drainage, percussion, and vibration are often employed with coughing and breathing retraining (breathing exercises) to maintain and promote patency of the airway through removal of secretions and improved overall ventilation of the lung. Such procedures may be employed in acute respiratory dysfunction as well as chronic obstructive airway disorders. The performance of this procedure may be directed by the inhalation therapist, the physical therapist, or the nurse.

HUMIDIFICATION THERAPY

Humidity refers to a quantity of water vapor in a gas mixture. A humidifier is a device which adds water vapor to a gas. The most common mechanism is bubbling gas through water, thereby, providing a maximum surface area of water to come in contact with the gas and promoting the movement of water molecules into the gas.

Humidifiers

The most common humidifier used in hospitals is a bubble type which is attached to an oxygen delivery system. Oxygen is a dry gas and thus its administration requires a humidifying source. If oxygen is not humidified prior to delivery, the mucous membranes of the upper respiratory tree become dry and irritated. Accumulated secretions also tend to become more viscous and difficult to expectorate.

Humidifiers may be prescribed to a client for home use. A cold-mist type room humidifier is usually employed. The room air in winter climates has a low relative humidity. Individuals susceptible to upper respiratory infections or persons who have chronic lung dysfunctions may be encouraged to provide a source of humidity in the home. The purpose is to promote more liquefied secretions and to assist in maintenance of an intact mucous membrane.

Proper education of clients who have room humidifiers includes: (1) always empty old water from

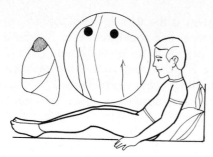

FIGURE 36-7. Upper lobes—apical segment: client should be placed in a sitting position on a bed, or this position may be done while the client is in a chair. The client should lean back on a pillow at approximately a 30 degree angle. Clapping is done over the area between the clavicle and the top of the scapula on each side.

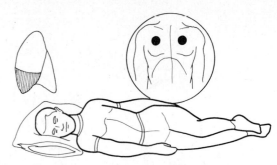

FIGURE 36-10. Left upper lobe—lingular segment: client lies on right side at a 45 degree angle. Pillows may be placed behind the shoulder and hips. Knees should be flexed. Percussion is done over the nipple area.

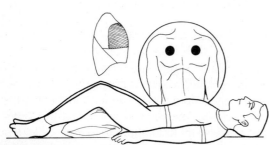

FIGURE 36-8. Upper lobes—anterior segment: the client is in a flat position on his back with a pillow placed under the knees. Percussion is done between the clavicle and the nipple on each side of the chest.

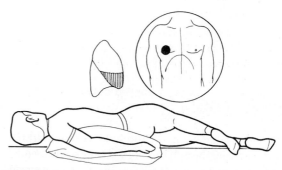

FIGURE 36-11. Right middle lobe—lateral and medial segments: client has head down on the left side and rotates body at 45 degree angle. Pillows may be placed behind the client at the shoulder and hip. Percussion is done over the nipple area.

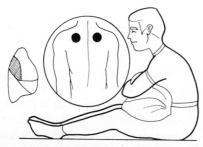

FIGURE 36-9. Upper lobes—posterior segments: client is placed in a sitting position and leans forward over a folded pillow. Percussion is done over the upper back on each side of the chest.

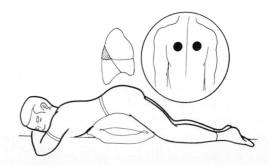

FIGURE 36-12. Lower lobe—superior segment: client lies flat on abdomen. Pillows are placed under the hips. Percussion is done over the middle third of the back (below scapula and on either side of the spine).

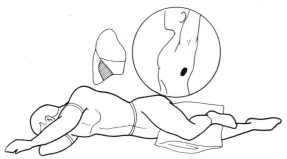

FIGURE 36-13. Lower lobes—anterior basal segment: provision is made to elevate the foot of the bed about 30 degrees. The client lies on side with head down and a pillow under the knees. Percussion is done over the lower ribs beneath the axilla.

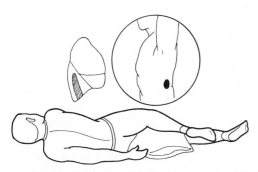

FIGURE 36-14. Lower lobes—lateral basal segment: provision is made to elevate the foot of the bed about 30 degrees. The client lies on the abdomen and rotates the body about 45 degrees. The upper leg may be flexed and supported over a pillow. Percussion is done over the uppermost part of the lower ribs.

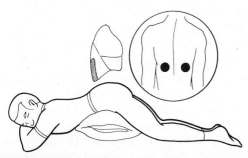

FIGURE 36-15. Lower lobes—posterior basal segment: provision is made to elevate the foot of the bed about 30 degrees. The client lies on his abdomen with the head down with a pillow under the hips. Percussion is done over the lower ribs close to the spine on each side of the posterior chest.

the humidifier before adding fresh water; (2) clean the unit at least once a week with a mild detergent; (3) periodically soak the immersible parts in a dilute vinegar solution, rinse, fill with water, and run the unit about 30 minutes prior to use as the vinegar fumes can be very irritating; (4) if present, filters should be changed as recommended; and (5) avoid over-the-counter vaporizer preparations unless physician prescribed.

Aerosols

Aerosols are another method of adding humidity to ambient air in hospitals. An aerosol is any suspension of particulate matter, solid or liquid, in a gas. Water, normal saline, and certain medications are common suspensions. The most critical factor in maintenance of an aerosol is the size of the droplets. The larger the droplet size, the greater the tendency for the liquid to move out of suspension. Inhaled aerosols are utilized for three purposes: (1) to aid in liquefaction of secretions, (2) to humidify inspired gases, and (3) to deliver medications.

Mechanical generators and electrical generators are utilized to deliver the aerosol. Mechanical generators or nebulizers use a baffle system with a high velocity flow to create the droplets. These may be utilized with or without a heating element.

Electronic generators or ultrasonic nebulizers have incorporated into their construction a thin membrane which by its vibratory motion in the solution causes particles to break off from the surface of the liquid and be transported via tubing connections and face mask to the client for inhalation. Such an aerosol device is capable of producing a very heavy mist of fairly uniform size droplets for deposition into the airway. The equipment is set up by the inhalation therapy department and often monitored by them.

Nursing care responsibilities during aerosol administration include: (1) evaluation of client's ability to effectively mobilize secretions with this liquefaction process; (2) increased perception of dyspnea by the client; (3) noting increased wheezing and respiratory distress; and (4) monitoring the color, amount, and consistency of secretions expectorated.

An example of aerosol delivery is a mist tent, which is primarily utilized in pediatric situations such as a child with croup. A fine mist is delivered

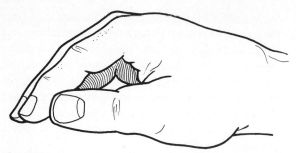

FIGURE 36-16. Percussion of the chest is performed by cupping of the hands as shown above and in an alternate manner clapping over prescribed area of the chest wall. Such areas are shown in Figures 36-7 and 36-15. If done correctly this procedure should not be painful.

by way of a tent setup. Such tents are designed for use where it is necessary to control the client's immediate atmosphere: (1) inspired oxygen concentrations, (2) temperature, and (3) amount of humidification. These mist tents can also be used to provide greater concentrations of oxygen than is in ambient air. Another example of this concept is seen in the use of Isolette incubators in nurseries. The oxygen tent, however, is not quite as popular today as in previous years.

Nursing concerns in the care of the client in an enclosed environment whether it be mist tent therapy or oxygen tent therapy are directed toward: (1) maintenance of the prescribed environment including oxygen concentration, humidity, and temperature; (2) monitoring client response to this method of treatment; and (3) prevention of electrical hazards and machine malfunctions.

Maintenance of the prescribed environment includes proper sealing of the tent around the client, tucking the bottom of the clear plastic canopy carefully under the mattress on the sides and top, and folding the bottom of the tent into the top of the bed linen over the client's chest. The tent should be flushed with 15 L of oxygen prior to opening and for 2–3 minutes after opening.

Air flow within the tent can create drafts and increase client discomfort. A towel may be wrapped turban style around the head. A shawl or towel can be draped around the shoulders. In croup tents, condensation and dampness may often be heavy and the child's clothing and linens have to be changed frequently.

The tent environment tends to be very restricting and some client's may experience a feeling of being trapped or may feel that they are suffocating. Check the air flow inside the tent and the connections for potential leaks. Look at the temperature gauge for excessive heat, and note any excess condensation on the inside of the tent. If the mist is too concentrated, the client may experience shortness of breath. In rare instances, bronchospasms may result.

Malfunctions do not often occur, but care must be taken to check the equipment at least once per shift. This is usually done by inhalation therapy personnel. Oxygen tends to support combustion; thus, any item with potential for electrical sparks (e.g., electric bed or electric call light), or smoking should not be permitted in the immediate environment.

INTERMITTENT POSITIVE PRESSURE BREATHING

Intermittent positive pressure breathing (IPPB) is a mechanical apparatus which provides a specific mixture of air/oxygen/air or air/oxygen/medication to the client utilizing increased delivery pressures. The client places a mouthpiece connected to tubing (which is connected to the machine) into his mouth and creates a tight seal around the mouthpiece. A preset inspiratory pressure is then dialed by the nurse or inhalation therapist. The machine forces a deeper inspiration by positive pressure inhalation. Exhalation is a passive process.

The use of IPPB is prescribed for two basic reasons: (1) as a modality for delivery of therapeutic aerosols topically to the bronchial tree and (2) to promote increased ventilation of the gas exchange units with decreased muscular work of breathing. Postoperatively, IPPB is utilized to prevent atelectasis and assist in clearance of secretions.

Monitoring the client is important. Attention to the client's ventilatory pattern facilitates improvement in the effectiveness of the therapy. Inspiration should be deep with breath holding (1–2 seconds) at the end of inspiration, followed by a slow expiratory phase with complete exhalation.

IPPB may be contraindicated in disorders such as: pneumothorax, hemoptysis, or impaired cardiovascular return. IPPB treatments can precipitate hyperventilation or excessive carbon dioxide exhalation by the client. Consequently, the client frequently feels dizzy or experiences the sensation of shortness of breath for a period of time after the treatment is completed. Assisting the client with a slow, controlled deep breathing pattern during the treatment helps minimize the tendency toward hyperventilation. The physician determines the amount of inspiratory pressure, medications if ordered, and the frequency of treatments. Timing of the treatments is important. Scheduling of therapy should be avoided within 1 hour postmeals as vomiting may be induced. Maximum respiratory effort is enhanced by the client assuming a sitting position. This position facilitates diaphragmatic movement and expansion of the thoracic cage. Treatments are sometimes ordered to precede postural drainage, percussion, and vibration to promote coughing and deep breathing.

Oxygen enriched atmospheres are utilized in the presence of persistent hypoxemia, to reduce the work of breathing needed to maintain a given oxygen tension and to reduce the work on the heart. Client parameters to monitor include: pattern of respiration, respiratory rate, blood pressure, pulse, and increased muscular work associated with the respiratory effort. Arterial blood gas analysis is an invaluable tool in monitoring the body's ability to meet tissue demands for oxygen.

Oxygen therapy is most beneficial in instances of hypoventilation, impaired diffusion capabilities and in disorders leading to venous admixture. Associated with alveolar hypoventilation is a rising carbon dioxide level which untreated can lead to respiratory acidosis.

Diffusion abnormalities which may be present in fibrotic conditions of the lung are benefited by increased concentrations of oxygen due to the associated increase in the alveolar oxygen tension.

The most common problem associated with hypoxemia (low oxygen tension) is venous admixture. In the instance of a true venous admixture or shunt (congenital heart defects) venous blood can bypass the gas exchange units (alveoli). An increase in oxygen concentration would not significantly affect the blood gases and correct the hypoxemia. Where there is a ventilation-perfusion imbalance such as COPD, a portion of the gas exchange units do not undergo adequate aeration, and blood eventually bypasses these units in favor of more adequately venitilated alveoli. Additional oxygen is beneficial in such instances.

Ventilatory insufficiency is a major clinical indicator for oxygen therapy. Simply stated, in ventilatory insufficiency, the arterial oxygen tension can not be maintained at greater than 50 mm Hg. The etiology of ventilatory insufficiency varies. The cardiac and pulmonary systems are working harder to maintain adequate basal metabolic oxygen requirements and at the same time utilizing more muscular effort. The goal of oxygen therapy is to decrease the strain on the heart and the work of breathing by the muscles of respiration.

Acute ventilatory failure is a medical emergency and requires immediate ventilatory assistance. The arterial blood pH is often less than 7.3 and metabolic acidosis with lactic acidosis is often present. In this situation, the body is deprived of adequate alveolar ventilation. The indications for impending ventilatory failure include: (1) sudden apnea; (2) severe chest trauma with resultant flail chest; (3) ineffective alveolar ventilation as reflected by blood gas analysis; and (4) increased fatigue with the work of breathing.

OXYGEN THERAPY

Nursing concerns in the care of the client receiving oxygen therapy are: (1) to understand why oxygen is ordered; (2) to be knowledgeable about the mode of administration; and (3) to be knowledgeable about the effects of oxygen therapy. The physician makes the initial decision to place a client on oxygen.

Oxygen therapy is essentially administered using one of two methods. The first employs the low flow oxygen system, which incorporates room air to deliver the prescribed oxygen concentration. The fraction of inspired oxygen (F_IO_2) is affected by changes in the client's tidal volume and ventilatory rate and pattern. The second method employs a high flow oxygen system, in which the client's total environment is controlled from the gas source. The advantages of this system of oxygen delivery include: (1) delivery of oxygen concentrations; (2) the inspired oxygen concentrations do not vary regardless of ventilatory pattern; and (3) the humidity and temperature of the delivered gas can be controlled more precisely.[15]

Determination of the necessary F_IO_2 is necessary prior to selection of the mode of therapy. Each piece of equipment has its limitations and advantages.

The oxygen source within the hospital setting can

be either piped into the room from a central gas source or may be brought to the client's room in an oxygen tank or cylinder. Cylinders must be handled very carefully as the gas is compressed and under as much as 2200 pounds of pressure per square inch, abbreviated as psi. Accidental rupture of the oxygen outlet on the cylinder may cause the tank to act like a jet propelled missile. Thus the tank must be secured in an upright position and chained to a stationary object. Most tanks are delivered in a portable stand for ease of mobility. The oxygen tanks are equipped with an oxygen outlet valve. An oxygen regulator must be attached to this outlet to regulate the oxygen flow rate from the cylinder. When the tank is initially being set up, the outlet valve should be opened slightly to allow a brief escape of oxygen. This clears the outlet valve and stem of accumulated dust or foreign particles that could clog the apparatus. This procedure is called "cracking" the tank. A bubbling humidifier is attached to the oxygen flow meter providing the necessary humidity to the inhaled gas. The setup is pictured in Figures 36-17A and B.

Piped in oxygen or wall oxygen is much more convenient and safer to use. The average psi is 50–60 pounds. A flow meter connects to the wall outlet and the necessary oxygen flow rate can then be regulated. Again a bubbling humidifier is utilized to humidify the gas. Regardless of the method of oxygen delivery a "No Smoking" sign must be placed on the client's door.

Low Flow Oxygen Systems

Low flow oxygen therapy may be administered by nasal catheter, nasal cannula, mask, and mask with a reservoir bag. A nasal catheter is utilized for low flow oxygen delivery and often for pediatric clients who will not keep a cannula or mask in place. The recommended flow rates are 1–6 L. Oxygen concentrations of up to 44 percent can be delivered by this means. The use of this method of oxygen delivery is dependent upon patent nasal passages. It is recommended that the cannula be changed every 8 hours from one nostril to the other to reduce trauma to the nasal passages. The nasal catheter is

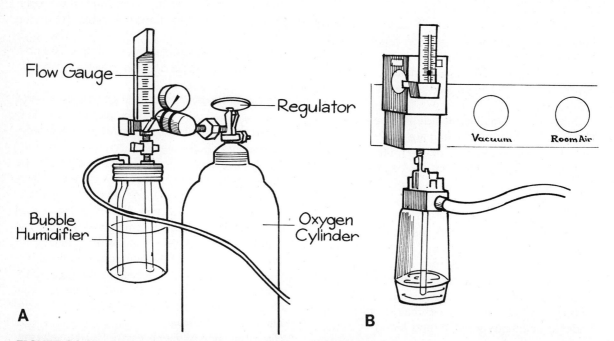

FIGURE 36-17. A, Oxygen cylinder. Oxygen cylinders are equipped with a regulator, oxygen gauge, and bubbling humidifier. The regulator and oxygen gauge allow the user to control the oxygen flow rate. The bubbling humidifier adds moisture to the otherwise dry gas (oxygen) before it reaches the client. B, Wall gauge oxygen Setup. Oxygen is also piped into clients' rooms. The outlet is located on the wall. Oxygen flow is regulated by a wall gauge inserted into the outlet. A bubbling humidifier provides humidity to the dry gas-oxygen.

positioned so that the tip of the catheter lies at the junction of the nasal and oropharynx. Care must be taken to see that the catheter does not extend beyond the uvula, as this can result in air passing into the esophagus causing gastric dilatation. If the catheter becomes displaced too far into the oropharynx, the gag reflex may be stimulated. The nasal catheter is taped into place as shown in Figure 36-18A.

The use of the nasal cannula or nasal prongs is the most common method for low flow oxygen delivery (Fig. 36-18B). There is minimal irritation to the nasal membranes from the equipment itself. The recommended flow rate is from 1−5 L. If greater flow rates than 6 L are used there is negligible benefit to the client as the anatomical reservoir is maximally saturated.[15] The anatomical reservoir consists of the nose, nasopharynx, and oropharynx. Thus, to provide higher oxygen concentrations, an increase in the anatomical reservoir is necessary. Oxygen concentrations of 24−44 percent can be achieved with the nasal prongs. For example, 2 L of oxygen flow delivers approximately 28 percent F_1O_2.[15] As with the catheter, the oxygen is bubbled through a humidifier with distilled water to add moisture to the dry gas. The most frequent complaint by the client is the sensation of dryness in the nose with subsequent nasal irritation. Application of a water soluble jelly just inside the nares is of some benefit in keeping the nares moist and preventing dry and crusted secretions. The oxygen tubing goes behind the ears and rubs against the area just behind the ear. Gauze padding over this pressure point is helpful.

The oxygen mask is employed when higher concentrations of oxygen are necessary. Concentrations of 40−60 percent can be achieved with the simple mask. The use of the mask increases the anatomical reservoir from 100 to 200 cc. Holes in the sides of the mask allow exhaled air to escape into the atmosphere. The normal flow rate for the oxygen mask is 5−8 L/minute. A mask should not be used at less than 5 L/minute as the flow rate will not be rapid enough to expel the exhaled carbon dioxide from the mask. Potential danger then exists for the client to rebreathe his own carbon dioxide.

One disadvantage in the use of the mask is that it must be removed for oral hygiene, eating, and talking. In addition, moisture builds up inside the mask and must be cleaned away. Clients do not always tolerate their nose and mouth being covered, thus frequently the nurse walks into the

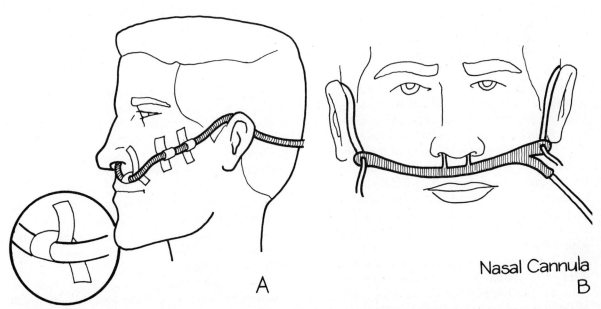

Nasal Cannula
B

A

FIGURE 36-18. A, The oxygen catheter is inserted into the nare (nostril) as described in the text. It is important to tape the cannula so that it is secure but does not interfere with the mouth or is in a position where the tape would be under strain. B, Nasal Cannula.

client's room only to find the mask propped up on the forehead.

When higher concentrations of oxygen are desired a mask coupled with a reservoir bag is utilized. The use of the bag increases the anatomical reservoir from 600 to 1000 cc with resultant oxygen concentrations of 60–95 percent and up to 100 percent in certain instances. The oxygen flow rate is set from 6–10 L/minute. The client inhales gas from the mask and reservoir bag with a minimum of room air in the mask. It is necessary to maintain high oxygen flow rates so that the reservoir bag is never completely emptied on inhalation.

A mask system which has recently become popular because of its more precise oxygen concentrations is the Ventimask or Venturi system; this mask incorporates a valve which mixes room air in the prescribed manner prior to reaching the client. The masks are designed to deliver oxygen concentrations of 24, 28, 35, and 40 percent. These operate regardless of the client's ventilatory pattern and thus technically fall into the category of high flow oxygen delivery systems.

In addition to watching for pressure areas, client tolerance, and the functioning of the equipment, it is also necessary for the nurse to be alert to signs of oxygen toxicity. Pulmonary oxygen toxicity is damage sustained to the lung secondary to prolonged exposure to high concentrations of inspired oxygen. The extent of lung damage is secondary to the duration and the concentration of the oxygen administration. The lung pathology indicates the presence of proteinacious fibrinous strands within the alveoli and alveolar ducts in the absence of acute inflammatory disease. Interstitial edema and fibrosis are also present. There is a resultant increase in physiologic dead space and a decrease in elasticity of the lung. Symptoms are vague and may only be perceived as a tightness of the chest and a dry cough. Arterial blood gases reveal a decreasing oxygen tension in spite of increased oxygen concentrations. Atelectasis or collapse of a number of gas exchange units (alveoli) is another potential complication of oxygen therapy. Nitrogen is washed out of the lung's alveoli being replaced by oxygen, carbon dioxide, and water vapor. If a transient airway obstruction occurs, the oxygen is continuing to be absorbed into the pulmonary capillary blood and eventually the alveolus collapses resulting in areas of atelectasis. A summary of the low flow oxygen system is found in Table 36-2.

High Flow Oxygen Systems

The most common type of high flow oxygen system employed is artificial ventilation. There are basically two types of ventilators: (1) pressure cycled and (2) volume cycled. Ventilation by the client may be classified as spontaneous, assist, assist-control, or controlled. Spontaneous ventilation occurs when the client initiates the device, including the respiratory rate and volume. Assisted ventilation is accomplished when the client initiates the respiratory effort, but the tidal volume is accomplished by the machine. In controlled ventilation, the client does not initiate the respiratory effort nor does he control the rate or volume of respiration. In assist-control, the client can initiate the respiratory effort, but if he does not, the machine automatically does it for him.

The pressure cycled ventilator is driven by a gas source, usually oxygen or room air. Upon initiation of inhalation gas flows into the lungs until a preset pressure is reached. At that point, the inspiratory valve on the ventilator closes, and the expiratory valve opens and passive exhalation begins. The tidal volume then is the variable. Thus, a client with increased resistance to air flow and stiff lungs would require high inspiratory pressure to deliver an adequate volume of gas to the alveoli. Therefore, effective tidal volume may not be insured if the lungs are stiff and there is increased resistance of the airways to gas flow. Examples of pressure cycled ventilators include the Bennett PR II and the Bird Mark II. These ventilators may also be utilized to give IPPB treatments. These ventilators can be set for assist or control. In assist, the inspiratory phase is concluded by reaching the preset pressure or by a preset time factor. Inspiration time can be controlled. The inspiratory time flow rate setting determines the duration of inspiration by regulation of the velocity of gas flow. The higher the flow rate, the sooner preset pressure is reached, and the shorter the inspiratory time. The lower the gas flow rate, the longer the inspiratory time. High flow rates produce turbulence with potential for shallow inspiration and uneven distribution of tidal volume. Low flow rates increase tidal volume and theoretically improve distribution of air.

Nursing observations of equipment include: (1) watching for leaks around the tracheal cuff, which is discussed in the following section; (2) a loose nebulizer jar which provides humidity; and (3) loose tubing connections to the client. Humidity

Table 36-2. Low Flow Oxygen Systems

Method	Recommended Liter Flow/% Concentration	Nursing Observations	Advantages	Disadvantages
Nasal prongs	1–6 LPM* 24–44% F_IO_2†	1. Watch for pressure points behind ears and under chin. 2. Complaint of dryness and patency of nasal passages. 3. Observe respiratory pattern.	1. Well tolerated by client. 2. Use in ambulatory situations.	1. Prongs tend to irritate nasal mucosa. 2. Pressure area may develop.
Nasal cannula	1–6 LPM 24–44% F_IO_2	1. Tip of catheter should be barely visible past uvula. 2. Excess irritation to nares. 3. Watch for gastric distension which means catheter is misplaced.	1. Alternate to nasal prongs without going to mask.	1. More uncomfortable for client. 2. Must be taped in place and repositioned as necessary. 3. Increased irritation to nasal passageways.
Oxygen mask	5–8 LPM 40–60% F_IO_2	1. Recommended liter flow not less than 5 as mask may not be flushed making CO_2 rebreathing possible. 2. Pressure points. 3. Respiratory pattern.	1. Fairly comfortable for client, yet can deliver up to 60% concentration of oxygen.	1. Fits over nose and mouth—remove while eating, sputum expectoration. 2. Condensation inside of mask; client's nose and mouth must be wiped off frequently.
Oxygen mask with reservoir	6–10 LPM 60–95% F_IO_2	1. Recommended liter flow not less than 5 as mask may not be flushed making CO_2 rebreathing possible. 2. Alert to signs of oxygen toxicity 3. Alert to signs of increased respiratory distress.	1. Fairly comfortable for client, yet can deliver up to 60% concentration of oxygen. 2. Can deliver oxygen concentrations of more than 60% without controlled oxygen therapy (i.e., ventilator)	1. Potential for excess oxygen delivery if used over period of time. 2. Have to maintain high minute ventilation and high oxygen flow rate to maintain concentration of oxygen. 3. Client often does not tolerate well.
Venturi mask	Liter flow specified on each mask: 24–28%; 35–40% F_IO_2	1. Specific LPM flow rate must be maintained which is marked on mask. 2. Client's tolerance.	1. Maintains a known oxygen percentage regardless of client ventilatory pattern. 2. No humidification device.	

*Liters/minute.
†Fraction of inspired oxygen.

must be added as the body's natural humidification apparatus is bypassed with the introduction of an artificial airway. The high humidity passing through the tubing causes condensation inside the tubing. It is necessary to periodically disconnect the tubing and empty the accumulated water into a receptacle. A reservoir bag is usually connected about halfway between the client and the machine. Condensed vapor accumulates in this bag. A plug in the bottom of the bag provides an outlet to drain the water. This prevents bacterial contamination and the need to disconnect the tubing. The entire tubing is changed once per shift by the inhalation therapist.

The volume cycled ventilator is usually electrically powered and operates by delivering a preset volume of gas to the lung. The volume that is delivered is less affected by changes in the pulmonary mechanisms as is a pressure variable machine. A volume cycled ventilator exerts whatever pressure is necessary to deliver the preset volume. A sudden increase in the inspiratory pressure can be indicative of an increase in airway resistance. The most common cause is accumulation of secretions. Suctioning is then necessary. A sudden decrease in the peak airway pressure or inspiratory pressure and a fall in the exhaled tidal volume (less than the preset inspired tidal volume) may indicate a leak in the system. Two examples of volume cycled ventilators are the Bennett MA-1 and the Ohio 560.

Nursing responsibilities for the client on the ventilator requires an organized team effort. The physician, inhalation therapist, physical therapist, nurse, client, and the client's family are all members of the "health care team." The nurse should be knowledgeable of the underlying pathophysiology, be familiar with the method of ventilation used, make pertinent observations regarding the client's changing respiratory status, provide for patent airway measures, and be alert to changes in vital signs and level of consciousness.

Two measures of adjunct ventilatory support currently employed in clients with acute ventilatory dysfunction on mechanical ventilation are: (1) PEEP and (2) IMV. PEEP or positive end expiratory pressure is utilized to keep the alveoli open during the expiratory phase of breathing. A positive end expiratory pressure of 5–15 cm water is maintained at end expiration instead of allowing the pressure to return to 0 cm water. PEEP is utilized to treat acute ventilatory failure resulting in persis-

tent hypoexmia despite administration of high concentrations of oxygen. It is thought that arterial oxygenation is increased by the prevention of collapse of terminal airways and alveoli during expiration. It is also thought to be beneficial in reducing the number of atelectatic alveoli and thus maintain adequate oxygenation without sustaining high concentrations of oxygen (greater than 60 percent).[15,16] Complications include the potential for: pneumothorax, mediastinal emphysema, and presence of air in subcutaneous tissue (subcutaneous emphysema).

Intermittent mandatory ventilation (IMV) is utilized to facilitate weaning from the ventilator. IMV allows the client to breathe spontaneously at his own rate. However, at intermittent and preset intervals a mechanical hyperinflation is delivered. Clinically the IMV assists in the prevention of atelectatic areas caused by alveolar hypoventilation and therefore minimizes the tendency for the client to develop peripheral infiltrates with the deep breathing maneuver.[15]

In summary, then, oxygen should be considered as a potent drug. It is the drug of choice in hypoxemia. The dosage and route of administration is dependent upon the underlying cause of the hypoxemia and the concentration of oxygen to be delivered and the status of the client. The action of the drug is to increase oxygen tension in the arterial blood and to promote tissue oxygenation. In addition, adequate oxygenation reduces the work associated with breathing and reduces the work of the heart. Side effects of the drug include: (1) pulmonary oxygen toxicity, (2) atelectasis, and (3) potential for respiratory depression. The effects of oxygen are best reflected and monitored by arterial blood gas analysis.

ARTIFICIAL AIRWAYS

In the absence of a patent airway, it may be necessary to insert a temporary airway for a brief period of time or an artificial airway for a prolonged period of time. The *oropharyngeal airway* is a device inserted between the posterior pharynx and the root of the tongue, thus maintaining patency of the airway. Such an airway is beneficial for short periods of time, such as temporary occlusion of the airway by the tongue and is best tolerated by the unconscious client as its presence tends to stimulate the gag reflex in the conscious client. Figure 36-19 shows an oropharyngeal airway.

The *S-tube* is another short-term emergency airway. This tube as pictured in Figure 36-20 is shaped like an S with one end inserted in the client's mouth over the tongue and the other end is utilized by the rescuer to blow air into the client's lungs. The wide rim or flange assists the rescuer in creating a seal over the mouth. The rescuer is positioned at the client's head and tilts the client's head back as far as possible. With both hands positioned on either side of the flange and both thumbs sealing the nose, the rescuer blows into the tube and watches for the rise in the chest. When the chest rises, the rescuer's mouth is removed from the tube and passive exhalation occurs. Other resuscitative measures are discussed in Chapter 37.

When the simple maneuvers just described do not provide for a sustained airway, then the placement of a more substantial artificial airway is necessary. An artificial airway bypasses the oropharynx and laryngeal structures and thus the obstruction caused by edema of soft tissue, such as the tongue, or of the larynx is relieved. Placement of an artificial airway is also utilized to protect the lower airway from aspiration in a situation where the gag reflex, laryngeal reflex, and tracheal reflexes are not functioning. Central nervous system (CNS) depression is one example. An artificial airway may also be considered in the case of a client who has copious secretions that cannot be adequately handled by any other means. Artificial airways are necessary when a client is placed on supportive ventilation by machine.

The *endotracheal tube* is one example of an artificial airway used in conjunction with a ventilator. If this tube is placed via the nasal route, it is termed a nasotracheal tube. If the tube is passed via the oral route it is termed an orotracheal tube. Placement of this airway is accomplished by an anesthesiologist or some other person equally skilled. When possible, a nasotracheal tube is preferred. Stabilization of the nasotracheal tube is increased as it is placed in the canal of the nose and can then be firmly taped to the nose and face. Proper securing of the nasotracheal tube decreases the potential for accidental extubation and displacement of the tube. Curvature of the endotracheal tube is less severe when placed through the nose than through the mouth. This facilitates greater ease in

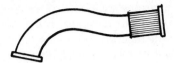

FIGURE 36-19. Oropharyngeal airway is a simple airway inserted into the mouth over the tongue. This prevents the tongue from occluding the airway.

suctioning the client. Nursing responsibilities with a nasally placed tube include observation of: pressure areas developing within the nasopharynx; blockage of sinus drainage which can result in acute sinusitis; and blockage of the opening of the eustachian tube on that side resulting in a middle ear infection.[13,15]

An *orotracheal tube* is more easily placed and may be the method of choice in nasal obstructions, facial trauma involving the middle third of the face, and in situations where acute sinusitis is a factor. Stabilization of the tube is more difficult than in the nasotracheal tube. Kinking of the tube is a greater potential problem and positional changes of the client affects the placement of the tube. Frequent mouth care is very important as secretions tend to pool around the tube and in the mouth. It is almost impossible for the client to drink or eat as the tube is in the way. It is often recommended that the tube be moved from one side of the mouth and retaped every 8 hours. This is potentially dangerous as accidental extubation becomes a key factor as well as

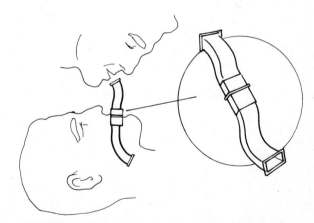

FIGURE 36-20. S-tube is an artificial airway shaped like an "S." One end of the "S" is suitable for insertion into a small child's mouth. The other end fits an adult size mouth. The holes in the ends of the tube facilitate the rescuer giving artificial respiration.

the tube being improperly placed, causing uneven distribution of air to the lung. For example, it is possible for the tube to slip into the right mainstem bronchus thus completely occluding air to the left lung, which would result in a collapse of that lung.

If placement of an endotracheal tube is not feasible or the client does not tolerate the endotracheal tube, placement of a *tracheostomy tube* may be necessary. A tracheotomy is the creation of an opening in the trachea. This procedure should be done under meticulously clean and preferably sterile conditions by a skilled surgeon or equally skilled individual. The necessity may arise under certain emergency conditions but should not be undertaken by untrained personnel. The tracheostomy or resultant opening is maintained by the placement of a tracheostomy tube. For the first 24 hours following the procedure, the nurse needs to be alert for: (1) increased bleeding; (2) development of a subcutaneous emphysema (air in subcutaneous tissue); and (3) increased secretions.

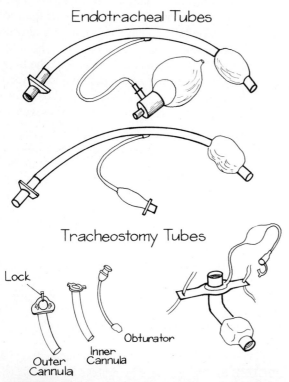

FIGURE 36-21. Tracheostomy tubes and endotracheal tubes are examples of artificial airways inserted by the physician to maintain an open airway for periods of time from a few days to several weeks.

Tracheostomy tubes can be made of metal or synthetic material (e.g., polyethylene and silicone). The more compliant and soft the material is, the more the tube tends to conform to the contours of the tissue through which it passes, resulting in less trauma to the tracheal mucosal tissue lining.

Endotracheal and tracheostomy tubes made of synthetic materials are equipped with inflatable cuffs as pictured in Figure 36-21. The purpose of this cuff is to provide an air seal around the tube and thus prevent a large air leak in clients on controlled ventilation. The cuff should be made of a very soft flexible material and be a large diameter with a large residual volume cuff. A large residual volume cuff even when inflated to the prescribed pressure will not be fully distended and will exert less pressure on the tracheal wall.[17,18] The contour of the tracheal wall is also followed more easily. An overinflated cuff can result in ischemia and necrosis of the tracheal wall. The potential for stenosis (narrowing) of the trachea is also increased. Periodic cuff deflation has been recommended in the past. The purpose of this maneuver is to restore blood flow to the tracheal mucosa. At this time, the literature does not totally support this theory.[15] A minimal leak technique is used in many institutions. The cuff is inflated to a point where a minimal leak exists around the tube. In controlled ventilation, this technique results in the least possible pressure on the tracheal mucosa during the expiratory phase. If it becomes necessary to deflate the cuff, the area above the cuff is suctioned as thoroughly as possible through the pharynx and the trachea prior to deflation. The cuff is then deflated followed by suctioning of the airway so that any secretions which may have lodged above the cuff are suctioned out of the airway.

In summary, artificial airways are utilized when there is an obstruction of the airway or collapse of the respiratory system. The type of airway selected is the prerogative of the physician. Selection is based in part on the underlying pathophysiology and the requirements for adjunctive oxygen and ventilatory support. Endotracheal tubes are used in ventilatory failure and in conjunction with ventilatory support. Tracheostomy tubes may be utilized with ventilatory support or without ventilatory support. Nursing responsibilities for artificial airways include: (1) monitoring equipment for air leaks or malfunction; (2) securing a patent airway; (3) monitoring changes in vital signs and levels of consciousness; and (4) knowledge of policy regarding tracheal cuff deflation procedures.

Suctioning and Care of Artificial Airways

Care of the tracheostomy tubes and endotracheal tubes is directed toward maintaining a patent and secure airway. Integral to airway care is suctioning. Techniques for suctioning of the airway have been discussed extensively in the nursing literature. Specifically, incidence of mucosal damage related to the type of suction catheter used and the technique of suction application; the amount of negative pressure applied during suctioning; and the use of preoxygenation and postoxygenation to prevent hypoxemia.

Selection of the suction catheter size varies with the presence of an artificial airway. The external diameter of the suction catheter should be no greater than half the internal diameter of the artificial airway used. Generally a 12 French or 14 French tube will suffice with an average length of 22 inches. In the absence of an artificial airway, the catheter size again should not be greater than one half the diameter of the airway. A 12 French, 14 French, or 16 French catheter is acceptable. Various catheter designs are currently in use. The design selected for use should be least traumatic to the mucosal wall. A coudé catheter with a slightly angled tip is often used to facilitate entrance into the left mainstem bronchus.

Considerations for insertion of the suction catheter into the airway are directed toward ease of insertion, promotion of the cough reflex, and removal of secretions. In the presence of an artificial airway, a thin coating of water soluble jelly will facilitate ease of insertion into an endotracheal tube. Gently, insert the catheter. The suction catheter should pass easily. If the catheter does not pass easily, there may be a sharp angle in the orotracheal tube offering resistance to the catheter. Reposition the client and try again. The head should not be flexed forward but rather in a neutral or slightly hyperextended position.

If there is not an artificial airway in place, position the head to facilitate the path of least resistance. A client may need to be positioned at a 45 degree angle or higher (as condition of client allows). If the client is able, ask him to stick out his tongue and insert the catheter into the lower airway during the inspiratory phase. If there is a persistent problem with passage of the catheter, notify the appropriate personnel.

Expect the client to cough when the suction catheter enters the lower airway. In the presence of an artificial airway, a cough is generated by touching of the carina (point of bifurcation of the mainstem bronchus). If the purpose of the suctioning is to promote an effective cough, then introduction of the catheter into the trachea will stimulate the tracheal reflex. If the client does not generate a cough at this point, bronchial suctioning may need to be done. This is not always recommended in every hospital because of the danger of laryngospasm. The policy and procedure varies from institution to institution as to the extent of suctioning allowed to be done by various levels of personnel.

Application of suction is measured relative to time and pressure. A total suction attempt should not last more than 15 seconds. Time spent in actual suctioning is only 5–10 seconds. One total suction attempt is defined as: (1) passage of the suction catheter; (2) application of suction; and (3) complete removal of the catheter. After insertion, the catheter is rotated and intermittent suction applied while removing the catheter. Between suctioning attempts, the client should be encouraged toward slow deep breathing with an increase in oxygen concentration. The oxygen concentration is determined by the physician. Five or six deep breaths is recommended. Bagging the client between suctioning attempts with an AMBU bag is suggested for those clients who have difficulty deep breathing spontaneously. Evaluate the client's response to the suctioning attempt and monitor the pulse rate. Pulse rates of greater than 150 can precipitate cardiac dysrhythmias. Be certain to chart the type of secretions suctioned: (1) the amount; (2) color; (3) odor; and (4) consistency. In some institutions (with a physician's order), 5 to 10 cc of normal saline are introduced into the artificial airway (in the adult client) to induce coughing and to aid in mobilization of secretions, however, the effectiveness of this procedure has not been adequately documented. Procedures for aspiration of the nose and mouth and suctioning of the lower airway in the presence of an artificial airway are found on Tables 36-3 and 36-4.

TABLE 36-3. Aspiration of the Nose and Mouth without Artificial Airway to Remove Secretions from Nasopharyngeal and Oropharyngeal Cavities

Anticipated Accomplishments	Scientific Principles/ Rationale	Specific Considerations
1. Determine that client requires suctioning.	Introduction of a foreign body into airway has potential for causing mucosal damage, increasing tissue irritation with resultant edema, and contributing to client discomfort. Increased potential of introduction of bacteria.	Partially obstructed airway decreases breathing effectiveness. Underlying pathology which would compromise client's condition. Client does not have an effective cough mechanism.
2. Conservation of time and energy. Organization.	Client will feel more confident and less anxious if nurse is organized and efficient.	
3. Decrease possibility of spreading infection.	Reduce transmission of bacterial contaminants since running water and friction remove many microorganisms from skin.	
4. Explain procedure to client.	Increase cooperation, decrease fear of unknown.	
5. Position the client on either side or with head slightly elevated.	Decrease danger of aspiration; lying flat on back can precipitate aspiration if client gags during procedure.	
6. Pour sterile irrigating saline into two paper cups.		
7. Turn on suction device.		
8. Decrease possibility of spreading infection.	Reduce transmission of bacterial contaminants since running water and friction remove many microorganisms from skin.	

Implementation	Recommendations	Observations
Make observations regarding client status.		Note increased restlessness, increased respiratory rate, increased apprehension, attempts to cough out secretions, and noisy respirations.
Assemble equipment at bedside: suction device (wall gauge with tube and vacuum bottle) or portable device, connecting tube. Tray with: sterile suction catheter, unsterile examining gloves, paper cups, sterile normal saline, and mouth swabs.		
Wash hands thoroughly using aseptic technique.		
Tell client what procedure is, why it is being done, and how he can help.		
Position client with pillows as necessary. If on back put head of bed at 45 degree angle and slightly hyperextend neck.		Check client's tolerance of positional change.
Place holding cups on work area; fill cups with saline or distilled water from pour bottle.		
Turn wall suction to pressure 80–140 cm. Turn portable suction machine switch on.		
Wash hands thoroughly using aseptic technique.		

Table 36-3. Continued

Anticipated Accomplishments	Scientific Principles/ Rationale	Specific Considerations
9. Reduce possibility of contaminating nurse's hands.	Use for aesthetic reasons. Use in cases of gross contamination of nose or mouth.	
10. Attach catheter to aspirating unit.		
11. Check functioning of vacuum of aspirating unit.	Ineffective vacuum will cause decreased efficiency of suctioning; client apprehension will be increased.	
12. Determine approximate distance catheter may be inserted.	Stimulation of laryngeal reflex could result in gagging or potential laryngospasm.	
13. Suction nasopharyngeal cavity allowing 3–5 min. between suction attempts.	Rest between suction attempts allows reaccumulation of air in anatomical reservoir which is also suctioned out. Decreases hypoxia. Rotation of catheter minimizes attachment to mucosal lining by vacuum and decreases mucosal damage. Forcing catheter can cause it to jam up against nasal turbinates and result in nasal irritation, minor bleeding, and edema.	Long periods of suctioning tend to increase potential of damage to mucosa.
14. Clear catheter lumen of any mucus.	Patency of catheter and tubing is assured when mucus is not plugging lumen.	
15. Suction oropharyngeal cavity.	Mucus also accumulates in mouth, especially severely debilitated clients. Suctioning too deeply into pharynx may cause stimulation of larynx and produce laryngospasm. Client usually coughs first.	

Implementation	Recommendations	Observations
Can use unsterile examining gloves.		
Attach catheter by connecter to tubing from suction machine.		
Place thumb over thumbport on catheter. Place catheter in cup of saline and suction small amount of irrigating saline from cup.		
Measure distance between tip of client's nose to ear and add 2 in for those clients over 10 years old.	The usual distance is 8–10 in.	
Insert appropriate catheter tip into nostril. Do not apply suction while inserting catheter. Gently advance catheter by letting it slide straight back along floor of nasal cavity to pharynx (about 8–10 in). Apply suction and gently rotate while withdrawing catheter. Suction should be applied no longer than 10 seconds. Repeat procedure for other nostril.	Be certain to find out if there is a septal defect or some other obstruction, making it difficult to pass catheter into nostrils. Application of a thin film of water soluble jelly facilitates insertion. Ask client to inspire when inserting catheter.	Be alert to increased apprehension by client. Note any obstructions in passage of catheter.
With clean cloth, wipe exterior of catheter. Place catheter in cup of irrigating solution and apply suction.		
Gently ease catheter tip into adult pharynx about 6 in. Apply suction. Rotate catheter and aspirate all areas. Withdraw catheter while aspirating. Clean catheter and repeat suction as necessary.	Comatose client tends to clamp down on catheter. Guide catheter along side of gum line and thread to back of mouth cavity. It may be necessary to insert oral airway to facilitate suctioning.	Note any effects such as profound shortness of breath.

Table 36-3. Continued

Anticipated Accomplishments	Scientific Principles/ Rationale	Specific Considerations
16. Turn off aspiration machine.		
17. Discard disposable equipment, including catheter, upon completion of procedure.	Proper disposal of equipment minimizes transfer of microorganisms.	
18. Facilitation of client cooperation during next performance of this procedure.	Reinforcement of desireable behavior encourages further cooperation when repeating procedure.	
19. Decrease possibility of spreading infection.	Reduce transmission of bacterial contaminants since running water and friction remove many microorganisms from skin.	
20. Record results in nurses' notes.		

It is appropriate at this point to briefly discuss sputum collection. One method of assessing the status of the respiratory system is to examine sputum for aberrant cells or organisms. The mucous membrane of the respiratory tract is responsive to foreign bacteria with resultant inflammation and increasing flow of secretions. Cytologic or cellular examination of sputum via the microscope can assist in defining causative disease organisms. This test is called a sputum smear. Sputum is also cultured. A sensitivity test determines the antibiotic to which the causative organism is most sensitive.

It is the nurse's responsibility to instruct and assist the client to obtain a good specimen. Sputum should be raised from deep within the bronchi as opposed to saliva from the mouth and mucus accumulated in the throat. Good coughing techniques are essential. Specimens should be collected early in the morning for several reasons. Secretions tend to accumulate overnight and are more abundant and hopefully easier to expectorate. Bacteria also tend to accumulate overnight as secretions are more stagnant as the client sleeps. Finally, obtaining the sputum specimen prior to breakfast eliminates the chance for food particles becoming mixed with the sample. Generally 4 ml are adequate for most studies.

Presence of artificial airways whether endotracheal or tracheostomy have certain commonalities. The normal upper airway defense mechanism of the lung is bypassed, and bacterial contamination is the rule rather than the exception. The presence of an artificial airway removes the effectiveness of the cough mechanism as the vocal cords are either bypassed (tracheostomy tube) or prevented from approximating (endotracheal tube). Interruption of the proper functioning of the vocal cords also prevents the client from talking which can be most

Implementation	Recommendations	Observations

Turn off suction apparatus.

Place disposable suction kit and catheter in paper bag. Discard.

Reassure client and provide positive reinforcement for cooperative behavior.

Wash hands thoroughly using aseptic technique.

Note: condition of client, type and amount of drainage, and changes in vital signs.		Frequency of suctioning. How client tolerates procedure. Any unusual findings.

frightening as well as very frustrating. Several methods have been utilized to increase the client's ability to communicate. These include: (1) pad and pencil; (2) magic slate; (3) visual aids; (4) sign language; (5) an electronic larynx; and (6) a device which attaches to a trachesotomy tube called a "trach talk."

Care of an artificial airway includes provision for cleansing of the airway site and the tube itself. One suggested procedure for the care of a tracheostomy is found in Table 36-5. In the event that the client does not have an inner cannula, as is common with some synthetic materials, then cleansing of the tracheostomy site at least every 8 hours is recommended. This is a sterile procedure. The soiled tracheostomy dressing is removed and the skin around the site is examined for redness, secretions, and presence of foul-smelling drainage. The area is cleansed with hydrogen peroxide and water using

a sterile dressing. The use of cotton applicators is discouraged as strands of the cotton fiber may remain at the tracheostomy site and be a source of potential infection. The skin is then dried thoroughly, and an antibiotic ointment is applied, unless contraindicated, followed by application of a tracheostomy dressing. Changing the twill tape which secures the tracheostomy tube is also completed at this time. Care should be taken not to tie the knot too tightly as this can cause pressure on the jugular veins. If the knot is too loose, then the tube can slide up and down in the trachea.

Occasionally a client is discharged with a permanent tracheostomy. Two examples are the client with radical neck dissection for carcinoma and the client with copious secretions as a result of a chronic obstructive lung disease. The client is generally sent home with a metal tracheostomy tube and an inner cannula. The client is often taught a clean tech-

TABLE 36-4. Tracheal-Bronchial Suctioning in Adults with Artificial Airways to Maintain Patency of Airway, Prevent Contamination of Secretions within the Tube, Decrease the Potential for Infection from Accumulated Secretions

Anticipated Accomplishments	Scientific Principles/ Rationale	Specific Considerations
1. Conservation of time and energy. Organization.	Client will feel more comfortable and less anxious if nurse is organized and efficient.	Determination of client's needs for suctioning.
2. Make certain duplicate tracheostomy tube is at head of bed (not necessary in endotracheal tube).	For emergency use in case tracheostomy tube is dislodged.	
3. Explain procedure to client.	Decreases client's apprehension and promotes cooperation.	Even if client is comatose, explanation is given.
4. Decrease possibility of spreading infection.	Running water and friction remove many microorganisms from skin, reducing transmission of bacterial contaminants.	
5. Prepare suction tray at bedside.		
6. Regulate suction.	High vacuums suck out increased quantities of gas in airway, cause trauma to mucosal wall and increase mucosal secretion.	Least amount of suction should be used to draw up secretions.
7. Reduce possibility of contamination.	Suctioning of tracheobronchial tree is sterile procedure. Sterile technique decreases contamination to lower airway.	

Implementation	Recommendations	Observations
Check size of current tracheostomy tube. Secure either same size or one size smaller. Be sure to have obturator taped to wall, current tube, and head of bed.	Collect: a sterile disposable suction kit, or sterile towel, sterile gloves, sterile bowl, sterile suction catheter, suction machine (wall or portable) with connecting tubing, resuscitation bag, and bottle sterile distilled water.	Client demonstrates increased mucus accumulation by ausculation of breath sounds. Sounds noted: coughing with "rattling" sound from airway. Increased inspiratory pressure readings on ventilator.
Tell client what you intend to do and why.		Look for signs of client understanding when communication is impaired by artificial airway. Use of paper and pencil or other device is helpful in communication process.
Wash hands thoroughly using aseptic technique.		
Place in a convenient location while still maintaining a sterile field. Emply catheter and glove on sterile field. Open bottle of sterile water and pour approximately 50 cc into disposable tray (sterile bowl is on tray).	Place equipment on stand over bed; move close to working area.	
Turn gauge to read 80−120 mm Hg, and portable vacuum to 3−5 in.		
Grasp disposable sterile glove by cuff and put on hand.	Both hands can be sterile gloved; however, only hand contacting catheter need be sterile.	

Table 36-4. Continued

Anticipated Accomplishments	Scientific Principles/ Rationale	Specific Considerations
8. Attach catheter to suction tubing with gloved hand.	Catheter is sterile, connective tubing is not.	Be certain not to touch unsterile part of tubing with sterile hand.
9. Lubricate catheter with sterile water from tray.	A lubricant increases ease of insertion into airway.	

Tracheal Suctioning

10. Insert catheter, without suction, into airway.	Potential for mucosal damage increases with amount and length of time vacuum is applied.	Catheter diameter should be less than ½ internal diameter of artificial airway used.
11. Creation of suction.		
12. Rotate catheter and remove while suctioning.	Chance of mucosal damage is decreased.	
13. Allow for deep breathing between attempts. Bag (AMBU) client as necessary.	Prolonged aspiration can produce hypoxia and promote cardiac dysrhythmias.	Allow 3-5 minutes between attempts. Hyperoxygenate as necessary.
14. Clear suction catheter and tubing.	Secretions become hardened and obstruct flow of air into connective tubing.	

Implementation	Recommendations	Observations
Clean hand holds connective tubing. Sterile hand holds catheter.		
Place catheter tip into sterile water tray. Aspirate fluid.	It is sometimes necessary to use a small amount of water soluble lubricant to facilitate passage of catheter (K-Y jelly).	Check to be certain to have adequate suctioning of fluid.
Tracheostomy tube: insert catheter 15 cm (or 6 in) in adults. Endotracheal tube: insert up to ¾ length of suction catheter. Suction catheter: should be 22 inches in length. Unsterile thumb placed over vents. Sterile gloved hand guides catheter. Apply suction for no more than 5–10 seconds. Apply intermittent suction while aspirating mucus.	Carefully "thread" catheter; do not try to jam it down. "Beaded" type of catheter may cause less mucosal damage. Multiple side holes in catheter.	Evaluate ease of passage of catheter. Does it meet with obstruction? It should pass with ease.
If client is on mechanical ventilation, bag with up to 100% oxygen entrained for several breaths. If on spontaneous ventilation, provide oxygen source, and assist with hyperinflations with AMBU bag.	Most desirable to have two people present during suction procedure.	Be alert to gasping attempts by client; air flow is significantly decreased during suction procedure. Observe nature of secretions aspirated. Take vital signs prior to and after suction attempts. Be alert to pulse rate greater than 150. Be alert for excessive bleeding.
Place catheter tip in bowl of sterile water; apply suction.		

Table 36-4. Continued

Anticipated Accomplishments	Scientific Principles/ Rationale	Specific Considerations
15. After tracheal suctioning, aspirate nasal and oral cavities as necessary.		Never aspirate nasal and oral cavities with same catheter before aspirating trachea.
16. Clean tubing; detach catheter and discard.	Use of new catheter each time reduces hazards of infection.	
Bronchial suctioning	Secretions may be copious and can not be adequately removed by tracheal aspiration.	Should be done by physician or skilled nurse.
17. Assemble equipment as per steps 1–8.		
18. Insertion of catheter.	Cough stimulus generated when catheter touches carina or point of bifurcation of mainstem bronc'·us (right and left).	Note obstructions. Check for any known cardiac dysrhythmias. Be prepared to bag client as necessary.
19. Catheter removal. (See step 12.)		
20. Repeat procedure as necessary.		

Implementation	Recommendations	Observations
See procedure on aspiration of nose and mouth.		
Place used catheter in paper bag with remainder of disposable equipment. Discard.		
Selection of curved tip catheter or coudé catheter. Secure assistance of another individual.	Turning head from left to right does not increase chance of suction catheter entering left mainstem bronchus. Two people suggested in case of complications, need to bag during procedure, if airway dislodges, and to help position client.	
Gently insert catheter without suction until coughing is stimulated. Withdraw catheter 1-2 cm, and gently angle catheter into right or left mainstem. Apply suction. Gently rotate catheter and apply intermittent suction for 5-8 seconds, while withdrawing catheter. Auscultate chest before and after suctioning attempts.	When inserting, concentrate on visualizing which direction curved tip is facing and when attempting to insert into right or left mainstem. Aim curve in that direction.	Be aware of client's tolerance, increases in combativeness, gasping attempts, pulse rate greater than 150, and cyanosis around mouth. Note nature and amount of secretions; chart color, viscosity, odor, and amount; note changes in character of breath sounds.
Upon removal of catheter, hyperoxygenate client with AMBU bag as necessary.		
Wait 3-5 min between attempts.		Watch for profuse perspiration, increased respiratory effort, redness of face, apprehensive facial expression; if present, discontinue suction attempt, provide oxygenation before reinsertion of catheter.

Table 36-4. Continued

Anticipated Accomplishments	Scientific Principles/ Rationale	Specific Considerations
21. Completion of procedure.		
22. Record and report procedure.		

nique rather than a sterile technique. Boiling the inner cannula once or twice a week is sufficient to keep it clean. Cleaning the inner cannula every day with hydrogen peroxide and water is essential in maintaining airway patency and preventing crustation of secretions within the airway. Each client should have an extra tracheostomy tube. After removal of the inner cannula for cleaning, the client is encouraged to cough and clear secretions from the airway. It may be necessary for the client to suction his own airway. Teaching a family member how to suction as well as how to care for the tracheostomy site is beneficial. Keeping the tracheostomy site clean and dry is encouraged.

Suctioning can be taught as a home procedure utilizing the principles outlined previously. The client again uses a clean technique and can obtain disposable suction kits or use a red rubber type catheter. If a nondisposable catheter is used, it is kept in a clean towel and thoroughly cleansed after use with hydrogen peroxide and water and then placed in boiling water for about 5 minutes once a day. Use of a mirror facilitates the self-suctioning maneuver. Teaching a family member or significant other is advised. The client should be instructed in measures to protect the tracheostomy site from entrance of foreign bodies, such as dust particles when he is outside. This can be accomplished by a scarf or a small knitted square of loosely woven fabric which covers the tracheostomy site, ties in the back, and allows for free movement of air. The body's natural humidification process is bypassed, so the client is instructed to drink plenty of fluids and note any change in the character of secretions.

The client is taught to communicate by placing his finger over the tracheostomy opening (there is no cuff on the tube) which then allows air to flow through the vocal cords or to use an artificial larynx if the voice box has been removed.

WATER-SEAL DRAINAGE

Pneumothorax, hemothorax, and trauma to the chest wall with a penetrating injury or surgical incision into the thorax may necessitate the placement of chest tubes to water-seal drainage. The purpose of the chest tube is to remove accumulated air and fluid from the chest cavity and restore the subatmospheric pressure which normally exists.

Water-seal drainage may be accomplished with or without suction. The one bottle water-seal drainage system provides no direct suction but effects drainage by gravity. Briefly, the system functions as follows: A catheter is introduced into the chest cavity by the physician. The catheter is connected to rubber tubing which attaches to a long underwater-seal tube inside a transparent drainage bottle as pictured in Figure 36-22. The short glass tube protruding from the stopper is the air vent. The top of the long glass tube is under water by approximately 2 cm. Greater than 2 cm of positive pressure within the chest cavity causes air and fluid to flow out of the chest tube and into the bottle. The air bubbles to the top and escapes out the air vent. The fluid continues to accumulate in the bottle. The amount of fluid accumulated in the bottle is recorded each shift or more often as the situation dictates. The color and consistency of the drainage is noted in

Implementation	Recommendations	Observations

Discard catheter and disposable
tray into paper bag and discard.
Turn off suction apparatus.

Note condition of client, type
and amount of drainage, and
changes in vital signs.

the charting. If the system is functioning properly,
the column of water in the long glass tube rises on
inspiration and falls on expiration. Bubbling signifies an air leak. When the bubbling ceases either
the lung has re-expanded or there is a leak in the
system.[13] Under most conditions chest tubes are
inserted for 24–72 hours. A simple pneumothorax
will usually re-expand within 24 hours.

If suction is necessary, a second bottle is added
to the water-seal bottle as shown in Figure 36-23.
The short tube which functioned as the air vent in
the single bottle system is now connected to a second bottle which again has a long glass tube which
is underwater and a third short tube which exits the
stopper and is connected to the suction source. The
amount of suction applied is directly related to the
depth of the water in this second bottle. For example, if the glass tube is submerged by 20 cm, the
negative pressure applied would be 20 cm. The
three bottle water-seal system as shown in Figure
36-24 incorporates a special collection bottle as
well as the water-seal and suction control bottle.
Otherwise, the principles are the same.

Water-seal bottles are not used as frequently
since the development of a disposable, light-weight
plastic chest suction unit called Pleur-evac. Essentially this unit can function as a water-seal only or
as a water-seal with suction. It has a collection
chamber, water-seal chamber, and suction control
chamber. The suction control and water-seal chambers are calibrated in centimeters to facilitate accurate readings of drainage amounts. Van Meter[19]
discusses the Pleur-evac unit and chest tube drainage in greater detail.

Nursing responsibilities include: (1) monitoring
for air leaks; (2) maintenance of a patent channel
from the client to the collection apparatus; (3) client
response to therapy; and (4) encouragement of
deep breathing and coughing. Occasional bubbling
in the water-seal chamber is expected as well as a
rise and fall in fluid levels as has been noted. Large
amounts of bubbling in the water-seal may indicate

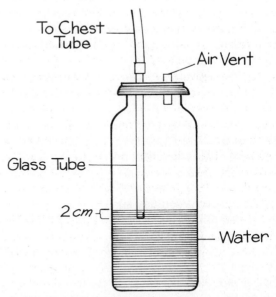

FIGURE 36-22. Water-seal drainage. Simple one bottle water-seal system. Such a setup may be used in uncomplicated pneumothorax. Air inside the chest escapes
through the tube into the bottle and out the air vent on
expiration. The column of water prevents air from rising
back up the tube.

TABLE 36-5. Tracheostomy Care for Maintenance of a Patent Airway and to Decrease Contamination of Tracheostomy Site to Prevent Systemic Infection

Anticipated Accomplishments	Scientific Principles/ Rationale	Specific Considerations
Cleaning Inner Cannula:		Procedure should be done a minimum of every 8 hours.
1. Decrease possibility of spreading infection.	Running water and friction remove many microorganisms from skin, reducing transmission of bacterial contaminants.	
2. Conservation of time and energy. Organization.	Client will feel more confident and less anxious if nurse is organized and efficient.	
3. Explain the procedure to client.	Reduces anxiety. Promotes co-operative atmosphere.	
4. Prepare work surface.	Maintaining sterile work area reduces contamination.	
5. Assemble equipment on sterile area.		Be careful not to contaminate work surface.
6. Prepare suction tray and materials for use.		Will need to suction client after removal of inner cannula.
7. Unlock inner cannula.		Be certain not to touch shaft of inner cannula. Support outer cannula with thumb and forefinger while gently removing inner cannula.

Implementation	Recommendations	Observations

Wash hands using aseptic technique.

Assemble equipment at bedside: a disposable tracheostomy care tray or the following items: gloves, small bottle brush, dressings, twill tape ties, gauze, sponges, sterile towel, pipe cleaners, tracheostomy dressing, sterile forceps, sterile scissors, sterile bowl, hydrogen peroxide, and normal saline. Have available: suction equipment, AMBU bag, duplicate tracheostomy tube.

Think through procedure first so that you do not have to run in and out of room.

Explain what you intend to do.

Place waterproof drape on overbed table.

Use of overbed table placed over client's lap provides a work surface close to the tracheostomy site.

Place assembled equipment on sterile drape.

Open disposable suction tray; attach catheter to suction source; and turn wall suction on.

Turn "key" on outer cannula that holds inner cannula in place.

If cannula is hard to remove, gently try to ease out by quarter turn to left and right. If secretions thick and crusted, may be necessary to suction prior to trying to remove inner cannula.

Table 36-5. Continued

Anticipated Accomplishments	Scientific Principles/ Rationale	Specific Considerations
8. Removal of inner cannula.		
9. Maintenance of patency and cleanliness of inner cannula.	Hydrogen peroxide is an antiseptic which loosens thick secretions and crusts.	
10. Aspiration of outer cannula	Suctioning removes secretions from airway.	
11. Prepare for removal of hydrogen peroxide and secretions from inner cannula.		
12. Reduction of spread of infection.	Contamination of inner cannula is reduced when sterile gloves are worn.	
13. Maintenance of patency and cleanliness of inner cannula.		Be certain all crusted secretions are removed.
14. Suction outer cannula again if necessary.	The cleanest environment possible, facilitates reinsertion of the inner cannula.	
15. Insertion and locking of inner cannula securely in place.		Tell client to take several deep breaths prior to insertion.

Implementation	Recommendations	Observations
Grasp outer flanges of inner cannula with sterile 4 × 4. Place cannula in sterile bowl.		
Pour hydrogen peroxide solution over inner cannula to completely immerse it.		Note condition of tube, amount of secretions attached, and consistency of secretions.
See procedure on tracheal aspiration described elsewhere in chapter.		
Pour sterile water into sterile bowl.		
Remove sterile gloves used while suctioning outer cannula. Replace with another pair of sterile gloves.		
With brush and pipe cleaner, wash out inner cannula. Rinse in bowl of sterile water. Inspect for any remaining secretions.		Inspect for cleanliness.
See procedure for suctioning with artificial airway in place.		
Gently slide inner cannula into tracheostomy tube. It should slide easily.	If inner cannula moist, this sometimes facilitates insertion. Allow adequate light. Helpful to sit client up at 45° angle.	Make notation if inner cannula does not slide easily into place.
Lock inner cannula in place. Check to be certain it is secure.		

Table 36-5. Continued

Anticipated Accomplishments	Scientific Principles/ Rationale	Specific Considerations
Dressing and Ties:		
1. Organization of necessary equipment.		
2. Decrease possibility of spreading infection.	Bacterial contamination is decreased by running water and friction which reduces number of microorganisms on hands.	If infection is present, use gloves and adhere to wound and skin isolation technique.
3. Removal of old dressings.	Reduction of media for bacterial growth.	Care must be taken to prevent dislodgement of the tracheostomy tube.
4. Decrease possibility of spreading infection.	Reduce number of microorganisms on hands by use of running water and friction.	
5. Cleanse skin around tracheostomy stoma.		Do not exert a lot of pressure. Be careful not to use cotton tipped applicators or dressings with loose cotton fibers as these can lodge at stoma site and provide a media for bacterial growth.
6. Decrease possibility of spreading infection.	Reduce number of microorganisms on hands by use of running water and friction.	
7. Replace tracheostomy dressing.		Sterile pre-packaged tracheostomy dressings with bound edges are most suitable.
8. Prepare new ties to secure dressing in place.		If unable to secure assistance, do not remove old ties until new ties are in place.

Implementation	Recommendations	Observations
Have a small paper bag ready to receive old dressings and used equipment.		
Wash hands using aseptic technique.		
Place fingers of one hand on outer rim of tracheostomy tube and with other hand, gently remove soiled dressing.	Asking client to turn head to side allows better visualization of stoma site. Be certain to have adequate light.	Note: presence of odor, color of secretions, redness and induration around stoma, and presence of pus.
With a sterile 4 × 3 dressing, moistened with ½ strength hydrogen peroxide and water, wipe stoma area clean.		Note: any bleeding, condition of stoma, edema, redness, presence of pus, and skin breakdown.
Wash hands using aseptic technique.		
Carefully place tracheostomy dressing under flange of outer cannula around tracheostomy tube from bottom to top. Bulk of dressing thus under tube.	Sterile gloves may be used.	Inspect skin prior to replacing dressing. Note any areas of redness or breakdown.
Remove soiled ties. Thread new twill tape ties through opening in flanges and draw free end of twill tape through a slit in tape.	Do not secure dressing with tape. Necessary to have another person present to secure tracheostomy tube in case client	

Table 36-5. Continued

Anticipated Accomplishments	Scientific Principles/ Rationale	Specific Considerations
9. Assure security of twill tape.	If tie becomes undone, tracheostomy tube may be coughed out; therefore, tie must be knotted.	Tie should be secure enough to prevent outer cannula from sliding up and down. Tie at side to prevent pressure area at back of neck. If tape is too tight, potential for impingment on jugular vein exists in addition to tape abrasion.

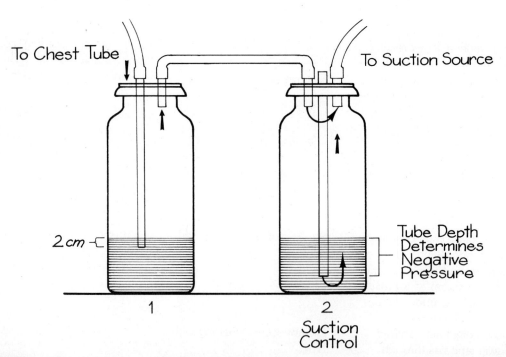

FIGURE 36-23. Water-seal drainage with suction bottle. If resolution of a pneumothorax cannot be controlled by one bottle drainage, suction may need to be applied by addition of a second bottle as shown. This assists in removal of air from the chest cavity.

Implementation	Recommendations	Observations
	should cough in some instances. The client can hold tracheostomy tube in place while you are preparing the new ties.	
Tie tape in knot at side of neck. Leave at least ½ inch end as any shorter could result in knot untying itself as pressure applied (i.e., by positional change or expulsive cough).	Tie should be just tight enough that one finger fits between skin and twill tape tie.	Charting should include: condition of skin, any unusual observations, how client tolerated procedure, and character of secretions.

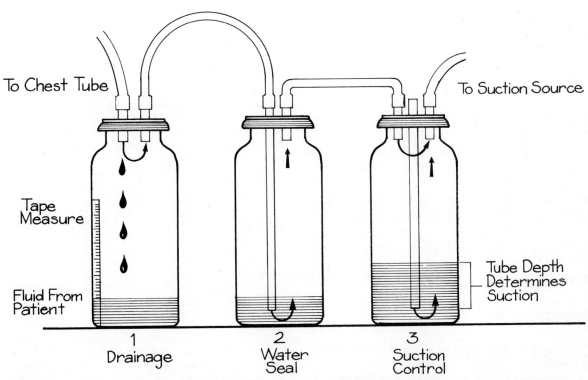

FIGURE 36-24. Water-seal drainage with collection bottle and suction. Pneumothorax may be complicated by accumulation of fluid and pus in the chest cavity. A third bottle (collection bottle) is used to collect fluid which exits via a tube inserted below the fluid level in the chest. A second chest tube may be inserted into the chest at the air level within the chest cavity. Thus, air and fluid can be removed to allow for re-expansion of the chest wall.

an air leak. Check the system for breaks in the tubing connections. This may be accomplished by clamping the tubing starting from the proximal end of the tubing and working down to the distal end. If no leak is found then it may be necessary to remove the dressing and check to be certain that the chest tube has not become displaced.

If a client becomes short of breath or complains of severe discomfort or a sensation of pulling inside the chest, then there may be an air leak or the negative pressure may be too high. The client should be allowed to assume a position of comfort unless contraindicated. Coughing and deep breathing at intervals creates an increase in the intrapleural pressure and assists in expulsion of air from the chest. Milking or stripping the tubing helps remove any accumulated clots. This is accomplished by pinching the proximal end of the tubing with the thumb and forefinger of one hand while using the thumb and forefinger of the other hand to apply pressure and slide down to the distal end. If the water-seal setup should break or become disconnected, a Kelly clamp should be applied to the chest catheter closest to the point of insertion and a physician notified immediately.[13]

SUMMARY

Nursing care measures in monitoring the client with respiratory dysfunction is directed toward: (1) maintenance of a patent airway; (2) removal of accumulated secretions; (3) monitoring oxygen therapy measures; and (4) measures to restore optimal lung expansion. Education of the client is critical as optimal success of nursing interventions are related to the client's knowledge and subsequent cooperation. Support, both physical and emotional, assists in relieving the fear and anxiety that accompanies respiratory distress.

REFERENCES

1. West, J. B.: *Respiratory Physiology—The Essentials,* Baltimore, Williams and Wilkins Co., 1974.
2. Baum, G. L.: *Textbook of Pulmonary Diseases,* 2nd ed. Boston, Little, Brown and Co., 1974.
3. Plum, F., and Posner, J. B.: *Diagnosis of Stupor and Coma,* 2nd ed. Philadelphia, F. A. Davis Co., 1972.
4. Burke, D. C., and Murray, D. D.: *Handbook of Spinal Cord Injuries Medicine.* New York, Raven Press, 1976.
5. Rogers, R. M., and Juers, J. A.: Physiologic considerations in the treatment of acute respiratory failure. *Basics RD* 3:1, 1975.
6. Bergersen, B. S.: *Pharmacology in Nursing,* 12th ed. St. Louis, C. V. Mosby Co., 1973.
7. Chusid, J.: *Correlative Neuroanatomy of Functional Neurology,* 16th ed. Los Altos, Calif., Lange Medical Publications, 1976.
8. deGutierrez-Mahoney, C. G., and Carini, E.: *Neurological and Neurosurgical Nursing,* 4th ed. St. Louis, C. V. Mosby Co., 1965.
9. Chopra, S. K., et al.: Effects of hydration and physical therapy on tracheal transport velocity. *Am. Rev. Respir. Dis.* 115:1009, 1977.
10. Fitzgerald, L. M.: Mechanical ventilation. *Heart and Lung* 5:939, 1976.
11. Schumer, W., and Nyhus, L. M. (ed): *Treatment of Shock: Principles and Practice.* Philadelphia, Lea and Febiger, 1974.
12. Giammona, S. T., Redding, J., and Snively, W. D.: Keeping the 'saved from drowning' saved. *Patient Care* 10:81, 1976.
13. Bushnell, S. S.: *Respiratory Intensive Care Nursing.* Boston, Little, Brown and Co., 1973.
14. Lawless, C. A.: Helping patients with endotracheal and tracheostomy tubes communicate. *Am. J. Nurs.* 75:2151, 1975.
15. Shapiro, B. A., Harrison, R. P., and Trout, C. A.: *Clinical Application of Respiratory Care.* Chicago, Ill., Year Book Medical Publishers, 1975.
16. Stackhouse, J.: Myasthenia Gravis. *Am. J. Nurs.* 73:1544, 1973.
17. Baier, H., Begin, R., and Sackner, M.: Effect of airway diameter, suction catheters, and the bronchofiberscope on airflow in endotracheal and tracheostomy tubes. *Heart and Lung* 5:235, 1976.
18. Selecky, P. A.: Tracheal damage and prolonged intubation with a cuffed endotracheal or tracheostomy tube. *Heart and Lung* 5:733, 1976.
19. Van Meter, M.: Chest tubes—basic techniques for better care. *Nurs. '74* 4:48, 1974.

BIBLIOGRAPHY

Ayres, S. M.: Cigarette smoking and lung diseases—an update. *Basics RD* 3:1, 1975.
Bageant, R. A.: Humidification terminology. *Respir. Ther.* 7:23, 1977.
Barlow, P. R: Treatment of tuberculosis. *Basics RD* 5:1, 1976.
Bartlett, R. H., and Allyn, P. A.: Pulmonary management of the burned patient. *Heart and Lung* 2:714, 1973.
Beland, I. L., and Passos, J. Y.: *Clinical Nursing Pathophysiological and Psychosocial Approaches,* 3rd ed. New York, Macmillan Publishing Co., 1975.
Bennett, R. M.: Drowning and near-drowning etiology and pathophysiology. *Am. J. Nurs.* 76:919, 1976.
Best, C. H., and Taylor, N. B. (eds.): *Physiological Basis of Medical Practice.* Baltimore, Williams and Wilkins Co., 1973.

Bredenberg, C. E.: Acute respiratory distress. *Surg. Clin. North. Am.* 54:1043, 1974.

Burrows, B., Knudson, R. J., and Kettel, L. J.: *Respiratory Insufficiency.* Chicago, Year Book Medical Publishers, 1975.

Carr, D. T., and Rosenow, E. C.: Bronchogenic carcinoma. *Basics RD* 5:1, 1977.

Clarke, E. B., and Niggemann, E. H.: Near-drowning. *Heart and Lung* 4:946, 1975.

Comer, P. B.: The use of muscle relaxants in respiratory failure. *Respir. Ther.* 7:31, 1977.

Cook, W. A.: Shock lung—etiology, prevention, and treatment. *Heart and Lung* 3:933, 1974.

Driscoll, J. M., and Mellins, R. B.: Idiopathic respiratory distress syndrome of infancy. *Basics RD* 1:1, 1973.

Farer, L. S.: Preventative treatment of tuberculosis. *Basics RD* 2:1, 1973.

Farney, R. J., et al: Oxygen therapy—Appropriate use of nebulizers. *Am. Rev. Respir. Dis.* 115:567, 1977.

Geelhoed, G. W., Kotch, A., and Petty, T. L.: Forestalling acute respiratory distress. *Patient Care* 11:58, 1977.

Gold, W. M.: Asthma. *Basics RD* 4:1, 1976.

Goldsmith, J. R.: Health effects of air pollution. *Basics RD* 4:1, 1975.

Guyton, A. C.: *Textbook of Medical Physiology.* Philadelphia, W. B. Saunders Co., 1971.

Kealy, S. L.: Respiratory care in Guillain-Barré syndrome. *Am. J. Nurs.* 77:58, 1977.

Kramer, J., Manoguerra, A., and Schnoll, S. H.: Treating the acute-overdose victim. *Patient Care* 11:76, 1977.

Likoff, W.: *Atherosclerosis and Coronary Heart Disease.* New York, Grune and Stratton, 1972.

Lloyd, J. R.: Thermal trauma-therapeutic achievements and investigative horizons. *Surg. Clin. North Am.* 57:121, 1977.

Mauss, N. K., and Mitchell, P. H.: Increased intracranial pressure—an update. *Heart and Lung* 5:919, 1976.

Moser, K. M.: Diagnostic measures in pulmonary embolism. *Basics RD* 3:1, 1975.

Najarian, J. S., and Delaney, J. P.: *Critical Surgical Care.* Miami, Symposium Specialists, 1977.

Oliver, M. F.: The metabolic response to a heart attack. *Heart and Lung* 4:57, 1975.

Parsons, L. C.: Respiratory changes in head injury. *Am. J. Nurs.* 71:2187, 1971.

Pierce, A. K., and Saltzman, H. A.: Conference on the scientific basics of respiratory disease. *Am. Rev. Respir. Dis.* 110:1, 1974.

Powaser, M. M., et al.: The effectiveness of hourly cuff deflation in minimizing tracheal damage. *Heart and Lung* 5:734, 1976.

Powers, S. R.: The use of positive end-expiratory pressure (PEEP) for respiratory support. *Surg. Clin. North Am.* 54:1125, 1974.

Pruitt, B. A., Erickson, D. R., and Morris, A.: Progressive pulmonary insufficiency and other pulmonary complications of thermal injury. *J. Trauma* 15:369, 1975.

Rau, J., and Rau, M.: To breathe or be breathed—understanding IPPB. *Am. J. Nurs.* 77:613, 1977.

Redher, K., and Sessler, A. D.: Intrapulmonary gas and blood flow distribution in awake and in anestherized man. *Surg. Clin. North Am.* 53:823, 1973.

Rosenow, E. C.: Spectrum of drug induced pulmonary disease. *Ann. Inter. Med.* 77:977, 1972.

Selecky, P. A.: Tracheostomy—a review of present day indications, complications, and care. *Heart and Lung* 3:272, 1974.

Shapiro, B.: *Clinical Application of Blood Gases.* Chicago, Year Book Medical Publishers, 1973.

Silver, D.: Pulmonary embolism. *Surg. Clin. North Am.* 54:1089, 1974.

Smith, B.: After anesthesia. *Nurs. '74* 4:28, 1974.

Smulyan, H., Gilbert, R., and Eich, R. H.: Pulmonary effects of heart failure. *Surg. Clin. North Am.* 54:1077, 1974.

Stevens, P. M.: Positive end expiratory pressure breathing. *Basics RD* 5:1, 1977.

Taber's Cyclopedic Medical Dictionary, 13th ed. Philadelphia, F. A. Davis Co., 1977.

Thorp, G. D.: Shock—the overall mechanisms. *Am. J. Nurs.* 74:2208, 1974.

Thurlbeck, W. M.: Chronic bronchitis and emphysema—the pathophysiology of chronic lung disease. *Basics RD,* 3:1, 1974.

Tong, T. G.: Poisoning and it's treatment. I. Incidence and clinical signs of poisoning and toxic overdose. *Nurse Pract.* 2:35, 1976.

Tong, T. G.: Poisoning and it's treatment. II. Treatment of poisoning and toxic overdose. *Nurse Pract.* 2:29, 1977.

Traver, G.: Symposium on care in respiratory disease. *Nurs. Clin. North Am.* 9:97, 1974.

Tysinger, D. S.: Oxygen (Part I). *Respir. Ther.* 7:74 (May–June), 1977.

Tysinger, D. S.: Oxygen (Part II). *Respir. Ther.* 7:50 (July–August), 1977.

Williams, M. H.: Symposium on Pulmonary Disease. *Med. Clin. North Am.* 61:1163, 1977.

Wilson, R. F., Murray, C., and Antonenko, D. R.: Nonpenetrating thoracic injuries. *Surg. Clin. North Am.* 57:17, 1977.

Wood, R. E., Boar, T. F., and Doersuk, C. F.: Cystic fibrosis. *Am. Rev. Respir. Dis.* 113:833, 1976.

Ziskind, M. M.: The acute bacterial pneumonias in the adult. *Basics RD,* 3:1, 1974.

CHAPTER 37

GLOSSARY

acidosis. A disturbance in the body's acid-base balance where acids accumulate and an excessive loss of bicarbonate occurs; this condition can be the result of retention of carbon dioxide as in the case of decreased respiration.

anoxia. Deficiency of oxygen; may be due to reduced oxygen supply, respiratory obstruction, inadequate respiratory movements, cardiac failure, shock, or conditions that result in reduced circulation of blood.

aspiration. The drawing into the throat or lungs of a foreign body on inspiration.

bolus. A mass of food that has been masticated and is ready to be swallowed.

costochondral separation. The separation of a rib and its cartilage.

cricothyrotomy. A division of the thyroid and cricoid cartilage.

defibrillation. Stopping rapid and ineffectual contractions (fibrillation) of the heart by using

EMERGENCY MEASURES IN RESPIRATORY OBSTRUCTION AND ARREST

Arlyne B. Saperstein, M.N., R.N., and
Margaret A. Frazier, M.S., R.N.

physical means (such as electrical countershocks) or drugs.

dysrhythmia. An abnormal or disturbed cardiac rhythm.

insufflation. To blow a vapor (such as air) into a cavity (as the lungs).

intubation. The insertion of a tube through the glottis into the larynx.

laryngoscopy. The examination of the interior of the larynx.

When any interference with respirations occurs, a life-threatening situation is present. The most crucial factor involved here is time, since the brain becomes irreversibly damaged after only 4–6 minutes without oxygen. In some cases, damage may occur very rapidly, especially in clients with cardiovascular disease. However, infants often survive longer periods of anoxia without permanent damage. One explanation for this is that at birth roughly 75 percent of the circulating hemoglobin is of the fetal type, and fetal hemoglobin binds more oxygen at a given plasma pO_2 than adult hemoglobin.[1] (Fetal hemoglobin is gradually replaced by adult hemoglobin.) Therefore, under conditions of relative anoxia, there will be a higher proportion of fully oxygenated hemoglobin in an infant than in an adult. This bound oxygen becomes available to the cells as it is released from the hemoglobin. Drowning and hypothermia victims are also less likely to suffer the ill effects of anoxia due to the decrease in their body temperature and thus a diminished metabolic need for oxygen.[2]

Many victims of heart attacks or accidents, such as choking, drowning, suffocation, drug intoxication, electrocution, and automobile and industrial accidents, might be saved if immediate and properly applied emergency care were instituted. Over 350,000 deaths occur annually from "heart attacks" before the victim is transported to a hospital. If the victims had received proper care immediately (i.e., within 2 minutes of the onset of symptoms), many might have survived.[3] It seems quite probable that many deaths each year are preventable if a victim is entered promptly into an organized and effective system of appropriate emergency treatment.[4]

This chapter focuses on measures utilized in specific types of respiratory emergencies: the person who is choking and the victim of a respiratory and cardiac arrest.

RESPIRATORY OBSTRUCTION

The American Heart Association made the following statement concerning respiratory obstruction:

Foreign body obstruction of the airway accounted for 3100 deaths in 1975 according to the National Safety Council .... Any structure forming the airway can either itself block the airway or become blocked by a foreign body. The tongue blocking the airway is the most common cause of airway obstruction, because the tongue is attached to the jaws. Any condition that leads to unconsciousness or loss of tone in the muscles of the jaw can cause the tongue to fall towards the back of the pharynx and obstruct the airway. Other causes include foreign body obstruction, trauma, swelling of the tissues of the airway (infections, burns, gas and smoke inhalation, and anaphylactic reaction), bilateral vocal cord paralysis, strangulation, and drowning.[5]

Café Coronary

Partial or complete obstruction of the trachea by a food bolus is one of the most common causes of respiratory emergency. The term *café coronary* has been coined to indicate a choking emergency, since it is most often associated with dining and is frequently seen in restaurants. In many cases, the condition has been confused with a cardiac problem; in others, the victim simply ceases to talk while eating, therefore attracting little attention until he collapses; or the victim may look frightened, grab for his throat, and try to indicate that he cannot breathe. In addition, his eyes may bulge and his face may become cyanotic. In all cases, a victim of a café coronary is unable to speak, a symptom which differentiates him from cardiac victims.

It is possible for anyone to choke; however, predisposing factors are inebriation, excitement, gorging while talking, and dentures,[6] especially those that fit poorly. The difficulty may also occur when several teeth are missing and food is, therefore, not chewed properly.[7] A pattern of repeated episodes of choking in adults may be due to heavy drinking, chronic disease, and certain nervous system disorders, as well as tracheoesophageal fistulas in children.[8] According to the American Heart Association:

Foreign bodies may cause either partial airway obstruction or complete airway obstruction. With partial airway obstruction, the victim may be capable of either "good air exchange" or "poor air exchange." With good air exchange, the victim can cough forcefully, although frequently there is wheezing between the coughs. As long as good air exchange continues, the victim should be allowed and encouraged to persist with spontaneous coughing and breathing efforts. At this point, *the rescuer should not interfere with the victim's attempts to expel the foreign body.*

Poor air exchange may occur initially, or good air exchange may progress to poor air exchange, as indicated by a weak, ineffective cough, high-pitched noises while inhaling (such as crowing noises), increased respiratory difficulty, and possibly cyanosis (bluish color of skin, fingernail beds, and inside mouth). At this point the partial obstruction should be managed as though it were a complete airway obstruction.[9]

Heimlich Maneuver

A remarkably simple, yet very effective technique for alleviation of respiratory obstructions, especially those caused by food or foreign bodies, was described by Dr. Henry J. Heimlich in the 1970s.[10] This method which is now called the *Heimlich maneuver*, is particularly useful in cases of cafe coronary because it can be done by anyone (professional or lay) who is familiar with the procedure.

While the standing victim leans forward, encircle his waist from behind, placing one fist below the rib cage and above the umbilicus. With the other hand grasp the fist and in a smooth movement push inward and upward sharply against the diaphragm (Fig. 37-1A). This is also referred to as an abdominal thrust. If the victim is seated, encircle the chair back as well as the victim when doing the procedure. If necessary, repeat the thrusts several times.[8] The usual result of this action is the expulsion of the foreign object from the trachea as a result of the pressure that is created in lungs by pushing up on the diaphragm (Fig. 37-1B). Cases have been reported of clients successfully performing this maneuver on themselves while leaning over a chairback and compressing their diaphragm with their fists.

In the case of an unconscious victim or one who is unable to stand, straddle the hips of the victim while he is in supine position. The heel of one hand is placed above the umbilicus, below the rib cage. The other hand is placed on top of the first (Fig. 37-1C). Quick upward thrusts are used as described above.[11] Chest thrusts can be used alternatively in victims with extremely large abdominal girth. The position of the rescuer is the same as that used in the Heimlich maneuver with the exception of arm and hand placement. The rescuer's arms are held under the axillae thus encircling the chest. Pressure of the hand and fist is placed on the sternum rather than below it. The mouth should then be checked and cleared of any material expelled by the procedure. If vomiting occurs, the victim should be turned to the side with his face down to prevent aspiration of the vomitus.[10] After successful completion of this maneuver, mouth-to-mouth resuscitation should be initiated if respirations have ceased.

Other Procedures

In the event that the Heimlich maneuver fails to dislodge the material obstructing the trachea, other methods should be attempted. Sharp blows to the area of the back between the scapulae, applied in an upward direction while the victim is in prone position with the head lower than the chest, may prove to be effective.[11] Infants and children may be placed in a similar position across the arm or knee or held upside down while blows (gentler than with an adult) are applied.[11]

If the obstruction can be seen at the back of the throat, try sweeping the mouth with the index finger to remove it. However, some authorities feel that this can be dangerous in that the bolus may be pushed further down, causing a partial obstruction to become complete.[11]

Other controversial techniques for the removal of an obstruction are devices that are inserted directly into the pharynx to extract the foreign body. For example, the ChokeSaver, a pair of plastic forceps, grasps and extracts the bolus from the throat.

However, this device could be dangerous in the hands of an unskilled person, particularly since tissue rupture is a very real possibility. The second device is the Throat-E-Vac, a pumplike apparatus with three mouthpieces (designed to fit infants, children, and adults) and a nose clip (for pinching the nostrils) attached to it. When pumped, it creates a suction effect which literally pulls the obstruction out of the throat. However, not only is it often difficult to get a tight seal when this is inserted in the mouth but also to keep the nostrils clamped while using the pump. In addition, unless the rescuer knows how to use this device it can be complex or confusing, and valuable time would be wasted in learning the application and implementation.

Some procedures that can be utilized to remove obstructions can be done *only* by qualified persons. They may attempt to remove the foreign body through direct laryngoscopy by using forceps and intubation;[11] a cricothyrotomy or tracheostomy may be performed to create an artificial airway in an emergency.[11]

CARDIOPULMONARY ARREST

Lungs

When confronted by a person whose respirations (and possibly heartbeats) have ceased, it is important to remain calm and organized. It must be remembered that the main goal of all interventions is to keep the brain oxygenated. Therefore, working with precisionlike timing and accuracy is essential.[12] There is absolutely no time to waste on frivolous gestures, such as taking a radial pulse for 30 to 60 seconds, looking for a stethoscope or a sphygmomanometer, or reassuring others who may be present not to worry. The presence of another person can be an asset. If knowledgeable in cardiopulmonary resuscitation (CPR) techniques, he can participate as an assistant; if not, he can be sent to obtain help. If the rescuer is alone, it is advisable to shout for help, or if in a hospital setting, to turn on the call signal. However, the victim should never be left unattended in order to seek help.

VENTILATION

The steps to be followed in the initiation of cardiopulmonary resuscitation vary according to

THE HEIMLICH MANEUVER

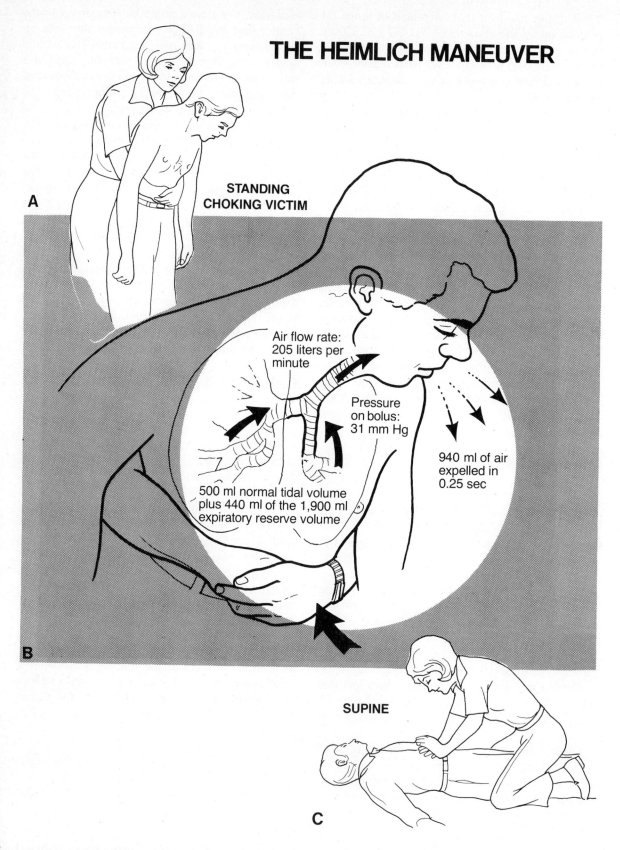

A

**STANDING
CHOKING VICTIM**

Air flow rate:
205 liters per
minute

Pressure
on bolus:
31 mm Hg

940 ml of air
expelled in
0.25 sec

500 ml normal tidal volume
plus 440 ml of the 1,900 ml
expiratory reserve volume

B

SUPINE

C

whether or not the victim's collapse was witnessed, his age, size, and condition. In any case, after noting the time, always determine first if a respiratory arrest has in fact occurred. Shake the victim's shoulder and call out, "Are you all right?" A person who has merely fainted may respond to these actions.[13] If there is no immediate response, observe the chest and upper abdomen for respiratory movement, and place an ear directly above the mouth and nose, listening and feeling for the exchange of air. This is most readily done with the victim in a supine position, although there are instances when this is not possible, such as the unconscious victim who is trapped behind the wheel of an automobile. If breathing does not appear to be present, turn their head to the side and remove any foreign material that is readily seen from the mouth. Use a crooked finger and sweep from the side and back of the mouth forward. If the tongue has fallen back, pull it forward while clearing the mouth. Do *not* worry at this point about any possible lower tract obstructions that cannot be visualized. Immediately hyperextend the head by tilting it back with one hand, supporting the back of the neck with the other (Fig. 37-2).[12] This maneuver will open the airway. In many cases where respirations have ceased, this action alone is enough to stimulate the restitution of breathing.[12] It is important to remember that in cases of suspected neck or cervical spine injury (such as in an automobile accident), the thrusting forward of the jaw without hyperextension of the head* is indicated, as the more exaggerated position can further complicate the already present condition.[15] Also, in infants, the

*The American Heart Association recommends that jaw thrust be done by "grasping the angles of the victim's lower jaw and lifting with both hands, one on each side displacing the mandible forward while tilting the head backwards. The rescuer's elbows should rest on the surface on which the victim is lying."[14]

head is not tilted as far back as the adult's, since this often closes the soft, flexible immature airway rather than opens it.[16]

If breathing has not spontaneously begun when the airway is opened, artificial ventilation is then instituted.[16] There are several acceptable methods for performing this procedure: mouth-to-mouth breathing; mouth-to-nose breathing; mouth-to-mouth-and-nose breathing (done with infants and small children); mouth-to-tracheostomy (or stoma) breathing; and in certain situations, the use of supplementary devices such as airways or a self-inflating bag-mask (AMBU bag). Mouth-to-mouth breathing is the most frequent method of choice. If dentures are present and appear to fit properly, they should not be removed as they maintain the shape and rigidity of the victim's mouth.[17] If the victim's mouth is injured, cannot be opened, or a tight seal cannot be easily applied (e.g., the victim who is wearing *poorly* fitting dentures), mouth-to-nose breathing is used.[16] In persons with a temporary tracheostomy or a permanent stoma (due to laryngectomy), ventilations must be given directly into the tracheostomy tube or stoma. In these cases, the head tilt and jaw thrust are unnecessary.[16] In each of the methods listed above, the expired air of the rescuer contains sufficient oxygen to keep the victim's brain oxygenated. (There is 16.3 percent oxygen and 4.0 percent carbon dioxide in expired air).[18]

To initiate mouth-to-mouth ventilation, keep one hand behind the victim's neck to keep the head hyperextended and the airway patent. With the other hand, pinch the nostrils together. After taking a deep breath, cover the victim's entire mouth with yours, creating a tight seal, and blow into the mouth (Fig. 37-3). Allow the victim to exhale *partially* by lifting your mouth between breaths and turning your head so that your ear is directly above the

FIGURE 37-1. A, The Heimlich maneuver with standing choking victim. B, In studies of conscious, healthy adult volunteers, the maneuver produced an average air-flow rate of 205 L/min and a pressure of 31 mm Hg. This is sufficient to explain the clinical observation that a bolus even partially obstructing the airway is ejected with some force by the procedure. The test was done at midpoint of tidal expiration with less than the 500 ml normal tidal volume present in the lungs. Yet an average volume of 940 ml of air was expelled in about a quarter of a second, which meant that additional air was being obtained from the expiratory reserve volume of 1,900 ml. The food-choking victim is in a normal tidal respiration phase when the bolus lodges and is not likely to be swallowing food at the end of a maximum respiration, so the respiratory reserve volume is the key. C, Application of the Heimlich maneuver with victim in supine position. (Adapted with permission from *Patient Care*, March 15, 1976. Copyright © 1976, Miller and Fink Corp., Darien, Conn. All rights reserved.)

Emergency Measures in Respiratory Obstruction and Arrest

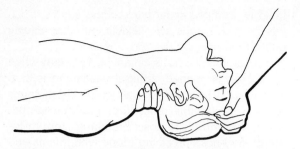

AIRWAY — HYPEREXTENSION OF THE HEAD

FIGURE 37-2. Head tilt method of opening airway. (Adapted by permission of the American Heart Association, Inc. Standards for Cardiopulmonary Resuscitation (CPR) and Emergency Cardiac Care (ECC). JAMA (Suppl.) 227(7):843, 1974.)

mouth. This position will enable the rescuer to observe the chest fall during expiration and both listen and feel for an air return. Repeat the process until four quick and full breaths have been administered,[16] being alert for any resistance felt while attempting to inflate the lungs. For aesthetic reasons, the rescuer may use a single thickness of handkerchief or cloth between the victim's mouth and his own, especially in cases where communicable disease of the victim is suspected or when vomiting has occurred.

The American Heart Association's *Manual for In-*

BREATHING

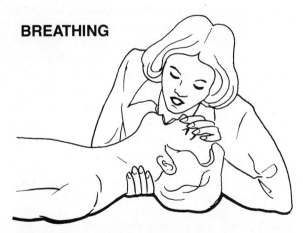

FIGURE 37-3. Mouth-to-mouth resuscitation. (Adapted by permission of the American Heart Association, Inc. Standards for Cardiopulmonary Resuscitation (CPR) and Emergency Cardiac Care (ECC). JAMA (Suppl.) 227(7):844, 1974.)

structors points out that a rescuer who wears dentures may have some difficulty with their dentures coming loose. It suggests that this problem often can be minimized by learning to make very light mouth-to-mouth contact, thus not putting pressure on the dentures which would loosen them.[19]

In the mouth-to-nose method, the victim's mouth is closed tightly with one hand on the lower jaw while the other hand tilts the head back. Air is blown into the nostrils, rather than the mouth, and exhalation is allowed to take place by opening the victim's mouth between breaths.[16]

In the mouth-to-mouth-and-nose method, cover the infant's entire mouth and nose with your mouth, creating a tight seal, and administer four quick and shallow puffs of air, again breaking the seal between breaths. Naturally, in infants and smaller children, the amount of air needed to inflate the lungs is much less than that needed to inflate an adult's. In addition, too great a volume of air used for insufflation can result in the rupturing of an infant's lungs.

The mouth-to-tracheostomy or stoma method requires breathing into the tracheostomy tube (after removal of the inner cannula) or stoma opening in the neck while the nostrils and mouth are sealed with your hands. The seal is then broken between breaths to allow for exhalation.

According to the American Heart Association, "Individual ventilation should be limited to that required to see the chest rise. In most adults, this is usually a minimum volume of 800 [ml of air] and adequate ventilation does not need to exceed 1200 [ml]. Below 800 [ml] ventilation is probably inadequate."[20]

OBSTRUCTIONS

If, when attempting to inflate the lungs, the chest fails to rise and fall or resistance is felt, make certain that the procedure was done properly with correct positioning of the victim, placement of the mouth creating a tight seal, and inflations of sufficient force or depth. If this has been done adequately, and the chest still fails to rise, then the possibility of an obstruction in the trachea is present. A series of four sharp blows given rapidly directly over the spine and between the scapulae should be attempted first, using the heel of the hand. These can be administered with the victim in a standing, sitting, or supine position.[21] Then attempt the Heimlich maneuver or chest thrusts. This can be done with the victim in the supine position by straddling the victim or kneeling at his side, and pushing on the diaphragm up to four times as discussed earlier. The combination of back blows and manual thrusts appears to be the most effective method of clearing upper airway obstruction, rather than the isolated use of one technique, according to the American Heart Association.[22] Hyperextend the head after removing from the mouth or upper airway any foreign objects which may have been expelled from the trachea and repeat the four ventilations. If this does not succeed, turn the victim on his side and deliver a few sharp blows between the scapulae with the heel of the hand. With two fingers, check the mouth and upper airway for foreign material as before.[15] Return the victim to supine position with the head hyperextended, and attempt the four ventilations once again. (With complete airway obstruction in infants or small children, hold them upside down or turned over your arm, and give gentle blows between the scapulae. Gravity will assist the dislodging of a foreign body in these cases. Clear the mouth, and proceed again with the ventilations).[15]

In cases where none of these interventions succeed, continue with ventilations anyway, as some air may pass around the obstruction and enter the lungs. Do not stop ventilations! In these instances, a qualified person may perform a laryngoscopy and endotracheal intubation to remove the object; an emergency cricothyrotomy or tracheostomy is usually performed if all else has failed.[15] The incision is made below the level of the obstruction, and ventilations are then done through this opening. Tracheostomy is a last resort and should only be attempted by a person skilled in this procedure.

EVALUATION OF VICTIM'S STATUS

Following the administration of the four ventilations, check the victim for spontaneous breathing. If this occurs, give no further respiratory assistance. If not, check for a carotid pulse by locating the victim's larynx, sliding the fingers laterally into the groove between the trachea and the sternocleidomastoid muscle at the side of the neck.[15] Locate the femoral pulse (groin) in the case of neck injuries, lacerations, or burns. An apical pulse can be taken if a stethoscope is directly at hand; do not interrupt the procedure to get one. In infants, a carotid pulse may be obtained by turning the head to the side, exposing the pulse on the short, flabby neck; however, this may be difficult to locate. The femoral pulse is a suitable alternative, or an apical pulse often can be felt by placing a hand directly against the precordium (chest wall).[23] It should be noted that although respirations have ceased, the heart can continue to contract for a number of minutes. This continues until the level of oxygen in the blood is reduced to the point at which cardiac depression, and thus cardiac arrest, follow.[24]

If the arrest was unwitnessed, the pupils of the eyes can be checked at this point, although many authorities believe this is to be unnecessary. The circular muscle fibers of the iris are innervated by a portion of the third cranial nerve, the oculomotor. Normally, these muscle fibers contract to constrict the pupil of the eye when the retina is brightly illuminated. When anoxia causes this reflex to dysfunction, the pupil no longer constricts in response to retinal illumination. Dilation of the pupils can be used as an indication of the approximate amount of time the victim's brain has gone without oxygen. The pupils begin to dilate shortly after anoxia occurs (in approximately 45 seconds); at approximately 1–2 minutes, they are fully dilated; after 4–6 minutes, they become fixed and nonreactive to light. The failure of the pupils to react to light usually indicates that brain damage is about to or already has occurred,[25] although in the cases of the elderly[25] or persons having taken certain drugs,[26] the dilation and light reaction may be altered or deceiving (Fig. 37-4). Noting the status of pupillary response can later be a useful piece of data for the physician and the family of the victim in planning long-term care or in making the decision to withdraw life-supporting measures. This is especially true in cases where, according to pupil dilation and fixation, it is known that interventions were not instituted until after the brain damage had already occurred. When the arrest is witnessed, the pupils do not have to be checked at this time as the length of time from the arrest to the beginning of cardiopulmonary resuscitative measures can be established.

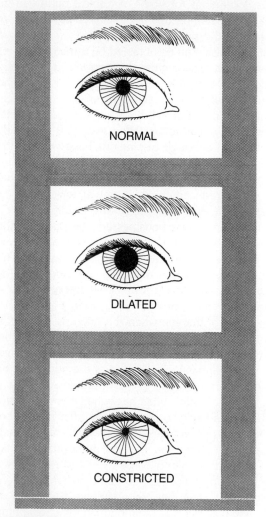

FIGURE 37-4. Pupilary response to light.

NORMAL

DILATED

CONSTRICTED

Heart

COMPRESSION

The next step in CPR is the initiation of external cardiac compressions. At this time the victim *must* be placed in supine position if this has not been done previously. This position is necessary for chest compressions to squeeze the heart between the sternum and the spine enough to force blood from the left ventricle into the circulatory system.[27] The horizontal position is also necessary in the performance of external cardiac compressions since there is no blood flow to the brain during a cardiac arrest

when the body is vertical, even when compressions are performed properly.[23] The victim should be on a very firm surface, such as the ground or floor. If the victim is in bed, then a hard board (cardiac board), or even a tray, can be placed under the back. If none is immediately available and the victim cannot be moved easily to the floor, begin compressions anyway, as no delay in the procedure should take place.[23]

With the adult victim in bed, CPR can be given while the rescuer stands at the bedside or kneels on the bed.[28] Many persons find that the latter position, (i.e., kneeling close to the side of the victim with the knees apart) facilitates the administration of cardiac compressions. Naturally, if the victim is on the floor, kneeling is the only plausible position. The heel of one hand is placed along the lower half of the sternum, approximately 1–1½ inches above the xiphoid process. The heel of the other hand is placed over the first hand, increasing the amount of pressure which can be applied. The arms must be kept straight with the shoulders above the victim's sternum[23] so as to apply 80–120 pounds of pressure vertically downward on the chest. By depressing the sternum 1½–2 inches,[23] enough pressure is placed on the heart to maintain a systolic pressure of 90–100 mm Hg.[29] Compression time should equal release (relaxation) time.[23] During the relaxation phase after each compression, the hands should not leave the sternum.[23] This eliminates the possibility of uneven, jerking movements and returning of the hands to an incorrect position. If pressure were to be applied to the xiphoid process, it could very well be fractured, increasing the likelihood of lacerating the liver, thereby causing internal hemorrhage. The possibility of causing fractured ribs (which might puncture a lung) or costochondral separation increases if pressure is applied to the rib cage.[28] To avoid this, interlock[23] or keep the fingers in an upward position during each compression. If compressions are done smoothly and accurately as described above, injuries to the victim will be minimal and fatigue in the rescuer reduced.[28]

When working alone, compress and release the adult victim's sternum 15 times and quickly inflate the lungs twice at the end of each cycle of 15 (Fig. 37-5A). Allow the lungs to deflate partially between breaths by breaking the seal and lifting your mouth. The two inflations should take not more than 5–6 seconds.[25] Compressions should equal 80/minute,[25] and respirations, 10–12/minute. When working with a partner, deliver compressions at a rate of 60/minute,[23] and ventilations, 8–12/minute. At the end of every fifth compression the partner delivers one ventilation (Fig. 37-5B). The pause between compressions is not lengthened; the partner doing the breathing must have perfect timing and be prepared to deliver the lung inflation in between compressions.[23] This is best achieved by having each partner on opposite sides of the victim and having the person doing compressions count aloud as he depresses the sternum. Saying, "One and two and three and four and five and one and two," *at one second intervals* facilitates inflating the victim's lungs precisely when the "and" between five and one is stated. This is known as a mnemonic. (Any other mnemonic, such as "one-one thousand, two-one thousand, three-one thousand . . .," accomplishes the same purpose.[30] If one partner becomes fatigued then the roles can be switched. An effective method of signaling the desire to reverse

roles is to have the partner doing compressions (who usually tires first) state, "Next time switch on three," instead of the one through five count. Note that this statement has five words. Each word can be said in time with a compression and the steady beat and cycle of five is not lost. The switch is then accomplished by having the partner who has done the ventilations give one final inflation. He then moves into position to take over compressions. The other partner compresses the chest twice, removes his hands and prepares to do the next inflation after the fifth compression. The new "compressor" smoothly places his hands on the sternum and completes the remaining three compressions of the cycle without missing a beat.

With small children, the administration of CPR is somewhat modified. Rather than two handed compressions, one hand is placed under the back for firm support while the heel of the other hand is placed on the *midsternum*.[25] This placement is used since the ventricles of the heart are higher in the chest, and a portion of the liver is located di-

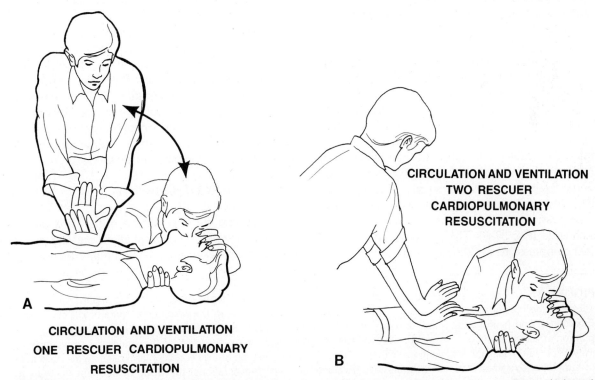

A CIRCULATION AND VENTILATION ONE RESCUER CARDIOPULMONARY RESUSCITATION

CIRCULATION AND VENTILATION TWO RESCUER CARDIOPULMONARY RESUSCITATION

B

FIGURE 37-5. A, 15 chest compressions to 2 lung inflations. B, 5 chest compressions to 1 lung inflation. (Adapted by permission of the American Heart Association, Inc. Standards for Cardiopulmonary Resuscitation (CPR) and Emergency Cardiac Care (ECC). JAMA (Suppl.) 227(7):846, 1974.)

Emergency Measures in Respiratory Obstruction and Arrest **739**

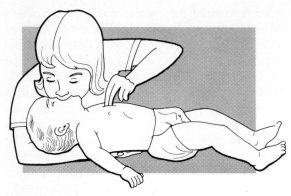

FIGURE 37-6. Cardiopulmonary resuscitation of an infant. Note, one hand is placed under the back, and the tips of the middle and index fingers of the other hand are used to compress the midsternum, approximately 100 times per minute.

rectly beneath the lower sternum and xiphoid process.[25] The chest is compressed ¾–1½ inches, depending upon the size of the child, at a rate of 80–100/minute.[25] One ventilation is given after every five compressions resulting in a ratio of 80 compressions to 16 ventilations or 100 compressions to 20 ventilations. Since mouth-to-mouth-and-nose technique is used and the head is not hyperextended, the placement of both hands does not have to be interrupted during the procedure.

When the victim is an infant, one hand is placed under the back and the tips of the middle and index fingers of the other hand are used to compress the midsternum ½–¾ inches,[25] approximately 100 times per minute. An alternate method is to compress the midsternum with both thumbs while the hands encircle the chest.[25] This gives firm support under the back as well. One small puff of air should be used to inflate the lungs after every five compressions, using mouth-to-mouth-and-nose technique (Fig. 37-6). This will produce a ratio of 100 compressions to 20 ventilations.

In both infants and small children, the procedure is done by one rescuer as it is not as tiring as with the adult, and considering the small size of the victim, a partner would most likely impede the progress of the procedure.

DISTENSION OF THE STOMACH

A problem which frequently arises while doing CPR on infants and children is the distension of the stomach. The causes of distension are airway obstructions, too much air pressure used for lung inflations, and the lack of hyperextension of the head, allowing some air to enter the esophagus and the trachea. If distension is minimal, it can be ignored.[15] However, if it becomes marked, the danger of regurgitation and gastric rupture results. Also, distension elevates the diaphragm, reducing the volume of the lungs and making the CPR procedure less effective.[15] Further, this distension increases vagal tone which, in turn, can lead to reflex bradycardia and hypotension.[31] To relieve gastric distension, the victim's head can be turned to the side and firm, yet gentle, pressure applied over the epigastric area with one hand.[15] There is a strong possibility that regurgitation will occur at this time, thus the American Heart Association is discouraging use of this procedure except where suction equipment is readily available. In those cases, check the mouth and upper airway before reinstituting CPR to minimize the possibility of aspiration of vomitus. This problem also occurs in adults, although not as frequently as in the younger victim and the same recommendations and constraints hold true.

EVALUATION OF CPR

To determine the effectiveness of the CPR procedure, the carotid pulse, respirations and the pupils should be checked after 1 minute and then every

---

FIGURE 37-7. The steps of assessment, diagnosis, immediate (or short-term) objectives, interventions, and evaluation can be readily seen in the use of CPR. Assessments are made as to the respiratory (breathing), circulatory (heartbeat), and neurological (pupil dilation) status of the victim. From that, the diagnosis of respiratory and cardiopulmonary arrest can be determined. The objectives (goals) will be oxygenation of the brain and prevention of irreversible brain damage. Interventions (CPR) are aimed at alleviating the anoxic condition and meeting the objectives of supplying oxygenated blood to brain cells. Evaluations (and re-evaluations) are done at frequent intervals to determine the effectiveness of the procedure. (Adapted with permission of the American Heart Association: Standards for cardiopulmonary resuscitation (CPR) and emergency cardiac care (ECC). *J. Am. Med. Assoc. (Suppl.)* 227(7):842, 1974.

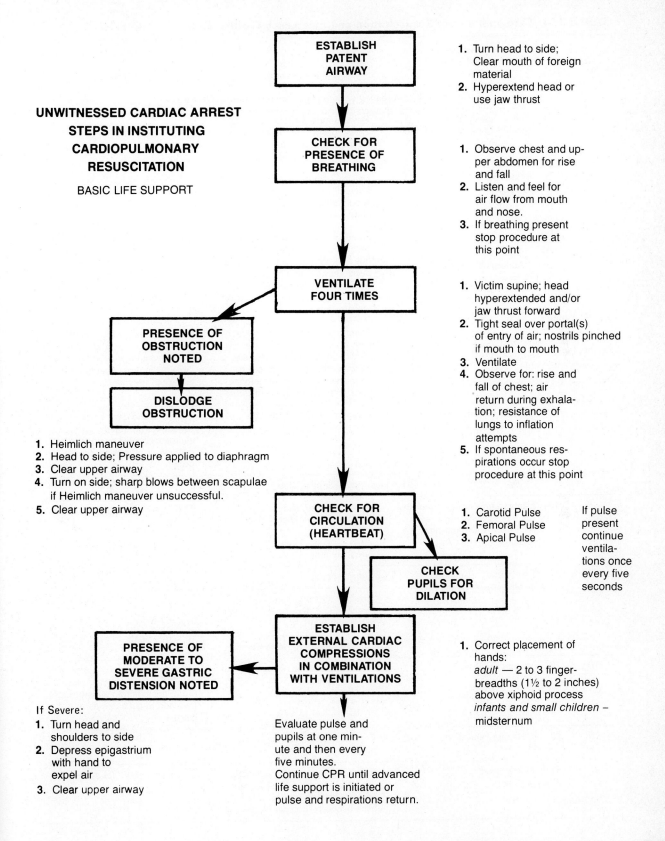

UNWITNESSED CARDIAC ARREST
STEPS IN INSTITUTING
CARDIOPULMONARY
RESUSCITATION

BASIC LIFE SUPPORT

ESTABLISH PATENT AIRWAY

1. Turn head to side; Clear mouth of foreign material
2. Hyperextend head or use jaw thrust

CHECK FOR PRESENCE OF BREATHING

1. Observe chest and upper abdomen for rise and fall
2. Listen and feel for air flow from mouth and nose.
3. If breathing present stop procedure at this point

VENTILATE FOUR TIMES

1. Victim supine; head hyperextended and/or jaw thrust forward
2. Tight seal over portal(s) of entry of air; nostrils pinched if mouth to mouth
3. Ventilate
4. Observe for: rise and fall of chest; air return during exhalation; resistance of lungs to inflation attempts
5. If spontaneous respirations occur stop procedure at this point

PRESENCE OF OBSTRUCTION NOTED

DISLODGE OBSTRUCTION

1. Heimlich maneuver
2. Head to side; Pressure applied to diaphragm
3. Clear upper airway
4. Turn on side; sharp blows between scapulae if Heimlich maneuver unsuccessful.
5. Clear upper airway

CHECK FOR CIRCULATION (HEARTBEAT)

1. Carotid Pulse
2. Femoral Pulse
3. Apical Pulse

If pulse present continue ventilations once every five seconds

CHECK PUPILS FOR DILATION

ESTABLISH EXTERNAL CARDIAC COMPRESSIONS IN COMBINATION WITH VENTILATIONS

1. Correct placement of hands:
   adult — 2 to 3 finger-breadths (1½ to 2 inches) above xiphoid process
   infants and small children – midsternum

PRESENCE OF MODERATE TO SEVERE GASTRIC DISTENSION NOTED

If Severe:
1. Turn head and shoulders to side
2. Depress epigastrium with hand to expel air
3. Clear upper airway

Evaluate pulse and pupils at one minute and then every five minutes. Continue CPR until advanced life support is initiated or pulse and respirations return.

TABLE 37-1. Cardiopulmonary Resuscitation and Emergency Cardiac Care and Rationale.

Elapsed Time (Seconds) Min.	Max.	Activity and Time (Seconds)	Critical Performance	Rationale
		A. Conscious Victim (Sitting or Standing); Complete Airway Obstruction		
2	3	Rescuer asks: "Can you speak?" Look, listen and feel for breathing (2–3 sec).	Rescuer must identify complete airway obstruction by asking victim if he is able to speak.	
5	8	4 Back blows (3–5 sec).	Deliver 4 sharp blows rapidly and forcefully to back between shoulder blades; support victim's chest with other hand.	Continually check for success.
9	13	4 Abdominal thrusts (4–5 sec).	Stand behind victim and wrap your arms around his waist. Grasp one fist with your other hand and place thumb side of your fist between breastbone and navel. Press fist into abdomen with quick upward thrusts.	The sequence of back blows and abdominal or chest thrusts may be more effective than either maneuver used alone.
		or		
		4 chest thrusts (4–5 sec).	Stand behind victim and place your arms under victim's armpits to encircle the chest. Grasp one fist with other hand and place thumb side of fist on breastbone. Press with quick backward thrusts.	Chest thrusts are more easily delivered than are abdominal thrusts when abdominal girth is large, as in gross obesity or in advanced pregnancy.
		Verbally indicate repeat of above sequence until effective.	Verbalize alternating above maneuvers in rapid sequence.	Time is of the essence: two techniques are rapidly repeated alternatively until obstruction is relieved or unconsciousness occurs.
		B. Unconscious Victim, Supine; Obstructed Airway		
4	10	Establish unresponsiveness and call out for help. Allow 4–10 sec if face down and turning is required.	Shake shoulder, shout, "Are you OK?" Call out, "Help!" Turn if necessary.	This initial call for help is to alert bystanders.
			Adequate time.	
7	15	Open airway. Establish breathlessness. Look, listen, and feel (3–5 sec).	Kneel properly.	
			Head tilt with one hand on forehead and neck lift or chin lift with other hand.	
			Ear over mouth, observe chest.	
10	20	Attempt to ventilate (3–5 sec).	Attempt ventilation. Airway remains obstructed.	Complete airway obstruction by a foreign body is assumed present, but at this point an attempt must be made to get some air into lungs.
13	25	Reattempt ventilation (3–5 sec).	Reposition head, airway remains obstructed.	
17	31	4 back blows (4–6 sec).	Roll victim toward you, using your thigh for support. Give 4 forceful and rapidly delivered blows to back between shoulder blades.	Continually check for success.

Elapsed Time (Seconds) Min.	Max.	Activity and Time (Seconds)	Critical Performance	Rationale
		4 Abdominal thrusts (5–6 sec).	Position yourself with your knees close to victim's hips. Place heel of one hand between lower breast bone and navel and second hand on top. Press into abdomen with quick upward thrusts.	Kneeling at victim's side gives the rescuer greater mobility and access to airway.
22	37	*or* 4 Chest thrusts (5–6 sec).	Same hand position as that for applying closed chest cardiac compression. Exert quick downward thrusts.	Chest thrusts are preferred in presence of large abdominal girth (advanced pregnancy and obesity). Downward thrusts generate effective airway pressures.
28	45	Check for foreign body using finger (6–8 sec).	Turn head to side, open mouth with jaw-lift technique and probe deeply into mouth along cheek with hooked finger.	A dislodged foreign body may now be manually accessible if it has not been expelled.
31	50	Attempt to ventilate (3–5 sec).	Reposition head. Airway remains obstructed.	By this time another attempt must be made to get some air into lungs.
		Verbally indicate repeat of above sequence until effective.	Verbalize, alternating above maneuvers in rapid sequence.	Persistent attempts are rapidly made in sequence to relieve obstruction.

C. For One and Two Rescuer CPR

4	10	Establish unresponsiveness and call out for help. Allow 4–10 sec if face down and turning is required.	Shake shoulder, shout, "Are you OK?" Call out, "Help!" Turn if necessary.	Frequently victim will be face down. Effective closed chest heart compression can only be provided with victim flat on back on hard surface.
			Adequate time.	Accurate diagnosis is important. 4–10 sec gives time to do that and to review mentally the sequence of CPR.
7	15	Open airway. Establish breathlessness. Look, listen, and feel (3–5 sec).	Kneel properly.	
			Head tilt with one hand on forehead and neck lift or chin lift with other hand.	Airway must be opened to establish breathlessness. Many victims may be making respiratory efforts that are ineffective because of obstruction.
			Ear over mouth, observe chest.	
10	20	4 Ventilations (3–5 sec).	Ventilate properly 4 times and observe chest rise.	
15	30	Establish pulse and simulate activation of EMS system (5–10 sec).	Fingers palpate for carotid pulse on near side (other hand on forehead maintains head tilt).	This activity should take 5–10 sec because not only does it take time to find right place, but pulse may be very slow or very weak and rapid.
			Know local EMS number.	
			Adequate time.	

TABLE 37-1. Continued

Elapsed Time (Seconds) Min.	Max.	Activity and Time (Seconds)	Critical Performance	Rationale
69	96	4 Cycles of 15 compressions 2 ventilations (54–66 sec).	Proper body position.	
			Landmark check each time.	
			Position of hands.	Precision in hand placement is essential to avoid serious injury.
			Vertical compression.	
			Says mnemonic.	Necessary to establish rhythm.
			Proper rate.	Should attempt to accomplish 60 compressions and 8 ventilations per minute.
			Proper ratio.	
			No bouncing.	
			Ventilates properly.	
72	101	Check for return of pulse and spontaneous breathing; pupil check optional (3–5 sec).	Check pulse and breathing; pupil check optional.	Pupil size helps to monitor changes in client.
80	111	Minimum of 2 cycles of 5 compressions and one ventilation (8–10 sec). Switch and repeat until examiner is satisfied.	Changes rate of compression.	
			Says mnemonic.	Necesary to establish rhythm.
			Interposes breath.	
			No pause for ventilation.	
			Calls for switch.	Signal for change must be clear.
			Switches.	
			Switches back.	
			Checks pulse (by ventilator).	
			(Pupil check—optional)	Pupil size helps to monitor changes in patient.
			Technique as above.	

D. Infant Resuscitation

3	5	Establish unresponsiveness and call out for help, including turning (3–5 sec).	Shake shoulder, shout, "Are you OK?" Call out, "Help!" Turn if necessary. Infant horizontal. Adequate time.	Diagnosis must be equally accurate in children and infants. With this emotionally charged situation, time must be taken to establish the diagnosis of cardiac arrest. Horizontal position aids effective circulation.
6	10	Open airway. Establish breathlessness (3–5 sec).	Tip head back. Do not hyperextend.	Hyperextention can collapse trachea.
			Put ear over mouth to feel for breathing.	
9	15	4 Ventilations (3–5 sec).	Use small breaths to ventilate.	

Elapsed Time (Seconds) Min.	Max.	Activity and Time (Seconds)	Critical Performance	Rationale
14	25	Establish pulse and simulate activation of EMS system (5–10 sec).	Fingers palpate for carotid or precordial pulse. Know local EMS number.	
44	55	8 Cycles of 5 compressions and 1 ventilation. Continue uninterrupted (30 sec).	Two fingers (midsternum) for compressions. 80 to 100 compressions/min.	Small children and infants need a more rapid cardiac compression rate (80 to 100/min) with breaths interposed every 5 compressions. Alternate technique is to encircle chest with hands, using both thumbs to compress.

Reprinted with permission of the American Heart Association: *A Manual for Instructors of Basic Cardiac Life Support.* Dallas, Sept. 1977.

4–5 minutes thereafter.[26] Constriction of the pupils upon exposure to light may indicate adequate flow of oxygenated blood to the brain.[25] Checking the pulse indicates effective circulation during compressions or the return of spontaneous beating of the heart.[26] At no time should the procedure be interrupted for longer than 5 seconds except when endotracheal intubation is being performed by a skilled person and then only a 15 second break should occur.[28] If the victim is to be transported to a more suitably equipped location, CPR should be maintained throughout the transport. Again a break of 15 seconds to maneuver staircases is a permissible reason for a slight lapse in the procedure.[28] CPR should be continued until the victim responds or until more advanced life supports can be instituted. According to the American Medical Association, advanced life support consists of the following elements:

1. Basic life support (Fig. 37-7).
2. Using adjunctive equipment and special techniques, such as endotracheal intubation and open chest internal cardiac compression.
3. Cardiac monitoring for dysrhythmia recognition and control.
4. Defibrillating.*

5. Establishing and maintaining an intravenous infusion lifeline.
6. Employing definitive therapy, including drug administration (a) to correct acidosis and (b) to aid in establishing and maintaining an effective cardiac rhythm and circulation.
7. Stabilization of the patient's condition.[33]

WARNING: The practice of CPR technique should be limited to manikins. Resuscitation and cardiac compressions performed on a person with normal respiratory and cardiac functioning can be hazardous to their well-being.

REFERENCES

1. Schmidt-Nielsen, K.: *Animal Physiology.* London, Cambridge University Press, 1975, p. 89.
2. Committee on Cardiopulmonary Resuscitation: *A Manual for Instructors of Basic Cardiac Life Support.* Dallas, American Heart Association, September 1977, p. 22.
3. *Ibid.* p. 23.
4. American Heart Association and National Academy of Sciences—National Research Council: Standards for cardiopulmonary resuscitation (CPR) and emergency cardiac care (ECC). *J. Am. Med. Assoc.* (Suppl.) 227(7):838, 1974.
5. *A Manual for Instructors, op. cit.,* p. 15.
6. Friberg, H. (ed.): Choking emergency "get a doctor quick! he's choking!" *Patient Care* March 15, p. 24, 1976.
7. Henderson, J.: *Medical Emergency Guide,* 3rd ed. New York, McGraw-Hill, 1973, p. 110.
8. Friberg, *op. cit.,* p. 28.
9. *A Manual for Instructors, op. cit.,* p. 16.

*According to the American Heart Association the most frequent cause of sudden death or cardiac arrest is ventricular fibrillation. CPR can keep the victim of ventricular fibrillation induced cardiac arrest alive but cannot convert the abnormal rhythm to a normal heartbeat unless defibrillation is utilized.[32]

10. Heimlich, H. J.: Death from choking prevented by a new life saving maneuver. *Heart and Lung* September/October, p. 755, 1976.
11. Friberg, *op. cit.*, p. 26.
12. American Heart Association Standards, *op. cit.*, p. 841.
13. Committee on Cardiopulmonary Resuscitation: *CPR in Basic Life Support.* New York, American Heart Association, 1974, p. 2.
14. *A Manual for Instructors, op. cit.*, p. 43.
15. American Heart Association Standards, *op. cit.*, p. 844.
16. *Ibid.*, p. 843.
17. Pribble, A. H., and Tyler, M. L.: Emergency! I. On-the-spot cardiopulmonary resuscitation. *Nurs. '75* 5:48, 1975.
18. Harmer, B., and Henderson, V.: *Textbook of the Principles and Practice of Nursing.* New York, Macmillan Co., 1960, p. 285.
19. *A Manual for Instructors, op. cit.*, p. 45.
20. *Ibid.*, p. 44.
21. *Ibid.*, p. 56.
22. *Ibid.*, p. 59.
23. American Heart Association Standards, *op. cit.*, p. 845.
24. *A Manual for Instructors, op. cit.*, p. 22.
25. American Heart Association Standards, *op. cit.*, p. 846.
26. *Ibid.*, p. 847.
27. Pribble and Tyler, *op. cit.*, p. 47.
28. American Heart Association Standards, *op. cit.*, p. 848.
29. Gordon, A. S., and American Heart Association: *Prescription for Life* (film). New York, Bandelier Films, distributed by American Heart Association, 1967.
30. *A Manual for Instructors, op. cit.*, p. 53.
31. Pribble and Tyler, *op. cit.*, p. 45.
32. *A Manual for Instructors, op. cit.*, p. 21.
33. American Heart Association Standards, *op. cit.*, p. 852.

BIBLIOGRAPHY

Committee on Cardiopulmonary Resuscitation: *Cardiopulmonary Resuscitation: A Manual for Instructors.* New York, American Heart Association, 1967.

Enarson, D. A., and Gracey, D. R.: Complications of cardiopulmonary resuscitation. *Heart and Lung* September/October, p. 805, 1976.

Taylor, G. J., et al: Importance of prolonged compression during cardiopulmonary resuscitation in man. *N. Eng. J. Med.* (June)30:1515, 1977.

CHAPTER 38

Food is composed of organic and inorganic substances called nutrients, which are essential to the maintenance of the human body. Nutrients provide energy, promote growth and development, maintain and repair tissues, and regulate the body's processes. There are six classifications of nutrients: carbohydrates, fats and lipids, proteins, vitamins, minerals, and water. While each nutrient fulfills a specific need in the human body, the nutrients cannot function independently of one another. Also, no two foods are alike in their nutrient makeup. Proper nutrition involves the complete and balanced intake of all nutrients to provide for good health.

NUTRIENTS

Carbohydrates

Carbohydrates (i.e., starches and sugars) provide the most economical energy source in human diets worldwide and comprise approximately 50 percent

BASIC PRINCIPLES OF NUTRITION

Dorothy C. Silver, M.Ed., R.D.

of the total caloric intake of the average American diet, the remainder being supplied by proteins and fats. Meeting the energy needs of the body takes priority over all other bodily functions. When a sufficient amount of carbohydrate is ingested, the body automatically employs it as its major energy source. Thus, carbohydrates have a regulatory effect on protein and fat metabolism which is termed *protein-sparing* or the allowance of the major portion of the protein to be used for tissue building (its major function) rather than energy.

Carbohydrates are broken down metabolically into *glucose* which enters the blood stream and becomes a major fuel source to the body and the only energy source for the central nervous system and the brain. The brain does not contain a reserve supply of glucose and is, therefore, dependent on a constant supply of glucose from the blood stream. Carbohydrates are indispensable for the functional integrity of nervous tissue.

Starches are carbohydrates that are stored as energy in plants, such as potatoes, yams, rice, wheat, corn, carrots, and cassava. The sugars in fruits or stems (sugar cane) are also a source of stored energy. Humans who eat these items store this energy in the form of *glycogen,* or animal starch, in the liver, and skeletal, cardiac, and smooth muscles. The glycogen, which can be mobilized more quickly than glucose, provides an emergency source of contractile energy for the muscles, including the heart.

Cellulose and *hemicellulose* are the structural components of plants. Cellulose is a carbohydrate found in fruits, vegetables, pulp, skin, stalks, and leaves, and the outer coverings of grains, nuts, and legumes. Although this material is primarily indigestible, it is extremely valuable in providing the roughage and bulk necessary for proper bowel function and for stimulation of peristaltic movement in the gastrointestinal tract.

Lactose, or milk sugar, promotes the growth of bacteria in the small intestine. Some of these bacteria are important in the synthesis of certain B-complex vitamins. Lactose also amplifies the absorption of calcium in the body. Milk and milk products are among the best sources of calcium. Milk is the only dietary source of lactose.

In addition to the functions already mentioned, the carbohydrates play another significant role. They provide flavor, color, texture, and variety to the meals in our diet.

Fats and Other Lipids

The term "lipid" is often used interchangeably with the term "fat" to indicate those chemical compounds grouped together because of their wide distribution in nature and their insolubility in water. Fats and oils are essential constituents of the body. They provide both the body's major storage source of energy and the transport system of the fat soluble vitamins. Lipids, including cholesterol and phospholipids, provide structural components to the body.

Fats that are fluid at room temperature are called oils; those that are solid at that temperature are called fats. Both fats and oils are composed of varying proportions of fatty acids and alcohol. The type and configuration of the fatty acids in each fat are responsible for the differences in flavor, texture, melting points, and absorption. *Saturated fatty acids* contain as many hydrogen atoms as the carbon chain can hold, whereas *unsaturated fatty acids* contain double bonds. A fatty acid having one double bond on the carbon chain is termed *monounsaturated.* Two or more double bonds on a fatty acid carbon chain is a *polyunsaturated* fat. The polyunsaturated fatty acids have been shown, in certain instances, to decrease blood cholesterol levels, while saturated fatty acids may actually raise serum cholesterol levels. Saturated fatty acids have higher melting points and tend to be solid at room temperature.

ESSENTIAL FATTY ACIDS

Certain polyunsaturated fatty acids, which are essential for human and animal health but cannot be synthesized in the body, must be supplied in the diet. The essential fatty acid, *linoleic acid,* occurs in high concentrations in edible vegetable oils, such as corn, cottonseed, safflower, peanut, and soybean. *Arachidonic acid,* another essential fatty acid, occurs in small quantities in animal fats; however, it can be manufactured by the animal from linoleic

acid. Therefore, linoleic acid *must* be present in a balanced diet. Symptoms of essential fatty acid deficiency include poor growth, dermatitis, poor reproductive performance, lowered caloric efficiency, decreased resistance to a number of stress conditions, and lipid transport impairment.

Essential fatty acids play an important role in the regulation of certain aspects of cholesterol metabolism and in the synthesis of hormonelike compounds. Diets that are high in essential fatty acids reduce hypercholesterolemia, or high serum cholesterol levels, in man.[1] However, it should be noted that the issue of cholesterol metabolism and regulation is one that is quite controversial.

LIPIDS

Lipids provide the most concentrated source of energy to the body. Like carbohydrates, lipids are composed of carbon, hydrogen, and oxygen, and in specialized lipids, phosphorus and nitrogen. However, fats and lipids have a smaller proportion of oxygen as well as various structures and formulas which produce more than twice the available calories than carbohydrates and proteins. Since fats go through more metabolic processes than carbohydrates and proteins in the production of energy, they are considered to be more of a storage form of energy. All tissues in the body, except those in the central nervous system, utilize fatty acids as a source of energy. Fats also provide a protein-sparing action, allowing the protein to be used for tissue synthesis.

Adipose tissue surrounds the vital organs of the body and protects them from physical injury. This subcutaneous layer of fat serves as an insulator and decreases loss of body heat during cold weather. Excessive amounts of subcutaneous fat, as seen in obesity, conserve heat during warm weather, contributing to increased discomfort.

Fats add to the palatability of food in the diet and contribute to a feeling of satiety because of the length of time it takes to leave the stomach. Fats and oils also have some value as a lubricant for the gastrointestinal tract.

PHOSPHOLIPIDS

All cells in the body contain phospholipids, with the highest concentrations found in the brain, liver, and nervous tissue. Phospholipids are emulsifying agents which have an affinity for water. They are essential in maintaining the structure of cells for the digestion and absorption of fats, and they assist in the uptake of fatty acids by the cells. Phospholipids comprise a proportion of the blood lipoproteins; however, their role in lipid transport is not clearly understood.

CHOLESTEROL

Cholesterol is found only in animal tissues and is an essential component of all cells in the body including structural membranes, brain, and nerve cells. Cholesterol may be synthesized in the liver to meet the body's needs regardless of the dietary intake. Cholesterol furnishes the nucleus for the synthesis of pro-vitamin D, the corticosteroids, sex hormones, and bile salts.

Oils, lard, butter, margarine, bacon, and salad dressing provide the most concentrated sources of fats in the diet. "Invisible" fats are those found in meat, fish, poultry, milk, cheese, eggs, and baked products.

Proteins

Proteins are complex compounds containing carbon, hydrogen, oxygen, and nitrogen. In addition to these elements, certain proteins may contain phosphorus, sulfur, iron, iodine, and cobalt. Protein is found in every cell in the body. The nature and function of protein in the cells of the various parts within a given living thing provide building materials of great diversity. Most protein is found in the muscle tissue, with the remainder in the soft tissue, bones, teeth, blood, and other body fluids.

Proteins are essential as structural components of the cells. They maintain cellular integrity by replacing worn out tissues lost by normal wear and tear of the body. Proteins supply building components for growth and development, thus the increased need for protein during pregnancy, lactation, infancy, and childhood.

Enzymes are proteins that monitor the digestion of food for energy and help in the synthesis of new compounds for the maintenance and repair of body tissues. When proteins are supplied in greater amounts than are needed by the body, the proteins contribute to the body's energy pool. Similarly, if carbohydrates and fats are not supplied in sufficient amounts to meet the body's energy requirements,

protein will be diverted from other functions to provide for these needs.

Proteins act as regulators of various functions of the body. Hormones are proteins. Proteins are necessary monitors of the body's osmotic balance. The protein in muscle not only allows for contractibility but allows the muscle to hold fluid which gives it firmness. Protein also regulates the acid-base balance in the body. Because proteins are buffers, too, they can act as acids or bases. Both the cellular and the blood proteins are part of the body's buffer system.

Antibodies are produced from protein. With adequate protein intake, antibodies help to assure the body's resistance against disease.

AMINO ACIDS

Proteins are made up of 22 (or more) nitrogen containing substances called amino acids. Amino acids make up some of the compounds essential in the vital processes of the body. Among these are digestive enzymes and those that function in the oxidation of cells. Some hormones, including insulin, epinephrine, and certain pituitary gland secretions, are also constructed from amino acids.

Constituent amino acids are important in determining the nutritive value of a protein. While certain amino acids are synthesized in the body as the need arises, others must be supplied by the diet; these are called *essential* amino acids. The *nonessential* amino acids are not necessarily those of lesser value but are those which may be synthesized from other related amino acids in the body or may be supplied by ingested food. There are eight essential amino acids that are necessary for proper growth and the maintenance of health (Table 38-1).

NITROGEN BALANCE

Nitrogen balance is the measurement of protein utilization—that is, the ratio between the anabolism and catabolism of protein substances. Most food and body proteins are approximately 16 percent nitrogen; therefore, analysis of nitrogen provides a measurable indicator of protein increases and decreases in the body.

A healthy well-nourished individual is in nitrogen equilibrium. Because normal tissue breakdown continually occurs in the body, repair and replace-

TABLE 38-1. Essential and Nonessential Amino Acids

Essential	Nonessential
Threonine	Alanine
Isoleucine	Aspartic acid
Leucine	Glycine
Valine	Proline
Lysine	Glutaric acid
Methionine	Hydroxyproline
Tryptophane	Cystine
Phenylalanine	Cysteine
	Tyrosine
	Serine
	Arginine*
	Histidine*

*These two amino acids are essential during the growth period.

ment is constantly taking place. During periods of major tissue building such as pregnancy, lactation, growth in the young, and convalescence from an illness, the body retains more nitrogen than it loses. These individuals are said to be in positive nitrogen balance. When tissue breakdown (catabolism) exceeds tissue building (anabolism), a negative nitrogen balance results. Inadequate dietary intake of protein or a diet providing an insufficient number of calories increases the amount of stored protein utilized to meet energy needs. However, introducing carbohydrates and fats to the diet can lower the amount of protein needed for energy. Because excessive breakdown of storage protein also occurs during systemic diseases, injuries, burns, or surgery, it is important to provide more dietary protein during these times to counterbalance the protein losses in the body.

The quality of protein in a food is classified by the content of essential amino acids. Foods that contain all eight essential amino acids in the appropriate amounts and proportions for the formation of tissues, enzymes, hormones, and maintenance of nitrogen equilibrium are said to be *complete proteins* (of high biological value). Animal protein foods, such as eggs, meat, fish, poultry, and milk, are considered complete proteins.

Foods that do not provide all the essential amino acids in sufficient quantities are termed *incomplete proteins* (of low biological value). Vegetable and grain proteins are incomplete, and therefore, biologically inferior. However, these food items are useful in reducing the amount of expensive animal proteins required to meet the body's protein needs. Breads, cereals, dried beans, peas, and peanut butter, when combined with small amounts of animal protein, can provide equally as good an assortment of amino acids as animal protein. Incomplete protein foods should be combined in the same meal with complete protein foods to increase their palatability and decrease meal cost.

ENERGY

The body requires energy for the utilization of ingested food, for physical activity, and for the maintenance of body temperature. Carbohydrates, fats, and proteins are the only nutrients that can furnish energy, but the energy releasing processes from the three nutrients requires the contributing activity of many vitamins, minerals, and other body substances.[2]

Energy is expended whenever an activity is executed by the body. The activity may be voluntary, such as walking, reading, or any other activity performed during daily living, or involuntary, such as circulation of blood, respiration, digestion, or the transportation of nutrients across cell walls.

Energy is a perpetual cycle. The ultimate source of energy for human beings is the sun. In the process of photosynthesis, with the union of water and carbon dioxide, plants transform the sun's energy into the storage forms found in man's food. Once in the body, food is digested, and stored energy is converted to glucose, the basic unit of energy. This then is oxidized making possible the liberation of energy. Water and carbon dioxide are the end products of this oxidation.

In nutrition, the unit of energy measurement is the calorie, (cal) or kilocalorie (kcal), which is the amount of heat required to raise the temperature of 1 kg of water 1°C. Caloric values have been determined for the major nutrients (carbohydrates, proteins, and fats) and the foods containing them. The average caloric value of a carbohydrate is 4 cal/g; proteins, 4 cal/g; fats, 9 cal/g; and alcohol, 7 cal/g. The amount of carbohydrate, protein, and fat in a food item determines its energy value.

Basal Metabolism

Basal metabolism is the minimum amount of energy needed by the body at rest, in the fasting state, to carry out life sustaining processes such as respiration, digestion, blood circulation, and maintenance of body temperature. Basal metabolic rates are measured in percentages above and below a set standard derived from the area of body surface of the individual. A variation of approximately 10 percent above or below this standard basal metabolic rate is considered normal.

Many factors influence individual metabolic rate. For example, during periods of growth, especially during the first and second years of life, and again during adolescence, the basal metabolic rate is high. As an individual matures and physical activity decreases, the basal metabolic rate slowly declines. The sex of an individual also influences the basal metabolic rate. In general, men at the same height, weight, and age as women tend to have a metabolic rate higher by 5 to 10 percent. Females, however, may show an increase in the basal metabolic rate during pregnancy and lactation. The greater the body surface area, the greater the amount of heat loss and, therefore, the greater the amount of heat produced. Athletes tend to have a higher basal metabolic rate, as muscle tissue requires more oxygen than adipose tissue. The secretions of the endocrine glands are the primary regulators of metabolic rate. Their hormonal variances may significantly increase or decrease the basal metabolic rate. The status of an individual's nutrition may also affect the basal metabolic rate. In a starvation state, or during periods of malnutrition, the metabolic rate may show decreases due to a reduction in the amount of active tissue.

BASAL ENERGY REQUIREMENTS

The energy requirements are the number of calories that are necessary to replace the daily metabolic loss from voluntary and involuntary activities, plus a small increment for the specific dynamic action of food. Meeting energy requirements takes priority over all other body needs.

The basal metabolic needs of the body represent about 50 to 70 percent of the total caloric needs. In addition, the type and amount of physical activity are important influences on the body's caloric needs. Since man is an active animal, calories must be supplied for daily life and health maintenance. Calculations may be based on sedentary, light, moderate, or heavy activity levels. Mental work

does not require a large caloric expenditure, but metabolic rate is influenced by stress and illness (physical and mental).

The body meets its caloric requirements by the ingestion of foods. A varied diet with fuel foods containing differing amounts of carbohydrates, proteins, and fats, as well as water, vitamins and minerals is essential to sustain life.

Vitamins

Vitamins are potent organic compounds other than carbohydrates, proteins, fats, and minerals. They are found in minute quantities in foods and are essential for specific functions within the cells and tissues of the body. Vitamins are needed for enzyme systems which facilitate the metabolism of amino acids, fats, and carbohydrates. Vitamins assist in the formation of bones and teeth and in the prevention of associated deficiency diseases that occur in their absence or improper absorption. Man cannot synthesize vitamins in adequate amounts; therefore, they must be supplied by the diet. Each vitamin has specific functions. They differ from each other in physiologic function, chemical structure, and in their distribution in food. They cannot substitute for one another. Many reactions in the body require the presence of several vitamins, and a lack of any one of them can interfere with the functions of the other.

Vitamins are classified into two groups on the basis of their solubility. The *fat-soluble vitamins* (A, D, E, and K), which are found in foods in association with lipids, are fairly stable in normal food preparation—that is, they are not lost in the cooking process. *Water-soluble vitamins* (B-complex and C), however, may be destroyed by overcooking and are easily dissolved in the cooking water.

Under normal conditions, a well-balanced diet, including foods from all the Basic Four Food Groups (Fig. 38-1), provides the necessary vitamins needed by the body. Vitamin deficiencies may occur if the total food intake is inadequate, if a particular food is constantly omitted, or if economic conditions are such that the purchase of foods for a well-balanced diet is restricted.

Vitamin supplements are not generally necessary for healthy individuals. Vitamin D supplements for infants, children, and pregnant or lactating women are the only exceptions, as the diet usually does

DAILY FOOD GUIDE
THE BASIC FOUR FOOD GROUPS

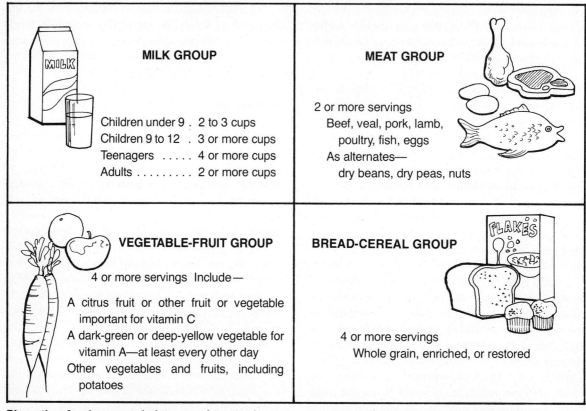

MILK GROUP

Children under 9 . 2 to 3 cups
Children 9 to 12 . 3 or more cups
Teenagers . . . . . 4 or more cups
Adults . . . . 2 or more cups

MEAT GROUP

2 or more servings
  Beef, veal, pork, lamb,
    poultry, fish, eggs
  As alternates—
    dry beans, dry peas, nuts

VEGETABLE-FRUIT GROUP

4 or more servings Include—

A citrus fruit or other fruit or vegetable
  important for vitamin C
A dark-green or deep-yellow vegetable for
  vitamin A—at least every other day
Other vegetables and fruits, including
  potatoes

BREAD-CEREAL GROUP

4 or more servings
  Whole grain, enriched, or restored

Plus other foods as needed to complete meals and to provide additional food energy and other food values

FIGURE 38-1. A well-balanced diet will include foods from all four of the Basic Food Groups. (From *Food for Fitness—A Daily Food Guide.* Reproduced by permission, Consumer and Food Economics Institute, Hyattsville, Md.)

not supply sufficient amounts of this vitamin unless fortified foods are included.

Minerals

Mineral elements comprise only a small proportion, (approximately 4 percent) of the body tissues. However, 17 minerals have been identified as essential to optimum human nutrition. The mineral elements have a number of necessary functions in both the vital processes and structural components of the body. The balance of mineral ions in body fluid regulates the metabolism of several enzymes. Electrolytes, of which sodium and potassium are the most important, are the primary factors in the osmotic control of water metabolism. In many instances, minerals are found in association with proteins: potassium binds with protein in the cell; iron is found in hemoglobin; and phosphorus is a compound of phospholipids. Minerals assist in the regulation of the transmission of nerve impulses and in the contraction of muscles, including the heart muscle. They are also important in the formation of hard tissue, such as bones and teeth.

Each of the four food groups supplies varying amounts of minerals. Fats and sugars are practically free of minerals, and highly refined cereals and flours are poor sources of most minerals. Only calcium, iron, and iodine require special attention in the planning of diets for healthy individuals. Diets which are adequate in proteins and calories and include normal amounts of fruits and vegetables can be expected to supply all other minerals in satisfactory quantities.

Table 38-2 provides a summary of selected nutrients discussed above in relation to their functions in the body and major food sources.

Water and Electrolytes

There is probably no human activity in which water, a necessary nutrient, does not play a critical role. The presence or absence of water can set limits on the amount of daily activity possible. Water is essential to the body's life sustaining processes; it is important in any febrile state and in many intestinal diseases. Although man can live for weeks without food, he can survive only days without water.

Water makes up approximately 60 percent of the body weight of the adult male. It serves as a transporter, carrying nutrients and disposing of wastes; it aids in digestion, absorption, circulation, and excretion. Water is essential in the regulation of body temperature, and serves as a lubricant for the joints, muscles, and viscera.

Blood is a component of extracellular fluid, enclosed in vessels, and kept moving by the pumping action of the heart. Circulation cannot be maintained unless there is a sufficient volume of blood. Carbohydrates, fats, and amino acids are all transported via the blood to various tissues. Blood also transports oxygen to the cells, where it provides energy to the tissues.

Body water is used as a temperature controlling device to keep the body cool. When environmental temperature increases, man may give off more than 2 L of water an hour during bursts of activity. Evaporation of water is important in maintaining normal body temperature in hot climates and for dissipating the excess heat produced by physical exercise or fever.

The average adult metabolizes approximately 3 L of water per day. There is a constant balance between intake and output of water. The basic regulators of the intake and output are the kidneys (Fig. 38-2).

Water is taken into the body by fluids which man drinks including water, beverages, soups, and solid foods. An additional source is the water produced in the body as a result of metabolic processes. Solid foods contain substantial amounts of water—from 5 percent in dry foods, such as cereals and crackers, to 90 percent in fruits and vegetables, such as tomatoes and watermelon.

Water is excreted from the body through the kidneys, as urine, from the lungs as water vapor in the expired air, and from insensible perspiration. Lesser amounts are eliminated through the feces. Though the major water loss is through urination, in hot weather a larger amount of water may be evaporated by perspiration to keep body temperature regulated.

Body water is classified as intracellular or extracellular fluid. Both contain electrolytes. The intracellular fluid is high in potassium and phosphorus, and contains more magnesium, sulfur, and protein than the extracellular fluid. The extracellular fluid contains large amounts of sodium chloride, some bicarbonate, and small amounts of potassium, calcium, sulfur, and magnesium.

The relationship of body water and electrolytes regulates the distribution of water between the cells and the extracellular fluid. This fixed osmotic pressure of the extracellular fluid stabilizes the cell volume. Cells will shrink if the extracellular fluid becomes concentrated and swell if it is diluted. Dehydration results when excessive amounts of sodium are lost from the body; edema is excessive sodium retention. The constant balance of sodium and water is maintained by the kidneys.

DIETARY GUIDES

Recommended Allowances

Good nutrition advocates an adequate intake of the proper types and quantities of nutrients to meet the needs of the body. Scientists have made significant advances toward the understanding of nutrient utilization and the identification of amounts required under varying conditions.

In 1940, the National Research Council established the Food and Nutrition Board and mandated as one of their primary objectives a set of standards for human nutritive requirements. The results of this task were the Recommended Dietary Allowances (RDAs) initially published in 1943. These rec-

TABLE 38-2. Summary of Selected Nutrients

Nutrients	Functions in Body	Major Food Sources
Carbohydrates	Major energy source Utilization of other nutrients	Fruits, vegetables, breads, cereals, grains, and root vegetables
Fats and other lipids	Energy source Supply essential fatty acids	Butter, margarine, cooking oils, fats, milk and dairy products, meat, fish, poultry, eggs, and nuts
Proteins	Build and maintain body tissues Regulate body processes Fundamental structural element Supply energy	Milk and dairy products, meat, fish, poultry, eggs, breads, cereals, legumes, seeds, and nuts
Fat-Soluble Vitamins:		
Vitamin A	Constituent of visual pigments Maintains epithelial cells	Green and yellow vegetables, yellow fruit, liver, milk products, and eggs
Vitamin D	Absorption of calcium and phosphorus Mobilization of calcium from bone Builds bones and teeth	Fortified milk, fatty fish, eggs, liver, and butter
Vitamin E	Protects cell structure Prevents destruction of certain enzymes and intracellular components	Vegetable and seed oils
Vitamin K	Essential in blood clotting	Dark green leafy vegetables
Water-Soluble Vitamins:		
Vitamin C	Collagen formation Metabolic reactions of amino acids Protects against infection Wound healing	Citrus fruits, melon, strawberries, tomatoes, potatoes, and dark green leafy vegetables
Thiamine	Coenzyme in carbohydrate metabolism	Pork, organ meats, green leafy vegetables, whole or enriched cereals, berries, nuts, and legumes
Riboflavin	Coenzyme for carbohydrate, protein, and fat metabolism	Organ meats, milk, cheese, dark green leafy vegetables, and enriched cereals
Niacin	Coenzyme for tissue oxidation	Organ meats, poultry, fish, whole grain and enriched breads and cereals, dried peas, beans, nuts, and peanut butter
B_6-pyridoxine	Protein metabolism	Meats, whole grain cereals, lentils, and nuts

ommendations are continually being revised as new research and data become available. The latest revision appears in Table 38-3. The Recommended Dietary Allowances are estimates of the amounts of essential nutrients that each person in a healthy population must consume in order to provide reasonable assurance that the physiological needs of all will be met.[3] The recommendations are listed in terms of reference individuals of constant body size for each age group. Adjustments must be made for individuals who differ in size from the standard. The recommendations should not be confused with the daily minimum requirements. In addition, it should be remembered that they do not consider the body's additional needs during periods of disease or abnormality.

Basic Four Food Groups

The Recommended Dietary Allowances for daily use are quite complex; for this reason, the Basic Four Food Groups were designed to simplify them for both nutrition education programs and daily meal planning. The Basic Four Food Groups, as shown in Figure 38-1, suggest the number of servings from four broad categories of foods that will provide a sound foundation for an adequate diet. These foods are rich sources of the essential food nutrients (except calories and iron for the premenopausal woman). Additional food choices from the Basic Four Food Groups and selections of fats, oils, and sugars, are used to increase calories to meet energy needs. Daily recommendations are given for

TABLE 38-2. Summary of Selected Nutrients (Cont.)

Nutrients	Functions in Body	Major Food Sources
B_{12} cobalamin	Production of red blood cells Protein synthesis Nervous tissue metabolism	Organ meats, nonfat dry milk, seafood, and eggs
Folic acid	Protein metabolism Red blood cell formation	Organ meats, green leafy vegetables, whole grain cereals, meat, and fish
Pantothenic acid	Constituent of coenzyme A	Organ meats, eggs, legumes, and whole grain cereals
Minerals: Calcium	Main structural element (such as bones and teeth) Blood clotting Regulates functioning of nerve tissue Activates enzymes	Milk, dairy products, shellfish, and green leafy vegetables
Phosphorus	Rigidity to bones and teeth Energy metabolism Nervous tissue metabolism	Meat, fish, poultry, milk, eggs, cheese, nuts, and legumes
Magnesium	Constituent of bones and teeth Carbohydrate and protein metabolism Muscle and nerve action	Whole grains, legumes, nuts, milk, and meat
Sodium	Water balance, osmotic pressure Acid-base balance Muscle contraction Glucose absorption	Table salt (NaCl), milk, meat, fish, poultry, eggs, baking soda, and baking powder
Potassium	Water balance Acid-base balance Muscle contraction Nerve action Protein synthesis	Whole grains, legumes, meat, fruits, and vegetables
Iron	Hemoglobin formation Oxidizing enzymes	Organ meats, meat, fish, eggs, poultry, whole grain and enriched cereals, legumes, nuts, and dark green vegetables
Iodine	Synthesis of thyroid hormone	Iodized salt, seafood
Fluorine	Prevention of dental caries	Fluoridated water

the number of servings and portion sizes that an adult should eat from each food group. It is important, also, that an increased number of servings and portion sizes aid the increased nutritional needs of children, adolescents, and pregnant and lactating women.

The employment of the Basic Four Food Groups can aid in the maintenance of good nutrition practices by providing a variety of foods to meet the body's need for nutrients.

FACTORS AFFECTING FOOD PATTERNS

Man chooses the food he eats, not because of its nourishing effect, but because of the environmental influences which shape his eating behavior. Initiated during infancy, these cultural, social, psychological, and economic influences affect the food preferences of an individual throughout his life cycle. The health team member, in dealing with individuals, must remember that these food patterns are deeply rooted and must be considered when planning nutritious meals or counseling clients.

Cultural Influences

To understand the food patterns of an individual, one must examine the cultural background, including values, attitudes, habits, and customs that are acquired through learning—a process which begins

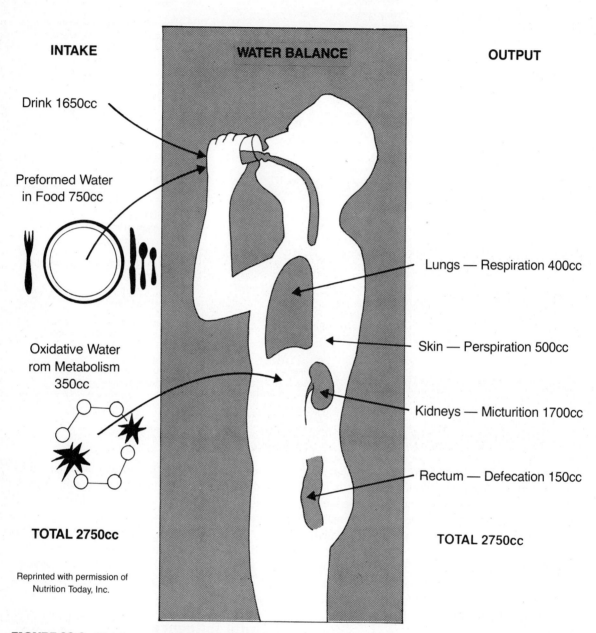

FIGURE 38-2. Maintenance of the body's water balance. (Reproduced with permission of *Nutrition Today* magazine, Spring, 1970, 101 Ridgely Ave., Annapolis, Md.)

TABLE 38-3. Food and Nutrition Board, National Academy of Sciences–National Research Council Recommended Daily Dietary Allowances* (Revised 1974)

	Age	Weight		Height		Energy	Protein	Fat-Soluble Vitamins				Water-Soluble Vitamins							Minerals					
								Vitamin A Activity (RE)‡	(IU)	Vitamin D (IU)	Vitamin E Activity‖ (IU)	Ascorbic Acid (mg)	Folacin# (μg)	Niacin** (mg)	Riboflavin (mg)	Thiamin (mg)	Vitamin B₆ (mg)	Vitamin B₁₂ (μg)	Calcium (mg)	Phosphorus (mg)	Iodine (μg)	Iron (mg)	Magnesium (mg)	Zinc (mg)
	(years)	(kg)	(lbs)	(cm)	(in)	(kcal)†	(g)																	
Infants	0.0–0.5	6	14	60	24	kg × 117	kg × 2.2	420§	1,400	400	4	35	50	5	0.4	0.3	0.3	0.3	360	240	35	10	60	3
	0.5–1.0	9	20	71	28	kg × 108	kg × 2.0	400	2,000	400	5	35	50	8	0.6	0.5	0.4	0.3	540	400	45	15	70	5
Children	1–3	13	28	86	34	1,300	23	400	2,000	400	7	40	100	9	0.8	0.7	0.6	1.0	800	800	60	15	150	10
	4–6	20	44	110	44	1,800	30	500	2,500	400	9	40	200	12	1.1	0.9	0.9	1.5	800	800	80	10	200	10
	7–10	30	66	135	54	2,400	36	700	3,300	400	10	40	300	16	1.2	1.2	1.2	2.0	800	800	110	10	250	10
Males	11–14	44	97	158	63	2,800	44	1,000	5,000	400	12	45	400	18	1.5	1.4	1.6	3.0	1,200	1,200	130	18	350	15
	15–18	61	134	172	69	3,000	54	1,000	5,000	400	15	45	400	20	1.8	1.5	2.0	3.0	1,200	1,200	150	18	400	15
	19–22	67	147	172	69	3,000	54	1,000	5,000	400	15	45	400	20	1.8	1.5	2.0	3.0	800	800	140	10	350	15
	23–50	70	154	172	69	2,700	56	1,000	5,000		15	45	400	18	1.6	1.4	2.0	3.0	800	800	130	10	350	15
	51+	70	154	172	69	2,400	56	1,000	5,000		15	45	400	16	1.5	1.2	2.0	3.0	800	800	110	10	350	15
Females	11–14	44	97	155	62	2,400	44	800	4,000	400	12	45	400	16	1.3	1.2	1.6	3.0	1,200	1,200	115	18	300	15
	15–18	54	119	162	65	2,100	48	800	4,000	400	12	45	400	14	1.4	1.1	2.0	3.0	1,200	1,200	115	18	300	15
	19–22	58	128	162	65	2,100	46	800	4,000	400	12	45	400	14	1.4	1.1	2.0	3.0	800	800	100	18	300	15
	23–50	58	128	162	65	2,000	46	800	4,000		12	45	400	13	1.2	1.0	2.0	3.0	800	800	100	18	300	15
	51+	58	128	162	65	1,800	46	800	4,000		12	45	400	12	1.1	1.0	2.0	3.0	800	800	80	10	300	15
Pregnant						+300	+30	1,000	5,000	400	15	60	800	+2	+0.3	+0.3	2.5	4.0	1,200	1,200	125	18+††	450	20
Lactating						+500	+20	1,200	6,000	400	15	80	600	+4	+0.5	+0.3	2.5	4.0	1,200	1,200	150	18	450	25

*The allowances are intended to provide for individual variations among most normal persons as they live in the United States under usual environmental stresses. Diets should be based on a variety of common foods in order to provide other nutrients for which human requirements have been less well defined.

†Kilojoules (kJ) = 4.2 × kcal.

‡Retinol equivalents.

§Assumed to be all as retinol in milk during the first six months of life. All subsequent intakes are assumed to be half as retinol and half as β-carotene when calculated from international units. As retinol equivalents, three fourths are as retinol and one fourth as β-carotene.

‖Total vitamin E activity, estimated to be 80 percent as α-tocopherol and 20 percent other tocopherols.

#The folacin allowances refer to dietary sources as determined by *Lactobacillus casei* assay. Pure forms of folacin may be effective in doses less than one fourth of the recommended dietary allowance.

**Although allowances are expressed as niacin, it is recognized that on the average 1 mg of niacin is derived from each 60 mg of dietary tryptophan.

††This increased requirement cannot be met by ordinary diets; therefore, the use of supplemental iron is recommended.

Reprinted with permission of Food and Nutrition Board, National Academy of Sciences, National Research Council, Washington, D.C.

with the earliest experiences during infancy.[4] As one's experiences grow out of culture, that culture has a strong, suggestive influence upon him. The small culture of the home and the larger cultural settings, such as school, community, race, and church, are equally strong conditioning influences.[5] Through these cultural settings, traditions and values are passed from one generation to another.

Food patterns reflect the cultural influences of a people. How food is acquired, which foods are selected, how they are prepared, who eats them, with whom, when and how, and in what quantity are dictated by the individual's culture.

Regional Influences

Regional variations in food patterns are affected by the availability of food and the ability of the land to produce food. A food readily available to one area, such as fish to coastal regions, may be unavailable to others. Crops, such as wheat, grow easily in the midwestern United States climates, but not in the cold climate of the northeast. Individuals become accultured to foods available in their geographic regions. Food preparation practices and food terminology also vary among regions.

Modern technology has decreased much of the regional variances in the United States today. Improved transportation and advances in food preservation enable the consumer to purchase foods from distant locations.

Religious Influences

Almost all religions of the world have certain rituals involving special foods. Primitive religions offered food and sacrificed animals to the gods for reasons of appeasement. Eating certain foods often symbolizes the past history of a religion. The prohibition of certain foods in some religions was protective in nature. In both instances, following these food rituals was a demonstration of faith in that religion.

The Jewish dietary laws were a protective measure against assimilation into other larger societies. The laws were a means of service to God and had a probable hygienic basis. The present dietary laws apply specifically to the selection, slaughter, and service of meat, milk, fish, and eggs. Pork products are omitted completely. Many special feast days commemorate historical events.

The Mohammedans fast for a month each year as commanded in the Koran. During this month food is not ingested from dawn to sunset, after which time feasting may take place. In the Mohammedan religion, pork is omitted, and other meats are slaughtered according to ritual.

Holy communion in the Christian church symbolizes past events and demonstration of faith. For example, during the period of Lent, before Easter, light meals are served; at this time, many Catholics omit meat from their diets on Fridays and on Ash Wednesday. Dietary restrictions vary markedly among the Protestant denominations, but they are generally more liberal than the Catholic practices.

Social Influences

Food plays an important role in the socialization of man. Food represents security, affection, communication, friendliness, and social acceptance.

A mother feeding an infant imparts feelings of security and affection toward her child. The infant begins to form food patterns which associate these earliest emotions with food. As the child grows and joins the family at the dinner table, the establishment of food patterns continues. The food served represents the traditions and preferences of the family. Adults may use food as a reward or as punishment for a child.

There is a distinct relationship between food and friendship. The offering to share one's food with another connotes offering of one's self. Eating with friends demonstrates the individual's acceptance into a social group and provides opportunities for communication and relaxation. Social occasions, such as weddings and parties, almost always involve food. Food may also be offered as a gift by which various emotions such as gratitude, affection, and sympathy may be expressed.

Psychological Influences

Eating is a highly emotional experience for many individuals. The simple act of satisfying the need for food may unleash a variety of emotions from pleasure to anxiety, stress, and fear.

Some people are overly concerned with the healthfulness of the food they eat. These individuals tend to follow fad diets, frequent health food stores, and ingest large quantities of nutritional supplements. Other individuals suffer from feelings of guilt, as in the obese person who sneaks food behind closed doors.

Food patterns are a part of an individual's behavior. Before attempting to modify a food pattern, or behavior, the health team member must understand that an individual is motivated to act according to what he perceives as necessary to meet his personal needs. Therefore, although the health team member may spend considerable time and effort in instructing the individual in good nutrition practices or on a special diet, a change in behavior will not occur unless the individual accepts the need for change and is motivated to do so.

Economic Influences

Food patterns reflect the economic status of an individual. People with higher incomes are able to purchase more expensive foods, such as meat, more frequently than a person with a lower income. The lower the income, the more likely one will find inexpensive, filling foods, such as starches in the daily diet.

As the income of a family decreases the percentage of the budget spent on food increases. At a low or middle income level, food may represent the largest percent of the budget. With the increase in food costs and food shortages, it is a challenge for the family food buyer to provide nutritious meals within the given budget. Nutrition education is important to ensure the best buy for the food dollar.

NUTRITION DURING THE LIFE CYCLE

Lewis[6] states, "Nutrition is an important environmental influence affecting the physiological and psychological development during each phase of the life cycle, since both the nutritional needs and responses to food change as the individual progresses through the life cycle. Knowledge of these cycles is necessary to provide the required nutrients in an atmosphere that contributes to optimum physiological and psychological development."

Infancy

Infancy is a period of rapid growth and development. In relation to body size, the nutritional requirements of an infant are higher than those of a child or an adult. Calories and nutrients, in sufficient amounts, are necessary for the infant to achieve optimum physical and intellectual development.

During the first months of life, the mother's milk is an excellent nutritional source. Commercially prepared formulas that approximate the nutrient composition of human milk are also available. The mother, at her discretion, can determine whether or not she wishes to breast-feed her baby.

Of greater importance than the method of feeding are the emotions developed between mother and child. From birth, food symbolizes love, security, and comfort. Being held and fed is the infant's first experience at socialization and communication. As the infant grows, the nutritional needs increase. At approximately 2 months of age puréed foods are usually introduced, with cereals and fruits added to the diet first. During the third and fourth month vegetables are included, and meat is added to the diet during the fourth to sixth months. By 6 months, infants are eating foods from each of the Basic Four Food Groups. During this period, the infant begins to experiment with new foods. Toast, breads, and teething biscuits, which can be grasped, may be added to the menu, especially when the child is teething.

By the time the infant is 9 months old, junior or chopped foods usually replace puréed foods. New foods should be introduced gradually and in small amounts to enable the child to adjust to them. The appetite may fluctuate as the teeth erupt.

Childhood

Beginning in the second year of life the rapid growth rate of infancy starts to decline. The appetite of the toddler and preschooler naturally diminishes. Although growth is now slower, it remains steady, and the child should be offered foods from the Basic Four Groups to provide the necessary calories and nutrients. Often, children will adapt readily to eating smaller meals served more frequently. Between-meal snacks, wisely chosen, can provide for the child's high energy needs and will help to avoid excess hunger at meals.

The child begins to explore the environment during this period. Loss of interest in food and a shorter attention span are frequently observed. Eating utensils are now introduced.

At this stage children will often go on particular "food jags." These periods will not last long if the parents do not attach too much importance to them. The child continues to form food patterns as a result of the social and emotional experiences of eating.

Food habits continue to develop as the child grows. As children become part of the family group eating at the table together, they become accultured to their ethnic, religious, and economic background.

By the time the child begins school, his food preferences may have increased. However, skipped meals and shorter meal periods may make it difficult to maintain optimum nutrition for growth. Snacks, chosen from the Basic Four food groups provide both the additional calories needed for the child's increased activity and the nutrients necessary for his continued growth.

As the child joins other children for lunch, he becomes aware of new foods. The child learns to accept the new and different from other children. Food habits and preferences continue to develop as the child's exposure to new foods continues.

Adolescence

Adolescence is the second period of rapid growth. Increased activity levels and the adolescent growth spurt stimulate the appetite. Adolescents are often fatigued and under emotional stress. These factors can have adverse effects on the retention of nutrients. Good nutrition practices are especially important during this period. Snacks chosen from the Basic Four augment meals and decrease the consumption of empty-calorie foods.

Adolescence is a period of personality development and a time when opportunities become available for decision-making. The adolescent usually determines his own food preferences from food habits established earlier in life. Since at this stage there is a need for peer approval, adolescents frequently follow food fads.

Pregnancy

The quality of the nutritional program throughout pregnancy is of primary importance to the mother and the fetus. The nutritional status of the mother, both prior to, and during pregnancy, has been shown to be directly related to the success of the pregnancy and the ultimate well-being of the infant. Toxemia and prematurity may occur due to an inadequate diet. Mothers with well-balanced diets tend to have fewer complications and easier labor.

The diet for the pregnant woman must be determined individually. Her current physical and nutritional status, as well as her living pattern, all influence the diet prescription. For the normal, healthy, pregnant woman, the Recommended Dietary Allowances should provide the proper guidelines for planning and evaluating the diet. Pregnant women should receive nutritional counseling as early in the pregnancy as possible to effect an understanding about the kinds of foods needed to meet their increased caloric and nutrient needs.

During the first trimester of pregnancy there is no need for additional nutrients for the growth of the fetus. The pregnant woman should consume a well-balanced diet to preserve and build up her physical well-being. It is usually during this period that a pregnant woman experiences nausea, vomiting, or gastrointestinal disturbances. This is usually due to adjustments of the woman's body to the fetus. Fat may be one of the intolerable foods. By changing to nonfat milk, omitting butter or margarine from toast, and by eliminating fried foods from the diet, nausea may be decreased. Smaller meals eaten more frequently are often recommended as well as eliminating liquids from meals and having them at other times during the day. Eating a few dry crackers before rising may also help to control nausea.

The appetite and digestive abilities of the mother should return to normal during the second trimester. The Recommended Dietary Allowances suggest increases for almost all essential nutrients during pregnancy, including 300 additional calories and 30 grams of protein per day. This provides for the tissue building of the fetus and maintenance and repair of the mother's tissues. As the pregnancy progresses during the second trimester, the mother begins to store fat which will protect the fetus against the possible poor nutrition of the mother.

During the final months of pregnancy the mother's diet must contain the additional nutrients needed for fetal growth. The additional needs should be met by foods of high biological value, protein, vitamins, and minerals.

Lactation

During lactation, the nutritional needs of the mother are increased more than they were during pregnancy due to the physiological stress of this period. An increase in calories, protein, vitamins, and minerals is suggested for the lactating woman.

The energy requirements of lactation are proportional to the amount of milk produced. A caloric increase of 500 calories per day is suggested for the first 3 months of lactation. These extra calories allow the maternal body fat stores to readjust after gestation.

The amount of additional protein is also dependent on the quantity of milk produced. Twenty grams of protein per day, *over* normal recommendations, is suggested in the Recommended Dietary Allowances. Additional vitamins and minerals are necessary to protect against maternal tissue depletion. Sufficient fluids are necessary to replace the water secreted in the milk.

As the weaning process occurs, the mother should return to a well-balanced dietary intake to protect against weight gain.

Maturity

Nutritional requirements for the mature individual and the older adult are not fundamentally different from the young adult. However, because the process of aging gives each age group unique characteristics, nutrition in later life is worth separate consideration.[7]

Elderly persons, with many special nutritional needs, constitute a rapidly growing segment of the population. The nutritional needs of the elderly are not much different from those of the younger adult, with the exception of a decrease in caloric needs influenced by decreases in activity and basal metabolic rate. Proteins, vitamins, and minerals remain the same except for a decrease in iron requirements for the postmenopausal woman.

It is the physiological, social, psychological, and economic influences which make the elderly population susceptible to malnutrition. Physical problems such as decreased activity, dental problems, joint disorders, diminished eye sight, and weakening sense of smell and taste acuity, can adversely affect nutrition maintenance. An increased incidence of disease and ill health can lower the efficiency of digestion, absorption, and metabolism and impair nutrient utilization.

Food fads are a problem among the elderly. Promises of eternal youth and miracle cures for disease states are tempting, however false. Nutrition education should be directed towards improving dietary habits.

Changes in living conditions can have a significant effect on the nutrition of the elderly. The elderly person may find himself living alone out of the family setting. Elderly persons who live alone may have little desire to shop or cook for themselves. Decreased mobility may add to the difficulty of shopping for food. The elderly person who is institutionalized, or on a modified diet due to a disease state, may find it difficult to give up food habits and preferences of earlier years.

Economic limitations present additional nutritional problems for the elderly. Inexpensive food items may be empty-calorie foods. The elderly should be encouraged to spend their food dollar wisely so as to include foods from the Basic Four Food Groups.

Currently, nutrition education programs and feeding programs for the elderly are attempting to provide better nutritional care for this growing segment of our population.

REFERENCES

1. Alfin-Slater, R. B.: Fats, essential fatty acids, and ascorbic acids. *J. Am. Diet. Assoc.* 64:168, 1974.
2. Stevenson, G. T., Miller, C.: *Introduction to Foods and Nutrition.* New York, John Wiley and Sons, Inc., 1962.
3. Harper, A. E.: Recommended Dietary Allowances: are they what we think they are. *J. Am. Diet. Assoc.* 64:151, 1974.
4. Fathauer, G. H.: Food habits—an anthropologist's view. *J. Am. Diet. Assoc.* 37:335, 1960.
5. Rathbone, F. S., and Rathbone, E. T.: *Health and the Nature of Man.* New York, McGraw-Hill Book Co., 1971.
6. Lewis, C. M.: *Nutrition of the Toddler and Preschool Child.* Unpublished manuscript.
7. Anderson, L. et al.: *Nutrition in Nursing.* Philadelphia, J. B. Lippincott Co., 1972, p. 165.

BIBLIOGRAPHY

American College of Surgeons, Committee on Pre- and Postsurgical Care: *Manual of Surgical Nutrition.* Philadelphia, W. B. Saunders Co., 1975.

Babcock, C. G.: Attitudes and the use of food. *J. Am. Diet. Assoc.* 38:546, 1961.

Blackburn, M. W., and Calloway, D. H.: Basal metabolic rate and work energy expenditure of mature, pregnant women. *J. Am. Diet. Assoc.* 69:24, 1976.

Bogert, L. J., Briggs, G. M., and Callahan, D. H.: *Nutrition and Physical Fitness.* Philadelphia, W. B. Saunders Co., 1973.

Burton, B. T.: *The Heinz Handbook of Nutrition,* 2nd ed. New York, McGraw-Hill Book Co., 1965.

Calloway, D. H.: Recommended dietary allowances for protein and energy. *J. Am. Diet. Assoc.* 64:157, 1974.

Committee on International Nutrition Programs: Relationship of nutrition to brain development and behavior. *Nutr. Today* 9:12, 1974.

Cosper, B. A., and Wakefield, L. M.: Food choices of women. *J. Am. Diet. Assoc.* 66:152, 1975.

Cottom, H. R.: The world food conference. *J. Am. Diet. Assoc.* 66:333, 1975.

Deutsch, R. M.: *The Family Guide to Better Food and Better Health.* Iowa, Meredith Corp., 1977.

Field, H. E.: *Foods in Health and Disease.* New York, Macmillan Co., 1964.

Food and Nutrition Board: *Recommended Dietary Allowances,* 8th ed. Washington, D.C., National Academy of Sciences, 1974.

Gifft, H. H., Washbon, M. B., and Harrison, G. G.: *Nutrition, Behavior and Change.* Englewood Cliffs, N.J., Prentice-Hall, Inc., 1972.

Goodhart, R. S. and Shills, M. E. (eds.): *Modern Nutrition in Health and Disease-Dietotherapy,* 5th ed. Philadelphia, Lea and Febiger, Inc., 1973.

Guthrie, H. A.: Concept of a nutritious food. *J. Am. Diet. Assoc.* 71:14, 1977.

Harper, A. E.: Those pesky R.D.A.'s. *Nutr. Today* 9(2):15, 1974.

Hegstead, D. M.: Dietary standards. *J. Am. Diet. Assoc.* 66:13, 1975.

Hegstead, D. M.: Protein needs and possible modifications of the American diet. *J. Am. Diet. Assoc.* 68:317, 1976.

Inkeles, A.: *What is Sociology—An Introduction to the Discipline and Profession.* Englewood Cliffs, N.J., Prentice-Hall, Inc., 1964.

Jacobson, H. N.: Nutrition in pregnancy—a critique. *J. Am. Med. Assoc.* 225:634, 1973.

Justice, C. L., Howe, J. M., and Clark, H. E.: Dietary intakes and nutritional status of elderly patients. *J. Am. Diet. Assoc.* 65:639, 1974.

Kaufman, N. A., Posnanski, R., and Guggenheim, K.: Eating habits and opinions of teenagers on nutrition and obesity. *J. Am. Diet. Assoc.* 66:264, 1975.

Leverton, R. M.: The R.D.A.'s are not for amateurs. *J. Am. Diet. Assoc.* 66:9, 1975.

Lewis, C. M.: *Basics of Nutrition.* Philadelphia, F. A. Davis Co., 1976.

Lowenberg, M. E., and Lucas, B. I.: Feeding families and children—1776–1976—a bicentennial study. *J. Am. Diet. Assoc.* 68:207, 1976.

Lowenberg, M. E.: The development of food patterns. *J. Am. Diet. Assoc.* 65:263, 1974.

Martin, E. A.: *Roberts' Nutrition Work with Children.* Chicago, Ill., University of Chicago Press, 1954.

Mitchell, H. S., et al: *Nutrition in Health and Disease,* 16th ed. Philadelphia, J. B. Lippincott Co., 1976.

Morse, E. H., et al: Comparison of nutritional status of pregnant adolescents with adult pregnant women. I. Biological Findings. *Am. J. Clin. Nutr.* 28:1000, 1975.

Murphy, G. H., and Wertz, A. W.: Diets of pregnant women: influences of socio-economic factors. *J. Am. Diet. Assoc.* 30:34, 1954.

Nutrition Reviews: *Present Knowledge in Nutrition,* 4th ed. New York, Nutrition Foundation Inc., 1976.

National Dairy Council: *Dairy Council Digest* 48:1, 1977.

Palmer, S., and Thompson, R. J.: Nutrition: an integral component in the health care of children. *J. Am. Diet. Assoc.* 69:138, 1976.

Pitkin, R. M. (ed.): Nutrition in pregnancy. *Diet. Curr.* 4:1, 1977.

Read, M. S.: Malnutrition, hunger, and behavior. I. Malnutrition and learning. *J. Am. Diet. Assoc.* 63:379, 1973.

Robinson, C. H.: *Normal and Therapeutic Nutrition.* New York, Macmillan Co., 1971.

Robinson, J. R.: Water the indispensable nutrient. *Nutr. Today* 5:16, 1970.

Schaefer, R., and Yetley, E. A.: Social psychology of food faddism. *J. Am. Diet. Assoc.* 66:129, 1975.

Shifflit, P. A.: Folklore and food habits. *J. Am. Diet. Assoc.* 68:347, 1976.

Sorenson, A. W., et al.: An index of nutritional quality for a balanced diet. *J. Am. Diet. Assoc.* 68:236, 1976.

Thompson, M. F., Morse, E. H., and Merrow, S. B.: Nutrient intake of pregnant women receiving vitamin-mineral supplements. *J. Am. Diet. Assoc.* 64:382, 1974.

Williams, S. R.: *Nutrition and Diet Therapy.* St. Louis, C. V. Mosby Co., 1973.

Wilson, E. D., Fisher, K. H., and Fuqua, M. E.: *Principles of Nutrition.* New York, John Wiley and Sons, Inc., 1967.

CHAPTER 39

Impaired health can significantly affect nutritional requirements and eating habits as disease states often impair the body's ability to digest, absorb, and utilize food, either as a primary consequence of the organic disease or as a secondary consequence of the accompanying anxiety, fear, and lack of physical exercise or treatment modalities. Providing and maintaining adequate nutrition for the person with impaired health may present a significant problem to the health team. The severity and the duration of the disease or injury, the previous state of nutrition of the individual, and the nutrients consumed during convalescence must be considered.

The first section of this chapter discusses the effects of common conditions on nutritional requirements and eating habits. The second section concerns ways in which nurses can assist the client with nutrition.

EFFECT OF IMPAIRED HEALTH ON NUTRITIONAL REQUIREMENTS AND EATING HABITS

Dorothy C. Silver, M.Ed., R.D.

COMMON CONDITIONS AFFECTING NUTRITION

Fevers and Infections

Individuals experiencing a febrile state face alterations in their nutritional requirements and eating habits. Acute febrile conditions are accompanied by an increase in energy and protein metabolism. The longer the duration of the fever and the higher the temperature, the greater will be the loss of protein from the body's tissues. Vitamin requirements are increased, especially B-complex, ascorbic acid, and vitamin A. As the caloric need increases, thiamine, riboflavin, and niacin requirements also increase. Body fluids and electrolytes are lost through increased diaphoresis. An increase in fluids is necessary to assist in both the regulation of body temperature and the prevention of dehydration.

Infections also increase the basal metabolic rate, paralleling the increase in body temperature. Bacterial invasion may lead to destruction of tissue protein; in turn, there is an increase in protein metabolism. A decrease in protein absorption from the gastrointestinal tract sometimes accompanies infections that decrease gastrointestinal functioning. Additional protein, above the recommended allowances, must be provided to counterbalance protein losses.

In individuals who have acute infections, fluids may be lost through the skin, lungs, and gastrointestinal tract. Without fluid replacement, dehydration, and electrolyte imbalance can occur. The additional fluids assist in removing toxins from the body.

During periods of fever and infection, there may be a loss of body weight largely due to loss of appetite, intolerance for food, and the body's catabolic response to the noxious or toxic mechanical agents which produced the condition.[1]

Maldigestion and Malabsorption

Maldigestion and malabsorption are associated with many diseases of the gastrointestinal tract. Protein and vitamin depletion are common. Individuals with acute illnesses are frequently unable or unwilling to ingest food. Complications of infection, starvation, fluid and electrolyte imbalances, and skin erosion are sometimes observed. In addition, excessive weight loss, marked reduction of serum albumin, and delayed wound healing may develop.

Stress

Stress is caused by a variety of internal and external factors which generate pathological effects on the body. Trauma, wounds, fractures, burns, surgical procedures, extreme heat or cold, starvation, pain, fear, and anxiety are examples of stressors to the body.

The body's need for calories increases during periods of stress. Severe stress increases the quantitive need for certain nutrients, including carbohydrates, proteins, C and B vitamins, and certain electrolytes beyond the recommended allowances for nonstressed individuals.

Stress results in an increase in catabolism of muscle protein with respect to synthesis, leading to the transportation of the amino acids away from muscle and peripheral tissues to the liver where they are converted to glucose for energy. This process creates a protein deficit.[2]

Protein may also be lost from draining wounds, such as burned surfaces, and in the accumulation of serous fluids, as in ascites. Chronic abscesses, decubiti, or osteomyelitis may be accompanied by an extreme loss of protein. The loss of protein-containing fluid represents a loss from the body not only of protein, but of vitamins, minerals, water, and other substances. The effect on the body will depend in part on the suddenness with which the losses occur, the causative conditions, and the length of time they persist. Sudden large losses of fluids into serous cavities may, by decreasing blood volume, lead to shock. Smaller losses over a period of time, may lead to malnutrition with decreases in weight, strength, and ability to respond to stress.

When decubiti form, they resist treatment unless and until protein and other nutritional deficiencies are corrected; recovery depends on the restoration of any inadequate nutritional elements.

Intense emotions, even pleasurable ones, interfere with digestion, inhibiting the flow of saliva, gastric, intestinal and pancreatic juices, slowing the peristaltic activity of the alimentary tract. Pain or violent emotions involve the autonomic nervous system which also exerts control over alimentation.

SECONDARY CONDITIONS

There are many conditions which may develop secondarily to disease states or stressful situations that severely affect an individual's nutritional requirements or his eating patterns. The most common are anorexia, vomiting, and diarrhea.

ANOREXIA. Anorexia, or loss of appetite, may accompany many illnesses or result from medication or certain treatments. Provided there are no contraindications, small amounts of foods and fluids should be encouraged but not forced.

VOMITING. Nausea and vomiting are symptoms accompanying many medical and surgical conditions. In severe cases of vomiting, dehydration and electrolyte imbalance may become evident. If the vomiting is persistent, interference with nutrition is quite possible. The nurse must record intake and output data carefully to assess the status of the client's fluid balance. When possible, oral feedings of hot or cold fluids should be initiated.

DIARRHEA. Diarrhea is a symptom of many gastrointestinal disturbances. Severe and prolonged diarrhea leads to a depletion of body fluids, electrolytes and nutrients, producing a loss of weight and strength. Here, too, a record of fluid balance should be maintained. Replacement of fluids and electrolytes is usually initiated intravenously. When oral feedings are feasible, a liquid diet should be introduced.

Hospitalization

The ill person when entering the hospital experiences many distressing emotions, including fear, guilt, anger, and helplessness. "The sense of separation from family and friends, economic concerns, alteration of roles, temporary and permanent changes in body functions or appearance, loss of self-esteem, and fear of the outcome of his or her illness may result in limited food intake and nutritional requirements as a result of these stresses."[3]

The hours of meal service in the hospital may be quite different than those the client is accustomed to in his home setting. Meals may be missed as a result of tests which must be administered during a fasting state or the failure of the client to be in his room at the time of meal service.

The client brings to the hospital his cultural, ethnic, and religious food preferences. All too frequently, the food served to a client does not consider these preferences, and unfamiliar foods are offered. If the diet has also been modified, the client may not find the different flavors and textures of the prescribed food particularly appealing.

The task of eating a meal, including the manipulation of a tray or utensils, can also present a problem for the bedridden client. It is frequently difficult for a client to admit the need for assistance.

The individual who is confined to bed, even if healthy, experiences a loss of protein during the first few days without ambulation. The nitrogen balance will then be restored to normal unless additional clinical problems exist. Calcium is lost following extended periods of bedrest or fractures. The lack of exercise with resultant decrease in muscle tone and reduction in the body's metabolic rate will also diminish caloric requirements.

Radiological Examinations and Treatments

Radiological examinations and treatments may alter nutritional requirements and eating patterns. Test meals, prior to specific diagnostic radiologic examinations, often are quantitatively and qualitatively precise to ensure accurate test results. The tests rarely consider a client's food preferences or eating patterns. Radiological treatments, including cancer therapy, have been found to cause nausea, impair nutrient intake, destroy the sense of taste, and damage the bowel with diarrhea and malabsorption.

Treatment and Medication

As the various disease modalities affect an individual's nutrient requirements and eating patterns, so do the treatments and medications employed as part of the medical care regimen. The nurse, as a key member of the health team, must be cognizant of all factors which might have an effect on the client's nutritional status.

A common side effect of pharmacological therapy is gastrointestinal disturbance. Among the most familiar pharmaceuticals causing these disturbances are aspirin, potassium salts, tetracycline (an antibiotic), prednisone (an anti-inflammatory agent), and chlorpromazine (a tranquilizer).[4]

A decrease in taste acuity and dysgeusia accompany therapy with some drugs such as D-penicillamine, and lincomycin (antibiotics), and several tranquilizers.[5]

Malabsorption, with clinical symptoms of anemia, steatorrhea and malnutrition, is frequently seen in conjunction with drug therapy. However, occasionally drug induced malabsorption is a desirable effect. Antimicrobial agents, antimitotic agents, cathartics, antacids, hypercholesterolemics, diuretics, and oral contraceptives can cause malabsorption in certain individuals.[6]

Chemotherapy presents many drug induced problems for the client with cancer. Loss of interest in food owing to taste impairment and depression of appetite secondary to the toxic effects of chemotherapy are typical. Chemotherapy often causes gastrointestinal disturbances such as nausea, vomiting, and diarrhea. Clients may also develop stomatitis, an inflammation of the mouth with oral ulcerations, making the ingestion of food painful, if not impossible.[7]

ASSISTING CLIENTS WITH NUTRITION

Diet Therapy

Diet therapy is that component of the treatment of an individual with an acute or chronic illness which involves the modification of food intake.[8] This might be the primary mode of therapy for a specific condition or may be used to supplement therapeutic agents and other supportive modes of therapy. Among the major aims of diet therapy are the achievement and maintenance of adequate nutrition, the adjustment of the ratio and balance of nutrients and foodstuffs, the alteration of body weight, the allowance of rest to the body's systems, and the varying of the number, type, or frequency of meals.

THERAPEUTIC OR MODIFIED DIETS

Therapeutic or modified diets are those that have been adjusted from the normal, well-balanced diet to compensate for altered nutritional requirements during disease states or injuries. The modified diet is designed to meet the requirements for essential nutrients, based on the Recommended Dietary Allowances of the National Research Council, (see Chapter 38). If the dietary modifications are so restrictive that the diet does not provide adequate nutrients, the physician should be notified so that appropriate adjustments in the diet or medications can be made.

Modified diets may be therapeutically correct and contain well-balanced food plans, but if they do not consider the client's established food patterns, the possibility of noncompliance is significant. Careful planning with the client and his family, based on interviews to obtain information regarding cultural, religious, social, and economic factors, as well as food preparation practices, will assist the client in adjusting to the diet modification.

If the modification is required for only a short time, it may not be difficult to plan. Clients may, in some facilities, select their own menus. Care should be taken to encourage and assist clients in this activity. If the diet modification is one to be followed at home after discharge from the health care facility, cost and availability of food, ease of preparation, and relationship to the family's food requirements must be considered.

Diet Prescriptions

A diet prescription is based on the knowledge of the nutritional status of the individual and the modifications dictated by the nature of the illness. If no constraints have been imposed by the disease state or nutritional status, a normal, regular, or "house" diet is prescribed. A house diet is not considered a modified diet as the latter is one which varies in some way from normal.

If a client is known to have a condition which requires the modification of his diet as part of his treatment or if diagnostic procedures indicate a disease which can be treated by diet therapy, a modified diet will be ordered. A client's diet prescription is usually ordered by his physician at the time of admission to the health care facility. The diet prescription is adjusted as the client's diagnosis or condition changes. Both the client and his family must be assisted to understand the diet prescription and its translation into food choices; any failure to comply with this could result in alteration of the client's health status.

DIET MANUAL

The diet manual is a compilation of routine and modified diets approved for use in a health care facility. The manual generally includes statements of rationale, nutritive evaluations, food allowances with detailed lists of foods to use and avoid, and sample meal patterns for each diet. The manual (1) eases communication among health professionals; (2) guides physicians in prescribing diets; (3) provides a reference for the nurse; (4) is a procedure manual for the dietary staff; and (5) serves as a teaching tool for professional personnel. A copy of the diet manual is usually available in each clinical unit for the convenience of the health team members.

The manual achieves standardization of procedures, yet allows ample opportunity for the individualization of a client's diet regimen. It is also the basis for the development of client educational materials.

Team Concept

The physician, dietitian, and the nurse form the core of the health team sharing the responsibility for nutritional care of clients. Each brings to this responsibility his own professional orientation and functioning, but for each, the focus is on the client.[9] Through independent and collaborative efforts, the team members reinforce each other in an attempt to attain and maintain an optimal level of nutrition.

In most health care facilities, the physician guides the team members, prescribing the diet to meet the individual requirements of the client. The dietitian provides the knowledge and expertise for the team since they are educated in assessing, interpreting, and determining an individual's nutritional needs in health and disease. The dietitian makes recommendations regarding an individual's meal plans, designs meals to meet his eating patterns and diet therapy, and provides counseling for the client and his family.

The role of the nurse in the nutritional care of the client is multifaceted. Depending on the sophistication of the facility, the nurse may assume the duties of the dietitian as well as her own. As the nurse has the most constant contact with the client, her role in his nutritional care is vital.

ASSESSMENT

The nurse is frequently the first member of the health team to visit the client. At this time an initial health appraisal is usually conducted including a nutrition assessment. Common elements of this assessment are: current, usual, and ideal body weight; food intolerances or allergies; appetite; physical factors affecting nutrition (e.g., the ability of the client to chew or swallow); and previously prescribed diets. If a dietitian is available, this information is communicated to her; the dietitian uses this information as the basis for an in-depth assessment of the client's nutritional status, including interviews with the client for a diet history, evaluation of laboratory data, and diagnostic test results. The dietitian, after consulting with the health team members, develops a nutrition care plan for hospitalization and home management.

INTERPRETATION

In most situations, the dietitian is responsible for translating the client's diet prescription into food and meal patterns and supervising food preparation and delivery. The nurse plays a vital role in assisting the client to accept his food and diet; she reinforces the explanation of the diet and prepares the client for what to expect if the food or meal plan differs from his typical eating pattern. In some facilities, the nurse helps the client select his foods.

If the client is on a modified diet, the nurse answers questions regarding the diet prescription and its relationship to his diagnosis, thus allaying his anxiety and confusion. The nurse has the opportunity to explain and support the nutrition counseling conducted by the dietitian during her contact with the client.

COORDINATION

Meeting a client's nutritional needs requires coordination of medical, nursing, and dietary personnel. The nurse is essential in the coordination of the team members' activities with the client in an endeavor to decrease duplication of effort and services.

If a diet prescription has not been ordered, the nurse has the responsibility of obtaining it from the physician and notifying the appropriate dietary personnel. The nurse may plan with the dietary staff to ensure that the client receives foods that are designed to meet his diet prescription and eating patterns.

The scheduling of the client's treatments and examinations are important factors in his food intake. Long waiting periods for radiological examinations, laboratory tests, and physical therapies tend to keep the client away from his room during meal service. Meal trays delivered to the client during an examination do not retain the correct temperature and are frequently unappealing and left uneaten. The nurse should be cognizant of these factors when scheduling examinations or treatment for the client.

Assisting with Eating Regimens

The nurse plays an important role in assisting a client to achieve optimum nutrition. By applying her knowledge of the principles of nutrition and nursing care, the nurse has the ability to increase appropriate food intake for clients of all ages. She may alter the environment, provide emotional support, and actually assist or feed a client.

The client's environment must be conducive to eating. Before the meal is served, every effort should be made to ensure a clean, orderly, and well-ventilated area. The appetite is easily depressed by disagreeable odors and increased by pleasant ones. Clients with foul smelling wounds often find eating difficult. Before providing the client with his meal tray, his face and hands should be washed, oral hygiene practices performed, and he should be offered the bedpan or urinal; however, bedpans should be removed prior to meal service.

The usual eating position for humans is upright necessitating the ability to sit up and control head balance. Proper positioning decreases the possibility of aspiration of food or fluids and increases the comfort of the client.

The meal tray should be clean with the dishes

attractively arranged and the food well presented. The portion sizes should meet the client's appetite. The temperature and condition of the food at the time of meal service is also important—that is, hot foods should be hot, and cold foods, cold.

The type of assistance needed by a client must be assessed on an individual basis considering specific needs, age, and stage of development. Clients with a partial handicap or with sight problems, including the blind, frequently prefer to feed themselves. Trays should be placed within easy reach, with utensils near the correct hand and with covers or lids removed. When necessary, the meat should be cut, bread buttered, and the beverage prepared. The client with sight problems needs to be oriented to the location of the tray and the position of foods on it to provide him with a clear mental image. The face of a clock is frequently used to explain the position of food on a plate. The nurse should not leave the client until she is certain that he is comfortable about eating.

When complete assistance is required, the nurse begins by sitting next to the client's bed or chair. The tray is placed within the client's visual range. Pleasant conversation and, at times, silence tend to put the client at ease. The client should be told what he is about to receive. The nurse must remember that many clients may feel embarrassment at having to be fed. She must present an attitude of caring and provide emotional support. It is important that the nurse submerge her own feelings about the foods being served so as not to discourage the client from eating. For example, the nurse who dislikes puréed meat should not grimace or comment on her own intense aversions while feeding this food to a client.

Small amounts of food should be offered to the client in the proper sequence. Sufficient time must be allowed for proper chewing, swallowing, and resting between mouthfuls. The desire for liquids must be anticipated. The client should be encouraged to hold any foodstuff which he is capable of handling. Face and hands are wiped as necessary.

The feeding period provides the nurse with the opportunity to observe the client's ability to eat and his appetite, food preferences, and attitudes. It also affords time for the nurse to answer any questions regarding his diet and care or to reinforce nutrition education. Any information gleaned at this time should be communicated to the dietitian and other health team members so that the care plan can be adapted as necessary.

The feeding and feeding training of the handicapped requires a great deal of ingenuity and planning on the part of all involved. These training programs restore the client's dignity and self-respect, prevent mental and physical deterioration, and increase strength and coordination. The handicapped client does not necessarily require a diet modified in texture except when alterations will make self-feeding easier or if dentition and swallowing are problems. The diet should be well balanced and include sufficient quantities of all essential nutrients unless contraindicated by other clinical conditions. Caloric requirements may vary from those of a nonhandicapped individual, depending on the mobility of the person. If there is a decrease in energy expenditure, the emphasis of the diet would be placed on increasing the nutritive value while decreasing caloric intake. However, it must be remembered that a significant amount of energy is expended in trying to get about. Parts of the handicapped person's body may be in constant involuntary movement or carrying a heavy piece of supportive apparatus. In these situations, the caloric requirements would then be increased accordingly.

Care must be taken that the handicapped client does not become dehydrated or overhydrated if he is also receiving intravenous therapy. Accurate records of intake and output are an important element of the nutritional care plan. Adequate fluid intake is required to prevent urinary tract infection and for some clients, to prevent the formation of renal calculi.

Immobilization promotes a negative nitrogen balance, and the loss of nitrogen is primarily from the muscle mass. Immobility also promotes calcium loss from the long bones. Muscular activity, combined with weight bearing on long bones can reverse these imbalances. The physically handicapped client, therefore, requires daily activity programs for effective utilization of nutrients.

Mealtime ought to be a normal social experience. Adaptive equipment may be used initially, but the objective is to progress to independent skill as soon as possible. For some individuals, such as the quadriplegic or neurologically handicapped, adaptive equipment becomes a part of their daily life. The basic areas in which adaptive devices are most often required are difficulty in sucking, poor grasp, poor upper extremity strength, and poor coordination of hand to mouth feeding.

All liquids are placed in plastic cups which are easier for the client to handle. The use of finger foods requires less energy than employing a spoon or fork. Finger foods should not be cut up into small pieces as this procedure tires the client. When necessary, feeding devices such as rocking knives and spoons should be used.

OBSERVATION AND COMMUNICATION

All clients should be observed for any indication of inadequate nutrition. These indications should be investigated, reported, and when necessary, treated by appropriate measures. The nurse, because of her continual contact with the client, should make observations of physical or psychological characteristics which may affect the ability to reach optimal nutrition. The adequacy of the client's food and fluid intake is reported, evaluated, and altered if necessary.

A client may have dentition problems, such as ill fitting or misplaced dentures. The nurse should observe the client's ability to chew the foods served to him. Altering the consistency, such as ground and puréed foods, is sometimes advantageous. Clients with wired jaws or facial injuries are apt to receive their food in liquid form through a straw. Observing the client's ability to accept this feeding system and identifying the need for a modification in the amount of liquid offered is a responsibility of the nurse.

Many medical conditions affect the swallowing and gag reflexes of an individual. Clients with these symptoms should be closely observed during mealtime to prevent aspiration and to identify the return of these reflexes.

In most instances, observation of food and fluid intake and output is sufficient to determine if a client is receiving adequate nutrition. This information indicates that the client is ingesting foods and fluids to meet his assessed needs as prescribed.

There are certain medical conditions, however, in which nutrients are lost from the body or inadequately utilized—for example, vomiting, diarrhea, or renal disease. It may be necessary for the nurse to maintain a record of exact food and fluid intake and output so that any nutrient or caloric deficiency may be determined, evaluated, and treated.

Nutrition Education

Nutrition education through the media has recently created in the American public an awareness of food and its nutritional value.[10] The American Dietetic Association defined nutrition education for the public in a 1973 position paper as "the process by which beliefs, attitudes, environmental influences, and understanding about food lead to practices that are scientifically sound, practical, and consistent with individual needs and available resources. And that it is needed, regardless of income, location, or cultural, social or economic practices or level of education."[11]

To reach people of varying backgrounds with nutrition education and to motivate them to change their eating behavior requires various educational techniques. The professional counselor must develop skills in interviewing, planning, educating, and evaluating with the focus on the client. Effecting behavioral change in dietary habits through counseling is, at best, difficult and complex. The highest degree of compliance is achieved through individualized, long-term, realistic programs in which the client becomes involved.

Nutrition education is a multidisciplinary process that involves all members of the health care team. As in other aspects of nutritional care, counseling roles will change in relation to the context of clinical practice. The major objective of the health team is to achieve and maintain adequate nutritional status of the population it serves. The nutrition counselor translates nutrition information into terms the client can accept and adopt.

The physician plays a leading role in nutrition education. During his visits with clients, he sees diseases or injuries in which nutrition may be involved. He may counsel the client or refer him to a dietitian. In the hospital, the physician is frequently the team member that orders diet counseling.

The dietitian is the nutrition education expert of the health care team. The knowledge of foods, nutrition, and education qualifies the dietitian as a counselor of individuals and groups.

Nutrition education cannot be separated from total nursing care. With increasing awareness of the role of nutrition in the maintenance of health and the treatment of disease, the nurse's role in nutrition education is significant. The nurse, whether in the hospital, clinic, doctor's office, or community is in a position to influence client behavior in relation to food and diet.

The nurse in the hospital or extended care facility has closer and more frequent contact than the other members of the health team and is, therefore, able to influence or alter a client's eating behavior. The nurse is able to discover a client's attitudes, knowledge, and readiness for instruction through her skills in listening, observation, and interviewing. All members of the health care team must anticipate a client's need for nutrition education. The client on a modified diet may need to continue this diet in the home setting. Instruction of the client and his family by the dietitian or nurse must be initiated early and re-evaluated as the client's condition changes. The nurse reinforces this education during her time spent with the client.

Current public awareness of the importance of nutrition and its relationship to health and disease has provided greater opportunities for nutrition education in the community setting. The nurse may practice in public health programs, doctor's offices, schools, or home care settings. The nurse in the community provides guidance to clients and their families for the establishment of realistic nutritional goals. The dietitian works with the nurse providing skills and techniques in adapting her counseling to meet the individualized needs of clients. The dietitian also supports the nurse in teaching normal and therapeutic nutrition.

REFERENCES

1. Krause, M. V., and Hunscher, M. A.: *Food, Nutrition and Diet Therapy,* 5th ed. Philadelphia, W. B. Saunders Co., 1972, pp. 327-334.
2. Scrimshaw, N. S., and Young, V. R.: The requirements of human nutrition. *Sci. Am.* 235:51,1975.
3. Moos, R. H.: *Coping with Physical Illness.* New York. Plenum Medical Book Co., 1977, p. 7.
4. Visconti, J. A.: *Nutrition in Disease—Drug Food Interactions.* Columbus, Ohio, Ross Laboratories, 1977, pp. 11-16.
5. *Ibid.,* p. 17.
6. *Ibid.,* pp. 22-24.
7. *Ibid.,* p. 18.
8. Mitchell, H. S., et al.: *Nutrition in Health and Disease,* 6th ed. Philadelphia, J. B. Lippinicott Co., 1976.
9. Anderson, L., et al.: *Nutrition in Nursing.* Philadelphia, J. B. Lippincott Co., 1972.
10. Robinson, C. H.: Nutrition education—what comes next? *J. Am. Diet. Assoc.* 69:126, 1976.
11. American Dietetic Association: Position paper on the scope and thrust of nutrition education. *J. Am. Diet. Assoc.* 72:302, 1978.

BIBLIOGRAPHY

American Dietetic Association: Position paper on nutrition education for the public. *J. Am. Diet. Assoc.* 62:429, 1973.

Beland, I. L., and Passos, J. Y.: *Clinical Nursing-Pathophysiological and Psychological Approaches.* New York, Macmillan Co., 1975.

Bosley, E. B.: Nutrition, human welfare, and economics *J. Am. Diet. Assoc.* 67:104, 1975.

Brown, E. L.: *Newer Dimensions of Patient Care.* New York, Russell Sage Foundation, 1967.

Bruch, H. (ed): Anorexia nervosa. *Diet. Curr.* 4(2):7, 1977.

Calvert, S., and Davies, F.: Nutrition in children with handicapping conditions. *Diet. Curr.* 4(3):13, 1977.

Cornelius, M. A.: Feeding handicapped patients. *J. Am. Diet. Assoc.* 67:136, 1975.

Cornely, P. B.: Community concern for total health care. *J. Am. Diet. Assoc.* 60:105, 1975.

Crenshaw, C.: Nutrition support for burn patients in intake: perspectives in clinical nutrition. New York, Eaton Laboratories, 1973.

Danish, S. J.: Developing helping relationships in dietetic counseling. *J. Am. Diet. Assoc.* 67:105, 1975.

Diet Therapy Committee, American Dietetic Association: Guidelines for diet counseling. *J. Am. Diet. Assoc.* 66:571, 1975.

Fielo, S. B., and Edge, S. C.: *Technical Nursing of the Adult.* New York, Macmillan Co., 1970.

Gailbraith, A., and Hatch, L.: Diet manual in a large teaching hospital: philosophy and purpose. *J. Am. Diet. Assoc.* 62:643, 1973.

Gifft, H. H., Washbon, M. B., and Harrison, G. G.: *Nutrition, Behavior and Change.* Englewood Cliffs, N. J., Prentice-Hall Inc., 1972.

Gimble, J. G.: Identifying the nurse practioner. *J. Am. Diet. Assoc.* 70:282, 1977.

Goodhart, R. S., and Shills, M. E. (eds.): Modern nutrition in health and disease dietotherapy. Philadelphia, Lea and Febiger, Inc., 1973.

Gragg, S. H., and Rees, O. M.: *Scientific Principles of Nursing,* 7th ed. St. Louis, C. V. Mosby Co., 1974.

Green, J. M.: Nutrition in nursing—a bookshelf review. *J. Am. Diet. Assoc.* 37:38, 1960.

Hanlon, J. J.: *Public Health-Administration and Practice.* St. Louis, C. V. Mosby Co., 1974.

Hein, E., and Leavitt, M.: Providing emotional support to patients. *Nurs. '77* 7(5):39, 1977.

Joint Commission on Hospital Accreditation: What's in a manual? *Hospitals* 45:16, 1971.

Kurtz, C.: Patient nutritional care—a dilemma for the hospital nurse. *J. Am. Diet. Assoc.* 67:367, 1975.

Lapointe, G.: A nutritional course for nurses. *Can. Nurse* 71:30, 1975.

Leverton, R. M.: What is nutrition education? *J. Am. Diet. Assoc.* 64:17, 1975.

Ling, L.: Guidelines for counseling. *J. Am. Diet. Assoc.* 66:571, 1975.

Manning, A. M., and Means, J. G.,: A self feeding program for geriatric patients in a skilled nursing facility. *J. Am. Diet. Assoc.* 66:275, 1975.

Melasanos, L., et al.: *Health Assessment.* St. Louis, C. V. Mosby Co., 1977.

Matheney, R. V., et al.: *Fundamentals of Patient Centered Nursing,* 3rd ed., St. Louis, C. V. Mosby Co., 1972.

Mayer, J.: The dimensions of human hunger. *Sci. Am.* 235:04, 1975.

McDaniel, J. M.: Diet therapy in the nursing school curriculum. *J. Am. Diet. Assoc.* 70:285, 1977.

National Nutrition Consortium: Guidelines for a national nutrition policy. *J. Am. Diet. Assoc.* 65:57, 1974.

Nutrition in cancer patient. *Dialog. Nutr.* 1(4):1, 1976.

Nutrition in stress and starvation. *Dialog. Nutr.* 1(3):1, 1976.

Nutrition in trauma and burns. *Dialog. Nutr.* 2(1):1, 1977.

O'Connell, S.: The nutrition consultant for visiting nurses. *J. Am. Diet. Assoc.* 68:247, 1976.

Ohlson, M. A.,: The philosophy of dietary counseling. *J. Am. Diet. Assoc.* 63:13, 1973.

Ohlson, M. A.: Uses of the dietary manual to promote communication. *J. Am. Diet. Assoc.* 62:534, 1973.

Peck, E. B.: The "professional self" and its relation to change processes. *J. Am. Diet. Assoc.* 69:534, 1976.

Peck, E. B.: The public health nutritionist-dietitian: a historical perspective *J. Am. Diet. Assoc.* 64:642, 1974.

Public Health Education Section, Committee on Educational Tasks in Chronic Illness, American Public Health Association: *A Model for Planning Patient Education.* Washington D.C., U.S. Department of Health Education and Welfare, 1975.

Robinson, C. H.: *Normal and Therapeutic Nutrition.* New York, Macmillan Co., 1971.

Rocchio, M. A., and Randall, H. T.: Nutrition in inflammatory bowel disease of the bowel, in *Intakes: Perspectives in Clinical Nutrition.* New York, Eaton Laboratories, 1974.

Schneider, H. A., Anderson, C. E., and Coursin, D. B.: *Nutritional Support of Medical Practice.* New York, Harper and Row Publishing, 1977.

Shafer, K. N., et al.: *Medical, Surgical Nursing.* St. Louis, C. V. Mosby Co., 1971.

Sloboda, S.: Understanding patient behavior. *Nurs. '77,* 7(9):74, 1977.

The patient who can't eat. *Dialog. Nutr.* 1(2):1, 1976.

The patient who won't eat. *Dialog. Nutr.* 1(1):1, 1976.

Tobias, A. L. and Van Italie, T. R.: Nutritional problems of the hospitalized patient. *J. Am. Diet. Assoc.* 71:253, 1977.

Treadwell, D. D.: Planning the nutritional component in long term care. *J. Am. Diet. Assoc.* 64:56, 1974.

Williams, C. D.: Grassroots nutrition-or consumer participation. *J. Am. Diet. Assoc.* 63:125, 1973.

Williams, S. R.: *Nutrition and Diet Therapy,* 3rd ed., St. Louis, C. V. Mosby Co., 1973.

Zifferblatt, S. M., and Wilbur, C. S.: Dietary counseling: some realistic expectations and guidelines. *J. Am. Diet. Assoc.* 70:591, 1977.

CHAPTER 40

Malnutrition is defined as a "lack of necessary or proper food substances in the body or improper absorption or distribution of them."[1] Malnutrition involves numerous disease modalities, ranging from the client who is morbidly obese to the client who is *cachectic** as a result of severe anorexia. Included are clients with single and multiple nutritional deficiencies.[2]

This chapter considers a specific aspect of malnutrition that affects hospitalized individuals termed protein-calorie malnutrition. This category of malnutrition results from a continued inadequate intake of nutrients or from the body's inability to digest, absorb, or utilize ingested nutrients.

Current research indicates that protein-calorie malnutrition is prevalent in American hospitals.[3,4] Many, and probably most, clients become malnourished prior to hospitalization as a result of illness-induced anorexia and the catabolic response

---

*A state of ill health, malnutrition, and wasting, which occurs in many chronic diseases.

ENTERAL AND PARENTERAL NUTRITION

Dorothy C. Silver, M.Ed., R.D.

to the stress of disease, but some also become malnourished after admission as a consequence of severe catabolic stress, particularly from surgery, infection, or the semistarvation regimens (e.g., clear liquid diets) employed with the very ill. The undesirable practices affecting the nutritional health of the hospitalized client as cited by Butterworth are listed in Table 40-1.

The malnourished client has an increased incidence of medical complications (Table 40-2). Malnutrition leads to loss of muscle protein accompanied by progressive weakness and debility. The malnourished individual becomes continuously less active. Subcutaneous fat is lost, and there is a breakdown of skin with decubiti. Clients with severe malnutrition do not have the same quality of recovery as the well-nourished individual. For example, debilitated clients have poor wound healing, and decreased immune response with a consequent increase in infections.[6,7] Fluid and electrolyte problems are more severe and difficult to handle. These complications often lead to prolonged hospitalization and contribute to morbidity and mortality.

ASSESSMENT OF NUTRITIONAL STATUS

It is now generally accepted that the prevalence of malnutrition significantly affects the clinical course of such clients and has direct bearing on morbidity and mortality. To formulate a regimen for nutritional support of the depleted client, it is essential to first establish the nature and extent of malnutrition.[8]

Anthropometric Measurements

Anthropometric measurements are used to identify normal and malnourished clients in an uncomplicated manner. These measurements are simple and easy to perform, identifying physiologically important tissues that are available to meet energy re-

TABLE 40-1. Undesirable Practices Affecting the Nutritional Health of Hospital Patients

1. Failure to record height and weight.
2. Rotation of staff at frequent intervals.
3. Diffusion of responsibility for patient care.
4. Prolonged use of glucose and saline intravenous feedings.
5. Failure to observe clients' food intake.
6. Withholding meals because of diagnostic tests.
7. Use of tube-feedings in inadequate amounts, of uncertain composition, and under unsanitary conditions.

Reprinted with permission from *Nutrition Today,* 101 Ridgely Avenue, Annapolis, Maryland 21404, © March/April 1974.

quirements in the semistarved state. These tissues are generally present in the ill client.

Measurement of height and weight is an effective measure in the hospital to diagnose chronic malnutrition. Weight loss usually reflects caloric inadequacy and a loss of protein from body cell mass. In a hospitalized adult with protein-calorie malnutrition, however, gross abnormalities caused by disease reduce the reliability of weight as an index of protein depletion. Disease states or therapies that cause fluid retention also make weight an inaccurate measure of nutritional status.[9]

The mid-upper arm circumference, which is easily measured with a standard tape measure, and the triceps skin-fold are used to calculate the mid-upper arm muscle circumference (Fig. 40-1). As

TABLE 40-2. Complicating Effects of Chronic Malnutrition (Protein-Caloric Deprivation)

1. Progressive weight loss.
2. Progressive weakness and apathy.
3. Decreased activity with delayed physical rehabilitation.
4. Decubiti at pressure points.
5. Depressed cell-mediated immunity with increased infection, particularly gram-negative sepsis.
6. Depressed ventilatory response to hypoxia.
7. Impaired wound healing, wound infections, wound disruption, and bowel fistula.
8. Increased incidence of pneumonitis and urinary tract infection.
9. Endocrine changes.
10. Decreased response to chemotherapy for infection and cancer control.
11. Delayed response in the completion of radiotherapy.
12. Increased difficulty with fluid, electrolyte, and acid-base management.
13. Increased and prolonged use of critical care facilities with expensive drugs and excessive requirements for hospital support services.
14. Delayed discharge and delayed ability to return to work.

Reprinted with permission from *Dialogues in Nutrition,* © Health Learning Systems Inc., Bloomfield, N.J.

skeletal muscle protein is utilized fairly uniformly during periods of caloric deprivation (except heart, diaphragm, and intercostal muscle), the mid-arm muscle circumference is a good indication of the general state of skeletal muscle protein. These measurements are compared to a table of norms to determine variations.

The triceps skin-fold provides an estimate of subcutaneous fat reserves. By pinching the skin and subcutaneous tissue at a point over the triceps muscle, midway between the head of the humerus and the olecranon, the triceps skin-fold can be measured by applying a caliper to the tissue to measure its thickness (in millimeters). This number is compared to a table of norms to get an approximation of loss of subcutaneous fat (Fig. 40-1).

Biochemistry

Serum albumin and transferrin levels are employed in determining protein-calorie malnutrition and depressed levels suggest significant visceral protein deficit in adults. Serum albumin is an indicator of visceral protein states as it is frequently supported by the erosion of skeletal muscle and conversion of released amino acids for the purpose of albumin production during chronic illness. In the catabolic state albumin is rapidly depleted. Transferrin, also a measure of visceral protein, is rapidly depleted during acute illness. Transferrin, an iron-carrying protein, may have significance in terms of immune competence as bacteria need iron for metabolism.

Laboratory Studies

BLOOD. Common hospital laboratory tests are useful in the determination of malnutrition. Among the hematology data used as diagnostic tools are changes in red blood cell counts to evaluate anemia and differential and total lymphocyte counts to identify lymphopenia.

URINE. Analysis of 24-hour and 48-hour urine samples for sodium, potassium, urea nitrogen, and creatinine is helpful in assessing the nutritional status of the client and the effect of therapy. The electrolyte balance information assesses renal function and metabolic response to infused electrolytes; urea nitrogen indicates utilization of exogenous protein, and rate of catabolism or anabolism. The

Measurement of Mid-Upper
Arm Circumference

Assessing Midpoint of Upper Arm
(Halfway between the Acromial
Process the Scapula and the
Olecranon Process of the Ulna)

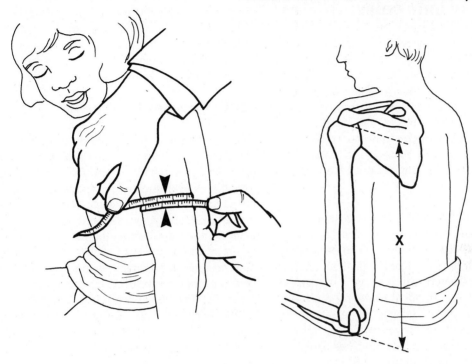

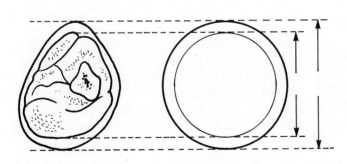

Calculation of Mid-Upper Arm
Muscle Circumference

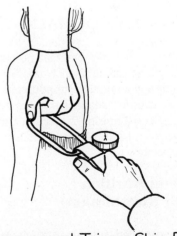

Measurement Triceps Skin-Fold
with Harpenden Calipers

FIGURE 40-1. Measurement of mid-upper arm circumference and triceps skin-fold. (Adapted with permission from Jelliffe, D.B.: *The Assessment of Nutritional Status of the Community.* W.H.O., Geneva, 1966.)

Enteral and Parenteral Nutrition 779

measurement of urea nitrogen can be used in the calculation of nitrogen balance and approximate net protein utilization.

CREATININE-HEIGHT INDEX. Many diseases are accompanied by or produce a retention of fluid; therefore, body weight may not be a good indicator of lean tissue erosion. Urine creatinine is a product of protein metabolism. Using a client's height, which remains relatively stable even during prolonged illness, and the 24-hour urine product of creatinine, a creatinine-height coefficient can be developed. Comparing these against controls, serial determination on a weekly basis gives a reasonable estimate of erosion and repletion of lean tissue mass.

IMMUNE COMPETENCE. Malnourished individuals have been shown to have a depressed cellular immunity.[7] Cellular immunity is important as a host defense mechanism against infection, and its depression is associated with increased morbidity and mortality. One method of assessing a client's immune competence is delayed hypersensitivity skin testing. A client who is anergic does not respond to usual intradermal tests and has a higher morbidity or mortality rate if he is subjected to the stress of a major surgical procedure or acute catabolic illness. Several antigens are used for this testing procedure including Candida, mumps, and streptokinase-streptodornase (SK-SD).

CATEGORIES OF MALNUTRITION

With these nutritional parameters, classification of protein-calorie malnutrition is possible and necessary to design a nutrition support plan for a specific client. Blackburn[9] identified three categories of protein-calorie malnutrition: visceral attrition (adult kwashiorkor), adult marasmus-cachexia, and intermediate states.

Visceral Attrition (Adult Kwashiorkor)

A well-nourished individual in whom the combination of severe catabolic stress and semistarvation diets combine to selectively depress the levels of visceral protein and immunologic competence is classified as being in the visceral attrition state or

having adult kwashiorkor. Because of the sudden onset of the condition, these clients maintain their anthropometric measurements despite severe depression of serum albumin and transferrin levels.

Associated with this visceral protein depletion is depression of cellular immune function. In visceral attrition, fat stores and skeletal muscle reserves are sufficient to maintain the client's calorie and protein requirements but are unavailable for use.[9]

Adult Marasmus-Cachexia

This condition is characterized by chronic hypocaloric intake, resulting in diminished fat and protein stores with preservation of visceral protein. Anthropometric measurements are diminished, indicating that *endogenous* fat and skeletal muscle are utilized to meet basal energy needs. Serum proteins remain relatively normal reflecting the maintenance of the viscera at the expense of skeletal muscle. Clients often present on admission with symptoms of marasmus-cachexia produced by a long-term inadequate diet associated with mild catabolic stress. Clients with anorexia or depression, geriatric clients, and those who cannot ingest sufficient nutrients are found in this classification.

Intermediate States (Marasmus/ Kwashiorkor)

The marasmic-cachectic client, as previously discussed, has markedly diminished fat and protein reserves. As this condition progresses, visceral proteins decrease and a depression of cellular immunity is found. When this client is unable to digest sufficient nutrients or when the client is maintained on a semistarvation regimen, he is less able to withstand additional stress or trauma. Immediate sophisticated support is required as further hypercatabolism makes recovery from this protein-calorie malnutrition difficult.

DETERMINATION OF THERAPY MODALITIES

The appropriate mode of nutritional support for an individual is determined by careful consideration of the complete nutrition assessment, the type of protein-calorie malnutrition involved, and the individual's nutrient requirements.

Therapeutic recommendations are based on objective data and the ability of the client to tolerate enteral or parenteral nutrition. Many individuals are unable to ingest, on a normal diet, sufficient nutrients needed during periods of catabolic stress. In this situation, the client can be provided with a defined formula liquid diet, either orally or by tube. In other instances, when the use of the gastrointestinal tract is not advised, parenteral hyperalimentation may be recommended. In certain circumstances, a combination of techniques provides for the restoration of visceral protein compartments of lean body mass and improves wound healing, increasing the client's strength and general sense of well-being.[10]

Figure 40-2 depicts a scheme of possible nutritional feeding modalities. Consideration must be given to whether the goal of treatment is a "fed"

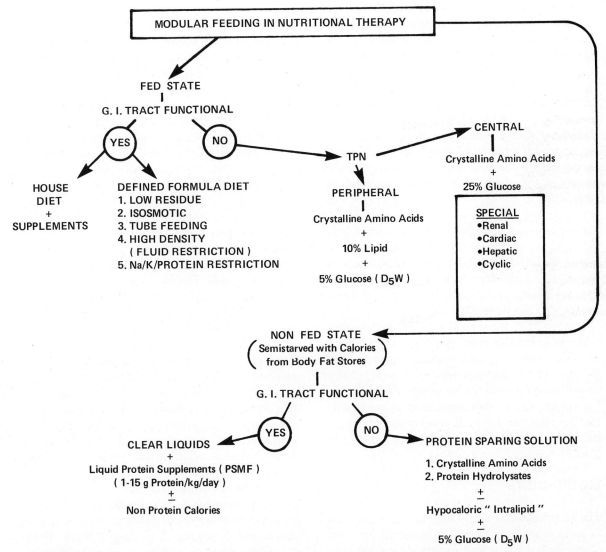

FIGURE 40-2. Modular feeding. In all available therapies, consideration is given to two nutritional states (fed and semistarved), and two possible means of delivery (enteral and parenteral). The use of this concept is depicted in this algorithm which allows a systematic approach to nutritional support. PSMF = protein-sparing modified fast. (Reprinted with permission from Blackburn, G. L., et al: *Manual for Nutritional/Metabolic Assessment of the Hospitalized Patient.* Boston, Mass., Nutrition Support Service, New England Deaconess Hospital, Harvard Medical School, 1976.)

or "nonfed" state and the route of administration, enteral or parenteral. Combinations of the various feeding categories are implied from this figure as, in many instances, both parenteral and enteral feedings are used to obtain the "fed" requirements.[11]

Enteral Nutrition

SUPPLEMENTAL FEEDINGS

A supplemental feeding is employed to augment the diet of an individual who otherwise would not receive adequate nutrition. The candidate for routine supplements may be able to ingest food orally, but essential nutrients are not being ingested in adequate quantities. Trauma from injuries, disease, surgical procedures, mastication, and emotional problems can increase the necessity for supplemental nutrition. The selection of the type of product, or food used to supplement the diet, depends on the client's ability to digest and utilize nutrients as well as the ability of the feeding to meet the client's needs.

If the client has the ability to eat, the simplest method of augmenting the diet is to provide regular food and to modify the diet with nutritional supplements. The addition of between meal snacks to increase the caloric intake may be employed. Foods that can be kept at the bedside and eaten throughout the day can be tried.[12]

Commercially formulated supplemental feedings that supply specific nutrients or meet special needs are given orally or by tube in liquid or powder form. Included in this category are high calorie, protein based, pure fat, pure carbohydrate electrolyte solutions, low sodium, and renal preparations.[12] If the client is able to ingest food, these preparations can be added to regular foods to increase nutrient intake.

LIQUID DIETS

The client with difficulty in ingesting large amounts of solid foods may benefit from liquid formulas. These diets are designed to provide enteral nutrition for clients who must be tube-fed or who are unable to chew or swallow. Clients with long-term gastrostomy, major surgery of the head and neck, radical surgery of the alimentary tract, neurological problems, psychological problems, and those requiring forced feeding beyond their voluntary intake, are candidates for a liquid diet.[13]

Frequently, a few servings are provided in a bottle and left on ice by the client's bedside. He is then encouraged to sip the supplement throughout the day. Palatability may be enhanced by the addition of flavorings. In some circumstances, supplements can be administered in the same manner as a medication.

There is a whole category of complete nutritional feedings. These preparations are designed to meet all nutritional requirements of the client when caloric needs are satisfied. These feedings may be supplied orally or by tube. If the client has the ability to ingest sufficient quantities of liquid orally, preparing a determined quantity of formula, leaving it in an ice bath beside the bed, and encouraging the client to sip the formula usually meets the nutrient requirements if all of the feeding is consumed.

TUBE FEEDINGS

When it is necessary to intubate a client for feeding, careful attention must be given to the selection and administration of the feeding. Tube feedings are prepared by mechanically processing regular foods into a thin purée. The foods used in these feedings are readily available and inexpensive. However, the consistency and coagulability necessitates the use of large lumen feeding tubes, which must be flushed after use. In addition, a sufficient volume of water must be provided to prevent a *solute overload* and *hypertonic dehydration*. It is often difficult to maintain a high degree of sanitation in the preparation and storage of these feedings.

The aforementioned commercially prepared complete liquid diets may be tube-fed. These are sterile and also relatively inexpensive. For those clients with a lactose intolerance, commercial lactose-free products are available.

Clients' tolerance to tube feedings can be maximized by diluting the initial feedings and beginning with a limited volume of feeding. If there are no side effects, nausea, vomiting, or diarrhea, the concentration and the volume can be slowly increased until the desired level of each can be reached. Water (50–75 ml) should be flushed through the tube before and after each feeding and should be administered between feedings to provide adequate hydration.

The evaluation of a client's progress from less concentrated to more concentrated and increased volume feedings is determined by client tolerance and by monitoring laboratory data, weight, and fluid intake and output. Physician's orders should include diet, caloric intake, and fluids. Close cooperation among the health team members is mandatory to assess client's nutritional needs, and to plan, implement, and evaluate appropriate feedings to ensure sound nutrition.[13]

CHEMICALLY DEFINED FORMULAS

Chemically defined formula or ''elemental'' diets provide nutrients in an easily digestible and absorbable form, particularly for clients with alimentary tract diseases. Chemically defined diets provide an intermediate step between high calorie intravenous nutrition and oral ingestion, or tube-feeding, of normal food.

There is a wide variety of disease modalities in which chemically defined formula diets are indicated, including inflammatory bowel disease, bowel fistulas, short bowel syndrome, acute pancreatitis, vascular disease, trauma, neurologic disturbances, accelerated metabolism, and protein-calorie malnutrition.[14]

Chemically defined formula diets furnish essential and nonessential L-amino acids. Some contain protein hydrolysates, simple sugars, minimal fat (essential fatty acids), electrolytes, minerals, and trace elements excluding cobalt, water, and fat-soluble vitamins (except vitamin K). These diets have several advantages over high calorie, high protein supplements or tube feedings. The bulk-free and virtually fat-free composition requires minimal digestion, thereby bypassing the digestive need for most pancreatic and biliary secretions. Because of the absence of digestible material, stool volume is reduced.[15]

Chemically defined formula diets may be administered orally or by feeding tube. All of these diets are hypertonic in normal dilution. Oral feedings are flavored to increase palatability of the amino acid solutions. The diets should be ingested slowly in small amounts due to the high osmolality of the

products. Tube feedings should be diluted and small in volume, again due to the high osmolality. If the client can tolerate the feeding without nausea, vomiting, or diarrhea, the concentration and then the volume can be increased until the desired caloric and protein intake is reached.

These diets have fixed compounding of products which make it necessary to have many products available. The concept of modular feeding was designed for this reason. The selection of one or two basic diets which provide maintenance nutrition appears adequate. These products can be supplemented with a variety of single nutrient compounds: carbohydrates, proteins, and fats. Indications for the modified and the standard defined formula diet are derived from protein utilization.

Parenteral Nutrition

Parenteral nutrition concerns the administration of nutrients by routes other than the gastrointestinal tract. Standard solutions of fluid and calories can be supplied by routine intravenous therapy for temporary situations, such as postoperative care. Each liter of 5 percent dextrose in water yields 50g of carbohydrate or 200 calories. However, this conventional intravenous therapy does not provide sufficient calories to permit utilization of administered amino acids unless very large volumes of water are used. Continued negative caloric and nitrogen balances result in gradual losses of tissue and if prolonged, in debilitation. Standard intravenous feeding is unable to improve the nutritional status of the already malnourished client.[16]

Parenteral nutrition may be partial or total. In many instances the client is able to sustain himself only partially by the oral route and needs some assistance through an alternate means. When the client is unable to eat normally, and not sustain himself nutritionally, total parenteral nutrition may be implemented.

The concept of total parenteral nutrition (TPN) or hyperalimentation was demonstrated by Dudrick.[17] To support protein synthesis, in the absence of oral intake, it is necessary to provide sufficient calories to permit utilization of amino acids. This requires a high concentration of glucose given simultaneously with amino acids. The resulting hyperosmolar solution can cause sclerosis of peripheral veins, so it must be introduced into a central vein.

The primary purpose of total parenteral nutrition is to maintain or improve nutritional status. It is indicated only when oral or tube feedings are contraindicated or insufficient, or when conventional intravenous therapy is no longer sufficient.[16]

Total parenteral nutrition can provide nutrition support for the client during various complex illnesses and under such circumstances that the nutrition can be thought of as a secondary modality, such as in preoperative weight loss, postoperative support, short gut syndrome, acute pancreatitis, burns, chemotherapy, radiologic therapy, coma, central nervous system disorders, or anorexia nervosa. In other instances, total parenteral nutrition can be considered a primary therapy. In such cases, oral intake usually ceases, and nutritive needs are provided by the parenteral route as in enterocutaneous fistulas, inflammatory bowel disease, acute renal failure, cardiac failure, and hepatic failure.[18]

The decision to institute total parenteral nutrition is a clinical one and should be made after consideration of many factors. When the clinical situation is such that prolonged maintenance or improvement in nutritional status assists in the recovery of the client, total parenteral nutrition should be considered. TPN is used only on carefully selected clients. In most cases it is not employed to extend the life of the hopelessly ill client or used in routine care.

Each prospective client must be evaluated. Total parenteral nutrition may be considered if the client's edema-free body weight falls approximately 10 percent below ideal body weight, if there is no apparent prospect for improvement, or if standard intravenous feedings have been utilized for about 10 days as the primary nutrient source, and there is no immediate prospect for improvement.[16] Prior to the start of total parenteral nutrition, the client's nutritional requirements, tolerance for fluid, nitrogen, glucose, and minerals must be assessed.

Once the decision has been made to institute total parenteral nutrition, the insertion of a superior vena cava catheter is necessary for the infusion of hypertonic solutions. The catheter permits the administration of solutions into a high blood flow rate where rapid dilution occurs and therefore reduces the occurrence of phlebitis and thrombosis. In pediatric clients the jugular vein is used as the superior vena cava is too small. Catheter placement is a surgical technique and should be done under rigid aseptic conditions. Following catheter placement, a slow infusion of 5 percent dextrose in water solution is administered until a chest x-ray confirms placement.

The solution used for total parenteral nutrition should contain nutrients equivalent to those of a well-balanced diet. The solution itself contains calories, nitrogen, minerals, vitamins, electrolytes, and water. Concentrated dextrose is the most common calorie source. The typical solution contains approximately 25 percent dextrose and 4-5 percent protein hydrolysates or crystalline amino acids in water. Vitamins, minerals, micronutrients, and water constitute the remainder of the solution. The clinical needs of the client determine the protein, electrolyte and glucose loads. Water is administered according to the renal and cardiovascular requirements and should replace normal fluid loss. Each client's needs are considered individually. For those clients with renal or hepatic disease, specially formulated solutions are available.

Generally, each liter of solution contains 1000 calories and 6.25 g of nitrogen. The solutions for pediatric clients require slight modification from the adult formula. The glucose concentration varies from 10 to 30 percent, depending on the needs of the child. Calcium, phosphorus, iron, trace elements, and all vitamins must be added to the solution of growing children because of the lack of reserve stores of these nutrients.[19]

As the nutritional solution is hypertonic a large bore vein with a high flow rate must be catheterized to dilute the solution and prevent thrombophlebitis. The insertion carries a small but definite risk. The heart and major vessel may be perforated, with extravasation of blood or solutions, blood vessel obstruction, pneumothorax, and air embolism.

Catheter related sepsis, bacterial or fungal, is one of the most dangerous complications related to total parenteral nutrition. Strict aseptic technique should be maintained during care of the catheter (and the site), solution preparation, and dressing changes.[20]

Hyperglycemia may present a problem, particularly in the client with glucose intolerance. Hyperglycemia can lead to osmotic diuresis, dehydration, and nonketotic hyperosmolar syndrome leading to coma. By gradually increasing the quantity of solution, endogenous insulin is usually increased and

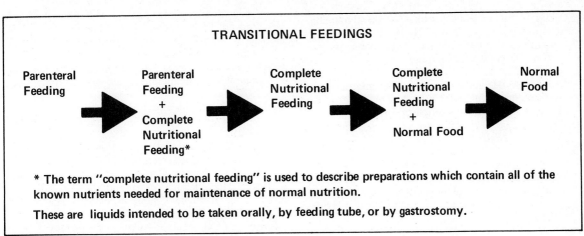

FIGURE 40-3. Transitional feedings. (Reprinted with permission from Dialogues in Nutrition. Health Learning Systems, Inc., Bloomfield, N.J., 1977.)

an induced hyperinsulinemic state occurs. When total parenteral nutrition is discontinued, the infusion rate is tapered and the client is monitored for glucose intolerance, and if necessary, insulin is added.[20]

TRANSITIONAL DIETS

Once the decision has been made to discontinue total parenteral nutrition and to institute oral or tube feedings, the client is not always able to tolerate or ingest sufficient calories to meet his needs for the first few days. It is necessary to overlap the parenteral and enteral feedings for several days prior to discontinuing the total parenteral nutrition. Figure 40-3 represents the transition from each of the various treatment modalities to the next. Failure to consider this transition may lead to the client's not receiving adequate amounts of calories and protein. These principles apply to the transition from tube feedings to oral feedings as well.[21]

REFERENCES

1. *Taber's Cyclopedic Medical Dictionary,* 13th ed. Philadelphia, F. A. Davis Co., 1977.
2. Malnutrition in the hospital. *Dialog. Nutr.* 2(2):1, 1977.
3. Bistrian, B. R., et al.: Protein status of general surgical patients. *J. Am. Med. Assoc.* 230:858, 1974.
4. Bistrian, B. R., et al.: Prevalence of malnutrition in general medical patients. *J. Am. Med. Assoc.* 235:1567, 1976.
5. Butterworth, C. E., Jr.: Malnutrition in the hospital. *J. Am. Med. Assoc.* 230:879, 1974.
6. Law, D. K., Dudrick, S. J., and Abdou, N. I.: The effects of protein-calorie malnutrition on immune competence. *Surg. Gynecol. Obstet.* 139:257, 1974.
7. Bistrian, B. R., et al.: Cellular immunity in semistarved states in hospitalized adults. *Am. J. Clin. Nutr.* 28:1148, 1975.
8. Blackburn, G. L. et al.: Manual for nutritional/metabolic assessment of the hospitalized patient. Presented at the Clinical Congress of the American College of Surgeons, Chicago, Ill., 1976.
9. Blackburn, G. L., and Bistrian, B. R.: Nutrition support resources in hospital practice, in *Nutrition Support of Medical Practice,* edited by Schneider, H. A., Anderson, C. E., and Coursin, D. B., New York, Harper and Row Publishers, 1977.
10. Wade, J. E.: Role of a clinical dietitian specialist on a nutrition support service. *J. Am. Diet. Assoc.* 70:185, 1977.
11. Blackburn, G. L., and Bistrian, B. R.: Curative nutrition: protein calorie management, in *Nutrition Support of Medical Practice,* edited by Schneider, H. A., Anderson, C. E., and Coursin, D. B., New York, Harper and Row Publishers, 1977.
12. The patient who can't eat. *Dialog. Nutr.* 1(2):2, 1976.
13. Randall, H. T.: Enteral nutrition, in *Manual of Surgical Nutrition,* edited by Committee on Pre- and Postoperative Care, American College of Surgeons, Philadelphia, W. B. Saunders, Company, 1975.
14. Kark, R. M.: Liquid formula and chemically defined diets. *J. Am. Diet. Assoc.* 64:476, 1974.
15. Randall, H. T.: Diet in the care of surgical patients, in *Modern Nutrition in Health and Disease,* edited by Goodhart, R. S., and Shills, M. E., Philadelphia, Lea and Febiger, 1977.

16. Shills, M. E.: Guidelines for total parenteral nutrition. *J. Am. Med. Assoc.* 220:1721, 1972.
17. Dudrick, S. J., et al.: Long term total parenteral nutrition with growth, development and positive nitrogen balance. *Surgery* 64:134, 1968.
18. Abbott, W. M.: Indications for parenteral nutrition, in *Total Parenteral Nutrition,* edited by Fisher, J. E., Boston, Little, Brown Company, 1976.
19. Dudrick, S. J., et al.: Intravenous hyperalimentation. *Med. Clin. North Am.* 54:577, 1970.
20. Meng, H. C.: Parenteral nutrition, in *Nutrition Support of Medical Practice,* edited by Schneider, H. A., Anderson, C. E., and Coursin, D. B., New York, Harper and Row Publishers, 1977.
21. Nutrition in stress and starvation. *Dialog. Nutr.* 1(3):7, 1976.

BIBLIOGRAPHY

Bistrian, B. R.: Nutritional Assessment and therapy of protein-calorie malnutrition in the hospital. *J. Am. Diet. Assoc.* 71:393, 1977.

Blackburn, G. L., and Bistrian, B. R.: Iatrogenic malnutrition. II. A report from Boston. *Nutr. Today* 9:30, 1974.

Blackburn, G. L., et al.: Nutritional and metabolic assessment of the hospitalized patient. *J. Enteral Parenteral Nutr.* 1:11, 1977.

Bollet, A. J., and Owens, S. O.: Evaluation of nutritional status of selected hospitalized patients. *Am. J. Clin. Nutr.* 26:931, 1973.

Bury, K. D., Stephens, R. V., and Randall, H. T.: The use of chemically defined liquid, elemental diet for nutritional management of fistulas of the alimentary tract. *Am. J. Surg.* 121:174, 1971.

Butterworth, C. E., Jr.: Iatrogenic malnutrition: the skeleton in the hospital closet. *Nutr. Today* 9:2, 1974.

Chernoff, R., and Bloch, A. S.: Liquid feedings: considerations and alterations. *J. Am. Diet. Assoc.* 70:389, 1977.

Committee on Pre- and Postoperative care, American College of Surgeons: *Manual of Surgical Nutrition,* 2nd ed. Philadelphia, W. B. Saunders Co., 1975.

Cooley, R., and Phillips, K.: Helping with hyperalimentation. *Nurs '73* 3:6, 1973.

Cowan, G., Jr., and Scheetz, W.: *Intravenous hyperalimentation.* Philadelphia, Lea and Febiger, Inc., 1972

Dudrick, S. J., and Ruberg, R. L.: Principles and practice of parenteral nutrition. *Gastroenterology* 61:901, 1971.

Duke, J. H., and Dudrick, S. J.: Parenteral feeding, in *Manual of Surgical Nutrition,* by Committee on Pre- and Postoperative Care, American College of Surgeons, Philadelphia, W. B. Saunders Co., 1975.

Fisher, J. E. (ed): *Total Parenteral Nutrition.* Boston, Little, Brown Co., 1976.

Greenberg, G. R., et al.: Protein-sparing therapy in postoperative patients—effects of added hypocaloric glucose or lipid. *N. Engl. J. Med.* 297:1104. 1977.

Goodhart, R. S., and Shills, M. E. (eds.): *Modern Nutrition in Health and Disease,* 5th ed. Philadelphia, Lea and Febiger, Inc., 1973.

Jelliffe, D. B.: *The Assessment of Nutritional Status of the Community.* Geneva, World Health Organization, 1966.

Law, D. K.: Total parenteral nutrition. *N. Eng. J. Med.* 297:1104, 1977.

MacFadden, B. V., and Dudrick, S. J. (ed): Total parenteral nutrition of the critically ill patient. *Diet. Curr.* 5(1):1, 1978.

Melling R. L.: Iatrogenic malnutrition. III. The institutional system. *Nutr. Today* 9:34, 1974.

Nutritional Principles of Nasogastric Tube Feeding. Columbus, Ohio, Ross Laboratories.

Schnieder, H. A., Anderson, C. E., and Coursin, D. B. (eds.): *Nutrition Support of Medical Practice.* New York, Harper and Row Publishers, 1977.

The patient who won't eat. *Dialog. Nutr.* 1(1):1, 1976.

Thiel, V.: *Clinical Nutrition.* St. Louis, C. V. Mosby Company, 1976.

Tobias, A. L., and Van Italie, T. B.: *Nutritional problems of hospitalized patients. J. Am. Diet. Assoc.* 71:253, 1977.

Total parenteral nutrition. *Pediatr. Curr.* 24:66, 1975.

CHAPTER 41

GLOSSARY

Blakemore-Sengstaken tube. Oral-gastric tube used for the specific purpose of stopping bleeding from esophageal and gastric varices by tamponade.

decompression. Removal of gas and fluid from the gastrointestinal tract by nasogastric or intestinal tube by gravity drainage or suction.

distention. Bloated or inflated gastrointestinal tract.

gastrointestinal tubes. Tubes used for drainage or instillation of fluids or air within the gastrointestinal system inserted through normal anatomical orifices or incisional opening into the gastrointestinal tract.

gastrostomy tube. A rubber or plastic tube used for decompression or feeding; inserted into the stomach through an incision in the abdominal wall.

gavage. Introduction of liquids, food, or medication into the stomach through a tube passed through the nose or mouth by way of the esoph-

CARE OF THE CLIENT WITH GASTROINTESTINAL INTUBATION

Barbara Bihm, M.S.N., R.N., and
Major Faith Sterling, M.S., R.N.

agus into the stomach or portions of the small intestine.

intake and output record (I and O). A form used to record the client's fluid intake, the route of ingestion (mouth, vein, or rectum), the dosage of fluid, and waste within a given period of time.

intubation. Insertion of a tube into the body.

lavage. Washing out a cavity. In this chapter, it pertains to the removal of substances from the stomach or intestine by tube.

lumen. Opening diameter of a tube.

NPO. Nothing per os, usually stated in relation to no oral intake permitted.

parotitis. Inflammation of the parotid glands.

peristalsis. The alternating, involuntary, contraction and relaxation of the alimentary tract which propels material through the gastrointestinal tract.

replacement therapy. Intravenous solutions given in equal amounts to the quantity of contents withdrawn from the stomach or intestine when a client's GI tract is being decompressed.

sump tube. A tube used primarily for decompres-sion which has an air line incorporated into its structure as well as its primary lumen for drainage. The purpose of the air vent is to prevent the tube from adhering to the lining of the gastrointestinal tract and occluding the drainage lumen.

tamponade. The production of pressure against an object (such as the esophagus) by insertion of a tube surrounded by a balloon which is then inflated.

tube feeding. Administration of nutrients in liquid form through a tube into the gastrointestinal tract, most commonly through a nasogastric or gastrostomy tube.

varices. Tortuous (twisted) dilated veins.

The gastrointestinal system, commonly referred to as the alimentary canal, is essentially a hollow muscular tube extending from the oral cavity to the anus. The churning and forward propulsion of food, the secretion of digestive juices and enzymes, the absorption of the resultant elemental nutrients, and the elimination of solid wastes are the life sustaining processes accomplished in the gastrointestinal tract.

Interruption of these normal functions or the presence of abnormal conditions in the alimentary canal may warrant *intubation,* that is, insertion of a tube into the gastrointestinal system. There are two types of tubes, gastric and intestinal, utilized in gastrointestinal intubation. *Gastric tubes* are introduced into the stomach by way of the nose or nasopharynx (nasogastric tubes) and occasionally the oropharynx (mouth). Gastric tubes, also referred to as *short tubes,* are utilized when intubation of the stomach is required, because they are long enough to reach the stomach (and possibly the duodenum) but not the bowel.[1] They may also be introduced by a gastrostomy, which is a surgical opening in the abdominal wall, through which a tube is introduced into the stomach; it is then sutured in place. *Intestinal tubes* extend past the stomach into the intestines. These tubes, commonly referred to as *long tubes,* are of sufficient length to extend into a portion of or the entire length of the small intestine. The reasons for gastrointestinal intubation—diagnostic procedures, decompression, gavage, and lavage—are discussed in detail in this chapter.

EQUIPMENT

Types of Tubes

To provide optimal care, the nurse must be familiar with the numerous types of tubes utilized in gastrointestinal intubation, the intended purpose of intubation, and other important general characteristics. The size of the lumen and the diameter of the tube are measured by the universal term "French" (abbreviated F). Gastrointestinal tubes generally range from 5 French (small) to 30 French (large). The length of the tube is determined by its destination; gastric tubes range from 36 to 50 inches, while intestinal tubes range from 6 to 10 feet for adults. The composition of the tube may be plastic, silastic, or silicone, in which case the tube is clear, or rubber, in which case it is opaque. Another important characteristic to consider is the number of lumens; a tube may be a one, two, or three lumen tube. A one lumen tube has only one exterior opening, usually for drainage. A double lumen tube has two exterior openings, one for drainage and one which serves as an air vent or as an opening

to allow inflation of a balloon. The air vent reduces the possibility of occlusion of the drainage lumen by sucking the stomach or intestinal mucosa into the lumen. Tubes which have air vents are called sump tubes; both gastric and intestinal tubes can be sump tubes. Triple lumen tubes have three exterior openings, and like the double lumen, these appear as a single tube (Fig. 41-1).[2]

By far the most common gastrointestinal tube is the *Levin* tube. This short tube is used for gastric lavage, gavage, and aspiration of gastric contents. The *Ewald* tube is another short tube that is used primarily for washing out poisons and aspiration of large quantities from the stomach. This tube has a larger lumen than the Levin tube and is usually inserted in the stomach via the oral cavity. Both the Levin and the Ewald are single lumen tubes.[3]

The plastic *Salem sump* tube is a double lumen, short tube which can be used for aspiration of gastric contents, gavage, or lavage. One lumen is for the removal of gastric secretions while the second lumen serves as an air vent to prevent the build-up of excessive negative pressure when attached to suction.[4]

Long tubes are used in the treatment of intestinal problems. The *Miller-Abbott,* used primarily for decompression, is the most common intestinal tube. This is a double lumen tube with a metal tip and a balloon on the end. One lumen is for the introduction of air, water, or mercury (instilled after insertion) to inflate the balloon. The other lumen is for drainage of intestinal contents. As the inflated balloon moves through the gastrointestinal tract, it stimulates peristalsis and prevents, locates, or breaks up obstructions. Aspiration of intestinal contents occurs at the end and side of the Miller-Abbott tube (Fig. 41-2).

The *Harris* tube is a single lumen mercury weighted tube with metal sleeves on each end of a small rubber bag. Approximately 4 ml of mercury are instilled in the rubber bag before insertion. The weight of the mercury carries the bag by gravity through the intestinal tract. The purposes of the Harris tube are decompression and lavage of the intestinal tract (see Fig. 41-2).

The *Cantor* tube is another single lumen, long intestinal tube. In this tube, the mercury filled balloon is at the extreme end of the tube. Depending on the age, size, and condition of the client, between 1.5 to 10 ml of mercury are injected into the

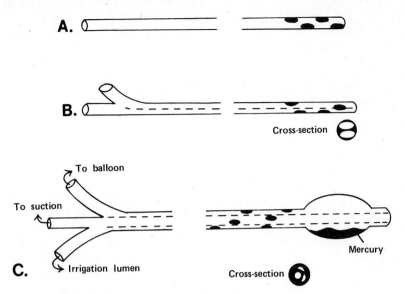

FIGURE 41-1. Lumen tubes. A, single; B, double; and C, triple.

balloon prior to insertion. Numerous large holes are along the sides of the tube to allow for the removal of gas and fluids (Fig. 41-2).

The *Blakemore-Sengstaken* is a naso- or oral-gastric tube which is used to stop bleeding esophageal or gastric varices. The underlying pathology associated with esophageal varices is portal hypertension, which is related to numerous medical conditions but is commonly seen with cirrhosis of the liver. The Blakemore-Sengstaken tube is a triple lumen tube with three distinct features: (1) an elongated balloon placed in the esophagus; (2) a small balloon placed in the stomach against the cardioesophageal junction; and (3) the catheter portion used to decompress the stomach as well as to offer an avenue for the instillation of iced saline. These outlets should be clearly marked as esophageal balloon, gastric balloon, and gastric lumen (drainage) (Fig. 41-3). Refer to a medical-surgical textbook for the care of a client with a Blakemore-Sengstaken tube.

Suction Devices

A thorough understanding of the scientific principles related to the functioning of various other kinds of equipment associated with gastrointestinal tubes is critical. The creation of a vacuum, and consequently suction, is essential for effective decompression. There are several types of suction devices available, ranging from the simple siphon suction to electrical suction pumps. Regardless of the type of equipment utilized, the general objective is the same—removal of fluid and air from the gastrointestinal tract.

The *siphon* method of removing gastric or intestinal contents is dependent upon air pressure gradients or differences in atmospheric pressure. A siphon is a bent tube with arms of unequal length, where the short arm is in the stomach and the long arm extends outside the body (Fig. 41-4). Since gastric contents exert pressure because of their weight, if the long arm of the gastrointestinal tube contains some fluid and is positioned below the level of the stomach, gastric contents will flow out through the long arm.[5]

If gastric contents can be extracted by lowering the long arm of the gastrointestinal tube, then it follows that if the long arm is elevated above the level of the stomach, fluids (food and medications) can be instilled. The law of gravity is the basic underlying principle here.

Several methods of creating gastric suction are dependent on a form of hydraulic suction, which in turn is based on the principle that a vacuum can be created when a column of fluid is allowed to

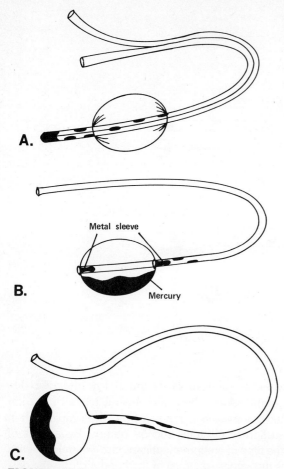

FIGURE 41-2. Intestinal tubes. A, Miller Abbott; B, Harris; and C, Cantor.

flow from a higher level to a lower level. Simple *gravity suction* is one method of creating a vacuum, utilizing the principle of hydraulic suction. As seen in Figure 41-5, a bottle partially filled with fluid is suspended above the level of the client's stomach. A rubber connecting tube extends from the suspended bottle to a similarly sized bottle, which is placed below the level of the stomach. The flow of the fluid from the suspended bottle to the lower bottle creates a vacuum;[6] thus, subatmospheric pressure exists. Since gastric contents are normally at atmospheric pressure, the direction of flow of the gastric contents will be from an area of higher pressure to an area of lower pressure, or into the upper bottle.[7] This type of set-up presumes an air-tight system. The force of the suction may be modified by increasing or decreasing the distance between the stomach and the lower bottle. If the lower bottle is raised, the force of the suction decreases.[3]

The *three bottle method* of gravity suction is merely a modification of the set-up just described. The principle is exactly the same, except a third bottle is introduced to collect the gastric contents (Fig. 41-6). This third bottle allows for easy examination and measurement of extracted gastric contents.[3]

Both the simple gravity suction and the three-bottle method are used when electric power is not available. These methods have been replaced by safer and more reliable electric suction pumps (Fig. 41-7), which function on the principle that by varying the temperature of air and thus the pressure of air, a vacuum can be created. Air is heated in a compartment in the electric pump. Some air is allowed to escape, and the remaining air is cooled, thus creating a vacuum.[3] The Gomco-Thermotic pump is a suction pump that operates on this principle. This device provides intermittent suction and some degree of control over the force of suction (high-low).

Many institutions have suction outlets over the client's bed, which provide continuous suction that can be regulated according to the client's needs and the physician's orders. Optimal negative pressure is considered between 75 to 100 cm of water.

In general, only low pressure intermittent suction is used for decompression because excessive negative pressure causes the gastric or intestinal mucosa to be sucked into the drainage holes of the gastrointestinal tube. Salem sump tubes should be used with continuous suction. Intermittent suction should be avoided with these tubes since the air vent continuously allows air to enter the stomach; therefore, it must be kept free of secretions at all times if the Salem sump tube is to function effectively.[8]

REASONS FOR GASTROINTESTINAL INTUBATION

Gastrointestinal intubation may be performed for the following four reasons: diagnostic procedures, decompression, gavage, and lavage.

Diagnostic Procedures

In general, all types of tubes can be utilized for a diagnostic procedure. When a specimen is required from the gastrointestinal tract, an irrigating syringe or some type of suction apparatus is needed. Di-

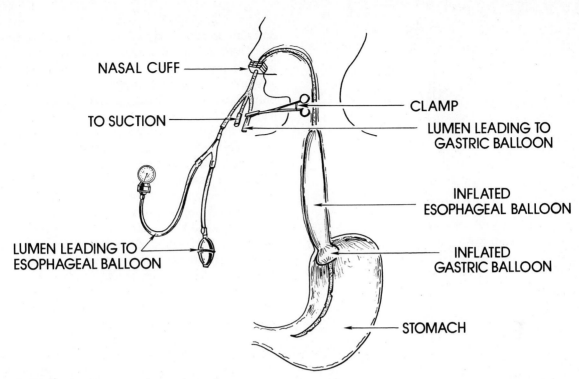

FIGURE 41-3. Blakemore-Sengstaken tube.

agnostic procedures may include: (1) collecting specimens for cytologic and gastric analysis; (2) determining the secretory ability of the stomach by measuring the volume output of gastric secretions at specific time intervals; and (3) visualization of various segments of the gastrointestinal tract under fluoroscopy by instillation of radiopaque material via the tube.

The nurse's responsibility varies with each procedure performed. However, an understanding of the medical orders and thorough explanations to the client and his family concerning the intubation are essential. Specific points to consider are: (1) knowing when the procedure is required and the length of time needed to accomplish the procedure; (2) type of equipment required; (3) recognizing the signs and symptoms that the client may experience indicating complications; and (4) recording data (see Chapter 44, "Diagnostic Tests").

Decompression

The use of gravity drainage or suction to remove fluid and air from the gastrointestinal tract is known as decompression. The absence or slowing of peristalsis causes fluid and gas to collect in the gastroin-

testinal tract resulting in abdominal distention and vomiting. Decompression is used with clients presenting overt signs of interrupted peristalsis and clients who may develop obstruction; for example, decompression may be used preoperatively to circumvent potential problems. Decompression is

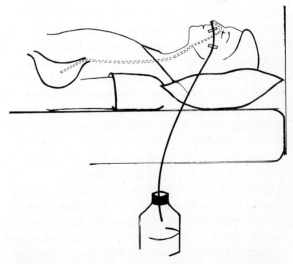

FIGURE 41-4. Drainage by the siphon method is attained by positioning of the gastric tube below the level of the stomach.

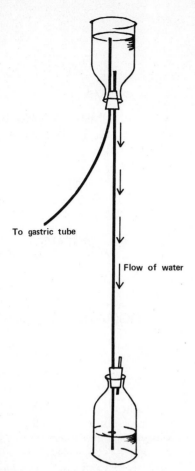

a mouth breather due to the occlusion of one nostril. Oral and nasal hygiene, therefore, are extremely important for the client's comfort and safety. Good oral hygiene prevents mucous membrane crustation, halitosis, parotitis, and oral distaste. A client who is not permitted anything by mouth (NPO) may still use a toothbrush, mouthwash, and toothpaste provided he does not swallow any of the substances. Nostrils should be inspected for tissue trauma due to the irritation from the tube. The nostrils should be kept clean and well lubricated. If tape is anchoring the tube to the face, the tape should be removed and replaced every 2 days and the skin underneath inspected and cleaned. This nursing care can be applied to any client with a gastrointestinal tube in place.

FIGURE 41-5. Gravity suction.

commonly used postoperatively when peristalsis is interrupted following surgical manipulation of the bowel, after general anesthesia, and in the early postoperative phase of gastric or intestinal surgery.[1]

The Levin and Salem sump tubes are most commonly utilized for gastric decompression while the Miller-Abbott, Cantor, and Harris tubes are most frequently used for intestinal decompression. (See previous discussion of the different types of tubes.) Some type of suction apparatus is necessary to remove secretions from the gastrointestinal tract.

An intake and output record is always kept on the client who has a gastrointestinal tube in place for decompression to monitor his physiological state in regard to fluid balance, volume, and composition of drainage material. The client is not usually allowed oral intake, particularly if the tube is in the stomach. Because the client is intubated, most commonly through the nose, he will probably be

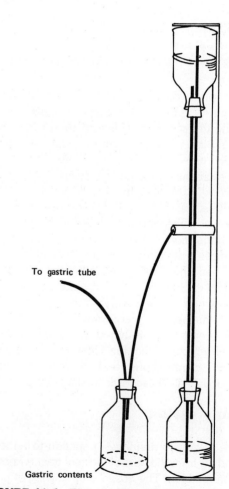

FIGURE 41-6. Three bottle method of gravity suction.

IRRIGATION

Normally, a client with gastrointestinal intubation has a medical order for irrigation of the tube to keep it patent and draining (see Table 41-2 on lavage procedures). Normal saline is usually used for irrigation; sterile or distilled water should not be used since frequent irrigations may contribute to hyponatremia (sodium depletion). The amount of solution ordered varies, but in most cases it is between 30 and 50 ml. There are two ways to do the irrigation. With the first method, 30–50 ml of normal saline are instilled through the drainage lumen of the tube which has been disconnected from the suction equipment. After instillation of the irrigating solution, the tube is reconnected to the suction machine. In the second method, 30–50 ml of normal saline are instilled through the drainage lumen, and the fluid is aspirated into the syringe by drawing back on the plunger of the syringe. In both cases, the irrigation should be reflected on the client's intake and output record.

With the advent of the sump tube used for decompression, the nurse may use the air vent for irrigation; thus, she may not need to disconnect the tube from the suction machine during this procedure. One problem frequently encountered is that the air vent may begin to drain even though the tube is connected to suction; this is due to siphoning. Thus, if the air vent is used for irrigation, the nurse must follow the fluid irrigation with 10–15 ml of air to clear the air vent of fluid and counteract the siphoning effect. The nurse should never tie off the air vent to prevent drainage, otherwise the sump tube becomes identical to the single lumen tube and counteracts the purpose of the air vent.[9]

REPLACEMENT THERAPY

The client who has a gastrointestinal tube for decompression is usually given replacement therapy of intravenous solution in amounts equal to the quantity of the contents withdrawn from the stomach or intestine. The solution is ordered by the physician, but the nurse must make constant adjustments to the intravenous fluid rate. Take for example the client who is to receive 5 percent dextrose and water (D5%W) at 125 ml/hour as *basic maintenance*. In addition, an order is written for "cc for cc replacement" of stomach or intestinal

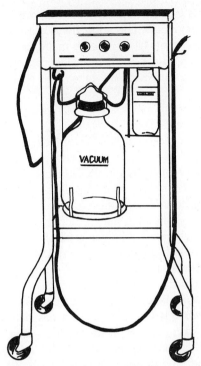

FIGURE 41-7. Electric suction pump. Adaption from Gomco Thermotic Pump.

drainage. Specifically, for a client who has 600 ml drainage in 6 hours, the replacement order is 5 percent dextrose and half normal saline with 20 mEq of potassium chloride "cc for cc" of drainage. The client now receives 125 ml of D5%W (basic maintenance) plus 100 ml of D5%1/2 NS with 20 mEq of potassium chloride (replacement) each hour for 6 hours or a total of 225 ml/hour. Each time decompression contents are measured, replacement therapy must be accounted for and the intravenous rate readjusted. The nurse must keep accurate intake and output records reflecting maintenance therapy and replacement therapy.

MONITORING THE CLIENT

The client with a gastrointestinal tube in place for decompression must be constantly monitored. The following discussion relates to electric suction pumps (Gomco-Thermotic pumps) since these are most frequently used. Decompression can be accomplished by attaching the gastrointestinal tube to intermittent suction via a 5 in 1 connecting adapter. The gastrointestinal tube should never be clamped unless this is ordered by the physician to test the client's tolerance.[10] The nurse may utilize a variety of indicators that will alert her to malfunction of the decompression set-up. If the client becomes distended, vomits around the tube, or if no drainage appears in the suction bottle after 1 hour, this would indicate a malfunction which must be investigated immediately.

The first checkpoint is to determine whether or not the suction machine is operational by checking the presence of suction in the drainage bottle. If it is operating correctly, as the bottle is disconnected and the vacuum is broken, there will be a "hiss" as air rushes into the bottle. If there is no "hiss" of air, the machine is inadequately functioning; therefore, it should be checked to determine whether or not it is turned on and the setting is correct. Also, a firm connection of the machine to the power source should be checked. Next, note whether the tube is connected properly or if it has been inadvertently clamped off. If these steps have been taken and all functions are operational, it is time to irrigate the tube to assure tubal patency. As a last resort, the tube may be advanced or withdrawn about an inch to be certain it has not adhered to the wall of the stomach or intestine. Be sure to retape the tube securely. If these measures fail to make the system operational, the physician should be notified. It may be necessary to insert a new tube. Caution: *This technique of advancement and withdrawal should not be employed if decompression is being performed to protect the suture line following gastric or intestinal surgery.*

RECORDING DATA

A final nursing responsibility is the accurate recording of pertinent data. The points to consider are: (1) the size and type of tube used and the nostril used for insertion; (2) client's symptoms and the effect of decompression; (3) description of the stomach or intestinal drainage; (4) output volumes recorded at specific time intervals; and (5) specimens collected along with specifics about any diagnostic procedures performed.

The gastrointestinal tube usually is removed once bowel function has returned to normal. Improved peristalsis will be indicated by flatus, defecation, or decreased drainage of secretions from the gastrointestinal tube.[10]

Gavage

Gavage is the process of introducing liquid feedings or medications through a gastric or intestinal tube. It is utilized when the functions of digestion, absorption, and elimination are intact. For example, gavage would be utilized with an infant who had a retarded sucking and swallowing reflex. The nasogastric tube is a temporary means of providing essential nutrients, while the gastrostomy is for long-term use.[11] The Levin (#16 F for adults) is the most frequently used tube for gastric gavage.

ADULTS

The procedure of intubation of the gavage tube is the same as for all other nasogastric tubes (Table 41-1). Either of two methods can be used to introduce feedings into the gastrointestinal tract. Feedings may be allowed to flow through a syringe by the force of gravity. The flow of the feeding can be altered by raising or lowering the syringe. If the distance between the stomach and syringe is increased, the flow increases, and if the distance is reduced, the flow decreases.[12] This method is frequently used when the client is on a meal-type feeding schedule. The second method is used when continuous gradual feeding is necessary. The nourishment is placed in a gavage bag that is suspended above the level of the client's stomach. The flow rate of the feeding can be regulated by adjusting the drop regulating clamp (similar to those on intravenous tubing). Mechanical pumps may be employed to provide more accuracy in regulating these continuous feedings.

Commercially prepared feedings are available; however, many institutions prepare nutritionally sound "blendorized" liquid diets. Generally, the client should receive between "2500 to 3000 ml of fluid through the tube daily."[13] Feedings should contain no more than 1 kcal/ml since feedings with a higher caloric concentration may precipitate the tube feeding syndrome (discussed later in this chapter).

The major responsibilities of the nurse in the care of a client receiving tube feedings are to: (1) check the tube placement to determine if it is in the desired position before each feeding; (2) correctly position the client into the semi-Fowler's position to reduce the possibility of aspiration pneumonia, should the client regurgitate during the feeding; (3) introduce the feeding media at room temperature (remove from the refrigerator for 1 hour) and at a safe and tolerable rate (gravity) to reduce the possibility of distention or diarrhea; (4) insure patency of the tube by flushing with approximately 30 ml of sterile water before and after feeding; (5) observe the client for dehydration from inadequate water intake in relation to client needs and osmolarity of the feeding media; and (6) cleanse and change equipment at least every 24 hours to reduce the occurrence of high bacterial counts within the equipment. If contaminated equipment is used bacterial diarrhea may occur and become an additional medical and nursing concern.

INFANTS AND CHILDREN

Nursing care specific to premature infants, neonates, and small children receiving gavage feedings is similar to that for the adult client except for the following points. The reservoir should be no higher than 6 to 8 inches above the infant's head during feeding. The rate and time should approximate normal bottle feeding (average is about 1 ml/minute). Following the feeding, the tube should be flushed with a small amount of sterile water to cleanse the tube and decrease the potential of bacterial growth. The infant should be held and burped during and following the feeding. Before beginning the next feeding, the tube should be checked for residual feeding medium in the stomach. Depending on the client's condition, the physician's preference, and the policy of the agency, the residual medium that is withdrawn may be subtracted from the feeding to be given; note that the residual feeding is always reinjected into the stomach to preserve the delicate balance of fluids and electrolytes. Occasionally, the physician prefers that the next feeding be temporarily withheld if one quarter or more of the amount of scheduled feeding is aspirated from the stomach. Following the feeding, the infant should be placed on his right side to minimize the potential of aspiration and regurgitation. If the gavage tube is removed and reinserted with each feeding, the tube must be clamped or pinched off so that media do not escape during withdrawal and accidently go into the lungs causing pneumonia. If the tube is left in place, it should be changed every 2 to 4 days.

TRACHEOTOMY CLIENT

There is a special problem involved with tube feeding a client who also has a tracheotomy (or tracheostomy) tube in place. Before introducing gavage feeding, the cuff of the tracheotomy tube should be inflated to prevent aspiration of the feeding media into the lung. After the feeding is completed, the cuff should remain inflated for an hour. If there is a question of aspiration during the feeding, the nurse should suction the client before deflating the cuff to prevent the collected feeding media from entering the lungs as the cuff is deflated.

After the administration of the gavage feeding, the nurse is responsible for charting and recording the intake and output. The notes entered should include such points as amount of media, type of media, method of administration, and the client's response to the feeding.

Lavage

Lavage is the process of washing out or irrigating the gastrointestinal tract, usually the stomach (gastric lavage), following the ingestion of various substances or prior to surgery (Table 41-2). The Ewald tube is frequently used for gastric lavage, particularly if large quantities must be aspirated from the stomach or if noxious substances (poisons) must be removed quickly. This tube has a larger lumen than the Levin tube and is usually inserted via the oropharynx (refer to Table 41-3). The Levin tube may also be used for gastric lavage. During episodes of gastric hemorrhage, lavage is performed with a solution of normal saline at 0°C (32°F) to promote hemostasis.[14]

The procedure for lavage, although relatively simple, is usually considered an emergency procedure. The prescribed irrigating solution is allowed to flow into the stomach by the force of gravity. After a portion of the irrigating solution has been instilled, the external portion of the tube is inverted to allow gastric contents to be removed utilizing the siphoning principle. Frequently suction is applied to the tube by means of an aspirating syringe or some other kind of suction apparatus, usually an electric suction pump (Gomco-Thermotic pump).

The nursing care related to managing a client undergoing lavage is similar to that of other procedures associated with gastrointestinal tubes. In

TABLE 41-1. Gavage (Tube Feeding or Medicating) When Client Refuses or Is Unable to Take Feeding Orally as a Result of Surgery, Treatment, or Physiologic Condition

Anticipated Accomplishment	Scientific Principles/ Rationale	Specific Considerations
1. Prepare client and equipment for intubation procedure.	In infants, oral passage is used because it prevents nasal membrane trauma, causes less airway interference, and reduces gag reflex.	With infants, oral passage is preferred. With adults nasal passage is usually preferred.
2. Select and assemble appropriate equipment.	Syringe is used to check placement of tube and may be used as receptacle for feeding media. Media should not be more osmolar than 1 kcal/ml or will cause diarrhea and dehydration.	
3. Ascertain location of nasogastric tube.	Tube must be in stomach to prevent feeding media from being instilled into lungs, causing aspiration pneumonia.	Three standard methods (aspiration, air and water) to check tube placement are discussed in this chapter.
4. Position client for tube feeding.	Correct position lessens chances of regurgitation and aspiration.	
5. Determine absorption of previous feeding.	If residual feeding remains, feedings are being administered at a faster rate than absorption is occurring.	
6. Administer gavage feeding.	Irrigation of tube insures patency.	Enough water should be given during feeding to prevent dehydration.

Implementation	Recommendations	Observations
Follow preparation and insertion procedure of nasogastric tube in Table 41-3 to point of gastric placement.	Generally nasogastric tube in infants is removed after each feeding, whereas tube is usually left in place in the adult client.	Restraints may be necessary with infants and children.
Assemble following equipment: Gavage set. Irrigation syringe.		
Feeding media that has been prescribed by physician.	Feeding media may be obtained from pharmacy or diet kitchen.	
Check placement of tube.		
Position client into semi-Fowler's position (conscious); lateral elevated position (comatose).		
With a syringe aspirate and then reinstill gastric contents to determine volume of previous feeding that has not been absorbed.	Generally if more than ¼ of previous feeding can be aspirated, next scheduled feeding is temporarily withheld for 1 hr and then rechecked for residual volume.	Palpate client's abdomen for distention.
Begin procedure by instilling 30–50 ml of distilled water into tube, via syringe.		Observe client for cramping.
Before system (syringe and tube) empties, pour in prescribed feeding media.	Rates/volume: adults: give maximum amounts of feeding, 500 ml over 15–30 min (average feeding consists of 150–200 ml); infants: 1ml/min; infant should be burped during and after feeding.	

Table 41-1. Continued

Anticipated Accomplishment	Scientific Principles/ Rationale	Specific Considerations
	Slow feedings help to prevent nausea, vomiting, and diarrhea. Air in stomach causes distention and discomfort.	Allow the media to flow in by gravity; regulate rate of flow by raising or lowering system. If system empties of feeding media, air pockets will form in tubing, causing air to enter gastrointestinal system.
7. Maintain patency of tube.	Flushing tube with sterile water keeps the system patent, clean and also decreases medium for bacterial growth.	
8. To maintain integrity of mucous membrane, administer oral and nasal hygiene.	There is diminished salivation in oral cavity, thus there is dryness and unpleasant taste in mouth. Nasal hygiene helps to prevent nasal irritation.	Even if client is NPO, he is allowed to use mouthwash and to brush his teeth if nothing is swallowed.
9. Prevention of cross-contamination.	Cleaning or disposing of equipment reduces the occurrence of bacterial contamination into feeding media resulting in medical complications (i.e., diarrhea).	
10. Report and record observations.	Client's record is a legal document which should include nursing activities, client's response to therapy, and status during hospitalization.	

Implementation	Recommendations	Observations
Feeding should be given slowly being careful not to allow air to enter stomach, causing distention and discomfort.	Reservoir of feeding media should be held no higher than 18 in above stomach of adult. Reservoir of feeding material should be held no higher than 6 to 8 in above stomach of infant. Tube feedings are usually administered every 3–4 hr., although continuous infusion is possible.	
Flush system with approximately 30–60 ml of sterile water. Clamp tubing, remove syringe while taking care not to allow air to enter stomach.		
Administer good oral and nasal hygiene to prevent irritation, decrease possibility of upper respiratory infection, and for comfort.	Lubricate inside of nostrils.	Observe for dryness of oral and nasal membranes.
Clean or dispose of equipment after use according to hospital policy.	If reusable equipment, date and time should be noted on equipment to insure that it is replaced every 24 hr.	
In client's record, note type of procedure (gavage), date, time, amount and type of feeding. Client's tolerance of procedure should be recorded.		

Anticipated Accomplishment	Scientific Principles/ Rationale	Specific Considerations
1. Prepare client and equipment for intubation procedure.		
2. Select and assemble additional equipment.	Ewald tube has a larger lumen than the Levin tube.	
	Many times Ewald tube is used when washing out or aspirating large quantities from stomach.	
	Antidote or solution to neutralize stomach may be used if procedure is treating poisoning.	
	Syringe may be used to check placement of tube and may be used as a receptacle for lavage solution.	Sometimes nasogastric tubes are attached to funnels rather than irrigating syringes.
	Intermittent or gravity suction decompresses stomach or intestine.	
3. Ascertain location of nasogastric or gastrointestinal tube.	Tube must be in proper location so as not to instill fluid into lungs, causing aspiration pneumonia.	Three standard methods (aspiration, air and water) to check tube placement are discussed in this chapter.
4. Position client for lavage.	Correct position lessens chance of regurgitation and aspiration.	Client positioned on side with head low in case of vomiting.
5. Perform lavage procedure.	Irrigation of tube insures patency.	

Implementation	Recommendations	Observations
Follow preparation and insertion procedure of nasogastric tube in Table 41-3 or Table 41-4 to point of gastric or intestinal placement.		With infants and children, restraints may be necessary during this procedure.
Assemble the following additional equipment:		
Levin or Ewald for gastric lavage.		
Solution for irrigation as prescribed by physician.		
Irrigation syringe and basin for aspirated material.		
Suction machine.	Continuous suction is *never* used—it damages mucosa.	Check suction machine to be sure it is working properly.
		If tubing is connected to suction machine, note color, amount, and consistency of drainage, in the drainage bottle.
Check placement of tube. Tube must be in stomach for gastric lavage or in intestines for intestinal lavage. Aspirate gastric contents with syringe before instilling water or antidote.	Do not reposition tube after gastric surgery. Contact physician if tube seems to have been dislodged.	
Position client in semi-Fowler's position if conscious and lateral elevated position if comatose.		Obtain specimen of gastric contents for analysis, particularly if poisoning is suspected.
Begin procedure by instilling 30 to 50 ml of normal saline into tube.		Observe during the procedure if the client has cramps, becomes distended or vomits. If this oc-

TABLE 41-2. Continued

Anticipated Accomplishment	Scientific Principles/ Rationale	Specific Considerations
	Physicians determine type and amount of solution to be used in lavage.	In poisoning, 500 to 1500 ml of solution or antidote may be used to remove or neutralize stomach contents.
	Iced saline promotes hemostasis by vasoconstriction of perforated gastric vessel.	In gastric hemorrhage, normal saline at 0°C (32°F) is commonly used.
	Slow lavage helps to prevent nausea, vomiting, and diarrhea. Air in stomach causes distention and discomfort.	Allow the solution to flow in by gravity; Regulate rate of flow by raising or lowering system.
		If system empties of solution, air pockets form in tubing, causing air to enter gastrointestinal system.
6. Apply suction.	Intermittent suction or gravity drainage (siphonage) empties contents of cavity.	Siphonage is difficult to obtain if there is no solution in system.
		Sometimes nasogastric tubes and gastrointestinal tubes are attached to intermittent suction.
7. Discontinue lavage.		
8. Removal of lavage tubing.		
9. Maintain integrity of mucous membranes and comfort of client by administering oral and nasal hygiene.	There may be diminished salivation in oral cavity, thus there is dryness and unpleasant taste in mouth after this procedure. Nasal hygiene helps to prevent nasal irritation.	Even if client is NPO, he is allowed to use mouthwash, and to brush his teeth if nothing is swallowed.

Implementation	Recommendations	Observations
Before system (syringe/funnel and tube) empties, begin to pour prescribed amount of solution.	Approximately 150–500 ml of solution may be instilled before being allowed to return by siphon method.	curs, suction machine and tube should be checked.
		Observe client for signs of shock due to hypovolemia (excessive blood loss).
Lavage solution should be given slowly being careful not to allow air to enter stomach, causing distention and discomfort.	The reservoir of solution should be no higher than 18 in above stomach of adult.	
	Reservoir of solution should be held no higher than 6–8 in above stomach of infant.	
After a portion of prescribed solution has been instilled, pinch tubing, invert system, and allow solution to siphon back by gravity.	Alternate this procedure until return becomes clear or until prescribed solution has been administered.	Note consistency of return. Be aware that vomiting may occur, if tube becomes occluded.
Clamp tubing, remove syringe or funnel while care is given to prevent air from entering stomach.		
Clamp tubing and withdraw tubing rapidly.		
Administer good oral and nasal hygiene to prevent irritation, decrease possibility of upper respiratory infection and provide comfort.	Although tube may be inserted a short time, lubrication of inside of nostril is recommended.	Observe for dryness of oral and nasal membranes.

TABLE 41-2. Continued

Anticipated Accomplishment	Scientific Principles/ Rationale	Specific Considerations
10. Prevention of cross-contamination.	Clean or dispose of equipment to reduce the occurrence of bacterial contamination into feeding media resulting in medical complications (i.e., diarrhea).	
11. Report and record observations.	Client's record is a legal document which should include nursing activities and client's status during hospitalization.	

addition, principles of emergency nursing apply to the lavage procedure.

INTUBATION PROCEDURES

Nasogastric Tubes

The insertion and care of nasogastric tubes are usually a nursing responsibility; however, in some institutions this procedure is performed by a physician. The nurse should refer to the procedure manual of the employing institution prior to initiating this procedure. The following discussion is based on the assumption that the nurse will be inserting the nasogastric tube and that she has reviewed the procedure manual of the agency (Table 41-3).

Prior to initiating this procedure, the nurse must check the physician's orders regarding the client's name, room number, type of procedure, and rationale for insertion. (This information may be found in progress notes.)[15]

The insertion of the nasogastric tube is not a sterile procedure; however, handwashing prior to insertion and adherence to principles of aseptic technique are required. The following equipment is assembled to assure a safe and expedient insertion.

1. Emesis basin as the client may vomit during the procedure. Stimulation of the glosso-pharyngeal nerve endings in the posterior pharynx by the tube activates the medulla oblongata, the vomiting center in the brain.[16]

2. Facial tissues as passage of the tube through the nasopharynx stimulates tearing and nasal secretion.

3. Appropriate nasogastric tube. A rubber tube is made firmer by chilling it in a bowl of chipped ice for 15–20 minutes. This prevents the tube from curling and kinking in the back of the throat. A plastic tube is made softer by placing it in a bowl of warm water for 5–10 minutes. This reduces the possibility of trauma to the mucous membranes by a rigid tube.

4. Waterproof and absorbent cover to drape the upper torso of the client.

5. Water-soluble lubricant to aid in passage of the nasogastric tube. The lubricant must be water-soluble to avoid serving as a focal point for pneumonia should the tube and lubricant be incorrectly placed into the lung.

6. Irrigating syringe (Asepto, or large syringe with adapter) to check for placement of the nasogastric tube.

7. Hypoallergenic tape to secure the tube to the skin. Hypoallergenic tape will help to prevent trauma to the skin which is subjected to frequent changing of the tape.

Implementation	Recommendations	Observations
Clean and dispose of equipment after use according to hospital policy.		
In client's record, note date, time, amount of solution used for lavage, and amount, color, and consistency of solution returned. Client's tolerance of procedure should be recorded.		

8. Stethoscope is necessary for checking the proper position of the tube.
9. A glass of water and straw (optional) can be used to assist during the insertion of the tube. These also offer an alternate method of checking the proper position of the tube.
10. Depending on the purpose of the intubation, suction equipment, irrigating solution, tube feedings, may need to be gathered.

PREPARATION OF THE CLIENT

Once the equipment has been assembled, the client must be prepared for the procedure. For many clients this will be an unfamiliar and anxiety-producing event. It is advisable to allow sufficient time for explanations and questions; however, avoid informing clients about the procedure too far in advance, as the client may become overly anxious. Additionally, instructions may need to be repeated to ensure client cooperation. The nurse should approach the client in a calm, reassuring, and confident manner. Ascertain the client's level of understanding and previous experience with this procedure. Preparing the client should include a thorough explanation of the procedure. Individualized explanations should be given (i.e., some clients may need to know each step of the procedure, whereas other clients may want only basic information). Attempt to alleviate anxiety by answering the questions of the client, family, and significant others. In terms appropriate for the client's level of understanding, explain the purpose of the procedure and the approximate length of time the tube will remain in place. Identify specific ways that the client can assist during the procedure, (e.g., mouth breathing and swallowing assist in easy passage of the tube).[15] Establish a communication system with the client to be used during insertion (e.g., if the client raises his left hand, this means he is experiencing discomfort, in which case the nurse should temporarily stop advancement of the tube).[17] Instruct the client to remove glasses or contact lenses before initiating the procedure.

Once the procedure has been explained to the client and the equipment is assembled, the nurse is ready to proceed. The client is placed in a high-Fowler's position (if conscious and not contraindicated by his condition). A clean waterproof and absorbent cover should be draped over the client's chest. The nurse then measures the tube by placing the end to be inserted next to the client's earlobe and extending it to the bridge of the nose using her index finger as a reference point. By adding the distance from the bridge of the nose to the xiphoid process at the lower end of the sternum, the required length of the tube to reach the stomach is determined (Fig. 41-8). The average adult requires 20 to 24 inches (55 to 60 cm) of inserted tube to reach the stomach. The tubes are marked at spe-

TABLE 41-3. Insertion and Removal of Nasogastric Tube for Diagnostic Procedures, Decompression of Gastrointestinal Tract, Gavage (Instillation of Medications and Feedings), and Lavage (Washing Out of Stomach)

Anticipated Accomplishment	Scientific Principles/ Rationale	Specific Considerations
1. Minimize spread of microorganisms by cleansing of nurse's hands.	Resident bacteria and other microorganisms are found on hands. These can be transmitted by direct contact with client or with objects that will come in contact with client.	
2. Select and assemble appropriate equipment.	Tube may stimulate glossopharyngeal nerve endings, causing vomiting and stimulation of gag reflex.	Passage of tube may stimulate vomiting.
	Eyes and nose will water as a response to passage of tube through nasopharynx.	Remove glasses or contact lenses before insertion.
	A rubber tube is made firmer by chilling in a bowl of chipped ice for 15–20 min; a plastic tube is made softer by placing it in a bowl of warm water for 5–10 min.	Size and type of tube is determined by size of client and purpose of the intubation: adult: 12 F to 16 F (14 F average); children: 8 F to 12 F (12 F common for children); and infants: 3 F to 10 F (6 F to 8 F average).
	Waterproof and absorbent cover protects client from minor spills.	
	Water-soluble lubricant facilitates passage of tube, (see text).	
	Syringe is used to check placement of tube by aspiration of gastric contents and by instillation of air.	
	Hypoallergenic tape helps to prevent trauma to skin that is subjected to frequent changing of the tape.	

Implementation	Recommendations	Observations
Wash hands thoroughly using aseptic technique.		
Assemble following: Emesis basin.		If vomiting should occur, note amount and character of emesis.
Facial tissue.		
Gastric tube.	Gastric tube may need to be chilled or warmed before insertion.	Before inserting, check gastric tube for damages by irrigating it with normal saline
Waterproof and absorbent cover.		
Water-soluble lubricant.		
Irrigating syringe.		
Hypoallergenic tape—1 in width.		

TABLE 41-3. Continued

Anticipated Accomplishment	Scientific Principles/ Rationale	Specific Considerations
	Stethoscope is used to check placement of tube as air is injected into stomach.	
	Water aids in passage of tube and may be used to check placement of tube.	Client should be allowed to drink water only if not contraindicated by his condition.
3. Decrease client's anxiety by providing explanation of procedure.	Fear of unknown or lack of information and knowledge can be major factors in production of or increase in anxiety.	Assess client's level of understanding, age, and previous experience with this procedure.
4. Prepare client for insertion of gastric tube.	With client in a sitting position, tube advances more easily and is less likely to go into trachea.	If client is unable to sit, he may lie on his back or side.
5. Determine amount of tubing necessary for insertion.	Length of tube must be adequate to reach destination (nose to stomach or mouth to stomach).	Measure from earlobe to nose and nose to xiphoid process. (See text for measurement procedure in infants and children.)
6. Ascertain site of insertion.	Nostril insertion preferred to oral insertion in reducing movement of tube and lessens stimulation of gag reflex in adult.	Previous trauma to nose may occlude nostril(s).
	Oral insertion preferred with infants because it causes less trauma to delicate nasal passages and decreases possibility of aspiration.	
7. Lubricate tube for insertion.	Lubrication aids in passage of tube.	Water-soluble lubrication should be used to prevent lipid pneumonia in event tube is accidentally inserted into lung.
	In cytology specimens, interference with cell visualization may occur if water soluble lubrication is used.	

Implementation	Recommendations	Observations
Stethoscope.	Use diaphragm portion of stethoscope.	
Glass of water.		
Explain to client in understandable terms reasons for doing, and steps of procedure.	Explanation of procedure should be given to family members and significant others to decrease their anxiety and enhance their cooperation.	Note verbal and nonverbal behavior.
Position client in high-Fowler's position.	Pillows placed behind shoulders facilitate hyperextension of head.	
Measure tube to determine length of tube to be inserted. Mark reference point with tape.	For oral intubation use same measurement technique.	
Determine orifice through which tube will pass.	Nasal route is usually used when tube is to be in place for an extended period of time.	
	Oral route is used when tube is to be in place a short time, when a nasal deformity is present, or the tube is too large to pass through nostril.	
Lubricate distal 8 in of tube for insertion.	Oily substances should not be used because of danger of aspiration.	
	Water-soluble lubrication should not be used if the procedure is for diagnostic purposes.	

TABLE 41-3. Continued

Anticipated Accomplishment	Scientific Principles/ Rationale	Specific Considerations
8. Intubation of gastric tube.		Dentures that fit properly need not be removed during the procedure unless client requests removal.
		The tube should follow natural contour of naso-oropharynx.
	Once tube reaches pharynx, sips of water facilitate passage.	Head should be in a natural position during swallowing. Client may be instructed to flex his head until his chin rests on his chest when tube passes into pharynx.
	Swallowing interrupts inhalation, decreases possibility of tube being passed into trachea. Flexing head forward assists gravity.	
9. Determine placement of tube.	Tube must be in stomach for successful gavage, lavage, or aspiration of gastric contents.	Three standard methods (aspiration, air, and water) to check tube placement are discussed in this chapter.
10. Prevent distention of stomach.	Air in stomach causes distention and discomfort.	Air will enter the stomach via the tube causing abdominal distention.
11. Secure tube.	Gastric tube should be properly taped to prevent accidental dislodging.	Tape tube in manner shown in Figure 41-10 to prevent pressure on the nostril or impair vision.

Implementation	Recommendations	Observations
	Infants and children should be restrained as necessary.	
Nasal intubation: tube should be held in one hand, while other hand is elevating tip of nose to expose selected nostril.		
Oral intubation: tube should be passed over middle of tongue.		
Tube should be guided downward and backward. Instruct client to swallow as tube is advanced.	Advance tube gently and steadily as client swallows. Do not rush intubation process.	
Check placement of tube.		Fluoroscopy is another way of determining tube placement. If client is unable to hum or speak, tube is incorrectly placed.
Once correct placement of tube is determined, clamp tube to prevent entrance of air into stomach.		
Tape tube in place.	Hypoallergenic tape should be used to secure tube. Tube should be positioned to avoid an upward pull or pressure against the tip of the nares.	Observe during daily activity so that there is no pulling or jerking of tube.
Once tube is secured, initiate procedure for which tube was intended. See text on decompression, lavage, gavage, and diagnostic procedures.		

TABLE 41-3. Continued

Anticipated Accomplishment	Scientific Principles/ Rationale	Specific Considerations
12. Administer oral and nasal hygiene to maintain integrity of mucous membranes.	Good oral hygiene prevents mucous membrane crustation, halitosis, parotitis, and oral distaste. Nasal hygiene prevents nasal irritation.	Even if client is NPO, he is allowed to use mouthwash, and to brush his teeth as long as nothing is swallowed.
13. Removal of gastric tube.	Clamping tube cuts off air pressure in tube and prevents fluid from escaping and causing aspiration.	
14. Prevention of aspiration.	During exhalation, possibility of fluid aspiration (pneumonia) decreases.	
15. Prevention of cross-contamination.	To reduce possibility of bacterial contamination and crossinfection, equipment must be cleaned and disposed of properly.	
16. Report and record observations.	Client's record is a legal document which should include nursing activities, client's response to therapy, and status during hospitalization.	Insertion of gastric tube may be performed for decompression, gavage, lavage, or for diagnostic procedures.

cific points, but the required lengths may fall between these markings. It is advisable for the nurse to use a piece of tape to mark the point to which the tube is to be inserted (Fig. 41-8).

The nurse must determine which nostril is to be used for insertion. To decide this, the client should be asked if he has ever had nasal trauma or other abnormality affecting his nose. If there are no contraindications for either nostril, the client should be permitted to make the decision. There are times when a client may not be able to remember or identify nasal complications. The nurse may then ask the client to occlude one nostril and exhale through his nose, while she (nurse) is listening for occlusion or other evidence of obstruction. If either nostril is occluded, the nurse should insert the tube into the unaffected side.

INSERTION

At this point the nurse is ready to insert the tube. The tube should be lubricated with a water-soluble

Implementation	Recommendations	Observations
Good oral hygiene should be administered frequently while tube is in place.	Lubricate inside nostrils.	Observe for dryness of oral and nasal mucous membranes.
Clamp tube, remove tape, and withdraw tube rapidly in a gentle motion. Have receptacle ready to receive tube. Client should take deep breaths while exhaling slowly during removal. After use, clean or dispose of equipment according to agency policy.	Administer good oral and nasal hygiene after procedure to eliminate unpleasant taste.	Observe for skin breakdown where tape was attached.
In client's record, note type of procedure, date, time, size of tube and other characteristics of the tube. Amount of intake and output, characteristics of drainage and client's tolerance of procedure should also be recorded.		

lubricant along the first 8 inches of the tube. The lubricant effectively reduces surface friction between mucous membranes and the tube. The client should hyperextend his head during the insertion. When the tube has reached the oropharynx, the client may return his head to its normal position. Swallowing is much easier when the head is in its normal position. Unless contraindicated, the nurse may now permit the client to sip from the glass of cool water. Instruct the client to swallow the water continually during the steady advancement of the tube. This encourages the client to concentrate on verbal instructions rather than concentrating on the discomfort caused by the tube. Additionally, swallowing initiates peristaltic waves that encourage forward advancement of the tube. With each swallow, the tube should be more easily inserted. As the tube is advanced the client may begin to gag. The nurse should stop and encourage the client to deep breathe through his mouth. Once the gag reflex is quiet, advancement of the tube should be resumed until the preinsertion measurement is reached. If

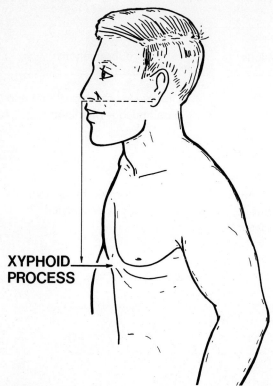

the irrigating syringe to the gastric tube and pull back on the plunger until stomach contents are visible in the tube or syringe if an opaque tube is used. If there is no return of gastric contents, this may mean that the tube is not in contact with gastric secretions. Advance or withdraw the tube approximately 2 inches and pull back on the plunger again until gastric contents appear in the syringe. This method of checking tube placement is the most reliable of the three methods.

A second method requires an irrigating syringe and a stethoscope. Fill the irrigating syringe with 5–10 cc of air and connect the syringe to the tube. Place the stethoscope over the epigastric region and rapidly inject the air into the tube. Listen for a "hissing sound" simultaneous with the injection of air (Fig. 41-9). This indicates that the tube is in the stomach.

A third method of checking tube placement is to place the external end of the tube in a glass of water and observe for air bubbles when the client exhales. If bubbles occur the tube is probably in the lung and should be removed immediately. This last method is controversial in that aspiration of the water into the lungs can occur if the client inhales rather than exhales during the procedure. Besides

XYPHOID PROCESS

FIGURE 41-8. Technique for measurement for proper positioning of the nasogastric tube. Place the end of the gastric tube to be inserted next to the client's earlobe and extend it to the bridge of the nose. To this measurement add the length of the tube as it is extended from the bridge of the nose to the tip of the xiphoid process. This technique will insure that the tube is of sufficient length to reach the stomach.

resistance to advancement of the tube occurs, *do not force* the tube forward. Attempt to gently rotate the tube. If this technique is unsuccessful, remove the tube, and insert in the other nostril. Signs of respiratory difficulty such as coughing, gasping, and cyanosis indicate that the tube has entered the trachea rather than the esophagus. The tube should be removed immediately and reinserted when respiratory difficulty abates. When the gastric tube is in place, it is essential to check its placement *before* taping.

CORRECT PLACEMENT

Three standard methods are used to insure that the gastric tube is indeed in the stomach. First, connect

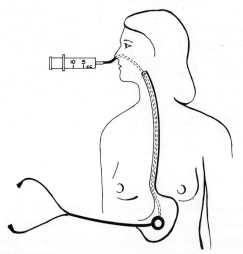

FIGURE 41-9. One technique for determining correct placement of a gastric tube. Fill an irrigating syringe with 5-10 cc of air. Connect the syringe to the tube. Place a stethoscope over the epigastric region while rapidly injecting the air into the tube. Listen for a hissing sound. This indicates correct placement of the tube in the stomach.

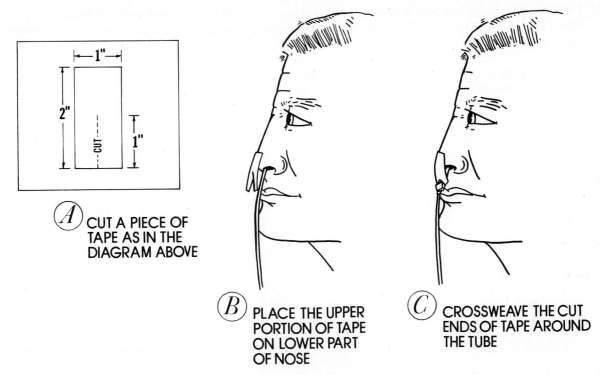

(A) CUT A PIECE OF TAPE AS IN THE DIAGRAM ABOVE

(B) PLACE THE UPPER PORTION OF TAPE ON LOWER PART OF NOSE

(C) CROSSWEAVE THE CUT ENDS OF TAPE AROUND THE TUBE

FIGURE 41-10. Correct method of securing a nasogastric tube.

being potentially dangerous, this is not a particularly reliable evaluation measure.

Once correct placement of the tube is ascertained, it should be taped as illustrated in Figure 41-10. Tape that leaves an adhesive residue on the skin and tube should be avoided.[18] In securing the tube, the nurse must remember not to allow the tube to pull up against the nares since continuous pressure may cause irritation necrosis. Additionally, the client's vision should not be obstructed by the tape edges. The gastric tube is now ready for its prescribed use.

INFANTS AND CHILDREN

The above discussion is relevant to the adult client. Special considerations must be taken into account for infants and children during insertion of the tube. Slight variations in procedures related to decompression, gavage, and lavage are also necessary for infants and children. These variations have been discussed in detail under the appropriate headings.

The following guidelines should be utilized when performing gastrointestinal intubations on infants and children. (1) Infants: measure the tube from the bridge of the child's nose to the umbilicus to determine length for insertion both orally and nasally. The tube size will be 3, 5, 8, or 10 French. The smallest diameter tube that will perform the needed function should be used. No more than 1–3 cc of air should be injected into the stomach to check correct positioning. With infants the oral passage is preferred because it prevents breakdown of the nasal membrane, lessens the chance of aspiration, and reduces the gag reflex.[19] (2) Children: the tube is measured in the same manner as stated in the procedure for the adult client although the tube size will vary from 8 to 12 French.

Intestinal Tubes

As discussed earlier, intestinal tubes are designed to extend past the stomach into the small intestines. The Miller-Abbott, Cantor, and Harris tubes are examples of tubes commonly used in intestinal intubation. The purpose of intestinal intubation is to stimulate peristalsis and to locate, break up, and prevent obstruction. Obviously, decompression is a major function of intestinal tubes (Table 41-4).

TABLE 41-4: Insertion and Removal of Intestinal Tube to Locate and Relieve Intestinal Obstruction, to Stimulate Peristalsis, for Decompression Therapy, and to Aid in Diagnostic Procedures.

Anticipated Accomplishment	Scientific Principles/ Rationale	Specific Considerations
1. Prepare client and equipment for intubation procedure.		
	Intestinal tube is longer and weight of mercury helps to carry balloon(s) through the GI tract by gravity. Anesthetic administered topically to pharynx to minimize discomfort.	Equipment varies slightly. Intestinal tube Mercury for instillation into balloon(s). Topical anesthetic (optional). Suction machine
2. Position client for advancement of intestinal tube.	Position allows peristalsis and gravity to aid in passage of tube through pyloric sphincter.	Place client on right side for 2 hr and advance tube 2–4 in. Place client in Fowler's position for 2 hr, advancing tube 2–4 in. Place client on his left side for 2 hr and advance tube 2–4 in more. If tube needs further advancement, advance maximum 4–6 in/hr and check placement by x-ray. Tape when tube in desired position.
3. If appropriate, connect intestinal tube to suctioning.	Suction occurs when there is a negative pressure strong enough to remove contents in cavity.	Decompression therapy (see text for details).
4. Administer oral and nasal hygiene to maintain integrity of mucous membranes.	Good oral hygiene will prevent mucous membrane crustation, halitosis, parotitis, and oral distaste. Nasal hygiene will prevent nasal irritation.	Even if client is NPO, he is allowed to use mouthwash and to brush his teeth if nothing is swallowed.

Implementation	Recommendations	Observations
Follow preparation and insertion procedure of nasogastric tube in Table 41-3 to point of gastric placement.		
Clamp suction tubing once suction has been established.		Check suction apparatus to be sure it is working before tube insertion.
Client's position is rotated and changed to aid advancement of tube through anatomical structure of stomach and intestine.	Client may not have a pillow. Foot of his bed may be elevated 12 in. Tube must not be advanced faster than physiological movement, otherwise tube will coil and further obstruct gastrointestinal tract. Tube should be advanced no more than 2–4 in every 30 min to 1 hr.	
	Do not tape until tube has reached final destination. Avoid pressure on nostril. Client should be able to move through activities (e.g., turning in bed without dislodging tube).	Most accurate method to determine if tube correctly positioned is x-ray.
Tubing may be connected to suction by means of a connecting adapter.	Suction machine must be turned "on" before connecting to the intestinal tube.	
Good oral and nasal hygiene should be administered frequently while tube is in place.	Lubricate inside nostrils.	Observe for dryness of oral and nasal mucous membranes.

TABLE 41-4. Continued

Anticipated Accomplishment	Scientific Principles/ Rationale	Specific Considerations
5. Removal of intestinal tube.	Clamping cuts off air pressure. Prevents fluid in tube from escaping and causing aspiration.	
6. Prevention of aspiration.	During exhalation, possibility of fluid aspiration (pneumonia) decreases.	
7. Prevention of cross-contamination.	To reduce possibility of bacterial contamination and cross-infection, equipment must be cleaned and disposed of properly.	
8. Report and record observations.	Client's record is a legal document which should include nursing activities and client's status during hospitalization.	Insertion of gastrointestinal tube may be performed for decompression, lavage, diagnostic procedures, to locate and relieve intestinal obstructions, or to stimulate peristalsis.

The insertion process for intestinal tubes is essentially the same as for the gastric tubes. The following discussion is related to the insertion procedure of the intestinal tube after it has reached the stomach.

When the selected intestinal tube has reached the stomach, it is *not* taped. For the first 2 hours after insertion, the client is placed on his right side with his face turned downward toward the bed. This is to encourage passage of the tube through the pyloric sphincter. Occasionally the tube must be threaded through the pylorus under fluoroscopy. During these first 2 hours the tube is advanced 2–4 inches. The client may now be x-rayed to determine the location of the tube. Once the tube has reached the duodenum, the tube is advanced 2–4 inches every 1–2 hours. The presence of bile in the aspirated fluid is an indicator that the tube has reached the duodenum.[20] If the tube is in the desired position, the client is placed in a Fowler's position for 2 hours with further advancement of the tube 2 to 4 inches. Again, the position of the tube may be checked by x-ray, and if it is in proper position, the client is placed on his left side, remaining in that position for 2 hours with continued advancement of the tube 2–4 more inches. The client may again be x-rayed to determine if the tube is in the desired position. If the tube needs further advancement, a rule of thumb is to insert the tube not more than 4 inches per hour or it may coil within the intestine and block function. Since these tubes are extremely long (6–10 feet), excess tubing should be neatly coiled and loosely attached to the bed, allowing ample slack for easy advancement. Once the tube is in proper position it will be taped as shown in Figure 41-10.

Implementation	Recommendations	Observations
To remove tube, deflate balloons, clamp lumens, remove tape, withdraw slowly, a few inches each at 10 min intervals. Once tube reaches stomach, tube may be withdrawn more rapidly in a steady motion.	Administer good oral and nasal hygiene after the procedure to eliminate unpleasant taste.	Observe for skin breakdown where tape was attached.
Client should take deep breaths while exhaling slowly during removal.		
After use, clean or dispose of equipment according to hospital policy.		
In client's record, note type of procedure, date, time, amount of intake and output, and characteristics of drainage. Client's tolerance of procedure should be recorded.		

Since the primary purpose of this tube is decompression, suction must be available. The suction apparatus must be checked prior to insertion of the tube to make certain it is functioning properly. If an electrical pump (Gomco-Thermotic) is used, test the suction power of the machine by determining if the electric pump can draw up water from a bowl into the collection bottle. If hydraulic suction is used, test for suction by allowing water to flow from the upper bottle into the lower bottle. Regardless of the method used, once suction is established, clamp the tubing of the suction device that will be connected to the intestinal tube.

Intestinal tubes are usually mercury-weighted to aid in the propulsion of the tube down the gastrointestinal tract. The amount of mercury used in the balloon is determined by the physician, but it usually ranges from 4–10 cc. If a Miller-Abbott tube is used, the mercury is instilled into the balloon after the intestinal tube has passed the pyloric sphincter. If a Cantor or Harris tube is used, the mercury is instilled prior to insertion.

GASTROSTOMY AND OTHER TUBES

The gastrostomy tube is a rubber or plastic tube inserted into the stomach through an incision in the abdomen. The tube is sutured or taped to the abdominal wall and requires daily dressing changes using sterile technique. The equipment used for wound care will be a cleansing solution, as prescribed by the physician, a hypoallergenic tape, and a sterile 4 × 4 gauze pad. The skin around the gastrostomy tube should be cleansed every 4 hours since this skin is particularly vulnerable to excoriation if gastric secretions seep out around the tube.

Aluminum paste or karaya powder may provide added protection to the skin.[21] Because the primary use of a gastrostomy tube is for feeding, the tube is generally clamped to prevent drainage and loss of feeding media. The procedure of gavage via gastrostomy tube is exactly the same as with the nasogastric tube (refer to Table 41-1).

If the gastrostomy tube is used for decompression, it is connected to a drainage setup. The method of drainage will be created by gravity or a suction apparatus.

Tubes may be introduced into the various segments of the small intestine through abdominal incisions. The name of the tube is correlated to its location in the gastrointestinal tract, (e.g., duodenostomy and jejunostomy).

The insertion of these tubes is performed by the physician in the operating room under sterile conditions. The nursing care specific to these tubes centers around care of the incisional site, drainage system, and accurate recording of intake and output. The tubes are normally sutured to the abdomen and require daily dressing changes using sterile technique. In addition to the nurse's responsibility for wound care, she is required to keep accurate intake and output records and observe for electrolyte and fluid imbalances. There is usually a large amount of drainage from these tubes. The further the tube is advanced into the intestinal tract, the more of a problem odor will be; therefore, additional consideration must be given to deodorization and handling of drainage to reduce the client's feelings of disgust and embarrassment.

Duodenostomy tubes or jejunostomy tubes may be used to introduce feedings into the duodenum or the jejunum, respectively. Jejunal feedings must be in a predigested form since the digestive processes of both the stomach and the duodenum have been bypassed. Liquid elemental diets provide "nutrients in a form ready for absorption so that little or no chemical transformation is needed."[22] These diets are essentially bulk-free and provide minimal stimulation for the secretion of intestinal, pancreatic, or biliary juices.

POTENTIAL PROBLEMS

Regardless of the type of tube inserted or the intended purpose of the intubation, a variety of problems may arise whenever a tube is inserted into the gastrointestinal tract. The problems associated with gastrointestinal tubes vary in degree of complication and medical management, but they all have an effect on client comfort and length of the client's stay in the health care agency.

Aspiration pneumonia, seen most frequently when gastrointestinal tubes are used for gavage, is a condition which may result from dislodging of the gastrointestinal tube from its correct position. When the tube is dislodged, instead of resting in the stomach, it slips into the trachea or lung and feedings are instilled into the lung rather than the stomach. This condition is most likely to occur with the comatose client who has diminished reflexes, specifically the gag and cough reflex. Aspiration pneumonia is by no means restricted to comatose clients receiving gavage. All clients with a gastrointestinal tube are at risk. The incidence of aspiration pneumonia can be reduced by elevating the head of the bed to 30 degrees during feedings and for an hour following feeding. The risk can be further reduced by always aspirating stomach contents prior to feeding and by checking the position of the gastrointestinal tube with air instillation and a stethoscope.

The problems of dehydration and electrolyte imbalance are common complications seen primarily when decompression and gavage are the intended purpose of the tube. With the removal of gastric or intestinal contents, the loss of potassium, chlorides, sodium, and water, there must be close monitoring of serum electrolytes and observation of the client for signs of fluid and electrolyte imbalance. To compensate for fluid and electrolyte loss through suction, clients are given replacement therapy intravenously. Typically, the adult client will be given maintenance fluid in the range of 3 L/day with added electrolytes based on the client's current laboratory values. An additional order of "cc for cc replacement" of a prescribed solution for fluid and electrolytes is usually the method used to manage dehydration and electrolyte disturbances. This "cc for cc replacement" means that if 1000 cc of gastric contents are aspirated, these 1000 cc must be replenished in the form of prescribed intravenous fluid in addition to the prescribed maintenance fluid. This additional amount may be in the range of 0.5 to 2 L/24 hours.

Clients receiving gavage feeding may develop dehydration and electrolyte disturbances caused by administering feeding with excessively high solute loads without providing an adequate volume of water. Clients with compromised renal function are particularly susceptible to developing this fluid and electrolyte disturbance, commonly called the *tube feeding syndrome.*

Clients with prolonged gastrointestinal intubation are at a higher risk of developing parotitis than the client with oral intake. This condition occurs as a result of limited stimulation of the parotid gland when the client is placed on NPO status. The nurse's responsibility is to provide the best oral hygiene possible a minimum of every 2 hours and more frequently if indicated by the client's condition.

Client discomforts associated with gastrointestinal tubes, such as sore throats, are more difficult to counteract because the tube is a foreign object and acts as an irritant. Measures that may help reduce discomfort are: changing the client's position frequently, the use of an anesthetic agent in the throat, limited client conversation, and optimal oral hygiene.

Associated with client discomfort and the use of gastrointestinal tubes are pressure points caused by poor positioning of the tube against the nares. This problem can be alleviated by correct taping of the tube as demonstrated in Figure 41-10. If pressure points do develop, the tube may need to be alternated from one nostril to the other at specific time intervals. This particular problem should not occur with vigilant nursing care.

REFERENCES

1. Luckmann, J., and Sorensen, K.: *Medical-Surgical Nursing: A Psychophysiologic Approach.* Philadelphia, W. B. Saunders Co., 1974, p. 1059.
2. Henderson, V., and Nite, G.: *Principles and Practice of Nursing,* 6th ed. New York, Macmillan Publishing Co., 1978, p. 1216.
3. *Ibid.,* p. 1214.
4. *Clinical Considerations in the Use of the Argyle Salem Sump Tube.* St. Louis, Sherwood Medical Industries, Inc., 1977.
5. Elhart, D., et al.: *Scientific Principles of Nursing.* St. Louis, C. V. Mosby Co., 1978, p. 556.
6. Henderson and Nite, *op. cit.,* p. 1213.
7. Elhart et al., *op. cit.,* p. 558.
8. Luckmann and Sorensen, *op. cit.,* p. 1060.
9. McConnell, E.: Insuring safer stomach suctioning with the Salem sump tube. *Nurs. '77* 7(9):57, 1977.
10. Scipien G., et al.: *Comprehensive Pediatric Nursing,* New York, McGraw-Hill Book Co., 1975, p. 643.
11. Beland, I., and Passos, J.: *Clinical Nursing: Pathophysiological and Psychological Approaches,* 3rd ed. New York, Macmillan Publishing Co., 1975, p. 706.
12. Lewis, L.: *Fundamental Skills in Patient Care.* Philadelphia, J. B. Lippincott Co., 1976. p. 204.
13. Luckmann and Sorensen, *op. cit.,* p. 1063.
14. Henderson and Nite, *op. cit.,* p. 1225.
15. Ellis, J., Nowlis, E., and Bentz, P.: *Modules for Basic Nursing Skills.* Boston, Houghton Mifflin Co., 1977, p. 188.
16. Dugas, B.: *Introduction to Patient Care: A Comprehensive Approach to Nursing.* Philadelphia, W. B. Saunders Co., 1977, p. 513.
17. Brunner, L., and Suddarth, D. (eds.): *The Lippincott Manual of Nursing Practice.* Philadelphia, J. B. Lippincott Co., 1974, p. 383.
18. Moidel, H., Giblin, E., and Wagner, B.: *Nursing Care of the Patient with Medical-Surgical Disorders,* 2nd ed. New York, McGraw-Hill Book Co., 1971, p. 743.
19. Scipien et al., *op. cit.,* p. 642.
20. Henderson and Nite, *op. cit.,* p. 1223.
21. Barber, J., Stokes, L., and Billings, D.: *Adult and Child Care: A Client Approach to Nursing.* St. Louis, C. V. Mosby Co., 1977, p. 634.
22. Luckmann and Sorensen, *op. cit.,* p. 1062.

BIBLIOGRAPHY

Chinn, P.: Infant gavage feeding. *Am. J. Nurs.* 71:1964, 1971.
Dison, N.: *Clinical Nursing Techniques.* St. Louis, C. V. Mosby Co., 1975.
Elhart, D. et al.: *Scientific Principles of Nursing.* St. Louis, C. V. Mosby Co., 1978.
Fuerst, E., Wolff, L., and Weitzel, M.: *Fundamentals of Nursing,* 5th ed. Philadelphia, J. B. Lippincott Co., 1974.
Jones, D., Dunbar, C., and Jirovec, M.: *Medical-Surgical Nursing: A Conceptual Approach.* New York, McGraw-Hill Book Co., 1978.
Leifer, G.: *Principles and Techniques in Pediatric Nursing,* 3rd ed. Philadelphia, W. B. Saunders Co., 1977.
Literte, J.: Nursing care of patients with intestinal obstruction. *Am. J. Nurs.* 77:1003, 1977.
Long, G.: G.I. bleeding: what to do and when. *Nurs. '78* 8(3):44, 1978.
McConnell, E. A.: All about gastrointestinal intubation. *Nurs. '75* 5(9):30, 1975.
Shafer, K. N., et al.: *Medical Surgical Nursing,* 6th ed. St. Louis, C. V. Mosby Co., 1975.
Sutton, A. L.: *Bedside Nursing Techniques in Medicine and Surgery.* Philadelphia, W. B. Saunders Co., 1969.

CHAPTER 42

GLOSSARY

albuminuria. The presence of albumin (protein) in the urine. Usually a sign of renal impairment but may be found in normal individuals following rigorous exercise or after standing for a length of time (*orthostatic* or *postural albuminuria*).

anuria. The complete suppression of urine secretion by the kidneys.

bowel movement. The passage of feces.

burning. A hot, irritated feeling at and around the meatus when urinating.

calculus (pl. calculi). Pathological formation of mineral salts (usually calcium) within the urinary tract. Also known as stones.

carminative. An agent removing flatulence from the intestine.

cathartic. A medication that causes the passage of feces.

MAINTENANCE OF URINARY AND INTESTINAL ELIMINATION

Arlyne B. Saperstein, M.N., R.N., and
Margaret A. Frazier, M.S., R.N.

catheter. A tube used for the removal of instillation of fluids.

colonic irrigation. The filling of the colon to capacity with large quantities of solution to flush it.

constipation. The passing of a hard, dry stool. When due to weakness of intestinal musculature, it is called *atonic constipation*; when due to hypertonicity of the intestine, it is called *spastic constipation*.

cystocele. A downward displacement and pouching of the bladder into the vagina.

defecation. The passage of feces.

diaphoresis. Profuse perspiration.

diarrhea. The passage of watery, unformed stools.

distention. Intestinal: the accumulation of flatus in the intestines; urinary: the accumulation of urine in the bladder.

diuresis. The production and excretion of abnormally large quantities of urine.

dysuria. Difficulty or pain on urination.

enema. The instillation of a solution or fluid into the rectum and lower portion of the large intestine.

enuresis. Involuntary urination, particularly at night; bedwetting.

fecal impaction. A hard, dry mass of fecal matter in the rectum causing partial or complete obstruction.

feces. Waste material (excreta) from the gastrointestinal tract.

flatulence. Excessive gas in the stomach and intestines.

flatus. Gas in the digestive tract.

frequency. Urination at very frequent intervals.

glomerulonephritis. A form of nephritis involving the glomeruli of the kidney.

glycosuria. The presence of detectable amounts of glucose in the urine often due to hyposecretion of insulin (diabetes mellitus). After ingestion of large amounts of carbohydrate, it is called *alimentary glycosuria*.

hematuria. The presence of blood in the urine.

hydronephrosis. Accumulation of urine in the kidney pelvis distending and damaging the kidney.

incontinence. Lack of sphincter control causing involuntary expulsion of urine or feces.

laxative. A medication used to cause passage of feces.

melanuria. Darkly pigmented urine.

melena. Black, tarry stools due to the presence of blood.

micturition. The passage of urine; voiding.

motility. The spontaneous movement along the gastrointestinal tract.

nephritis. Acute or chronic inflammation of the kidney.

nephrosis. Degenerative changes in the kidneys without inflammation.

nocturia (nycturia). Excessive urination during the night.

oliguresis. Scanty or infrequent voiding.

oliguria. Decreased formation of urine.

peristalsis. Wavelike motion along the gastrointestinal tract caused by contraction and relaxation of musculature pushing its contents forward.

polyuria. Excessive production and excretion of urine.

proctoclysis. Infusion of solution into the rectum and colon by a continuous drip.

purgative. A cleansing agent causing evacuation of stool.

pyuria. The presence of pus in the urine.

reflux (vesicoureteral). The flow of urine backward from the bladder into the ureter.

residual urine. Urine remaining in the bladder immediately after voiding.

retention. The inability to urinate when the bladder contains urine. Dribbling of urine due to increased pressure in the distended bladder is called *retention with overflow* or *paradoxical incontinence*.

sphincter. A ring of muscle which opens and closes an orifice, as the urethra or the anus.

stasis. Stagnation of the flow of urine.

stool. Excreta from the gastrointestinal tract.

suppository. A cone, bullet, or pencil-shaped sub-stance which may or may not contain a medication. After insertion into the rectum or urethra, it dissolves and is absorbed.

suppression. Complete lack of production of urine.

tenesmus. Painful and ineffective straining to empty the bowel or bladder.

tidal drainage. Periodic draining of the bladder to promote bladder tone and function by use of irrigation apparatus.

tympanites. Abdominal distention caused by gas in the intestines (also known as meteorism).

urgency. Extreme need to void immediately.

urinalysis. Laboratory testing (analysis) of the urine for the presence of abnormal substances.

urination. The passage of urine.

urine. Excreta from the urinary tract.

voiding. Evacuation of the bladder.

Elimination of waste from the body occurs through four routes: the respiratory system (lungs), the integument (sweat glands), the gastrointestinal tract, and the urinary tract.

Although the physiological processes by which the body produces urine and feces are the same in all individuals, the *patterns* of their elimination (especially from the gastrointestinal tract) often vary. Many factors influence these elimination patterns, including illness, stress, diet, activity, exercise, and medications. Alterations in normal activities of daily living may bring about elimination problems (such as constipation), which can lead to serious problems unless resolved. The nurse in dealing with clients must understand the process of elimination, the functions of the anatomical structures involved, the possible malfunctions or problems that can occur, the conditions under which the process can be affected, and the treatments, both preventive and restorative, which promote and maintain normal elimination of waste products. She must also be aware of the embarrassment and guilt most people experience (and the misconceptions most people have) when they are forced to publicly concern themselves with the processes of elimination and the urogenital area of the body, particularly when these areas are exposed and touched.

This chapter deals first with urinary elimination and then with intestinal elimination. After reviewing the anatomy and physiology of elimination, common problems and treatment measures are discussed. Nursing responsibilities in relation to prevention are also examined.

URINARY TRACT

Function

The function of the urinary system is to eliminate wastes (end products) of cellular metabolism and to regulate fluid, electrolyte and acid-base balance in the body. (See Chapter 35 on maintenance of fluid and electrolyte balance). The *kidneys* form and excrete a waste solution, *urine*, through the processes of *filtration* and *reabsorption*. Solid inorganic salts and organic compounds which constitute nitrogenous waste from the metabolism of protein make up 5 percent of the urine, with water totaling the other 95 percent. Organic substances include urea (comprising about half of the solid material), hippuric acid, uric acid, creatinine, indican (indoxyl), urobilin or bile pigment (giving urine its characteristic pale yellow color), fatty acids, carbonates, mucin, cystine, sugar, white blood cells, and epithelial cells. Most of these are found only in trace amounts; if found in quantity (e.g., sugar), a pathological state may be present. The inorganic components (salts) are ammonia (the most abundant of these compounds), which is eliminated as ammonium salts, and chlorides, sulfates, bicarbonates, and phosphates of sodium, potassium, calcium, and magnesium. (Sodium chloride constitutes approximately a fifth of the urine's solid material). In addition, trace amounts of iron may be found.

To be eliminated by the kidneys, the solids must be in solution; the larger the amount of solid waste to be handled by the kidneys, the more water is required for its elimination. The quantity of water, which is reabsorbed by the kidneys, is regulated by antidiuretic hormone (ADH) and influenced by aldosterone (a mineralocorticoid hormone secreted by the adrenal cortex), which causes changes in osmotic pressure by affecting sodium, chloride, and potassium (electrolyte) balance. The specific gravity of the urine may vary from 1.005 to 1.040 (usually, 1.010 to 1.030)*, depending upon the amount of

---

*Sources vary on the ranges given for specific gravity of urine.

solid waste it contains. Usually the more urine excreted (causing it to be dilute), the lower the specific gravity. An instrument called a urinometer is used to measure the specific gravity of the urine, or the comparison of the weights of equal volumes of water and urine. Water is represented by the weight 1.000.

The pH of urine when the diet is normal is slightly acid. When meat is excluded from the diet and fruit and vegetable consumption increases, the urine may become alkaline. Medications also affect the pH. Upon standing, urine cools and becomes alkaline due to bacterial action causing production of ammonia; as this occurs, urates and phosphates precipitate and the urine becomes cloudy. If the urine were returned to the prior state, that is, back to the temperature of the body and to the acidic state by the addition of an acid, it would become clear again. Urine in a healthy individual is clear since there is no bacterial action on the urine. No bacteria are present in the urinary tract except in a diseased state. In addition to microorganisms, albumin, glucose, blood, pus, casts, calculi ("stones"), and ketone (acetone) bodies, produced during fatty acid oxidation, are not normally found in the urine. Table 42-1 contrasts normal and abnormal characteristics of the urine in relation to color, odor, transparency, and quantity.

Anatomy

KIDNEYS

The kidneys are two bean-shaped organs, each weighing 4–6 ounces and approximately 4 inches long, 2–3 inches wide and 1 inch thick in the average adult. They are located on each side of the retroperitoneal aspect of the abdominal cavity (lumbar region). To perform their function of filtering specific constituents out of the blood for excretion, the kidneys must have an abundant blood supply; this is provided by the *renal artery*. The blood is transported via arterioles and capillaries into the *nephrons*, the basic structural and functional unit of the kidney. Each kidney contains over a million nephrons. A central capsule, the malpighian capsule or renal corpuscle, is found in each nephron; within this is a glomerulus (a mass of capillaries) and a capsule (Bowman's capsule) which

TABLE 42-1. Normal and Abnormal Characteristics of Urine

Normal	Abnormal	Significance
A. Quantity		
1−2 L (95% water; average 1.5 L/day)		Depends upon water and fluid-foods consumed, exercise, temperature, and kidney function
	High (polyuria)	Diabetes mellitus, diabetes insipidus, certain types of chronic nephritis, or diuretics (drugs causing increased urinary excretion)
	Low (oliguria)	Acute nephritis, heart disease, fevers, diarrhea, or vomiting
	None (anuria)	Uremia (urinary substances in the blood), acute nephritis, metal poisoning, e.g., bichloride of mercury
B. Color		
Yellow to amber		Depends upon concentration of pigment in urine
	Pale or colorless	Diabetes insipidus, granular kidney, or very dilute urine
	Milky	Fat globules or pus corpuscles in genitourinary infections
	Reddish (and red-orange)	Blood pigments, drugs (such as Pyridium), or food pigments
	Greenish	Bile pigment with jaundice
	Brown-black	Poisoning (mercury, lead, phenol), or hemorrhages
	Black	Melanuria, malignant pigmented tumor, melanotic cancer, or carbolic acid poisoning
	Blue	Presence of methylene blue or indigo
C. Transparency		
Clear		No significance
Cloudy on standing		Precipitation of mucin from urinary tract; contamination by bacteria in environment; not pathological
Turbid		Precipitation of calcium phosphate; not pathological
	Milky	Presence of fat globules; pathological
	Turbid	Presence of pus as result of inflammation of urinary tract; pathological
D. Odor		
Faintly aromatic		No significance
Peppermint		Menthol ingestion
Acrid		Asparagus in diet
Spicy		Ingestion of sandalwood oil or saffron
	Pleasant (sweet, overripe apple)	Acetone bodies in urine, may be associated with diabetes mellitus (ketonuria)
	Unpleasant (ammoniacal)	Decomposition products or ingestion of certain drugs or foods
	Fecal	Fistulous communication between urinary and intestinal tracts
	Fishy	Cystitis
	New mown hay	Diabetes mellitus
	Violet	Turpentine

Adapted from *Taber's Cyclopedic Medical Dictionary*, 13th ed. Philadelphia, F. A. Davis Co., 1977. pp. U-14—U-16.

leads to a tubule, or collecting channel. The blood is filtered through the capillaries into the malpighian capsule. Blood cells and proteins are retained within the capillaries. The glomerulus allows plasma to pass through by acting as a semipermeable membrane. It is then channeled through the tubules where water, sugar, and salts needed for body functioning are reabsorbed. From there it is re-turned to the renal vein and finally back into the circulatory system. Waste products and water in excess of body needs remain behind (in the tubules) as urine. From the nephrons, urine is emptied via a duct system (papillary ducts) into the calyces of the pelvis of each kidney. It is then carried by peristaltic movements and gravity through the two *ureters* to the *bladder*. A membranous fold within the bladder keeps the ureters closed, preventing the backflow of urine into the kidneys when the pressure of a full bladder increases.

The kidneys are capable of filtering approximately 1 L of blood every minute. Under normal conditions, they can remove approximately 180 L of fluid each day, returning all but about 1 percent of this.[1] Approximately 1−2 L of urine are excreted daily in an adult (the average amount being 1.5L). The amount varies with fluid intake, composition of the diet, activity, vital signs, blood pressure, the velocity of the flow of blood, and pathological conditions.

BLADDER

The bladder is a sac made up of mucous membrane and three layers of muscle tissue—an inner and an outer longitudinal layer and a circular middle layer. These three layers comprise the *detrusor muscle*. The circular layer forms the *internal* (involuntary) *sphincter* (trigonal muscle) at the point where the *urethra* joins the base of the bladder. This sphincter remains contracted (closed), keeping the urine within the bladder, until the process of voiding or micturition occurs. Sensory (stretch) receptors found in the wall of the bladder are stimulated when there is a pressure of 200 to 500 ml of urine in the adult or 100 to 200 ml of urine in the child. At this point, the individual feels an urge to void and the micturition reflex is initiated. The voiding reflex is controlled by the autonomic nervous system. The stimuli from the receptors in the bladder responding to the pressure of increased urine volume are carried to the voiding center in the spinal cord. The parasympathetic nervous system causes the detrusor muscle to contract and the internal sphincter to relax, allowing the urine to enter the urethra. Contraction of the bladder wall, or detrusor muscle, forces the urine out and is maintained until the bladder empties.

The entire process should involve no pain. Discomfort occurs, though, when the bladder is greatly distended and the desire to void becomes urgent. An adult bladder is quite distensible, being capable in some persons of holding up to several liters before rupturing. In others, the capacity is much less. Because it is located in the anterior pelvic cavity (anterior to the upper portion of the vagina and the uterus in the female and to the rectum in the male)

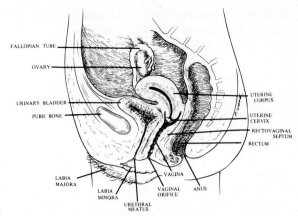

FIGURE 42-1. Sagittal section of female reproductive organs. (Reprinted with permission from Leitch, C. J., and Tinker, R. V.: *Primary Care*. Philadelphia, F. A. Davis Co., 1978, p. 243.)

and is drawn into folds when not filled with urine, it cannot be palpated when empty. As the bladder fills it expands upward and when full or distended can be palpated as a smooth oval above the symphysis pubis in the hypogastric region. (See Figures 42-1 and 42-2 for location of bladder, urethra, and meatus, and related structures in males and females.)

URETHRA

The urethra, which is approximately 1½−2½ inches long in the female and 5½−7 inches long

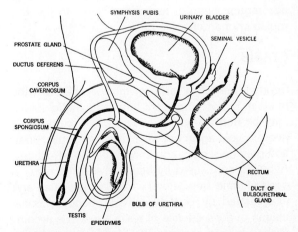

FIGURE 42-2. Male urinary tract. (Reprinted with permission from *Taber's Cyclopedic Medical Dictionary*, 13th ed. Philadelphia, F. A. Davis Co., 1977, p. G-19.)

in the male, is surrounded by a striated (voluntary) muscle ring below the bladder just beyond the portion of the urethra that passes through the prostate gland in the male and at midurethra in the female. This *external sphincter* remains contracted except during micturition when it is relaxed. Initiation or inhibition of voiding is controlled by centers in the cortex of the brain after the approximate age of 2 when the individual develops neuromuscular control and can relax or contract the external sphincter at will. However, in certain situations, such as extreme fear, hearty laughter, sneezing, coughing, certain diseases, injuries, or traumatic conditions, voiding can occur involuntarily. Prior to the age of 2, external sphincter relaxation is involuntary; voiding in infancy is, therefore, entirely a reflex process. In children the abdominal muscles assist urination more than in the adult since the bladder is not as much a pelvic organ as it is in later life; urination then, is often quite forceful in the child. After passing through the urethra, the urine exits the body through the *urethral meatus*.

Problems

A number of problems related to the functioning of the urinary tract are seen fairly frequently. Many have a direct relationship to extended periods of confinement in bed. Some can be prevented, and those that cannot often respond positively to a variety of nursing care measures. Identification of the client's needs, after assessing his health status, taking into consideration the complications known to accompany bedrest, assists the nurse in the formulation of an effective plan of care.

STASIS

Residual urine is a problem that occurs when the bladder is not emptied completely. Fluid intake may be normal, and the client often expresses a need to void again just after urinating. This condition may be seen in conjunction with obstructions. Although not caused by bedrest itself, the result is *stasis of urine* (see below) which is aggravated and exaggerated by periods of recumbency. Confirmation of the existence of residual urine is accomplished by catheterizing the bladder immediately after voiding to determine the amount of urine re-

maining in the bladder. Under normal conditions only a few ml of urine should remain in the bladder after micturition. (Catheterization is discussed later in this chapter.)

Urinary stasis is a slowing of the flow of urine, causing stagnation to take place. When this occurs, the possibility of *urinary tract infection* increases. The urine becomes more concentrated within the bladder which is warm and dark. This combination is conducive to the proliferation of bacteria. Because the mucous membrane of the urinary tract is continuous from the meatus to the kidney pelvis, the pathogens can readily travel from the meatus to the bladder and from the bladder to the kidneys causing more serious problems. *Escherichia coli*, found in the intestinal tract is frequently the causative organism, although *Staphylococcus* and *Streptococcus* and others are also seen. The client with a urinary tract infection may exhibit symptoms such as smaller amounts of urine with increased *frequency* and *urgency* of voiding, pain or a burning sensation during micturition, pus or blood in the urine, chills, fever, and aching or pain in the flank or lower back region or in the suprapubic area.

Stasis also predisposes the urinary tract to the formation of *calculi* (*urolithiasis*). Most calculi (stones) are composed of calcium or magnesium along with phosphorus or oxalate. Alterations in pH of the urine causing its alkalinity, concentrated urine caused by dehydration, and immobilization of the individual causing changes in the mobilization of calcium from the bone also contribute to precipitation of particles in the urinary tract. Stones can obstruct the flow of urine, can cause infection, and can damage the kidneys by destroying the tissue.

Treatment

Since many of the problems stated above are not as apt to occur if (1) the urine remains dilute, (2) mobility of the client is promoted, (3) good aseptic technique and hygiene are practiced, and (4) the diet is carefully planned, then preventive and restorative nursing measures become fairly obvious. Accurate monitoring of *fluid intake and output* reveals the need for fluids. Unless contraindicated, the client should be encouraged to remain well hydrated by the consumption of sufficient amounts of fluid. This will keep the urine from becoming concentrated and the solutes diluted, and will naturally "flush out" the urinary tract. Urinary output should also be maintained at at least 1 L/day. If catheterization or clean catch urines (see Collection of Specimens later in this chapter) are to be done, careful sterile or *aseptic technique* is used during the procedure and for the duration of time the catheter is in place. Clients should be taught to improve *hygienic practices*, such as wiping or cleansing from the anterior to the posterior after voiding (women) and washing hands well after urinating or defecation to prevent the introduction of microorganisms into the meatus. Passive and active *exercises* and positioning of the body in good anatomical alignment helps to prevent stasis of urine for the client on bedrest. *Ambulation*, when possible, even for short periods of time promotes gravity drainage of urine, also decreasing the possibility of stasis, infection, and calculi precipitation. A reduction in the diet of the minerals known to cause stones is an important part of the client's management. Usually diets low in calcium and phosphorus are prescribed for the individual with renal calculi. Urine is often strained to collect particles for laboratory analysis. This aids the physician in the determination of a suitable diet.

RETENTION

There are numerous circumstances in which an individual will be unable to void even though fluid intake is adequate and the kidneys and ureters are functioning normally. Urine enters the bladder as it is produced by the kidneys, but rather than being eliminated through the urethra, it accumulates in the bladder. Eventually the full bladder rises above the symphysis pubis causing some abdominal distention; its height in the abdomen can be palpated manually. The client with *urinary retention* may feel the need to void but is unable to do so. In some instances, sphincter tone is lost due to the pressure of the large quantity of urine in the bladder. When this occurs, small amounts of urine may dribble continuously until the pressure is reduced and muscle tone (sphincter control) is regained. This condition is known as *retention with overflow* or *paradoxical incontinence*. Retention of urine is seen in many clients following surgery as a result of the

effects of anesthesia, when ambulation is not instituted early in the postoperative period and when fluid intake is inadequate. It is also commonly found in a variety of conditions obstructive to urination, such as an enlarged prostate gland, urethral anomalies (i.e. strictures), and trauma to and swelling of the meatus (e.g., after childbirth). These as well as psychological factors, such as anxiety, may cause temporary retention of urine. Certain injuries involving the spinal cord may cause permanent problems with retention. If allowed to continue, retention can cause pain and lead to stasis and urinary tract infection.

Treatment

When clients are having temporary, nonobstructive difficulty with voiding, a number of nursing measures which are conducive to or stimulate micturition can be employed before resorting to catheterization. These include the provision of both privacy, whenever possible, and conditions allowing for gravity drainage of urine. Because females are accustomed to voiding in a sitting position, voiding in the dorsal recumbent position may be extremely difficult for some women. If the toilet can be used, this is naturally the location of choice. A portable bedside commode or placement of the bedpan on a chair are also usually satisfactory if walking to the bathroom is not possible. If the bedpan in bed is the only choice, then barring any contraindications, the client can be placed on the bedpan at the edge of the bed with her feet supported on a chair and the overbed table in front of her to lean upon. When this is not possible, the client is placed on the bedpan as comfortably as possible. The head should be elevated (Fowler's position is recommended). Having the woman lean slightly forward while seated on the bedpan may put pressure on the bladder and assist with sphincter relaxation. A small pillow or folded towel at the small of the back may increase comfort. Before use, metal bedpans should always be warmed by warm water and then carefully dried. The shock of sitting on an icy bedpan is not at all pleasant or helpful in encouraging voiding. Male clients usually void in a standing position but can also void while seated. Other measures that should be attempted, include pouring warm water over the perineum, stroking the inner aspect of the thigh, running water nearby, immersing the hands in warm water, and placing gentle pressure on the bladder in the direction of the urethra. Emotional support should also be given to the client since the tension that he experiences due to the inability to void may make urination even more difficult.

URINARY INCONTINENCE

Urinary incontinence, or loss of voluntary control of voiding, occurs for many of the same reasons as retention of urine. In fact, retention with overflow is a form of incontinence. These include surgery, inflammation, irritation or trauma of the urinary tract, bladder spasms, loss of consciousness, and various conditions causing damage or improper functioning of the brain or spinal cord. Incontinence can be temporary or permanent, and the incontinent client may or may not be aware of the need to void. In either case, the client is usually extremely disturbed by this condition, which after toddlerhood, is considered improper and socially unacceptable. In addition to the support and understanding that is needed, the client must be kept clean, dry, and free of odor. Bedclothes and linens that are moistened or saturated with ammoniacal urine irritate and break down the skin, causing dermatitis and subsequently, decubitus ulcers. Therefore, methods of keeping the client and his bed dry must be found. Linen protector pads and specially made waterproof underwear help to keep the bed dry and decrease the embarrassment of the client when the urine is contained within the garment; however, these must be changed as often as necessary to keep the skin dry. It is recommended that clients *not* be diapered as a measure for maintaining dryness. For male clients, appliances such as condom catheters (Texas condoms) are available. These are worn on the penis and collect the urine externally in a bag. Devices such as these can be adapted for use by ambulatory and bedridden clients. Skin care is still an important aspect of client management when using these appliances.

Other methods used in the treatment of certain incontinent clients include surgical urinary diversions (See Chapter 43 on ostomy care) when obstruction is present and catheterization. The latter, discussed below, is often a last resort due to the hazards involved in initiating the procedure and in its maintenance.

Bladder Training Program

A bladder training program may be initiated by the health team when careful assessment of the client and his condition determine that his level of neurological and muscular functioning will support some form of bladder control. The client must be willing and able to cooperate in the program and whenever possible, actively participate in setting goals for himself and in planning the program. Careful explanations are necessary. The client must realize that the process may be an extended one and that results may not occur for a period of time.

The program is based on regularity and habit. Fluids are provided at specific intervals from morning through evening. Large amounts of fruit juices, which alkalize the urine, and carbonated beverages, which cause bladder irritation, should be avoided. Usually, fluids are limited later in the evening to decrease the possibility of nocturnal incontinence. Provisions for voiding (using the toilet, commode, bedpan, or urinal) in privacy and in a comfortable position are scheduled at regular times. As most people void upon awakening and prior to retiring at night, these times should be taken into consideration. If there has been a pattern to the times of incontinence, this information can also be helpful in planning the schedule at these times. Note that the repetition of the time; for example, 9:00 AM each day is more important than the exact intervals between attempts to void. Usually 20 minutes are sufficient for an attempt. Prolonged periods of time may discourage the client if he feels that he is spending too much time trying to void. The nursing measures for encouraging voiding discussed above are also applicable in the bladder training program. If one method appears to work, for instance hearing running water, then this should be used by the client as a means of stimulating the voiding reflex. Clients need to concentrate on being able to recognize the sign (stimulus) that they may experience when voiding is imminent. These may include feelings of fullness of the bladder, restlessness, chills, goose flesh, perspiration, and muscular twitches.

In cases of bladder flaccidity, urine is often removed by manual expression or firm downward pressure over the abdomen and bladder. This is known as the Credé maneuver. For clients with neurological and muscular damage or paralysis, the training program will be much more of a challenge to plan and employ. The client will need a great deal of encouragement, especially when many attempts are not successful.

The bladder training program is considered a success when the client can empty the bladder by conscious effort, using one particular method. If voiding occurs accidentally or not in conjunction with his chosen method, then the client is not considered to have bladder control.

CATHETERIZATION

Catheterization is the introduction of a tube (catheter) into the bladder, by way of the urethra, to remove urine. The purposes of the procedure are: (1) to completely empty the bladder prior to surgery or childbirth, (2) to keep the bladder decompressed during certain surgical procedures, (3) to empty the bladder and prevent distention after surgery or delivery when the individual is unsuccessful in attempts to void, (4) to empty the bladder when the individual should not void due to a specific treatment or surgical procedure, (5) to relieve urinary retention by gradual decompression of the overly distended bladder, (6) to measure the amount of a residual urine, (7) to intermittently drain and irrigate the bladder, (8) to instill medication into the bladder, (9) for certain incontinent clients, and rarely, (10) to obtain a sterile urine specimen. This last instance is usually not utilized today because of the hazards inherent in the catheterization procedure. In its place, *clean catch urine collection* has become popular. This method is discussed under Collection of Specimens later in the chapter.

The two main dangers of catheterization are *trauma* and *infection*. Trauma can occur when: (1) the catheter is introduced harshly or forced into the urethra, especially if there is a narrowing or stricture present; (2) the procedure is done improperly, as when the catheter is too large for the urethra; (3) too little or no lubricant is used causing friction and subsequent irritation; and (4) the angle of insertion is incorrect; this is more likely in the male whose urethra is longer and more curved than that of the female.

Trauma of the urethra or bladder can predispose the client to infection. The fact that the individual is in a stressed state with lowered resistance also increases the possibility of infection. As stated previously, the mucous membrane that lines the urinary tract is continuous from the meatus up through the pelvis of each kidney, microorganisms can readily travel from one point to the other. The meatus is very close in proximity to the anus (and vagina in the female). Since the skin cannot be sterilized, any time catheterization is done, although the most scrupulous care is taken to implement aseptic technique, introduction of bacteria by the catheter through the meatus is a distinct possibility. It is for this reason that clients are catheterized only when it is absolutely necessary. See Table 42-2 for the steps in catheterization.

Clients who have indwelling catheters must be taught the principles of gravity drainage, including the importance of keeping the collection receptacle below the level of the bladder at all times and keeping the tubing from becoming kinked or compressed. It must be stressed that the catheter and the tubing should never be clamped without the specific orders of the physician, nor should they ever be disconnected from one another. When being disconnected, both ends of the catheter and the tubing should be protected with sterile covers or plugs to prevent contamination. An antiseptic solution is usually used to clean the tubing each day. Hygienic care is also reviewed with the client. The meatus is cleansed daily or more often as needed. In addition, antiseptic or antibiotic ointments may be ordered for application after cleansing.

The intake and output of the catheterized client is usually measured at the end of each shift; however, in certain very seriously ill clients, urine may be measured hourly, using a specially calibrated collection device called a urometer. In cases of minimal output (as in renal failure), the urine may have to be measured with a syringe to maintain accuracy. Unless contraindicated, the catheterized client should be encouraged to drink fluids, ensuring adequate intake and producing urine having a specific gravity low enough to keep flowing freely. (The more dense the urine, the slower it will flow.)

TABLE 42-2. Urethral Catheterization of Bladder as an Assessment Tool, to Prevent Distention, to Keep Bladder Decompressed, to Keep Client from Voiding, and to Irrigate Bladder and Provide for Intermittent or Continuous Drainage

Anticipated Accomplishment	Scientific Principles/ Rationale	Specific Considerations
1. Decreased possibility of spreading infection.	Friction and running water remove many microorganisms from skin.	
2. Conservation of time and energy. Organization.	Client will feel more confident and less anxious if nurse is organized and efficient. Much time is saved if several trips to obtain equipment are eliminated.	Where is procedure to be done? (In treatment room or client's room?) What type of catheter set is necessary? What is purpose of procedure?

Implementation	Recommendations	Observations
Wash hands using aseptic technique.		
Collect all equipment necessary for procedure: a. Additional light source (e.g., goose neck lamp). b. Drapes for client and linen protector pad for bed. c. Sterile catheterization set: antiseptic cleansing solution; gauze pads; cotton pledgets or cotton balls in receptacle or small basin; forceps; water-soluble lubricant; receptacle for collection of urine; specimen container with lid; and catheter (see below).	Disposable catheter sets are economical and safer than others since they are used only once and discarded; there is no need for sterilization. Drape can be sheet or bath blanket which provides warmth as well as privacy.	
d. Sterile gloves.	Sterile gloves are usually included in disposable catheterization sets. If possible, additional package of sterile gloves should be convenient in case of contamination.	
e. If retention catheter, materials for inflation of balloon (see below), collection bag and tubing, and adhesive tape.	Set up collection bag and tubing if using retention catheter; do not remove sterile protective sheaths or plugs at this point. Cut appropriate lengths of adhesive tape to be used later. Set aside.	

TABLE 42-2. Continued

Anticipated Accomplishment	Scientific Principles/ Rationale	Specific Considerations
	If too small a catheter is used, emptying time is extended unnecessarily; if a retention catheter is used, urine may leak around it, or it may slip out. If too large, pain and trauma to urethra can occur, increasing risk of infection or pressure necrosis of meatus.	
	While most catheters are made of latex, rubber, or plastic, finely woven silk catheters are occasionally used in male clients because they are both flexible enough to follow curvature of urethra and firm enough not to collapse. Many catheters are coated with silicone which inhibits collection of sediment around walls, maintaining their patency longer.	What is the purpose of procedure? A straight catheter is used to empty bladder or remove residual urines or specimens. An indwelling (Foley) catheter is used for continuous or intermittent drainage and irrigations.
3. Reduction of anxiety in client.	Fear of unknown and of pain increases anxiety and decreases cooperativeness of client.	What is client's level of understanding about his condition? Has he ever been catheterized before?
	Exposure and handling of the genitalia is often anxiety and guilt provoking.	Is room cool or drafty? Does client have elevated temperature? Does he feel chilled?

Implementation	Recommendations	Observations
f. Select proper catheter for procedure. (Catheters are graded according to lumen (diameter) size on the French (Fr) scale. The larger the number, the larger the lumen. (Fig. 42-3).	Usual catheter sizes: for children: sizes 8 or 10 Fr; for adult females: sizes 14 or 16 Fr (although a 12 Fr is used if these are too large); for adult males: sizes 18, 20, and 22 Fr (although a 16 Fr is used if these are too large). Most often, physicians order catheter size.	What is condition and size of urethra?

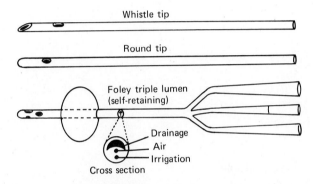

FIGURE 42-3. Types of catheters.

For indwelling catheters select correct materials needed to inflate balloon; instructions are always printed on packaging or on catheter. These materials *may* include: syringe (sterile), needle (sterile), sterile water or sterile saline, and clamp.

If there is a choice, sterile water is preferred to saline as latter may deteriorate latex over time.

Explain procedure and purpose to client in understandable terms.

Tell client that procedure may cause some discomfort or a feeling of pressure, but should not be painful. Client may experience desire to void when catheter is inserted.

Provide for privacy by closing door to room and using appropriate draping.

Hold sheet or bath blanket at a diagonal to client if in dorsal recumbent position (see below).

Is client chilled? Is client embarrassed?

TABLE 42-2. Continued

Anticipated Accomplishment	Scientific Principles/ Rationale	Specific Considerations
	When anxious, muscles tense and insertion of catheter is more difficult than when client is relaxed.	
4. Provide for good visualization of meatus and proper anatomical positioning.	Bladder, when located above meatus, allows for drainage by gravity.	
	Sim's position is more tolerable to clients with difficulty flexing knees or hips (as in severe arthritis). It also limits exposure of genitalia, decreasing anxiety or embarrassment.	
	Artificial lighting in addition to overhead light increases visualization by decreasing shadows and providing high illumination of area.	If right-handed, stand to client's right (left side of bed) and vice versa if left-handed.
5. Decrease possibility of spreading infection to client.		

Implementation	Recommendations	Observations
	Wrap two opposite points of diamond around client's feet. The third point at bottom fits between legs and can be lifted when ready to assemble sterile field.	
If in bed, place female client in dorsal recumbent position with flexion of knees and abduction of the legs.	A modification of position in which client's legs are wide apart is sometimes used. To facilitate this position, place client on back, and ask her to flex knees keeping ankles together; then spread knees apart, resting the bottoms of feet together. Another helpful method for maintaining positioning is to support thighs of client with pillows, holding them apart.	
If this is not possible, Sim's (side lying) position may be used for females. In treatment room, female client is placed in lithotomy position on examination table, using stirrups to hold legs and feet in place. The male client is placed in back-lying position with knees slightly apart.	In Sim's position, client lies with buttocks close to edge of bed and the knees pulled up toward chest. Upper knee is higher than lower knee.	
After positioning client properly, provide adequate lighting.	A gooseneck lamp with a bright bulb placed on opposite side of bed (when dorsal recumbent or lithotomy position is used) does not interfere with procedure and helps to locate meatus.	
Open outside (nonsterile) wrapper of catheterization set. If retention catheter is to be used, peel open package of indwelling catheter, but do not touch contents.		

TABLE 42-2. Continued

Anticipated Accomplishment	Scientific Principles/ Rationale	Specific Considerations
	Reduction in number of micro-organisms on hands.	
	Gloves maintain sterility by blocking passage of microorganisms from hands to sterile equipment.	
6. Preparation of materials for use during procedure.	There is a reduction in possibility of contamination since materials are placed in a manner that eliminates reaching over sterile field. Organization of materials facilitates ease and expediting of procedure.	
	Lubrication decreases friction and trauma to urethra and increases ease of insertion.	Occasionally physician orders catheter tip lubricated with antibiotic ointment as a prophylactic measure, or in presence of infection.
	Coiling catheter in receptacle facilitates picking it up with one hand without dragging the end risking contamination.	

Implementation	Recommendations	Observations
Wash hands using aseptic technique.		
Place sterile drape under hips of client.	Pick up sterile drape by one corner and remove from catheter set. Holding two corners only, place under hips of client, leaving large area of sterile drape in area between legs as sterile field. Avoid touching client's skin.	
Put on sterile gloves. (See Chapter 31, "Asepsis")		
Place sterile catheter tray on sterile field formed by sterile drape.	If using disposable set, place in such a way that items to be used first (e.g., forceps and cotton balls) are nearest and those used last are at distal side of sterile field (e.g., specimen bottle).	
Carefully add catheter from opened package to catheter tray without contaminating glove.	Wind catheter around gloved hand so it does not drag when removed from interior package.	
Pour solution (if sterile container within set) over cotton balls.		
Lubricate 1½−2 in of catheter tip, and leave it coiled in sterile receptacle.	Open lubricant and squeeze into bottom of sterile receptacle. Lubricate 1½−2 in of catheter tip. Do not get lubricant into holes in catheter, if possible.	

TABLE 42-2. Continued

Anticipated Accomplishment	Scientific Principles/ Rationale	Specific Considerations
7. Decrease possibility of contamination of gloves and spread of infection.	Drape provides a further barrier between client's body and sterile materials.	Some people prefer not to use upper drape as disposable paper drapes tend to slip or fall off during procedure. If not used, care must be taken to avoid contamination of objects by contact with client's body.
8. Expose meatus.	Possibility of trauma is minimized with good visualization. By spreading labia minora, meatus may be visualized. Perpendicular elevation of penis straightens cavernous portion of urethra.	Retract foreskin (prepuce) if present in male.
9. Decrease possibility of contamination and infection.	Cleansing from "clean" to "dirty" area reduces possibility of contamination of meatus and reduces number of microorganisms which can be transmitted from anus (and vagina) to urethra. Use of forceps minimizes possibility of contaminating right glove. Using a separate cotton ball for each stroke prevents transference of microorganisms from posterior area of perineum to anterior aspect (including meatus). Cleansing strokes are gentle since vigorous action can be traumatic to meatus.	In some institutions, initial cleansing is done with soap and water prior to catheterization. Care must be taken to remove all soap from area before beginning. If female client has a large amount of discharge or blood, extra pledgets may be used to cleanse area.

Implementation	Recommendations	Observations
Place a sterile drape over female's perineum or over penis.	Center opening in middle of drape over genitalia.	
In female, separate labia minora. In male, straighten urethra.	If right handed, place thumb and forefinger of left hand between labia minora and spread apart. Once separated, do not move fingers allowing tissue to return to normal position (Fig. 42-4). Using left hand, hold penis at coronary sulcus with thumb and forefinger and elevate penis perpendicular to body keeping foreskin retracted.	Observe female perineum for a "dimple" or pucker in tissue between clitoris and vestibule. This is the usual appearance of meatus.
Cleanse labia from anterior (above meatus) to posterior (toward anus). Cleanse penis from meatus outward.	With right hand, use forceps to hold each cotton ball or pledget. Use each cotton ball once and discard to corner of sterile drape (or into appropriate waste container) being careful not to contaminate forceps.	Observe for location of meatus while cleansing area if it has not yet been visualized. Also, observe for any anomalies, unusual physical characteristics, odors, or discharge.
	Usually approximately 3–4 pledgets are used for cleansing. Pressure of strokes should be enough to cleanse area; however, gentleness should always be used.	

TABLE 42-2. Continued

Anticipated Accomplishment	Scientific Principles/ Rationale	Specific Considerations

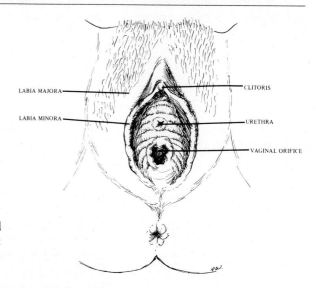

FIGURE 42-4. External female genitalia. (Reprinted with permission from Leitch, C. J., and Tinker, R. V.: *Primary Care.* Philadelphia, F. A. Davis Co., 1978, p. 241.)

	Microorganisms from surrounding area are kept away from meatus by maintaining separation of labia and elevation of penis with retraction of foreskin.	If labia close or the foreskin is not kept retracted with penis elevated, consider area contaminated. Cleansing must be repeated.
10. Insertion of catheter.	Avoidance of "dragging" end of catheter minimizes risk of contamination.	
	Focusing on a specific task may encourage client to relax, facilitating insertion. Tension or anxiety cause muscular tightening of sphincter, making insertion more difficult.	
	Female urethra is approximately 1½−2 in long; the male urethra is approximately 5½−7 in long.	

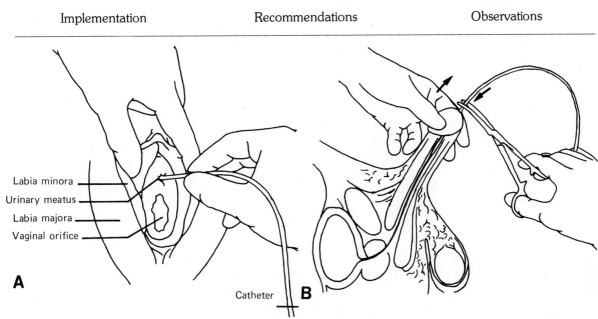

Labia minora
Urinary meatus
Labia majora
Vaginal orifice

A

Catheter   **B**

FIGURE 42-5. A, Catheterization of urinary bladder in female. B, Technique for catheterization in male.

Do not permit labia to close or foreskin to cover glans penis. Keep the penis elevated. Some people prefer to use cotton balls under the thumb and forefinger to prevent them from slipping when spreading labia.

Insert catheter into urethra until urine begins to flow. Allow urine to flow into sterile receptacle (Figs. 42-5A and B).

Make certain that drainage receptacle is close to perineum; use caution to avoid contamination by touching body with receptacle.

Have client take deep breaths through the mouth.

Insert catheter into urethra, approximately 2–3 in in females and approximately 7–9 in in males. With indwelling catheters, advance catheter approxi-

TABLE 42-2. Continued

Anticipated Accomplishment	Scientific Principles/ Rationale	Specific Considerations
	The catheter occasionally pushes against fold of mucous membrane.	
	Withdrawal and advancement of catheter increases chance of introducing microorganisms into bladder.	Do not force catheter in; if extreme pain occurs or resistance or obstruction is noted, discontinue procedure and notify physician.
11. Allow bladder to drain.	Gradual decompression of overly distended bladder avoids loss of bladder tone with resultant trauma and damage to bladder. When emptied too quickly, chills, fever, and shock can occur due to rapid change of internal bladder pressure and distention of blood vessels.	After 750 to 1000 ml (agency policies, physicians, and authorities vary), remove catheter; do not decompress bladder any further. Always collect a sterile specimen while client is catheterized. If not needed, it can be discarded.
(Go to step 13 if an indwelling catheter is being inserted)		
12. Removal of catheter (if not an indwelling catheter).	Slow removal avoids both trauma and discomfort.	
	If foreskin is left retracted, glans can become edematous, causing difficulty in voiding.	Be certain that foreskin is replaced over glans penis. Send specimen (correctly labeled) to laboratory if ordered.

Implementation	Recommendations	Observations
	mately 1 in further after urine begins to flow to be sure that balloon is beyond urethra and in bladder.	
	If resistance is felt, wait momentarily, then gently twist catheter while advancing it slowly. In males, increased traction and slightly lowering penis helps while advancing catheter, to pass it through membranous and prostatic portions of urethra which is a fixed curvature.	
	Do not withdraw and advance catheter. If no urine begins to flow in female client, catheter may be in vagina. Leave it in place and when inserting sterile replacement catheter, this will serve as a landmark to avoid.	
Hold catheter in place until flow of urine ceases.	Do not allow catheter to change position while urine is draining. Penis may be lowered while drainage takes place.	
		Observe urine for color, odor, and any unusual characteristics.
Withdraw catheter quite slowly.	After withdrawal of the catheter, gently cleanse meatus of any lubricant. Gently dry area well.	
Measure amount of urine obtained. Record and report procedure in manner appropriate to agency.		

TABLE 42-2. Continued

Anticipated Accomplishment	Scientific Principles/ Rationale	Specific Considerations
13. Indwelling catheters: maintain position of catheter in bladder.	When inflated, balloon is wider in diameter than urethra, preventing catheter from sliding out.	Balloons are inflated with 5 to 30 ml of air or sterile water or saline. Catheters will have a side arm for inflation which requires using tip of a sterile syringe with or without a needle. A clamp may or may not be needed for the side arm, depending upon style.
14. Provide for gravity (straight) drainage.	Drainage bag must always remain below level of bladder to insure gravity drainage and prevent flow of urine back into bladder. Rate of drainage is affected by distance from bladder to drainage receptacle as well as size of lumen of catheter. Taping in place prevents tension on catheter and possibility of its being pulled out. Compression of drainage tubing by client's body causes drainage to stop, and increases chance of both stasis and infection. Closed drainage systems are least hazardous since urine flows from bladder to receptacle via an unbroken sterile system. Entrance of microorganisms is prevented since system is not disconnected or interrupted.	When the client is ambulatory, a leg bag can be strapped to his thigh or he can carry drainage receptacle. Client must be taught to keep collection bag lower than bladder.
15. Recording of output.		A record of intake and output (I & O) is kept on most clients with indwelling catheters. Amount of drainage is usually measured at end of each shift; this can be done more fre-

Implementation	Recommendations	Observations
Inflate balloon according to manufacturer's directions.	Read manufacturer's instructions carefully before beginning procedure.	If pain occurs during inflation balloon may be in the urethra. Deflate balloon and slowly advance catheter approximately 1 in farther. Reinflate.
	Very gently pull back on catheter after inflation of balloon to ascertain its placement in bladder.	
Connect end of catheter to sterile tubing and drainage receptacle (Fig. 42-6).	Secure drainage receptacle to bed frame.	Observe for uninterrupted flow of urine. Avoid kinking of tubing.
Tape catheter in place (Figs. 42-7A and B).		
	Place drainage tubing over client's thigh. Tubing should be just long enough to allow client to have freedom of movement in bed.	
Record intake and output on appropriate record form.	Gradations on most drainage bags are not very accurate. For precise measurements, urine should be drained from bag into a calibrated measuring device.	Observe color, odor, transparency, volume, and any unusual characteristics of urine. Also note any complaints, such as burning or pain.

TABLE 42-2. Continued

Anticipated Accomplishment	Scientific Principles/Rationale	Specific Considerations

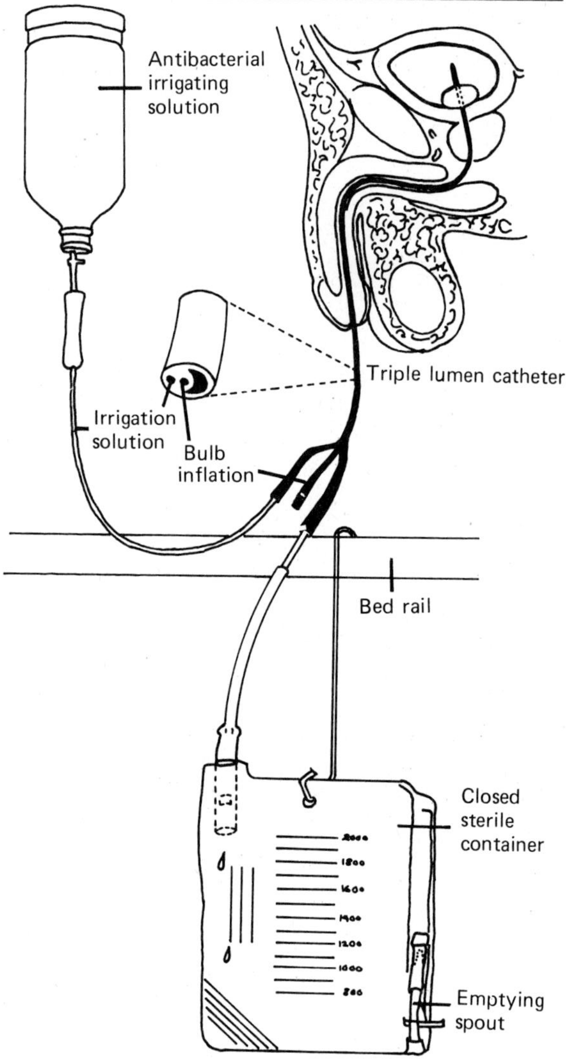

FIGURE 42-6. Closed sterile drainage system.

quently if necessary, when amounts are either large or physician wishes an hourly output record.

16. Removal of catheter.   See step 12 above.

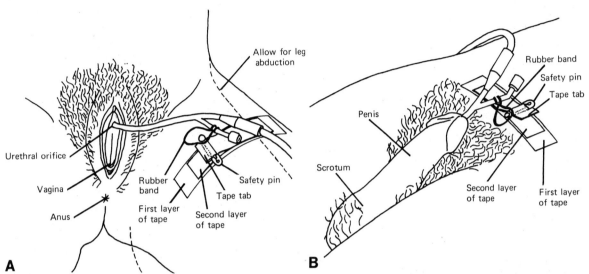

FIGURE 42-7. A, Taping a Foley catheter (female). The objective is to prevent extension of the catheter when the balloon is inflated. The catheter is taped to the thigh when the leg is abducted to allow sufficient length of catheter to permit leg mobility without putting stress on indwelling portion of catheter. B, Taping a Foley catheter (male). The object is to straighten the urethral curve at the penoscrotal area to reduce the chance of pressure necrosis within the urethra and to prevent additional force on the catheter and urethra in the event of erection. Positioning the Foley catheter against the thigh would frustrate this objective; therefore, the catheter is anchored on the abdomen instead. (Adapted from Jones et al.: *Medical Surgical Nursing—A Conceptual Approach.* New York, McGraw-Hill Book Co., 1978, pp. 1150–1151.)

Remove tape. Deflate balloon according to manufacturer's instructions. Slowly withdraw catheter. See step 12 above.

Observe for difficulty in voiding and symptoms of urinary tract infection, such as burning, frequency, cloudy urine, or pus or blood in urine.

Irrigation

For the same reasons that catheterization is avoided unless absolutely necessary, irrigations too, are used judiciously. The possibility of trauma and of the introduction of microorganisms into the bladder is increased with this procedure. Irrigation—that is, the instillation of a solution through the catheter into the bladder—is used when there is a problem with the patency of the catheter. In essence, the catheter is flushed out by introducing sterile saline or a sterile antiseptic solution into the catheter. An Asepto or bulb syringe, a receptacle for the solution, and a collecting container are needed. Needless to say, all equipment must be sterile, although the collecting container may be clean rather than sterile. Approximately 90–120 ml of solution are gently instilled (never forced) 30 ml at a time. Each instillation of solution is allowed to drain out into the collecting container before adding more.

To irrigate the catheter, it often must be disconnected from the tubing to insert the tip of the syringe into the end of the catheter. Both the end of the catheter and the end of the tubing must be protected against contamination when using this method. Preferable to this is the use of indwelling catheters that have an additional side-arm for irrigation purposes, eliminating the necessity of disconnecting the tubing, thus minimizing the risk of infection.

Also utilized for irrigation of catheters is an intermittent closed system where the solution is dripped into the catheter at approximately 30–60 drops per minute. The rate of flow and the height of the solution container are determined by the physician. Usually very low pressure is used. In most instances, a physician's order is needed to irrigate an indwelling catheter. (See Figure 42-6).

GASTROINTESTINAL TRACT

Function and Anatomy

Mechanical and chemical processes in the gastrointestinal tract break down food and convert it into forms which can be absorbed and utilized by the body. The *enzymes* ptyalin, pepsin, trypsin, lipase, amylase, and invertase bring about the chemical actions; churning and rhythmic waves along the musculature of the gastrointestinal tract (*peristalsis*) provide mechanical propulsion of the contents.

Digestion begins in the *mouth*; food is moistened, softened, and a part of it dissolved. The breakdown of starches into sugar begins here. The food enters the *stomach* through the *cardiac sphincter* via the *esophagus*. The enzymes in the gastric juices, in conjunction with hydrochloric acid, begin to act on proteins (breaking them down into peptones) and on certain emulsified fats.

Depending upon the amount and type of food ingested, the stomach empties in 3 to 6 hours. At this point, the food bulk is a thick, almost liquid, multicolored acid mass called *chyme*. Chyme enters the *duodenum*, the widest portion of the *small intestine*, through the *pyloric sphincter (pylorus)* and is mixed with *intestinal juices, pancreatic juice*, and *bile*. While traveling the length of the small intestine, including the *jejunum* and *ileum*, the intestinal and pancreatic juices break all starches and sugars into monosaccharides, convert peptones into amino acids, and fats (which have been emulsified by the bile) into fatty acids and glycerol (glycerin). These nutrient substances are then absorbed into the bloodstream through the walls of the small intestine.

The remaining residue and products of digestion which are not needed by the body for nutrition then enter the *cecum* of the *large intestine* through the *ileocecal valve* in a nearly liquid state. This valve permits movement in one direction, preventing backflow of the waste into the small intestine. In the 4½ to 5 foot *colon*, which includes the *ascending colon, hepatic flexure, transverse colon, splenic flexure, descending colon*, and *signoid flexure* (see Fig. 43-5 in Chapter 43), *bacterial action* and *reabsorption of water* occur, causing the waste (feces) to become firm or semisolid in consistency. (Up to a liter of water is absorbed from the intestinal tract each day.) Microbial action on carbohydrates in the alimentary canal causes their decomposition. This results in *fermentation*, a chemical process which produces hydrogen and carbon dioxide. Likewise, the breakdown of undigested proteins results in *putrefaction* and liberation of hydrogen sulfide.[2] The end products of fermentation and putrefaction are amines, ammonia, and organic acids, which chemically stimulate contraction of the intestinal musculature. Food bulk or gas volume mechanically irritate the muscle tissue, causing it to contract. This contraction moves the fecal matter downward. Feces in the large intestine are propelled into the *rectum* by a mass peristaltic movement which may occur once a day (or more) and is often associated with consumption of food. This reflex movement is often seen after breakfast before which the stomach had been empty for several hours. If the feces (stool) pass through the colon too rapidly, water absorption is decreased considerably, causing the stool to be watery and poorly formed (*diarrhea*). On the other hand, if the stool is moved too slowly or is retained in the colon, too much water will be absorbed and the stool becomes hard and dry (*constipation*).

When the feces stimulate sensory nerve endings by distending the rectum, a desire to expel the material is experienced and the defecatory reflex occurs. The smooth muscle of the *internal sphincter* in the *anus* is relaxed involuntarily by the autonomic nervous system while the striated muscle of the *external sphinter* in the anus voluntarily relaxes. The abdominal muscles and the levator ani, which form the floor of the pelvis, contract voluntarily, along with increased pressure (also voluntary) of the diaphragm on the abdominal viscera, increasing intra-abdominal pressure and assisting the process of defecation. Since the external sphincter of the anus is normally under voluntary control from the age of 2 on, it can be constricted if the individual desires to delay defecation. This may cause the defecatory reflex to be suppressed in a short amount of time. Its reappearance usually occurs hours later. When the person continuously ignores or inhibits the reflex, irregularity of bowel habits occurs and difficulties with defecation result (constipation is the most common problem) since the large intestine and rectum eventually lose their sensitivity to mechanical and chemical stimulation.

The stool is composed at the time of expulsion of any undigested materials, residue from the digestive process, epithelial cells, mucus, water, inorganic salts and bacteria, such as the colon bacilli, *E. coli, Staphylococci,* and others. Having been mixed in the small intestine with bile pigment excreted by the liver, the feces have a characteristic brown color. When erythrocytes disintegrate in hemoglobin breakdown, bilirubin (a red pigment) is formed; this in turn can be oxidized to biliverdin

(which is green) and finally broken down to sterobilin (brown).[2] A change in the color of the stool may indicate an impaired function or abnormal condition in the body; clay-colored stools (absence of bile) may be a symptom of altered liver function, while black, tarry stools (melena) can be due to either blood in the feces or the ingestion of iron compounds (medication).

The odor of stools is due primarily to bacterial decomposition (putrefaction) of tryptophan (an amino acid found in protein), resulting in indole and skatole, malodorous solid substances. Diet and drugs can influence the odor and the color of the stool. The pH of stools is normally neutral or slightly alkaline, although in infancy, it is usually acid.

In most instances, the shape of a formed stool consistently remains the same, since it is "molded" by the rectal wall. When this changes significantly, it may indicate an altered condition of the colon or rectum, such as when a tumor narrows the diameter of the colon causing very thin stools.

Problems

Problems involving the lower gastrointestinal tract are usually related to prolonged bedrest, surgery in which a general anesthetic has been used, diseases, drugs, unbalanced diet, emotional influences, and the practice of undesirable bowel habits. Lack of exercise, long periods of inactivity, such as bedrest, and the effects of anesthesia decrease peristalsis, upsetting bowel function. Stress, illness, and dietary insufficiency can result in irregularity. When conditions under which a bowel movement is attempted are altered or interfered with, difficulties in the elimination process may arise. These conditions might include lack of *privacy*, which most people, especially in our culture, find difficult to overcome. The majority of Americans are accustomed to carrying out elimination processes alone, behind a closed (often locked) door. They find the normal sounds of urination, defecation, and the passage of flatus embarrassing, unrefined, and discourteous, and will often suppress the stimulus to go to the bathroom if others are in the immediate or an adjacent area. *Familiarity of the environment* and *positioning* may also affect the ability to have a bowel movement. To have a bowel movement on a bedpan rather than in the toilet may be extremely difficult, and this difficulty is further compounded when the client cannot assume the natural sitting posture that not only feels correct but assists anatomically in passing the stool. These habits are lifelong and thus extremely difficulty to modify, even when one understands the reason why the change is necessary.

NURSING CARE

After assessment of individual needs, nursing measures in conjunction with medical management are aimed at restoring and maintaining normal elimination patterns and relieving hypermotility and hypomotility and the conditions that may ensue. In determining the appropriate nursing measures, data about the client's usual patterns and habits of elimination must first be identified.

How often does the client have a bowel movement? While most people have one bowel movement each day, some normally have one every 2 or 3 days and others more than once every day. Normalcy and disturbances should only be compared to the client's usual pattern, not to the patterns of others.

Is defecation usually at a particular time or is it related to a certain event, such as breakfast? Since peristalsis is increased after consumption of food, especially the first meal of the day, passage of stool is frequently seen immediately following the meal.

Does the client routinely rely on specific methods of stimulating a bowel movement, such as laxatives, enemas, suppositories, or others? Many people because of employment situations and other daily activities have become accustomed to ignoring the urge to have a bowel movement (the defecation reflex); thus, the lack of stimulation from the presence of the fecal mass (sensory adaptation) occurs, forcing them to resort to other means of being "regular." Soon dependence on outside stimulation is established, and the individual is unable to have a bowel movement without it. This is frequently seen in geriatric clients who are very concerned with their elimination processes and are thus very "bowel conscious."

How active is the client and how much daily exercise does he get? Adequate activity and exercise increases general well-being by improving muscle tone (assisting the defecatory process) and the functioning of the gastrointestinal tract (digestion and motility).

What is the client's normal food and fluid intake? Because the gastrointestinal tract lacks enzymes that can digest *cellulose*, the residue from foods eaten that contains this substance will supply bulk and increase peristalsis. This can assist the elimination process if consumed in appropriate amounts. If too much bulk is present in the diet, motility is stepped up and frequent watery stools (diarrhea) may occur. To keep stools normal in their consistency, a balanced combination of foods with high fluid content and liquids in the daily intake maintain softness and consequently, ease of passage.

HYPERMOTILITY

A large number of conditions may cause temporary or chronic *hypermotility* of the lower gastrointestinal tract: various *diseases* or conditions within and outside of the gastrointestinal tract, such as allergies, inflammation, tumors, and glandular disturbances; *irritants*, such as medications and cathartic drugs, certain foods and beverages (e.g., coffee and alcohol), and microorganisms; and *emotional or stressful conditions*. Normally the mucous membrane of the large intestine is lubricated and protected from injury by the secretion of mucus. When intestinal irritation occurs, such as in bacterial invasion, the body protects itself by secreting more of the mucus to dilute and counteract the irritant. This in turn liquefies the intestinal contents. With hypermotility, water, electrolytes, and nutrients cannot be absorbed well from the intestinal contents because passage through the lower gastrointestinal tract is too rapid. When this occurs, *diarrhea*, or evacuation of poorly formed, possibly liquid stools, is the result. Defecation is at fairly frequent intervals, although frequent passage of normally formed stools would not be considered diarrhea. Abdominal (intestinal) cramps, weakness, nausea, vomiting, weight loss, and stools containing blood or mucus may accompany diarrhea. Since diarrhea is a symptom rather than a disease, the total clinical picture for each client and the medical and nursing management will vary with the causative condition. When diarrhea is severe, dehydration, inadequate nutrition, and electrolyte and acid-base imbalances can occur. This can be serious in the adult client, but in infants and small children, it can rapidly become life-threatening.

Treatment

In cases of excessive fluid depletion, parenteral (intravenous) fluid replacement is usually instituted. Correction of the nutritional and chemical imbalances must also be implemented. In less serious cases, treatment usually consists of increased fluid intake, a liquid or bland diet, and the administration of antidiarrheal agents such as paregoric (camphorated tincture of opium), Kaopectate or kaolin, Lomotil, and others.

Usually bedrest is suggested as this decreases peristalsis and provides rest while the client is in a weakened condition. If the client is too debilitated to get to the toilet, the provision of a portable bedside commode and ready assistance in getting in and out of bed or easy access to a bedpan are basic necessities. The signal light should be within easy reach of the client and answered immediately. The client may find the inability to control the defecation reflex and the associated sounds and odor embarrassing. Occasionally, accidents occur, and the bed and clothing are soiled. Emotional support is thus a vital part of nursing care. Often the skin around the anus becomes irritated and sore. Thorough cleansing with soap and water and gentle drying after each bowel movement are helpful in preventing skin breakdown. Application of powder or soothing, protective ointments or creams may also be utilized as a comfort and preventive measure. If the bed linens become soiled, they should be changed immediately. This not only removes the possibility of skin irritation but also reduces the psychic pain of incontinence. The client's intake and output as well as the number and character of all stools should be reported and recorded according to agency policy.

FECAL INCONTINENCE

Fecal (anal) incontinence, or lack of sphincter control in the passage of feces, can occur temporarily as in diarrhea or unconsciousness or chronically as in certain diseases or neuromuscular disorders. Nursing measures and factors to be considered are much the same as those that were stated previously under urinary incontinence. With all incontinent clients conscientious skin care to prevent decubitus formation is mandatory.

Bowel Training Program

A bowel training program is planned and implemented with the cooperation and participation of the client after a careful assessment of his past and present elimination patterns and status and personal needs for scheduling. Attempts to defecate of approximately 20 minutes in length are tried at the chosen time each day. Conditions (privacy and positioning) that are conducive to defecation are provided. If the client has a particular personal habit that has a customary place in his daily elimination practice (i.e., a glass of prune juice, a cup of coffee, or reading), it is often helpful to include this in the program. Activity and exercise, especially of the abdominal and pelvic musculature, are planned and encouraged in a manner realistic to the client's abilities. Food and fluid intake are reviewed and regulated according to individual need. The necessity for and use of laxatives, enemas, and suppositories are determined on an individual basis, but regular usage is discouraged in most cases. In some cases of paralysis, the use of mechanical stimulation (suppository or digital stimulation) may be needed. As in any program in which progress is slow and often discouraging, a great deal of emotional support is needed to keep the client from feeling like a failure and ultimately giving up.

TYMPANITES

Up to 10 L of gases are formed in the large intestine of an adult every day. The gases formed in the intestines and the stomach (*flatus*) include oxygen, nitrogen (from air swallowed during consumption of food and fluids), carbon dioxide, hydrogen, and methane (from the metabolism of protein and carbohydrates). When *flatulence* (excessive gas) accumulates due to lack of expulsion, it is known as *tympanites* or *distention*. Normally, most of the gas produced in the intestines is absorbed through the intestinal walls, while the gas in the stomach is eliminated by belching (eructation) before reaching the small intestine. When motility increases, absorption of gases is reduced, thus causing larger amounts of flatus to be passed. This is seen with diarrhea. When peristalsis is slowed, as with use of certain drugs and after surgery, distention is promoted. In addition, certain foods are irritating and when acted upon by bacteria, have a tendency to cause flatus.

Treatment

Distention, which often causes cramping pain and protrusion of the abdomen can at times be relieved by encouraging activity and ambulation. Medications (antiflatulents) may also be ordered for relief. A *rectal tube* is a mechanical means of removing flatulence, although the results may only be temporary, since the cause of the distention is not being relieved by this measure. With the client in side-lying position, a well-lubricated tube is inserted into the anus in the same manner as in an enema (Table 42-3); if no resistance is felt, it can be very slowly and gently advanced a bit farther into the rectum. The tube, which is connected to plastic tubing leading down below the level of the rectum into a container with air vents or a disposable bag, is left in place for approximately 20 minutes. It may be reintroduced every few hours. Periods of longer than 20 minutes may produce spasms of the sphincter muscle and its eventual relaxation or unresponsiveness. The addition of water to cover the end of the tubing in the container helps to assess whether or not gas is being evacuated as bubbles appear when the flatus is expelled. A physician's order is needed for use of rectal tubes. The order usually includes the size of the tube, which in adults ranges from 22 to 32 Fr; with children, naturally, the size is decreased.

A *Harris flush*, or *return flow enema*, irrigates the lower portion of the bowel and helps remove flatulence. It is different from other enemas in that the solution used is allowed to flow out of the rectum (through the enema tube) by gravity drainage; the tube is not removed as it is in cleansing enemas. Alternating periods of allowing the solution to flow in and then out encourages expulsion of the flatus by stimulating peristalsis.

CONSTIPATION

As stated earlier, when motility slows, intestinal contents remain in the colon for longer periods of time, allowing larger amounts of water than usual to be absorbed and causing the stools to become hard and dried. *Constipation*, or the presence of stools with this abnormal consistency, may be acute or chronic and can be the result of a number of conditions or circumstances, such as conscious retention of feces to avoid pain on defecation as when hemorrhoids are present, repeated ignoring of the defecation urge, chronic use of and dependence upon laxatives or enemas, prolonged periods of inactivity (bedrest), lack of exercise, inadequate intake of fluids, dehydration, low residue diets or those that are low or lacking in cellulose or fibrous foods, certain drugs, stress, extreme weakness, diseases that obstruct or cause problems with motility of the gastrointestinal tract, and interference with either innervation or the functioning of the smooth or voluntary muscles needed for defecation.

Symptoms that may accompany constipation are general malaise, headache, lethargy, abdominal distention, pain, cramping, a feeling of fullness in the rectum, loss of appetite (anorexia), coated tongue, an unpleasant or foul breath, expelling of flatus or *small amounts* of dry, hard stool, liquid feces, or the complete lack of defecation.

Treatment

Treatment plans are directed toward elimination of the original source of the problem. In some cases this requires all or selected steps of a bowel training program as previously described and education of the client, including giving up poor bowel habits and learning healthy new practices (i.e., balanced diet, fluid intake, or increased activity). Palliative or symptomatic relief of temporary constipation may include the oral administration of fecal softening agents; oral cathartics; laxatives, purgatives or suppositories that soften stools, stimulate peristalsis, or provide bulk (see Chapter 34, "Administration of Medications"); oil retention enemas that lubricate and soften the feces, promoting ease of expulsion; soap and water; hypotonic (tapwater), physiologic (isotonic), or hypertonic saline enemas that distend or irritate the colon and rectum, stimulating peristalsis and the expelling of feces and flatulence. (See Table 42-3 for the steps in the administration of enemas.) A physician's order is needed for all of these medications and treatments. The order will include type, amount, and frequency of the treatment. Indiscriminate use of any of these methods should be avoided. Explanations should be given to the client, clarifying that use of over-the-counter agents should be limited to selected situations and only on the recommendation of a qualified health professional.

FECAL IMPACTION

Several factors can cause fecal material to be retained and then hardened into an obstructing mass in the rectum: constipation, prolonged bedrest, certain drugs, instillation of barium into the rectum, and foods containing a great deal of fiber. The fecal impaction can totally or partially obstruct the passage of stool, causing the individual pain in the rectum and a feeling that he has to defecate. When the obstruction is not total (which is the usual occurrence), small quantities of liquid feces, which seep around the impaction, are expelled.

All efforts should be made to prevent the occurrence of a fecal impaction. Observation and recording of all client's bowel movements, describing color, frequency, consistency, and amount, should be made on a *daily* basis, especially if they may be prone to the condition (i.e., on bedrest). A fecal impaction can develop with great rapidity—within a 24-hour-period—thus the importance of careful monitoring.

Treatment

Treatment of impaction is usually an oil retention enema followed by a cleansing enema a few hours later. As a last resort, digital manipulation may be attempted. After placing the client in Sim's position, draping and using a protective pad under the hips, the nurse or the physician (in some agencies and in certain states nurses are not permitted to do this procedure) inserts a well lubricated gloved finger gently into the anus and carefully breaks up the mass. As pieces are removed they are placed into a bedpan. The finger is lubricated with each insertion to reduce friction and irritation and to facilitate insertion and manipulation. If the impaction is particularly hard to remove, it may have to be done in stages with the addition of oil between attempts. This procedure is extremely uncomfortable, and the client will almost certainly require rest after its completion. Again, a physician's order is needed to perform this procedure.

COLLECTION OF SPECIMENS

Urinalysis

Included as part of a complete physical examination, upon admission to the hospital, prior to surgery and the performance of certain procedures, and as a diagnostic tool, urine testing is routinely done. *Urinalysis* is the most frequent examination, looking for the presence of any unusual substances, such as protein, blood, pus, casts, sugar, and acetone. *Cultures* are done when the possibility of a urinary tract infection exists and knowledge of the causative pathogenic organism is needed to determine the correct treatment modality.

For the urinalysis, a simple voided specimen is obtained in a clean collection container; however, some institutions require an uncontaminated specimen. For the culture, an uncontaminated specimen is always needed to differentiate between organisms that have actually invaded the bladder or kidneys and those that may have entered the specimen from the container, hands, or adjacent structures, as the anus or the vagina. In the past, catheterized specimens were usually obtained for a urine culture, but with the reduction in the frequency of catheterizations due to the hazards involved, this is only performed in instances where the client already has an indwelling catheter in place. The urine is obtained from the catheter, rather than from the tubing or the collection bag where stasis occurs. In place of catheterized specimens, an alternate technique for obtaining the urine sample is usually utilized. The *clean catch* or *midstream urine* specimen is a fairly good substitute; although not sterile, the number of microorganisms present is markedly reduced when the collection is performed properly. In this method, which can be done on the toilet, the perineum is cleansed in the same manner as with catheterization: the labia minora are separated (and maintained in this position throughout both cleansing and voiding) or the foreskin in the uncircumcised male is kept retracted through the entire procedure. Women who are menstruating should be asked to wear a tampon to avoid contamination of the urine with blood. Cleansing is done with soap and water or with an appropriate antiseptic solution, such as benzalkonium chloride. A minimum of three sterile cotton balls or pledgets saturated with solution are used;

TABLE 42-3. Enema Administration for Relief of Constipation and Fecal Impaction (Early); to Avoid Expulsion or Contamination with Fecal Matter while under Anesthesia or during Childbirth; to Cleanse Lower Gastrointestinal Tract for Diagnostic Procedures, X-rays, or Surgery on Colon or Abdomen, and after Barium Sulfate Instillation; and to Lower Body Temperature (Rarely)

Anticipated Accomplishment	Scientific Principles/ Rationale	Specific Considerations
1. Preparation of materials for procedure. Organization.	Enema procedure is often anxiety provoking in clients. Having all equipment ready and organized when initiating procedure raises client's confidence in nurse and avoids anxiety (as when interruptions to locate forgotten equipment occur).	What is purpose of procedure? What type of enema and amount of solution have been ordered?
	The larger the lumen the greater the amount of solution flowing in, and the greater the stimulation of the sphincters upon insertion.	Physician usually orders tube size. Children's sizes are smaller.
		Disposable sets do not use a separate rectal tube and tubing. Distal end of length of tubing has holes at side for solution flow.
		Equipment if not disposable is sterilized between each use. Commercial products when packaged are sterile. Procedure, however, is clean rather than sterile.
		The bedpan is kept nearby for client on bedrest or who, for any reason, cannot ambulate to bathroom or bedside commode.

Implementation	Recommendations	Observations
Gather equipment: Bag or enema can large enough to contain the maximum amount of solution that might be given.	Note, read instructions on all commercially prepared products carefully before preparing for administration of enema.	
Rectal tube sizes: 18 to 22 Fr (retention enemas); 26 to 32 Fr (for soap, saline, tap water cleansing enemas which are not retained). Two to three feet of tubing.	Viscous solutions such as oil, need tube with larger lumen to permit flow.	
A clamp for compression of tubing to control flow of solution and lubricant.	Many commercial or disposable sets come with prelubricated tips. This will be stated on package.	
Bath thermometer for measurement of solution temperature.		
A bedpan and toilet paper.	Keeping bedpan nearby is a good preventive measure in rare case that a client who can ambulate is unable to reach bathroom and prematurely expels enema solution.	
Clean disposable glove and materials for solution.	Glove is optional; it is recommended to protect nurse's hand from contamination in case of	

TABLE 42-3. Continued

Anticipated Accomplishment	Scientific Principles/ Rationale	Specific Considerations
	If solution is too hot, burns can result. Cold solutions will cause muscle contractions and cramping. Changes in temperature in colon stimulates peristalsis to occur.	
	Average adult colon can hold up to approximately 1 L of solution. This is determined by condition of musculature. Some adults can receive 2 L while others can receive 750 ml or less. Fluid bulk stimulates peristalsis by distending walls of intestine.	
	When large quantities of hypotonic solution (tap water) are given (especially when enemas are given repeatedly), absorption through colon may increase blood volume and cause water intoxication and electrolyte imbalance.	Care must be taken with the client who has congestive heart failure.
	Physiologic saline (sodium chloride solution 0.9%) is isotonic with human blood and therefore, nonirritating.	

Implementation	Recommendations	Observations
	leakage of fecal matter from rectum around tube, or premature expulsion of solution.	
Connect container, tubing, and rectal tube. Place clamp on tubing.		
Preparation of the solution: solution temperature should range between 100-110°F (37.8-43.3°C) for adult and 100°F (37.8°C) to no higher than 105°F (40.6°C) for pediatric client. (In cases where temperature is to be lowered, physician will order amount and temperature of solution.)	Use a bath thermometer to measure temperature. For prepackaged sets, solution can be at room temperature, but it is advisable to place bag of solution into a basin of warm water to bring it up to body temperature.	
0.5−1 L is the usual adult amount for water, saline or soap and water enemas, although more or less may be ordered or tolerated.	It is safest to request that physician order maximum amount of solution that he wishes instilled.	
For infants: 150 to 250 ml; 18 months to 10 years: 250 to 500 ml; 10 to 14 years: 250 to 750 ml.[3] Oil retention enemas usually contain 4−6 oz of oil (usually mineral oil).	Usually no more than 300 ml are given to child unless otherwise ordered.	
	It should not be assumed that tap water is to be used for an enema unless specified by physician.	
One teaspoon of table salt is added to each pint of water to make normal saline solution.		

TABLE 42-3. Continued

Anticipated Accomplishment	Scientific Principles/ Rationale	Specific Considerations
	Soap acts as an irritant to intestinal mucosa and lowers surface tension of water, facilitating its combination with feces. Quantity of solution distends colon. Too much soap, or too irritating a kind of soap can cause damage to mucous membrane.	
	Hypertonic solutions which are mildly irritating to intestinal mucosa cause fluid to be drawn into bowel from tissues by osmosis causing increased bulk in colon and a more liquid stool.	Due to small amount of solution, it is usually not tiring for client nor does it cause great distress or discomfort. It is quite desirable for clients who are weak, or unable to retain large amounts of solution. It is seen frequently in community or home settings.
		Other types of enemas include: cleansing—sodium bicarbonate and water or hydrogen peroxide and water; carminative—(to remove flatulence) glycerin and water or milk and molasses or 1-2-3 (magnesium sulfate, 1 oz; glycerine, 2 oz; and water, 3 oz); softening—oil (retention enemas).
	Air in tubing increases pressure in colon and interferes with effectiveness of instillation and retention of solution.	
	Lubricant decreases friction and eases insertion of tube into sphincter.	

Implementation	Recommendations	Observations
For soap and water enemas (usually referred to as soap solution enemas), a gentle (bland) soap such as castile is used for solution. (Approximately 1 tsp of concentrated liquid soap per liter of water or 1 oz of normal strength liquid soap per liter is used).	Measure water into container first; then add soap. Do not shake vigorously. (If water is added to soap, it gets extremely sudsy and although not harmful to individual, can increase distention.) Commercial sets usually contain packets of concentrated liquid soap. Small disposable enemas, for instance, Fleets, contain about 4½ oz of hypertonic solution (16 gm sodium biphosphate and 6 gm sodium phosphate per 100 ml) and 2¼ oz for pediatric size.	
After correct amount of solution is in container, expel air from tubing.	Holding end of tubing over sink or basin (at a level lower than that of enema can or pouch), open clamp. Fluid runs through tubing forcing air out. When air has been removed, clamp tubing to stop flow.	
Lubricate approximately three inches of rectal tube (if not pre-lubricated).	End of tube can be placed into opened end of individual disposable packet of lubricant or the lubricant can be squeezed out of the tube onto a 4 × 4 gauze square and the tube lu-	

TABLE 42-3. Continued

Anticipated Accomplishment	Scientific Principles/ Rationale	Specific Consideration
2. Preparation of client.	Knowledge of what is expected of client and progression of steps in procedure helps him to relax, facilitating ease of administration.	
a. Provision of privacy	Anxiety and embarrassment are increased when genital area is exposed and handled.	
b. Positioning of client.	Some authorities believe left side-lying position to be position of choice because it allows solution to reach descending colon on left side of body. Others disagree.	
	Knee chest position facilitates distribution and flow of solution further into lower portion of large intestine.	Knee chest position may be too difficult or uncomfortable for some clients.
	When sitting, solution must flow against gravity, needing higher amounts of pressure to administer solution. Less solution can be instilled since distention of lower portion of intestine occurs rapidly with an urge to defecate before effective amount of solution can be instilled.	
c. Draping of client	Draping increases feeling of privacy and decreases possibility of becoming chilled.	

Implementation	Recommendations	Observations
	bricated with this. Do not get. lubricant into opening of tube if possible.	
Give thorough explanation of purpose of procedure. Review steps so client understands that he is to retain fluid (with retention enemas) for specified amount of time, and so he knows quickest route to bathroom or bedside commode.	Have shoes or slippers at bedside (and robe if needed). Have bedpan available for emergencies.	
Provide for privacy.	Close door, pull curtains, or place screens around bed.	
Knee chest position and side-lying are most effective positions for enema administraton. Infants and children are placed in side-lying or recumbent position. Rectal tube must be held in place entire time (Fig. 42-8).		
	Do not give enemas in a sitting position. For client who has little or no sphincter control, however, enema may be given to client while on bedpan by elevating head of bed *slightly*. For comfort, a folded towel or small pillow can be placed at small of back.	
After positioning, drape client with bath blanket, exposing buttocks.	Place a moistureproof pad under client's buttocks to protect linens from soilage.	

TABLE 42-3. Continued

Anticipated Accomplishment	Scientific Principles/ Rationale	Specific Considerations
child's position		
knee-chest position		
Sims' position		
position for self-administration		

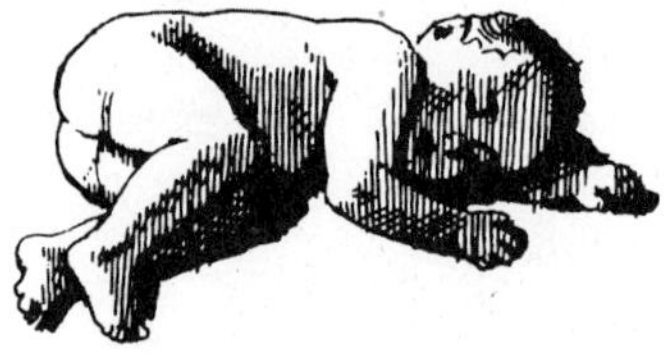

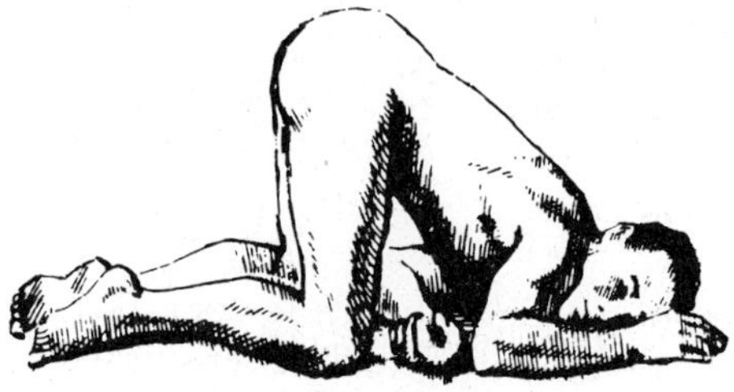

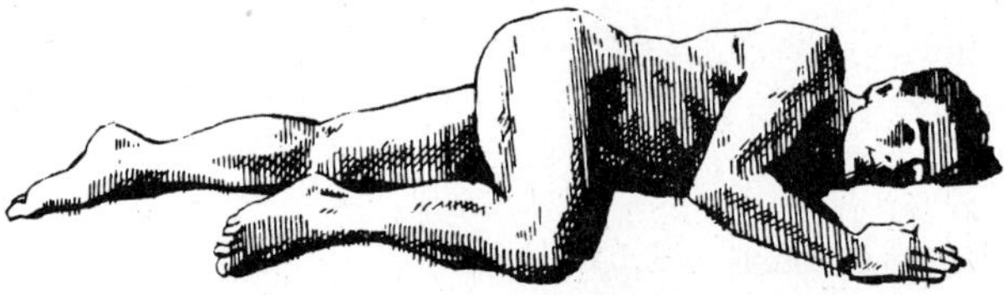

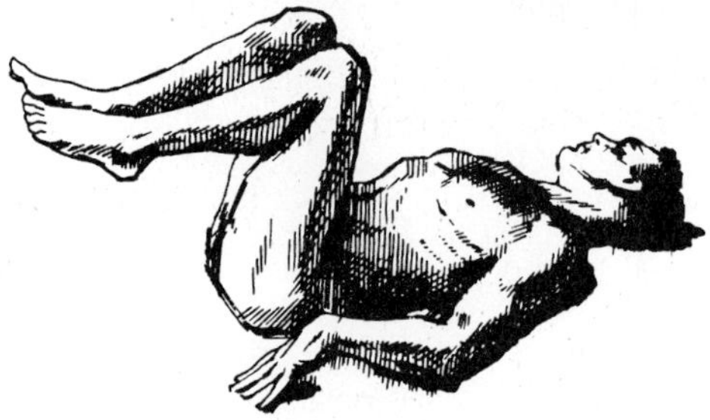

FIGURE 42-8. Positions for enemas. (Reprinted with permission from C. B. Fleet Co., Inc., Lynchburg, Va.)

3. Administration of enema

Anus is approximately 1 in long and rectum approximately 6–8 in long in adults. Tube should be inserted beyond internal sphincter, allowing solution to reach cecum by force of solution, but not far enough to damage or perforate wall of intestine at splenic flexure or to curl up on itself.

Implementation	Recommendations	Observations

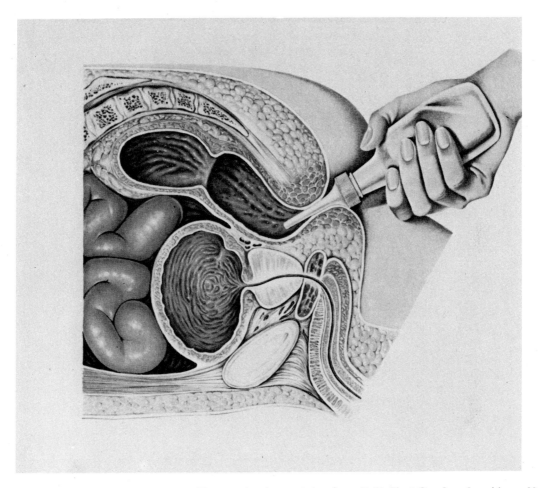

FIGURE 42-9. Administering an enema. (Reprinted with permission from C. B. Fleet Co., Inc., Lynchburg, Va.)

Implementation	Recommendations	Observations
Gently and slowly insert tube 2–4 in in direction of umbilicus in adult and approximately 1½ in in small children.	Wear glove on hand inserting tube (optional). Ask client to take a couple of deep breaths during insertion of tubing to assist him in relaxing.	Note presence of external hemorrhoids (varicosities of rectal veins) when inserting tube.

TABLE 42-3. Continued

Anticipated Accomplishment	Scientific Principles/ Rationale	Specific Considerations
	Gentleness of insertion is vital since hemorrhoids may be present and pain on insertion will cause contraction of sphincters. Force can damage or perforate intestinal wall.	
	Solution may push folds of mucous membrane away from tip of tube if it has pushed up against wall of intestine. It also may dislodge any feces that have lodged in opening of tube upon insertion.	
	The solution flows into colon by gravity. The higher the level of the solution, the faster and more vigorous the flow. High pressure and rapidity stimulates peristalsis (possibly causing cramping) and desire to expel solution before enough has been instilled to be effective.	Pressure can be decreased by lowering container and by tightening clamp on tube.
	Rolling up of plastic bottle may prevent the aspiration of solution back into bottle as it re-expands.	
	Pressure applied externally to anus may minimize sphincter spasms and facilitate retention of solution.	

Implementation	Recommendations	Observations
	Never use force to insert tube or solution. If resistance is met, withdraw tube slightly, and allow some solution to flow in and advance tube again.	
Open clamp and elevate enema can or bag slowly until solution flows. Allow solution to flow in slowly until client expresses an intense need to defecate.	An elevation of 12 to 18 in above anus is usually adequate to permit flow of solution. Use no greater pressure than is necessary to instill solution. By using clamp, allow solution to flow for 5 to 10 sec and then shut off for approximately 5 sec. Extend instillation time to about 10 min. Have client take deep breaths through mouth to help him relax if necessary. Clients vary in amount of solution that they can tolerate and retain. *Never* force client to take more than he feels he can accept, but encourage relaxation which may result in increased amount tolerated.	Is client feeling any discomfort or pain?
With small (4–6 oz) commercial enemas, squeeze bottle and roll it up as fluid flows into the rectum (Fig. 42-9).		
Remove tube and apply pressure over anus with toilet paper if solution is one that is to be retained.	Cleansing enemas should be retained for 5 to 10 min if possible, although many clients have difficulty with this.	

TABLE 42-3. Continued

Anticipated Accomplishment	Scientific Principles/ Rationale	Specific Considerations
	Sitting or standing promotes peristalsis and gravity drainage causing distention of rectum and a desire to expel solution. Infants and small children cannot voluntarily retain solution.	
4. Expulsion of enema solution and the lower intestinal contents.	Sitting is a comfortable and natural position for defecation.	
	The fluid is siphoned out by gravity drainage.	If the solution is not expelled, physician may order it removed via a rectal tube.
5. Prevent contamination and spread of infection.	Equipment is contaminated with fecal material and associated microorganisms.	
6. Recording and reporting.		Note any unsual responses to procedure, i.e., pain, difficulty in instillation of solution, or blood or mucus in stools.

Implementation	Recommendations	Observations
	With retention enemas, have client remain in a flat or side-lying position while holding in solution until evacuation time. With infants or children, apply pressure over anus, while solution is being retained.	
Assist client to bathroom, bedside commode, or on to bedpan.	A sitting position is preferable to assist expulsion of solution and intestinal contents.	
	After insertion of lubricated tip of tube, it is lowered to approximately 18 in below anus and solution allowed to flow out into a receptacle such as a bedpan.	
Dispose of equipment in appropriate manner and wash hands well.		
Record and report procedure and results according to agency policy.		Observe color, odor, amount, and character of feces and expulsion of flatus. Also record type and amount of solution instilled, date and time of administration.
	If physician has ordered enemas until clear, no more than three should be given (providing client tolerates this well). If stool is still present in evacuation, physician should be consulted for further instructions.	

after *one* stroke from anterior to posterior, the cotton ball is discarded and a new one used for the next stroke. The labia on each side are cleansed first, and then the central area, including the meatus, is cleansed. The glans penis is cleansed in the same manner from the meatus outward using a circular motion. In certain agencies, sterile gloves are required for the clean catch procedure.

After cleansing, the client is asked to void forcefully approximately 2–3 ounces into the toilet. This will flush out most organisms that are located at the urethral opening. (The voiding process itself, is one of the body's natural defenses against invasion of microorganisms, carrying bacteria away from the meatus at regular intervals each day.) The client then voids approximately 3–6 ounces forcefully (in order to keep the stream away from the female perineal tissues) directly into a sterile specimen container. After removal of the bottle, the foreskin and the labia can be replaced in the normal position, and the client may finish voiding into the toilet. This is important in males since some prostatic fluid may be combined with the urine at the point when the bladder is almost emptied. Most responsible clients can be taught to do this procedure by themselves. Infants and young children will not be able to cooperate; therefore, other means of collection must be utilized. After cleansing the perineal and anal areas with soap and water and drying carefully, either a special disposable plastic urine bag is affixed to the perineum or a disposable cellophane collection diaper is used. For either method, the infant is placed in Fowler's position to facilitate gravity drainage. The former type of collector has an adhesive strip which adheres to the skin around the labia majora or the penis. A diaper may be applied over the bag. The bag collects the urine as the infant voids and is gently removed as soon as the required amount is obtained. The child should be observed frequently to avoid leaving the bag in place for long periods of time. The cellophane collector is applied in the same manner as a diaper and removed when the specimen is voided into the collection portion. Specimens are then placed into appropriate containers, labeled, and sent to the laboratory. When all methods have proven unsatisfactory, the physician may perform a *suprapubic urine aspiration* (percutaneous bladder puncture) rather than catheterizing an infant. Using sterile technique, urine is withdrawn from the bladder through the abdominal wall with a sterile syringe and needle.

For diagnostic testing, the collection of a *24 hour urine specimen* is sometimes called for. It the client is ambulatory, instructions must be given as to the method used for collection. The first specimen voided is discarded and the time noted. All voidings are collected for exactly 24 hours and usually kept in a large glass or plastic opaque bottle. Often a preservative has been added to avoid deterioration of the urine. In some cases, the bottle is either refrigerated or kept in an ice bath for the 24 hours.

Urine specimens are observed for color, odor, transparency, presence of sediment, and particles (Table 42-1). Usually the early morning specimen is concentrated, making it desirable for sediment analysis, but this may possibly be undesirable for other tests.

Stool Analysis

Stool specimens are obtained from a clean or sterile bedpan (adult) or from the diaper of an infant or small child. Tongue depressors can be used to transfer the feces into a waxed and covered specimen container. The stool should not be contaminated with urine or menstrual blood. In some cases the stool is refrigerated, but when parasites are suspected, the specimen is kept warm to ensure that the organisms are kept alive.

Testing of stool specimens is usually for occult blood (guaiac reaction), urobilinogen, ova, parasites, protozoa, bacteria, fat, and nitrogen content. Specimens should be observed for amount, color (brown, black, green, yellow, or bloody), odor (foul, putrid, or sour), mucus, pus, consistency (hard, fluid, unformed, or greasy), and the presence of parasites, such as tapeworms.

All specimens should be labeled properly, including the client's name, room and bed number, type of specimen, analysis ordered by the physician, and the date and time of collection. Specimens should be delivered to the laboratory as rapidly as possible to prevent a change in pH or deterioration of the excrement.

SUMMARY

In caring for all clients attention must be given to elimination processes, both urinary, intestinal, and that of the integumentary and respiratory systems. Diaphoresis and changes in the rate and character of the respirations should be looked for and noted, especially when there are disturbances in voiding or defecation.

Assessment of the client's daily bladder and bowel habits and patterns give information as to what concerns and problems may exist. Data to be gathered include his customary diet, fluid intake, activity, exercise, and life style. In addition, difficulties with urination or defecation, including dependency on any of a variety of methods to induce elimination must be explored. A plan of care is then developed in cooperation with the client, his family, or significant others when appropriate to meet his individualized needs. The goal of any plan should be the return to and maintenance of as normal a pattern of elimination as possible. Included are measures to promote regularity of bladder and bowel functioning without the necessity of catheterization, enemas, or excessive and possibly habitual use of laxatives or suppositories. The provision of comfort, hygienic and safety measures, as well as emotional support and encouragement are necessary through the planning and implementation of all bladder and bowel management programs. The client's level of understanding, need for information and teaching, and his physiological potential must be considered in setting realistic objectives and strategies. Naturally, evaluation of any plan must take place to determine its effectiveness or lack of success. Revisions in the plan are made as needed to ensure the desired outcome.

REFERENCES

1. Miller B. F., and Keane, C. B.: *Encyclopedia and Dictionary of Medicine, Nursing, and Allied Health,* 2nd ed. Philadelphia, W. B. Saunders Co., 1978, p. 553.
2. Nordmark, M. T., and Rohweder, A. W.: *Scientific Foundations of Nursing,* 3rd ed. Philadelphia, J. B. Lippincott Co., 1975, p. 150.
3. Leifer, G.: *Principles and Techniques in Pediatric Nursing.* Philadelphia, W. B. Saunders Co., 1977, p. 76.

BIBLIOGRAPHY

Baker, R. B.: Constipation and the geriatric patient. *Nurs. Care* 8(10):21, 1975.
Bass, L.: More fiber—less constipation. *Am. J. Nurs.* 77:254, 1977.
Beaumont, E.: Urinary drainage systems. *Nurs. '74* 4(1):52, 1974.
Blackwell, A., and Blackwell, W.: Relieving gas pains. *Am. J. Nurs.* 75:98, 1975.
Caldwell, K. P.: Sphincter stimulators to prevent incontinence. *Nurs. Times* 69:1524, 1973.
DeGroot, J., and Kunim, C.: Indwelling catheters. *Am. J. Nurs.* 75:448, 1975.
Delehanty, L., and Stravino, V.: Achieving bladder control. *Am. J. Nurs.* 70:312, 1970.
Dison, N.: *Clinical Nursing Techniques,* 3rd ed. St. Louis, C. V. Mosby Co., 1975.
Elhart, D., et al.: *Scientific Principles in Nursing,* 8th ed. St. Louis, C. V. Mosby Co., 1978.
Falconer, M. W., et al.: *The Drug, the Nurse, the Patient,* 6th ed. Philadelphia, W. B. Saunders Co., 1978.
Fuerst, E., Wolff, L., and Weitzel, M.: *Fundamentals of Nursing,* 5th ed. Philadelphia, J. B. Lippincott Co., 1974.
Garner, J.: Urinary catheter care: doing it better. *Nurs. '74* 4(2):54, 1974.
Guyton, A. C.: *Textbook of Medical Physiology,* 5th ed. Philadelphia, W. B. Saunders Co., 1976.
Habbet, M., and Kallstrom, M.: Bowel program for institutionalized adults. *Am. J. Nurs.* 76:606, 1976.
Lewin, D.: Care of the constipated patient. *Nurs. Times* 72:444, 1976.
Maney, J. Y.: A behavioral therapy approach to bladder retraining. *Nurs. Clin. North Am.* 11:179, 1976.
McGuckin, M.: Microbiologic studies: urine cultures—key to diagnosing urinary infections (Part I). *Nurs. '75* 5(12):10, 1975.
Taber's Cyclopedic Medical Dictionary, 13th ed. Philadelphia, F. A. Davis Co., 1977.
Willington, F. L.: Incontinence V. Training and retraining for continence. *Nurs. Times* 71:500, 1975.
Winter, C. C., and Morel, A.: *Nursing Care of Patients with Urologic Diseases,* 4th ed. St. Louis, C. V. Mosby Co., 1977.

CHAPTER 43

GLOSSARY

appliance. A device which is secured to the abdomen and used to collect the urine or feces which drain from the stoma.

colostomy. An artificial opening from the colon through the abdominal wall.

distal. Farthest from the center, from a medial line, or from the trunk (opposite of proximal).

diverticulitis. Inflammation of a diverticulum or of diverticula in the intestinal tract, especially in the colon, causing stagnation of feces in little distended sacs of the colon (diverticula).

effluent. Urine or fecal matter which exits through a stoma.

enterostomal therapist. A nurse with expertise in ostomy client care, who has completed a program in enterostomal therapy certified by the International Association for Enterostomal Therapy.

fistula. An abnormal tubelike passage from a nor-

CARE OF THE CLIENT WITH AN OSTOMY

Pamela Gaherin Watson, M.S., R.N.,
and Robin Young Wood, M.S., R.N.

mal cavity or tube to a free surface or to another cavity. May be congenital due to incomplete closure of parts or may result from abscesses, injuries, or inflammatory processes.

flatus. Gas in digestive tract.

hypokalemia. Extreme potassium depletion in the circulating blood, commonly manifested by episodes of musuclar weakness or paralysis, tetany, and postural hypotension.

hyponatremia. Decreased concentration of sodium in the blood.

ileostomy. Artificial opening of the small intestine through the abdominal wall.

karaya. A gum from the bark of a tree in India used as an accessory product in ostomy appliances. Karaya has adhesive properties.

ostomy. An abdominal stoma. It may be a colostomy, ileostomy, urinostomy, ureterostomy, or cecostomy.

peristomal. The area of skin which surrounds a stoma.

proximal. Nearest the point of attachment, center of the body, or point of reference (opposite of distal).

stoma. Greek word for mouth; in surgery, a permanent artificial opening; in the lower neck, a tracheostomy; in the abdominal wall, a colostomy or ileostomy.

tenesmus. Spasmodic contraction of anal or vesical sphincter with pain and persistent desire to empty the bowel or bladder, with involuntary, ineffectual straining efforts.

urinary diversion. An opening into some part of the urinary tract which directs urine from an obstructed or diseased area to an external opening (stoma or nephrostomy tube) or into the gastrointestinal tract for elimination (ureterosigmoidostomy).

Each year approximately 100,000 persons undergo surgery which alters the normal pattern of elimination and results in the creation of an ostomy, an artificial opening in the abdominal wall. Who is the ostomy client? The ostomy client may be male or female, married or single, young or old. He may have been sick or healthy prior to the time of ostomy surgery. Each ostomy client faces a "mutilating" surgical procedure; thus, each client must learn technical skills to enable him to manage the altered pattern of elimination.

Providing nursing care for the ostomy client through the application of the nursing process is a challenging and rewarding undertaking. This chapter has been divided into four sections. The first section outlines the steps of the nursing process as it applies to ostomy client care. The second section discusses the care of the colostomy client. Care of the ileostomy client is described in the third section, and the fourth section presents the care of the client with a urinary diversion.

APPLICATION OF NURSING PROCESS IN OSTOMY CLIENT CARE

Assessment

A thorough assessment which considers all aspects of the client's stoma experience is essential if one is to formulate a plan of care which will meet the client's needs. Relevant data must be carefully collected, analyzed, and interpreted to determine problems for which the nurse must establish goals and appropriate nursing interventions. Assessing ostomy client needs is a continuous process; as the needs change all the time. One must be prepared to re-examine baseline data and to deal with the day-to-day changes in the client's situation. Ostomy client assessment guidelines are presented here to assist in the determination of pertinent data which must be collected.

GUIDELINES

Pathophysiologic Aspects

What is the nature of the underlying condition which has necessitated the creation of a stoma?
How has the pathophysiologic problem involved affected the client's general health?
What is the client's prognosis?

Psychosocial Aspects

What are the client's strengths, coping mechanisms, and family relationships?
Does he appear to have the ability to adapt to the realities of the situation at hand?
What are the client's goals, expectations, interests, and hopes?
How old is the client? In which stage of the life cycle is he?
What is the client's educational background, occupational history, and career goals?
What is the meaning of the underlying condition and the stoma to the client and family?
Are client and family knowledgeable about the client's condition?
To what extent has the client's family been included in the client's plan of care?
What is the family's attitude toward the individual and the stoma?
How does the client refer to the stoma?
What is the client's emotional reaction to the presence of a stoma?
Does the client fear recurrent illness?

Activity Level

Is the ostomy client independent in activities of daily living?
Does he move about freely?
Are there other physical and emotional problems present which may affect the ostomy client's ability to care for the stoma?
How can ostomy management be incorporated into the client's customary routine of daily living?

Nutrition

Are there specific dietary recommendations associated with the client's particular type of diversionary procedure?
Is the client on a therapeutic diet because of a medical condition unrelated to the stoma?
What is the client's understanding of nutritional aspects?

Fluid and Electrolyte Status

Is the client adequately hydrated?
Are fluid and electrolyte problems anticipated with the client's particular kind of ostomy procedure?

Elimination

Does the client have bowel or bladder problems unrelated to the presence of a stoma?

What has been the client's lifelong pattern of elimination?

Is the stoma functioning adequately at present?

Has a satisfactory routine been established for ostomy care?

What type of stoma care equipment is being used?

Skin Condition

What is the overall condition of the client's skin?

Is the peristomal skin area intact?

Has a skin care routine been established for the peristomal skin area?

What preparations are being used for skin care?

Does the client have a healing incision site or a wound which interferes with the application of an ostomy appliance?

Is there a perineal wound to consider in planning client care?

Drug Therapy

What medications have been ordered for the client?

Is the client on drug therapy unrelated to the present condition?

Is the client receiving chemotherapy?

Have medications specifically related to the stoma been ordered (e.g., odor control preparations or ascorbic acid)?

Is the drug therapy being employed apt to adversely affect stoma function?

Once the baseline data have been collected and organized, inferences can be made about the facts obtained. Basically, the nurse is sizing up the client's situation and making educated guesses about what his problems are. It is then necessary to validate or confirm these observations. Validation is not limited to verbal corroboration with the client. Current literature, the client's chart, other members of the health care team, and family members must be utilized.

EXAMPLE. Mr. M appeared very anxious about the prospect of ostomy surgery. When asked about this, he confirmed the observation and

mentioned that a relative had had a bad experience with an ostomy. Mr. M seemed unwilling to elaborate further. The physical examination report in Mr. M's chart noted that Mr. M's father had died of cancer of the rectum. Further validation with members of the nursing staff and the attending physician revealed that Mr. M's father had lived with a colostomy for 5 years and that he never left his house after the ostomy surgery. When interviewed, Mrs. M stated that Mr. M is now fearful that he will experience the same problem as his father. Reading the current literature, one finds that anxiety and fear are very normal for the ostomy client in the preoperative period.

In the example cited, an observation has been wholly validated. The nurse has a good understanding of what had been observed, and a client problem has been identified. Thus, the entire assessment is composed of observing, validating, and evaluating.

Nursing Diagnosis

Having completed the assessment, the nurse can now formulate a meaningful nursing diagnosis. An important component of the diagnosis is a summary statement in which the ostomy client's strengths and weaknesses are identified. This is very helpful in terms of the rehabilitation process. It enables the nurse to know client strengths on which to build and areas of weakness in which the client will need more help.

A list of client problems can now be constructed. A problem is any client issue, need, or question for which the nurse proposes a solution or intervention. The word problem should not necessarily have a negative connotation.

EXAMPLE. Mr. M does not understand the nature of the ostomy surgery to be performed.

The fact that Mr. M lacks information concerning the surgical procedure is a problem. However, there is nothing negative about this problem. It is a normal situation which can be dealt with by the nurse.

As the problem list is constructed, every problem identified should be thought of in terms of what can be done to facilitate a solution. An efficient way of organizing client problems is to consider them with regard to the following areas:

1. Problems which relate to the underlying pathophysiologic condition and the client's general health status; examples: phase of illness, fluid and electrolyte balance, pain, wound healing, and cardiovascular status.
2. Issues concerning the technical management of the stoma; examples: appliance selection, peristomal skin care, leakage, and odor.
3. Problems associated with the process of adapting to the presence of the stoma; examples: grief and loss, depression, dependence, anger, and acceptance.

Organizing client problems in this way also helps in determining long and short-range needs.

Plan of Care

OBJECTIVES

Short and long-term objectives or goals must be established for each problem identified. Sometimes it is helpful to think of the long-term objective first— that is, what is it that you and the client want to accomplish ultimately? Next consider what must take place in the interim to achieve the long-term objective.

> *EXAMPLE.* Long-term objective: Mr. M will apply his ostomy appliance independently. Short-term objective: Mr. M will begin to participate in the care of his ostomy by: washing the peristomal skin area and cutting the appropriate size stoma opening in the adhesive backed face plate of the appliance.

Thus, having determined where the client is to go, one can identify successive steps to reach the objective. Considerable thought should be given to the process of setting objectives. These must be realistic and attainable. Perhaps more important, the objectives must be mutually established with the client; otherwise there is little chance of achievement.

INTERVENTIONS

Nursing interventions are intended to move the client toward the successful achievement of his rehabilitation objectives. Every intervention proposed must be based on a scientific rationale. Attention should be directed to the areas discussed below.

Preoperative Teaching

Every preoperative teaching program should include careful review of the disease entity and the nature of the surgery planned for the ostomy client. Anatomical explanations, supplemented with drawings or charts, are imperative. Ostomy appliances and a stoma facsimile should be shown to the client and his family. A stoma site should be marked on the client's abdomen by a nurse skilled in this area or by the surgeon. Guidelines for stoma site marking are shown in Figure 43-1.

The value of information obtained in the preoperative period cannot be overestimated. It is an important intervention particularly in terms of helping to alleviate fears and anxieties. By the time the client goes to surgery, he and his family should be fully prepared for what to expect postoperatively.

Stoma Management

Central to the concept of stoma management is the fact that the ostomy client must be provided with a suitable ostomy appliance which adheres to the abdomen and allows the client to remain dry and odor free. As shown in Figure 43-2, selection of an appropriate appliance requires consideration of a number of important criteria. A great variety of disposable ostomy appliances are on the market. Ostomy appliance catalogues are available in most hospitals. It is now possible to find an effective appliance for nearly every stoma created.

Although skin care is discussed in the following sections, it is useful to note here, that the following basic principles apply regardless of the type of stoma with which one is dealing:

1. Prevention is the keystone of peristomal skin care.
2. Peristomal skin should be carefully examined each time an appliance is removed. Any

problems found should be treated immediately. Table 43-1 lists common skin problems and effective remedies.

3. Skin should be washed gently with plain warm water. Soap is best avoided as it leaves a filmy residue which may interfere with appliance adherence. Remnants of karaya or other skin barriers should not be rubbed off.

4. After washing, skin should be allowed to dry thoroughly. The ostomy client should be encouraged to indulge in an air bath, allowing the skin to remain open to air for as long as possible. If the stoma emits effluent continously, the stoma opening can be wicked, with a rolled up face cloth or gauze pad to keep drainage off the skin while an appliance is not in place. The use of a hair dryer is sometimes encouraged to insure absolute drying of the peristomal skin area.

5. A skin barrier, such as a karaya preparation, Stomahesive, or Reliaseal, should be used for any ostomy which drains liquid or corrosive effluent. In addition, a skin barrier should be considered for anyone whose skin is sensitive naturally or because of chemotherapy or radiation therapy.

6. If there is hair growing on the peristomal skin area, it should be cut with a scissors or shaved carefully.

Prevention of Leakage

Leakage of effluent from an ostomy appliance usually does not occur if the following guidelines are followed:

1. Apply an appropriate appliance to absolutely dry skin, making sure that the adhesive disc has been smoothed out across its width and height.

2. Be certain that the disc opening for the stoma does not exceed the one-eighth inch border on all sides.

3. Use a skin barrier whenever indicated.

4. Do not allow the appliance to become more than one-third full before emptying.

5. Do not leave the appliance on until it leaks.

6. Picture frame the adhesive disc or use a belt to hold the appliance in place.

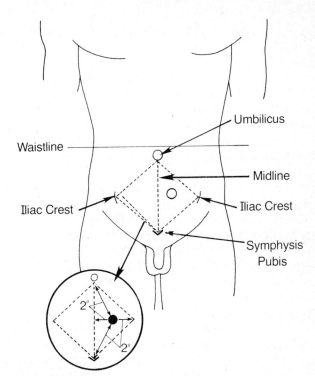

FIGURE 43-1. Marking a site for stoma placement. A site for stoma placement should be marked after the abdomen has been observed with the client in a supine, sitting, and standing position. (1) With the client lying flat draw a diamond on the right and left lower quadrants, extending from the umbilicus to both iliac crests and down to the symphysis pubis. (2) Note the client's waistline and mark it. (3) Observe the client in the positions indicated above. While the client is standing, have him bend down and flex the hips. (4) The stoma site selected should be somewhere within the diamond. Either the right or the left side of the abdomen may be used depending on the surgery to be performed and the client's physical structure. Be sure there is enough smooth skin around the site selected to accommodate the adhesive disc of the appliance. The stoma site should be approximately 2 in away from the landmarks noted on the diagram (i.e., umbilicus, midline, iliac crest, and symphysis pubis).

Important guidelines: (1) Do not select a site near scars or irregular surfaces of the abdomen which will interfere with the adherence of an appliance. (2) Do not mark a site which is too close to the inguinal fold, as movement may dislodge the appliance. (3) Mark the stoma site on the upward slope of the abdomen if at all possible. This will make self-care easier for the client. (4) Colostomy stomas are usually placed on the left lower quadrant. Ileostomy and urinary diversion stomas are generally located on the right lower quadrant.

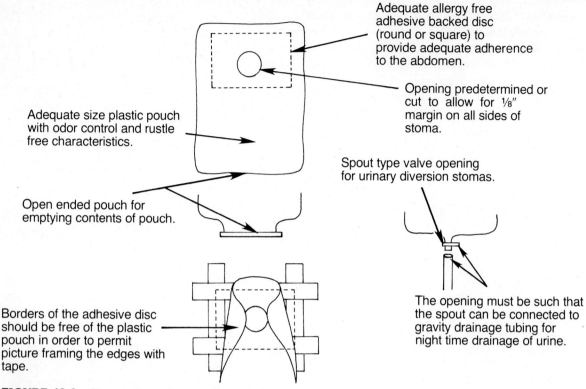

Adequate allergy free adhesive backed disc (round or square) to provide adequate adherence to the abdomen.

Opening predetermined or cut to allow for ⅛″ margin on all sides of stoma.

Adequate size plastic pouch with odor control and rustle free characteristics.

Spout type valve opening for urinary diversion stomas.

Open ended pouch for emptying contents of pouch.

Borders of the adhesive disc should be free of the plastic pouch in order to permit picture framing the edges with tape.

The opening must be such that the spout can be connected to gravity drainage tubing for night time drainage of urine.

FIGURE 43-2. Characteristics of an appropriate appliance.

Odor Control

The control of odor is discussed in depth in the other sections; however, it is important to note here that the issue of odor is of tremendous importance to the client. Guidelines for odor control include:

1. Dietary recommendations should be made so that the client will be aware of foods which cause odorous effluent and flatus.
2. Only those appliances with odor control characteristics should be used. Pinholes to emit flatus must not be made in the appliance as this negates the odor control properties of the appliance.
3. Deodorants which can be inserted into the pouch should be suggested.
4. In some instances, preparations which can be taken by mouth may also be recommended for clients with certain kinds of diversionary procedures.

5. Appliances should be emptied frequently and rinsed thoroughly.

Teaching Self-Care of the Stoma

From the outset, substantial effort should be directed toward assisting the ostomy client to become independent in self-care. Even if the client's participation in stoma care is minimal at first, the fact that he is actually involved will help him to begin to gain a sense of independence. When teaching self-care, it is important to do so under conditions which simulate the client's home environment. The stoma care regimen should be as simple as possible. It should be individualized to fit into the client's customary daily routine at home. Once a satisfactory routine is established, it should be followed by all who care for the client. The routine should be put in writing and communicated to members of the nursing staff. The client's progress in learning self-care should be noted daily. One should always be working toward having the client do more of the stoma care. Every client should be afforded the opportunity to care for the ostomy independently while still in the hospital setting.

Meeting Psychosocial Needs

Learning to accept the stoma is a very difficult task. The nurse is in a key position to assist the client and his family to adapt to the presence of a stoma. One of the most important interventions in meeting psychosocial needs is the creation of an environment in which the client feels free to express his feelings with regard to grief, loss, mutilation, self-esteem, and the myriad of other emotions associated with the ostomy experience. Information, acceptance, and understanding are essential in meeting psychosocial needs.

Dependence and anger are normal responses to stoma surgery. However, when these behaviors are exhibited, the client is often greeted with a negative response on the part of his caretakers. Certainly, it is not easy to deal with the dependent or angry client, but we should understand that the client must be allowed time to work through stages of adaptation if he is to make a positive adaptive response to the presence of a stoma.

Ostomy Association Visitor

The United Ostomy Association is an ostomy client self-help organization with chapters across the United States, Canada, and some parts of Europe. One service provided by the Ostomy Association is that of sending rehabilitated members to visit new ostomy clients either in the hospital or at home. Every ostomy client should be made aware of the association and the Ostomy Visitor program. Frequently, it is very helpful for a new ostomy client to be able to see and talk with someone who has undergone a similar experience. Just seeing the person dressed in normal clothing, looking healthy, and active is often very reassuring to both the client and his family. An ostomy visitor may be called at any time. If the client does not wish to see the visitor during hospitalization, the Ostomy Association telephone number should be given to the client as he may feel differently at a later date.

Discharge Planning

Planning for the ostomy client's return to the community is an activity which should take place early in the hospitalization period. Assessment of the home environment should be done to be sure facilities are available for stoma care. The nurse must work closely with the family concerning the client's return home. The client will need to know where ostomy care equipment can be obtained in the community.

A Community Health Agency referral should be made for every ostomy client who leaves the hospital. This will provide for continuity of care in the community. The nurse who visits the client in the home will be able to evaluate the progress being made in self-care. Any problems in transferring stoma management skills to the home environment can then be quickly noted and remedied before serious setbacks occur. Many clients require a visiting nurse for only a 2 or 3 week period. Other clients require home supervision and assistance for a longer period of time. Specific arrangements for follow-up care in the community should be made. This means that the stoma itself should be examined periodically along with an overall assessment of the client's health status.

Most important, the ostomy client and family should not feel abandoned in the community. The Ostomy Association is one resource, and the Community Health Agency is another. In addition, the telephone number of a resource person at the hospital should be given to the client.

IMPLEMENTATION

The person with a newly created ostomy can be expected to be acutely aware of and sensitive to the reactions of the nurse toward the ostomy. Every nurse who works with an ostomy client should examine her own feelings about the presence of an ostomy. It is extremely important that the ostomy client plan of care be implemented in a positive accepting manner. A negative response on the part of the nurse can confirm a client's suspicions about being offensive or unacceptable because of the ostomy.

The plan of care to be implemented must be one which is mutually acceptable to both the client and

TABLE 43-1. Colostomy and Ileostomy Appliance Application to Contain Effluent from Abdominal Stomas

Anticipated Accomplishments	Scientific Principles/ Rationale	Considerations
1. Select appropriate appliance.	An appliance not specifically designed for type of stoma present and its effluent will not function properly.	*Adhesive disc* must be large enough to accommodate stoma and still allow for an adequate adhesive margin on all sides. *Odor resistant properties* are necessary in a colostomy appliance.
2. Select a peristomal skin barrier.	Stoma effluent must not come in contact with peristomal skin. Preventive skin care is best means of reducing skin irritation problem. Peristomal skin is vulnerable because it is sealed under a disc and continuously deprived of air. Fungi can grow readily in this environment.	A skin barrier should fit snugly around stoma. Client must not be allergic to barrier's composition. Barrier should be one which permits healthy skin to grow beneath it.
3. Remove old appliance.	Appliance must be changed when bond is no longer effective or when odor cannot be eliminated by rinsing appliance.	
4. Wash peristomal skin area with warm water.	Perspiration, bacteria, and effluent residue must be eliminated to insure skin integrity. Soap is avoided because it leaves a residue which interferes with ostomy appliance bonding.	For loop colostomies, hold on to bridge while washing to avoid dislodging rod.
5. Allow peristomal skin area to dry thoroughly.	Absolute drying is imperative to discourage growth of skin bacteria and to assure adherence of ostomy appliance.	If stoma continues to drain, wick it with a piece of gauze so effluent stays off peristomal area.
6. Measure stoma size.	An accurate stomal measurement is necessary to assure a properly fitting appliance.	Measuring a loop or double-barreled colostomy is often challenging and may require use of a large index card to make a suitable guide.

Implementation	Recommendations	Observations
Appliance is selected from an ostomy supply catalogue and ordered from hospital's supply system.	Appliance must be open-ended. The opening should be large enough to emit formed stool (sigmoid colostomy), and to permit adequate rinsing after emptying. During early postoperative period, a clear appliance is used so that stoma and effluent can be observed.	
Karaya may be used either in sheet or disc form. Some appliances are constructed with karaya rings. *Stomahesive* is available in wafer form. Most skin barriers are ordered separately from appliance.	Karaya is suitable for any type of fecal stoma. Stomahesive is usually only needed for loop or double-barreled stoma.	
Ease appliance off slowly while holding client's skin taut. Dispose of used appliance in a plastic bag.	Before old appliance is removed, all equipment for applying new appliance should be assembled and ready to use.	Note amount and character of effluent.
Gauze pads or a face cloth dipped in warm water are used to wipe around stoma.	Do not be afraid to touch stoma or wash around it. Rubbing should be avoided. Small remnants of previous skin barrier can be left on the skin if they do not come off easily.	Examine stoma carefully. Observe for healthy color. Note any problem areas (i.e., abscess formation or bleeding).
Dry area with a towel, then allow it to remain open to air for as long as possible.	A hair dryer is sometimes used to facilitate drying.	If karaya is used as skin barrier, peristomal skin should be sprayed with Skin Prep after drying.
Slide the appropriate size hole in guide over stoma. Note stoma size.	Measuring guides come with ostomy appliances. If unavailable, any guide for measuring circles can be used.	Note any increase in stoma size which indicates possible problems, such as edema or prolapse.

TABLE 43-1. Continued

Anticipated Accomplishments	Scientific Principles/ Rationale	Considerations
7. Prepare skin barrier and adhesive disc.	Skin barrier and adhesive disc must fit snugly around stoma to avoid leakage of effluent onto skin.	Opening in adhesive disc should be ⅛ in larger than stoma. Skin barrier should be cut to stoma size.
8. Place skin barrier over stoma.	More effective appliance adherence is possible if skin barrier is in place first.	
9. Place appliance over skin barrier.	Appliance can be applied with more accuracy if barrier is already in place.	Appliance must be centered over stoma. Application is facilitated if one inserts one's hand into pouch to guide it over stoma.
10. Picture frame adhesive disc.	Placing tape on four edges of adhesive disc assures adequate adherence of appliance.	
11. Place liquid deodorant in pouch.	Use of topical deodorant reduces odor complications.	Many companies supply ostomy deodorants. Deodorant should be used for all colostomy clients.
12. Remove air from pouch and close off bottom.	Air in pouch prevents appliance from lying flat on client's abdomen.	

Implementation	Recommendations	Observations
On paper covered side of skin barrier, trace a circle the size of stoma. Follow same procedure for adhesive disc except that circle will be ⅛ in larger than stoma. Cut out both circles.	Save paper backings with stoma patterns on them. Date these and leave with client's supplies.	Check to see that both circles fit properly before applying skin barrier and ostomy appliance.
Slide barrier down over stoma. For a loop stoma, ease barrier under bridge and around stoma. It is best to slit skin barrier at top to facilitate fitting around loop rod.	Remove protective backing before applying skin barrier.	Note whether skin barrier is flat without any air bubbles beneath it. Skin around stoma should not be visible.
Slip pouch over stoma. Ease over upper end of rod first for a loop stoma. Press adhesive down flat.	Apply appliance so that opening is toward the client's feet.	Be sure adhesive is pressed flat without wrinkles or air bubbles.
Tape across all sides as shown in Fig. 43-2.	Micropore or paper tape should be used. Do not use adhesive tape. A nonallergic tape must be used.	
Insert a piece of tissue soaked with appropriate amount of deodorant into bottom of bag.	Never use aspirin or other irritating substances as deodorant.	Be sure deodorant is not in direct contact with stoma.
Smooth pouch down from top. Fold up end of pouch three times and then fan fold bottom and place rubber band around it.	Some appliances come with a clamp for bottom of pouch. Save clamp if this is case.	Be sure appliance is not sticking to stoma itself. Note whether end of pouch is adequately secured.

nurse. Recently, it has become popular in some hospitals for client and nurse to sign a contract concerning what the client is to learn and what the nurse is to teach. An example of such a contract is shown in Figure 43-3. In any event, a well-organized plan of care is essential if implementation is to be carried out in an orderly fashion. A sample care plan tool is shown in Figure 43-4. Pencil should be used to fill out the client's care plan so that changes consistent with the client's progress can be made on the plan. The written plan of care should be shared with the client. This will help him to gain a sense of control over the ostomy care. In addition, this action facilitates the notion that the client is in control of his own destiny and retains the right to make decisions about his care.

As the plan of care is implemented, frequent health care team conferences should be held concerning the client's progress; whenever possible, these conferences should include his family as well. The ostomy client requires positive reinforcement as the plan of care is being implemented. He must be kept apprised of the progress being made.

EVALUATION AND REVISION

A plan of care should not be considered static. Ostomy client care needs are always changing, and the plan of care should be modified according to changes in his status. The client and family's reaction to the plan of care should be evaluated continuously. Whenever a nursing intervention falls short of achieving its objective, an alternative intervention must be proposed.

In addition to revising the plan of care according to normal changes in the client's status, the nurse must be alert to possible complications which may occur following various types of ostomy surgery.

OSTOMY CARE CONTRACT

It is agreed that _____ will be independent in the care of
             patient's name
_____ ostomy as evidenced by the following demonstration of
   his/her
self-care skills:

1. Emptying the pouch whenever it becomes 1/3 full. _____ date
2. Determining when the appliance should be changed. _____ date
3. Removing the old appliance and discarding it. _____ date
4. Cleaning peristomal skin area. _____ date
5. Assessing peristomal skin condition. _____ date
6. Measuring stoma size. _____ date
7. Making and cutting out stoma hole pattern on the adhesive
   disc of appliance and skin barrier. _____ date
8. Applying ostomy appliance. _____ date
9. Closing open end of pouch. _____ date
10. Other related treatments, i. e. incision site and/or wound care. _____ date

Patient's Signature _____

Signature of Primary Nurse _____

FIGURE 43-3. An example of an ostomy care contract, which concerns what a client is to learn and what the nurse is to teach. Any patient problem which requires self-care skills should be addressed in the contract. If the patient has had a proctectomy, self-care of the perineal wound should be included in the contract. If the patient has a colostomy which is to be irrigated, the steps of that procedure should be listed in a manner similar to the other aspects of stoma care listed above. (The procedure for irrigating a colostomy is shown in Fig. 43-11).

OSTOMY CARE PLAN

Name _____ Age _____

Date of admission _____ Admitting Diagnosis _____

Date of ostomy surgery _____ Surgical Procedure _____

Type of ostomy created _____

Locate stoma and incision site on the diagram:

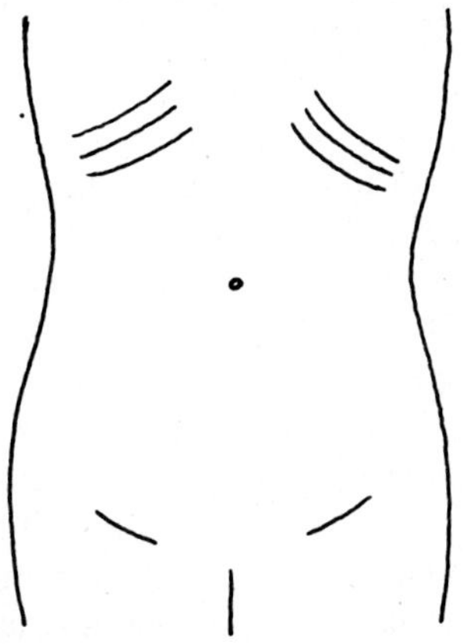

Date _____
Stoma measurement _____

Draw any open wounds ie. perineal wound, or
other problems ie. drain sites, fistulae.

Ostomy Care Routine

Peristomal skin care: _____
_____
_____
_____

Skin barrier in use: _____
_____

Size and type of ostomy appliance: _____
_____
_____

Special ostomy treatments: _____
_____
_____
_____

Suggested time for carrying out routine: _____
_____

Wound or Incision Site Care Routine

FIGURE 43-4. An example of a care plan tool.

Definitive evaluation of the overall plan of care requires that the nurse refer to the ostomy client objectives which have been defined. This procedure emphasizes the necessity for clearly defined objectives. When these have not been clearly defined, it becomes very difficult to evaluate the extent to which they have been achieved.

CARE OF COLOSTOMY CLIENT

A colostomy is an opening into the colon which provides for the elimination of fecal material through an aperture on the abdominal wall. Colostomies are created more frequently than any other type of ostomy. Any portion of the colon may be involved. A colostomy may be temporary or permanent. The stoma may be located anywhere on the abdomen; however, it is most frequently found on the left lower quadrant or right upper quadrant.[1]

Functional Considerations

The colon is considerably wider and shorter than the small intestine. Its total length is approximately 4½ feet. The functions of the colon are to absorb water and electrolytes and store feces. The proximal portion of the colon is primarily concerned with absorption, and the distal portion with storage. Thus, the nature of the effluent which exits from a colostomy is determined by the portion of the colon which has been entered. As shown in Figure 43-5, the large intestine is composed of the cecum, ascending colon, transverse colon, descending colon, sigmoid colon, and rectum.

The ascending colon extends upward from the short pouchlike cecum. Fecal material in this section is liquid and high in enzymes. The transverse colon continues across the abdominal cavity from right to left. Although some water has been absorbed, the fecal mass in this area is of a mushy consistency. Beginning near the spleen, the descending colon passes downward on the left side of the abdomen to become the S-shaped sigmoid colon. The fecal mass in this region ranges from semisolid to solid. The rectum which is contiguous with the sigmoid colon terminates in the narrow anal canal. The solid fecal mass is contained in the rectum until it is expelled in the act of defecation. Mucus, the only significant secretion in the colon, protects the intestinal wall against excoriation from the fecal mass and bacterial activity. It also serves as an alkaline barrier to keep acids formed deep in the feces from attacking the intestinal wall.[2] In addition, mucus helps to hold the fecal mass together.

Types of Colostomies

A colostomy may be described according to the construction of the stoma, such as loop, double-barreled, or end colostomy. It is also identified according to anatomical location along the colon (i.e., ascending, transverse, descending, or sigmoid colostomy). Here a description of the common structural types of colostomy stomas is presented. This is followed by a discussion of the significance of the anatomical location.

LOOP COLOSTOMY

As shown in Figure 43-6, a *loop colostomy* is one in which a loop of bowel is exteriorized on the abdomen. A glass rod or plastic device is then inserted underneath the bowel to hold it out on the abdomen. Two openings are made into the bowel. The proximal opening discharges fecal material and the distal opening emits a mucous discharge. Approxi-

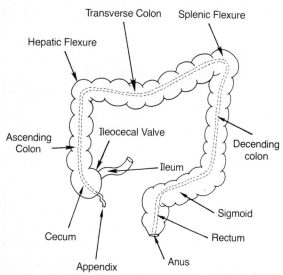

FIGURE 43-5. Large intestine. Note the last portion of the small intestine, the ileum, as it joins the cecum at the ileocecal valve. The short pouch like cecum is only 2–3 in long. The entire length of the colon is approximately 4½ feet. It terminates with the rectum which is about 7 in long.

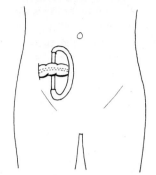

LOOP COLOSTOMY USING GLASS ROD

Glass rod inserted under loop of bowel. Rubber tubing is attached to maintain the position of the rod.

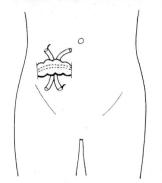

LOOP COLOSTOMY USING PLASTIC DEVICE

Plastic device inserted underneath the loop of bowel, and sutured at two points.

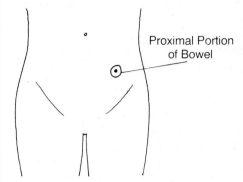

END COLOSTOMY

Proximal Portion of Bowel

Only one stoma is present on the abdomen. The colon distal to the stoma has been removed.

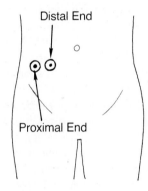

DOUBLE–BARRELED COLOSTOMY

Distal End

Proximal End

Both stomas are together.

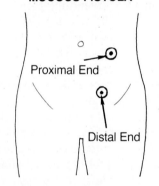

DOUBLE–BARRELED COLOSTOMY OR END COLOSTOMY WITH MUCOUS FISTULA

Proximal End

Distal End

Separated stomas showing proximal end and distal end (mucous fistula).

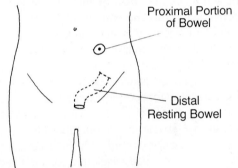

END COLOSTOMY AND HARTMANN POUCH

Proximal Portion of Bowel

Distal Resting Bowel

One stoma is present on the abdomen. The resting distal bowel is in the intra-abdominal space.

FIGURE 43-6. Various types of colostomies.

mately 7 days after surgery, the bowel becomes sufficiently adherent to the abdomen to permit the removal of the glass rod or plastic device. This type of colostomy is rather large, and its use is usually confined to emergency situations.

DOUBLE-BARRELED COLOSTOMY

A *double-barreled colostomy* (Fig. 43-6) is one composed of two separate stomas, which may be immediately adjacent to one another or somewhat far apart. When the distal stoma is placed away from the proximal stoma, the colostomy is usually referred to as an end colostomy with a mucous fistula. Technically, in either case, the colostomy is double-barreled with a functioning proximal opening through which fecal material exits. The distal opening (resting colon), regardless of its location, drains mucus and is correctly termed a mucous fistula.

END COLOSTOMY

End colostomy usually means that a proximal portion of the bowel has been exteriorized as a stoma and the remaining distal portion of the bowel has been removed (Fig. 43-6). However, as mentioned above, the term may be used when the distal portion of the colon is still in place.

Occasionally, the terms end colostomy and Hartmann pouch are seen. This is the same as an end colostomy except that the distal resting portion of the colon is sutured closed and returned to the intra-abdominal space (Fig. 43-6).

Anatomical Location of Colostomy

ASCENDING COLOSTOMY

The ascending colon is used infrequently for the location of a colostomy, as this portion of the colon is not easily mobilized. It may be used when the ascending or transverse colon is involved in trauma or a malignancy. Any of the variations in stoma construction may be employed (Fig. 43-7). An ascending colostomy is very similar to an ileostomy in terms of the character of its effluent. For this reason, it is managed in the same manner as an ileostomy. The reader is referred to the section on the ileostomy for specifics concerning skin care and appliance application. However, in contrast to the ileostomy, special attention must be paid to the problem of odor control with the ascending colostomy. The appliance selected to contain the effluent must have odor resistant properties. The appliance must be rinsed meticulously when emptied and should be changed at least every 48 hours. If a belt is used with the appliance, this should also be changed frequently. A deodorant product should be placed in the pouch of the appliance. Many types of appliance deodorants are available from the manufacturers of ostomy equipment. Lastly, dietary recommendations should be given with regard to foods which are likely to produce odor and flatus, and those which are said to decrease odor. Information concerning diet therapy is found at the end of this section.

Irrigation should not be employed as a method of regulation. An ascending colostomy cannot be regulated. Liquid feces can be expected to drain frequently from the stoma. Occasionally, an irriga-tion may be ordered postoperatively to stimulate peristalsis or as preparation for a diagnostic procedure. When this is the case, normal saline is usually used in amounts not exceeding 500 ml. If the colostomy is double-barreled, only the proximal opening is irrigated if the intent is to stimulate the bowel. Preparation for diagnostic procedures, such as x-rays, usually requires that both openings be irrigated to provide for adequate visualization of the bowel. The procedure for stoma irrigation is shown in Table 43-2.

TRANSVERSE COLOSTOMY

A transverse colostomy may be constructed as a curative, palliative, or healing measure. When constructed for curative or palliative reasons, the transverse colostomy carries with it the concept of permanence. As a healing measure, it may have different connotations. Traditionally, the transverse colostomy has been thought of as a temporary intervention. However, experience with ostomy clients has revealed that the word "temporary" is best avoided. Not infrequently, the pathology which necessitated the creation of the transverse colostomy is such that colostomy closure becomes impossible. In situations where colostomy closure is possible, the client must still learn to live with the colostomy in the interim. Often the colostomy is present for a protracted period of time. When colostomy closure does take place, it is a major surgical procedure often followed by complications. Thus, the person with a transverse colostomy should be assisted to adapt to the presence of the stoma without regard to its possible impermanence.

Congenital anomalies (imperforate anus or rectovaginal fistula), Hirschsprung's disease, colonic trauma, diverticulitis, fistulae, and obstructing or perforating colon carcinoma constitute the major reasons for creating a transverse colostomy. Either the right or left transverse colon may be used. If the right side is used, the effluent will be more liquid. A left sided transverse colostomy will emit feces of a mushy consistency. Generally, the right transverse colon is selected because of its mobility. Also, it leaves a large amount of mobile distal bowel for subsequent surgical interventions. Depending on the reasons for its creation, the transverse colostomy may be loop, double-barreled, or end (Fig. 43-7). The loop is the easiest stoma to construct

THE ASCENDING COLOSTOMY

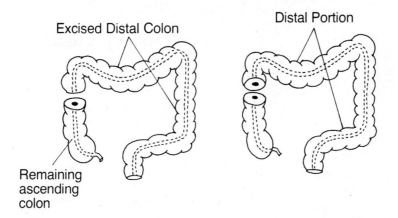

End ascending colostomy. Distal portion of the colon has been removed.

Double-barreled ascending colon. Distal portion of colon is resting.

THE TRANSVERSE COLOSTOMY

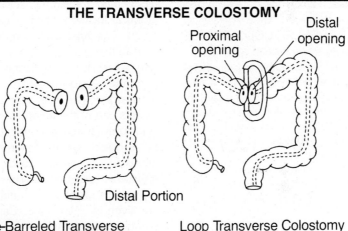

Double-Barreled Transverse Colostomy. Distal portion is resting.

Loop Transverse Colostomy

FIGURE 43-7. The ascending colostomy and transverse colostomy.

and is sometimes used in emergencies. The double-barreled colostomy is frequently constructed. A transverse end colostomy is seen somewhat less often.

Although some shrinkage will occur, the loop colostomy and the double-barreled colostomy with adjacent stomas are large and can be cumbersome to manage. Both have irregular configurations which make technical ostomy appliance management difficult. An appliance must be selected with an adhesive disc large enough to accommodate all

of the exteriorized colon (Fig. 43-8). The appliance should be open-ended to permit frequent emptying. Odor control is necessary as the effluent is quite malodorous. The appliance must have odor control properties. It should be carefully rinsed after each emptying. A deodorant product developed for ostomies should be instilled into the pouch. Dietary recommendations related to odor control are discussed later in the chapter. Because the effluent contains digestive enzymes, a *skin barrier* such as karaya or Stomahesive should be used to protect

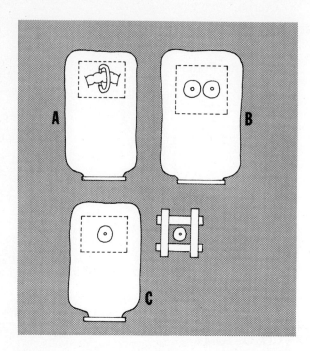

LOOP AND DOUBLE BARRELED COLOSTOMIES

FIGURE 43-8. A, A loop colostomy with glass rod contained within an open-ended disposable appliance. The Hollister and Marsan manufacturing companies have each produced a special device for managing the loop ostomy. Either of the devices may offer an alternative to the appliance shown above. B, A double-barreled colostomy with adjacent stomas is contained in a similar appliance. C, The proximal functioning end of a double-barreled colostomy in an open-ended disposable appliance. The mucous fistula (distal nonfunctioning end) is covered with a 4 × 3 gauze pad to collect the mucous drainage.

the skin. Table 43-1 outlines the steps required for the proper application of an ostomy appliance.

A transverse colostomy cannot be regulated. Attempts to do so by irrigation are frustrating for nurse and client. Further, a situation is created in which the client cannot achieve success and often becomes depressed at the failure to do so. Irrigation is only indicated postoperatively to stimulate peristalsis or as preparation for a diagnostic procedure. See Table 43-2 for the steps to follow in irrigating a colostomy. If a double-barreled or loop colostomy is being irrigated, it is necessary to ascertain whether both ends of the colostomy are to be irrigated. Normal saline should be used in amounts not to exceed 500 ml. When the purpose of the

irrigation is to stimulate peristalis following surgery, only the proximal functioning end would be irrigated.

DESCENDING COLOSTOMY

A colostomy may be created in the descending region of the colon as a permanent or transient measure. The stoma is usually located on the lower left side of the client's abdomen. Underlying conditions which necessitate surgery resulting in a descending colostomy are as follows: (1) trauma to the sigmoid colon or rectum below the descending colon, (2) colorectal cancer, (3) congenital anomalies, (4) fistulae, (5) perforating diverticulitis, and (6) colorectal abscesses.

In terms of function, the descending colostomy is similar to the sigmoid colostomy. However, the consistency of effluent is usually less solid with the descending colostomy. This is attributed to its anatomical location which is closer to the transverse colon. The type of descending colostomy stoma constructed may be loop, double-barreled, or end (Fig. 43-9). If the colostomy is not intended to be permanent, a double-barreled stoma is generally constructed. The loop type of stoma is rarely used for this part of the colon. A permanent descending colostomy stoma is constructed as the end type. For a double-barreled stoma, appliance considerations will be similar to those mentioned under transverse colostomies. The instructions for applying an appliance to a double-barreled colostomy are given in Table 43-1. Care of an end type descending colostomy is the same as for an end sigmoid colostomy. For this reason, it has been included in the discussion of end sigmoid colostomy care. Odor control is an important consideration regardless of the type of stoma created. The appliance selected must have odor resistant properties. It should be open-ended to allow for emptying as soon as effluent collects in the pouch. After emptying, the pouch should be rinsed very carefully. An appliance deodorant should always be present in the pouch. Dietary recommendations are indicated to help control flatus production and odor. For further information, refer to the dietary information at the end of this section.

Stomal irrigation as a method of regulation is not generally indicated for the descending colostomy. Attempts to regulate a descending colostomy by

DESCENDING END COLOSTOMY

DESCENDING DOUBLE-BARRELED COLOSTOMY

SIGMOID END COLOSTOMY

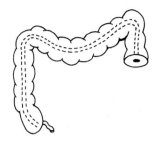 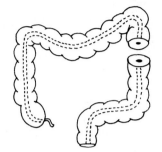 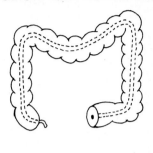

FIGURE 43-9. Descending end colostomy, descending double-barreled colostomy, and sigmoid end colostomy.

irrigation are not usually successful. The reader is referred to the sigmoid colostomy discussion for further information concerning the issue of colostomy irrigation.

SIGMOID COLOSTOMY

The sigmoid colostomy is the most common colostomy created. Although various nonmalignant rectal problems can result in a sigmoid colostomy, rectal cancer is the underlying causative factor in most instances. When rectal cancer is present and considered amenable to a surgical cure, the rectum is removed. The surgical procedure is called an abdominal perineal resection. In this procedure, the sigmoid colon is detached from the rectum and its end is brought to the surface of the abdomen as an end sigmoid colostomy (Fig. 43-9). The rectum is then removed through a perineal incision. Following surgery, the client must learn colostomy care and also perineal wound care. Recommendations for the care of a perineal wound are given in Figure 43-10. For men, the abdominal perineal resection carries with it a high incidence of impotence. This is a problem which requires supportive sexual counseling on the part of the health professional. In situations where the rectum has not been removed, impotence is not related to the presence of a colostomy.

When the rectum is left in place following the construction of an end sigmoid colostomy, it can be expected to produce a malodorous discharge consisting of dead cells and mucus. Meticulous perineal care is required to deal with this problem.

Although the origin and experiencing of the sensations are different, both types of clients may continue to feel the need to defecate for a period of time; this is often a very upsetting experience. Explanations concerning the reasons for these sensations must be provided. The client whose rectum has been removed experiences what is called phantom rectal pain. One whose rectum is still in place often experiences a tenesmuslike sensation. Both are related to nervous innervation of the rectum and will subside in time. Sitz baths several times daily may help to alleviate the problem.

Stoma and Skin Care

The end sigmoid colostomy stoma is usually located in the left lower quadrant of the abdomen. The stoma should protrude slightly from the surface of the abdomen. During the early postoperative period, the effluent from the stoma is watery. However, as peristalsis returns to normal and the client resumes his customary dietary habits, the colon functions in the same manner as it did prior to the creation of the colostomy. The output from the colostomy can then be expected to resemble the client's usual bowel movements. In most instances, this will mean formed stools. During the postoperative period an open-ended appliance is used to allow for emptying the watery drainage. Once the output from the stoma becomes formed, a closed-end pouch is often recommended because the person can simply remove and discard it when output occurs; therefore, emptying and rinsing of the pouch are avoided. The disadvantage of this

CARE OF THE PERINEAL WOUND

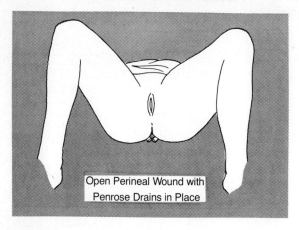

Open Perineal Wound with
Penrose Drains in Place

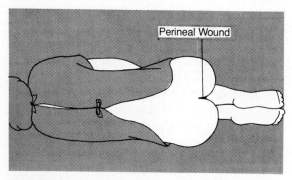

Perineal Wound

FIGURE 43-10. (1) During surgery Penrose drains are usually placed in the perineal wound. These are removed approximately 7 days after surgery. The pressure caused by the drains, particularly on the wound margins, often makes the client very uncomfortable. (2) Perineal wound irrigations with normal saline are usually started within the first week after surgery. The wound must be irrigated thoroughly and vigorously to eliminate sloughing tissue and to promote the growth of healthy granulation tissue. During irrigation it is important not to touch the wound margins with the tip of the irrigating syringe as this is often painful to the client. (3) Generally the wound is not packed between irrigations. It is covered with a generous dry sterile dressing, sufficient to absorb rectal drainage and keep the client dry. The location of the perineal wound makes the application of a dressing a challenge. The most effective means of securing the dressing is to use the Flexi-knit tubular dressing cut to form mesh-underpants, which can be pulled on just like underwear. (4) The client should be provided with a foam cushion as sitting down will be very uncomfortable. (5) Careful home care instructions are necessary as perineal wounds take several months to heal.

method is that an appliance change is required each time output occurs. This means that wherever the person is, he must change the appliance to get rid of the stool in the pouch. The possibility of skin irritation increases with frequent appliance changes. With the open-ended pouch, the person is required to empty and rinse when output occurs. This procedure brings the person in closer contact with odor and feces. Further care must be taken when selecting an open-ended pouch to be sure that the opening in the end of the pouch is wide enough to permit the passage of formed stools. The advantage of the open-ended pouch is that the person may empty and rinse the appliance as needed. Less wear and tear is put on the skin. Fewer ostomy appliances are used, which makes this method more economical. In any case, disposable appliances are always recommended rather than the reusable appliance which tends to retain fecal odor.

The steps in colostomy appliance application are outlined in Table 43-1. Whatever type of ostomy appliance is selected, a skin barrier should be used with it. Most often karaya rings, which are manufactured by many companies, are used. The use of a skin barrier is an important preventive measure in skin care. In addition, most appliances are constructed so that a rigid plastic ring with belt attachments surrounds the stoma. When a skin barrier is in place, it prevents the rigid plastic from traumatizing the stoma. For persons allergic to karaya, other skin barriers are available. Emphasis on skin care is a crucial aspect of colostomy client teaching. The use of a skin barrier by itself will not prevent skin irritation. Peristomal skin should be washed carefully with warm water. Rubbing should never be used as a method of cleaning the peristomal skin area. Absolute drying should follow, allowing the skin to remain open to the air for as long as possible. Any hair growing in the area where the appliance is applied should be cut with scissors or shaved carefully.

Use of a belt with the colostomy appliance is best avoided whenever possible. Belts are known to cause pressure areas, and to pull upon the appliance causing trauma to the stoma. Many clients, however, insist upon the security of a belt, and it is their right to do so. If a belt is going to be worn, the client must be instructed on the hazards involved and the need for examining the stoma each time the appliance is changed.

Odor Control

Containment of odor is an important consideration for the colostomy client. Effective odor control can be achieved if attention is directed to the following:

1. Selection of an appliance with odor resistant properties.
2. Use of an ostomy deodorant preparation in the stoma pouch (Table 43-1).
3. Thorough rinsing of the pouch after each emptying.
4. Changing the pouch at least every 4 days.
5. Frequent washing of the ostomy appliance belt.
6. Avoiding pinhole perforations of the pouch to allow for gas to escape.
7. Dietary recommendations concerning eating habits and foods to avoid. Dietary aspects are discussed later in this section.

When the subject of odor control is discussed, it is particularly important to clarify the fact that everyone produces odor at the time of defecation. Odor is expected to be present when the appliance pouch is opened for emptying or when it is being changed. Because the stoma is located on the front of the client's body, he is brought into closer contact with fecal odor than the person who defecates through the rectum. This often leads the client to conclude that the odor is greater than it was before surgery and that it is present all the time. Performing stoma care only in the bathroom helps to alleviate this problem, as it allows the client to leave the odor behind in the bathroom. Whereas, when stoma care is done with the client in bed, he must remain with the lingering odor. Supportive encouragement is also necessary to help the client cope with odor anxiety.

Irrigation

For many years, irrigation was employed routinely as a method of sigmoid colostomy regulation. Clients were encouraged to irrigate to achieve enough control so that feces would only exit from the stoma at irrigation time and the use of an ostomy appliance would be eliminated. While many people have achieved considerable success with irrigation, a significant number of people never have much success and are left with a sense of failure.

When irrigation is considered as part of the colostomy care regimen, the client should be carefully assessed with regard to ability to irrigate and access to bathroom facilities. Irrigation is contraindicated for people with: (1) physical disabilities for whom the acquisition of the required manipulative skills is too difficult, (2) limited comprehension (i.e., confused, senile, mentally retarded, or alcoholic clients), (3) psychological problems, (i.e., depression, obsessive compulsive traits, psychoses, irrigation fears, or anxiety).

Every potential candidate for irrigation should be given adequate information concerning all aspects of irrigation. The final decision to irrigate or not to irrigate should rest with the client. If a decision is made to irrigate, the procedure should be taught under conditions which simulate the client's home environment. Irrigation should not be started until the client is well enough to use the bathroom. It is not necessary to begin irrigation in the immediate postoperative period unless it is necessary to stimulate peristalsis or as a preparation for a diagnostic procedure. The client should be an active participant in the procedure from the outset. He must be competent in independent stoma irrigation at the time of discharge. If the client's condition is such that he is unable to irrigate, it is best to omit irrigations as a routine intervention, rather than to teach a family member to do the procedure. A detailed procedure for colostomy irrigation is presented in Table 43-2 and Figure 43-11. Briefly summarized, the advantages and disadvantages of irrigation follow:

Advantages

1. Feces are only eliminated at irrigation time.
2. Odor and gas are reduced.
3. A collecting device is not required.
4. Body image assault is reduced. Person appears more like other people.

Disadvantages

1. Leakage often occurs between irrigations.
2. People with previously irregular bowel habits find that irrigation does not regulate the bowel.
3. Colostomy care regimen is more complex and time consuming.

TABLE 43-2. Colostomy Irrigation to Regulate a Sigmoid or End Colostomy, Reduce Number of Colostomy Movements, and Decrease Gas and Odor

Anticipated Accomplishments	Scientific Principles/ Rationale	Considerations
1. Select appropriate schedule for irrigation.	Best time schedule for irrigation is one which allows client to participate in customary daily activities without interruption. Client's previous bowel habits should also be determinant.	Privacy and availability of bathroom facilities must be assured.
2. Irrigate at same time each day.	Promote regulation of colon evacuation.	
3. Advance time schedule.	Allow client freedom from irrigation, while continuing to maintain colostomy regulation.	Remember that irrigation schedule must be tailored to fit into client's life style.
4. Select irrigation equipment.	Irrigation equipment should be easy for client to assemble and use.	Cost of irrigation equipment is an important factor. Irrigation set which contains only essential items should be selected. Remember that carrying cases raise price of irrigation set.
5. Assemble equipment with client.	Client should be an active participant in irrigating procedure.	Be sure all equipment is within easy reach of client.
6. Fill container with approximately 600 ml of tepid water and hang up on hook.	Water is intended to stimulate bowel to empty. Cold water causes cramping. Water which is too warm may also cause cramping or injure bowel.	

Implementation	Recommendations	Observations
Interview client to determine work schedule and other daily routines.	Irrigation is best scheduled at times when family bathroom facilities are available. Some people find that irrigating 1 hr after a large meal is most effective.	Note the length of time it takes the client to irrigate colostomy. Share this information with client's family. Approximately 1 hr is required to complete irrigation.
Continue with daily regimen until client is free of spillage for 24 hours.	When colostomy becomes regulated, same general time period should be followed. One need not irrigate at exactly same time.	
When evacuations do not occur for 24 hour periods, advance irrigation schedule to every other day.		Note variation in returns with each daily irrigation. Days on which minimal returns occur are best selected as days for omitting irrigation.
Cone tip irrigation tip is safest.	Many types of irrigation sets are available. Ostomy equipment catalogs should be reviewed to determine best irrigator for individual client.	The client's ability to use equipment selected should be carefully assessed.
Set up equipment as though client were doing procedure alone. 　a. H_2O container with clamp and tubing. 　b. Cone irrigating tip. 　c. Irrigating sleeve with belt, faceplate, and clamps.	Irrigation should take place under circumstances which simulate home conditions.	Note client's manipulative skills and emotional reaction to irrigation procedure.
Use warm tap water. Height of hook should be such that bottom of water container is level with client's shoulder when he is in position for irrigating.	Encourage client to be relaxed and to carry out procedure in an unhurried manner.	Be sure overflow water clamp is closed. Irrigation bag should be visible to client when in a sitting position so that water level can be observed.

TABLE 43-2. Continued

Anticipated Accomplishments	Scientific Principles/ Rationale	Considerations
7. Expel air from tubing and attach irrigating cone.	Air in tubing may cause cramping. Use of cone rather than catheter eliminates possibility of perforating colon during irrigation.	Cone must be firmly attached to irrigating tubing.
8. Remove old appliance from stoma.	Stoma must be easily accessible for irrigation.	
9. Place irrigation sleeve over stoma using belt to secure it.	Effluent must have direct efficient passageway to toilet.	
10. Have client sit on toilet or on chair in front of toilet.		Provide for client warmth while he is performing the irrigation (i.e., blanket on lap or bathrobe over shoulders).
11. Lubricate cone tip and insert it through top of drain sleeve and into stoma.	Lubricant will facilitate cone insertion and eliminate trauma to stoma.	
12. Open water outflow clamp and allow all water to flow in.	All water must flow into colon to stimulate colon. Water introduced too rapidly may cause cramping.	Water must run in slowly.
13. Remove cone and allow stool and water to flow into toilet.	Water and fecal matter must be able to exit freely from colon.	

Implementation	Recommendations	Observations
Open outflow clamp allowing all air to leave tubing, then re-close clamp.		
Carefully remove pouch and place in plastic bag for disposal.	Client should wear garment which opens in front so that stoma is easily accessible and modesty is not compromised.	Note appearance of stoma and peristomal skin condition. If effluent present in pouch, note character and amount. Assess client's response to stoma appearance.
Connect belt to plastic ring of irrigating sleeve, and place around waist. Belt must be tight enough to prevent leakage of water under plastic ring.		Note client's ability to apply belt and sleeve.
	Use pillow or rubber ring as cushion if client has difficulty sitting due to perineal wound.	
Press cone gently into stoma. Do not try to push it in farther than it will go easily.	Lubricant or water may be used. If uncertain of location of stoma opening insert a gloved finger into stoma.	
Client should adjust water flow regulator clamp so that cramping or nausea are not experienced from water flowing in too rapidly.	If water will not flow, rotate cone to be sure it is not lodged against colon wall.	If back-flow occurs, (water escaping around cone) apply more manual pressure on cone. If water will neither go in nor come out, remove cone and try massaging abdomen; start again. Do not force water into colon.
Center irrigating sleeve over stoma. Have clamps handy to close off top of irrigating sleeve.	Close top of sleeve down as stool and water may gush out suddenly. Rinse out irrigating sleeve after initial drainage of stool and water.	Most of water will be expelled in approximately 15 min. If fluid does not return, replace ostomy appliance and try irrigating again next day.

TABLE 43-2. Continued

Anticipated Accomplishments	Scientific Principles/ Rationale	Considerations
14. Close off bottom of drain sleeve. Wait 20 min for bowel evacuation to complete itself.	Bowel will continue to respond to water stimulation and will evacuate for an additional period of time.	
15. Empty drain sleeve. Rinse and remove.	Irrigation is now completed. Further spillage should not take place.	
16. Apply new appliance.	Appliance protects against unexpected spillage between irrigations.	Skin must be absolutely dry at time appliance is applied.

4. People who cannot achieve control feel they have failed.
5. More attention is focused on the disability.
6. Ritualistic behavior associated with the irrigations often occurs.

Dietary Recommendations

A distinction should be made between a therapeutic diet and dietary recommendations. *Therapeutic diets* are not ordered for colostomy clients per se, except during the immediate postoperative period when liquid and low residue diets are used until the bowel recovers from surgery. The person with a colostomy may be receiving a therapeutic diet for other medical reasons. For example, the elderly colostomy client may also have congestive heart failure and be on a low sodium diet. Therapeutic diets are an important part of many health care programs and must be considered when dietary recommendations are made. This should be clarified for the client.

Dietary recommendations consist of food suggestions that reduce odor and gas. Eating habits are also reviewed. When dietary recommendations are discussed, it is essential to bear in mind that food

and eating should be enjoyable. Undue attention should not be focused on the subject of food. The client needs to feel that he can eat the same foods which were enjoyed preoperatively; however, it is necessary to remind him that foods which were gas producing or created intestinal problems before surgery will continue to do so now that a colostomy is present. Some clients may wish to pay close attention to foods selected to reduce gas and odor; others will not. Every client should be given a written list which includes the following information:

1. Certain foods and beverages are known to be gas producing (e.g., cabbage, garlic, onions, scallions, Brussels sprouts, turnips, beans, peas, beer, and other alcoholic beverages).
2. Foods with characteristic end product odors are: fish, eggs, cheese, onions, prunes, cucumbers, and coffee.
3. Parsley, spinach, yogurt, and fruit juice are thought to reduce odor.
4. A well-balanced diet, which includes fruits, vegetables, and adequate amounts of fluid, is essential for healthy colostomy functioning.
5. Food should be eaten slowly and chewed well to avoid air swallowing.

Implementation	Recommendations	Observations
Use clamps which come with irrigation set. Fold up end of sleeve and apply clamps.		All returns should be completed in 30 min. Observe client for signs of fatigue. Client may return to bed or engage in other activities while waiting for bowel to empty.
Wash off abdomen with soap and water. Dry abdomen and peristomal area thoroughly.	Client may wish to shower while appliance is off.	The total irrigation procedure will take approximately 1 hr.
Apply appliance following steps identified for application of colostomy appliance in Table 43-1.	Use disposable open-ended pouch with a skin barrier.	Note stoma appearance and peristomal skin condition.

6. Gum chewing is associated with air swallowing and results in increased amounts of gas.

Complications

A variety of complications are associated with colostomies. *Stomal strictures* are commonly seen with sigmoid colostomies. Strictures are caused by circular scar tissue. If the stricture is such that it inhibits stool evacuations, surgical excision of the scar tissue may be necessary.

Prolapse of the colon occurs most often with the loop type stoma construction. A segment of the bowel protrudes through the colostomy opening. This is a frightening occurrence for the client. Correction requires cutting off the protruding bowel and creating a new stoma.

Parastomal hernias are often seen in ostomy clients. They are not painful. Large hernias require surgical correction. Smaller ones are generally managed by the use of a supportive garment.

Colon perforation has been seen less frequently since the advent of the use of the cone type apparatus for colostomy irrigation. Perforation of the colon generally requires surgical intervention.

Stoma fistulas are usually associated with ab-

scesses or appliance trauma. Superficial fistulas may heal spontaneously with the use of topical antibiotics and a change in the type of appliance used. More extensive fistulas may require surgical intervention and stoma revision.

CARE OF THE CLIENT WITH AN ILEOSTOMY

An ileostomy is an opening into the ileum which provides for the elimination of small bowel contents through a stoma on the abdominal wall. An ileostomy is always constructed as a permanent fecal diversion. Most often, the colon and rectum are removed, and the terminal ileum is matured as an abdominal stoma. The stoma is generally located on the lower right quadrant of the abdomen. Ileostomies are usually performed for inflammatory bowel disease which does not respond to conservative medical management.

In contrast to colostomy clients, the illness experience of the person with an ileostomy is significantly different. The ileostomy client has probably suffered a long and debilitating disease prior to surgery and creation of a stoma. To him, surgery brings relief from symptoms and often a cure of the

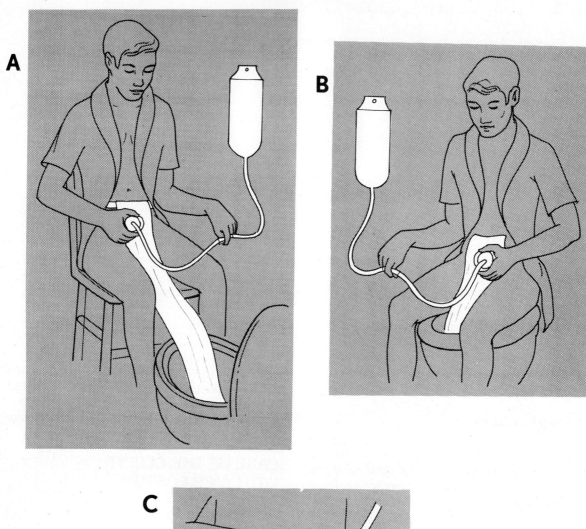

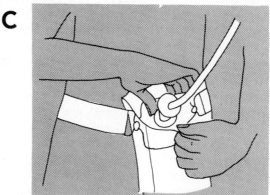

FIGURE 43-11. A, The person in position to irrigate while positioned on a chair in front of the toilet. B, The person is shown ready to irrigate while sitting on the toilet. C, A close-up of the cone being inserted in the stoma.

underlying disease. Although ileostomy is a permanent diversion, the client views the surgery as a positive gain since his illness experiences have been so devastating that even radical surgery is preferable to continued disease. However, the person with a colostomy most often has to deal with the catastrophic diagnosis of cancer. Surgery may or may not be a cure for the disease. The colostomy client is usually asymptomatic prior to surgery and has little time to adjust to the concept of radical surgery. The colostomy client is usually forced to deal with diagnosis of cancer, fear of multilation, death, and altered body image as he is coping with the real loss of body part and function (i.e., colon and control of elimination). Additionally, the factor of age is a significant variable in the two groups. The ileostomy client is most often a young adult (average age, 29–31). This client may have numerous stressful life experiences ahead of him—education, beginning a career, courtship, marriage, childbirth, and childrearing. The colostomy client is most often over 60-years-old; perhaps he may already feel social and familial usefulness is spent. The client may be retired from vocational or occupational responsibilities. Surgery for the creation of a colostomy may be one more indication to this client that his health is failing and that he is becoming regressed or dependent. Family support systems also vary in these two groups. The person with an ileostomy may have alienated family members by using the illness as a negative attention-seeking form of manipulation. Reversal of roles in the family may have occurred as the client was unable to meet his former responsibilities. The colostomy client may have strong support by significant others as families tend to band together to protect threatened members in a time of crisis. Role reversals are less likely to occur as chronic illness is usually not a precursor to colostomy surgery.

Functional Considerations

The small intestine is comprised of approximately 22 feet of duodenum, jejunum, and ileum. The ileum is the end portion of small intestine, which is attached to the cecum of the colon at the ileocecal valve. The primary function of the small intestine is assimilation of food products. Iron is absorbed in the duodenum and ileum. Absorption of fat-soluble vitamins (A, D, E, and K) occurs throughout the small intestine. Absorption of vitamin B_{12} occurs exclusively in the distal segment of the ileum, called the terminal ileum. Food products are passed from the stomach into the small intestine where they are synthesized by a process of segmental (mixing) activity into an end product of food digestion called chyme. Assimilation of food is accomplished by the two processes of digestion and absorption. Digestion occurs when enzymes secreted by intestinal glands break down food particles into smaller particles. Absorption of these small food particles occurs when they are transferred across the intestinal wall to vascular and lymphatic circulations which carry them to body cells. The small intestine is constructed in such a way that 4 to 5 million small fingerlike projections are present in the mucosal lining of the intestinal wall. These projections, called villi, greatly increase the absorption surface and aid in assimilation of chyme. The small intestine also maintains fluid and electrolyte balance by absorption of water, calcium, sodium, and potassium.[3] However, discharge from the ileum has a high water content because reabsorption of water (and some sodium) is the primary function of the proximal colon. Therefore, the characteristics of ileal effluent are watery discharge high in sodium and enzymes.

An ileostomy is usually created in the terminal end of the ileum to relieve the client of disease distal to the ileostomy (Fig. 43-12). Ileostomy surgery is usually accompanied by removal of the colon (colectomy) and rectum (proctectomy) to remove disease which occurs in those organs. Therefore, the person with an ileostomy has symptoms characteristic of absence of colon (high water and sodium loss, water discharge from ileostomy) but should not have symptoms of malabsorption (malnutrition and avitaminosis) unless large segments of small intestine are removed for disease proximal to the colon. The ileostomy is created by pulling the terminal ileum through a circular opening in the lower right abdomen. The ileum is pulled out and everted into one-half to one inch protrusion on the skin. This slightly protruding stoma is essential for facilitating placement of an appliance which can contain the highly enzymatic ileal effluent. Clients with ileostomies also have midline incisions and perineal wounds as a result of removal of the colon and rectum. (For details, see previous section.)

Ileostomy and total colectomy with proctectomy

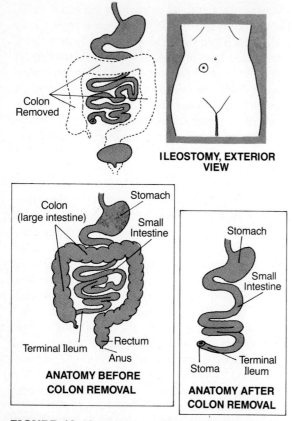

Colon
Removed

**ILEOSTOMY, EXTERIOR
VIEW**

Colon
(large intestine)

Stomach

Small
Intestine

Stomach

Small
Intestine

Terminal Ileum

Rectum

Anus

Stoma

Terminal
Ileum

**ANATOMY BEFORE
COLON REMOVAL**

**ANATOMY AFTER
COLON REMOVAL**

FIGURE 43-12. Ileostomy: The terminal ileum is resected from the colon and pulled through the abdominal wall to create a stoma for elimination of small bowel contents. Usually the colon and rectum are removed.

is the surgical intervention for ulcerative colitis, regional enteritis (Crohn's disease), and familial polyposis. The first two disease processes are generally chronic and surgery is preceded by lengthy medical management of the client. Ulcerative colitis and regional enteritis are inflammatory bowel diseases of unknown origin. Factors which precipitate the disease are speculative—that is, they may be viral, chemical, or bacterial in origin. Further, stress-related factors may be significant. However, specific causes are unknown. Both diseases are characterized by exacerbations and remissions. Ulcerative colitis is inflammation of the mucosal lining of the large intestine. Crohn's disease can effect muscle and mucosa and can occur anywhere in the gastrointestinal system from mouth to anus. It is most important to note that ulcerative colitis can be cured

by total colectomy and ileostomy. Crohn's disease may recur.

Familial polyposis is a genetically determined pathological process in which multiple polyps form throughout the colon and rectum. The polyps are premalignant lesions of which 100 percent become malignant if allowed to progress. In the unfortunate families which carry this disease, approximately one in four family members contract polyposis. Ileostomy with colectomy (and usually proctectomy) is the only effective treatment.

Preoperative Care

Preoperative considerations for the ileostomy client are similar to those for other stoma clients described previously. Special attention should be given to the marking of a stoma site as the client will be wearing an appliance for a lifetime, and good stomal placement is crucial for management of the appliance. Poorly placed ileostomy stomas result in inadequate appliance adherence to skin, resulting in leakage and skin excoriation. In addition, it is essential that ileostomy stomas be constructed in such a way that they are everted or protrude about one-half to one inch to facilitate appliance placement and containment of the drainage. Ileostomy clients generally respond very positively to visits from members of local ostomy clubs who have learned how to live with the ileostomy stoma. Enterostomal therapists are also helpful in educating the client before surgery.

Postoperative Care

A collecting device should be applied in the operating room. This appliance should be of clear, disposable plastic to allow observation of the color and consistency of ileal drainage. Initially, drainage will be minimal since the small intestine has been devoid of food and fluid. The initial output will be serosanguinous for about 24 hours. As ileal function returns, output will increase and become dark brown in color. After the client resumes oral intake, drainage will become more copious and thicker. Normal ileostomy effluent is light brown in color and has a consistency similar to toothpaste or applesauce. An output of about 500 ml/day is normal. The nurse should maintain responsibility for observing and measuring the ileostomy drainage, recording her observations, and reporting deviations from normal. Complications which are specific to the client with an ileostomy are described in Table 43-3.

Stoma Care

The corrosive digestive enzymes present in ileal effluent are considerably more excoriating to skin than other less enzymatic fecal drainage from colostomies. Therefore, skin must be carefully protected from ileostomy drainage and appliances should fit well. A peristomal seal, such as karaya ring, Colly-Seel, or Stomahesive is essential to protect the skin surrounding the stoma. Since stoma edema will subside progressively in the immediate postoperative period, the stoma should be measured every 2 to 3 days, and the opening to the appliance cut to the correct size. The peristomal barrier should approximate the stoma; the appliance opening should be cut about one eighth inch larger than the stoma. The step-by-step procedure for affixing the appliance is described in Table 43-1.

A variety of appliances are commercially available to the person with an ileostomy. These appliances are diverse in relation to durability, color, size, cost, and convenience. Clients should always use clear, disposable appliances in the immediate postoperative period. However, they should be given the option for reusable equipment and educated regarding the differences between the two types. Most disposable appliances are light-weight plastic and odorproof; these appliances should be worn approximately 7 days then discarded as the materials begin to retain odor after that time. Reusable equipment is manufactured from vinyl or rubber which is more durable than plastic. These appliances may be worn for 7 days then washed and reapplied. Vinyl appliances may last 4−6 months, rubber appliances 6−12 months before the materials become brittle or retain odor. They should be discarded when these problems develop.

Reusable appliances require careful evaluation to determine correct fitting and ease in handling for each individual. Enterostomal therapists are trained in the intricacies of reusable equipment, and the client should seek consultation from one of these specialists before buying permanent equipment. Since a custom-made faceplate must be designed

for reusable equipment, clients should wait about 3 months postsurgery to order the appliance. By that time, the stoma size will have stabilized, and a proper size opening can be determined. Reusable appliances are more costly to purchase than disposable appliances; however, since the equipment can be used many times before requiring replacement, cost may be comparable over time. Clients should always be encouraged to view the cost of appliances over a period of 1 year when evaluating the economics of various types of equipment.

All stoma appliances for ileostomies are open-ended or drainable. The patient must be able to empty the appliance 4−5 times per day without removing the appliance. The semiliquid consistency and constantly draining nature of the ileostomy effluent absolutely preclude the use of closed-end nondrainable appliances. The nurse should empty the appliance every 3−4 hours postoperatively explaining to the client how and why it is done. The client should be encouraged to assume this task as soon as he can manage it. This is an important step in the progression to self-care.

Clients should also be instructed in methods of rinsing out the appliance after emptying, but prior to closing the appliance. This can be accomplished by pouring tepid tapwater from a cup into the bottom of the appliance, gently rinsing the appliance, draining, and closing it. This step is aesthetically desirable if feasible; however, many persons with ileostomies find it too complicated to carry out when emptying appliances in public toilets.

Odor Control

Normal ileostomy effluent is nonodorous or has a slightly sweet odor which is not offensive. However, as bacteria proliferate in pooled ileal contents, the odor may be a problem when the client drains the appliance. Clients should be educated that odor in the bathroom is normal and unavoidable. Using odorproof appliances and preventing leakage or soiling of clothes by the ileal effluent prevent odor outside of the bathroom. For those persons who are particularly sensitive to odor, ostomy deodorants can be purchased. These deodorants are bacteriostatic and prevent odor by retarding the growth of bacteria while neutralizing the ileal effluent. Ostomy deodorants must be reinserted into the appliance each time it is emptied. Vanilla extract is a

TABLE 43-3. Complications of Ileostomy

	Causes	Effects	Intervention
I. Obstruction **A. Stomal** 1. Volvulus	Torsion of small intestine around a fixed point, usually where ileum passes through abdominal wall.	Severe obstruction evidenced in significant decrease in ileal output, cramping; eventual perforation or rupture of small intestine.	Surgical intervention. (*Emergency*)
2. Prolapse	Abdominal opening for ileum is too large and mesentery of the small intestine has not been secured to abdominal wall.	Any increase in intra-abdominal pressure (sneezing, coughing, sexual intercourse, or vigorous peristalsis) forces ileal segment out *several* inches; unaesthetic; fearful to client; may lead to necrosis.	1. Have client lie down to decrease intra-abdominal pressure. 2. Cover prolapsed intestine with warm, damp cloth. 3. Manual reduction (i.e., replace ileum by gentle manipulation). 4. Prolapse guard or elastic girdle may be worn to prevent recurrence. 5. Surgical repair in recurrence of prolapse.
3. Edema of stoma	Appliance opening is too tight; fits too snugly around stoma leading to swelling	1. Blockage. 2. Difficult to remove appliance (if faceplate is inflexible).	Provide client with an appliance at least 1/8 in larger than stoma
4. Adhesion	Scar tissue forms at point where ileostomy passes through abdominal wall; usually takes time to develop (i.e., several months).	Stomal stenosis leads to obstruction.	1. Progressive dilatation.* 2. Surgical reduction (minor procedure).
B. Ileostomy dysfunction	Ileal segment is brought through stab wound or incisional line instead of through a round abdominal opening. Pressure on ileum leads to lymphedema, peristomal scarring, and stenosis.	Food products become trapped in dependent segments of ileum; bacterial overgrowth occurs leading to the following: 1. Functioning sporadically in spurts and rushes (i.e., noisy); 2. Foul odor; 3. Thin liquid output with occasional large particles; and 4. Output increases to more than 1 L/day.	Passage of time may reduce edema. Periodic dilatation to decrease stenosis.* Gentle irrigation of ileostomy to remove trapped food particles.
C. Food blockage (very common)	Foods that absorb water (e.g., dried fruits, corn, and popcorn) and fibrous food products (e.g., mushroom, celery, coconut, Chinese vegetables, white fibers of oranges, and grapefruit) are	Undigested food products obstruct stoma leading to: 1. Cramping, abdominal pain; 2. Vomiting; 3. Decreased flow from ileostomy; and 4. Dehydration.	1. Oral enzymes. 2. *Gentle* irrigation. 3. Surgical intervention (last resort). 4. *Never give laxatives.*

*Treatment by progessive dilatation is controversial. Experts feel that dilatation breaks down the structures which secure the ileum to facia. Scar tissue will further develop. Some claim that teaching stoma dilatation will aid clients to accept the change in body image—that is, putting one's finger into the stoma encourages the client to identify the new body orifice as his own. However, one must be aware that, to some persons, dilating a stoma is as aesthetically unacceptable as putting one's finger into the anus. Allowances should be made for individual feelings.

TABLE 43-3. Continued

	Causes	Effects	Intervention
	poorly digested in small intestine. Inherent enzymes cannot decompose these foods to small enough particles to pass through ileostomy stoma.		
II. Fluid and electrolyte imbalance	The person with an ileostomy loses large amounts of sodium and water which are primarily absorbed in large intestine. Flu, dysentery, and other gastrointestinal disorders cause diarrhea and vomiting.	The patient may *very* quickly become dehydrated and go into electrolyte imbalance. With diarrhea, he may increase ileal effluent to many times normal amount; may have to empty appliance every 30 min instead of 4–5 times/day.	1. Antidiarrheal agents. (calcium carbonate, bismuth subgallate, Metamucil) 2. Force fluids high in electrolytes (orange juice, bouillon, Coke, tea, and Energade). 3. Intravenous fluids with electrolyte replacements (*extreme* but not uncommon).
III. Kidney stone formation	Dehydration and electrolyte losses common to person with ileostomy leads to acidic urine. Uric acid kidney stones are precipitated, causing incidence of kidney stone formation approximately twice that of a normal population.	Kidney stone obstruction in urinary system leads to: 1. Abdominal cramping; 2. Vomiting; 3. Cessation of ileostomy flow (due to secondary ileus); 4. Urinary bleeding.	1. Prevention: maintain consistently high fluid intake; oral intake; of sodium bicarbonate if prone to stone formation. 2. Treatment: routine for persons with renal calculi. Medications: a. Analgesics (Demerol); b. Antispasmodics (Atropine); c. Antibacterial (Gantrisin); and d. Sodium bicarbonate. Strain all urine (to determine stone composition). Increase oral intake (to dilute urine and facilitate "passing" of stone).
IV. Retraction	Scar tissue develops around stoma; as supporting structures at the facia layer shrink, the stoma is pulled inward.	Stoma becomes flush with skin or retracted into skin. Consequently more difficult to manage. Skin irritation develops at point where ileal effluent contacts skin surface. Fitting client with appropriate appliance is more difficult.	1. Use an appliance with *convexity* of faceplate to force stoma outward. 2. Use only thin karaya rings under faceplate. 3. Simple surgical procedure to release adhesions (i.e., stoma revision preferable).
V. Fistula	Recurrence of original disease (Crohn's disease), or mechanical injury to stoma (rubbing of faceplate), or damage to ileum during the surgical procedure. Enzymatic drainage from ileum leads to local tissue damage; false passages develop through intestine to outside of bowel wall.	Above skin level: poor adherence of appliance if fistula close to stoma, resulting in leaking and skin excoriation and irritation of stomal mucosa. Below skin level: abscess formation and infection. Significant fluid and electrolyte losses can occur.	1. Medical treatment to encourage spontaneous healing. a. Client is kept NPO to decrease ileal flow through fistula and possibly placed on hyperalimentation therapy (TPN). b. Medications to decrease intestinal motility.

Care of the Client with an Ostomy 907

TABLE 43-3. Continued

	Causes	Effects	Intervention

			2. Surgical treatment.
			  a. Incision and drainage of abscess.
			  b. Excision of fistulous tract.
			  c. Possible revision of ileostomy.

VI. Hernia	Weak abdominal muscles, inadequate postoperative healing or poor surgical technique in securing supportive structures of stoma lead to interstitial protrusion of ileum into subcutaneous layers of skin surrounding stoma.	Obstruction of stoma. Poor adherence of appliance to bulging skin surface.	Surgical revision. Use very flexible appliance; disposable appliances conform best to irregular abdominal contours.

household item that is an effective ostomy appliance deodorant and can be used safely; an aspirin tablet, although an effective ostomy appliance deodorant, should *not* be used since it may ulcerate the stoma if the stoma is bathed in the ileal effluent when the client is prone. Oral preparations to retard fecal odor are not necessary for persons with ileostomies. Most intestinal gas is generated in the colon. Therefore, persons with normally functioning ileostomies should not experience problems with flatus. (See previous section for description of flatus control.)

Dietary Recommendations

The most common nutritional problem postoperatively for the person with an ileostomy is *excessive weight gain*. This phenomenon occurs because the client can consume favorite foods previously denied. Frequently, the underlying pathological process has meant years of strict adherence to a low-residue diet. Chronic diarrhea has led to weight loss, malnutrition, and avitaminosis. Consequently, resolution of the problem by ileostomy means a return to normal eating habits. The client may be immediately restricted to low-residue (low fiber) diet to prevent trauma to the operative site. However, psychological and physical advantages are gained by putting the client on a regular diet as quickly as possible. The psychological advantages are in assisting the client to feel as normal as pos-

sible and compensating for the losses of colon and control of defecation by reinstating normal diet. Physiological advantages are in promoting weight gain and rebuilding of tissue through optimum nutrition.

Dietary considerations are important for the ileostomy client in regard to preventing some complications (Table 43-3). Food blockage is the most common complication following ileostomy. Humans do not have the enzymes necessary to completely digest high-cellulose foods. Therefore, foods such as Chinese vegetables, corn, the white parts of grapefruit and oranges, mushrooms and celery pass through the gastrointestinal system relatively unchanged. Also foods that absorb water such as dried apricots, raisins, and popcorn are poorly digested. When these foods are ingested in large quantities, they may become blocked at the point where the ileum passes through the abdominal wall creating the stoma. The ileum cannot expand to expel the food products as the rectum can. The symptoms of food blockage are vomiting, cramping abdominal pain, and decreased ileal output. Treatment is aimed at breaking up the food particles. Drinking warm tea may help to break up food blockage. However, gentle irrigation is usually necessary and should *only* be carried out by a physician or qualified enterostomal therapist. The best approach to food blockage is prevention. Clients must learn to ingest foods associated with problems one at a time in small quantities. They should be cautioned to masticate food thoroughly, eat slowly, wear properly fitting dentures, and practice good dental care.

Fluid and electrolyte imbalance is another major problem of the person with an ileostomy. Since he lacks a colon, which is responsible for reabsorption of water and some sodium, the ileostomy client tends to lose large amounts of water and sodium in the ileal effluent. Therefore, when the person experiences the vomiting and diarrhea caused by flu or dysentery, he may quickly become dehydrated and hyponatremic. The person will know he has diarrhea if: (1) the ileal output substantially increases in excess of 1 L/day; (2) the effluent is hot from increased body temperature; and (3) the consistency of the effluent is watery. Treatment is aimed at restoring and maintaining fluid and electrolyte balance. The person with an ileostomy should be taught the following steps to treat diarrhea:

1. Ingest large volumes of fluid high in sodium and potassium, such as tea, Coke, orange juice, bouillon or broth, Energade, or Gatorade.
2. Eat foods high in potassium and sodium, such as bananas and salted crackers.
3. Seek emergency treatment quickly if oral feedings are impossible due to nausea and vomiting.

The ileostomy client can become severely dehydrated within 12 hours after onset of diarrhea if replacement of fluids is not immediate.

Avitaminosis is usually not a problem for the ileostomy client unless large amounts of the small intestine have been removed due to Crohn's disease. However, since vitamin B_{12} is absorbed exclusively in the terminal ileum, the person with an ileostomy may be unable to synthesize that vitamin from ingested food. Pernicious anemia results from vitamin B_{12} deficiency. The liver has an impressive capacity to store vitamin B_{12}. Therefore, the problem will not develop for several months postsurgery. It may never develop if attempts are made to preserve most of the terminal ileum at the time of surgery. However, all persons with ileostomies should be tested for B_{12} absorption and the vitamin replaced through weekly intramuscular injections as needed.

Medications

Special considerations must be given to the person with an ileostomy who is being treated for other pathological processes. For example, ileostomy clients are rarely placed on a restricted sodium diet for cardiovascular conditions and high blood pressure. Ileostomy clients naturally lose high amounts of sodium in effluent which precludes need for sodium restriction. In addition, fluid retention is usually not a problem as water is eliminated with the sodium in ileostomy effluent. Therefore, diuretics are seldom used by persons with ileostomies. When diuretics are used, caution should be taken to order only potassium-sparing diuretics. The thiazides cause severe potassium excretion or hypokalemia. The client may develop digoxin toxicity if he becomes hypokalemic while maintaining pre-existing levels of digoxin ingestion. As oral potassium solutions are hypertonic, they will increase the ileal output and lead to severe hypovolemia or water loss. Therefore, potassium must generally be replaced intravenously for the ileostomy client.

Enteric-coated tablets and time-released capsules or tablets should be avoided by the person with an ileostomy. At least part of these medications pass through the small intestine relatively unchanged and undissolved as they are constructed for absorption in the ascending colon. The ileostomy client, who no longer has a colon, will not derive full benefit from the drug. The physician can most reliably prescribe for the ileostomy client syrups or elixirs—solutions in which the active compound is dissolved and easily absorbed. Oral contraceptives are completely absorbed in the small intestine and can be prescribed for women with ileostomies.

Activity

The person with an ileostomy frequently experiences a renewed vigor and mobility in pursuing activities of daily living. He was probably severely debilitated prior to surgery, and activities were restricted by a constant need for immediate access to bathrooms. With surgery, comes increased health and energy. The client can return to occupational and leisure activities in which he participated before the illness. This is one of the major objectives of surgical intervention, and every effort should be made to allow the client any activities which may be enjoyed.

Persons with ileostomies are employed in a diverse range of professions, vocations, and jobs. Employment should not be restricted by the presence of a stoma. Physicians and nurses can be useful client advocates in educating employees regarding the functional restrictions necessitated by an ileostomy stoma. The only significant limitation is on tasks involving heavy lifting which may predispose the client to hernia formation. In fact, the person who has experienced a stoma can return to his former occupation, and this person is often a most desirable employee as he re-enters the work force with enthusiasm and a desire to make up for lost time.

Leisure activities are possible and beneficial to the client with an ileostomy stoma. He can participate in all sports as he regains strength and feels able to participate. Contact sports such as hockey, soccer, basketball, and football should be played with some caution to prevent damage to the stoma. Plastic stoma guards are commercially available for this purpose. Water sports such as swimming, diving, and water skiing are enjoyed by many persons with ileostomies. An appliance must be worn while swimming, and it should be secured to the skin with waterproof adhesive strips or tape. The well-placed ileostomy stoma will accommodate an appliance that will not show under even the briefest swimming apparel.

An ileostomy should not interfere with sexual activity. Males maintain potency, erection, and ejaculation postoperatively. Females are able to experience orgasm and bear children. In the past few years, surgical techniques for proctectomy have been perfected in such a way that minimal pelvic damage affecting sexual functioning results. Suggesting to a man that he may be impotent following surgery to create an ileostomy may create a self-fulfilling prophecy. These clients should be well informed of the actual facts—that is, that physiological sexual functioning is not diminished for most ileostomy clients. In fact, increased vigor and health frequently enhance sexual functioning postoperatively. Clients may be inhibited by their real or imagined perceptions of the feelings a sexual partner has regarding the ileostomy. A supportive, caring mate can do much to foster self-confidence in the client's sexual attractiveness. Many clients feel more attractive wearing special coverings which hide the appliance. These cloth covers can be made or purchased in a variety of colors and designs. Clients inevitably feel more confident in resuming intimate relationships if they are free from fear of appliance leakage. A securely-fitting reliable appliance is an absolute prerequisite to sexual intercourse. As illness may have interfered with the client's role as sexual partner, time may be necessary to re-establish formerly meaningful relationships. Talking with other persons of the same sex and age who have an ileostomy is often helpful to the client and his sexual partner. If sexual problems persist, sexual counseling by a trained professional may be helpful.

Discharge Planning

The person who has experienced ileostomy surgery has multiple new experiences to incorporate into his daily activities and self-concept. Educating the client regarding these changes is essential to his successful rehabilitation. The nurse who is aware of what new experiences the client will have and what he must learn can be very helpful in assisting him to adapt. Clients should be given as much experience as possible in caring for the stoma in the hospital. They should be encouraged to empty and change appliances in the bathroom as that is what they will be doing at home. They should also be encouraged to talk frequently about the complications and special considerations for ileostomy. Their conversations regarding diet, stoma management, odor, and activity may reveal misconceptions which could lead to later problems in adjustment. The process of resocialization begins in the hospital where the client may begin to feel confident relating to family members, visitors, personnel and other clients. Social contact should be encouraged. Consultation with a social worker may relieve anxiety regarding hospital bills and payments for equipment outside the hospital setting. Significant others should be included in the client teaching to reinforce and encourage the client in the first anxious days at home. Community resources should also be mobilized to help the newly discharged client. A hospital visit from the community health nurse will enhance the nurse's understanding of the client and foster the client's sense of security in the visiting nurse who will assist him at home. The adjustment to radical changes in body image and functioning caused by ileostomy surgery is monumental. A knowledgeable, understanding nurse can greatly assist the client in making the adjustment.

CARE OF THE CLIENT WITH A URINARY DIVERSION

A urinary diversion is an opening into some part of the urinary tract which diverts urine from an obstructed or diseased area through an external abdominal opening to a urine collecting device. Any malfunctioning part of the urinary system may necessitate temporary or permanent diversion of urine. Table 43-4 describes pathological conditions which may necessitate urinary diversion. Table 43-5 describes various types of urinary diversions, and Figure 43-13 depicts the types of diversions. Urinary diversions have unique considerations because of their constantly draining nature. Urine flows continuously from any urinary stoma because the sphincteral mechanisms of the urethra are lost in surgical diversion.

Functional Considerations

The normal urinary tract contains two kidneys, two ureters, one bladder, and one urethra (Fig. 43-14). The primary function of the urinary tract is to eliminate from the body waste products of metabolism such as urea, uric acid, creatinine, ketone bodies, and fluid. The kidneys are concerned with the homeostatic functions of conserving or eliminating fluids and electrolytes present in the blood plasma that passes through them. Through the processes of glomerular filtration and tubular reabsorption, secretion, and excretion, kidneys continually adjust osmotic pressure, volume, and ionic structure of body fluids essential to preserving life. The remainder of the urinary system, ureters, bladder, and urethra, serve to transport, store and eliminate urine. Only the bladder is functionally equipped to store urine.

Approximately 1–2 ml of urine per minute flows into the bladder creating the normal adult volume of urine of about 1200–1500 ml per day. Roughly, twice as much urine is excreted during waking hours as during sleep. Urine is usually acidic but pH varies with dietary intake and body needs and may also be alkaline.[4]

TABLE 43-4. Pathological Conditions Leading to Creation of Urinary Diversions

Chronic
  Neurogenic bladder
  Intractable cystitis
  Urinary incontinence
  Diabetes insipidus (hydronephrosis)
  Polycystic kidney disease

Acute
  Neoplasms
    Cancer of bladder
    Metastatic cancer of cervix, prostate, and colon
  Fistula
    Colovesical fistula
    Vesicovaginal fistula
  Trauma—injury to bladder or ureters
    Gun shot wounds
    Stab wounds
    High velocity impacts
    Spinal cord injuries (incontinence and retention)

Congenital
  Exstrophy of bladder, epispadias
  Spina bifida
  Myelomeningocele
  "Prune belly" (congenital absence of abdominal muscles)

Urine must flow freely through the urinary system if renal functioning is to be preserved. Obstruction of urine at any point in the urinary tract will cause back-flow to the kidneys which will, subsequently, cause diminished production of urine and damage to the renal parenchyma. Obstruction of either ureter by congenital or pathological conditions necessitates immediate relief by surgical intervention. A tube may be inserted directly into the involved renal pelvis (nephrostomy) or the ureter maybe redirected to the skin surface above the point of obstruction (ureterostomy). Both procedures allow urine to flow from the kidney to the outside until measures can be taken to permanently rectify the situation. Some congenital and pathological conditions interfere with bladder functioning either through retention of urine in the bladder or inability of the bladder to store urine. These conditions require less immediate surgical intervention to redirect urine from the bladder. Urine may be shunted from ureters to the outside through ureteral openings (ureterostomy), artificially created conduits (ileal and sigmoid loops), or bladder opening (vesicotomy). All of these procedures may be temporary or permanent depending on the underlying pathological condition.

TABLE 43-5. Types of Urinary Diversions

Type	Pathological Condition	Surgical Intervention	Advantages	Problems
Ileal conduit (loop)	Neoplastic lesions Neurogenic bladder Congenital anomalies	Ureters implanted into isolated segment of ileum which functions as conduit for urine. Ileal segment is brought through abdominal skin opening and a matured (everted) stoma is created.	Management facilitated by urine draining from the "spout" of an everted stoma. Excellent vascular supply of ileum.	Complex surgical procedure. Requires two surgical teams. Stomal stenosis. Pyelocystitis. Leakage of urine at ureteral anastomosis.
Sigmoid conduit (loop)	Neoplastic lesions Congenital anomalies	Ureters implanted into isolated segment of sigmoid colon which functions as conduit for urine. Sigmoid segment is brought through abdominal skin opening and a matured (everted) stoma is created. Ureters can be tunneled into walls of colon in such a way that muscular contractions of peristalsis prevent reflux of urine to kidneys.	No stomal stenosis. Antireflux procedure. Larger stoma (pediatric).	Complex surgical procedure. Requires two surgical teams. Poor vascular supply of colon may lead to necrosis (death of segment).
Vesicostomy	Urethral stricture Epispadius Exstrophy of bladder	Opening into bladder to bypass urethra. Bladder flap used to create opening.	Simple surgical procedure. No stomal stenosis.	"Proud flesh"—a painful granulation tissue develops in hair follicle of skin exposed to constant urine contact. Difficult to contain drainage. Cystitis common.

Procedure	Indications	Description	Advantages	Disadvantages/Considerations
Transuretero-ureterostomy	Neoplasms / Trauma	One ureter implanted into other ureter below the skin level. Longer ureter is brought to skin surface to drain as single flush stoma.	No intestinal surgery required.	Difficult to contain drainage with flush stoma. Ureteral stenosis.
Bilateral ureterostomy	Neoplasms / Trauma	Each ureter resected from bladder brought to skin surface to drain as single stoma.	No intestinal surgery required; simple surgery.	Difficult to contain drainage; client must wear two appliances. Ureteral stenosis.
Loop ureterostomy	"Prune belly" / Spina bifida	Ureters brought to skin surface, sutured in place and opened as single stomas flush with skin. Ureters remain implanted into bladder.	Temporary diversion. Simple procedure to relieve acute problems in pediatric anomalies.	Difficult to contain drainage; client must wear two appliances.
Nephrostomy	Neoplasms / Trauma	Silastic or Teflon catheter inserted directly into pelvis of kidney, sutured to skin surface, and connected to leg urine collecting appliance.	Palliative; simple surgical procedure (temporary).	Tube easily dislodged; must be reinserted as emergency procedure. Renal infection.
Ureterosigmoidostomy	Neoplasms / Exstrophy of bladder	Ureters implanted into sigmoid colon which remains intact. No stoma created. Client urinates and defecates from rectum with continence from sphincter control.	External appliance not needed. Less body image loss. Continency possible.	Chronic pyelonephritis caused by reflux of urine. Electrolyte disturbances caused by hyperchloremic acidosis. Requires excellent external anal sphincter control.

Types of Urinary Diversions

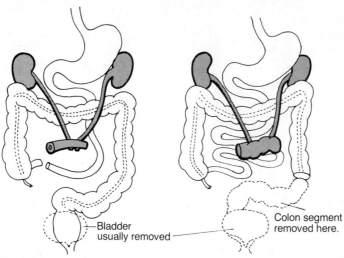

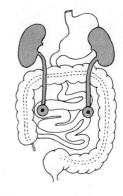

Bladder usually removed

Colon segment removed here.

Ileal Conduit: (Surgical Intervention) Ureters implanted into an isolated segment of ileum which functions as a conduit for urine.

Sigmoid Conduit: (Surgical Intervention) Ureters implanted into an isolated segment of sigmoid colon which functions as a conduit for urine.

Bilateral Ureterostomy: (Surgical Intervention) Each ureter resected from bladder brought to skin surface to drain as single stomas.

LOOP URETEROSTOMY

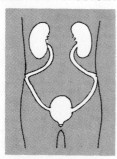

NEPHROSTOMY

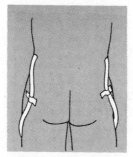

URETERO SIGMOIDOSTOMY

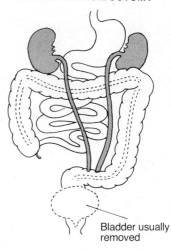

Loop Ureterostomy: (Surgical Intervention) Ureters brought to skin surface, sutured in place and opened as single stomas flush with skin.

Nephrostomy: (Surgical Intervention) Silastic or teflon catheter inserted directly into pelvis of the kidney, sutured to the skin surface and connected to leg urine collecting appliance.

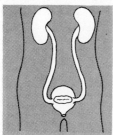

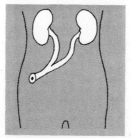

Bladder usually removed

VESICOSTOMY

TRANSURETERO URETEROSTOMY

Vesicostomy: (Surgical Intervention) Opening into bladder to bypass urethra.

Transuretero Ureterostomy: (Surgical Intervention) One ureter implanted into other ureter below the skin level.

Uretero Sigmoidostomy: (Surgical Intervention) Ureters implanted into sigmoid colon which remains intact.

FIGURE 43-13. Various urinary diversions.

Psychoemotional Considerations

The ability of the client to accept the alteration in urinary elimination depends greatly on his previous illness experiences and perceptions of the pathology involved. Children with congenital anomalies usually have no prior elimination practices upon which to formulate strong attachment. As these children learn from birth how to live with the diversion and incorporate it into body image, acceptance will not be an immediate problem. The feelings of parents who have produced imperfect children are often complex and may be reflected onto the child as growth and maturation occur. When the child begins to recognize his differences in relation to peers, anger toward the parents (who caused the problem and made decisions for surgical correction) is common. As with any physically disabled child, understanding and open discussion of facts on the part of parents is essential.

The person who has suffered the chronic, disabling condition of incontinence of neurogenic bladder may welcome surgery as a relief. Physical and social mobility may have been limited by years of being wet from incontinency and never being able to stray far from a bathroom. Persistant urinary tract infections may have further incapacitated the client. As with the client inflicted with inflammatory bowel disease, chronic illness may have interfered with work and interpersonal relationships. Role reversals may have occurred, and family members may have been alienated. Surgical intervention may bring a cure of disease or at least permanent relief of symptoms. Former life activities can be resumed.

For the client with cancer, few symptoms may have been experienced prior to diagnosis. This person has probably enjoyed wellness and full pursuit of life activities up to surgical intervention. The client is forced to deal with the catastrophic diagnosis of cancer; mutilating, painful surgery; and radical changes in body image after surgery. Loss of urinary control and loss of sexual functioning are expected outcomes. Virtually all men are rendered impotent by the dissection around the prostate necessary to perform cystectomy for cancer of the bladder. In addition, the client will feel weak and ill postoperatively. Family relationships are likely to be strong as families tend to be supportive in times of crisis. Role reversals are more likely to occur

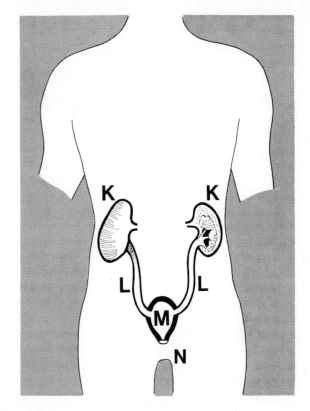

K = Kidneys
L = Ureters
M = Bladder
N = Urethra

FIGURE 43-14. Normal urinary tract.

postoperatively as the client is forced to depend on others for assistance. This is particularly true if the disease is not cured and the client is forced to deal with debilitating, terminal illness. Additionally, cancer is often a disease of older age, and clients may already be experiencing loss of other body functionings, social relationships, productivity in work, and significant others through death.

Regardless of the reason for urinary diversion, however, all clients experience significant loss both of a highly valued function (urinary continence) and of body image (external opening for urine). In addition, clients suffer the fear of loss of love and acceptance by others if they should be unable to keep themselves clean and dry. They are unable to avoid conflict with the social code of cleanliness which, in our culture, places great emphasis on bladder training.

Preoperative Care

Recognition of the psychoemotional trauma experienced by clients anticipating urinary diversion is crucial to effective nursing intervention. The nurse should assess the client's knowledge of his situation and the degree of his understanding. The nurse should review with him normal urinary functioning and how his functioning will be altered. As with all ostomy clients, his family or significant others should be included in the preoperative teaching. The nurse should be aware of cues the client and family members give which indicate fear, depression, concern, and confusion. As discussed in the beginning of the chapter, the routine preoperative considerations for demonstrating equipment, marking stoma site, securing an ostomy visitor, and setting postoperative expectations should be implemented when appropriate by the nurse.

Postoperative Care

An appliance is secured in the operating room. This appliance does not have to be sterile as it attaches to an external body surface to collect urine; the urinary stoma prevents reflux into the urinary tract. It should be connected immediately to gravity drainage. Measurement of hourly outputs are maintained on the client for about 24 to 48 hours. The urine should be observed for volume as well as for signs of bleeding and opacity. A volume of at least 30 ml of urine per hour is adequate. The urine may be pink-tinged, but gross bleeding is abnormal. Observations should be accurately recorded and immediately reported to the physician if abnormal.

The client with an ileal or sigmoid loop usually remains in an intensive care unit on bedrest for about 48 hours after surgery. He is observed for the routine complications of surgery, and measures are taken to maintain respiratory and circulatory functions. The appliance should be removed every day to observe the peristomal skin and the stoma. The peristomal skin should be free of excoriation, and the stoma should resemble the lining of the mouth and other mucous membranes. A dusky, pale, or necrotic stoma may be indicative of poor circulation to the operative site and should be reported to the physician.

Wire retention sutures are frequently used to close the midline incision, and a Penrose drain is placed in the lower abdomen to drain accumulated serosanguinous fluid. The incision requires no dressing, but the Penrose drain should be covered with a sterile dressing. This dressing should be changed as often as it becomes damp with drainage.

When the client's condition is stabilized and he returns to the surgical floor, his activities may be increased gradually. He should become involved in his own care as soon as he is ready. A first step in self-care for many clients is emptying the appliance. This activity will probably be nonthreatening to the client and a simple task that he can perform without difficulty. For this reason, and to increase mobility, the client should be disconnected from gravity drainage as soon as hourly output measurements are discontinued. He should be taught how to manipulate the spout of the appliance and shown how to empty the appliance into a measuring cup before disposing of the urine. The client may want to empty the appliance at his bedside. As soon as he is able to maneuver into the bathroom, he can be taught to empty the appliance into a measuring cup in the bathroom. After his output no longer needs to be measured on a daily basis, he can be taught to empty the appliance directly into the toilet. The nurse can be helpful in assessing the patient's readiness to look at his stoma. He should be encouraged to view his stoma in the first few postoperative days. This process facilitates his acceptance of the altered body part and allows him to progress more rapidly in a program of self-care. He should be reminded that his stoma will get smaller as time progresses and that the incision line will heal and the drains will be removed. If stents are in place, he should be informed that they will be removed before he is ready for discharge. He should be encouraged to touch his stoma shortly after he has viewed it.

MAINTENANCE OF ACIDIC URINE

Maintaining acidic urine is essential to the client with a urinary diversion. Alkaline urine produces urea-splitting organisms which proliferate in the urine collection bag. As the bacteria split, ammonia is given off, and the stoma which is bathed in the ammonia urine becomes irritated and prone to bleeding. Alkaline urine predisposes to urinary tract infection because of the proliferation of urea-splitting bacteria. Urine that pools around the stoma may reflux* into the loop, causing urinary tract infection. Alkaline urine also has a characteristic foul, strong odor caused by bacteria. Alkaline urine enhances the production of mucus which plugs up the spout of the appliances. Furthermore, alkaline urine leads to peristomal skin irritation problems. Since the skin surface is slightly acidic (pH 6.5), alkaline urine excoriates the skin. The aim should be to promote acidic urine in persons with urinary diversions. This can be accomplished by teaching them to ingest large doses of vitamin C (ascorbic acid). A dosage of over 3 g/day may be necessary for adults and over 2 g/day for children. Clients can be educated to test their urine with litmus paper to ascertain acidity. Attempting to acidify urine with cranberry juice is often futile. Many people cannot ingest enough cranberry juice to change the urine from an alkaline pH to an acidic pH, and cranberry juice often becomes unpalatable over time. There are very few side effects associated with ingesting high doses of ascorbic acid. However, there is some evidence that sulfa crystallizes in the kidney in the presence of highly acidic urine. Therefore, people who are attempting to acidify urine with ascorbic acid should use sulfa drugs with caution. In addition, acidic urine apparently leads to the rapid excretion of a few drugs such as quinidine and some tranquilizers. Testing for pH should be done when the appliance has been removed and urine can be obtained from the stoma.

Two other complications related specifically to urinary stomas are caused by alkaline urine. These are *calcium crystallization* and *pseudoepithelial hyperplasia*. Alkaline urine keeps uric acid in solution but precipitates out calcium. Therefore, calcium crystals form around the stoma and in the appliance. Accumulation of the crystals can obstruct the flow of urine from the stoma. Blockage of the emptying spout can also result from crystallization. Irritation and bleeding of the stoma may be caused by accumulated crystals in the appliance rubbing against the stoma. The treatment for crystallization is oral and topical acidification of urine. Oral acidification is accomplished by ingestion of ascorbic acid. Topical acidification is done by instilling a half-

strength vinegar solution into the appliance (1 cup vinegar: 1 cup water). The solution should be instilled into the spout of the appliance three to four times per day. Each instillation should remain in the bag for about 20 minutes while the client remains supine so the stoma will be bathed in the acidic solution. The appliance should be emptied after 20 minutes. This treatment will probably dissolve the crystals if it is carried out twice a day for 3 to 4 days.

Pseudoepithelial hyperplasia (PEH) is identified by the presence of wartlike thickenings on the peristomal skin caused by saturation of the skin with alkaline urine. It is generally associated with a stomal opening in the faceplate of the appliance which is too large. Peristomal skin is thus constantly bathed in the alkaline urine. Treatment is aimed at covering the hyperplastic areas with a properly fitting peristomal seal, such as karaya ring. Topically and orally acidifying the urine further assists in dissolving the hyperplastic area. Occasionally, hyperplastic skin may require surgical removal.

Candida albicans (monilia) commonly grows under urostomy appliances. This yeast is initially manifest on the skin as a pink, raised rash. If allowed to progress, it creates weeping and pustular formations. Skin excoriation is inevitable. Yeast grows in warm, moist, occluded areas and usually takes about 2 weeks to proliferate when cultured for laboratory identification. If *Candida albicans* is suspected, cultures can be taken (by skin scrapings); however, treatment should be instituted immediately to prevent proliferation of the yeast. Mycostatin powder is an effective antifungal agent. It should be dusted lightly over the absolutely dry peristomal skin, spread gently with the fingers to make a thin, uniform coating, then sprayed in place with an aerosol skin barrier (such as Skin Prep or Vi Drape). The last step provides a smooth, nonpowdered surface upon which an adhesive-backed appliance can be secured.

Odor Control

Urine is foul-smelling when infected or extremely alkaline. This odor is particularly apparent in clothing or appliances which are not meticulously cleaned. Clothing should always be clean and dry. After 5 to 7 days, appliances should be discarded if disposable or cleaned if reusable. Urostomy ap-

---

*Reflux occurs when urine flows backward from the appliance into the urinary conduit or ureters; usually occurs when urinary output is low so forward movement of urine is slow.

TABLE 43-6. Urostomy Appliance Application to Contain Drainage from Urinary Diversions, Prevent Leakage and Provide Securely Adhering Appliance, and Permit Maximum Socialization and Rehabilitation of Person Who Has Lost Urinary Continence

Anticipated Accomplishments	Scientific Principles/ Rationale	Considerations
1. Assemble necessary equipment at client's bedside.	Organization of equipment assists client's learning and allays anxiety.	If client has enough strength to ambulate to bathroom, equipment should be assembled there, as changing appliance will be done in bathroom at home.
2. Empty appliance and measure and record urine.	Urinary output should roughly equal fluid intake on daily basis in clients with normal renal function.	Note relationship between client's intake and output. Report to physician if output less than 30 ml/hr.
3. Gently remove appliance.	Epidermis protects skin from invasion of yeast and bacteria which can cause excoriation.	If appliance adheres tightly, use solvent in medicine dropper.
4. Wash peristomal skin.	Scrubbing skin removes epidermal surface; soap leaves film which interferes with appliance adherence.	Do not use soap.
5. Air bathe peristomal skin.	Urine which is trapped under an appliance excoriates skin and interferes with adequate seal.	Wick absorbs urine while skin thoroughly dries.
6. Measure stoma.	Stomal opening of appliance should closely approximate stoma to prevent pooling of urine on peristomal skin.	If opening is too large, peristomal skin will be exposed to urinary irritation; if opening is too small, the appliance causes stomal abrasion.
7. Decide which peristomal seal is appropriate for client.	Peristomal seals which remain intact in presence of urine prevent pooling of urine on peristomal skin.	Karaya products melt quickly in presence of urine.

Implementation	Recommendations	Observations
Equipment includes: temporary urostomy appliance, skin barrier (seal), measuring guide, scissors, paper tape, warm water, nonsterile gauze, and litmus paper.	Equipment should remain at client's bedside. Reorder equipment before supplies are depleted.	Assess client's interest in self-care and knowledge of why each item is necessary.
Open spout and allow urine to drain into measuring flask. Record on intake and output sheet.	If client is disconnected from gravity drainage when hourly outputs are no longer necessary, mobility should be encouraged.	Assess client's understanding of why urine is measured, how it is done. Can the client empty own appliance?
Slowly pull appliance off while pushing skin back with one hand.	Begin at an outer edge and work toward stoma.	Examine side of appliance which was close to skin for signs of where leakage occurred.
Wash peristomal skin gently with warm water; pat dry.	Washcloth may be used.	Is client able to look at or touch stoma?
Roll up nonsterile gauze (wick) and apply to stoma. Fan dry for 15 min.	At home clients may use Kleenex or Tampax for wick and blow dry skin with hairblower on cool setting. Oxygen (nonhumidified) can be used in hospital to blow dry skin.	Examine skin for signs of monilia, calcium crystals, PEH, or excoriation. Observe client's ability to hold wick for part of drying time. Is he dexterous, anxious, or too weak?
Using measuring guide, find the size that is ⅛ in larger than stoma.	If measuring guide is not available or the stoma is irregularly shaped, a pattern can be custom-made by cutting out proper sized hole in piece of paper.	Note if the stoma size has changed since previous measurement (leave pattern at client's bedside).
Try product which holds up well with urinary drainage and fits the contours of client's abdomen.	Products most effective with urine are: Colly-Seel, Reliaseal, and Stomahesive.	Did the seal used previously hold up well? How many days did it last?

TABLE 43-6. Continued

Anticipated Accomplishments	Scientific Principles/ Rationale	Considerations
8. Cut peristomal seal and adhesive backing on appliance.	Peristomal seal and appliance should have same size opening to prevent urine leaking between the two products.	Paper covering on adhesive backings of products should be left in place.
9. With litmus paper, pH test urine using urine from stoma.	Alkaline urine causes increased problems in skin excoriation, mucous formation, odor, calcium crystallization, and pseudoepithelial hyperplasia.	If urine is alkaline, client should be started on a regimen of oral acidification with vitamin C (ascorbic acid).
10. Treat monilia overgrowth.	Antifungal agents inhibit proliferation of yeast.	Use of antifungal agents which do not interfere with appliance adherence is essential with stoma clients.
	Topical cortisone inhibits growth of yeast.	Chronic use of topical steroids may lead to folliculitis.
11. Adhere appliance to seal.	If two products are together, application to skin will be faciliated.	Make sure product openings are well centered before affixing.
12. Prepare to secure appliance to skin.		Reliaseal and Stomahesive have adhesive backing. Colly-Seel does not.
13. Secure appliance to skin.	Appliance adhesives adhere to thoroughly dry skin.	Appliance must be well centered around stoma to prevent stomal pressure and abrasion by appliance.

Implementation	Recommendations	Observations
Using measuring guide, outline correct opening in pencil on seal and appliance.	Rub fingers around openings to smooth rough edges after cutting.	Do openings on two products fit exactly? Can client assist you in cutting?
Apply litmus paper to stoma. Read by comparing to color chart supplied with paper.	Place litmus paper quickly on stoma and immediately replace wick to prevent urine from contacting dry skin.	Observe for alkaline or acidic pH. Does the client know how to acidify alkaline urine? Does he know why urine should be acidic?
Apply thin coat of Mycostatin powder to absolutely dry peristomal skin. Brush away excess powder. Spray with protective skin barrier. Allow spray to thoroughly dry. Stoma must be constantly wicked to prevent urine from contacting peristomal skin.	Keep Mycostatin powder at client's bedside. Spray protective barriers include: Skin-Prep, Vi-Drape, and Rezifilm. Paint-on products such as Skin-Gel or Skin-Prep can be used if spray products are not available.	Presence of monilia: pink, raised rash on peristomal skin surface where old appliance was secured (warm, moist occluded area). If monilia advanced, pustular areas may develop or inflammation of skin causing weeping.
	Topical corticosteroid sprays (Kenalog) may be used for several days.	Has client been treated for monilia before? Has culture been sent? Does client understand what monilia is? How many days has steroid spray been used?
Remove paper backing on appliance and affix it firmly to seal.	Place seal on hard surface like a table to stabilize it.	Is appliance well centered on seal?
Remove adhesive backing if present on seal. Moisten skin side of Colly-Seel to promote tackiness. Air dry for 1 min to allow moisture to evaporate.	Do not touch adhesive backing after paper has been removed (oils from your fingers interfere with good seal). Use two fingers dipped in tap water to lightly moisten Colly-Seel.	
Remove wick and press appliance firmly into skin. Hold for several minutes until well secured.	Hold wick with left hand and appliance with right hand so appliance can be fixed to skin at same time wick is removed.	A good seal has been obtained if steam begins forming inside appliance around stoma.

TABLE 43-6. **Continued**

Anticipated Accomplishments	Scientific Principles/ Rationale	Considerations
14. Reinforce bond between appliance and skin.	As weight of appliance increases with urine filling it, adherence to skin is strained.	If client has been wearing a belt, he should continue since change may threaten his feeling of security.
15. Close drainage system.	Promote mobility and prevent leakage.	If client is ambulatory, he should not be connected to gravity drainage apparatus or leg bag as these inhibit mobility. Bedridden clients need gravity drainage bags. Wheelchair clients need leg bags.
16. Clean drainage tubing and overnight collection bottles.	Acidic solutions dissolve calcium crystals and reduce odor by inhibiting growth of urea-splitting microorganisms.	Reusable appliances should also be cleaned.

pliances and overnight drainage tubing should be soaked in a half-strength vinegar solution to remove odor (and calcium crystals). Appliances manufactured only from odorproof plastic or rubber should be used. Urine should be acidified to reduce odor. Few foods effect odor in urine; however, asparagus will give urine a characteristically musky odor. Highly acidic fruits and vegetables may reduce urine odor. Commercially prepared antibacterial agents (deodorants) can be instilled in appliances to retard odor. These products must be reinserted each time the appliance is emptied.

Skin Care

Meticulous care of skin around a urinary stoma is essential to maintain good skin integrity. The skin should be allowed to air dry thoroughly (about 15 minutes) before the appliance is reapplied. A wick, made by rolling a nonsterile gauze or toilet paper, can be applied to the stoma to absorb urine while the skin dries. The client can be taught to assist the nurse by holding this wick in place. If severe skin excoriation is present, nonhumidified oxygen can be blown across the skin to enhance the drying process. This technique has the added advantage of increasing peripheral circulation to the area, thereby promoting healing. At home, the client may use a hair blower (on a cool setting). Moisture-laden (water-logged) skin is the most common cause of excoriation around urinary diversions. Therefore, urine should never be trapped under an appliance. If leakage occurs under a urostomy appliance, it must be immediately removed, the skin completely air dried, and the appliance reaffixed. Table 43-6 describes a step by step procedure in affixing a disposable urostomy appliance. Disposable appliances are usually used in the immediate

Implementation	Recommendations	Observations
Apply porous paper tape to outer edges of four sides of adhesive backing or apply appliance belt.	"Picture-framing" appliance with paper tape causes less movement of appliance on skin than a belt which may move with client movement and dislodge appliance.	Is appliance securely attached to skin?
Securely close drainage spout or connect to gravity drainage or leg bag.	Connect all clients to gravity drainage at night. Otherwise, client will have to get up to empty appliance during night. At home, client should use nonsterile drainage tubing and old plastic bottle as sterile closed drainage system is difficult to attach to regular beds.	Can client open and close spout? Can he ambulate to bathroom to empty appliance? How often does he empty appliance?
Soak equipment for 1 hr in half-strength vinegar solution (1 cup vinegar : 1 cup tap water).	White vinegar prevents staining of plastic equipment. Equipment should be discarded when plastic becomes brittle or odor is retained in equipment after cleaning.	Does soaking remove calcium crystals and odor? Can client understand and assist in cleaning of his equipment?

postoperative period and continued for 2 to 3 months postoperatively until the stoma size stabilizes and edema has thoroughly subsided. At that time, clients should be consulted as to their preference for continuing the use of disposable appliances or being fitted for a reusable appliance. Clients should be apprised of the cost and time factors involved in making their decision. Reusable appliances may be comparable in cost to disposable appliances. Cost should always be analyzed in relation to time (i.e., a more expensive reusable appliance which can be worn for a longer period of time may be less costly than inexpensive disposable equipment which may only be worn for 4–7 days). However, disposable equipment is less time consuming to the client in terms of application and cleaning. The different types of disposable and reusable equipment are made by a variety of manufacturers. Many fine products are available. The most important points to consider in selecting an appliance are that the appliance itself is odorproof, that the adhesive used to secure it to the skin is nonexcoriating, that the appliance is made of a product that is rustle-free as the client moves, and that it is aesthetic to the client. A nurse skilled in enterostomal therapy should be consulted to assist the client in selecting a reusable appliance.

Discharge Planning

Activity is frequently a primary concern to people as they prepare for discharge. Certainly clients should not be sent home unless they have recovered enough strength to learn the skills of self-care and to realistically anticipate caring for themselves at home. Most clients are not limited in activity following surgery for the creation of a urinary diversion. As soon as their strength has returned following the surgery, they can resume former life activities, including work, sports, and leisure activities. Usually, it is the course of the disease which precipitated surgery for diversion that determines the outcome of the client's health status. If cancer is recurrent or metastatic, the client's life activities can be expected to become limited over time. However, if the chronic disabling condition of neurogenic bladder is cured, activity can be expected to increase as time progresses.

Sexual activity may be radically altered by surgery which results from cancer. Because of the extensive dissecting of lymphatics around the prostate in males who have cancer of the bladder, postoperative impotence is almost a certainty. Clients and their significant others should certainly have been informed of this side effect prior to surgery. Sexual counseling may be implemented. The client should be allowed to express his fears and frustrations. Often the full impact of this complication is not realized until the client has returned home and regained an interest in former life activities. Consequently, the client may not experience frustration in relation to his inability to function sexually until 6 months or more after surgery. At this time, clients who have attained a satisfactory state of health, may be interested in penile implant surgery. A prosthetic penile device can be inserted which will allow the client to be an active participant in sexual intercourse and which may enhance both his ability to perform sexually and the sexual gratification of his partner. Only those persons who have had extensive experience in sexual counseling should attempt to intervene with the client and his sexual partner at this level. However, all health care providers should be aware of the importance of sexuality in the human experience and should be prepared to deal with the questions which result when sexual expression is threatened by an altered body part. Referral to appropriate individuals trained in sexual counseling who can answer questions is a responsibility of all nurses.

SUMMARY

Nursing care of the client with a stoma has unique implications in regard to preoperative preparation, preventing complications and teaching self-care. The nurse who is knowledgeable about the various types of stomas and stoma care is well equipped to counsel clients about diet, activity, appliances, odor control, and skin care. An awareness of the client's rehabilitation potential is essential to assisting the client both in setting objectives and acquiring the knowledge and skills necessary to attain the objectives. As primary caregivers, nurses can systematically evaluate client learning and plan for discharge which allows maximum comfort and independence.

REFERENCES

1. Rowbotham, J. L.: Proper care of abdominal stomas. *Geriatrics* 29(10):56, 1974.
2. Guyton, A. C.: *Textbook of Medical Physiology,* 4th ed. Philadelphia, W. B. Saunders Co., 1971, p. 763.
3. Given, B. A., and Simmons, S. J.: *Nursing Care of the Patient with Gastrointestinal Disorders.* St. Louis, C. V. Mosby Co., 1971. p. 175.
4. Winter, C. C., and Barker, M. R.: *Nursing Care of Patients with Urologic Diseases,* 3rd ed. St. Louis, C. V. Mosby Co., 1972, p. 25.

BIBLIOGRAPHY

Dlin, B. M., and Pertman, A.: Sex after ileostomy or colostomy. *Med. Aspects Hum. Sex.* 62:32, 1972.

Hagihara, P. F., and Griffen, W. D.: Physiology of the colon and rectum. *Surg. Clin. North Am.* 54(4):797, 1972.

Happenie, S. D.: *Colostomy: A Second Chance.* Springfield, Ill., Charles C Thomas, 1968.

Hughes, B., and Wilson, F.: *Colostomy Care.* Sidney, Australia, Australian Medical Publishing Co., 1967.

Jacob, S. W., and Francone, C. A.: *Structure and Function in Man.* Philadelphia, W. B. Saunders Co., 1974.

Jensen, V.: Better techniques for bagging stomas. II. Colostomies. *Nurs. '74* 4(8):30, 1974.

Jeter, K. F., and Lattimer, J. K.: Common stomal problems following ileal conduit urinary diversion. *Urology* 3:4, 1974.

Katona, E. A.: Learning colostomy control. *Am. J. Nurs.* 67:3, 1967.

Lippincott, R.: Coping with the difficult ostomate. *Enterostomal Ther. J.* 4(2):9, 1977.

Mahoney, J. M.: *Guide to Ostomy Nursing Care.* Boston, Little, Brown and Co., 1976.

McGarity, W. C.: Colostomy—to irrigate or not to irrigate. *J. Med. Assoc. Georgia* 73:93, 1973.

Murray, B. S.; Elmore, J., and Sawyer, J. R.: The patient has an ileal conduit. *Am. J. Nurs.* 71(8):1560, 1971.

Sperberg, M.: *Ileostomy Care.* Springfield, Ill., Charles C. Thomas, 1971.

United Ostomy Association: *Sex and the Male Ostomate.* Los Angeles, 1973.

United Ostomy Association: *Sex and the Single Ostomate.* Los Angeles, 1973.

United Ostomy Association: *Sex, Pregnancy, and the Female Ostomate.* Los Angeles, 1972.

Vukovich, V., and Grubb, R. D.: *Care of the Ostomy Patient.* St. Louis, C. V. Mosby Co., 1973.

Watt, R. C.: Colostomy irrigation yes or no? *Am. J. Nurs.* 77(13):442, 1977.

Walker, F. C.: *Modern Stoma Care.* New York, Churchill Livingstone, 1976.

Watson, P. G.: Applying rehabilitation concepts in ostomy patient care. *ARNJ* 1(7):12, 1976.

Watson, P. G.: Comprehensive care of the ileostomy patient. *Nurs. Clin. North Am.* 2(3):427, 1976.

CHAPTER 44

A great challenge in nursing today is staying abreast of the many innovative applications of scientific findings to client care. It is in the area of diagnostic tests that some of the most dramatic changes have taken place. Diagnosis is the process by which scientific methods are used to establish the cause and nature of a person's illness. It requires the history of the illness, including the signs and symptoms, and laboratory data and special tests, such as an electrocardiogram or radiologic examination. Diagnosis is important because it provides a logical basis for both treatment and determination of the client's prognosis.

The purpose of diagnostic testing is to confirm or exclude a diagnosis which has been tentatively established. It may also be used for evaluation of client progress, detection of complications, or assessment of treatment. In the last two decades, the number and sophistication of available tests has greatly enhanced the diagnostic process.

This proliferation and increased complexity of

DIAGNOSTIC TESTS

Anita Giovannetti Galway, M.S., R.N., and
Ellen Christian, M.S., R.N.

diagnostic tests demands that the nurse assume responsibility for continually updating her knowledge. Some diagnostic tests are performed by the nurse, and some are performed with her assistance. The nurse often prepares the client for a test performed in another department and is responsible for his care after the completion of the procedure. This preparation is intellectual, emotional, and physical. Therefore, the nurse must fully understand the reason for the test and the steps it involves. A helpful guide for preparation is usually found in the procedure manual of the institution. This manual, which sequentially outlines the nurse's areas of responsibility during diagnostic procedures, should be referred to before approaching the client. Information concerning the intent of a test may be obtained from the laboratory or the physician performing the test. Since test results and values may differ among institutions due to variations in testing procedures and laboratory methods, the nurse must be familiar with the laboratory methods and standard "normal" values used in her own institution.

NURSE'S ROLE IN DIAGNOSTIC TESTING

Emotional Preparation of Client and His Family

The approach chosen to prepare the client and his family for diagnostic testing is influenced by many factors. When determining the intellectual capacity of the client to understand information about the test, the nurse should assess the client's (1) ability to comprehend, (2) educational level, (3) understanding of his body and its functions, (4) familiarity with medical procedures, and (5) other factors which affect intellectual functioning, such as medications or stress. When talking with the client and his family in preparation for the test, it is imperative to be selective—that is, to offer only information that will be most helpful. It is important to avoid medical jargon, abbreviations, and technical terms, as they lead to apprehension and misunderstanding, effectively intimidating the client and blocking communication. The client and his family should be encouraged to ask questions about the procedure, and these should always be answered. An explanation of exactly what is to be done, including details, in terms that are unlikely to be alarming, should be provided. It is important to discuss the sensations experienced at different points in the procedure, such as flushing, strange tastes, or discomfort, so the client knows what to anticipate. It is not necessary to tell the client about technical points, such as sterile procedures or draping if they do not involve the client or influence his perception of the experience.

It is necessary that the client understand the rationale for the test, how it will affect him, and how he can participate. It is important that significant family members be given information so they can be supportive.

In addition to the nurse's role in conveying information as part of client preparation, providing emotional support is critical in helping the client and his family successfully cope with the stresses imposed by the test. To provide this support effectively, the nurse must first assess the client's emotional status by collecting data concerned with: (1) family and cultural background, (2) prior experience with diagnostic tests, (3) amount and type of information relayed by the physician, (4) coping mechanisms used in previous stressful situations, and (5) primary support persons.

Some diagnostic tests, such as an upper gastrointestinal series, are lengthy and uncomfortable. Many require the client assume embarrassing positions throughout the test, such as in a sigmoidoscopy, where a knee-chest position must be maintained. Even the diagnostic tests that are performed in a short time can be physically and emotionally exhausting. Encouraging the client to express his concerns is a most effective nursing intervention.

During the procedure, supportive nursing intervention includes telling the client when special sensations are about to occur, showing him how to work with the examiner, and keeping him informed of the progress of the procedure. After the procedure, it is important to allow time for the client to express his feelings. For example, the man who cries during an uncomfortable procedure may need to talk about it and be reassured that his behavior was appropriate—that is, that his manhood was not compromised in the eyes of the health care team.

After the test, the client's emotional status may be affected by the results that he anticipates. Often several days elapse before the test results are known. This waiting period is an anxious time for the client and his family. When providing nursing care for clients and families in this transitional period, it is important to realize that, first, the test itself may have altered the client's image of himself by its intrusiveness or its potential for emotional scarring. Second, the definitive diagnosis which results from the test could determine medical treatment which drastically alters his life style. These factors greatly influence behavior during this time.

Physical Preparation of the Client

The client, once he understands what is to be done and has expressed his concerns adequately, is ready for specific physical preparation for the test. Most health care agencies and institutions have manuals which describe the physical preparation necessary for each diagnostic test. The nurse should be familiar with these manuals and if necessary, should request additional information from the department in which the test will be performed.

Physical preparation usually is implemented the day before or morning of the test. Specific preparations include fasting, special diets, or bowel cleansing procedures. If medications are also part of preparation, the nurse must assess the client's history of allergies and observe for allergic reactions following administration. Clients must be told of common untoward reactions, such as diarrhea after radiopaque tablets for a gallbladder series. Sedatives, tranquilizers, and drugs to minimize secretions may also be given. If the diagnostic test is an operative procedure, preoperative preparation, such as shaving for biopsy with or without special skin cleansing, may be necessary.

Several members of the health team may be involved in preparing a client for a diagnostic test. Therefore, it is essential that the nurse confirm that complete preparation has been properly carried out. The nurse should inform the department concerned if the preparation has not been completed so that the test can be postponed. This assures accurate results and saves time and expense for the client, his family, and department personnel.

Preparation of Equipment and Environment

Health agencies and institutions vary in their preferences of equipment for diagnostic tests. Some tests are performed in the inpatient area and require the nurse to prepare the equipment used by the examiner. For example, a lumbar puncture may be performed in the client's room, in an examining room, or in an inpatient unit. A comfortable and therapeutic environment should be provided for the procedure.

The nurse should refer to the agency's procedure manual for information concerning the equipment necessary for each procedure. Packaged disposable equipment labels must be examined for needed additions, such as gloves or catheters. Some institutions use only reusable equipment which must be assembled. Aseptic technique should be employed in preparing the equipment. Instruments with batteries or lights should be tested and extra lights and batteries available in case replacement is necessary during the procedure. Specimen containers and appropriate labels should be on hand. Emergency equipment should always be available in anticipation of an untoward reaction to the test or procedure.

The nurse should know where the procedure will take place and must provide for adequate privacy. Whether a treatment room or the client's room is used, a "Do Not Enter" or "Room Occupied" sign should be placed on the door. If the client's body is exposed, a warm room temperature must be maintained. Lighting should be adequate and chairs or stools available. If the client is to be in a recumbent position, a pillow should be provided if allowed. Additional support structures to help the client remain in a fixed position may be needed. A comfortable atmosphere will be more relaxing during a stressful procedure.

The nurse who has reviewed the procedure utilized by the agency and has gathered and checked

the equipment has done everything possible to assure that the procedure will be performed as quickly and smoothly as possible. This increases the client's confidence and enables him to cope with the procedure more effectively.

Assisting the Client and Examiner

Nurses frequently assist the client or the examiner during complex or uncomfortable procedures. The nurse who has prepared the client will rely on her assessment and plan to support the client according to his needs. It is often helpful for a nurse to observe a procedure prior to assisting with one.

The client may need physical and emotional support during a procedure. The nurse should help the client assume the prescribed position and maintain that position during the test using physical support when needed. If the client has difficulty coping, the nurse may provide support by using techniques which enhance coping. This may include slow, deep breathing to provide distraction, control and relaxation. Praise for coping up to this point with a word as to how much longer the procedure will last is helpful. Sometimes holding a client's hand provides excellent support. Reinforcement of prior preparation is helpful; for example, "If you remember, now the doctor is about to. . . ." The nurse who has prepared the client is the person who is best able to give support at these times.

The nurse must observe the client for reactions to the procedure and communicate them promptly to the examiner. She must also be familiar with and be prepared to use emergency equipment.

The nurse may also assist the examiner by passing needed instruments, holding them in place or holding lights on the area being examined. She is usually responsible for placing the specimens in the proper containers, accurately labeling, and arranging for their transportation to the proper laboratory.

The nurse who has anticipated the client's need for assistance during a procedure can help him cope with the situation more effectively. The nurse also helps by assuring that the procedure is performed as efficiently and smoothly as possible. This cooperation between client, nurse, and examiner reduces the anxiety and length of an uncomfortable procedure.

Collection of Specimens

The nurse often is responsible for the collection of specimens of body secretions and excretions such as urine, stool, or sputum. Essential knowledge necessary before specimen collection is attempted includes identifying: (1) rationale for collection, (2) special conditions necessary (i.e., fasting or aseptic technique), (3) role of the client in facilitating collection, and (4) necessary equipment (i.e., culture tube or sterile container). The reliability of the information gathered from these specimens depends upon the manner in which they are collected. Specimens should be:

1. Collected according to the accepted procedure of the institution.
2. Placed in correct containers.
3. Labeled with all pertinent data including:
   a. client's name and hospital number
   b. room number
   c. type of specimen
   d. amount of specimen collected
   e. date and time
   f. doctor's name
4. Transported to the laboratory promptly or kept under proper environmental conditions until transport (i.e., refrigeration or warmth).
5. Recorded in the client's chart, including a description of the specimen's appearance.

The nurse may delegate the task of specimen collection to other prepared personnel, such as a nurse's aide. However, it is the nurse's responsibility to validate that the above procedures have been followed by that designated person.

Preparation for Tests in Other Departments

Many diagnostic tests are not performed on a client's unit. The nurse must be familiar with the procedure as it occurs in another department before preparing a client. It is very helpful if the nurse observes such a procedure at least once so that she is familiar with the department, the personnel, and the test to be administered. If this is not possible, the nurse should discuss the procedure with the department personnel so she may adequately prepare clients with correct information.

LABORATORY TESTS

Excretions and Secretions

Body fluids provide important information about the functioning of body systems. Laboratory tests performed on body fluids yield very specific data that can be used in the diagnostic process. The accuracy of these data depends on the correct collection of the excretion or secretion. For example, microorganisms that are causing infection can be determined by taking a culture. If the culture is contaminated, the results will not identify the causative organism and treatment may be ineffective. Table 44-1 describes common tests of body excretions and secretions along with particular nursing considerations.

Blood

Many laboratory tests can be performed on capillary blood obtained from a finger prick. Sometimes a *venipuncture* must be performed when larger amounts of venous blood are required. Venipuncture entails entering a vein directly and withdrawing blood into a syringe or a vacuum tube. Although this is a relatively simple and painless procedure, it does provoke client anxiety. To decrease this anxiety, the nurse should provide a clear explanation of the procedure. It should include the fact that blood most probably will be taken from the antecubital space and that successful venipuncture can be facilitated if the client keeps his arm still during the procedure. Clients frequently fear that a large amount of blood is being taken from them when in fact most tests do not require more than 10 ml. The multisystem screening test is an advance in laboratory technology that has directly affected client care. One blood sample results in a complete biochemical profile. The results of the tests are arranged on easily readable graphs. Since there is considerable variation in laboratory testing procedures, results vary from one institution to another. The nurse must be familiar with the laboratory methodology and values in each given setting. Again note that test results always fall within a "normal" or "average" range. Table 44-2 gives normal values of diagnostic tests commonly performed on blood. For a more detailed discussion on individual tests and their nursing implications,

TABLE 44-1. Secretions and Excretions

Description of Diagnostic Test	Purpose	Nursing Considerations
A. Gastrointestinal Secretions		

Gastric Analysis

| Direct: A nasogastric tube is passed into stomach and its contents are aspirated. Drugs such as histamine may be given to stimulate gastric activity. | To analyze gastric contents for volume and acidity.

To aid in diagnosis of ulcers and anemia. | Prepare client for passage of a nasogastric tube which is an uncomfortable procedure. Suggest that swallowing during passage of tube is helpful.

8–10 hr of fasting are required prior to procedure.

Smoking is not allowed because it stimulates gastric secretions. Anticholinergic drugs should be omitted for at least 12 hr before test because they tend to decrease gastric secretions.

If histaminic drugs are given, it is important to warn client that he will be flushed when drug is administered. Observe client for allergic reactions. Have emergency drugs and equipment available. |
| Indirect (Diagnex blue test, tubeless method): A dye is given orally, absorbed by gastrointestinal tract and excreted in urine. Initial urine specimen is obtained. Then a dose of histamine is given. One hour later, after emptying bladder, granules of azure A are given in water. Two hours later another urine specimen is obtained and amount of dye excreted is determined. Urine appears blue if hydrochloric acid is present in stomach. | To determine presence or absence of free hydrochloric acid. | Prepare client for 8 to 10 hr of restricted food and fluids. 8–10 hr of fasting are required prior to procedure. Fasting continued until end of test.

Emphasize the importance of emptying bladder before test and of collecting all urine excreted after administration of granules until completion of test (2 hr.).

When histaminic drugs are given, nursing considerations discussed under direct gastric analysis apply. |

TABLE 44-1. Continued

Description of Diagnostic Test	Purpose	Nursing Considerations
B. Gastrointestinal Excretions: Stool		
Occult Blood		
A single specimen is tested with chemicals that detect presence of blood.	To detect bleeding in gastrointestinal tract.	If nurse performing test, carefully follow directions supplied with chemical test. Promptly communicate results to appropriate personnel.
Culture		
Specimen is collected on sterile swab and placed in sterile culture tube and promptly sent to bacteriology laboratory.	To identify specific pathogenic microorganisms as well as normal bowel flora.	Wash hands carefully to prevent spread of infection after collecting specimen. If client is unable to defecate, permission may be given by physician to introduce swab into rectum to obtain specimen.
Ova and Parasites		
A warm fresh stool is examined in laboratory.	To identify parasitic infestations, such as pinworms or roundworms.	Note that clients are often embarrassed about suspected infestation. Keep stool warm and send immediately to laboratory. Stools containing mineral oil or barium are not reliable specimens.
C. Nasopharyngeal Secretions		
Nasal Culture		
Specimen collected from nares on sterile swab, placed in sterile culture tube and promptly sent to bacteriology laboratory.	To identify specific microorganisms.	Maintain aseptic technique.
Throat Culture		
Specimen collected from pharynx on sterile swab, placed in culture tube and promptly sent to bacteriology laboratory.	Same as above	Advise client that a tongue blade will be placed on his tongue when culture is obtained and that this may stimulate gag reflex.

TABLE 44-1. Continued

Description of Diagnostic Test	Purpose	Nursing Considerations
D. Serous Fluids—Cerebrospinal Fluids		
Lumbar Puncture A sterile procedure performed under local anesthesia to obtain cerebrospinal fluid (CSF). The client is positioned on his side with head and body flexed, knees drawn up on abdomen and clasped with his hands. This position separates spinous processes and facilitates introduction of needle. After puncture is made, a manometer is used to measure pressure of CSF. At least three tubes of CSF are then collected. They should be numbered in sequence of collection. After test a sterile bandage is applied. Normal CSF Values: Pressure: 75–200 mm H_2O Color: Clear Cells: 0–5 lymphocytes pH: 7.32–7.35 Glucose: 45–85 mg/100 ml Protein: 15–45 mg/100 ml	To measure CSF pressure To identify specific microorganisms and chemical properties of CSF.	A consent form may be necessary since this is an intrusive procedure. Reassure client that the test will not cause paralysis of legs—a common misconception. Prepare client for injection of local anesthesia. After it takes effect, he will experience pressure rather than pain as spinal needle is inserted. Help client lie quietly in correct position. After test, client should be flat for several hours to prevent headache attributed to decreased volume of CSF. Encourage fluids to restore volume of CSF.
E. Sputum		
Culture Sputum is expectorated into a sterile container and sent promptly to bacteriology laboratory.	To identify specific microorganisms in respiratory tract.	First morning specimen is most productive. Teach client to breathe deeply and cough effectively to obtain sputum not saliva. Decrease viscosity of sputum by encouraging fluids.

TABLE 44-1. Continued

Description of Diagnostic Test	Purpose	Nursing Considerations
Smear		
Small amount is spread on microscope slide and stained.	To reveal casts, malignant cells, pathogenic organisms.	If client is unable to raise sputum, for instance, a child or debilitated person, a tube may be passed into stomach to obtain gastric washings for specimen of cells that have been swallowed.
F. Urinary Excretion		
Urinalysis		
A single specimen is examined. Normal Values: Color: Golden yellow Odor: None pH: 4.6−8 Specific gravity: 1.001−1.035 Glucose: None Acetone: None Protein: None Cells: Few RBC 1: 2 WBC 1: 2 Casts: Occasional	To determine bacterial, chemical and cellular components of urine.	Obtain a midstream urine in a clean container. If client is menstruating, a vaginal tampon may be inserted before cleansing the perineum. The pH should be measured promptly as urine becomes alkaline upon standing. A special plastic urine collector may be applied to obtain specimens from children who are not toilet trained.
Culture		
A midstream or catheterized specimen of urine is aseptically placed in a sterile container and sent to laboratory. Normally urine is sterile.	To identify specific microorganisms. To diagnose cause of urinary tract infections.	Maintenance of aseptic technique is *critical* to accurate results.
Timed Collection		
Specimens are collected over a designated period of time, usually 24 hr.	To measure quantity of urine and production and excretion of hormones or drugs.	Begin collection by having client void and discard that specimen. Save all subsequent urine voided for specified time. End collection by having client void at end of specified time.

TABLE 44-1. Continued

Description of Diagnostic Test	Purpose	Nursing Considerations
		Prominently displayed signs may remind client, family, and staff to avoid discarding any collections during collection period.
Pregnancy Test Detect presence of human chorionic gonadotrophin (HCG) during early pregnancy.	To detect pregnancy.	Collect first morning specimen. 95% reliable by 10th-14th day after expected date of menstruation.
Sugar and Acetone (S & A) A single fresh specimen is tested by a chemical reagent. The results are determined by color changes and compared to a specific chart.	To detect sugar and ketone bodies in urine.	Usually done by nurse or client. Instruct client to empty bladder ½ hr before specimen is needed. Have client void again to obtain fresh urine for test. If client has an indwelling catheter, urine must be obtained from catheter, not from collection bag or tubing.

G. Vaginal and Cervical Secretions

Description of Diagnostic Test	Purpose	Nursing Considerations
Culture Swab is introduced into vagina through a speculum.	To identify specific microorganisms especially gonococcus.	Instruct client not to douche prior to examination. Prepare client to assume lithotomy position and drape appropriately. Deep breathing during procedure lessens discomfort.
Smear Obtained same as culture.	To identify microorganisms, yeast infections, protozoans.	Same
Cytologic Test (Papanicolaou [Pap] smear) Cells are scraped off cervix with a wooden spatula and smeared on a slide.	To diagnose malignant lesions.	Advise client to have test performed at least once a year. Other nursing considerations are the same as above.

TABLE 44-1. Continued

Description of Diagnostic Test	Purpose	Nursing Considerations
H. Wound Discharge		
Culture		
A representative sample of discharge is aseptically obtained with sterile culture swab. Specimen is promptly sent to the bacteriology laboratory.	To identify specific microorganisms.	Maintain strict aseptic technique. Wound precautions may be indicated according to specific policy of institution.

TABLE 44-2. Normal Values of Common Laboratory Tests of Blood

Laboratory Tests	Normal Values
Complete Blood Count (CBC)	
Hematocrit (Hct)	Female: 36%–47%
	Male: 40%–54%
Hemoglobin (Hb)	Female: 12.0–16.0 gm/100 ml
	Male: 14.0–18.0 gm/100 ml
Red blood cell count	Female: 4,000,000–5,500,000/mm³
	Male: 4,500,000–6,000,000/mm³
Erythrocyte indicies:	
Mean corpuscular volume (MCV)	80–90 cu/μm
Mean corpuscular hemoglobin (MCH)	27–32 μg
Mean corpuscular hemoglobin concentration (MCHC)	33%–38%
White blood count (WBC)	5,000–10,000/mm³
White Blood Cell Differential	
Neutrophils	60%–70%
	3,000–7,000/mm³
Monocytes	2%–6%
	100–600/mm³
Lymphocytes	20%–40%
	1,000–4,000/mm³
Eosinophils	1%–4%
	50–400/mm³
Basophils	0.5%–1%
	25–100/mm³
Coagulation Tests	
Bleeding time (IVY)	1–6 min
Bleeding time (Duke)	1–3 min
Partial thromboplastin time (PTT)	60–70 sec
Prothrombin time (PT)	12–14 sec
Platelet count	150,000–450,000/mm³
Chemistries	
Amylase	60–160 Somogyi U/100 ml
Bicarbonate	21–28 mM/L
Calcium	4.2–5.2 mg/100 ml—ionized
	9.0–10.6 mg/100 ml—total
Carbon dioxide (CO_2)	22–26 mM/L—venous blood
Cholesterol (total)	150–250 mg/100 ml

TABLE 44-2. Continued

Laboratory Tests	Normal Values
Creatinine	0.6–1.2 mg/100 ml
Glucose, fasting	70–110 gm/100 ml
Glucose tolerance (oral)	Fasting: 70–110 mg/100 ml
	30 min: 30–60 mg/100 ml above fasting
	60 min: 20–50 mg/100 ml above fasting
	120 min: 5–15 mg/100 ml above fasting
	180 min: fasting level or below
Protein bound iodine (PBI)	4.0–8.0 mg/100 ml
Iron binding capacity	250–450 mg/100 ml
Ketone bodies	Negative
17-Ketosteroids	25–125 mg/100 ml
Lactic dehydrogenase (LDH)	80–120 Wacker U
Lead	0–50 mg/100 ml
Magnesium	1.5–2.5 mEq/L
Nonprotein nitrogen (NPN)	20–35 mg/100 ml (serum)
Phosphatase, alkaline	Adults: 1.5–4.5 Bodansky U
	Children: 5.0–14 Bodansky U
Phosphorus, inorganic	Adults: 1.8–2.6 mEq/L
	Children: 2.3–4.1 mEq/L
Potassium	3.8–5.0 mEq/L
Proteins:	
Total	6.0–7.8 gm/100 ml
Albumin	3.2–4.5 gm/100 ml
Globulin	2.3–3.5 gm/100 ml
Sodium	135–142 mEq/L
Transaminase:	
Serum glutamic-oxalacetic (SGOT)	12–36 U
Serum glutamic pyruvic (SGPT)	6–53 U
Urea nitrogen (BUN)	8–18 mg/100 ml

refer to the references given at the end of the chapter.

Tests of Electrical Activity

Diagnostic tests of electrical activity measure and record changes in electrical potential that take place in some organs, specifically, the heart, brain, and muscles. Electrical activity is picked up by sensors placed on the skin or scalp. It is relayed into a machine, such as an electrocardiograph, which is capable of visually recording the information on specially designed paper. The graphic tracing is analyzed to determine the electrical functioning of the organ (See Fig. 44-1). Table 44-3 describes the different diagnostic tests which measure electrical activity.

Endoscopy

Endoscopy is the examination of body organs through a hollow lighted instrument which is passed either through one of the body openings or a surg-

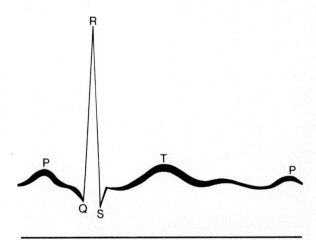

Normal ECG Deflections

FIGURE 44-1. The cardiac cycle is represented by: P wave which signifies atrial depolarization, QRS complex which signifies ventricular depolarization, S-T segment which signifies early beginning of ventricular repolarization, and T wave which signifies ventricular repolarization.

TABLE 44-3. Diagnostic Tests of Electrical Activity

Description of Diagnostic Test	Purpose	Nursing Considerations
Electrocardiogram (EKG, ECG)		
Electrodes are placed on extremities and across chest. They transfer electrical events of cardiac cycle into visible form on printout. This tracing represents depolarization and repolarization of heart muscle.	To evaluate heart's electrical activity. To detect disturbances in rate and rhythm and presence of injury to heart muscle.	Reassure the client that flow of electricity is from client to machine. He will not receive a shock during test as no electricity enters his body. Electrode paste is irritating and should be thoroughly removed from skin after EKG.
Electroencephalogram (EEG)		
Electrodes are placed on scalp and electrical activity of brain is recorded visually on printout.	To detect abnormalities in the electrical functioning of central nervous system and to diagnose brain death.	Hair should be shampooed to remove oils that interfere with good conduction. This test is best performed in a special laboratory.
		The client may be kept awake night before test to ensure sleep during test. Avoid stimulants (i.e., tea or coffee) before test. Medications are given only by special order on day of test since they may interfere with results.
		During test client may be asked to hyperventilate or look at a flashing light. After test, remove electrode paste and allow client to sleep.
		Observe for potential seizures and check to see if medications are to be restarted.
Electromyogram (EMG)		
Recording of electrical activity within individual muscle fibers by means of small needle or paste electrodes placed in muscle.	To evaluate inflammatory muscle disease, denervated muscle, and peripheral nerve injuries.	Explain procedure to client. Reassure client that he will not receive a shock during test as no electricity enters his body.

ical incision. There are two types of "scopes." The *rigid scope* is a metal or plastic tube which necessitates the straightening of the passageway into which it enters. A *flexible scope (fiberoptic scope)* is made of fiberglass and contains a bundle of fibers that reflect light. The flexible scope is more comfortable and more easily passed than the rigid scope. Scopes are usually equipped so that color photographs may be taken through them.

The passing of a scope into any body cavity is uncomfortable and sometimes quite painful. Tension and fear tend to increase the discomfort associated with the examination. These reactions are distressing to the client and can make it more difficult to complete the examination quickly and successfully.

Endoscopies are performed for confirmation of a diagnosis, therapeutic measures (i.e., removal of a foreign body), or evaluation of therapy. Small surgical procedures such as biopsy or cauterization may be performed through the lumen of the instrument. Endoscopic procedures are referred to by the name of the organ being visualized, such as bronchoscopy and cystoscopy. The physician examines all portions of the organ being scoped. For example, a colonoscopy will also include an anoscopy, proctoscopy, and sigmoidoscopy. Table 44-4 will help the nurse prepare clients and their families for endoscopic examinations.

Radiologic Testing

Radiologic testing constitutes one of today's most important diagnostic tools. This technique utilizes various sources of high energy radiation to visualize internal body organs and structures. Radiologic testing utilizes only a small segment of the very short wavelengths (gamma rays and x-rays) which are at one end of the electromagnetic spectrum.

Any structure of the body can be visualized by x-rays if the molecular density of that structure differs significantly from that of the adjacent structures. Relatively dense tissues such as bone tend to absorb x-rays and prevent them from passing through the body to the photographic plate. These areas are radiopaque and will appear light on the film. Less dense tissues, such as muscles, absorb less of the energy. This type of tissue is radiolucent and appears darker on the photographic plate.

To achieve the necessary degree of inequality in density where no such inequality exists, it may be necessary to introduce either an artificial high density "contrast medium" or a low density medium such as air or gas. This will delineate the lumen of any tube or hollow organ. Injections of air in the vicinity of a structure being examined renders the background translucent and thus outlines the structure.

FLUOROSCOPY

Fluoroscopy combines the use of contrast media and a specialized detection technique. Motion within the client's body can be observed, such as fluid moving through an organ. The image is transmitted on a screen covered with fluorescent chemicals. Fluorescent chemicals have the ability to absorb energy of one wavelength, such as that produced by x-rays, and transmit energy of another wavelength, such as visible light which can then be seen on a screen. The image may be photographed or videotaped and kept as a permanent record.

TOMOGRAPHY

Tomography, also called *body section radiography,* is used to attain focus of a specific plane of the body while the surrounding area is out of focus. It is accomplished by moving both the x-ray tube and the photographic plate on an axis so that the selected plane remains in focus through the entire movement. Even more precise recordings can be obtained during tomography by using a computer, rather than film, to record the x-rays which have passed through the client. This particular tomography is referred to as Computerized Axial Tomography or CAT scan. The final numerical results are transmitted on an oscilloscope in varying shades of grey, or even in color. A Polaroid film may then be taken for a permanent record. Currently CAT scans of the brain are the most fully developed technique. At the time of this writing, ongoing research is attempting to perfect techniques for using the CAT scan on other body structures.

XERORADIOGRAPHY

Xeroradiography is another recent advancement in imaging soft tissues. Using an electrostatic tech-

TABLE 44-4. Endoscopies

Description of Diagnostic Test	Purpose	Nursing Considerations
Anoscopy, Proctoscopy, Sigmoidoscopy, and Colonofiberoscopy		
Rigid scope may be used for passage to sigmoid colon. A fiberoptic scope enables visualization to splenic and hepatic flexures and ileocecal valve. Air can be pumped into bowel to distend lumen.	To confirm a diagnosis. To evaluate therapy. To perform a biopsy. To remove polyps.	Preparation includes low residue or liquid diet day prior to procedure. Client will have bowel cleansing procedure. May be performed in client's room, treatment room, or operating room. Usual position for procedure is knee-chest position. However, he may be on left side with head of table elevated about 15° and thighs flexed on abdomen. As the scope is advanced, client is asked to extend thighs and legs so that they are almost straight. Client needs to be prepared for feeling of pressure and urge to defecate as scope is passed. This is temporary. If air is pumped into bowel, client experiences gas pains. Room will be dark. After procedure, client should be observed closely for perforation of bowel.
Bronchoscopy		
Fiberoptic scope is passed into trachea and is directed into smaller airways. It may also include a bronchogram.	To confirm a diagnosis. To collect secretions for laboratory study. To determine if tumor can be resected surgically. To remove foreign bodies.	Client must be fasting. Medication to minimize secretions and provide sedation is usually given. May be performed under local or general anesthesia. Usually performed in operating room. Procedure is exhausting. After procedure wait for return of gag reflex. Observe closely for respiratory difficulty.
Culdoscopy		
A small incision is made in posterior cul-de-sac.	To visualize fallopian tubes, uterus, rectal wall, sigmoid, and	Preparation includes preoperative preparation. Anesthesia

TABLE 44-4. Continued

Description of Diagnostic Test	Purpose	Nursing Considerations
	small intestine. To confirm a diagnosis such as ectopic pregnancy. To cauterize fallopian tubes.	may be local, regional, or general. Client will be in knee-chest position. Incision heals without sutures. Client may have slight vaginal discharge.
Cystoscopy Scope is passed through urethra into bladder. A ureteral catheter may also be passed through ureter to kidney so a specimen can be obtained directly from kidney.	To provide a magnified illuminated view of bladder. To confirm a diagnosis. To obtain a biopsy. To remove calculi from either ureter, bladder or urethra. To evaluate each kidney function separately.	Preparation usually includes drinking one or two glasses of water prior to examination. Usually performed under local anesthesia but may have regional or general anesthesia. May experience urge to void as instrument is passed. After examination, client may experience bladder spasms, burning upon voiding, blood tinged urine, and perhaps frequency from trauma to mucous membrane. Comfort measures may include moist heat to lower abdomen or sitz baths. Observe for urinary retention caused by urethral edema.
Esophagoscopy, Gastroscopy, Duodenoscopy, and Jejunoscopy A rigid scope may be used if only an esophagoscopy is performed. Otherwise a fiberoptic scope is used. Client should be asked to swallow as scope is passed. He may be asked to turn on his right side as scope enters stomach.	To confirm a diagnosis. To remove a foreign body. To inspect lesions. To perform a biopsy. To evaluate treatment.	Preparation usually includes a radiologic examination (i.e., study of esophagus, stomach, and duodenum). Client must be fasting so that he does not regurgitate as scope is passed and so that food will not obscure visualization. Usually performed in operating room. Sedation with topical anesthetic spray is usually sufficient, but general anesthesia may be used. Position may be uncomfortable as client's head and shoulders extend over the end

Diagnostic Tests 941

TABLE 44-4. **Continued**

Description of Diagnostic Test	Purpose	Nursing Considerations
		of table. Client may be able to help during the procedure by swallowing. Comfort and rest should be provided following the exhausting procedure. A sore throat for a few days is expected. Severe pain may indicate injury to the esophagus.
Laparoscopy		
A small incision is made usually below umbilicus. Scope is introduced and carbon dioxide gas is injected in peritoneal cavity to separate intestines from pelvic organs.	To visualize pelvic organs. To cauterize fallopian tubes. To perform a biopsy. To confirm a diagnosis.	Procedure may be performed under regional or general anesthesia. Usually done in operating room. Prepare client for shoulder pain after procedure which is referred pain* from phrenic nerve. Client will have a very small scar from incision as well as a "puncture" scar from gas injection. A rare complication is a ruptured bowel.

*Pain felt in a part removed from its point of origin.

nique, x-rays which pass through the tissue are recorded on a plate coated with selenium. This produces an image which gives good delineation of soft tissue. The most popular example of xeroradiography is mammography. Breast tissue is examined radiologically for difference in density; thus, malignant and benign lesions are differentiated. The nurse should also be aware that controversy exists over the use of this procedure in women under 35.

The client should be reassured that the quantity of x-ray absorbed by the body is minimal. Ordinary exposure to this type of radiation is of small magnitude. However, the nurse who experiences repeated contact with x-rays should protect herself with appropriate shielding, such as a lead apron. Nurses who suspect that they are pregnant should never assist with a radiologic procedure.

Table 44-5 contains the description and purpose of commonly used radiologic tests and their nursing considerations.

Radionuclide Studies

Radionuclides are unstable substances which emit radiant energy. Diagnostically, they are given to clients orally or injected in tracer doses. These doses are small and pose no danger of radiation exposure to the client or the personnel caring for him.

As these substances circulate to the target organs, their concentration is registered by special machines called scanners. The presence of hot or cold spots is recorded by the scanner on a graphic tracing. Hot spots represent areas of increased concentration of the radionuclide, such as in areas of ma-

TABLE 44-5. Radiologic Tests

Description of Diagnostic Test	Purpose	Nursing Considerations
X-ray images of body parts (i.e., chest or bones).	To diagnose or detect masses, fractures or changes due to other factors.	Client should remove all metal objects from area to be examined. Nurse may remind client that it is important to remain motionless during procedure.
Angiogram Catheter is threaded into a proximal artery or vein and radiopaque dye is injected into organ's vascular system. Types include: pulmonaryangiogram, cardioangiogram, and cerebral angiogram.	To diagnose or detect malformation, tumors or defects in the vascular system of an organ.	Client must be fasting. Puncture site may be shaved. Skin test may be done for possible allergic reaction to dye. Client is usually sedated prior to test. Prepare client for changes in position during test to enhance concentration of dye in desired area. A pressure dressing covers puncture site and must be observed closely for bleeding. Peripheral pulses must be observed. Observe for complications related to organ under study. Observe for a delayed allergic reaction to the dye.
Arteriogram Catheter is threaded into a major artery and radiopaque dye is injected.	To make a diagnosis to outline arterial system in many organs. For example: heart, liver, or kidney.	Same as for angiogram.
Bronchogram (x-ray film of the bronchial tree) A topical anesthetic is sprayed into posterior pharynx to prevent gagging. A catheter is passed through nose or mouth into bronchi. Contrast medium is instilled. A series of films are performed. This procedure may be in conjunction with a bronchoscopy.	To identify anomalies of bronchial tree. (Especially important in diagnosis of bronchiectasis as involved segments cannot be outlined by any other method.)	Prepare client for bitter taste from topical anesthetic. Client is usually sedated prior to procedure. If client is unusually upset, procedure can be performed under general anesthesia. Postural drainage is usually performed morning of test to cleanse smaller bronchi of secretions. Good oral hygiene is necessary evening be-

TABLE 44-5. Continued

Description of Diagnostic Test	Purpose	Nursing Considerations
		fore and morning of test. Client assumes positional changes during test to distribute dye. Client will have increased secretions after test; therefore, observe for respiratory difficulty. Observe for return of gag reflex. May have postural drainage to aid in eliminating contrast medium.
Cystogram		
Involves injection of a radiopaque dye through catheter into bladder. In voiding cystourethrogram (VCUG), client will be asked to void during procedure.	To visualize bladder size, shape and irregularities by use of a contrast medium. (When voiding, reflux as well as strictures can be visualized.)	Reassure client that privacy will be provided during procedure. Client may be embarrassed to void during procedure. After test, encourage fluids to promote excretion and prevent stasis.
Cholecystogram (gallbladder series)		
Client is given radiopaque tablets evening prior to test. Client is fasting after medication. First films demonstrate concentration of dye in gallbladder. After a fatty meal, film shows contracting gallbladder and passage of contrast medium through common bile duct into duodenum.	To detect gallstones which are radiolucent. To estimate ability of gallbladder to fill, concentrate its contents, contract and empty in normal fashion.	Client must have fat free meal evening prior to test to enable gallbladder to concentrate dye. Radiopaque tablets also contain a laxative; therefore, prepare client accordingly. Additional bowel cleansing procedures may be necessary. If gallbladder is not visualized, test is usually repeated. Explain to client that this is not an unusual occurrence.
Computerized Axial Tomography of Brain (CAT scan)		
Scanner uses a narrow beam of x-ray in conjunction with a computer. Part of machine rotates slowly around client's head as x-ray readings are taken. Can be done on an	To produce a highly contrasted detailed study useful in diagnosis of both benign and malignant lesions. Can evaluate some areas not as accessible to other diagnostic measures.	Client's head will be held in snug-fitting restraints because movement makes images impossible to interpret. Women who use hair spray should wash their hair. Hairpins should

TABLE 44-5. **Continued**

Description of Diagnostic Test	Purpose	Nursing Considerations
outpatient basis, is noninvasive, and highly sensitive. Its increased use has resulted in less frequent use of pneumoencephalography.	Used frequently because it is reliable and has no side effects.	be removed. Client remains in street clothes for procedure. Client will be alone in room for procedure but can communicate through an intercom. Procedure takes about 20–30 min with actual scanning taking from 1 to 5 min.

Intravenous Pyelogram (IVP)

A baseline film is taken for a control. Then a radiopaque dye is injected intravenously. Films are taken at specific intervals; last at about 30 min after injection. A postvoiding film may also be taken.	To demonstrate size and location of kidneys, abnormalities within kidneys, filling of renal pelvis and outline of ureters and bladder.	Client must have a bowel cleansing procedure so that shadows do not obstruct view of kidneys. To produce slight dehydration and greater concentration of dye in kidneys and urinary system, client must be fasting. Check for allergy to iodine, a component of radiopaque dye. Prepare client for feeling of warmth, flushing of face, salty taste, and perhaps nausea with injection of dye. Deep breathing helps client at this time. After test, encourage client to drink fluids liberally. The test is exhausting; therefore, provide opportunity for rest. Observe for delayed allergic reactions to dye.

Upper Gastrointestinal Series
(upper GI or barium swallow)

The client swallows barium while radiologist does a fluoroscopic study. X-rays are then taken of stomach and duodenum. Client may be asked to assume various positions to help barium flow and outline structures. An additional film may be taken 24 hr after actual test.	To identify tumors, ulcerations or inflammations of esophagus, stomach, and duodenum. To reveal any abnormal anatomy or malposition of these organs.	Client must be fasting as food will obstruct view. Barium has a chalky taste but may be flavored. Client may eat as soon as test is completed. Client may be given a laxative after test to hasten elimination of barium.

TABLE 44-5. Continued

Description of Diagnostic Test	Purpose	Nursing Considerations
Lower Gastrointestinal Series (lower GI or barium enema)		
An enema of barium solution is administered to client in radiologic department. Client must retain enema while films are taken.	To identify presence of polyps, tumors or other lesions of large intestine. To demonstrate abnormal anatomy or function of large intestine.	Client will have low residue diet on day prior to test. Bowel cleansing is necessary. Client will be fasting day of test. Client needs to know that he must do his best not to expel enema during films, which takes about 10 min. Test is uncomfortable, and client may be embarrassed by procedure. Client will be asked to assume different positions to help distribute barium. Client may be given laxatives to help eliminate barium. Observe for constipation.
Myelogram		
Lumbar puncture is performed and a contrast medium is injected into subarachnoid space. Medium is removed after film by lumbar puncture because it causes serious irritation of meninges.	To identify lesions in intradural or extradural spaces, of spinal cord, or subarachnoid space.	Client needs to know that films are usually taken on a tilt table to help distribute the medium. Removal of medium may be uncomfortable. After test, client should be closely observed for signs of meningeal irritation.
Pneumoencephalogram		
Client is restrained in a special rotating chair. A lumbar puncture is performed and fluid withdrawn. Air is injected. Client is rotated to distribute air into ventricles as films are taken.	To study ventricular and disternal systems. To permit accurate localization of brain lesions. (The CAT scan is a preferred test because of its reliability, safety and lack of side effects.)	The client will have a severe headache during and after procedure which may remain for 24–48 hr. It is helpful if client remains flat during this time. Nausea and vomiting are common during and after procedure. Procedure is emotionally traumatizing. Client may hear noises in his head caused by air in ventricles. This is temporary. After test, observe for signs of increased intracranial pressure.

lignant growth. Cold spots represent areas of decreased radionuclide concentration, such as occurs in a hypofunctioning organ. Scanning techniques are generally safe, pain free, and cause little discomfort to the client. They are valuable diagnostic tests because they allow lesions in inaccessible organs, such as the spleen and pancreas, to be detected.

Preparation of the client for radionuclide studies should include how the substance will be given and what the time interval between its administration and the scan will be. A description of the scanner will allay anxiety. It resembles an x-ray machine and never touches the client. No special precautions are necessary to prevent contamination after the test because of the small dose. Table 44-6 con-

TABLE 44-6. Radionuclide Studies

Description of Diagnostic Test	Purpose	Nursing Considerations
Thyroid I^{131} Uptake		
I^{131} is given orally or intravenously. Thyroid is scanned 24 hr later to determine its concentration.	To assess thyroid structure and function.	Ascertain that medications affecting results of test have been properly discontinued. All urine may be collected during the 24 hr after administration of the I^{131} to determine what percent of radionuclide is excreted. Observe for possible allergic reactions to iodine.
Brain Scan		
Radionuclide given intravenously.	To diagnose brain tumors and vascular lesions.	Client must be still for procedure which takes 30–50 min.
Liver Scan		
Radionuclide given intravenously.	To evaluate hepatic function.	Explain test to client and prepare him for the intravenous infusion.
Lung Scan		
Radionuclide may be given intravenously or inhaled as a gas.	To evaluate structure and function of lungs. Helpful in diagnosis of pulmonary emboli or other lesions.	If gas is used, personnel should be protected from inhaling radionuclide.
Kidney Scan		
Radionuclide given intravenously.	To evaluate renal structures and function.	Takes 1–3 hr.
Bone Scan		
Radionuclide given intravenously.	Early detection of lesions.	Prepare client for intravenous infusion and explain test.

TABLE 44-7. Specialized Tests

Description of Diagnostic Test	Purpose	Nursing Considerations
Bone Marrow Aspiration		
After infiltrating iliac crest or sternum with local anesthesia, a needle is inserted into marrow. Discomfort occurs briefly when marrow is aspirated because of pressure changes.	To evaluate production of blood cells.	Prepare client for local anesthesia, site of puncture, and an uncomfortable sensation when marrow removed. Maintain pressure over site after test to minimize bleeding. Anticipate heightened anxiety about results.
Cardiac Catheterization		
A long flexible catheter is passed into heart through vein or artery in arm or groin. Radiopaque dye is injected so structures and blood flow can be visualized. Blood samples can be removed and analyzed. Pressures within heart can be measured. This test is performed in a highly specialized laboratory.	To evaluate structure and function of heart by visualization, pressure studies and measurement of blood oxygenation.	Client will fast before test. Ascertain site of catheterization (i.e., groin or arm), and explain to client. Tour laboratory with client before test if possible. Explain that client will be sedated but not anesthetized during test. Certain sensations are experienced during test such as a hot, flushed feeling felt at insertion site when dye is injected. Test takes 1–3 hr. After test, client should lie quietly for several hours. Catheterization site should be inspected for bleeding and pulses distal to site should be palpated frequently. Observe for emboli which produce symptoms of a stroke or pulmonary embolus. Clients are usually very concerned about results, especially if cardiac surgery is indicated.
Pulmonary Function Tests:		
Ventilation		
Measure ability to move air in and out of lungs.	To assess preoperative pulmonary function. To classify type of pulmonary disease. To evaluate therapy.	Explain that client will be asked to participate in some special breathing studies. Recognize that changes in the values of these tests are more helpful in diagnosis than individual val-

TABLE 44-7. Continued

Description of Diagnostic Test	Purpose	Nursing Considerations
		ues. Client will probably have repeated tests.
Vital Capacity Measures maximum amount of air that can be expelled in a forced expiration following a minimal inspiration.		
Maximum Breathing Capacity Measures ability of client to move air in and out of lungs.		
Blood Gas Studies Arterial blood is obtained in a heparinized syringe, placed on ice and sent immediately to laboratory.	To determine effectiveness of ventilation by measuring partial pressures of oxygen and carbon dioxide in arterial blood.	Pressure must be maintained over puncture site for 5 min to prevent hemorrhage.
Normal Values for Blood Gases pH: 7.37−7.44 pO_2: 80−90 mm Hg pCO_2: 35−45 mm Hg		

tains the description and purpose of commonly used radionuclide studies and their nursing considerations.

Specialized Tests

The following diagnostic tests are frequently used in specialized situations (Table 44-7). Although they do not lend themselves to any of the preceding categories, they represent important tests with which the nurse should be familiar.

THERMOGRAPHY

Thermography is another diagnostic measure which is noninvasive, rapidly performed, and relatively inexpensive. An infrared scanner is used to detect heat emissions from the body. Areas of increased vascularity and of a higher metabolic rate are readily detected. A heat "image" is produced by the scanning device which may be in shades of grey or in color.

Thermography is currently being used as a preliminary screening mechanism for breast malignancy because of its low cost, ease of administration, and safety. Clients with suspicious "hot" areas may then proceed to more definitive diagnostic testing measures such as mammography or biopsy.

SONOGRAPHY

Sonography, also called ultrasound or echography, involves the use of a transducer crystal and receiver usually contained in the one instrument. Sound waves which are above the upper limit of the audible sound range, are transmitted through the body. Sound waves change velocity as they travel through tissues of different densities. The change in velocity results in part of the sound energy being reflected back to the source. The reflected sound wave is connected into an electrical impulse and appears on an oscilloscope. A photograph is usually taken for a permanent record.

Sonography has many advantages for the client. It is a noninvasive procedure that can be performed rapidly, painlessly and with relatively low cost. Portable equipment is available so it can be done on the client unit.

Sonography may be used to detect changes in the cranial vault, detect masses, differentiate cysts from tumors, and detect changes in cardiac structure. Perhaps its most valuable contribution has been in the area of maternity care. It is safely used to detect pregnancy, monitor fetal growth, locate the placenta, and even detect congenital anomalies of a structural nature. Since most sonographic units are located in the radiology department, it is important for the pregnant client to know that sonography is not radiology and has no effect on the fetus. The only preparation for this specific sonography of the fetus is that the client have a full bladder. This elevates the uterus and helps transmit the sound waves. The pregnant client is usually given a photograph of the fetus to keep.

BIOPSY

Biopsies are tests done to obtain specimens for microscopic examination. An incisional biopsy is a surgical procedure in which tissue is removed and identified. The identification may be immediate, as when a frozen section is done, or the tissue may be examined at a later time. A punch biopsy is done by inserting a hollow needle into a cavity and removing a piece of tissue. Needle aspiration of body fluids can be considered nonsurgical biopsies when the fluid is examined for cells.

Any type of biopsy imposes great psychological stress on the client and his family, usually related to the fear of cancer. The nurse preparing the client must consider this and include a great deal of supportive intervention along with pertinent information about the procedure. Structures frequently biopsied include the breast, liver, kidney, and lung. After a biopsy, it is important to observe for internal and external bleeding. Emotional support for the client and his family is important during the anxious time of waiting for results of the test.

BIBLIOGRAPHY

Brunner, L. S., and Suddarth, D. S.: *Textbook of Medical-Surgical Nursing,* 3rd ed., Philadelphia, J. B. Lippincott Co., 1975.

Diagnostic Tests I and II, filmstrips with audio cassettes, Concept Media, 1500 Adams Avenue, Costa Mesa, Calif. 92626.

DuGas, B. W.: *Introduction to Patient Care,* 3rd ed. Philadelphia, W. B. Saunders Co., 1977.

Ellis, J. R., and Nowlis, E. A.: *Nursing: A Human Needs Approach.* Boston, Houghton Mifflin Co., 1977.

French, R. M.: *Guide to Diagnostic Procedures,* 4th ed. New York, McGraw-Hill Book Co., 1975.

Gragg, S. H., and Rees, O. M.: *Scientific Principles in Nursing,* 7th ed. St. Louis, C. V. Mosby Co., 1974.

Kelly, P.: Diagnostic tests: what should we tell the patient? *Nurs. '74* 4:15, 1974.

Pohutsky, L. C., and Pohutsky, K. P.: Computerized axial tomography of the brain: a new diagnostic tool. *Am. J. Nurs.* 75:1341, 1975.

Reeves, K. R.: This CAT is a revolutionary scanner. *RN* 38:40, 1976.

Shafer, K. N., et al.: *Medical-Surgical Nursing,* 6th ed. St. Louis, C. V. Mosby Co., 1975.

Smith, D. W., and Germain, C. P. H.: *Care of the Adult Patient,* 4th ed. Philadelphia, J. B. Lippincott Co., 1975.

Tilkian, S. M., and Conover, M. H.: *Clinical Implications of Laboratory Tests.* St. Louis, C. V. Mosby Co., 1975.

Widmann, F. K.: *Clinical Interpretation of Laboratory Tests,* 8th ed. Philadelphia, F. A. Davis Co., 1979.

CHAPTER 45

Discharge is an important event in a client's life. It is part of the transitional process which brings to a close the goals of hospitalization and prepares the client for the changes associated with returning to the community. Discharge generally occurs when a client no longer needs the level of care or range of services offered by a health care facility. Regardless of how routine a client's experience may seem, each individual requires the opportunity to prepare for the termination of his client experience. At the time of discharge, the client relinquishes his role as a recipient of care for a more independent life style. In most cases, the client's energies are mobilized to resume his former responsibilities. Where this is not possible, the assistance of the family or community is sought.

As an integral member of the health team, the nurse shares the responsibility for preparing and implementing a client's discharge. The nurse's role includes collaboration with the interdisciplinary team and community agencies, preparatory instruction of the client and family, and termination of the

THE DISCHARGE PROCESS

Kathleen F. Zagata, M.S., R.N.

nurse-client relationship. As in previous phases of the client's hospitalization, the nursing process is the method by which the nurse carries out these responsibilities.

ASSESSMENT

The first nursing task is assessment of the client's discharge needs. To do this, information is gathered about his physical, emotional, and social status. The purpose of this assessment is to gain an understanding of the client that extends beyond the walls of the hospital. In this way, the nurse can anticipate the changes a client will experience once discharged.

A client's post-hospital adjustment is directly affected by his equilibrium of health and illness. For many, discharge represents a return to a former level of wellness, but for others, it is the beginning of a lengthy convalescence in a compromised state of health. The effects of illness can be far-reaching. A person's family and community position may be

jeopardized along with his financial security, independence, and former residence. By assessing the extent of impairment, it is possible to determine how a client's former life style will change.

Self-supporting capabilities are equally important in determining a client's optimal level of functioning. If a person's autonomy has not been seriously impaired, an independent life style is possible. Such factors as motivation, general health, and personality influence the adaptation and resolution of losses associated with illness.

The transition from the hospital can further be influenced by the client's feelings about leaving. At the time of discharge, his dependency on the staff and hospital ends. For some, this may be a welcome change, but for others, it may be met with ambivalent feelings. To assess a client's emotional reaction, it is necessary to explore what the hospitalization meant and what he feels lies ahead. The client's answers may reveal realistic concerns as well as distortions and fears. For an accurate assessment, a client's statements need to be correlated with his behavior. If discrepancies occur, it may indicate ambivalent feelings about discharge. Because clients often are not consciously aware of the conflict that exists, client insight can not be assumed. By allowing the client to express his positive and negative feelings about discharge, the nurse can increase his awareness of the conflict and explore its possible meanings.

The third consideration in preparing a client for discharge is his social network. The presence or absence of significant others cannot be overlooked as a factor in a client's recovery. Family and friends may be a potential source of care-giving and emotional and financial support. During the hospitalization, the nurse can assess how the significant people contribute to the client's well-being. By including family and friends in the discharge preparations, the nurse acknowledges the central role they play in the client's recovery and facilitates their adjustment to his illness. Besides reducing their feelings of helplessness and anxiety, this intervention encourages their active involvement with the client following discharge.

By being alert to the possible family crises that are precipitated by discharge, the nurse can directly intervene or refer the family to the appropriate resources. In considering home care, a family may be anxious about their ability to assume responsibility for an ill person. Through discharge instructions, a family's responsibilities can be clarified and necessary skills taught. Arranging home visits for the client prior to discharge may be an added support. These visits allow the family to practice their newly acquired skills in the home setting. It may also be helpful to identify the community supports available to the family following the client's discharge. Many families are relieved when community services are offered to supplement their care.

Before a decision can be made about alternatives to home care, a family needs time to work through their feelings. Grieving the loss of the client as an independent and functioning family member may be the first step. Since a client and his relatives often experience similar reactions to the threatened separation, their ability to jointly discuss the discharge alternatives may be impeded. Frequently, family members feel caught between the client's wish to return home and the realistic needs that prevent home care from being a safe alternative. Thus, guidance is needed when making decisions about

placement in a long-term care facility. Since the nurse is familiar with the client's care, she is a resource for the family seeking to understand the need for placement. The nurse may also refer the family's questions to the social worker. In this way, the family can receive additional support and assistance. The social worker can provide information about the facilities under consideration and can assist the family with the application procedure and financial arrangements.

Lack of a social network can result from death, interpersonal conflicts, and distance. The absence of family and friends can limit the discharge alternatives available to a client. This is especially true when the combined loss of health and family impair a client's motivation for recovery. As discharge draws near, feelings of loneliness may intensify. Termination with the hospital staff may renew old conflicts concerning nurturance. A person's ability to grieve these losses can make the difference between acceptance and resignation of one's life situation. In planning discharge without social supports, counseling and community home care services may prove invaluable.

DISCHARGE PLANNING

Discharge planning is the shared responsibility of the client, hospital, and community. The purpose of planning is to maximize a person's potential for achieving independence and a meaningful life in the community. During this preparatory phase, a tentative plan of action is developed to assist the client's post-hospital adjustment. Planning has several advantages: for example, it helps to alleviate anxiety the client may have about being discharged. As with any change, discharge involves an element of uncertainty. Through anticipatory planning, a client's concerns can be identified and evaluated. The resulting plan of action may include measures to control the impact of the variables or to strengthen the client's coping skills. Planning also assures that the benefits received from the hospitalization will continue. Continuity of care is achieved by providing the client with the necessary instructions and community services. Finally, planning facilitates integration into the community. A brief hospitalization may represent a minor interruption in a person's life. However, an illness that required the full range of services and a lengthy stay is likely to make major changes in the client's life style. When this occurs, planning includes measures to help the client live within the limits of his illness.

The hospital staff is responsible for identifying the client's post-hospital needs and offering assistance. The staff's effectiveness in meeting this responsibility depends on their commitment to discharge planning and their ability to work collaboratively to achieve this end. Each hospital has its own structure for screening clients prior to discharge. In many facilities, the primary care team and the hospital's continuing care specialists hold weekly planning conferences at the unit level. Together, they review each client's progress and develop discharge plans. Since the continuing care specialists are familiar with the hospital and community resources, they can assist the primary team to coordinate the client's needs with the appropriate community services.

Discharge planning is dependent on the services offered by the community. The best laid plans can be rendered ineffective if the needed services are not available. The hospital staff needs to be knowledgeable about the availability, range, and quality of services offered by the community they serve.

To effectively coordinate a client's discharge, established channels of communication are essential between the hospital and community. Referrals are one communication link for providing continuity of care. Through the referral process, the availability and appropriateness of the community service is matched with the client's needs and eligibility. The hospital staff directly responsible for the client's care initiates the referral to insure that information is accurately communicated. Many community agencies require an admission's interview for acceptance into a program. Besides enhancing the success of the referral, the meeting introduces the client to the staff members of the new agency.

The timing of the client's departure deserves consideration during the planning phase. The day of the week can make a difference in the availability of the family and community supports. Delays in needed services and equipment can have serious consequences for the client's initial adjustment and safety. Setting a definite time permits the specifics of a discharge to be worked out. The tentative date should allow ample time to implement and evaluate the discharge plans.

IMPLEMENTATION AND EVALUATION

Implementing a client's discharge involves completing the discharge preparations as well as overseeing the actual departure. As the nurse implements the plan of care, it is important to evaluate its effectiveness in achieving the desired goals. Depending on the evaluation, the plan of care can be maintained or modified to meet the client's changing needs and responses.

In implementing a discharge, the nurse may be expected to complete the nursing portion of the referral form for follow-up services. The quality of the referral depends on the nurse's written and verbal communication. The nurse is responsible for providing the new agency with the pertinent information needed to continue the client's care with the fewest interruptions. Following the client's discharge, the nurse initiating the referral is in the best position to follow up with the community agency. In this way, the nurse can assess the referral's effectiveness in meeting the client's discharge needs and obtain a progress report on the individual's post-hospital adjustment. This type of feedback can serve as a self-assessment tool for improving the nurse's skills in planning future discharges.

Discharge teaching may be another aspect of the nurse's role in preparing the client to leave the hospital. To assume responsibility for self-care, the client must clearly understand what his responsibilities will entail and be able to perform the necessary skills safely. Before initiating the teaching plan, the nurse should evaluate the client's current knowledge, motivation, and attitude toward learning. It is also important for the nurse to know how the client feels the new knowledge and skills will help him cope with his changed life style. Whenever possible, the nurse should enhance the discharge teaching by allocating time for return demonstrations. These demonstrations are beneficial to both the teacher and learner. While the nurse evaluates the client's learning, the individual gains confidence in his performance skills prior to discharge. The nurse should also prepare written instructions outlining the discharge teaching. The written material later serves as a reference for the client at home.

The discharge instructions to family members will depend on their role in the client's care following discharge. If they are directly involved, the family members will actively participate in acquiring the necessary knowledge and skills. When the client is the primary learner, the instructions to the family will focus on supporting the client's learning.

Achieving a sense of closure to the nurse-client relationship is accomplished through termination. This process consists of the nurse and client reviewing the relationship's development with its established expectations and goals. It also involves a mutual sharing of feelings about the meaning of the relationship. In this way the relationship is brought to a close and former commitments concluded. Both are then free to say goodbye and form new relationships.

An important consideration is the nurse and client's readiness to terminate. A person's readiness is influenced by previous experience with separation and loss. As in earlier phases of the relationship, the nurse's awareness of her own feelings is a prerequisite to therapeutic work with her client. The nurse needs to develop an understanding of how her personal and professional experiences with separation both past and present influence her response to a client's discharge.

By assessing the client's readiness, the nurse can plan the intervention that facilitates the termination process. Learning about a client's style of saying goodbye can serve as a reference for evaluating a person's current reaction. During the initial discussions, the nurse can observe the client's willingness to reflect on the relationship. For example, does the client openly express or defensively deny the relationship's importance? By being alert to nonverbal expressions, the nurse can help the client put his feelings into words. Sometimes clients present gifts at the time of discharge. This gesture provides an opportunity to discuss the client's feelings. The nurse may question whether it is appropriate to accept presents. Each situation should be individually decided by taking into account the meaning of the client's behavior and the nurse's feelings about accepting gifts. Regardless of the decision, the gestures deserve acknowledgment. Another common expression of appreciation is the thank you note sent to a nurse following discharge. Although this permits expression of the client's feelings, it does not allow a mutual exchange of feelings. This situation can occur when a client feels overwhelmed by the approaching discharge or when he is un-

comfortable expressing his feelings directly. When a nurse actively pursues termination, she can provide the client with an opportunity for an expression of feelings prior to leaving the hospital.

Preparing the client for dismissal begins a few days prior to the actual discharge date. The aim of the nurse's interventions are to insure an uninterrupted and safe dismissal. Six basic steps in coordinating a departure follow:

1. Carry out the hospital's policies and procedures for discharging a client.
2. Finalize the details of the client's departure. Confirm the time of discharge and mode of transportation. Make sure the client's clothing is suitable for travel.
3. Once the discharge order is written, notify the hospital departments involved in the client's discharge and the community agencies responsible for the post-hospital care.
4. On the day of discharge, assemble the client's belongings and valuables. Provide assistance with dressing as needed.
5. Review the discharge instructions with the client and significant others. Make sure the client's written instructions about self-care, medication, and follow-up appointments, are accurate and complete. Assemble the supplies, equipment, and prescriptions needed for the immediate post-hospital period.
6. Enter a discharge nursing note in the client's record. Document the date, time, general condition of the client, and circumstances pertinent to the dismissal. When relevant, include the referral agency and contact person.

AGAINST MEDICAL ADVICE (AMA) DISCHARGE

When a client leaves the hospital against medical advice, it is commonly referred to as an AMA discharge. The reasons for requesting an AMA discharge vary. It may result from a client's misunderstanding or apprehensions about hospitalization. In other instances, it may represent a failure of the client and staff to form a trusting relationship in which the client can communicate his needs. Two additional factors that lead to an AMA discharge are dissatisfaction with treatment or a concurrent family crisis. Besides understanding the client's reasons for terminating a hospital stay, the staff and client must discuss the consequences and alternatives to an early discharge. As with all discharge planning, the post-hospital adjustment is a priority. As the circumstances permit, discharge planning as outlined in this chapter should be implemented. Prior to initiating the dismissal, it is important to consult the hospital's policies and procedures governing discharges against medical advice.

SUMMARY

Discharge is a transitional process in which the client terminates his hospital affiliation and begins his integration into the community. As an integral member of the hospital team, the nurse actively participates in preparing the client for discharge. Three aspects of the nurse's role include collaboration with the interdisciplinary team and community agencies, preparatory instruction of the client and family and termination of the nurse-client relationship. Through assessment of the client's physical, emotional, and social needs, the nurse develops a plan of care that prepares him for the changes associated with leaving the hospital. As the day of departure approaches, the nurse is responsible for overseeing the actual dismissal.

BIBLIOGRAPHY

Bristow, C., Stickney, C., and Thompson, S.: *Discharge Planning for Continuity of Care.* New York, National League for Nursing, 1976.

Department of Nursing: *Massachusetts General Hospital Nursing Procedures Manual.* Boston, Brown and Connally, Inc., 1976.

Fox, E., Nelson, M., and Bolman, W.: The termination process: a neglected dimension in social work. *Social Work* 14(10):53, 1969.

Kelly, H. S.: The sense of an ending. *Am. J. Nurs.* 69(11):2378, 1969.

Nehren, J., and Gilliam, N.: Separation anxiety. *Am. J. Nurs.* 65(1):109, 1965.

CHAPTER 46

The anticipated death of a loved one is one of the most serious crises occurring in family life. Families of dying clients who face the dissolution and final termination of a relationship need special preparation to mobilize their strengths and coping mechanisms to deal with the stress that ensues.

Preparation of the client and his family to face inevitable death is difficult, at best, and includes a repertoire of skills, knowledge, and experience on the part of health care personnel. Included in these is awareness of the ways in which grief is manifested, facility in dealing with reactions to grief, knowledge of available resources, and the ability to provide comfort measures. The extent to which the dying client and his family are prepared to cope depends upon their emotional resources and the skill of the health care workers, not only in interpreting their behavior, but in guiding them in the use of appropriate coping mechanisms.

Grief is a response to a loss or a series of losses. A loss which has meaning for the individual results in an observable response, grieving, which varies

DEATH, DYING, AND GRIEF

Beverly C. Fineman, M.Ed., R.N.

in intensity and in relation to the lost object. We would expect to see, therefore, a greater response to the loss of a person than to the loss of an animal. However, the significance of the lost object may differ from individual to individual. The death of a casual acquaintance may be of less significance than a family dog.

In general, it is possible to state that in normal grief the more significant the loss, as defined by the mourner, the more observable will be the grief reaction. Assessment of the meaning of a loss to an individual and observation of the grief response are primary functions of the nurse in dealing with clients who face death and their families.

GRIEVING

The work of grieving is so universal a manifestation that a common pattern can be identified in the bereaved. A variety of frameworks for identifying stages of grief have been constructed by Kubler-Ross,[1] Engel,[2] and others. These frameworks are valuable contributions and provide a means of classifying grief behavior, as well as diagnosing an individual's response to loss. Normal grieving is made up of three phases: (1) a short period of shock; (2) intense grief; (3) recovery and resumption of activities of daily living.

With clients who experience normal grief, it is important to realize that the stages of grief are not static; clients progress and regress through them; for example, individuals may appear to be recovering from their loss on one day and manifest intense grief on another.

Shock and Denial

The family of a dying individual when informed of a terminal prognosis will experience much of their grief ahead of time. The response of the family will be similar to that observed after a sudden or unexpected death has occurred. In anticipatory grieving, the client and his family begin to grieve the loss *before* the loss occurs. In this situation, the shock phase is often experienced and completed before death. Some individuals never complete this stage of anticipatory grieving and use the coping mechanisms of denial, intellectualization, and projection to prevent further awareness of reality.

The usual first response upon learning of a real or anticipated loss is to deny the loss. "No, it isn't true," or "There must be some mistake," are reactions expressed. The client who is told of a terminal illness may insist that an error was made. Shock and disbelief serve the purpose of counteracting the enormity of a loss by shielding the individual from total awareness. Disbelief is often followed by feelings of numbness or being out of contact with reality which protects the individual from overwhelming stress. Some individuals cope with the pain of realization by intellectually accepting the loss but emotionally denying the full impact. This mechanism further shields the person from full recognition of the loss.

The disbelief and shock phase may last hours, days, and in some situations, may be maintained by the client or his family up to the time of death. This occurrence is especially likely when the interval between shock and actual death is short, and time does not permit movement in the grieving process.

When disbelief is maintained for very long periods of time, critical assessment of the situation by the nurse is necessary to determine why the client and his family persist in the denial of reality. The nurse should always bear in mind, however, that denial may be the best adjustment the client can make; further progression in the grief process is too painful and produces overwhelming anxiety. In other situations, the client may continue to deny because he believes this behavior to be most valued by his family. The family may deny the implications of the diagnosis rather than the illness itself. It is important to remain open-minded, when dealing with clients and families using coping mechanisms designed to prevent stress, and to be always aware that defense mechanisms are not totally under the control of the individual. Full realization and acceptance are never accomplished all at once.

The nurse and other members of the health team must realize that denial is ego protective. Forcible confrontation with reality may precipitate disorganization and severe depression. Nursing decisions made at this time should be ego supportive.[3] Active

measures to relieve the client's anxiety should be instituted as well as a plan that recognizes the denial but does not reinforce it.[4] Maintaining a supportive relationship aids the client in moving toward acceptance of reality.

Why is it important for a dying client and his family to face the fact of his dying at some time in the terminal period? Perhaps it is not possible for everyone to face stark reality, but continuous denial does prevent the further progression of the grieving process. The individual is more or less "stuck" in the shock phase and may never complete mourning. Specifically, the dying client and his family who continue to utilize denial over a long period of time are cheated of the opportunity to express their true feelings, to maintain some control over their lives, and to share with each other the final termination of the relationship.

Intense Grief

Intense grief is the work of mourning and is an acute situation manifested by actual and measurable symptoms. Tearfulness and weeping are frequently seen; these can range from occasional crying to public lamentation. Collection of data about the individual's sociocultural background will often provide clues as to how grief is commonly expressed. The family of a more stoic culture may grieve by turning inward, leaving the client alone because they dare not give rise to public expression of mourning. The stoic client may tend "not to burden" anyone with his problems and may be lonely in his grief and unable to give full vent to his emotions. Providing a quiet room for the family to be together and understanding support of the client by the nurse may alleviate somewhat the feelings of aloneness and abandonment which can occur.

For some families the need to surround the client and openly express sadness may prove detrimental when client resources are weakened by shock and illness. Though the client may need to know that his entire family is available, the nurse may find it necessary to monitor the number of visitors to reduce fatigue. If this is the case, a place for the family to congregate should be provided, or the family should be asked to make frequent short visits in small groups.

Guilt and anger at the self, the dying individual, or the health care team are frequently manifested.

Frequently, the nurse bears the brunt of this anger because she is a ready and available target. "If only—" is often heard. It is necessary for the nurse to remember that these outbursts, no matter how guilty or angry, are necessary for the individual to carry out the grieving process. A calm, nonjudgmental, and attentive attitude on the part of the nurse will allow the client to give vent to his emotions. Families should be helped to realize that guilt and anger are normal and should not be suppressed. Families experiencing anticipatory grief are often shocked at their anger, especially when it is directed at the dying client. They should be helped to understand that this is a normal and expected reaction to their anticipated loss and is relatively short-lived. Guilt, especially in the case of a dying child, is concomitant with parental grief. It is difficult for parents to assuage guilt feelings if they become internalized. Parents can be guided to share with each other their feelings of responsibility to prevent repression of their anger, future blame and, recrimination.

A few individuals experiencing intense grief may find that crying is not possible, and there are many reasons for this. For example, if ambivalence is felt about the dying person, it may be difficult for the individual to express grief until he is able to sort out his feelings. The sorting-out process is difficult and time consuming, and failure at it may explain individuals who continue to be ambivalent for months or years after the death of a family member. For another, active grieving may be postponed until an appropriate environment is available in which to allow free emotional expression. Dying clients sometimes postpone active grieving until they pick up cues from their families that grieving is permissible behavior.

Lindeman[5] has described the period of active grief as one of emptiness in the chest and with waves of anguish occurring at intervals, particularly when the dying or deceased individual is mentioned or imagined. The dying client and his family may begin to experience frustration or loneliness as they perceive the environment without the dying person.

One way to help a person who faces death is to talk about his situation and what it means to him.[6] If the individual is realistic in his approach to his impending death, and if he is willing and able to verbalize his thoughts and feelings, the discussion of what the loss means to him as a person, as a family member, as a worker, as a social being will help to decrease the frustration felt as "why me?"

Anticipatory grieving is not always carried out in a usual manner. Lindeman[7] found that wives of servicemen who were sent overseas during World War II sometimes grieved so completely for their husbands that the husband returned to find nothing left of the original relationship. Anticipatory grieving occurs before death and will continue afterward on the part of the family. In anticipatory grief, the family may have completely experienced the stage of intense grief. No matter how completely this has been accomplished, the survivors will still manifest varying degrees of sorrow when the death actually occurs.

Recovery

The recovery phase includes the ritualistic expression of grief, the giving up of ties to the deceased, and full acceptance of the death. Ritualized expressions of grief, such as the funeral, wake, or burial service, serve a useful purpose—that is, at this point it is difficult, though not impossible, to maintain denial, and suppression of feelings is not encouraged. Indeed, the mourner is encouraged by friends and other mourners to give full vent to his feelings. Also, the attention of the others is geared to the mourner, so that he is not alone. Discussion of the deceased helps to put the past relationship into perspective and enables the survivors to consider the future. In considering the future without the deceased, the groundwork is laid for future relationships and the belief that life continues.

Grief can be delayed, but it's healthier not to postpone it indefinitely, for it will eventually need to be worked through. If grieving is not completed, it will be done later at greater cost to the individual. Such delayed reactions may be seen in the anniversary grief reaction. The individual experiences an episode of acute grieving and often acute distress on the anniversary of the death of a loved one. An anniversary reaction is often more intense than is the normal grief response experienced at the time of death because of the repression of feelings over a long period of time. With such a reaction the individual may suffer varying degrees of personality disorganization. Astute observation during the period of anticipatory grief and at the death of the loved one may help to prevent a later crisis from occurring.

If the dying client has had an opportunity to grieve for the impending loss of the self, he may reach acceptance and withdraw from his environment in anticipation of something else.[8] The family of the dying client that has a chance to grieve along with him over a period of time will recognize the necessity for letting go.

THE FAMILY

If the dying client is a child with siblings, assessment must be made of the role to which the siblings are relegated during the illness of the child. If possible, some way must be found to include the other children in the support given to the parents and other family members. Children often have fantasies about dying and misconceptions about what is happening to a sister or brother, and these fantasies can cause problems in the future if steps are not taken to aid the child early in the illness. One way to alleviate misconceptions about what is happening is to allow siblings to visit in the hospital. Parents do not always have the emotional strength to deal with a dying child, and at the same time, the complex needs of other children. Health team members can guide some other family member to take over these emotional duties until the parents are able to do so.

The responses of close family members to an impending loss of a loved one are those of helplessness and hopelessness. The family feel helpless because they see nothing constructive that they can do for their loved one. This is especially true once the client has been admitted to a hospital for terminal care. Hospital routine appears to be efficient and structured, and there seems to be no way for the family to take part in client care activities. As a result, relationships become altered by routine, policy, and scheduled treatments. Hopelessness occurs because family members believe there is nothing they can do to stop the progression of the disease and the terminal outcome.

For the family experiencing powerlessness, a plan for involved assistance can be instituted by the health care team. Usually the closest family members, or those who have been most attentive to the client, will feel the most helpless and will need to be aided to cope appropriately.

Support—A Nurse's Responsibility

Support of the family through the period of anticipatory grief and eventual death of the terminally ill client is largely the responsibility of the nurse because she has the most frequent contact with the family members during their visits. However, no one individual should be or can be completely responsible for mobilizing the resources to adequately deal with a protracted period of anticipatory grief. Rather, an interdisciplinary approach to the assessed needs of the family should be developed with the entire health care team who should be fully aware of the changing needs of the family and of appropriate methods of intervention. A team approach involves a group of concerned individuals who utilize skills of critical assessment and planning and are available to the client and his family. A method of communication for all team members should be instituted so that pertinent data are not lost and are shared readily during client care planning.

Because families and their needs differ, so will the types of support that can be offered each family. To achieve individualization of planned support, careful assessment of the family's method of interacting with each other will suggest the coping abilities and other emotional resources available. Assessment of the family's response to the anticipated loss will enable the observer to tentatively establish whether or not the response is adaptive or maladaptive and may suggest the need for counseling. The role of the client in the family group should be looked at critically to determine how the other family members perceive his role. If the dying client has been the backbone of the family unit, for example, there may be problems in unifying the group after his death.

Involvement in Client Care

Involvement in the actual care of the client helps to decrease the helplessness experienced by family members. This does not mean that relatives need to be taught to carry out technical procedures, but the opportunity to carry out simple comfort measures is often welcomed. Frequently, visitors to the hospital are hesitant to aid the client by doing simple tasks they may have performed for him at home. They see these acts as a nurse's responsibility and believe they would be encroaching on her territory. The nursing staff will also need to evaluate, at this time, their feelings about family members taking over some of their duties. It is important for nurses to realize that family members are helped and supported by being allowed to do these simple tasks, and this is a necessary aspect of the nursing care plan.

Family members can be taught to give a sponge bath without chilling the client and to give back massages correctly. They can learn to position the client in good alignment and to get him out of bed to sit in a chair or to take a walk. The strength of the individual carrying out these tasks must be assessed, as well as his ability to follow directions. Grieving family members can exhaust themselves emotionally and physically so that careful observation is necessary to prevent an untoward result. Family members also can be entrusted to feed clients and to chart intake and output correctly.

Planned involvement will only be valuable when the family appears to need this kind of intervention and seems to benefit by the resulting closeness with the client and interaction with the staff.

Families will feel supported by the health team if they are informed of new procedures and treatments as changes occur, along with careful explanation for the changes in routine. This will enable the family and the client to feel somewhat in control of the situation. "We would like to send Mr. J. to x-ray in the morning instead of the afternoon, because he's less likely to become fatigued," is an appropriate explanation of a routine change. Thus, the family is included in the decision to decrease fatigue in the client, and an opportunity for discussion is offered. Appropriate interpretation of recent laboratory studies can help family members to understand the client's condition or may explain a request for diminished visiting hours. The client and his family should be led to believe that they are not only participating in but planning the care along with health team members.

One must be carefully attuned to the number of stressors in process at any one time and with a particular family member. Dealing with anticipatory grief is a great stress, and for some individuals, multiple stressors occurring at the same time can result in collapse or physical illness. In supporting family members, one must be ready to intervene appropriately with them, perhaps even more than

with the client. The opportunity to talk out problems can be as helpful as referral to an appropriate counselor. What sometimes appears to be argumentative or rude behavior on the part of visitors often masks underlying feelings of fear, inadequacy, or guilt. "What can I do to help?" continues to be a valuable question when asked by a concerned health team member and may give the stressed family member the opening he needs to initiate discussion of his fears and inadequacies.

Sociocultural and Religious Background

Knowledge of the sociocultural and religious background of the client and his family will enable the nurse to predict certain behaviors and manipulate the environment to provide for others. Take, for example, an American Indian client and his family who were distressed to learn that hospital policy and routine would not allow their tribal medicine man or shaman to perform a tribal ritual at the client's bedside. Though the client and his family did not attribute curative powers to the ceremony, they were discomfited to learn that the ritual would be considered a disruption to the routine of the unit. With the help of a concerned nurse, the reason and need for the ritual and a description of what would occur was explained to the unit administrator. It became clear that the ritual would not be disruptive nor would it disturb the other clients. It was then an easy matter to arrange the client's treatments and procedures for a short period to allow the shaman to visit.

Awareness of the client's background can prove exceptionally valuable in planning care and in obtaining his cooperation in his treatment. A West Indian man had been hospitalized for a serious stomach disorder, but he insisted that the severe pain he was experiencing was caused by a curse. He believed that a jealous rival had caused an iguana to be present in his stomach, and as long as the iguana was present, no amount of medicine or surgery would help his condition. As a result, he refused all medications and food. As his health deteriorated, the nursing and medical staff became more concerned; but no amount of admonishments would move the client to accept medication and treatment. In desperation, a nurse questioned the family about the curse, keeping in mind that, to them, such a thing was real. The nurse, although not sharing the belief, was careful to let them know that she respected their belief. In discussion, a suggestion was made to find someone who could remove the curse. The family had been too distraught to think of this solution before, and the professional staff had not been willing to consider the client's strange beliefs. Yet, the client's sociocultural background was one in which belief in curses was commonplace. By listening and giving credence to the client's beliefs, support for the family was established and the client benefited by resulting treatment.

While these examples are unusual, there are many situations in which client care is inappropriate due to the incomplete or inadequate assessment of the religious or cultural background of the client and his family. The client who needs to be coaxed to accept certain comfort measures, such as a backrub or his evening glass of juice, because in his culture no one accepts the first time, will be shortchanged if the nursing staff is unaware of his orientation. The old Italian lady dressed in black could be labeled a "bother" or a "crock" by the staff if it is not known that, in her particular village in Italy, someone must sit up with the sick at all times to prevent bad spirits from taking the soul before it is ready.

Understanding is as important as direct intervention with the family by health team members. The client and his family and their unique perceptions must be considered when support is planned. Only by considering all aspects of the whole human being and attending to the diverse needs which result can an individual actually receive the solace and help which is offered.

NURSING APPROACH TO DEATH AND DYING

The basic needs of the dying client can be categorized into three areas: (1) security; (2) maintenance of hope; and (3) comfort. The nurse's approach to the dying patient, and her ability to meet his basic needs, are influenced by her attitudes, beliefs and feelings about death and dying. The nurse brings to client interactions unique life experiences which influence the way in which she perceives the client who is dying. The nurse's viewpoint is influenced by the way in which she has learned to deal with her own losses. The nurse who has not experienced a significant loss and, thus, has not needed to face her true feelings about death, may not be sensitive to this need in others. All the classes and information about death and dying the nurse has attended in the past are of no consequence if she does not consider the knowledge to be a necessary aspect of client care. Consider, also, the nurse, who in her family life, was taught to give no outward sign of grief, to keep her feelings to herself. This individual may find it difficult to be supportive of the dying client who expresses his grief publicly and involves others in its process. His manifestations of grief are more or less foreign to her and perhaps frightening. The nurse who has recently experienced a significant personal loss may also find it difficult to relate to the terminally ill client. In this situation, if her own grieving process is not yet completed, she does not possess adequate emotional resources for dealing with the grief of another individual.

Care of Terminally Ill Clients

The terminally ill individual's needs for security, comfort, and maintenance of hope are difficult to meet if the nurse's energies must be directed to the diminishment of her own anxieties about death and dying. Often, this process is manifested as a conspiracy of silence among nursing staff. Integral to this conspiracy is a repertoire of avoidance techniques and rationalizations used to prevent personal involvement with the dying client. Many nurses are not aware that such a goal underlies their motives and directs their plan of care. What appears to be concern for the client's privacy in placing him in a single room at the end of a corridor may actually be a means of preventing too frequent contact. The assignment of an ancillary worker to the client to give basic care while the nurse supervises at a distance further dilutes the nurse-client relationship and places the nurse in a "safe" situation. She is absolved of her responsibility to deal with questions and grief behavior as she is less likely to be available to pick up cues from the client as to his need to explore his feelings with someone. In some cases, the nurse does give the care, but the contact is infrequent, consisting of ritualized activities and conversation relegated to light or social topics.

COPING MECHANISMS

The easy way to handle a problem is to ignore it. The nurse who believes her actions are blocked by a diagnosis of terminal illness, and thus nothing she can do will be of consequence, may prefer to deal with her clients on a superficial level, giving necessary physical care without its emotional component. This decreases the frustration and conflict in what is perceived as a hopeless situation.

Both client and nurse suffer by the use of coping mechanisms designed to avoid, rationalize, or ignore real client needs. The client and his family have an incomplete outlet for feelings, and their sources of emotional comfort are severely curtailed. The message is clear that questions are not invited and, therefore, needed information may not be obtained. The client's need for help in moving through the grieving process may be thwarted. The nurse is also disadvantaged, as her personal and professional growth are stunted by her inability to function on all levels. Satisfaction with professional tasks is not derived easily, if at all, and the nurse is unable to use all of her professional skills to their best advantage.

To deal effectively and therapeutically with the dying client and his family, the nurse must possess an excellent background of skills and knowledge. No one particular skill is of prime importance; rather, one must be able to utilize a variety of skills built on an adequate knowledge base. Effective verbal and nonverbal communication skills and the ability to use them as needed is vital in caring for the terminally ill client. Part of communication includes the establishment of a trust relationship with the client. To do this the nurse must be aware of her own feelings and behaviors in the death and dying situation. It is necessary for the nurse to understand that her feelings will influence her approach to the client and his subsequent response to her. Dying persons, unless they are unusually anxious, needing to talk to anyone, are quite astute at identifying the hesitant or anxious nurse. The client will not wish to invest fully in a relationship which will prove inadequate for his needs, and a superficial interaction will result. The nurse may need help from an objective observer to recognize her avoidance behavior in particular situations. Recognizing the behavior for what it is and taking action to decrease anxiety in other less destructive ways will contribute greatly to the nurse's ability to care for dying clients. Self awareness, and the willingness to put into practice the lessons learned through introspection, will enable the nurse to be more accepting and open to client cues.

ASSESSMENT SKILLS

Recognition of normal grief patterns and knowledge of the grief response are necessary for the nurse who deals with dying clients. The amount of literature on grief is vast and readily accessible; familiarity with the variety of ways in which grief can be manifested will prevent the uninformed nurse from labeling a client as "uncooperative, apathetic," or as a "behavior problem." The nurse's experience and knowledge of grief behavior can easily set to rest the fears of a client and his family that certain behaviors signal the onset of insanity. "This too will pass" with an explanation of the dynamics of grief behavior will enable the client to recognize that he has not lost his faculties along with everything else.

It is necessary for the nurse to be possessed of excellent assessment skills and the ability to use these skills in client care. All information pertaining to the client should be collected by the nurse prior to planning care. The family of the client is also important, for they may be able to supply insight into the way the client has dealt with previous losses. This knowledge enables the nurse to predict some client behavior, as well as decrease the chance of unexpected behavior.

COMMUNICATION SKILLS

Does the client know he is dying is a pertinent question to be asked by the nurse. A client unaware of his diagnosis may ask questions the nurse believes can be answered only by "ask your doctor" and will add to her feelings of failure and to the client's disappointment in hearing another vague response. Yet, careful assessment of the client's situation may help the nurse to decide what he really wants to know when he asks questions which are difficult to answer. Often, clients do not wish to know all of the answers to their questions but only part of an answer. The unspoken, "Will I die from this condition?" may be preceded instead by, "What were the results of my lab tests?'' or ''What did the doctor find during surgery?'' The nurse's anxiety level will rise when questions asked are specific to a diagnosis or an aspect of illness and demand a response she is not prepared to give. In this situation it is the doctor or close family member who will inform the client. The nurse can respond by saying simply that she is not sure or she does not know, but such a vague response should be followed by a more positive answer. ''I'll remind your doctor to discuss his findings with you,'' or something similar will assuage the client's anxiety. He will be relieved of his fear that the nurse is not informing him because the news is too terrible to hear. It will be clear that, in this situation, the doctor is the better person to consult. Also, the client's trust in the nurse has not diminished because she has not left him with an unsatisfying response.

It may be necessary for the nurse to intervene with the physician and inform him of the kinds of questions his client is asking, so that he can prepare his discussion. If the physician or the family refuse information to the client, the nurse must obtain some guidelines as to how far she and the other members of the staff can go in discussing his particular disease condition. This sort of situation is always difficult. At present, most Nurse Practice Acts do not allow the nurse to inform the client of a diagnosis if such information is considered the express prerogative of the physician. What the nurse can do is to be aware of the needs of the client for information and, using communication techniques, allow him to discuss his feelings and beliefs about his illness. Consistency of the staff members in what information can be shared will also be helpful. The physician should be informed that the client is still requesting information and seems dissatisfied by what he has been told.

Dealing with dying clients and their families is challenging and rewarding, but it is also difficult and emotionally draining. It is difficult to physically avoid contact with the terminally ill client in most health care agencies, though many individuals find ways to avoid him emotionally. The nurse who is not aware and awake to her own feelings about death and dying will find it difficult to function appropriately when faced with a dying client. The methods used will also be carried over into other aspects of her nursing practice and will become a pattern of behavior to be used whenever a situation

becomes anxiety provoking or painful for her. It is never easy to look at ourselves and learn from what we find there, but such introspection is a necessary and essential part of the nurse's personal and professional growth.

PHYSICAL SIGNS OF APPROACHING DEATH

When death is a gradual cumulative process, there are definite physical signs that indicate its imminence. These are in addition to signs caused by specific pathology.

Level of consciousness varies a great deal. Some persons are alert, some are drowsy or stuporous, and others are comatose. During the process of dying, vision becomes blurred, and the eyes usually remain partly open. Hearing is believed to be the last sense lost. With loss of muscle tone, the person's facial muscles relax and speech becomes difficult. Inability to speak creates the impression that the dying client is unconscious, especially if his eyes are closed. Thus, even though the person may not be able to communicate in any way, he may still be able to hear and understand what is being said around him. Due to the general slowing of circulation, the feet become cold to touch and later the hands, ears, and nose. Although the skin may be cold the individual may feel warm. The person's temperature is usually elevated, and there is often excessive diaphoresis.

The pulse becomes fast, weak, and irregular, and the blood pressure falls. Respiration is rapid, shallow, irregular, or abnormally slow. There are often periods of rapid breathing separated by pauses; this is called Cheyne-Stokes respiration. The jaw may sag, and the person breathes through the mouth with flaccid lips and cheeks. Lips are dry, swallowing becomes difficult, and mucus collects in the throat, which may account for the noisy breathing spoken of as the ''death rattle.''

During the process, the person usually has little or no interest in food or drink. Taste and smell are frequently altered. Pace of eating is slow. Swallowing is difficult. The person may be nauseous, due to decreasing peristalsis and subsequent delayed emptying of the stomach. Dryness of mouth, which is often due to side effects of drugs or mouth breathing, is a frequent symptom which interferes with eating and talking.

Loss of muscle tone may produce urinary and rectal incontinence. Due to the decreased activity of the gastrointestinal tract, there may be an accumulation of flatus, causing abdominal distention and nausea. There may be retention and impaction of feces especially if the client is receiving narcotics, tranquilizers, or hypnotics as these decrease motility of the gastrointestinal tract.

As the slowing of the circulation and loss of muscle tone progress, reflexes are lost, the extremities lose sensation and become cyanosed; eventually the power of motion is lost.

It must also be remembered that, in old age particularly, the very sick seem to die more than once. The individual may suddenly recover and live for weeks or months.

Implications for Nursing

No one can predict how long the process of dying will take.

The needs of the person include cleanliness of the skin, clean hair, and cleanliness of the mouth. Wearing apparel may be daytime clothes if the person wishes, or whatever is comfortable or desired.

The nurse should keep the bed dry. Sweating may make frequent baths and linen changes necessary. Picking at bed linen is a typical behavior during the process of dying. This may be an indication that the client feels warm or that there is a need for oxygen.

Narcotics as ordered by a physician should be administered for pain relief every 3–4 hours. The decreased circulation may necessitate administration of analgesics by intravenous infusion rather than intramuscularly or subcutaneously.

Secretions may accumulate in the eyes and should be removed using cotton dipped in normal saline. If the eyes become dry, they should be lubricated with an ophthalmic ointment or solution. The eyes should be protected from bright lights, though the room should be comfortably illuminated.

Appropriate nursing actions should be taken to relieve respiratory difficulties, such as positioning and suctioning. Cough medicine for coughs, ephedrine and oxtriphylline for bronchospasm, or antibiotics for purulent sputum may be ordered by the physician. Humidity can aid respiration and relieve some of the dryness of the nose and throat.

Cold cream or petroleum jelly with vitamins A and D should be used on the nose and lips. Antihistamines, such as Benadryl, may decrease secretions. Benadryl may also relieve anxiety and thus act as a tranquilizer. Suctioning will help reduce the accumulation of mucus. Oxygen may aid respiration. However, oxygen tents can isolate the client and deepen anxiety. For hiccoughs or diaphragm spasms, administer small amounts of carbon dioxide. Iced water or possibly tube feedings may aid in dysphagia.

The dying person usually experiences anorexia. Antiemetics, alcoholic beverages, or small doses of steroids may help stimulate the appetite. A high caloric, high vitamin diet is used. If the person experiences nausea and vomiting, control the sights and smells, administer antiemetics; remember too much water can increase vomiting. The gag reflex must be present in order for the individual to swallow. This should be checked frequently.

The person's needs related to elimination must also be met. Ducolax often prevents constipation. For skin irritation due to diarrhea, use of a soothing ointment around the anus is helpful. Check the availability of the bed pan, toilet, or commode. Position the person on the bed pan or with the urinal frequently. Protection of the bed is also a consideration, and linens should be changed as often as necessary. If the client is incontinent, absorbent pads are used and should be changed frequently. Catheterization for retention may be necessary, or in some cases, an indwelling catheter may be inserted.

Movement and changes of position, including being out of bed if possible, are also important nursing considerations. The side-lying position is better than lying flat on the back. Fowler's or semi-Fowler's position may aid respiration. The person may not be able to maintain a comfortable position without support.

People differ in their desire to have family and friends present. If the person's family is present, the nurse must also be aware of their special needs at this time. Being supportive, keeping them informed of changes in the person's condition, and explaining what is being done to make the person as comfortable as possible, will let them know that you care and are doing your best to help the person and them during this difficult time. If family or friends are not present, the nurse should be available and willing to stay with the individual as needed.

POSTMORTEM NURSING RESPONSIBILITIES

Care of the individual who has died is carried out by the nurse after the client has been officially pronounced dead by the attending or staff physician. Until this pronouncement takes place, preparation of the body for discharge from the unit may not be initiated. The time and cause of death are noted on the death certificate, along with other pertinent information, which becomes a matter of record.

The major function of the nurse in caring for the body after death is to carry out legal requirements, protect the body tissues, and to discharge the body to an appropriate area for claim. It is at this time that the family of the deceased are usually given one more opportunity to see the body. The offer could be made to a waiting family member, or close relatives are sought by telephone. If family members wish to view the body, it should be made to look as familiar as possible. The eyes should be closed, the hair arranged in the usual style, dentures are inserted; stains and marks are washed from the face and, if possible, tubes and drains are removed. Low lights in the room soften the appearance of the corpse. Positioning the bedsheets and placing the head on pillows give a peaceful appearance. This is important to some family members who wish to come away with the perception that their loved one died easily and without pain. Family members appreciate being left alone with the body for a short period of time.

Someone on the nursing staff should be available at this time to comfort the family, as needed, to answer questions, and to give necessary information.

Legal Requirements

If an autopsy is required by law or requested by the physician, the family spokesman will be approached for permission at this time. Autopsy is governed by state law in cases where death is caused by the possibility of suicide or homicide, accident, illegal practices, or death within a specific number of hours of admission to hospital. If the client has died of an unusual or relatively unknown disease, however, the physician may request permission for the postmortem examination to obtain information that might help others. Reasons for the postmortem examination should be carefully explained to the family, keeping in mind that, unless a legal need prevails, the family has a right to refuse permission. Orthodox Jews strongly oppose autopsies or any form of human dissection. A part of Orthodox law calls for complete burial, based on the belief that the physical integrity of the body is a prerequisite for resurrection.[9] Autopies prescribed by law, however, take precedence over religious issues. It is helpful to inform the Jewish family in this situation that all organs will be returned to the body after autopsy, thus meeting religious requirements.

Organ Donations

It is also at the time of death that healthy organs donated before death are removed for transplant or other use. Individuals wishing to donate organs after death can contact their local chapters of the National Kidney Foundation or the Eye Bank For Sight Restoration. A wallet-sized card to be signed by the donor and two witnesses is given by both agencies. The cards allow the individual to be identified by others as a potential donor.

Donor eyes must be removed from the body preferably within 6 to 24 hours after death. Eyes removed before the 24-hour time limit can be used for corneal transplant. Eyes removed after 24 hours are used for research into eye diseases and physician training. Eyes are removed by physicians or trained technicians associated with the Eye Bank. In caring for the client who has donated his eyes after death, the nurse must be aware of the gift and make every effort to contact the required persons.

Donor kidneys, to be used for transplantation, must be removed within 1 hour after death. The deceased client's attending physician never removes the kidneys as this could give rise to speculation about the death.

The Body

Procedures for care of the body after death vary somewhat from agency to agency but are essentially similar. Many agencies utilize a procedure to guide the nurse in carrying out care. In caring for the body after death, there are several points for the nurse to bear in mind. (1) The body must be clean. A complete bedbath may not be necessary, but any stains, drainage marks, or other soiling should be removed with soap and water. (2) Sharp objects that could scratch the skin or cause pressure should be removed. After death the skin discolors with pressure. Dark areas on the skin, especially facial areas, will distress the family and should not be allowed to occur. This can be accomplished by making sure that the body is not left in a prone position. (3) Protection should be provided for the relaxation of bowel and bladder sphincters. This can be accomplished by padding the area well and pinning a diaper in place. Some agencies keep adult-sized disposable diapers handy for this purpose. (4) Wounds should be covered with clean dry dressings to prevent leakage. (5) Proper identification should be made to avoid error. Tags are attached to the big toe and one wrist. The tags should have the name and age of the client and any other information necessary for proper identification.

The body should be placed in good alignment. Most morticians recommend that the arms be tied loosely over the abdomen with padding to protect the wrists. The legs can be padded at the ankles and tied together loosely. Crossing the ankles over each other will result in pressure and unsightly tissue damage. A shroud or sheet is used to cover the body before it leaves the unit.

Valuables still with the client at the time of death should be safeguarded until they can be given to the family or sent to a designated place for claiming. Most agencies use a form on which valuables can be listed. Articles which remain with the body, such as the wedding ring, should be so designated on the form sheet. In most cases the mortician will return personal articles to the next of kin before burial.

While caring for a body, some nurses handle their high levels of anxiety by laughing, joking, or casual conversation with other staff members. The body is depersonalized in this way, but the nurse's anxiety is decreased and she is able to go about her business not fully aware of what the body signifies to her. Referring to the corpse as "it" or wearing an unnecessary gown and gloves also keep the nurse from conscious reality of the death. This behavior denies the body the respect and dignity it deserves. Hopefully, as the nurse becomes more experienced and more in tune with her feelings, the need to depersonalize the corpse will diminish.

The transfer of a body to the agency morgue is a procedure which differs from agency to agency and is a function of the available facilities. In some agencies the body may be transferred on a stretcher. In others a false bottom stretcher is used. This particular piece of equipment looks like a two-layered stretcher. The body is placed on the second layer. The top layer is covered by a sheet which hangs over the sides and hides the second layer, giving the appearance of an empty stretcher. The advantage of this is that the body can be transported to the morgue at any time of the day or night without distress to other clients and visitors.

In the morgue, the body is placed in a required area and written notation of its arrival is made. Again, proper identification of the body is of prime importance. The mortician, who may not know the individual personally, will be calling for the body. Proper identification can prevent further undue distress to family and friends when the body is later viewed.

REFERENCES

1. Kubler-Ross, E.: *On Death and Dying.* New York, Macmillan Co., 1967.
2. Engel, G. L.: Grief and grieving. *Am. J. Nurs.* 64:93, 1964.
3. Kiening, M. M.: Denial of illness, in *Behavioral Concepts and Nursing Intervention,* edited by Carlson, C., Philadelphia, J. B. Lippincott Co., 1970, p. 9.
4. Carlson, C.: Grief and mourning, in *Behavioral Concepts and Nursing Intervention,* edited by Carlson, C., Philadelphia, J. B. Lippincott Co., 1970, p. 95.
5. Lindemann, E.: Symptomatology and management of acute grief. *Am. J. Psychiatry* 101:141, 1944.
6. Ujhely, G. B.: Grief and depression: implications for preventions and therapeutic nursing care. *Nurs. Forum* 5(2):23, 1966.
7. Lindemann, *op. cit.,* p. 148.
8. Kubler-Ross, E.: What is it like to be dying? *Am. J. Nurs.* 71:54, 1971.
9. Hendin, D.: Death as a fact of life. New York, Warner Communications Co., 1974, p. 48.

BIBLIOGRAPHY

Wolf, L., et al: *Fundamentals of Nursing,* 6th ed. Philadelphia, J. B. Lippincott Co., 1979.
Henderson, V., and Nite, G.: *Principles and Practice of Nursing,* 6th ed. New York, Macmillan Publishing Co., 1978.
Luckmann, J., and Sorenson, K.: *Medical Surgical Nursing: A Psychophysiologic Approach,* New York, W. B. Saunders Co., 1974.

INDEX

Page numbers in italics indicate tables.

Compliance, 671
Comprehensive Health Planning Act, 202
Comprehensive Health Planning and Public Health Service Amendments of 1960, 166
Compresses
  cold, use of, 583
  packs and, application of moist heat and, 581
Compression, cardiopulmonary resuscitation and, 738-740
Computerized axial tomography of brain, *944*
Confidentiality, interviewing and, 272-273
Congenital anomalies, respiratory dysfunction and cardiovascular, 688-689
Congestion, cardiovascular disorders and respiratory dysfunction and, 687-688
Congrove v. Holmes, 252
Conjunctiva, examination of, 305-306
Conjunctivitis, 360
Consciousness, physical examination and assessing states of, 299
Consent, informed, 251-252
Consolidation, 290
Constipation, 856-857
  definition of, 825
Contract
  between client and nurse, 886
Contracting
  crisis intervention and, 105, 107
Contracture, 487
Control, hospitalization and loss of privacy and, 69-70
Controlled Substances Act, 588
Consultant, registered nurse as, 217-218
Consumer
  federal protection of interests of, 171-176
  of health care services, 152-177
Consumer movement, in health delivery service, 162-176
Consumer-users, public policy decisions and, 162-170
Contaminated materials, disposal of, in isolation technique to maintain medical asepsis, *530-531*
Contamination, 515
Contrast baths and packs, 584-585
Cooptation, citizen participation in health care delivery and planning and, 165

Coordination, testing of, 304-305
Coordinator, registered nurse as, 216
Coping mechanisms, care of terminally ill clients and, 965
Cornea, examination of, 306
Coronary, café, 732
Cor pulmonale, 671
Corrigan's pulse, 482
Cost, supply as factor in reducing medical, 157-160
Costochondral separation, 730
Costovertebral tenderness, 341
Coughing, maintaining patent airway and, 690
Counselor, registered nurse as, 216
Counterirritants, *602-603*
Cradle, footboard and, positioning of client and, 505
Cranial nerves, physical examination and, 300-302
Creams, 614
Creatinine-height index, 780
Credé maneuver, 833
Cremasteric reflex, 303
Crepitation, 328
Crepitus, 290
Cricothyrotomy, 730
Crime, 238
Crisis(es)
  classification of, 99
  components of, 103-104
  conceptual framework of, 98-99
  development of state of, 101
  duration of, 98
  individual manifestations of, *103*
  intervention and, 96-108
    guidelines in, *107*
    plan and techniques for, 105-107
  manifestations of, 102-103
  maturational, 99-100
  outcomes of, 99
  situational, 100-101
  theoretical concepts of, 96-101
Cross-contamination, 515
Croup, upper airway obstruction and, 675
Crutches, 507-509
Culdoscopy, *940*
Cultural factors, layperson's definition of health and illness and, 63-64
Cyclopegics, *602-603*
Cystic fibrosis, 678-679
Cystocele, 345, 825
Cystogram, *944*
Cystoscopy, *940*
Cytotoxic agents, *602-603*

DARLING case, 240
Data
  base of, for nursing care plan, 395-396
  collection of, 435-436
    interviewing as tool for, 268-279
Dead space
  anatomical, 671
  physiological, 671
Death
  brain, 253
  dying, grief and, 958-969
  nursing approach to dying and, 964-966
  nursing responsibilities concerning, 968
  physical signs of approaching, 966-968
  right to die and, 252-253
Debridement, 515
Decompression, 788
  gastrointestinal intubation and, 793-794
Decubitus ulcer, 548-549
Deep tendon reflexes, 303
Defamation, 238
Defecation, 825
Defendant, 238
Defervescence, 456
Defibrillation, 730
DeFillipo v. Preston, 252
Deformities, respiratory dysfunction and, 684
Dehydration and electrolyte imbalance, gastrointestinal intubation and, 822
Demulcents, *600-601, 604-605*
Denial, shock and, 959-960
Depressants, chemical, respiratory dysfunction and, 681-683
Developmental assessment, of child, 363-370
Developmental milestones, 7
Diagnosis
  medical and nursing, 388-389
  nature of any, 386
  nursing
    development of, 389-392
    health care problems and, 384-393
    tentative list of, *391*
Diagnostic tests, 926-950. *See also names of specific tests.*
  nurses role in, 927-930
Dialogical encounter, 234-237
Dialogue, 235
Diaphoresis, 825
Diaphragm, 325
Diarrhea, 854

Force, body mechanics and, 490
Forceps, transfer, in sterile procedures, 534
Foreign bodies, legal aspects of nursing and, 247
Fowler's position, 503
Frames, turning, moving of client with, 507
Fremitus, 291, 322
Frequency, 825
Friction, body mechanics and, 490
Friction rub
  pericardial, 333
  peritoneal, 338
  pleural, 322, 328
Funduscopic examination, 308-309
Fungicides, *596-597*
Fungistatics, *596-597*
Fungus
  definition of, 515
  lower airway obstruction and infection with, 677-678

Gait, inspection of, 292
Gallop sounds, 331-332
Ganglionic blocking agents, *596-597*
Gargles, 619
Gastric analysis, *931*
Gastrointestinal intubation. *See also names of specific procedures involving.*
  care of client with, 788-823
  equipment for, 790-792
  problems with, 822
  procedures for, 806-822
  reasons for, 792-806
Gastrointestinal system, review of systems and, 285
Gastrointestinal tract, 852-857
  function and anatomy of, 852-853
  problems involving, 853-857
    nursing care in, 854
Gastrointestinal tubes, 788
Gastroscopy, *941*
Gastrostomy tube
  definition of, 788
  procedures for, 821-822
Gavage, 796-797
  definition of, 788
  procedures for, *798-801*
General adaptation syndrome, 90-91
Generalist team, roles and educational preparation of members of, *208*
Generativity, 18
Genitalia
  female. *See* Female genitalia.

human sexuality and, 49-56
male. *See* Male genitalia.
newborn assessment and, 371
review of systems and, 285
Germicides, 515, *598-599*
Gestational age, determination of, 376
Gestures, assessment of nonverbal behavior and, 264-265
Gland(s)
  bulbourethral, 351
    rectal examination and, 352
  thyroid, 315
Glans penis, inspection and palpation of, 349-350
Glomerulonephritis, 825
Glossopharyngeal nerve, 302
Gloving, in isolation technique to maintain medical asepsis, *528-529*
Glucose, 749
Glycogen, 749
Glycosides, cardiac, *600-601*
Glycosuria, 825
Goals
  family, 34
  plan of care and establishment of, 398
Good Samaritan laws, 253-254
Government
  as purchaser of health care services, 156
  drug regulation agencies of, 588
  health care responsibilities of, 143
Gowning
  for sterile procedures, 533-534
  in isolation technique to maintain medical asepsis, *528-529*
Grasp reflex, newborn and, 376
Gravity, 487
  body mechanics and, 488
Grief
  death, dying and, 958-969
  intense, 960-961
  recovery from, 961-962
Grooming, assessment of nonverbal behavior and, 264
Group
  character of, 187-188
  primary, 189-190
Group process, 186-198
Growth and development, groups and, 189-191
Grunt, 361
Guardian ad litem, 239
Guillain-Barre syndrome, respiratory dysfunction and, 683
Gums, examination of, 312

Hair
  hygienic care of, 547-548
  physical examination and, 298
Hand, evaluation of, 356
Handwashing
  surgical, 532
  to maintain medical asepsis, 522-524, *522-523*
Harris flush, 856
Harrison Narcotic Act, 588
Harris tube, 790
Hartmann pouch, end colostomy and, 890
Hazards. *See also* Accident; Injury; Trauma.
  thermal and electrical, in hospital, 568-569
Head
  examination of, 305
  neck and, in physical examination, 305-316
  newborn assessment and, 371
  review of systems and, 284
Healing, wound, 535-537
Health
  assessment of, child, 360-382
  belief models and, 83-84
  concepts of, 84
  definition of, *80*, 112-113
  disease prevention and promotion of, 116-117
  general state of, health history and, 283
  illness and, 78-87
    behaviors in, 81-82
    concepts about, 77-138
    continuum of, 82-83
    definitions of, 79-81
    layperson's definition of, 63-65
  marketplace of, 155-160
  medical, and illness care services and, 141-142
  promotion and maintenance of, group process and, 192-193
  restoration of, 132-138
  right to, 146-147
Health care, 142
  as basic right, 155-157
  community approach to, 147-148
  community services providing, evaluation of, 144
  comprehensive, 201-202
  consumer of services providing, 152-177
  delivery of, 141-150
  individualizing needs for, 257-439

Ileostomy —*Continued*
definition of, 875
functional considerations with, 903-904
Illness
confrontation with, 66-67
definition of, 387
health and, 77-138
layperson's definition of, 63-65
Illness care, 142
Immune competence, nutritional status and, 780
Immune system, 515
Immunity
active, 514, 520
passive, 516, 520
Immunization, 515
Impaction, fecal, 825, 857
Incidence, 515
Incident reports, 250
Incision, 515
Incontinence
definition of, 826
fecal, 855
paradoxical urinary, 831
urinary, 832-833
Individual, restoration of health and, 133-134
Individuality, hospitalization and loss of, 70-71
Infant, 377-380
bathing of, *558-561*
children and
cardiopulmonary resuscitation and, 736, 739-740
gastrointestinal intubation and, 797
growth and development of, 4-7
health history of, 377
low birth weight, 376
nutrition and, 761
Infant respiratory distress syndrome, 686
Infarction, cerebral, respiratory dysfunction and, 681
Infection(s)
definition of, 515
epidemiology of, 517-519
fungus, lower airway obstruction and, 677-678
nosocomial, definition of, 515
nutrition and, 767
Infectious disease, control of, 519-521
Inflammation, 515
Informant, health history and, 282
Informed consent, 251-252
Infusions, intravenous, *650-667*

Inhalation therapy
drug administration by, 613-614
technicians for, 182
Injection, drug administration by, 611-613
Injury(ies). *See also* Accidents; Trauma.
chemical, in hospital, 569-576
spinal cord, respiratory dysfunction and, 681
Insufficiency, respiratory, 672
Insufflation, 731
Insurance
health, nurse and physician supply and, *159*
malpractice, 239
plan for national health, 146-147
Intake process, multidisciplinary team and, 205
Integument, physical examination and, 296-298
Intellectual development. *See* Cognitive and intellectual development.
Interactional patterns, family system and, 29-30
Intermittent mandatory ventilation, 702
Intermittent positive pressure breathing, maintenance of patent airway and, 696-697
Intervention, crisis, 101-105
plan and technique for, 105-107
Interview
beginning of, 271-272
termination of, 278
Interviewer
behavioral changes in, 275-276
perceptions of, 276
Interviewing, 270-278
as tool for data collection, 268-279
Intestinal and urinary elimination, maintenance of, 824-873
Intestinal tubes, procedures for, 817-821, *818-821*
Intraocular pressure, measurement of, 309
Intravenous infusions, *650-667*
Intravenous therapy, venipuncture and, 649
Introitus, 344
Intubation
definition of, 731, 789
gastrointestinal. *See* Gastrointestinal intubation.
Invasion of privacy, 250
Inversion, 487

Involvement
commitment to the nursing plan and, 403
hospitalization and loss of belonging and, 72
Irrigation
colonic, definition of, 825
colostomy, 895-900, *896-901*
ascending, 890
descending, 892
transverse, 892
gastrointestinal intubation and, 795
of urinary catheter, 852
of wound, 542
Isolation, *526*
definition of, 515
medical asepsis and, 525-532, *528-533*
social, 527-532. *See also* Sensory deprivation.
teaching client about, 527
Isotonic, 487
IVP, *945*

Jaundice, 361
Jejunoscopy, *941*
Joints, examination of, 354-355
Joint motion
exercises for, 495
range of, 495-500
Journals, major nursing, *227*
Judicial law, legal basis for nursing and, 243
Jugular veins, examination of, 314

Karaya, 875
Kardex, 419
Kassmaul's respirations, 459
Kayser-Fleischer ring, 306
Kefauver-Harris Drug Amendment, 587-588
Keloid, 515
Kidneys
anatomy of, 827-829
palpation of, 340-341
scan of, *947*
Kinetic behavior, assessment of nonverbal behavior and, 264
Knee, evaluation of, 357
Knee-chest position, 503-504
Knowledge, assessing mental status and manipulating, 299
Knowledge base, nursing care plan and, 399-400
K-pads, aquamatic, 582-583
Kwashiorkor, adult, 780

Monitoring,
    CVP, 668
    of client, gastrointestinal intuba-
        tion and, 795-796
Mons pubis, 342
Mood, assessing mental status and,
    299
Morbidity rate, 515
Moro reflex, newborn and, 376
Mortality rate, 515
Motility, 826
Motion
    body mechanics and, 489
    definition of, 487
Motor development, physical and.
        See Physical and motor de-
        velopment.
Motor function, assessment of,
    302-303
Mouth. See also Oral cavity; names
        of specific parts of mouth.
    aspiration of nose and, 706-711
    hygienic care of, 546
    newborn assessment and, 371
    throat and, in review of systems,
        284
Moving
    of clients, 491-494
        ambulating and, mechanical
            aids in, 506-512
    of objects, 491
Mucosa, oral, 312
Multidisciplinary team, 203-205
    dynamics of teamwork and, 208-
        209
    evolutionary development of,
        206-208
Murmur
    definition of, 291
    heart, 333-335
Muscles
    cervical, examination of verte-
        brae and, 313-314
    extraocular, examination of, 307-
        308
    inspection and palpation of, 355
Muscle-setting, 487, 495
Muscular dystropy, respiratory dys-
        function and, 683
Musculoskeletal disorders, respira-
        tory dysfunction and, 683-
        684
Musculoskeletal system, review of
        systems and, 285
Myasthenia gravis, respiratory dys-
        function and, 683
Mydriasis, 307
Mydriatics, 602-603
Myelogram, 946

Myocardial infarction, respiratory
        dysfunction and, 688
Mystique, medical, 160-162

NAILS
    hygienic care of, 548
    physical examination and, 297-
        298
Nares, hygienic care of, 547
Nasal culture, 932
Nasal medications, 618
Nasogastric tube
    insertion and removal of, 808-
        815
    procedures for, 806-817
Nasopharyngeal and oropharyngeal
        cavities, removal of secre-
        tions from, 706-711
Nasopharyngeal secretions, testing
        of, 932
Nasotracheal tube, 703
National health insurance plan,
        146-147
National Health Planning and Re-
        sources Development Act,
        166-168, 202
National League for Nursing, 225-
        226
National Student Nurses' Associa-
        tion, 226
N-CAP. See Nurses' Coalition for
        Action in Politics.
Nebulization, ultrasonic, 672
Nebulizer, 672
Neck
    newborn assessment and, 371
    physical examination and, 313-
        316
    review of systems and, 284
Needles, choice of, 625
Negligence
    definition of, 239
    malpractice and, 244-245
Neonate, 515
Nephritis, 826
Nephrosis, 826
Nerves(s), cranial, physical exami-
        nation and, 300-302
Neurological deprivation, respira-
        tory patterns and, 682
Neurological disorders, respiratory
        dysfunction and, 680-683
Neurological system
    physical examination and, 298-
        305
    review of systems and, 284
Newborn assessment, 370-376
New York State Regents External
        Degree Programs, 220

Nicking, 291
Nightingale, Florence, 218
Nipples, examination of areolar
        nodes and, 317
Nitrogen balance, 751-752
NLN. See National League for
        Nursing, 225-226
Nocturia, 826
Nodes, areolar, examination of nip-
        ples and, 317
Nonprofessionals, paraprofession-
        als, indirect providers and,
        182-183
Nonverbal behavior, observation
        of, 258-266
Nonverbal communication, verbal
        and, 269
Nose
    aspiration of mouth and, 706-
        711
    newborn assessment and, 371
    physical examination and, 311-
        312
    sinuses and, in review of sys-
        tems, 284
Nosocomial infection, 515
Note taking, interviewing and, 272
NSNA. See National Student
        Nurses' Association.
Nuclear family, 24
Nurse(s)
    as humanistic artist, 232-237
    codes for, 224, 225
    physician supply and, health in-
        surance coverage and, 159
    practical, 182
    registered, 212-231
        contemporary role of, 212-218
        earnings of teachers vs., 160
        educational preparation of,
            218-221
        specific duties of, 245-249
        supply and distribution of doc-
            tors and, 158
        visiting, 136
Nurse Practice Act(s), 223, 241
    California, 241
    New York, 241-242
Nurse practitioner. See also Pri-
        mary health care provider.
    independent, 207
Nurses' Coalition for Action in Poli-
        tics, 225
Nurse Training Act, 157
Nursing
    as foundation for diagnosing,
        386
    associate degree programs in,
        219-220

baccalaureate programs in, 219
codes for ethics of, 224-225
evolution of art of, 233-234
legal aspects of, 238-255
legal basis for, 240-243
primary, registered nurse and,
213-214
team, registered nurse and, 214
training and certification in, 181-
182
Nursing audit, 223
Nursing care, evaluation of, 434-
438
Nursing diagnosis(es). See also
Problem; names of specific
conditions for which nursing
diagnoses may be made.
classification of, 391-392
components of, 387-389
development of, 389-392
in formulating plan of care, 396
of health care problems, 384-
393
tentative list of, 391
Nursing education, collegiate, 219-
220
Nursing journals, major, 227
Nursing notes, in charting, 411-412
Nursing practice
American Nurses' Association
Standards of, 222-223
minimum preparation for, 220-
221
principles of body mechanics
and, 490-495
standards of, 221-224
Nursing problem, 387
Nursing schools, diploma, 219
Nursing services, community
health, provision of, 147-
150
Nursing unit, patient assignment to,
448-451
Nutrients, 748-752
functions and sources of, 756-
757
recommended allowances of,
755-756
Nutrition
assessment of status of, 292-293,
777-780
assisting clients with, 769-774
basic principles of, 748-764
common conditions affecting,
767-769
determination of therapy modalities and, 780-785
education about, 773-774
effect of impaired health upon

eating habits and requirements for, 766-775
enteral, 782-783
infant and, 5-6
life cycle and, 761-764
parenteral, 783-785
total, 649-668
Nycturia, 826
Nystagmus, 300, 308

OBSTRUCTION(S)
cardiopulmonary arrest and,
736-737
lower airway, 676-680
respiratory, 732-733
upper airway, 675
Occlusion, cardiovascular disorders
and respiratory dysfunction
and, 688
Occult blood, test for, 932
Occupational therapy, training and
certification in, 182
Oculomotor nerve, 300
Odor
breath, 312
control of
ascending colostomy and, 890
descending colostomy and,
892-893
colostomy client and, 895
ileostomy and, 905-908
ostomy client and, 880
transverse colostomy and, 891
urinary diversion and, 917-
922
Ointments, 614
Olfactory nerve, 300
Oligopnea, 458
Oliguresis, 826
Oliguria, 826
Ophthalmic medications, 616-617
Optic nerve, 300
Oral cavity. See also Mouth; names
of specific parts of oral cavity.
physical examination and, 312-
313
Oral medications, preparation of,
625
Oral route, drug administration by,
610-611
Organ(s)
donation of, 968
quadrant map and position of,
335
Organizations
group process in work of, 196-
197
professional nursing, 224-227

Oropharyngeal airway, 702
Oropharyngeal and nasopharyngeal cavities, removal of secretions from, 706-711
Orotracheal tube, 703
Ortalani maneuver, 361
Orthopnea, 322, 459, 672
Osmolarity, transport and, 643-645
Ostomy
appliance for
application of, 894
leakage and, 879
selection of, 893-894
assessment of client with, 876-
877
care of client with, 874-925
contract in, 886
nursing diagnosis and, 877-
878
nursing process in, 876-888
definition of, 875
Ostomy Association, United, visitor
from, 881
Otic medications, 617-618
Ova, parasites and, testing stool
for, 932
Ovary(ies), palpation of, 348
Ovulation, body temperature and,
455
Oxygen, low flow, 672
Oxygen therapy, 697-702
high flow systems for, 700-702
low flow systems for, 698-700,
701

PACKS and compresses, moist heat
application and, 581
Pain, sensory function testing and,
304
Pair-bonding, human sexuality and,
44
Palates, examination of, 313
Palpation
abdominal examination and,
338-342
examination of thorax and lungs
and, 322
physical examination and, 293
Pandemic, 515
Pansystolic murmur, 334
Papanicolaou test, 347, 935
Paraprofessionals, nonprofessionals, indirect providers and,
182-183
Parasite, 516
ova and, testing stool for, 932
Parasympathetic stimulants, 602-
603
Parasympatholytics, 594-595

growth and development of, 10-12

Prescriptions, 623
  diet, 770
Present problem, health history and history of, 282-283
Pressure
  blood. *See* Blood pressure.
  positive end expiratory, 702
    definition of, 672
Prevention
  definition of, 114-116
  health education and, 123-130
  levels of, 116-122
    within community, 145-146
  primary, 116-119
  secondary, 119-121
  screening and, 122-123
  tertiary, 121-122
  trend toward, 111-112
Preventive health care, 110-130
Primary care team, 205
Primary health care provider, 214-215
Primary nursing, 213-214
Privacy
  hospitalization and client loss of control and, 69-70
  invasion of, 250
Problem(s). *See also* Nursing diagnosis.
  formulating plan of care and list of, 396-399
  health, definition of, 387
  nursing, definition of, 387
  nursing approaches to solving of, 400-402
Problem-oriented system of charting, 414-418
Problem-solving approach, *397-398*
Process
  family 33-36
  group, 186-198
  intake, multidisciplinary team and, 205
Proctoclysis, 826
Proctoscopy, *940*
Prodromal, definition of, 516
Professional Standard Review Organization Act, 168-170
Progress notes, in problem-oriented system of charting, 415-416
Pronation, 488
Prone position, 501
Prostate gland, 351
  examination of, 352
Protectives, *604-606*
Proteins, 751-752
Providers

health care, 178-184
  expansion of group of, 178-181
  registered nurse as, 213-215
  indirect, paraprofessionals, non-professionals and, 182-183
Proximal, definition of, 875
Proximate, definition of, 239
Psychiatric clients, rights of, 251
Psychoanaleptics, *594-595*
Psychosocial development
  infant and, 4-5
  later maturity and, 20
  middle years and, 18
  preadolescence and adolescence and, 14-15
  preschooler and, 10
  schoolchildren and, 12
  toddler and, 8
  young adults and, 16-17
Public Health Service, 588
Pulmonary disease, chronic obstructive, 671
Pulmonary disorders, respiratory dysfunction and, 675-680
Pulmonary embolus, 688
Pulmonary functioning, maintenance of respiratory status and, 670-729
Pulmonary physiotherapy, 672
Pulse. *See also names of specific types of pulses.*
  apical, 329, 481
  apical-radial, 481
  blood pressure and, 480-483
    measurement of, 481-483
  peripheral, inspection and palpation of, 352-353
  terms describing, 482
Pulse pressure, 480
Pupils, examination of, 306
Pure Food and Drug Act of 1906, 587
Purgative(s), 826, *600-601*
Purulent, 516
Pus, 516
Psychic energizers, *594-595*
Pyelogram, intravenous, *945*
Pyrexia, 455
  treatment of, 457
Pyuria, 826

QUADRANT map, organ position within, *335*

RADIOLOGIC examinations and treatments, nutrition and, 769
Radiologic testing, 939-942, *943-946*

Radionuclide studies, 942, *947*
Rales, 327-328
  definition of, 291
Record(s)
  client, data found in, *413*
  intake and output, 789
Recording
  gastrointestinal intubation and, 796
  reporting and, of vital signs, 483-484
Rectal route, drug administration by, 616
Rectal tube, 856
Rectocele, 345
Rectum
  examination of, 349
  female genitalia and, 342-349
  male genitalia and, 349-352
Reflex(es)
  abnormal, testing for, 303-304
  accommodation, 300
  sensorimotor, newborn assessment and, 376
  testing of, 303-304
Reflux, vesicoureteral, 826
Regents External Degree Programs, New York State, 220
Regional Medical Programs of 1965, 166
Registered nurse. *See* Nurse, registered.
Regression, hospitalized client and, 71-72
Rehabilitation, 488
Religion
  death, dying and grief and, 963-964
  food preferences and, 760
  layperson's attitude toward illness and, 64
Replacement therapy
  definition of, 789
  gastrointestinal intubation and, 795
Reporting, recording and, of vital signs, 483-484
Reports, incident, 250
Reproduction
  evolution of sex and, 44-45
  versus sex, 42-45
Reproductive bias, 43
Researcher, registered nurse as, 216-217
Reservoir, infectious disease and, 517
Res ipsa loquiter, 239
Resistance, 516
Resonance, percussion of thorax and lungs and, 324

isolation technique to maintain medical asepsis and, *530-531*

Speculum examination, of female internal genitalia, 345-347

Speech, assessment of, 293

Spermatic cord, palpation of, 350

Sphincter, 826

Spinal cord injuries, respiratory dysfunction and, 681

Spleen, palpation of, 341

Splitting, of heart sounds, 331

Sponge baths, alcohol, 584

Sputum
    collection and examination of, 710
    testing of, *933-934*

Stadium, 456

Staff supplement strategy, citizen participation in health care delivery and planning and, 165

Standards of nursing practice, 221-224
    American Nurses' Association's, 222-223

Standing, 502-503

Stasis
    definition of, 826
    urinary, 830-831

State government, health care responsibilities of, 143

State Health Coordinating Council, 167

State Health Planning and Development Agency, 167

Stature, inspection of, 292

Statutory law, 239

Statute of limitations, 240

Stereognosis, testing of, 304

Sterile, 516

Sterile equipment, handling, *534-535*

Sterile field, 516

Sterilization, 524-525, *525*
    definition of, 516

Stertor, 459

Stertorous respiration, 322

Stimulants, *608-608*
    parasympathetic, *602-603*

Stoma(s). *See also* Colostomy, Ileostomy; Urinary diversion
    abdominal, colostomy and ileostomy appliance application and, *882-885*
    definition of, 875
    ileostomy and care of, 905
    management of, 878-879
    skin care and, 893-894

teaching self-care of, 880-881
    urinary, care of skin surrounding, 922-923

Stoma fistulas, 901

Stomal irrigation. *See* Irrigation.

Stomal strictures, 901

Stool, 826
    collection of specimen for analysis of, 872
    testing of, *932*

Strabismus, 308

Stress, 90-93
    assessment of, 94
    definition of, 387
    homeodynamics and, 88-95, 638-641
    nutrition and, 768

Stressor(s), 92

Stretchers, types and use of, 511-512

Stretch reflexes, 303

Striae, abdominal examination and, 337

Stridor, 459

Stroke volume, 480

S-tube, as temporary airway, 703

Submaxillary glands, examination of, 312

Subsystems, family system structure and, 28-29

Sucking reflex, newborn and, 376

Suction devices, for gastrointestinal intubation, 791-792

Sugar and acetone, testing urine for, *935*

Sulfonamides, *608-609*

Sump tube, 789

Superficiality, interviewing and, 273-274

Superficial reflexes, 303

Supervision, teaching, training and, role of health professional in, 195-196

Supination, 488

Supine position, 500-501

Support services, restoration of health and, 136-137

Suppositories, 616
    definition of, 826

Suppression, 826

Supraclavicular area, axillae and, in examination of female breast, 318

Surfactant, 673

Surgery, respiratory dysfunction and, 684

Susceptibility, 516

Suspensions, drug administration and, 611

Sutures
    definition of, 362
    wound healing and, 537

Symbiosis, 516

Symbols
    abbreviations and, in charting, 412-413
    chemical, electrolytes, functions and, *642*

Sympathetic amines, *590-591*

Sympathomimetics, *590-591*

Syndactyly, 362

Syndrome
    adult respiratory distress, 686
    general adaption, 90-91
    local adaptation, 91
    tube feeding, 823

Syringes, choice of, 625

Systole, 329, 480

Systolic clicks, 333

Systolic ejection murmurs, 334

Systolic murmurs, 334

TABLETS, 610

Tachycardia, 482

Tachypnea, 322, 362, 459, 672

Talipes equinovarus, 362

Tamponade, 789

Taste, assessment of nonverbal behavior and, 262

Teacher, registered nurse as, 215

Teaching
    legal aspects of nursing and, 247-248
    training, supervision and, role of health professional in, 195-196

Team
    health care, 205
    interdisciplinary health care, approach of, 183-184
    medical care, 205
    multidisciplinary, 203-205
    nutrition and concept of, 770
    primary care, 205

Team nursing, registered nurse and, 214

Team practice, 193-194

Teamwork, dynamics of, coordinating health service resources and, 203

Technicians, 182

Technology, trend toward disease prevention and, 112

Telangiectasis, 362

Temperature
    body, 453-457
        deviations in, 455-456, 457
        factors affecting, 454-455